# FUNCTIONAL
# NEUROANATOMY
# OF MAN

# FUNCTIONAL NEUROANATOMY OF MAN

being the Neurology section from Gray's Anatomy,
35th British edition

by

## PETER L. WILLIAMS
D.Sc., M.A., M.B., B.Chir.

## ROGER WARWICK
B.Sc., Ph.D., M.D.

Professors of Anatomy
Guy's Hospital Medical School, University of London

W. B. SAUNDERS COMPANY
PHILADELPHIA
1975

Exclusive distribution in the United States of America and Canada granted
to W. B. Saunders Company, Philadelphia and Toronto

© Longman Group Limited 1975

First published 1975


ISBN 0 7216 9450 0


Library of Congress Catalog Card Number 74-10038


Printed in Great Britain

# Explanation

When it was suggested that we should publish the Neurology Section from the 35th edition of Gray's Anatomy as a separate book there was a very enthusiastic response, and this volume is presented as an addition not only to medical literature but to that of the wider field of biology.

The separate, rigid disciplines of neuroanatomy and neurophysiology are merging and an integrated approach to what can be termed neurobiology is now favoured. Although the Neurology Section from Gray's Anatomy applies directly to human anatomy and physiology the principles apply to the wider field of mammalian neurology.

In the interests of economy certain decisions have had to be taken to ensure that the quality of the parent volume was preserved without involving the potential purchaser with a prohibitively high price. For this reason certain unusual elements will be found in this volume.

1. Pagination begins at page 746, as in the parent volume, and ends on page 1170.

2. Cross references to the parent work have not been deleted but their presence does not detract from the value of the book.

3. The co-ordinated bibliography is absent, but the footnote citations to the literature of the Nervous System will serve the needs of most readers.

A list of publications which appeared subsequently to the preparation of this book has been appended for the interest of readers.

PETER L. WILLIAMS
ROGER WARWICK

1975

# Preface

When our predecessor, Professor David Vaughan Davies, began his preface to the last edition, his first words were to regret the death of his co-editor (Professor Francis Davies) and to acknowledge, with characteristic generosity, the latter's editorial virtues. It is now our equally saddening task to record the death of an editor and friend for whom we shared, with so many others throughout and beyond the confines of human anatomy and medicine, a deep respect both as a scientist and teacher, and as a man of many accomplishments outside his profession. During a period of fifteen years he brought to this editorship the same unyielding standards of scholarship which he applied so outstandingly in his own discipline and school. For both of us his death had also immediate personal associations, for one (P.L.W.) had enjoyed twenty-five years as his student, colleague and companion, and for a number of years acted as his indexer, while the other (R.W.)—frequently a co-examiner—was expecting him on the second day of an examination of our own students when he was so suddenly stricken. We both regard it as an honour to carry forward his editorial obligations.

At the time of his death Professor Davies had completed a small number of revision notes, and these and his collection of references have been valuable to us. However, the decision had already been taken to modernize the format of this volume, with a complete resetting of the text; and it was therefore opportune to undertake a more extensive revision than would have been otherwise possible. The original role of *Gray's Anatomy* as a treasury of 'descriptive and applied' systematic human topography has become amplified through more than a century of usefulness by the early addition of histology and embryology, and by the gradual development of introductory sections to the various 'systems'. To many readers, both graduate and undergraduate, this elder textbook has, however, represented *in excelsis* the field of naked-eye or *dissectional* anatomy. We have neither disturbed nor curtailed this aspect of the volume: rather have we added to it—by the correction of errors, the addition of a host of new observations, the inclusion of hundreds of new references to cover details beyond the scope of even a large textbook, and by reinstatement of variations in respect of many structures. On the other hand we have endeavoured to reduce prolixities of language, as far as the shortened period of revision remaining to us has permitted; no page has escaped such attention, frequently extensive in degree. A considerable saving of space has been thus effected—to offset large additions of new writing and to keep this new edition within a single volume. To rewrite the whole text would have been an impossibly lengthy task, and there has inevitably resulted an increase in size. Subsequently we hope and intend to render all of the established text in a simpler and more succinct style, but to do this throughout with no loss of factual detail is a massive undertaking, and for our limited success in this regard we ask our readers' forbearance. Moreover, we were convinced that other tasks were more urgent and important.

Particularly in this century, the conviction has increased amongst anatomists that isolated observation and description is not enough, and that an experimental approach to problems of structure is as necessary as in other biological sciences. In addition, the great advances in technique—especially in the study of finer detail, in living and developing organs, tissues and cells—have enlarged the scope of anatomy far beyond the parent stem of macroscopic structure. These advances have engendered a spate of new specialities, such as histology, cytology, ultrastructure, embryology, neurology, electromyography, kinesiology, ergonomics, and so on, to a degree dependent only upon the choice of individual minds and the canalization of techniques. The expanding scope of structural knowledge and the exacting demands of more elaborate techniques do indeed dictate such specialization; but all such knowledge remains a continuum—except insofar as extensive gaps of ignorance and uncertainty persist. Unfortunately, and perhaps particularly in the medical sphere, the compartmentalization of anatomy into several disciplines or subjects—with attendant titles, individual chairs, and even separated departments—tends towards disintegration. To study some such region as a limb, in all its proportions, activities, and even evolution, and then its major structures—bones, joints, muscles, vessels and so forth—and to proceed to the microscopic, ultrastructural and ultimately biochemical details of its tissues and cells, appears to us a continuous process, and most desirably so to a balanced education for medicine, however elementary the standard. Unfortunately, these different levels of organization and function are perforce usually considered in separate laboratories, departments, lectures and books.

The defects of this compartmentalization are widely recognized, and have resulted in much effort to 'integrate' teaching. In this persuasion we have re-arranged certain contents of this volume, and in particular have transferred most of the existing section of histology to the appropriate systems. Hence, in *Myology* will be found not only a systematic description of the muscles of the human body, but also of muscle as a tissue. Moreover, there are certain general considerations such as, in this instance, the variable form and the mode of action of muscles and accessory structures—tendons, aponeuroses, bursae, and the like—which have already in recent editions been set out in introductory sections. It is precisely in these generalized aspects of human anatomy that the greatest interest often lies, attracting the major volume of research. We have concentrated special attention upon these sections, which are the more difficult to keep in accord with current progress in research. For this reason, and because the *significance* of structural data is more apparent in generalizations, we have found it necessary to rewrite all such introductory sections and to extend them—to a marked degree in most instances.

The accelerating tempo of enquiry in all respects of structure has a dual effect: there is not only a continuous correction and, more especially, accumulation of data, but also in the main a sharpening awareness of defects in knowledge and deficiencies in its interpretation. It is our belief that ignorance and uncertainty should be more prominently stated in textbooks than they usually are. We have tried to imbue this new edition with rather more of this attitude, not merely in introductory sections, but throughout the systematic text. Where the actions of a muscle are not convincingly demonstrable by direct observation or experiment, we believe uncertainty should be admitted; and where, for example, intricate central nervous organization has been investigated in another animal—perhaps quite remote from man—we consider that the need for caution in extrapolation to mankind should, in a textbook of human anatomy, be clearly appreciated.

It would be burdensome to categorize the changes and additions in this edition; approximately seven hundred pages of completely new writing have been contributed, covering all systems and a wide spectrum of topics. Doubtless our efforts have been uneven; we have, for example, not been able to revise some aspects of cardiac anatomy as thoroughly as we wished, but these and other defects will be remedied in the next edition. While hoping that many will welcome the substantial changes and additions in histology (and especially ultrastructure), in the sections on the teeth (completely rewritten), joints, muscles, lymphatic system, nervous system, special senses and endocrine organs, we also hope that our readers will freely and constructively criticize our mistakes, excesses and deficiencies. To keep abreast of all the new work reported is a formidable undertaking, and we trust that no one will hesitate to inform us of our shortcomings in this or any other regard.

In one particular this edition is unique; for the first time since the first edition, in 1858, this, the *direct* descendant of the original 'Gray', will be available in the United States side by side with the American scion, which has also persisted through almost an equal period, having begun in 1859 as a reprint of the first edition, but having diverged markedly in its evolution from the direct British descendant. The American parallel version ceased to refer to the British senior heir as long ago as 1896, though preserving the name of Henry Gray on its title-page. With subsequent editions, and particularly this, the divergence has become so great that the two books cannot be regarded as parallel versions; each has its own character.

Our editorial labours have been lightened by much help from others. Doctor Lawrence H. Bannister has contributed the new section on cytology and many of the histological and ultrastructural passages in the sections devoted to myology, neurology, and splanchnology. Doctor Jeffrey W. Osborn has recast the section on dental anatomy. Doctor Susan M. Standring has prepared the bibliography, which appears as a new feature at the end of the text, and has meticulously supervised all reference material. Doctor E. Lowell Rees has not only undertaken the complex revision of an expanded index, but has also provided many special dissections, histological prepara-

tions and advice. However, the majority of the revision remains the work of the editors, who are wholly responsible for any errors of judgment, incorrect terminology, omissions, misquotations, or lack of clarity throughout the volume. With the complete resetting of the text, index, illustration captions and tabbing, and the addition of a new bibliography, it is inevitable that, despite prolonged and repeated proof reading, some typographical errors will have eluded us; for these we apologize.

In accord with the comprehensive textual changes in this edition, the illustrations have also received much attention. More than 200 of the 1,305 figures of the 34th edition have been removed, with the addition of over 600 new items; thus, in this 35th edition almost a third of the illustrations are new. Moreover, new blocks have been prepared for all illustrations retained—from the original artwork wherever possible. Apart from those radiographs and reproductions from external sources, acknowledged below, all new illustrations have been prepared in our Medical Centre. We are much indebted to Doctor Aszal Riaz and Doctor John D. Dow (Department of Diagnostic Radiology) and to Mr. Kenneth Twinn and Mrs. Joy Taylor (Department of Physics) for much help with radiographs. In our own department Doctors E. Lowell Rees and Michael C. E. Hutchinson have produced many special dissections and other preparations, assisted in this by Doctors Andrew M. Seal and William J. Owen. Most of these have been photographed by Mr. Kevin Fitzpatrick, our photographer, to whom we are much indebted. Mr. Derek Lovell and Mr. David Ristow have provided skilled technical assistance in respect of electron microscopy and histology. Many other workers on our staff, past and present, have also helped with illustration material, including Doctors Mary Dyson, Murray Brookes, Karen Hiiemae, Wimal Jayaratnam and Kenneth J. W. Taylor; Doctors David R. Turner and Roy O. Weller (now in Pathology), Doctor David N. Landon (now in the Department of Neurobiology, National Hospital for Nervous Diseases, London), Doctor Eric W. Baxter, Mr. Eric C. Tatchell and Miss Hilary Phillip (Department of Biology) and Doctors J. P. Black and P. Barkhan (Department of Haematology) have all afforded us generous aid with preparations for photography. We also gratefully record the expert help of our School's Librarian, Miss Jean M. Farmer and her willing staff.

Mr. S. W. Woods had already prepared six new illustrations (chiefly in embryology), with the same high standards with which he embellished several previous editions while serving Professor Davies. Most of the new artwork, however—amounting to about 210 items—has been carried out by our colleague, Mr. Richard E. M. Moore, D.F.A.Lond., M.M.A.A., member of l'Association Internationale pour l'Etude de la Mosaique Antique, and Fellow of the Royal Society of Arts. His combination of meticulous draughtsmanship, a most unusual ability to comprehend the scientific intent of projected illustrations, and his extraordinary patience and stamina throughout two and a half years of continuous effort, have made our collaboration most fruitful and enjoyable.

Many other authorities in various fields have allowed us to reproduce, copy or adapt illustrations from papers and monographs, or have made special materials available for photography. It is a pleasure to acknowledge the generosity of Professor Janos Szentágothai (University of Budapest), Doctor Elizabeth Crosby (University of Michigan), Doctor W. J. W. Sharrard (University of Sheffield), Doctor Michael J. Hogan, Doctor Jorge J. Alvarado and Mrs. Joan E. Weddell (University of California), Doctor Alan M. Laties (University of Pennsylvania Medical School), Mr. Emanuel Rosen (Royal Eye Hospital, Manchester), Doctor N. A. Locket (Institute of Ophthalmology, London), Professor Alf Brodal (University of Oslo), Professor William J. Hamilton (Professor Emeritus, University of London), Professor Peter M. Daniel (Institute of Psychiatry, University of London), Professor J. André-Balisaux (University of Brussels), Doctors Keith E. Webster and A. Robert Lieberman (University College, London), Professor Don Fawcett (Harvard University Medical School), Professor N. Cauna (University of Pittsburgh), Professor Yves Clermont (McGill University), Doctor Max Levene and Mr. Emrys Turner (St. Helier Hospital, Surrey), Doctor Charles Levene (Sir William Dunn Department of Cellular Pathology, University of Cambridge), Doctor R. C. Edwards (University of Cambridge), Doctor A. F. Holstein (University of Hamburg), Doctor L. M. Franks (Imperial Cancer Research Fund, London), Doctor Don H. Tompsett (Royal College of Surgeons of England), Doctor M. A. Sleigh (University of Bristol), Professor Sir John O. Eccles (Laboratory of Neurobiology, State University of New York), Doctor Berta Scharrer (Albert Einstein College of Medicine, New York), Professor Paul D. Maclean (National Institute of Mental Health, Maryland), Doctor Walle J. H. Nauta (Massachusetts Institute of Technology), Doctor Webb Haymaker (Ames Research Center, N.A.S.A., California), Doctor Bror Rexed (Socialstyrelsen, Stockholm), Professor James M. Sprague (University of Pennsylvania), Doctor Ray S. Snider (University of Rochester, New York), Professor Clinton N. Woolsey (University of Wisconsin), Doctor Julia Fourman (University of Leeds), Professor David B. Moffat (University College, Cardiff), Doctor Alexander Barry (University of California), Professor Viktor Hamburger (Washington University, Missouri), Professor Setsuya Fujita (Prefectural University Medical School, Kyoto), Doctor Douglas R. Anderson (University of Miami), Professor Koji Uchizono (University of Tokyo).

We have had the benefit of special advice from many of the authorities acknowledged above, and in addition from Professor M. A. MacConaill (University College, Cork), Professor Jack J. Pritchard and the late Doctor James H. Scott (University of Belfast), Doctor F. Torrent Guasp (University of Barcelona), Professor John Z. Young (University College, London), Mr. D. G. Wilson Clyne, Professor Patrick D. Wall (University College, London) and Professor J. V. Basmajian (Emory University, Atlanta). Among colleagues in other departments in our centre we are especially indebted to Doctor R. T. Grant (late of the Department of Experimental Medicine) and Professor Paul E. Polani and his staff (Department of Paediatric Research) for much help respectively in regard to arteriovenous anastomoses and genetics. Similarly we have had the advantage of advice from many other colleagues in their own specialities, including Doctor Sidney Liebowitz (Immunological Pathology), Doctor John R. Henderson (Physiology) and Doctor David Watts (Biochemistry).

Although we have striven to acknowledge with punctilio the many publishers of scientific journals and books who have allowed us, with customary generosity, to use copyright material, we trust that any neglect in this respect of which we may have been guilty will be forgiven in the same generous spirit.

Throughout the ardours and pressures of this ambitious revision we have enjoyed the most cordial relationship with our publishers and printers, who have both given us the greatest freedom and encouragement. In particular we wish to mention Mr. John A. Rivers of Churchill, and Mr. William G. Henderson, Mr. Gerald J. Hooton and Mr. Alfred S. Knightley, of Churchill-Livingstone, who have been our companions in many anxious, sometimes convivial, and always protracted discussions.

We are most grateful to our departmental secretaries, Miss Margaret Collins and Mrs. Patricia Elson, for much sporadic and demanding help, and to our official secretarial assistant, Mrs. Peter Williams, who has patiently translated innumerable notes and drafts into immaculate typescript for the printers.

It is customary to eulogize the patience of wives—faint praise which is scarcely *galante*. Far from tolerating our preoccupation, our wives have supported us unfailingly with a true and critical interest and sympathy in our labours. To them and all our friends and colleagues, who have helped more than they know to sustain our enthusiasm, we remain profoundly grateful.

PETER L. WILLIAMS and ROGER WARWICK

# Contents

# NEUROLOGY

## Introduction

The dependence of living organisms upon environmental energy sources and the essentially dynamic nature of their life processes have been emphasized elsewhere in this volume (pp. 2–4). Many aspects of this dynamic state stem from the ability of organisms continually to interact with a fluctuating external environment whilst preserving their own structural integrity. Such effective adaptations to a varying environment can, as we have seen, be considered in relation to either long or brief time scales (p. 54).

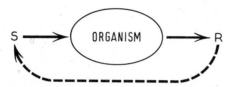

**7.1**   A diagram of the relationship between a stimulus (S) and a response (R) emphasizing its closed-loop nature.

Thus, over many generations, the forces of natural selection operate upon the genetic variants introduced by sexual reproduction and occasional mutation, resulting in species with an enhanced ability to adapt to changing or different environments. Alternatively, within the lifetime of a complex organism, such adaptive responses range from complicated behaviour patterns associated with mating, rearing of young, capturing of prey, avoidance or combat with predators, etc. to the innumerable transient readjustments, e.g. of posture, or the reaction and composition of the body fluids which constantly occur. The foregoing are examples of *homeostatic responses* which are a central feature of the behaviour of living organisms and which may be simply summarized as in illustration **7.1**.

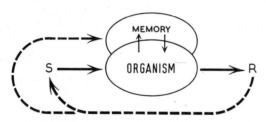

**7.2**   The stimulus-response loop with the added flexibility of a memory store.

When an environmental change (S or *stimulus*), to which the organism is capable of reacting, occurs in its vicinity, an appropriate response (R) follows. In general, the nature of the response is such that it tends to preserve the internal constancy of the organism within the fairly narrow limits necessary for the continued life of its cells and hence ultimately to preserve the whole organism and the species. It should be noted that because of the response, the relationship of the organism to the stimulus is altered (the broken arrow in the diagram), and that in this sense, the whole sequence of events is a *loop*, and not an *arc* with open ends. Further, in the simple case illustrated, the structural organization of the organism (the result of its phylogenetic history) limits the array of stimuli to which it can react, and also restricts the repertoire of its responses, which may be mechanical, chemical, photic or electrical. Accordingly, there are many environmental disturbances to which it is unable to respond,

or the disturbances may be of such an intensity that any responses are inadequate; the organism 'dies' and gradually undergoes dissolution (i.e. it merges with its environment). In the example quoted the *genetic memory* of the organism, which has emerged by natural selection over countless generations, has determined its receptivity of stimuli and its range of responses, and hence its degree of fitness for survival within some particular environment. However, such a system leads to a rather stereotyped set of responses, and in more complex organisms, selective processes have led to the addition of a second more flexible *memory system* which operates throughout the life of the individual (**7.2**). In the latter the general sequence of the stimulus–response loop is similar to the previous example, but in this case the information derived from a particular stimulus pattern is transferred to a memory store, where it is compared with a record of previous experiences. As a result of this comparison, a choice of a particular response is made (out of the many alternatives available), as the one with the highest probability of effectiveness under the circumstances prevailing. It is considered that once having occurred, the effectiveness of the response is somehow assessed, and the results of this assessment are transferred to the memory store, which is modified accordingly; the probability of the same response being chosen under similar conditions in the future being either raised or lowered. In this manner the memory store is continually modified, readjusted and refined as, with time, further experiences occur, i.e. the organism *learns*.

As implied above, homeostatic responses are a characteristic attribute of *all* living organisms, from simple unicellular forms to the most complex multicellular ones. However, with increasing complexity of structure there is a corresponding increase in the range and flexibility of the responses, and this has paralleled the emergence of a *nervous system*—the concern of the present section of this volume.

The human nervous system is, without question, the most complex, widely investigated, and least well understood system known to mankind. Its structure and activities are inseparably interwoven with every aspect of our lives, physical, cultural and intellectual. Accordingly, investigators of many different disciplines, methodologies, motivations and persuasions converge in its study. Similarly, depending upon the context, there are many more or less appropriate ways of embarking upon a study of nervous systems; for example the approach may be developmental, phylogenetic, physicochemical, energetic, structural—gross or cellular, cybernetic, behavioural or ethological.

For our present purposes, the detailed neuroanatomy of the various arbitrary but convenient divisions of the human nervous system is preceded by an account of some relevant experimental methods, the biology of its components in cellular terms, a brief review of some simple nervous systems, and introduced by comparing nervous systems with the information-processing, communication, and control systems of homeostatic machines. (For an extended discussion of the latter approach, the interested reader should consult footnote reference.[1])

### A SIMPLE HOMEOSTAT

It will perhaps prove helpful at this point to draw certain analogies with the main features of a simple man-made homeostatic device such as a thermostat (**7.3**).

In the thermostatic system illustrated, the *energy level* (temperature) of the water bath is continuously *monitored*

[1] J. Z. Young, *A Model of the Brain*, Clarendon Press, Oxford. 1964.

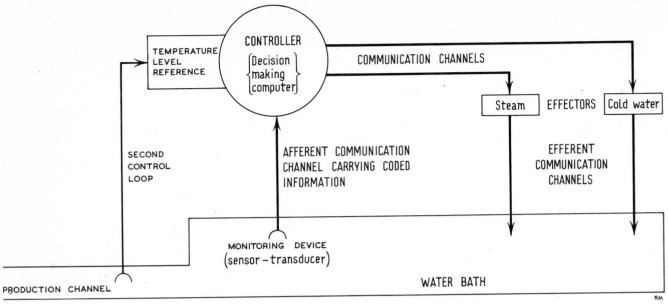

7.3 A diagram of the essential features of a thermostat coupled to an industrial production line. This is an example of a man-made homeostatic device; see text for further details and discussion. Modified from an illustration in: *A Model of the Brain*, by J. Z. Young, published by the Clarendon Press, with the permission of the author and the publishers.

by an appropriate *sensor* or *receptor* (in this case a thermocouple), and variations in this level are converted into variations in the flow of a *pattern of signals* or *coded information* (in this case current flow) along an *afferent communication channel* to a *controller*. The physical design of the latter is such that it combines or *integrates* the information flow along its afferent channel with that provided by the temperature reference level, and makes a *decision* between alternative patterns of activity (*responses*) of the *effectors* (steam or cold water). If, for example, there is a fall of temperature in the bath (of sufficient magnitude to be detected by the sensor), this change is transformed into signals in the afferent channel which, after comparison and computation in the controlling centre results in an increased flow of steam. It may be noted that it is inherent in the design of such a *control loop system* that there will not be a simple, smooth, immediate return to the reference level of temperature; some overshoot occurs and, with time, there follows a series of oscillations of decreasing amplitude, which gradually converge on the reference level. All the features described in this man-made homeostat have their counterparts in primitive nervous systems. These include the possession of a variety of sensors each capable of monitoring the rate and magnitude of some particular type of environmental change, communication channels carrying coded information (nerve fibres bearing temporo-spatial patterns of nerve impulses), integrative computing and decision-making centres (geometric patterns of contact between nerve cells), further communication channels (nerve fibres) and finally effectors (gland or muscle cells) which may be thrown into appropriate patterned responses. All these features will be considered in greater detail in subsequent sections.

As also indicated in illustration 7.3, simple control loops of the type described, which are a characteristic feature of all organisms (and widely used in engineering design), are frequently coupled with further loops, thus giving more complex responses. For example, the reference level of such a factor as the bath temperature may be continually readjusted to maximize the output of an industrial production line. As we shall see, many features of more complex nervous systems are conveniently considered in terms of an integrated hierarchial system of control loops.

## Cell Communication

Many aspects of intracellular and intercellular communication (7.4 A, B) have been mentioned elsewhere in this volume. Thus, consideration has been given to the selective interaction between cell surfaces, when in close apposition, and the phenomena of contact guidance and contact inhibition (p. 62). The structure and informational role of nucleic acids in cells has been discussed in some detail (p. 15), and brief reviews of current theories concerning how local cytoplasmic factors, or intercellular chemical messengers (embryonic organizers, hormones, etc.) may effect changes in genotropic control loops, and result in the enhancement or repression of different patterns of gene activity (p. 18). Where cells are in particularly close apposition (e.g. at 'tight' and 'gap' junctions) a variety of ions and molecules are able to pass selectively between the cytoplasms of the adjacent cells at such sites (p. 5). (However, much work remains to be carried out concerning the precise nature and variety, mechanisms of transfer, and informational role of the substances involved at these sites.) Alternatively, chemical messengers, such as the secretory products of endocrine glandular cells, pass into the blood circulation and then diffuse through the tissue fluid to reach groups of cells which may be quite remote from their site of production. Necessarily, such mechanisms operate upon relatively slow time scales.

### EXCITABLE TISSUES

More rapid mechanisms of both intracellular and intercellular communication have evolved in certain specialized *excitable tissues* (including receptor, neural, muscular and certain glandular cells). Some general features of an excitable cell are illustrated in 7.4 B. All cells possess a plasma membrane which separates the surrounding tissue fluid from the various intracellular compartments (p. 4, 1·1). By virtue of the permeability characteristics of this membrane, and its associated energy-dependent ionic pumping mechanisms, the ionic composition of the intracellular fluid contrasts sharply with that outside the cell, and consequently a large recordable difference in electrical

747

## GENERAL TISSUE CELLS

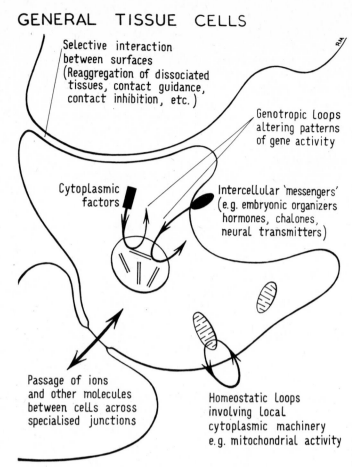

Selective interaction between surfaces (Reaggregation of dissociated tissues, contact guidance, contact inhibition, etc.)

Genotropic Loops altering patterns of gene activity

Cytoplasmic factors

Intercellular 'messengers' (e.g. embryonic organizers hormones, chalones, neural transmitters)

Passage of ions and other molecules between cells across specialised junctions

Homeostatic loops involving local cytoplasmic machinery e.g. mitochondrial activity

7.4A A diagram illustrating various forms of cellular and intercellular communication systems.

## EXCITABLE TISSUE CELL

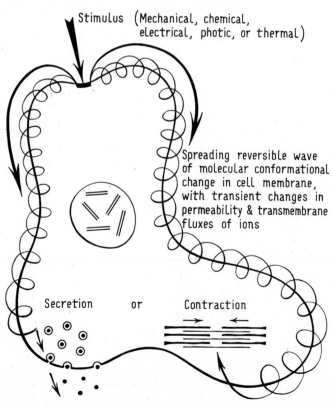

Stimulus (Mechanical, chemical, electrical, photic, or thermal)

Spreading reversible wave of molecular conformational change in cell membrane, with transient changes in permeability & transmembrane fluxes of ions

Secretion    or    Contraction

7.4B A summary of the main events which may follow the application of an effective stimulus to the surface of an excitable tissue cell.

potential exists between the two compartments across the membrane. Upon the receipt of an appropriate form of *stimulus* at some point upon its surface, a transient, reversible wave of change spreads over the surface of the excitable cell from this point. Whilst the details of the change in molecular terms (presumably involving conformational alterations in the membrane substructure) are not yet understood, changes in the permeability (conductance) of the membrane result. Accordingly there is a rapid local redistribution of ions across the membrane, as they flow down their concentration gradients; this soon ceases as the permeability returns to its resting state. These ionic fluxes may be recorded as variations in electrical potential using suitable equipment, and they are also accompanied by characteristic energetic (thermal) exchanges between the cell and its environment. These properties of excitable cells are discussed in greater detail elsewhere, as are the features which lead to *trains* or *volleys* of such *impulses* upon prolonged stimulation, and the relationship of stimulus strength to impulse pattern (number and frequency). The impulse, having spread over the surface of the cell, then causes, by some imperfectly understood process, either the release of a specific secretory product or the contraction of actin-myosin complexes, depending upon the type of cell involved. The different cells which cooperate in the functioning of nervous systems are modified in various ways, and exhibit these properties of excitable tissues to greater or lesser degrees (7.5 A, B, C). Thus, whilst in unicellular forms, and some primitive multicellular forms, *individual cells* are capable of reacting to stimuli, in the majority of multicellular forms possessing nervous systems, a *division of labour* occurs between the cells which make up the system. Thus, we see the emergence of cells specialized particularly for the reception of stimuli, or for the conduction and integration of information, or for the operation of responses. A more detailed account of the cytology, and theories concerning the functioning and evolutionary history of these cell varieties will be found elsewhere in this volume (pp. 766 *et seq.*); what follows is a brief introduction to certain features common to many types of nervous system.

## RECEPTOR CELLS

Within the various epithelial layers which clothe the body surfaces, and their associated sub-epithelial connective tissue, within the walls of some blood vessels, and incorporated into the structure of many of the solid and hollow viscera, and into muscles, tendons, ligaments, etc. are arrays of *receptor cells*. The latter possess specialized regions of their surfaces which enable them to monitor selectively changes in both the internal and external environment. Certain receptors are particularly responsive to mechanical deformation whilst others are sensitive to either thermal, chemical, electrical or photic variations. Views concerning the *degree of specificity* of action of individual 'types' of receptor cell have been modified on a number of occasions during the last one hundred and thirty years. Thus, since the first enunciation of a law of *specific nerve energies* by Johannes Müller in 1840, many investigators have held that any particular receptor reacted preferentially to only one type of energetic change, and this constituted its usual physiological role. A receptor was considered to exhibit a *low threshold* with respect to this form of stimulation, i.e. it reacted to small variations in energy level, whereas to all other types of change it exhibited a *high threshold*, only reacting if the stimulus strength was of relatively great, perhaps abnormal, intensity. Following experiments on cutaneous innervation in mammals, however, other investigators reached the opposite conclusion[2]—that the cutaneous receptors were *non-specific* and that sensory perception depended entirely upon the *spatio-temporal patterns* of nerve impulses in a common set of neural pathways. With more refined methods of recording from individual nerve fibres and nerve cell bodies, however, there has been a partial return to the specificity theory, but with many complexities, subtleties and grades of interaction, not envisaged in the earlier theories.[3,4,5] Thus, some nerve fibres have been identified which stem from receptors reacting to more

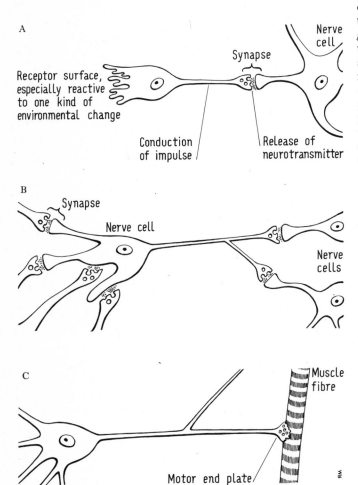

A

Nerve cell

Synapse

Receptor surface, especially reactive to one kind of environmental change

Conduction of impulse

Release of neurotransmitter

B

Synapse

Nerve cell

Nerve cells

C

Muscle fibre

Motor end plate

**7.5 A–C** The three main avenues of differentiation which may be followed by a primitive nerve cell: A a receptor neuron; B an interneuron; and C an effector neuron. See text for further discussion.

than one class of environmental change. Further, receptors may be *fast* or *slowly adapting*: the former respond to a brief stimulus with a sharp volley of nerve impulses which ends as the stimulus ceases, but if the stimulus is maintained the frequency of nerve impulse firing rapidly drops to the resting level. Slowly adapting receptors may continue to generate a volley of impulses for prolonged periods if the stimulus strength persists. Yet other varieties of receptor show a resting level of impulse discharge which may be either raised or lowered with different changes in the environment. These variants will be further considered with the anatomy of the individual receptor cells (p. 795).

The intimate molecular mechanisms whereby an environmental change, whether mechanical, chemical or thermal, causes an alteration in the receptor cell are imperfectly understood (although more is known concerning the activation of photosensitive pigments in retinal receptors— p. 1113). Nevertheless, electrophysiological recording from some varieties of receptor cell has

demonstrated that, when the cell is exposed to a stimulus of adequate strength, there follows a change of permeability to ions in its specialized receptor surface. Consequently, some of the ions which are differentially concentrated in the intra- and extra-cellular compartments flow down their concentration gradients across the specialized receptor surface; a microelectrode inserted into the cell records these ionic fluxes as variations in electrical potential—the so-called *receptor potential*. The circuit for this flow of ionic current is completed by a flow of ions in the opposite direction across the neighbouring non-specialized (but excitable) regions of the receptor cell membrane, where the resulting variations in potential are termed .the *generator potential*. The detailed consequences of fluctuations in the level of the generator potential have only been analysed in a few sites, but vary with the type and geometry of different receptors. In some situations, for example, the gustatory cells of the tongue, the generator potential may directly affect the level of activity of the points of synaptic contact between the receptor cell and the peripheral process of a neuron (*vide infra*). In other situations (the Pacinian corpuscle is a particularly well investigated example, p. 798), where the specialized receptor surface is the peripheral part of a long cytoplasmic conducting process (nerve fibre) which proceeds to the central nervous system, other events occur. If the variation in the generator potential reaches a critical threshold level, it causes a dramatic but rapidly reversible series of changes of ionic permeability in the regions of cell membrane which border the specialized receptor surface. The consequent ionic fluxes are recordable as an *action potential*, and they set in train a self-generating wave of similar changes which spreads along the conducting process as a *nervous impulse*. Maintenance of the generator potential at an adequate level results in a *volley of impulses* which passes centrally along the fibre. In this manner, receptors act as *transducers*, whereby fluctuations in various environmental energy levels are transformed into coded volleys of nerve impulses. Much work is currently in progress attempting to analyse the detailed mechanisms and quantitative aspects of their responses.

## SYNAPTIC CONTACTS

As we shall see elsewhere, the geometry of receptor cells varies enormously, but in all cases at one or more (sometimes many) points on their surface they form specialized intercellular contacts with one or a number of *nerve cells* or *neurons* (**7.5 A**). These contact points, and also those between neurons, are termed *synapses*.

In the synapses of certain invertebrates and lower vertebrates, and also at the specialized contacts between smooth muscle cells or between cardiac muscle cells, the cell membranes approach each other closely and a path of high conductance between the cells is formed. Accordingly, ions can flow easily between the cells, and when the spreading wave of permeability change and accompanying electrotonic current flow, which encompass one cell, converge upon its point of contact with its neighbour, these travel across to affect the latter directly. Such a cell junction is termed an *electrical synapse* and a number of types have now been recognized. They differ in the degree of polarization of action which they exhibit, and they may mediate either excitatory or inhibitory effects; these will

[2] G. Weddell, *J. Anat.*, **75**, 1941.
[3] V. B. Mountcastle and T. P. S. Powell, *Bull. Johns Hopkins Hosp.*, **105**, 1959.
[4] D. Sinclair, *Cutaneous Sensation*, Oxford University Press, London, New York, Toronto. 1967.
[5] P. D. Wall, *J. Physiol., Lond.*, **188**, 1967.

be treated more fully elsewhere (p. 775). To date, electrical synapses have only been identified within mammalian nervous systems in isolated locations.

In mammalian synapses (as in the majority of sub-mammalian and invertebrate synapses) *chemical transmission* occurs. The cell membranes are in this case separated by *synaptic clefts* and transmission occurs in one direction only, i.e. the synapse is *polarized* and is bounded by the membranes of a *presynaptic* and a *postsynaptic* cell. As the nerve impulse which has spread over the surface of the presynaptic cell (either a receptor cell, or a neuron) approaches the presynaptic membrane, it causes the release of a *neurochemical transmitter* which rapidly diffuses across the confines of the synaptic cleft and approaches the postsynaptic membrane, where it causes a change in its ionic permeability. The action of the transmitter is short-lived, as it is broken down almost immediately by the action of a specific enzyme. The character of the permeability change in the postsynaptic membrane, however, varies with the chemical nature of the transmitter substance at a particular synapse, and also with the nature of the membrane. In some cases the permeability change is such that the resulting flow of ions tends to *depolarize* the postsynaptic membrane, i.e. to *reduce* the level of the electric potential difference which reflects the asymmetric distribution of ions across the membrane of the 'resting cell'. Such synapses and their transmitters are said to be *excitatory* with respect to the postsynaptic cell (*vide infra*). In contrast, other varieties of neurotransmitter tend to *hyperpolarize* the postsynaptic membrane and are said to be *inhibitory*. These distinctive effects, as recorded by a microelectrode impaling the postsynaptic cell, are known as *excitatory postsynaptic potentials* (EPSP's) and *inhibitory postsynaptic potentials* (IPSP's) respectively. To understand some features of their interaction, the morphology of a common type of nerve cell must now be outlined.

## NEURONS

Neurons or *nerve cells* are essentially excitable cells which are specialized for the *reception, integration, transformation* and *onward transmission* of coded information.

Vertebrate neurons consist of a *cell body* or *soma*—a localized mass of specialized cytoplasm which carries a diploid nucleus and is bounded by an excitable membrane, from the surface of which project one or more *neurites*. The latter are delicate, branching, cytoplasmic processes, each enclosed by an excitable plasma membrane, which extend varying distances from the cell body. Accordingly, neurons may be classified as either *unipolar*, *bipolar* or *multipolar* (7.6 A–C). The neurites in each case may be divided into those which conduct broadly towards the cell body, namely one or more *dendrites* and another one which may branch more or less profusely, and conducts away from the cell body, the *axon*.

Neurons present a great range of shapes, sizes and interrelationships with other cells, both in different species and in different regions of the nervous system. Many of these variations will be treated in greater detail in subsequent parts of the present section. For our present introductory purposes it should be noted that the dendrites of a bipolar or unipolar neuron are either in synaptic contact with specialized receptor cells in the tissues of the body, or, by their dendritic terminals, themselves function as specialized peripheral receptor surfaces. In contrast, virtually all the nerve cells of the vertebrate *central* nervous system (brain and spinal cord) are of the multipolar variety (7.7).

It is clear that the surfaces of the dendritic tree and of the cell body provide a large area, which receives the synaptic terminals of other neurons. Such terminals may be relatively few in number, but usually they number many thousands, being derived from the axonal branches of some hundreds of neurons which are pre-synaptic relative to the one on to which they converge. Such pre-synaptic cells may be widely scattered in different regions of the nervous sytem; evidently there is a great *convergence* of information paths in such a case.

The synaptic contacts illustrated may thus be classified as *axodendritic*, or *axosomatic*, according to their site on the postsynaptic membrane; other less common varieties include *axoaxonic* synapses involving either the initial segment of the axon or the presynaptic terminals of the cell concerned, *dendrodendritic* sites of interaction, and finally synaptic *glomeruli*, in which a number of neurites are interrelated in complex geometrical patterns. The cytological details and possible modes of operation of these and other varieties will be described in later pages (pp. 773, 775).

Of the numerous synaptic terminals clustered over the dendrites and cell soma of a multipolar neuron, those from certain sources are *excitatory* whilst the remainder, from other sources, are *inhibitory*. Depending upon the

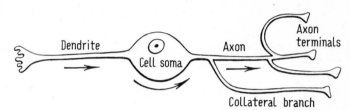

**BIPOLAR NEURON**

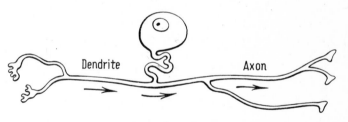

**UNIPOLAR NEURON**

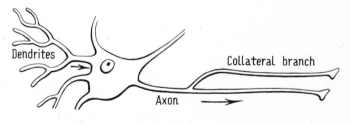

**MULTIPOLAR NEURON**

7.6 A–C Three broad morphological groups of neurons classified according to the number of neurites which arise from the surface of the cell soma: A bipolar neuron; B unipolar neuron; and C multipolar neuron. For a more detailed analysis of the branching patterns of neurites, see 7.15.

states of relative activity or quiescence of these different sources, the proportion of excitatory and inhibitory synapses which are active also varies continuously with the passage of time. Accordingly, their overall effect is summated (*integrated*) and the *excitatory state* of the cell, i.e. the relative level of depolarization or hyperpolarization of its cell membrane also fluctuates. Only when the depolarization reaches a critical *threshold level* are the local

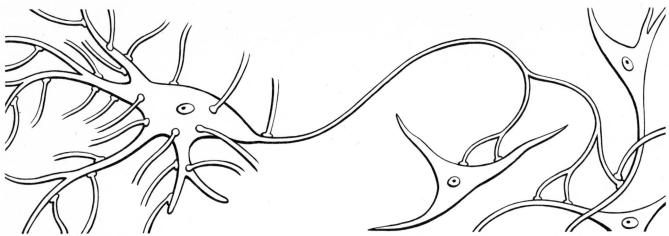

**7.7** A diagram to introduce the concept of the multipolar neuron and the parts of its surface upon which synaptic terminals from other neurons may converge. These include the surfaces of the dendrites, the cell soma, the initial segment of the axon, and the proximal surface of its own axonal synaptic terminals. For a more detailed representation of the cytology and surface contacts of a multipolar neuron see **7.17**.

electrotonic current flows, which encircle the dendritic tree and cell soma, sufficient so to alter the permeability characteristics of the *initial segment* of the axon, that an action potential is generated and spreads down the axon as a *nervous impulse*. If the threshold excitatory state continues to be exceeded, a volley of such impulses is discharged along the axon and its collateral branches. It is to be noted that, since the excitatory level of the neuron *continuously* reflects the innumerable variations in pattern of the information paths which converge upon it the nerve cell bears some similarity to the operation of an *analogue computing device*. In contrast, the outflow information channel, the axon, exhibits an *all or none* response. Thus, it is either quiescent, or carries one or more discrete, identical, intermittent nerve impulses—only their frequency varies. In this regard the axon is more like a *digital computer*.

The axon terminals of a particular neuron may be few in number and concentrate their effect on one or only a small localized group of postsynaptic cells. In other situations *collateral branches*, which may be numerous, arise from an axon at points throughout its course, and each of these may themselves arborize and *diverge* to many destinations. The 'many to one' *convergence* of information channels with the integration of their effects, and, in other situations, the 'one to many' *divergence* of channels, are essential features of all advanced forms of nervous system.

## INHIBITORY CIRCUITS

Some elementary inhibitory circuits, currently proposed as a result of microelectrode studies, are illustrated in **7.8 A–C.**

In **feed-forward inhibition** (**7.8 A**) an excitatory neuron (X) is functionally linked with two others (Y and Z). However, it is clear that the interposition of an inhibitory neuron on the second path causes the excitatory level of Z to fall whilst that of Y rises, during the period that X is active. Of course, in practice, many other local circuits are simultaneously active; nevertheless, the principle illustrated probably accounts in part for such examples as the ·increase in force of contraction of a muscle group during a particular activity, whilst, concurrently, the contraction level of a cooperative group of muscles is progressively reduced.

In **feed-back inhibition** (**7.8 B**) a volley of impulses initiated by a multipolar neuron (A) proceeds down its axon to its principal group of synaptic terminals (B).

However, the persistence of the volley is limited in time by the operation of a feed-back loop. A collateral branch leaves the axon and its excitatory terminals synapse with a single inhibitory neuron (X), the terminals of which pursue a recurrent course and synapse with the dendrites and soma of the original cell (A), where they hyperpolarizing effect terminates the volley. Such feed-back circuits may vary greatly in complexity, and in some situations two inhibitory neurons (Y and Z) may be interposed at some point in a recurrent loop. Evidently, some inhibitory effect on A by neuron Z, perhaps initiated by an alternative source (C), is diminished by the operation of inhibitory neuron Y. This release from an inhibitory effect by a second one, in series with the first, is termed, somewhat inelegantly, *disinhibition*.

In **7.8 C** one form of feed-forward inhibition known as **lateral inhibition** or **inhibitory surround**, of great importance in many neural pathways, is illustrated. A series of parallel pathways A–E which carry functionally similar types of information is shown. It may be imagined that all these channels are transmitting sporadically with a rather low information content. If, however, the excitatory state of one (e.g. channel A) rises significantly above the others, by the operation of neighbouring shells of inhibitory neurons, the activity in B–E is reduced. Consequently, the centrally activated channel becomes surrounded by a quiescent zone; there is less chance of confusion by random activity in the neighbouring channels, and the discriminative value of the central channel is greatly increased—a phenomenon termed *neural sharpening*. Many examples of this important process will be referred to in the subsequent sections.

Mention should also be made at this point of two further sites of inhibitory interaction between neurons (**7.9**). These forms are of less common occurrence, but they evidently have completely contrasting roles. An inhibitory terminal surrounding the initial segment of the axon is advantageously placed to *prevent* rapidly and completely an outflow from the neuron. On the other hand, *presynaptic inhibitory terminals* may *selectively diminish* the activity or effectiveness of some terminals whilst others continue to act unimpeded—a number of examples will be encountered in later sections.

It should be stated here, however, that our knowledge of the geometry of dendritic trees, cell somata and axonal branching, in quantitative terms, of the three-dimensional interconnexions between neurons, and the spatial distribution of synaptic types, is still in its infancy. So, too, is our knowledge of how individual neurons and cooperative

751

groups of neurons transform patterns of information flow, and how these relate to the operation of the whole nervous system and the overall economy of the organism. For the same reason, much research is currently concentrated upon investigations into the causal mechanisms which operate during neurogenesis, to determine which features of neurons, and neuron assemblies, are specified by the genome, and on what is the nature of the modifications which occur during the establishment of acquired memory traces during the lifetime of the organism. Some specific examples, where illuminating research is proceeding, will be mentioned in the appropriate sections.

*effectors*, such as the contractile cells which surround the pore-system of sponges, or the stinging organs of coelenterates, which can respond to direct mechanical or chemical stimulation of their surfaces.

Coelenterates are the simplest multicellular forms which possess a true nervous system: and in various types and bodily regions different orders of complexity can be recognized (7.10). In some sites specialized receptor cells situated between the general epithelial cells of the surfaces of the organism send a conducting process from their bases which is in direct functional contact with underlying effectors (muscle cells). Elsewhere, however, the

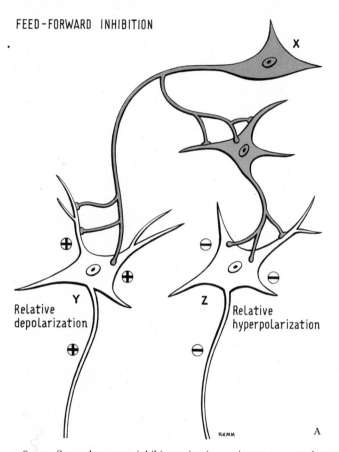

FEED-FORWARD INHIBITION

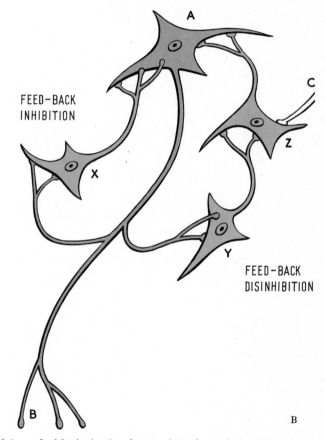

FEED-BACK INHIBITION

FEED-BACK DISINHIBITION

**7.8** A–C  Some elementary inhibitory circuits; excitatory neurons shown in red, inhibitory neurons in blue: A  a direct excitatory circuit (on the left) is compared with a simple feed-forward inhibitory circuit (on the right); B  feed-back circuits of two orders of complexity with one (on the left) and two (on the right) inhibitory interneurons interposed on the recurrent pathway; C  lateral inhibition. A central excitatory train of

## Some General Features of Neural Organization

What follows is an attempt to present some aspects of the organization of nervous systems, of varying intricacy, which may be of assistance before embarking upon a study of the complex nervous arrangements of vertebrates, and in particular mankind. It is in no sense intended to reflect a phylogenetic history, and no consideration will be given here to the distribution of inhibitory and excitatory neurons, to synaptic morphology, or chemical or behavioural studies; comments are limited to the elemental aspects of the arrangement of neurons.

In the unicellular protozoans, of course, the single cell constitutes the whole organism, and its various parts can act as primitive receptor, conductor and effector mechanisms. Some ciliated protozoans, for example, show coordinated beating of their cilia, so that the organism may advance towards or retreat from particular sources of stimulation (p. 11).

Simple multicellular forms possess many *independent*

processes from the receptor cells discharge into a sub-epithelial 'network' of nerve cells which are functionally interconnected in a tangential plane. From the latter, processes pass to the effectors. The interconnexions or 'synapses' between the cells forming the network are, however, not functionally polarized as they are in more complex systems; a strong stimulus applied to any point on the surface of the organism causes motor effects in all other regions. A superficial examination might indicate that the network of neurons is random (7.10c), but closer study shows that some regions have a greater density of receptor cell inputs, others have closer meshes in the network, and in yet others the conducting fibres are longer and have a distinct orientation. These features presumably subserve the more complex behavioural patterns associated with the capturing of prey, avoidance reactions, and other locomotor activities of these simple organisms. It should also be noted that these structural characteristics foreshadow similar fundamental arrangements which persist in more complex nervous sytems, including those of Mammalia.

In simple forms which exhibit bilateral symmetry we

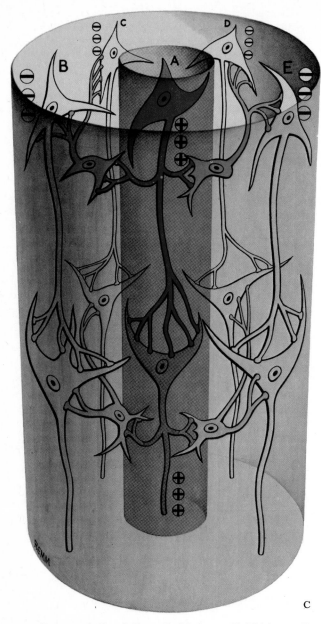

C

neurons is surrounded by a hollow cylindrical zone of inhibition, mediated by shells of inhibitory interneurons which are activated by the central column. See text for further discussion.

In the higher invertebrates, which exhibit metameric segmentation of the body, many of the same considerations apply. The receptor cells are still largely intra-epithelial in position and their centrally directed nerve fibres collect into bundles, or *sensory nerves*, within each segment, as they approach the central nervous system. The latter consists of masses of intercalated and motor neurons— usually a ventrally situated pair of masses (or 'ganglia') in each segment. Each pair is interconnected by axonal processes which cross the midline, and the masses are also interconnected longitudinally on both sides of the midline, so that a structure often likened to a rope-ladder is formed. The axons of the motor neurons emerge from the central nervous system as a series of bundles, *motor nerves*, within each body segment. The transverse communications also carry axonal processes of intercalated neurons and are responsible for cooperative responses involving both sides of the body. Similarly, short-axoned neurons interconnect adjacent body segments longitudinally in both directions. Others possessing longer axons inter-connect more distant segments, including the increasingly important 'head' end, whose specialized receptors must at times play a dominant role in behaviour.

As we have seen elsewhere (p. 83), during embryo-genesis in *Chordata*, including *Mammalia* and mankind, the central nervous system develops in the dorsal midline, as a hollow tube-like structure which contains a *central canal*, and expands cranially to form a *brain* containing extensions of the central canal termed *ventricles*. Throughout the vertebrates, the walls of the brain and spinal cord again consist of interneurons and, less numerous, motor neurons, together with associated non-nervous glial cells and blood vessels; but two quite distinctive tissue varieties can be recognized, namely *grey matter* and *white matter*, when freshly cut nervous tissue is examined.

**Grey matter** consists of the cell somata, dendritic trees and initial axon segments of the neurons, the terminal segments and synaptic endings of axons which are associated with them, together with varieties of glial cell and blood vessels. Some intercalated neurons have short axons that remain wholly within the grey matter. Many, however, possess longer axons and these leave the grey matter, where they course in functionally associated bundles termed *tracts*. Outside the grey matter each acquires a laminated lipo-protein sheath of *myelin* derived from certain varieties of neighbouring glial cells. The sheaths are essentially concerned with the functional efficiency

see the first appearance of a *central nervous system* (7.11). The receptor cells are still largely situated in the surface epithelial layers, but their basal conducting processes are longer, since they traverse the tissue layers to approach the region on each side of the plane of symmetry. Here, the nerve cell bodies are concentrated, and the synaptic terminals of the receptor cells end in relation to some of them. The somata of the motor (effector) neurons are sited within this concentration, and their axonal processes leave the central nervous system to reach the effectors. The remaining nerve cells are interposed between some of the receptor cell terminals and the motor neurons. They may possess short or longer axonal processes and are termed *intercalated* or *internuncial* neurons or simply *interneurons*. Thus, paths of varying complexity connect the receptor cell input and the motor neuron output; some paths are *polysynaptic*, with a number of neurons successively interposed, whilst in others a direct receptor-effector *monosynaptic* path exists. It is in such diversity of *connectivity*, that the variations in speed and complexity of behavioural responses to different environmental conditions reside.

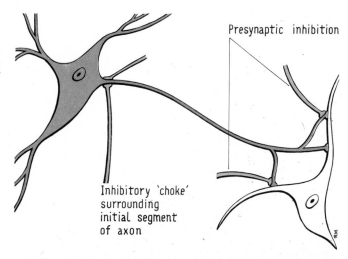

**7.9** The multipolar neuron shown in red has inhibitory synaptic terminals (blue) applied to the initial segment of its axon, and others to the surfaces of its own axonal synaptic terminals.

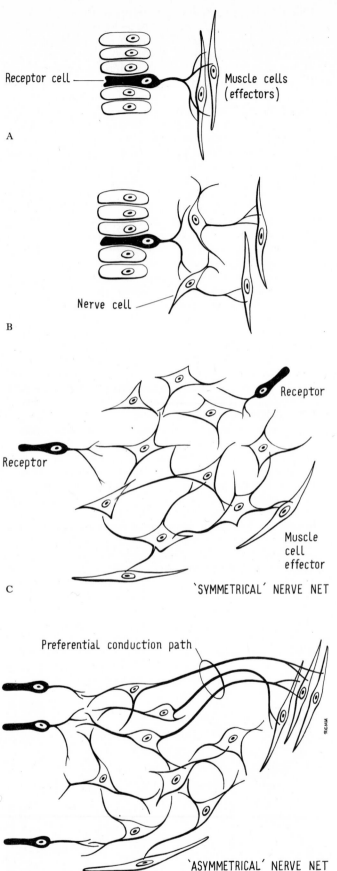

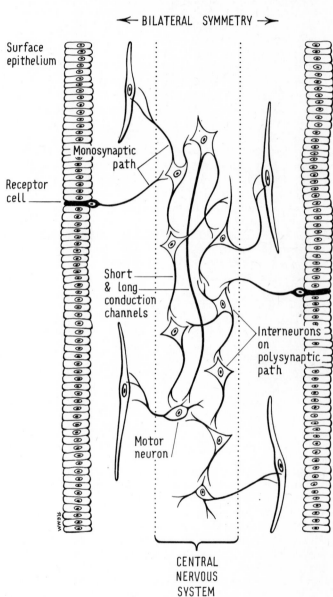

of the nerve fibres during impulse conduction, in terms of an enhanced conduction velocity for a given diameter, and a reduction in their energy requirements (p. 786). They impart a pinkish-white opalescence to the fresh tissue—hence the term **white matter**.

The vertebrate central canal is largely lined by a ciliated columnar epithelium termed *ependyma*, and during early embryogenesis the grey matter develops in a zone immediately surrounding the ependymal lining,

7.11 Some features of the nervous system in a primitive organism with bilateral symmetry. Note the intraepithelial positions of the receptor cells, and the aggregation of interneurons and motor neurons near the plane of symmetry as a central nervous system. Note also the different orders of complexity of the conduction pathways, and the possibility of cooperative actions involving both sides of the body.

7.10A–D Simple nervous systems. A direct interaction between a receptor cell and the muscle cell effectors. B interneurons which make functional contacts with each other are interposed between the receptor cell terminals and the muscle cell effectors. C receptor cell terminals feed into a fairly symmetrical network of interneurons which in turn makes contact with the effectors. D the interneurons between the receptors and effectors are organized where 'diffuse' multisynaptic conduction pathways predominate, and others where more direct routes are present.

whilst the white matter forms external to this. At first these relationships are present throughout the length of the neural tube, and, in the spinal cord, they persist to maturity. With the development and elaboration of hindbrain, midbrain and forebrain vesicles, however, whilst some masses of grey matter are retained in the primitive para-ependymal position, others migrate outwards to insinuate themselves between the developing tracts of white matter on the ventrolateral aspects of the tube. Most importantly, profuse secondary migrations of developing grey matter occur in the roof of each of the three vesicles, where they become arranged as a subsurface series of fibrocellular laminae, which are of the greatest significance in the functioning of the system.

Before embarking upon a detailed account of human neuroanatomy, methods which have been employed in neuroanatomical research and the cytology of nervous tissue will be reviewed.

## TECHNIQUES AND DEVELOPMENT OF NEUROANATOMY*

The previous section has been largely a consideration of the analytical philosophy of nervous systems—only possible on the results of a long historical process of accumulation of data, explanations, and hypotheses. These results, due to the efforts of a large succession of observers and experimenters,[6-10] have been primarily dependent upon perceiving relationships between observed phenomena, especially in the most effective contributions. Even these, however, were conditioned by the technical means available at the time. It is hence suitable at this point to examine the methods by which major advances leading to current levels of knowledge have been achieved. Inevitably such a survey must be brief, and while historical in approach, it is not intended as an account of neurological discovery, but of the neuroanatomical and other techniques involved. Hence, it is impossible here to cite more than a few examples of the fruits of the various methods included, nor can treatment of these subjects be exhaustive. In any case, other references to technique, and to the advances made by them, will appear in the general description of the nervous system which follows. Ideally, the names of innovators should be kept before us by habitual citation, but this is scarcely practicable in the textbooks of today. Perhaps the ensuing pages will help to correct this deficiency, though necessarily in a limited and irregular manner.

The development of neuroanatomy, as with any other corpus of knowledge, has been linked at every stage to contemporary means of observation and experiment. Hence, it was initially slow: a period of about two millennia separated the earliest recorded observations from the introduction of even simple magnifying lenses. The great accessions to knowledge during the nineteenth and twentieth centuries have coincided with the acceleration of technical innovation and improvement during this period. Until recent times physiology lagged centuries behind anatomy, a frustration to all who find function the chief interest in structure; but in the same explosion of technical progress functional studies have overtaken the purely structural in many fields, and have indeed carried concepts of function beyond structural observation in some. In neurology this has provided a much needed intellectual stimulus to morphologists.

### From the Greeks to the Renaissance

Granted the importance of technique, and hence the extremely simple means available, the paucity of neurological observation, or even speculation, recorded by earlier civilizations, prior to classical Greek times, is surprising. Opportunities presented by injury, sacrifice and mummification are obvious; yet the earliest records are limited to a description of the optic nerves by Alcmaeon (c. 500 B.C.) and a few statements in the Hippocratic Collection (c. 400 B.C.), amounting to little more than recognition of the cleft between the cerebral hemispheres and a belief that the brain is associated with intelligence. Even Aristotle (384–322 B.C.) confused peripheral nerves with tendons (with lasting effects visible in the term 'aponeurosis'); and he unaccountably set intelligence in the heart, unlike Plato (429–347 B.C.), who sited sensation and thought in the brain. Of course, biological thought was already permeated by the Four Elements of Empedocles (c. 493–433 B.C.) and the Four Humours of Polybus (c. 390 B.C.). The humoral concept in particular was to dominate and, indeed, obstruct biological thought for almost two thousand years, however improbable it now seems or how extraordinary that simple contradictory observations were ignored.

Human dissection began (as far as records support) with the rise of the Alexandrian School, whose leaders in biology, Herophilus and Erasistratus (c. 300–250 B.C.), are widely regarded as the 'father figures' of anatomy and physiology. (The possible debt of such dissectors to the embalmers of Egypt should not be overlooked, though how far this age-old source of practical knowledge influenced deliberate dissection cannot be assessed.[11]) Herophilus distinguished cerebrum and cerebellum, describing the fourth ventricle and even its calamus scriptorius; he also differentiated motor and sensory nerves. Erasistratus detailed the ventricles further, ascribing them functions entangled in humoral concepts, as was his entire physiological teaching, complicated further by the *pneuma*, or vital spirit, an intellectual impediment lingering long after the Renaissance. However, he also equated the more elaborate gyral pattern of the human brain with mankind's pre-eminent intelligence, a remarkably prophetic speculation.

With the Roman annexation of Egypt (50 B.C.) the Alexandrian School decayed; but Galen (A.D. 129–199) left his native Pergamon to study there, his most productive years being spent in Rome. His significance in medicine and biology, as a dissector and experimentalist, calls for no reiteration.[12, 13] He classified the cranial nerves, omitting the olfactory and trochlear and confusing others, though his description was not improved until some 1,500 years later. Much of Galen's voluminous and dogmatic writings was theoretical, but his work on spinal cord functions was directly based on experiment, and was not extended until Bell and Magendie added their observations early in the nineteenth century. Section between the first two vertebrae, he concluded, led to immediate death, between the third and fourth to respiratory arrest, and at lower levels to paralysis of bladder, intestines and legs. In contrast, most of Galen's prolific output was couched in humoral and vitalistic ideas which—in view of the

* Throughout this section references to earlier workers have been omitted, since they can be found in historical accounts such as:

[6] Anglo-American Symposium on *The Brain and its Functions*, Blackwell, Oxford. 1958.
[7] M. A. B. Brazier, in: *Handbook of Physiology*, vol. I, ed. G. J. Field and H. W. Magoun, American Physiological Society, Washington, D.C. 1959.
[8] C. Singer and E. A. Underwood, *A Short History of Medicine*, Clarendon Press, Oxford. 1962.
[9] E. Clarke and C. D. O'Malley, *The Human Brain and Spinal Cord*, University of California Press, Berkeley. 1968.
[10] A. Meyer, *Historical Aspects of Cerebral Anatomy*, Oxford University Press, London. 1971.
[11] A. J. E. Cave, *Proc. R. Soc. Med.*, 43, 1958.
[12] G. Sarton, *Galen of Pergamon*, University of Kansas Press, Laurence, Kansas. 1954.
[13] C. Singer, *Galen on Anatomical Procedures*, Oxford University Press, London. 1956.

veneration with which his teaching was held for many centuries—were a serious brake on progress.

After Galen, biological and medical thinking entered a long suspense. The classical legacy was all but extinguished in Europe during the ensuing 'Dark Ages'. Greek texts survived chiefly in Arabic translations, with little improvement in knowledge; in accord with the general intellectual lethargy, neuroanatomy marked time for a thousand years; indeed, anatomical accuracy degenerated. The rising popularity of astrology and the insistence of early Christian authority upon the unimportance, and even degradation of man's physical estate, displaced interest from his own true fabric.

From the eleventh century Greek medical manuscripts were being translated into Latin, at first from Arabic versions. Though this was the start of the rewakening of European science, progress was very slow, the ensuing centuries remaining barren of fresh anatomical or physiological advance. The opinions of Hippocrates, Aristotle, and especially Galen were the approved sources of anatomical knowledge in medieval times, with almost unchallenged authority. Even in the rising universities of the twelfth and thirteenth centuries, observation of natural phenomena was neglected; achievements were literary. Dissection reappeared, but at first as an exercise to confirm established dogma. Even Mondino of Bologna, whose *Anathomia* of 1316 is regarded as the first text in the modern period, ascribed the functions of antique teaching to the brain ventricles, and in sum he added nothing of significance to neuroanatomy. Though dissection continued in Bologna, spreading to other Italian centres and to Montpellier, the fourteenth and fifteenth centuries brought little more than translations from Greek, rather than Arabic texts. The anatomical Humanists of the sixteenth century were pre-occupied with the replacement of Arabic anatomical terms by Greek and Latin, but great exceptions from such drab polemics were at work, as we shall now see.

## From the Renaissance to the Nineteenth Century

The movement towards naturalism amongst artists of the Renaissance in the late fifteenth and early sixteenth centuries culminated in Leonardo da Vinci (1452–1519).[14] Like his great contemporaries, Dürer, Michelangelo and Raphael, he turned to dissection for direct information on human structure. The extent of his contemporary influence is uncertain, but he brilliantly epitomizes the revival of an inquiring spirit in Europe, reacting powerfully against traditionalism and the excesses of scholastic orthodoxy. His contribution to neuroanatomy was limited but impressive—some remarkable figures of the brain, depicting wax casts of the ventricles, a technique invented by him. The movement represented by Leonardo, together with the introduction of improved techniques of engraving, paved the way for Vesalius.

Vesalius (1514–64)[15] has received perhaps excessive medical adulation; his plates, starkly structural when compared with the functional inspiration of Leonardo's, nevertheless introduced an accuracy unrivalled in his time, marking a new era in medicine. Dissatisfied with Galenic inaccuracies, and with the near sanctity accorded them despite the ascertainable facts, and yet unable fully to emancipate himself from Galen's physiology, he revised the whole field of anatomy by his own dissections. In neuroanatomy he struck a new high level in detail and precision, though with lesser success in the peripheral nervous system. He illustrated the brain partly in a sectional manner (a technical innovation), going far beyond existing knowledge. He clearly indicated the basal ganglia,

hippocampus, fornix, internal capsule, pulvinar, colliculi, fourth ventricle, and many other details, with almost the accuracy of a modern atlas.

Eustachius (1550–74), a contemporary of Vesalius, has received less than just acclaim; his work, like Leonardo's, only became generally known long after his death. He left a brilliant depiction of the sympathetic nervous system (7.12), and he portrayed the cranial nerves more accurately than Vesalius and the pons (Varolii) than Varolius.

Vesalius' successors at Padua were less eminent, but exerted much influence on visiting scholars. Thus, Coiter of Montpellier (1534–76), a notable early comparative anatomist, studied under Fallopius, and he improved the work of Vesalius and Eustachius on the cranial nerves, describing the two roots of spinal nerves and distinguishing white and grey matter in the spinal cord. Fabricius, also a comparative anatomist, taught Harvey (1578–1657), whose celebrated discovery of the circulation was strangely combined with a veneration for Galen's views in other matters, sometimes almost servile. Nevertheless, Harvey rejected the flow of 'spirits' in hollow nerves, a break with dogma perhaps not unassociated with the influence of his contemporary, Bacon (1561–1626). Bacon's contempt for scholastic orthodoxy, and his inductive approach to experimentation and factual verification of hypothesis, have proved the first clear advance beyond the logic of Aristotle. This new scientific attitude, though a working philosophy rather than a practical technique, has perhaps influenced subsequent scientific endeavour as profoundly as Harvey's experimental genius. Thereafter the tempo of discovery has slowly augmented, with the focus upon humours in nerves or the blood, as avenues of control and communication, gradually turning towards the nervous system.

Until the times of Vesalius and Harvey the only techniques for study of the nervous system were dissection and the simplest experimentation, both observed with the unaided eye. No sudden changes occurred; but during the seventeenth and eighteenth centuries discoveries in parallel fields, especially in electrical phenomena and optics, have proved highly significant to nervous system investigation. The experiments of Gilberd (1540–1603) in electricity and magnetism foreshadowed the development of electrical stimulation of nerves by Galvani (1737–98) and Volta (1745–1827), which heralded the evolution of neurophysiology. Simple microscopes began to appear, enabling van Leeuwenhoek (1632–1723) to dispute the hollowness of nerves; the compound instruments which rapidly followed, though notably exploited by observers such as Hooke (1635–1703), were not applied extensively to neuroanatomy until the early nineteenth century.

Meanwhile, topographical neuroanatomy prospered, and such exponents as Willis (1621–1675) and Vieussens (1641–1716) hardened the brain, either by soaking it in wine or by boiling. They were hence able to dissect it, an advance over the slicing methods of their predecessors, enabling them to achieve a new level of excellence. Willis in particular was a pioneer of macroscopic dissection of nerve fibre bundles in the central nervous system, the only technique available for such investigation for nearly two

7.12 The brain and autonomic nervous system depicted by Bartolomeo Eustachio (1550–74), a contemporary and rival of Vesalius (1514–64), from *Tabulae Anatomicae*, published posthumously in 1714 by Lancisi. The copperplates of Eustachio (or Eustachius) are not only anatomically more accurate than the woodcuts of Vesalius, but also technically superior. (By courtesy of the Trustees of the British Museum.)

[14] E. Belt, *Leonardo the Anatomist*, University of Kansas Press, Laurence, Kansas. 1955.
[15] C. D. O'Malley, *Andreas Vesalius of Brussels, 1514–1564*, University of California Press, Berkeley. 1964.

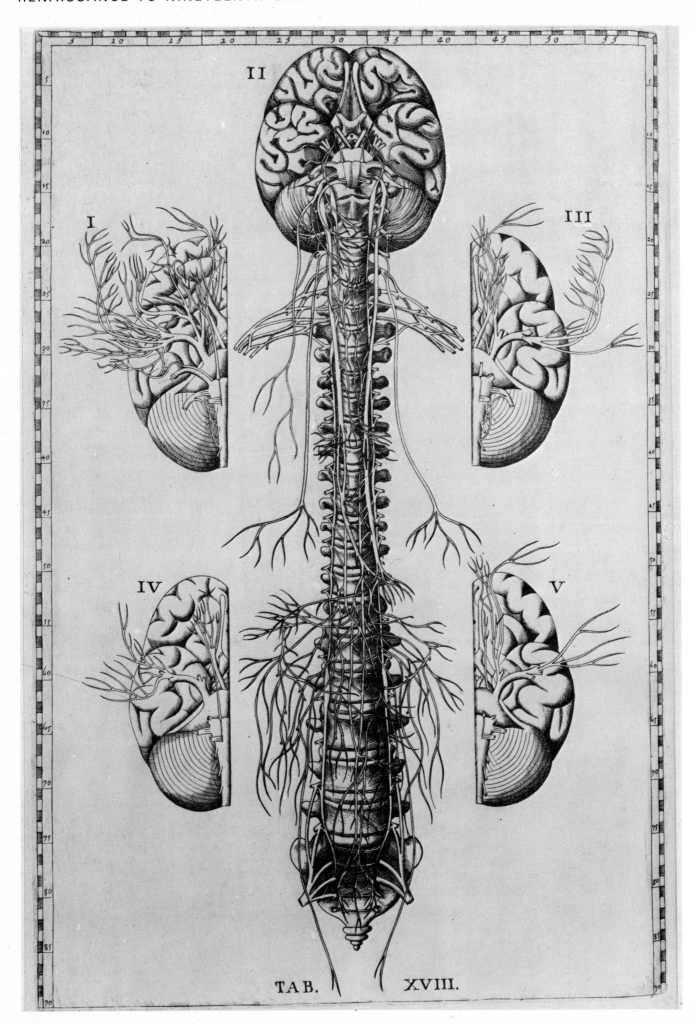

TAB. XVIII.

centuries after him. Naturally disposed towards experiment, he was also approaching modern concepts of reflex activity.

During the latter part of the eighteenth century the speculations of Willis, von Haller, Whytt and others regarding involuntary reactions to stimulation were beginning to emerge as realities in the experiments of the 'galvanists'. At the same time the compound microscope was coming into wider use; and during the first half of the nineteenth century the accessory supporting techniques of fixation, microtomy, and staining were also evolving. Neuroanatomists were turning from external features to internal structure, though the former diverged into a wide interest in comparative morphology. Many workers were becoming more specialized, and it is perhaps less confusing to consider further technical progress as a number of arbitrarily separated topics.

## Comparative Anatomy and Embryology

Though Erasistratus is sometimes regarded as the first comparative neuroanatomist, the modern movement stems from the observations of Willis.[16, 17, 18] At first the accent was on functional rather than evolutionary concepts; and in this Willis laid the foundations of nineteenth-century preoccupation with localization of function, especially in the cerebral cortex. Gall (1758–1828) and his pupil, Spurzheim (1776–1832),[19] though achieving a notoriety undeserved by the former through their erroneous theory of phrenology, nevertheless were initially responsible for the principle of cortical localization. In their massive publications[19] they much improved on Willis's comparative observations on cerebral gyri, and they also carried further his method of brain dissection. Tiedemann (1781–1861)[20] was a pioneer in description of the human fetal brain, and Reil (1759–1813)[21] concentrated on the development and comparative anatomy of the cerebellum and insula, advocating the technical value of combining such studies in functional interpretation. Owen[22] added the concept of brain weight and volume as a comparative technique, and he also linked the early developmental appearance of certain gyri with the regularity of their occurrence. Many others extended the series of animals studied, especially in respect of primates, and in this the advent of Darwinism was an additional spur. Throughout the nineteenth century a wealth of comparative and embryological observations were adduced in evidence of homologies in cortical pattern to support the polemics of the 'localizationists' and their opponents, a now almost forgotten controversy. All these contributions were based on macroscopic technique; but with Campbell, the Vogts and Brodmann,[23] at the end of the century and extending into the twentieth, microscopic investigation of the cortex on a comparative basis became established. The vast cytoarchitectonic investigations, familiar in the 'Brodmann maps' of many current texts, have never been equalled except by Conel's studies of developing cortex.

With the great advances in neurohistology and neurophysiology in the late nineteenth and twentieth centuries, interest in topographical comparative neuroanatomy has somewhat waned. Nevertheless, with the new morphological techniques classical work such as that of Herrick,[24] of Larsell[25] on the cerebellum, and Polyak[26] on the visual system, continued to appear. The great compendia of comparative neuroanatomy compiled by Ariëns Kappers[27, 28] and his collaborators must also be mentioned. (References to the work of others, including Tilney, Connolly, Bailey and von Bonin can be found in the recent text of Crosby and her pupils.[29])

The linkage between embryology and comparative anatomy was early established, as already noted. Arnold (1842), for example, described the early development of the hippocampal gyrus in primates; His (1874) distinguished 'complete' fissures, which appear first, and secondary cortical sulci; and Broca (1878) supported his concept of a speech centre as much by such considerations as by functional data.

More significant, however, have been embryological studies at the microscopic level. His (1887)[30] demonstrated stained preparations showing that axons grow from neuroblasts, thus providing positive evidence for the neuron doctrine, and in a sense foreshadowing the tissue culture studies of Harrison (1907).[31] The work of His was confirmed by Held (1897), who nevertheless concluded that synaptic gaps, as we would call them today, disappeared during maturation of neurons—evidence against the individuality of nerve cells. Flechsig (1876)[32] discovered that myelination proceeds—before and after birth—at different rates in various tracts, thus introducing a *myelogenetic technique* for investigation of fibre connexions.

## Neurohistological Technique and Light Microscopy[33 – 35]

Leeuwenhoek (1674) identified nerve fibres with a simple high-powered lens, and with a similar 'microscope' Swammerdam (1675) even dissected out the nervous system of the mayfly larva, a brilliant anticipation of microdissection. Jansen (1590) had already constructed the first compound microscope, put to practical but not biological use by Galileo. Kepler is also credited with a similar invention, carried into effect by Scheiner (1611). Huygens (*c.* 1684) introduced the compound eyepiece. Malpighi (1666) has been supposed to have been first to visualize nerve cells with a somewhat crude compound microscope, but a reconstruction of his observations with a similar instrument has neatly demolished this claim

[16] T. Willis, *Cerebri Anatome*, Martyn and Allestry, London. 1664.
[17] F. J. Cole, *A History of Comparative Anatomy*, Macmillan, London. 1944.
[18] J. Needham, *A History of Embryology*, 2nd ed., Cambridge University Press, 1959.
[19] F. J. Gall and J. C. Spurzheim, *Anatomie et physiologie du système nerveux en général, et du cerveau en particulier*, Schoell, Paris. 1810–19.
[20] F. Tiedemann, *Anatomie und Bildungsgeschichte des Gehirns im Foetus des Menschen*, Steinishen, Nuremberg. 1860.
[21] J. C. Reil, *Arch. Physiol. Halle*, **8**, 1807.
[22] R. Owen, *On the Anatomy of Vertebrates*, Longmans, Green, London. 1868.
[23] K. Brodmann, *Vergleichende Lokalisationslehre der Grosshirnrinde, in ihren Prinzipien dargestellt auf Grund des Zellenbaues*, Barth, Leipsig. 1909.
[24] C. J. Herrick, *Introduction to Neurology*, Saunders, Philadelphia. 1931.
[25] O. Larsell, *Archs Neurol. Psychiat., Chicago*, **38**, 1937.
[26] S. Polyak, in: *The Vertebrate Visual System*, ed. H. Klüver, University of Chicago Press, Chicago, Illinois. 1957.
[27] C. U. Ariëns Kappers, *Die vergleichende Anatomie des Nervensystems der Wirbeltiere und des Menschen*, Bohn, Haarlem. 1920–1.
[28] C. U. Ariëns Kappers, G. C. Huber and E. C. Crosby, *The Comparative Anatomy of the Nervous System of Vertebrates, Including Man*, Macmillan, N.Y. 1936.
[29] E. C. Crosby, T. Humphrey and E. W. Lauer, *Correlative Anatomy of the Nervous System*, Macmillan, N.Y. 1962.
[30] W. His, *Abh. Gesch. Math.*, **13**, 1887.
[31] R. G. Harrison, *Anat. Rec.*, **1**, 1907.
[32] P. Flechsig, *Die Leitungsbahnen im Gehirn und Rückenmark des Menschen auf Grund entwicklungsgeschichtlicher Untersuchungen*, Engelmann, Leipzig. 1876.
[33] R. S. Clay and T. H. Court, *The History of the Microscope*, Griffin, London. 1932.
[34] J. Brachet and A. E. Mirsky (eds.), *The Cell*, vol. I, Academic Press, New York and London. 1960.
[35] G. L. Clark (ed.), *The Encyclopedia of Microscopy*, Reinhold, New York. 1961.

(Clarke and Bearn, 1968).[36] Fontana (1781) described nerve fibres clearly, but failed to distinguish axon from sheath. Further advances were in fact impossible without improvement in microscopy. Lister (1827) and Amici (1827) manufactured *achromatic* objectives; however, Lister's pioneer efforts were sustained by no British successor, the centre of further development passing to Germany, where Abbé, working for Carl Zeiss, was able to construct *apochromatic* objectives in 1886, using the newly discovered Jena glasses. He also improved the condenser and devised compensating eyepieces. Dark-field condensers (Wenham, *c.* 1853) and immersion objectives (Tolles, 1874 and Abbé, 1878) further accelerated the refinement of the late nineteenth-century microscope.

The immediate result of even achromatic objectives was a flood of descriptions of animal tissues. Botanical *cells* had been portrayed long before, of course, by Hooke (1665) and so named. Nerve cells, a discovery at one time accorded to Schwann when enunciating the cell theory with Schleiden in 1839, are now considered to have been first satisfactorily recognized by Ehrenberg (1833).[37] However, there seems to be little doubt that Schwann first described the neurolemmal cell. These early achievements were rapidly surpassed with the new optical resources, but this progress rested equally upon development of adequate methods of preparation and staining of animal tissues.

## PREPARATION OF MATERIAL FOR MICROSCOPY

Early microscopists used teased or squashed preparations of either fresh or, at most, partially preserved biological material. Since fixation and hardening are essential to adequate sectioning, especially of animal tissues, Reil's introduction of alcohol for this purpose in 1809 was an important advance. Hannover added chromic acid as a fixative in 1840; and Stilling (1842) used both methods, sometimes coupled with freezing, in accomplishing his classical work on the spinal cord (1846), cutting it both transversely and in longitudinal section. He also advocated serial sections, as did Virchow (1846), in describing and naming neuroglia. Formalin fixation was introduced much later by Blum (1893). Stilling and Wallach (1842) devised a simple hand microtome, improved by Welcher (1856); machines of increasing accuracy were invented and improved throughout the second half of the nineteenth century, still linked with names such as Jung, Thoma, Cambridge Rocker, etc. Von Gudden and Catsch (1875) were able to cut whole sections of the cerebral hemisphere, and Rutherford and Cathcart (1873) introduced the first freezing microtome. By the 1880s semi-automatic microtomes, such as the Cambridge Rocker, were capable of producing ribbons of thin serial sections from wax-embedded material, paraffin wax having been introduced by Klebs in 1869. Embedding of tissue in collodion (Duval, 1879), celloidin (Schiefferdecker, 1882) and other materials followed, leading to such modern innovations as water-soluble waxes, freeze-drying, and cryostat techniques.

## TISSUE STAINING METHODS IN NEUROANATOMY

It is a source of surprise and admiration to note how much was achieved by the early nineteenth-century microscopists without staining techniques, though it would be misleading to overlook the sporadic use of colouring methods from the beginnings of microscopy.[38–40] Nevertheless, Remak's early description of axons and their sheaths in 1836 was based on unstained embryonic material,[41] and under similar difficulties Purkinje, a year later, confirmed these observations and identified the cerebellar nerve cells

named after him. Incidentally, Purkinje adopted acetic alcohol as a clearing agent and Canada balsam for permanent mounting of sections. It is nowadays difficult to believe that Waller's study of degeneration in nerve fibres reported in 1850 was conducted on teased nerves, unfixed and unstained; or that Kühne's discovery of motor endings in 1862 followed mere treatment with weak hydrochloric acid to clarify the sarcoplasm.

The first neurohistological stain was probably the carmine and gold method of Gerlach (1858), which enabled him to advance a *reticular* or *net* theory of neuronal continuity. The controversy between the protagonists of this and the rival *neuron theory* reverberated through the rest of the nineteenth century and into the twentieth. Though Faraday had discovered benzene in 1825, and Perkins had prepared the first aniline dye, mauveine, in 1856, the industrial development of dyes was quickly taken up in Germany, a by-product being a rapidly increasing range of such dyes available for histological use from 1862 onwards.[42] Carmine staining was applied by Deiters (1865)[43] in differentiating between dendrites and axons. Ranvier's (1871)[44] classical delineation of nerve fibres and their nodes depended upon a silver impregnation of chromic acid fixed tissue; and Golgi (1878)[45] further elaborated silver staining, thus rendering occasional whole neurons visible, from which preparations he described the cell types still known today by his name. Golgi emphatically supported the reticular theory, but Ramon y Cajal (1906),[46] who adopted Golgi's metallic impregnation methods and added his own refinements, was thus able to accumulate such an overpowering array of observations on neurons in all parts of the human nervous system, and in many other animals, that the neuron theory has prevailed. The accuracy and volume of this work was the chief factor in advancing the individuality of nerve cells, although the theory is often accorded to Waldeyer. Not until the advent of the electron microscope was it possible to adduce more convincing evidence in favour of Cajal's teaching; however, even as recently as 1933, a year before the appearance of the first electron microscope, he considered it necessary to re-emphasize his views.[47] Cajal also used Nissl's methylene-blue method for staining 'chromatin granules' (*vide infra*). Ehrlich (1886),[48] applying the same dye to living tissues and thus initiating vital staining, was thereby able to define peripheral nerve cell processes to their terminations; being an axonal stain, this technique has proved most valuable, in various modifications, for the demonstration of peripheral non-myelinated autonomic nerve fibres.

Nissl (1892)[49] discovered the *acute response* of a nerve cell body to damage of its axon, characterized by *chromatolysis*, a breakdown of the *Nissl* or *chromatin granules*, as well as other manifestations, such as swelling of the cell and eccentricity of its nucleus. (These, and other features of retrograde changes are described more fully elsewhere —pp. 793–794.) He thus provided further evidence of continuity of nerve cell and axon and also a most valuable

[36] E. C. Clarke and J. G. Bearn, *J. Hist. Med. allied Sci.*, **23**, 1968.

[37] C. G. Ehrenberg, *Poggendorf's Ann. phys. Chem.*, **28**, 1833.

[38] J. R. Baker, *Cytological Techniques*, 4th ed., Methuen, London. 1960.

[39] A. G. E. Pearse, *Histochemistry*, 3rd ed., Churchill, London. 1968.

[40] E. Gurr, *The Rational Use of Dyes in Biology*, Hill, London. 1965.

[41] R. Remak, *Arch. Anat. Physiol.*, 1836.

[42] H. J. Conn, *The History of Staining*, Biotech. Publications, Geneva and New York. 1948.

[43] O. F. K. Deiters, *Untersuchungen über Gehirn und Rückenmark des Menschen und der Säugethiere*, Vieweg und Sohn, Braunschweig. 1865.

[44] L.-A. Ranvier, *C. r. hebd. Séanc. Acad. Sci., Paris*, **73**, 1871.

[45] C. Golgi, *R. C. Inst. Lombardo Sci.*, 2nd ser., **12**, 1878.

[46] S. R. y Cajal, in: *Les Prix Nobel en 1906*, Norstedt, Stockholm. 1908.

[47] S. R. y Cajal, *Archos Neurobiol.*, **13**, 1933.

[48] P. Ehrlich, *Dt. med. Wschr.*, **12**, 1886.

[49] F. Nissl, *Allg. Zt. Psychiat.*, **48**, 1892.

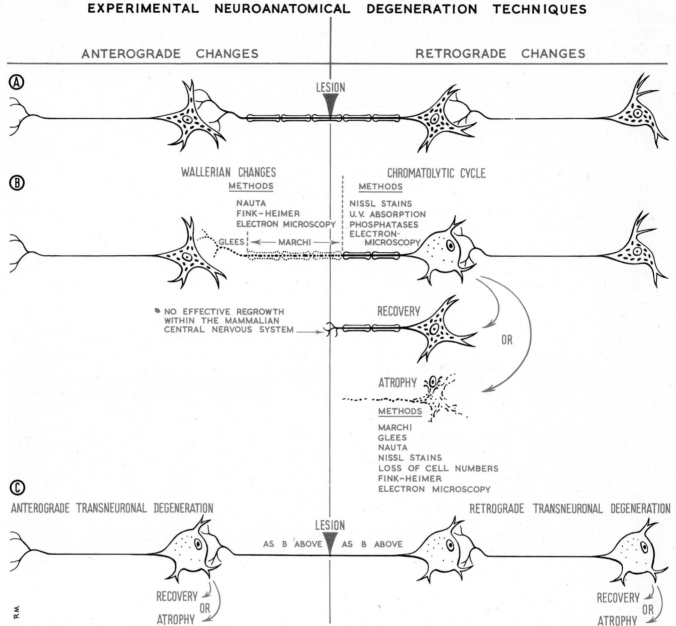

EXPERIMENTAL NEUROANATOMICAL DEGENERATION TECHNIQUES

ANTEROGRADE CHANGES · RETROGRADE CHANGES

Ⓐ LESION

Ⓑ WALLERIAN CHANGES · CHROMATOLYTIC CYCLE
METHODS · METHODS
NAUTA · NISSL STAINS
FINK–HEIMER · U.V. ABSORPTION
ELECTRON MICROSCOPY · PHOSPHATASES
GLEES ← MARCHI → · ELECTRON-MICROSCOPY

NO EFFECTIVE REGROWTH WITHIN THE MAMMALIAN CENTRAL NERVOUS SYSTEM · RECOVERY OR

ATROPHY
METHODS
MARCHI
GLEES
NAUTA
NISSL STAINS
LOSS OF CELL NUMBERS
FINK–HEIMER
ELECTRON MICROSCOPY

Ⓒ ANTEROGRADE TRANSNEURONAL DEGENERATION · RETROGRADE TRANSNEURONAL DEGENERATION
LESION
AS B ABOVE · AS B ABOVE
RECOVERY OR ATROPHY · RECOVERY OR ATROPHY

7.13 Diagram of the sequelae of interruption of the fibres of central nervous system neurons. As shown, regeneration or atrophy may follow the response to injury, both in the neuron primarily damaged and in those affected transneuronally. Transneuronal effects may occasionally supervene in neurons more remotely associated with the damaged neuron. See text for further details.

means of delineating the arrangement of neurons. Weigert (1882),[50] somewhat earlier, had elaborated a staining technique for *normal* myelin sheaths based on pretreatment with potassium bichromate, followed by acid fuchsin (haematoxylin is now more often used). It is interesting to note that he was already using collodion for embedding material, xylol for clearing, and balsam as a mounting medium. This innovation was quickly followed by Marchi's[51] osmic acid method for staining *degenerating* myelin, for which it is specific and hence an early example of histochemical technique. A few years before Nissl's description of the early response of neurons to damage, Gudden (1870)[52] had studied the later sequelae of these changes, finding that the injured cells commonly atrophied and ultimately disappeared; he also noted that the changes were more rapid and marked in young animals.

Both Gudden and Nissl made considerable personal contributions using their own techniques. The former's original experiments were an investigation of thalamo-cortical connexions, which his pupil von Monakow[53] carried further, also discovering the visual function of the lateral geniculate body. It is noteworthy that both problems have been reinvestigated by the same technique half a century later,[54, 55] an example of the continuing value of such degeneration techniques; these have continued in use throughout the twentieth century, and their application, together with certain other allied methods, is of such general importance in neuroanatomy that they must now be considered in more detail.

## Neuron Tracing Techniques

The researches of Waller, Gudden, Golgi, Weigert, Marchi, Nissl and Cajal were all published within the last thirty years of the nineteenth century, except for Waller's

[50] C. Weigert, in: *Gesammeete Abhandlungen*, **2**, 1882.
[51] V. Marchi and G. Algeri, *Riv. sper. Freniat.*, **11** and **12**, 1885–6.
[52] B. von Gudden, *Arch. Psychiat. NervKrankh.*, **2**, 1870.
[53] C. von Monakow, *Arch. Psychiat. NervKrankh.*, **12**, 1882.
[54] W. E. Le Gros Clarke and G. G. Penman, *Proc. R. Soc. B.*, **114**, 1934.
[55] W. E. Le Gros Clarke, *J. Anat.*, **70**, 1936.

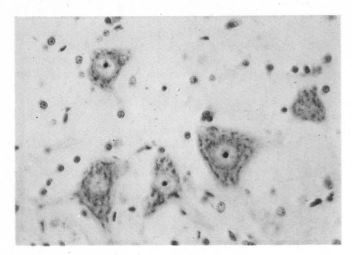

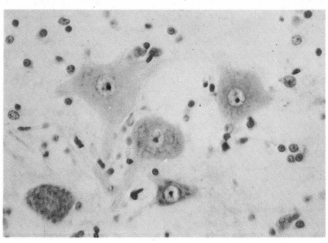

7.14 A–D   A   Large multipolar neuronal perikarya in the magnocellular part of the feline red nucleus, showing prominent Nissl's granules, bases of dendrites and axon hillocks. The nuclei are euchromatic and vesicular, with prominent nucleoli. The small nuclei scattered in the surrounding neuropil are characteristic of the various categories of neuroglial cells.

B   A field similar to that depicted in A, but after previous contralateral hemisection of the spinal cord at the level of the fifth cervical segment, thereby severing the rubrospinal tract. The section shows characteristic chromatolytic retrograde changes in the cytoplasm of three large neurons. Two smaller neurons are unaffected.

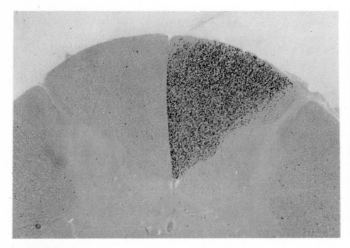

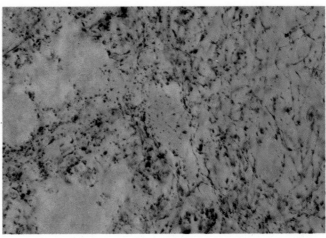

C   Transverse section through dorsal funiculi of feline cervical spinal cord, after unilateral dorsal column section at a more caudal level. Note anterograde Wallerian degeneration of ascending nerve fibres: degenerating myelin sheaths are stained black by Marchi technique. (Provided by Dr. E. W. Baxter, Dept. of Biology, Guy's Hospital Medical School.)

D   A high-power light micrograph showing preterminal degeneration of afferent axons ending in relation to neurons of the red nucleus of a rat, after the previous placing of a cerebellar lesion. The preparation was stained by the Nauta-Gygax method. (Kindly supplied by Dr. K. E. Webster of University College, London.)

basic observations in 1850.[56] His demonstration that damage to nerve fibres induces microscopically identifiable changes proved a most fruitful starting point in this brilliant period and, indeed, in neuroanatomy and neuropathology in general. His immediate successors established the broad basis of neuronal morphology and the major techniques for an enormous volume of investigation into the organization of the nervous system. Modifications and some additions have followed, as we shall see, but their methodology remains substantially unchanged, persisting up to the present in parallel with subsequently evolved techniques in neurophysiology, histochemistry and electron microscopy (*vide infra*).

The essential features of the use of degeneration techniques in tracing out the arrangements of nerve cells and their neurites are shown in illustrations 7.13, 14.

When the cell body is actually ablated or damaged to such an extent that it dies, all its neurites, including the whole of the axon and its sheath of myelin, degenerate and finally disappear (for further details *see* p. 793), and during this period the changes described by Waller can be distinguished by Marchi staining of the degenerating myelin. The axon's terminal branchings, including their terminal synaptic buttons (*boutons terminaux*), are equally involved

in their degenerative process, though this was not at first appreciated. Being devoid of myelin these degenerating terminals did not stain by Marchi's technique, and this often led to errors when interpreting their presumed destination. More recently, however, methods introduced by Glees (1946),[57] and by Nauta and Gygax (1951),[58] with various modifications by other workers, do stain these degenerating preterminal and terminal structures. More recently still, ultrastructural changes in *boutons terminaux* during degeneration have been utilized for fibre tracing.

However, as we shall see, there are many technical difficulties associated with the placing of small discrete experimental lesions within a mass of nervous tissue. Further, there is no known method of selectively ablating *cell bodies alone* within the central nervous system; in all experimental situations, their dendritic trees and the synaptic terminals from other functionally associated neuron groups, blood vessels, and often other structures, are involved simultaneously. In some respects a clearer

[56] A. V. Waller, *Phil. Trans. R. Soc.*, Ser. B., **140**, 1850.
[57] P. Glees, *J. Neuropath. exp. Neurol.*, **5**, 1946.
[58] W. J. H. Nauta and P. A. Gygax, *Stain Technol.*, **26**, 1951.

experiment results when axonal processes are interrupted at some point along their course, and various terms have been introduced to indicate the different situations in which degenerative changes occur following such focal damage. These are summarized here.

Firstly, the effects confined to the neuron that has been damaged—those affecting that part of the axon, and associated structures, which has been detached from the parent cell, i.e. *distal* to the lesion, are termed *anterograde*; those affecting the dendritic tree, parent cell body and that part of the axon still attached to the cell body, i.e. *proximal* to the lesion, are *retrograde*. Secondly, changes may follow in neurons which have suffered no direct damage, but are functionally associated with the damaged cell. These are *transneuronal* (or *transynaptic*) changes, and they may be *primary* or *secondary*, etc. depending upon their degree of separation from the damaged cell, and further they may be *anterograde* or *retrograde*, depending upon their position relative to the damaged cell in a functional train of neurons. These varieties are detailed further in the following pages, and elsewhere in the present section.

Following a focal lesion of the axon, anterograde degeneration (of the Wallerian type involving again both the axon, its terminals, and myelin sheath) occurs distal to the lesion. The changes do not occur simultaneously at all points, but spread as a 'wave-front' distally from the lesion. After suitable time intervals they may be followed experimentally using the methods of Marchi, Glees, Nauta, Fink-Heimer, and histochemical and ultrastructural methods.

The proximal part of the fibre often does not show any changes when stained by Marchi's method, and for long it was believed that no degeneration occurred there, although Cajal had described a process of retrograde degeneration of Wallerian type which extended backwards along the fibre, but only as far as the first node of Ranvier proximal to the site of damage. However, it has now been established that more extensive changes sometimes do occur in the fibre proximal to the injury, and that is when there occurs a *retrograde atrophy* of the nerve cell body in question (which is of course accompanied by degeneration of *all* its neurites). Such an atrophy of the cell soma is a later sequel of the *acute retrograde* (chromatolytic) *response* studied by Nissl (but as we shall see the latter is not followed in every case by the more chronic manifestations of atrophy). The degenerative changes in the nerve fibres are thus termed *retrograde* in the sense that they occur proximal to the lesion, but they proceed in a *centrifugal* direction, from the cell soma towards the lesion. Again, at suitable time intervals they may be studied using the methods of Marchi, Glees, Nauta and Fink-Heimer.

These various phenomena develop more rapidly and are more marked in degree in newborn or at least very young animals, as Gudden noted, whereas Nissl apparently did not. Brodal (1940),[59] who has worked extensively with these methods, has introduced a so-called *modified Gudden technique*, which depends upon using very young experimental animals, in which both the acute and chronic types of retrograde change occur much more rapidly, the former being more usually relied upon.

The application of such methods, and the selection of a particular one in a given problem, require careful consideration; and the control of timing between infliction of a lesion and inspection of the consequent degeneration is critical. Moreover, workers in this field have reported much variation in the extent and rate of degenerative sequelae in different kinds of neurons and in the same cells in different species. Critiques[60, 61] of these experimental difficulties should be consulted, as also the many publications of workers by whom these techniques have been employed.

The ultimate fate of neurons damaged deliberately for experimental purposes is not always the same, and the following remarks apply also to the long-term results of naturally occurring injury. As stated above, when the nerve cell is ablated or coagulated, or otherwise severely damaged as in the infliction of focal lesions (*vide infra*), the whole neuron, including all its processes, degenerates and disappears. However, where axonal injury is inflicted, the acute retrograde reaction which supervenes may be followed either by a gradual recovery extending over some weeks, or by chronic retrograde atrophy, a much slower process with ultimate disappearance of the cell and, of course, its processes. Quantitative aspects of these phenomena have been investigated in some respects by Turner (1943)[62] and Bodian and Mellors (1945),[63] amongst others. Where the nerve cell survives, its characteristic pattern of chromatin granules returns and the proximal, attached part of its axon recovers, whereas its severed part is finally absorbed, after passing through the changes of Wallerian degeneration. The time relations of the latter vary in different instances, and they may be very slow. In the spinal cord it has been possible to apply Marchi staining to identify degenerating tracts up to a year or so after injury (Smith, 1951).[64]

So far the retrograde and anterograde degenerative responses to injury *within a single neuron* have been considered. Early in the present century, however, it was recognized that experimentally induced degeneration in one set of neurons may be followed by similar changes in others, arranged in the same functional sequence, the phenomenon being termed *transneuronal* or *transynaptic degeneration*.

The best known example of *anterograde transneuronal degeneration* occurs in the visual pathway: selective lesions of the retina result in degeneration not only of the nerve fibres of the injured ganglion cells which travel thence to the lateral geniculate body, but also of the geniculate neurons with which these fibres form synapses. The process may extend even further, involving a second group of functionally associated neurons in the striate cortex. It is thus possible to speak of *primary* and *secondary* transneuronal degeneration. The potentiality of this finding for elegant experimentation has not been overlooked, but this kind of 'polysynaptic' degenerative response has not been discovered in more than a few instances. There are indications that it may be limited to situations where neurons receive their afferent impulses predominantly, if not exclusively, from a single source. However, ventral grey column cells in the spinal cord receive afferents from multiple sources, and yet it has been claimed that they exhibit transneuronal degeneration when appropriate dorsal spinal roots are cut; these claims have been severely criticized. However that may be, the technique offers obvious possibilities in tracing pathways, and it may be more widely applicable than is so far expected.

*Retrograde transneuronal degeneration* has received less attention, though its occurrence in Gudden's cortical ablation experiments is now regarded as undoubted. The damage inflicted caused not only degeneration in anterior thalamic neurons, whose axons reach the cortex, but also in other thalamic nuclei now known to be in a primary

[59] A. Brodal, *Archs Neurol. Psychiat.*, *Chicago*, **43**, 1940.
[60] P. Glees, *Experimental Neurology*, Clarendon Press, Oxford. 1961.
[61] A. Brodal, *Neurological Anatomy*, Oxford University Press, London. 1969.
[62] R. S. Turner, *J. comp. Neurol.*, **79**, 1943.
[63] D. Bodian and R. C. Mellors, *J. exp. Med.*, **81**, 1945.
[64] M. C. Smith, *J. Neurol. Neurosurg. Psychiat.*, **14**, 1951.

and secondary functional relation to the anterior thalamus.[65] In Gudden's investigations the destructive technique was surgical ablation, a method still used when applicable, and when no more accurate means is required. A number of other methods of making highly selective lesions have been devised.

## SELECTIVE LESIONS AND STEREOTAXIS

In using fibre-tracing techniques an appropriately accurate method of killing nerve cells or dividing their fibres is essential. Simple division may suffice in peripheral nerves or in superficial central tracts; crushing or repeated injury has been advocated as more effective in the former. Superficial targets, such as cerebral or cerebellar cortex, can be damaged by ablation or by simple removal of pia mater, which naturally devascularizes a considerable depth of tissue. Most targets, however, are at some depth, and the surgical approach may invalidate some experiments by undesired damage to other regions. This difficulty has prompted alternative techniques, such as the introduction of fine electrodes, which can be used for stimulation as well as electrocoagulation, or of a fine probe capable of producing intense cold at its tip. Implantation of destructive substances, including alcohol, hydrocyanide, carbon dioxide snow, or radioactive yttrium, has also been practised. Irradiation by focused ultrasound[66] or proton beam[67] offers the advantage of causing damage within the nervous system without entering it, thus obviating even the usually trivial damage entailed by the passage of an electrode or probe. The latter complication becomes more serious when large or irregular structures, such as nuclei or ganglia, are to be destroyed, because repeated overlapping lesions must be made, requiring repeated insertions. The use of antibody-antigen reactions has been suggested, and it is claimed that the caudate nucleus has been selectively destroyed in this manner.

All the methods commonly employed to make selective lesions of the central nervous system, usually some part of the brain, entail the complication of *stereotaxis*—some means of aligning an electrode, cold probe, transducer, or the like with respect to the target selected.[68] The usual method is to fix the head of the experimental animal in a rigid frame in relation to which the electrode, etc. can be adjusted in three planes according to the coordinates of a particular target. These coordinates are established by measurements of the position of the target structure in serial sections of the whole head prepared in three planes, or by the use of an X-ray guidance system, using such features as air-filled ventricles as reference points. Preliminary dissection down to the target for direct estimation of coordinates in preserved material has also been advocated. Since all such coordinate data vary a little from brain to brain, and with the method employed, the degree of accuracy obtainable is limited, but is acceptable for all but very small structures. Horsley and Clarke (1908)[69] constructed the prototype stereotactic apparatus, and a considerable succession of modifications have improved on this, particularly under the stimulus of neurosurgery.

## The Rise of Histochemistry, Electron Microscopy, and Neurophysiology

The morphological techniques so far discussed continue to be used and refined, and in parallel with them are electrophysiological methods which must also be mentioned.

With improving instrumentation in the early part of the twentieth century, the study of action potentials in nerve fibres has become increasingly accurate, and with continuous refinement in electrodes, smaller and smaller groups of fibres or nerve cells can be subjected to electrical recording. The technique of *evoked potentials* consists in controlled stimulation at one point with recording of the induced action potentials at another.[70] The stimulus may be applied at receptor organs and, for example, the recording terminal may be in the cerebral cortex, and the pathway may in fact involve a number of synapses. Another technique—*strychnine neuronography*[71]—is less applied at the present time; strychnine solution applied to small areas of the cortex, for example, causes rapid firing in subjacent neurons, and the recording of distant responses can be correlated with the area stimulated.

These two kinds of approach to fibre tracing are often differentiated as anatomical and physiological, but in fact each inescapably contains an element of the other, and they often provide complementary advantages and an important check on each other. With either, whenever relatively lengthy pathways are under investigation, precise details of the intermediate route between the points of stimulation or destruction and the sites of consequent distant effects may require repeated experiment for full elucidation. The distance between such experimental terminals may be contracted or extended, or intermediate blockage at suspected sites may abolish a response and thus reveal the pathway situation at that level. A useful combined technique consists in the use of the same electrode to produce electrocoagulation in neurons to set in train degeneration along fibres from which electrophysiological activity has just been recorded.

By combination of data from all these various methods a most impressive volume of knowledge of the interconnexions of the parts of the central and peripheral nervous system has now accumulated; and by further application of the methods most likely to give accurate and reliable information, and by combining them where appropriate, this knowledge will doubtless continue to grow. Of late, however, attention has been directed most intensively towards the finer details of interneuronal connexions.[72] By insertion of microelectrodes or micropipettes directly into individual neurons the activity of single cells has been recorded in a wide variety of situations in the central nervous system. By simultaneous recording from numbers of cells in small 'units' of interconnexion, and by combining the results of such experimentation with recent highly detailed studies of the morphology of the neurons involved and their synapses, a new era of analysis of nervous system function is beginning.[73] Earlier concepts of excitation, inhibition and facilitation are being expanded by disinhibition, disfacilitation, lateral, pre-, and post-synaptic inhibition, and the like, a somewhat inelegant neology, but perhaps necessary to the

[65] W. M. Cowan, in: *Contemporary Research Methods in Neuroanatomy*, ed. W. J. H. Nauta and S. O. E. Ebbesson, Springer Verlag, New York, Heidelberg, Berlin. 1970.

[66] R. Warwick and J. B. Pond, *J. Anat.*, **102**, 1968.

[67] L. I. Malis, R. Leovinger, L. Kruger and J. E. Rose, *Science, N.Y.*, **126**, 1957.

[68] M. B. Carpenter and J. R. Whittier, *J. comp. Neurol.*, **97**, 1952.

[69] V. A. H. Horsley and R. H. Clarke, *Brain*, **31**, 1908.

[70] H.-T. Chang, in: *Handbook of Physiology*, Sect. 1, *Neurophysiology*, ed. G. J. Field and H. W. Magoun, American Physiological Society, Washington, D.C. 1959.

[71] J. G. Dusser de Barenne, H. W. Garol and W. S. McCulloch, *Res. Publs Ass. Res. nerv. ment. Dis.*, **21**, 1942.

[72] G. A. Horridge, *Interneurons*, Freeman, London and San Francisco. 1968.

[73] K. Lissák (ed.), *Recent Development of Neurobiology in Hungary*, Akadémiai Kiadó, Budapest. 1967.

rapidly growing information on activity in the repetitive interneuronal patterns so characteristic of much of the central nervous system. The role of the synapse in these studies is basic, and in this regard the techniques of histochemistry and electron microscopy have mediated great progress.

## PHYSIOLOGICAL TECHNIQUES FOR TRACING NERVE FIBRES

By the end of the nineteenth century microscopes and supporting histological techniques were well advanced. The general appearance of nerve cells and their fibres were established, their diverse types had been described in some detail, and the neuron theory was widely accepted. The gross and microscopic arrangement of the nervous system, central and peripheral, including its autonomic moiety, had been defined in much detail and in sufficiently explanatory functional terms to be highly useful in clinical diagnosis, even though understanding of the basic mechanisms might still be elementary. It is appropriate to note here the considerable contributions to neuroanatomy made by neurologists, both in the nineteenth century, when a combination of clinical and laboratory activities was more usual and perhaps easier, and in the twentieth, despite the effects of specialization and the increasing technical complexity of experimentation. By this stage also, neurophysiological approaches were proving particularly successful in localization of function and reflex activity. The spectacular evolution of electronics has provided a continually increasing array of accurate instrumental techniques for the measurement of nerve fibre activities, the behaviour of synapses, and the electrical phenomena of integrated cerebral activity. The study of synapses has perhaps been even more potently stimulated by the discovery of transmitter substances (by Loewi, Dale, and others), such as acetylcholine and adrenalin, with immense physiological, biochemical and pharmacological consequences. In company with these brilliant advances morphological investigation has continued under the particular impetus of new light microscope techniques, new histochemical developments and the invention of the electron microscope.

## DEVELOPMENTS IN LIGHT MICROSCOPY

General development of the light microscope has produced a highly flexible instrument with refined optics, and with such alternatives as dark-field illumination for examination of living cells in tissue culture, polarization accessories allowing the definition of birefringent substances such as myelin, and the addition of a host of auxiliary equipment, including varieties of moving stage, warmed stages for tissue culture, recording cameras for still, ciné and time-lapse photography, devices for micromeasurement including microdensitometry, microdissection and micro-injection.

The introduction of the phase contrast microscope of the Zernicke type in 1935, and of its congener, the interference microscope by Francis Smith in 1947, has ushered in a new era in the examination of living cells. Phase microscopy has become a normal adjunct of tissue culture, which has been extensively applied in the study of nerve cells and neuroglia.[74, 75] Like the phase instrument, the interference microscope can be used to assess refractive index, even in different parts of the same cell, and the latter also makes possible measurements of concentration, water content and dry mass in living cells.[76]

Recently, incident illumination optics have been introduced as a method for studying myelinated nerve fibre populations *in vivo* by Williams and Hall;[77] the technique allows examination of the dynamics of the axon and its satellite cells under various experimental conditions such as osmotic stress, severance, varieties of trauma, and after the micro-injection of, for example, electron-dense tracers and substances which cause demyelination.

Ultraviolet microscopy offers two advantages—firstly, about twice the resolving power of the ordinary light microscope (now rendered less important by the advent of the electron microscope, especially since the latter's lowest magnification overlaps the highest in light microscopy) and, secondly, the selective absorption of particular frequencies in the ultraviolet spectrum by various substances and especially nucleoproteins. Caspersson (1936)[78] has evolved a technique of ultraviolet microspectrography applicable to single cells, and this has been widely applied in quantitative assessments of DNA and RNA. The amount, distribution and behaviour of these and other substances in various kinds of nerve cells have been studied extensively in normal, experimental and pathological situations.[79]

## NEUROHISTOCHEMISTRY

Phase, interference, and ultraviolet microscopy may be considered as adjuncts to histochemistry and, more especially, to cytochemistry. Histochemistry stretches back at least a century; Raspail, a botanist, published in this field as long ago as 1830;[80] but like other innovations of the nineteenth century, histochemistry has developed slowly and by an accelerating multiplication of individual identification methods for particular biological compounds, whose distribution in tissues and at the intracellular level has been recorded in innumerable studies, some of outstanding functional significance. A wide spectrum of such tests is available for nervous tissues and neurons both in normal and pathological states.[81] Of particular interest are the methods elaborated for the identification of transmitter substances and their associated enzymes, in nerve cells, fibres and synapses. These extend from the original chromaffin reaction of Henle (1865) and its modern modifications,[82] to the Gomori method (1943) and the more recently devised fluorescence techniques, including immunofluorescence. The application of fluorescence techniques in neuroanatomy have been recently surveyed.[83] Such methods have led to a classification of nerve cells into neurosecretory types, and a convenient, if inelegant jargon—NA neurons (noradrenalin containing) and so forth.

In the more general field of neurohistology other comparatively recent innovations must be mentioned. New staining methods such as those of Bodian (1936)[84] for nerve fibres, Glees (1946) and Nauta (1950) for terminal

---

[74] R. S. Geiger, in: *Neurobiology*, vol. 5, eds. C. C. Pfeiffer and J. R. Smythies, Academic Press, New York and London. 1963.

[75] M. R. Murray, in: *Cells and Tissues in Culture*, vol. 2, ed. E. N. Willmer, Academic Press, London and New York. 1965.

[76] K. F. A. Ross, *Phase Contrast and Interference Microscopy for Cell Biologists*, Arnold, London. 1967.

[77] P. L. Williams and S. M. Hall, *J. Anat.*, **107** and **108**, 1970–1.

[78] T. Caspersson, *Skand. Arch. Physiol.*, Suppl. **8** zum **73** Bd., 1936.

[79] H. Hydén, in: *The Cell*, vol. 4, ed. J. Brachet and A. E. Mirsky, Academic Press, New York. 1960.

[80] A. G. E. Pearse, *Histochemistry*, 3rd ed., Churchill, London. 1968.

[81] C. W. Adams (ed.), *Neurohistochemistry*, Elsevier, Amsterdam, London, New York. 1965.

[82] R. E. Coupland, *The Natural History of the Chromaffin Cell*, Longmans, Green, London. 1965.

[83] K. Fuxe, T. Hökfelt, G. Jonnson and U. Ungerstedt, in: *Contemporary Research Methods in Neuroanatomy*, ed. W. J. H. Nauta and S. O. E. Ebbesson, Springer-Verlag, New York, Heidelberg and Berlin. 1970.

[84] D. Bodian, *Anat. Rec.*, **65**, 1936.

degeneration in experimentally divided axons, Einarson (1932)[85] and Klüver (1953)[86] for 'chromatin granules' (Klüver's method also stains axons)—all these and others have augmented the neurohistologist's repertoire.

Of special interest, in view of the resurgence in the use of Golgi's technique,[183] are various modifications (e.g. Fox et al., 1951),[87] which have been employed widely of late in working out the morphological interrelationships of small groups of neurons, particularly interneurons. The Golgi type of staining has an unexplained peculiarity in that only a fraction of the cells are actually stained, and this makes the unravelling of their intricacies practicable, and often allows the application of quantitative histological methods, including those of microreconstruction. Studies of this kind, carried out in a wide variety of vertebrates and invertebrates, have led to a considerable *rapprochement* between current electrophysiological and anatomical investigation of small-scale neuron networks and individual neurons.[88] An equally potent technique in drawing together workers in separated disciplines in neuroanatomical studies has been the advent of electron microscopy.

## ELECTRON MICROSCOPY

Although practicable electron microscopes have been in use since the Ruska prototype in 1933, years elapsed before sufficiently thin sections of biological material could be reliably prepared. Pearse and Baker succeeded in doing this in 1948, using an adapted Spencer rotary microtome. Sjöstrand (1967)[89] has described these early struggles and the emergence of the ultramicrotome in its modern varieties. It must also be emphasized that biological electron microscopy would have been equally impracticable without the introduction of glass and diamond knives to cut the hard embedding media required. From the 1950s all the basic requirements were met, and from then onwards biological preparations could be submitted to the increasingly high resolutions and magnifications of continuously improving electron microscopes, the use of which has transformed the morphological approach to cytology. Two decades of application have shown great improvement and innovation in supporting techniques. Heavy metal shadowing, replication methods, the production of homogenate films, heavy metal staining including negative contrast, autoradiography, densitometry, microreconstruction, cell fractionation methods depending upon differential centrifugation (of fundamental importance in neurochemistry), electron diffraction and electron phase contrast optics, and many other techniques have enriched the basic potentialities of electron microscopy. Perhaps even more necessary has been the rapid improvement in the interpretation of the appearances of the greatly enlarged intracellular detail, and the growth of an experimental attitude and of quantitative methods in the use of electron microscopy; otherwise the singularly productive approximation of cytology, biochemistry and molecular biology, which is fast occurring, would have been improbable. In neuroanatomical research such bonds are developing with much effect. Elucidation of the structure of the myelin sheath and of synapses have been notable achievements. With improvement in microtomes and in the orientation of material, it is becoming possible to counter the two main criticisms of electron microscopy— the small scale of sampling and the difficulty in equating some of the findings of light and electron microscopy. Techniques have thus been developed by which adjoining thick and thin sections of the same block can be prepared, stained by contrasting techniques, and examined using the light and the electron microscopes respectively. Even short runs of serial ultra-thin sections can be produced, with the possibility, for example, of tracing the full complexities of part of a nerve cell process using reconstruction techniques. A number of further developments are being elaborated or projected,[90] and the potentialities of the scanning and high-voltage electron microscopes have yet to be exploited by neuroanatomists.

## OTHER MODERN TECHNIQUES

A number of other relevant techniques can be barely mentioned—autoradiography,[91] ciné and time-lapse photography,[92] microreconstruction,[93] microphotometry, micromanipulation,[94] neuron counting techniques,[95] morphotometric analysis,[96] and the elaboration of models to provide functional analogues.[97] Enough has been said, however, to illustrate the ever-growing dependence of neuroanatomical investigations upon technical development. Despite widespread misapprehension, neuroanatomy—and indeed anatomy in general—has at no stage been an entirely morphological, merely descriptive discipline, though it can descend, and frequently has so fallen, to this somewhat sterile level. However, there have always been those, such as Willis, Harvey, or Sherrington, who have disregarded the artificial separation of nervous structure and function. Unfortunately, levels of knowledge of one or the other have often been imbalanced. After a considerable period, early this century, of separation of disciplines concerned with morphology and function (perhaps chiefly due to the exigencies of teaching organization in medical schools), the consequent isolationism now shows signs of dissolution. This is particularly true of studies of the nervous system. Preoccupation with the minutiae of shape and of the nervous impulse have borne their separate fruit, and we can now pass on to more hopeful prospects. As morphologists become more experimental and the functionalists look more attentively at the arena of their experiments, instrumentation and outlooks are evincing an increasing similarity, and purposes a new cohesion. Doubtless we are still far from concepts of integrated brain activity; but, at simpler divisions or units of the whole, electrophysiological and anatomical inquiries into the behaviour of the individual neuron and synapse, and their associations in small functional networks, seem to afford a prospect of joint success. We may at least be much nearer to comprehending the 'miniaturized' basic units in central nervous mechanisms. It is to the individual elements at this level of organization that we must now turn our attention.

[85] L. Einarson, *Am. J. Path.*, **8**, 1932.

[86] H. Klüver and E. Barrera, *J. Neuropath. exp. Neurol.*, **12**, 1953.

[87] C. A. Fox, M. Ubeda-Purkiss, H. K. Ihrig and D. Biagoli, *Stain Technol.*, **26**, 1951.

[88] J. C. Eccles, M. Ito and J. Szentágothai, *The Cerebellum as a Neuronal Machine*, Springer-Verlag, Berlin, Heidelberg, New York. 1967.

[89] F. S. Sjöstrand, *Electron Microscopy of Cells and Tissues*, vol. 1, Academic Press, New York and London. 1967.

[90] H. E. Huxley and A. Klug (eds.), *New Developments in Electron Microscopy*, The Royal Society, London. 1971.

[91] A. W. Rogers, *Techniques of Autoradiography*, Elsevier, Amsterdam, London, and New York. 1967.

[92] G. C. Rose (ed.), *Cinematography in Biology*, Acadamic Press, New York and London. 1963.

[93] W. A. Gaunt, *Microreconstruction*, Pitman Medical, London. 1971.

[94] M. J. Kopac, in: *The Cell*, vol. I, ed. J. Brachet and J. Mirsky, Academic Press, New York and London. 1960.

[95] B. W. Konigsmark, in: *Contemporary Research Methods in Neuroanatomy*, ed. W. J. H. Nauta and S. O. E. Ebbesson, Springer-Verlag, New York, Heidelberg, Berlin. 1970.

[96] E. R. Weibel and H. Elias, *Quantitative Methods in Morphology*, Springer-Verlag, New York, Heidelberg, Berlin. 1969.

[97] N. Weiner and J. P. Schadé, *Prog. Brain Res.*, **2**, 1960.

The foregoing sections have been concerned with the organization and investigation of the nervous system. We shall now consider the cellular elements of the nervous tissue in more detail, since it is impossible to create a model of brain function without an appreciation of how the individual units work.[98]

## The Neuron

Neurons, although diverse in appearance and size, have many characteristics in common. All possess a large surface area compared with most other cell types, and this

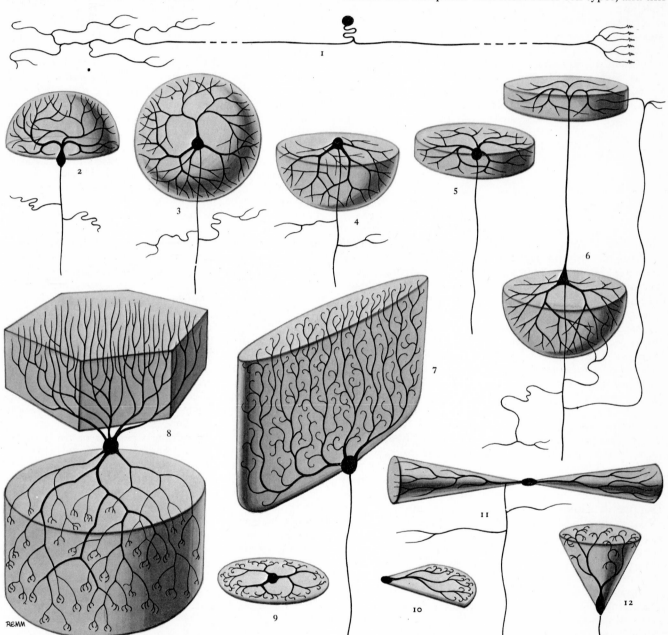

7.15 A–E A Schema showing pattern variations of neuronal geometry: (1) unipolar, sensory ganglionic neuron; (2) bipolar neuron; (3) stellate (isodendritic) neuron, with (4), (5), and (11) which are modifications of this pattern; (6) pyramidal neuron with an apical and a series of basal dendrites, and recurrent axon collaterals, from the cerebral cortex;

(7) Purkinje neuron from the cerebellar cortex; (8) Golgi neuron from the cerebellar cortex; (9) and (10) amacrine cells lacking axons; (12) glomerular neuron (mitral cell) from the olfactory bulb, showing recurved dendritic tips.

As already stated, nervous tissue is composed of two distinct sets of cells, the excitable cells or *neurons*, and the non-excitable cells which constitute the *neuroglia* and *ependyma* in the central nervous system, and the *Schwann cells* and associated elements in the periphery. Since our interest in terms of neural behaviour centres on the neurons, more space will be given to outlining their structure and behaviour.

surface is specialized for the reception, conduction and transmission of neural information by virtue of its molecular composition, and by the topographic specialization of the neuron. The branch-like extensions of its

[98] F. O. Schmitt, G. C. Quarton, T. Melnechuk and G. Adelman (eds.), *The Neurosciences, a Study Program*, Rockefeller University Press, New York. 1967.

periphery are termed *neurites*, and these may be divided into receiving processes or *dendrites*, and efferent processes termed *axons*. Usually there are many dendrites but only one axon extending from each cell. The protoplasm massed around and including the nucleus of the cell is termed the *soma*, *perikaryon*, or *cell body*; the cytoplasm of this structure is characterized by the presence of numerous strongly basophilic inclusions, the *Nissl bodies* or *granules* (7.14). The soma is often angular in shape (7.15), the projection which leads to the axon being the *axon hillock*, and its bare continuation the *initial segment* of the axon. Sometimes the axon emerges from the base of one of the main dendrites rather than directly from the soma. From the other angles of the soma spring a number of main or *primary dendrites* which branch repeatedly to form a *dendritic tree*. Each axon may also possess side branches or *collaterals*, usually much finer than the main axonal process. Axons at their termination

## HISTOLOGICAL DEMONSTRATION OF NEURONS

As stated previously (p. 759), what we know of neuronal structure is dependent upon the special methods which have been elaborated to show various aspects of neuronal cytology,[99] and it is useful to consider these methods further here. Although the standard methods of light microscope histology are valuable in showing their cell bodies, the neurites of neurons do not stain sufficiently well to allow them to be traced with any degree of confidence. Various types of impregnation of *blocks* of tissue with metallic salts, particularly those of silver, do, however, stain some or all parts of the cytoplasm. One of the most useful class of techniques, invented by Golgi (*see* p. 759), results in the precipitation of silver chromate or other metal salts within individual neurons, which can therefore be demonstrated in their entirety in thick sections; and, since only a small percentage of the total

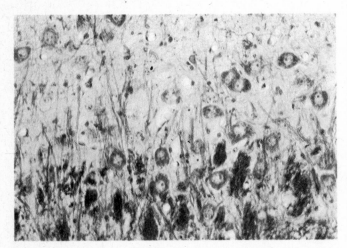

B  A high-power light micrograph showing part of a pyramidal neuron from the cerebral cortex of a rat, prepared by the rapid method of Golgi. The bases of several dendrites covered with dendritic spines, and a thin axon (left) are visible. (Preparations kindly supplied by Dr. A. R. Lieberman of University College, London.)

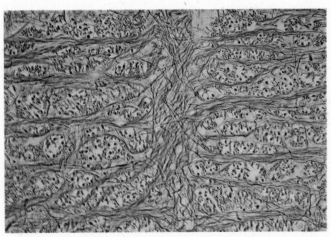

C  A low-power light micrograph of groups of interweaving axons from the medulla oblongata of a cat, stained by the Holmes' silver method. (Preparations C–E kindly supplied by Dr. E. L. Rees of the Anatomy Dept., Guy's Hospital, Medical School, London.)

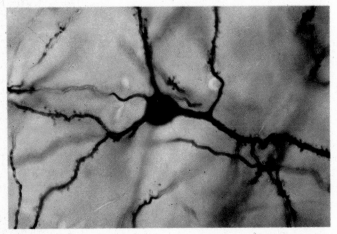

D  A group of neuronal perikarya (purple) amongst bundles of myelinated fibres (blue), from the brainstem of a rat. Stained by the cresyl fast violet—Luxol fast blue method.

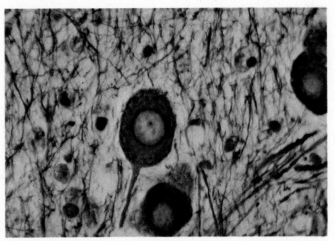

E  A section through the mesencephalic nucleus of the trigeminal nerve (rat), stained with the Holmes silver nitrate method to show large unipolar neurons from one of which a dendro-axonal process is emerging.

usually break up into several fine branches, the *axon terminals* or *telodendria*, which end in apposition, variously, with other neurons to form zones of interneuronal transmission or *synapses*, with effectors such as muscles (*neuromuscular junctions*) or with glands; adipose tissue also receives motor terminals (*see* p. 797). The plasma membrane of the axon is known as the *axolemma* and its internal cytoplasm the *axoplasm*.

cell population is affected, they are visible as black spidery profiles against a clear background (7.15B). Although the fidelity of the method has in the past been questioned, electron microscopy supports the view that the results obtained with the Golgi techniques are an accurate

[99] R. A. B. Drury and E. A. Wallington, *Carlton's Histological Technique*, 4th ed., Oxford University Press, London. 1967.

representation in even the finest of light microscopic details, so that now there is a resurgence of interest in this means of investigation. However, there has, so far, been no critical evaluation of the distortion introduced by either of these preparative techniques.

Next, there are the various techniques of staining *sections* with silver salts, some of which are specific for the neurofibrils within neurons (neurofibrillar stains),[100] and others which seem to stain the entire cytoplasm (7.15E). In this category are the ammoniacal silver nitrate methods of Bielschowsky and their subsequent modifications, the silver proteinate methods of Bodian, and the various silver nitrate techniques such as that of Holmes. The block staining methods of Cajal also give good results by a similar process. Various modifications of the silver reactions have also been used to demonstrate anterograde degeneration of axons (the Nauta methods) and of their terminals (such as the techniques of Glees) in sections, by chemically suppressing the staining of normal as opposed to degenerating axons (7.14, see also p. 761). Recently, important modifications of these degeneration techniques for use with the electron microscope (e.g. the Fink-Heimer method) have been introduced.

Numerous methods have been developed to demonstrate the sheaths of myelinated fibres (*vide infra*, p. 782), some based on osmium staining, and some on haematoxylin and allied stains such as luxol fast blue (7.15). A modification employing chromium salts has also been developed to demonstrate *degenerating* myelin sheaths (the method of Marchi) although this is now less widely used because of various difficulties of interpretation (p. 781). Added to these, there are modifications of normal cytological stains which demonstrate various organelles within the cytoplasm. The most useful of these, the Nissl stains, are basic substances which bind strongly to the nucleic acids which are abundant in neuronal nuclei and cytoplasm. Such stains as cresyl fast violet (7.14) and toluidine blue are widely employed by neuroanatomists for this reason. A number of stains also demonstrate mitochondria, particularly in axon terminals, and modifications show the *degeneration of axon terminals* after experimenting trauma.

More recently, electron microscopy has in many cases revolutionized our concepts of neuronal structure or, in some instances, has determined which of several alternative models is the correct one. However, since this discipline is restricted to the examination of ultra-thin sections, three-dimensional reconstruction of nervous tissue is laborious and limited in scope. It is therefore of great importance to correlate light and electron microscopy to obtain an understanding of neuronal organization.

All of the above methods involve the examination of dead material, but much may also be learnt from studies of neurons stained by supra-vital methods. Methylene blue was found by early neuroanatomists to stain the entire cytoplasm of neurons, giving a picture of individual cells as striking as those obtained with the Golgi methods. Because methylene blue is a vital stain, however, its use is restricted largely to thin or small whole tissue situations such as the peripheral and embryonic nervous systems, where penetration and staining are rapid. Many other techniques are also available for specific purposes.

## GENERAL MORPHOLOGY OF NEURONS

Neurons can be described in several ways according to the patterns of their neurites, their physiological action, the transmitter which they release and so on.[101, 102] Of these various descriptions, only the first is generally possible, since our understanding of the physiological and biochemical properties of neurons is limited to relatively few

instances, whereas the morphology of many neuron populations is well established. Even within the field of general structure, several types of classification are possible, mostly based on the patterns of ramification of the neurites. As mentioned previously (p. 750) a commonly used scheme distinguishes: (1) *unipolar neurons*, in which the cell body has a single extension giving rise to both dendritic and axonal branches, examples being dorsal root ganglion cells (sometimes termed *pseudo-unipolar* because this form is arrived at secondarily in development), and granule cells of the olfactory bulb; (2) *bipolar neurons*, with an extension at each end of the cell body, for example retinal bipolar cells, and cells of the cochlear and vestibular ganglia; (3) *multipolar neurons*, with several extensions of the cell body; most cells of the central nervous system are of this last type. Although this scheme of classification (7.15) is useful for descriptive purposes, it appears to have limited physiological significance. Of more importance is the classification of central neurons into relatively large, Golgi type I neurons which have long axons connecting different parts of the nervous system,[103] and small Golgi type II neurons (microneurons) in which the axon is short and terminates in the neighbourhood of the cell body, or else is entirely absent (7.15). The Golgi type II neuron is often present in inhibitory situations, an example being the periglomerular cells of the olfactory bulb (p. 932). A special category of microneurons, lacking an obvious axon, consists of *amacrine cells*; in these cells nervous conduction is apparently possible in either direction along their dendrite-like processes. Amacrine cells have long been known in the retina, where they lie in synaptic contact with ganglion and other cells (p. 1116), but their presence is also indicated in other parts of the central nervous system, including the olfactory bulb (granule cells) and, possibly, the lateral geniculate body. It is probable that they constitute a characteristic element of all the main sensory pathways. In some situations, at least, microneuron cell processes make reciprocal synapses with adjacent dendrites, so that *dendrodendritic transmission* occurs (*see* p. 750).

The small inhibitory neurons appear responsible for an important type of interaction between neurons, such as those of the sensory projection pathways, in which maximally excited cells can inhibit the activity of less excited, adjacent neurons, by means of intercalated inhibitory neurons, thus 'sharpening' the sensory patterns at various levels in the pathway (7.8 and p. 751), a process termed *lateral inhibition*[104] (see also pp. 751, 834).

Central neurons can also be classified according to the branching patterns and shape of their dendritic fields (7.15). Those with dendrites extending equally in all directions away from the cell body, to fill a roughly spherical volume with their smaller branches, are termed *stellate cells* (7.15), a type common in the cerebral cortex, and in reticular nuclei of the brain stem and spinal cord, amongst other locations. In *pyramidal cells*, the cell body is pyramidal or conical in shape, and *basal dendrites* emerge from the angles made by the base and the walls of the pyramid to fill a roughly hemispherical volume (7.15); an *apical dendrite* emerging from the apex of the cell may also be present to give a second dendritic field at some distance from the cell body, as in the pyramidal cells of the cerebral cortex (7.15). Spindle-shaped cell bodies with dendrites emerging at one or both ends are termed *fusiform*.

[100] E. G. Gray and R. W. Guillery, *Int. Rev. Cytol.*, **19**, 1966.

[101] H. Hydén (ed.), *The Neuron*, Elsevier, Amsterdam. 1967.

[102] G. H. Bourne (ed.), *The Structure and Function of Nervous Tissue*, vol. I, Academic Press, N.Y. 1968.

[103] S. Ramón y Cajal, *Histologie du Système Nerveux*, vols. I and II, Maloine, Paris. 1911.

[104] G. A. Horridge, *Interneurons*, Freeman, London. 1968.

Many variations of these basic patterns exist, of course, throughout the nervous system, depending upon the pattern of afferent fibres, their synaptic sites, and the mechanical constraints imposed by other cells and so on. One of the most remarkable dendritic fields is that of the cerebellar Purkinje cell (p. 866), in which a primary dendrite emerges apically and branches to form a complex two-dimensional fan-like array (7.15, 79, 80). *Glomerular neurons* are also known, in which there may be relatively few dendrites with highly convoluted branches at their tips (7.15, 79, 81) where most synaptic contact occurs, as in the mitral and tufted cells of the olfactory bulb (p. 933), in the lateral geniculate nucleus, in certain 'relay' nuclei of the thalamus (p. 895), and in the cerebellum (p. 869).

Several attempts have been made to classify dendritic patterns by their symmetry, but most of these schemes, although useful for descriptive purposes, seem to have limited functional significance. More important seems to be the mathematical analysis of the branching patterns of dendrites in terms of the frequency, angles and dimensions of the branches, the spatial distribution of cell surface and volume, and the frequency, type, and spatial location of synaptic endings, since all of these parameters are known to be significant in the electrical activity of neurons. Although such studies are still in their infancy, a number of important contributions to the field have already been made. The use of computers to collate such information holds out considerable promise for the future. Other biometric parameters, such as the ratio between nuclear and cytoplasmic volume have also been examined.

## STRUCTURAL PARAMETERS OF DENDRITES

When dendritic fields are examined, as for instance with the Golgi methods, the dendritic branching is seen to be largely dichotomous.[105, 106, 107] Where dendrites spread and branch symmetrically around the cell body, the *total number* of dendritic branches is, of course, dependent upon the number of primary dendrites and the number of sub-orders of branches. The *surface area* of cell membrane associated with the *dendrites* can be calculated from simple, although laborious, measurements of the diameters and lengths of the branches, and this can be compared with the *surface area* of the *cell body*. In spinal cord motor neurons and interneurons, up to 80 per cent of the total neuronal surface area is associated with the dendrites, emphasizing their important role as a receptive area for afferent stimuli (see also p. 829). Various methods of describing the dendritic tree have been used; the frequency of branching can be expressed by imagining a series of equally-spaced concentric spheres centred on the cell body; as the dendrites emerge and branch, the number of dendritic segments passing through the surface of each imaginary sphere can be counted and expressed as a function of distance from the cell body. In neurons of the cerebral cortex and spinal cord, the number of branches rises quickly to a maximum, and then tails off asymptotically or logarithmically, with increasing distance from the base of the primary dendrite.[105] Counts of the thorn-like extensions of the dendrite surfaces, the *dendritic spines*,[108] —an important index of numbers of incoming synapses (p. 774)—show that in some types of neuron there are often many thousands equally spaced over much of the dendritic tree.[107] Thus it follows that the number of synapses probably first increases, and then decreases asymptotically with distance from the cell body in the same manner as the number of dendritic branches. Careful measurements indicate that different populations of neurons, although showing the same general

mode, have their own peculiar relationships between cell body and dendritic surface areas, volumes, spine counts, and so on.[108]

The importance of these parameters, of course, lies in the numbers of afferent synapses made with the cell, their position, and the spreading patterns of electrical disturbance at the cell membrane which follow their activation. A vital feature is the relative distribution of excitatory and inhibitory synapses, but, as yet, this can only be estimated from electron micrographic studies, which are often statistically invalid (see, however, p. 867). Microelectrode studies are a possible means of analysis of dendritic action, but in most cases the dendrites are too small to be monitored individually, and elaborate mathematical techniques are necessary to extract any meaning from the records. There are, however, some functional observations indicating the general significance of dendritic branching patterns; for example when neonatal mice are made thyroid hormone-deficient to simulate the condition of cretinism in man, they show behavioural retardation, and the dendritic trees of their cerebral cortical neurons are also smaller, with fewer branches, than those in control animals.[109]

## PHYSIOLOGICAL PROPERTIES OF NEURONS

Neurons, as we have seen (p. 750), are characterized by their ability to receive, conduct and transmit *information*, which is coded in terms of transient electro-chemical changes in their plasma membranes.[110] These changes are associated with rapid fluxes of ions in and out of the cytoplasm, which occur against the background of a steady electrical potential difference maintained across this surface. The measurement of these changes by means of various electrophysiological instruments, and their analysis, provide a means of understanding the structure of the nervous system in functional terms, and progress in these two fields is coming more and more to depend on a close working relationship between them. A detailed survey of electrophysiology is beyond the scope of the present account and only a brief summary will be attempted.

**The resting potential** (7.16) of a neuron is in many respects similar to the membrane potential of non-excitable cells, consisting of a steady potential difference of about 80 mV which can be measured across the plasma membrane, the inside negative with respect to the outside. This bioelectrical potential is the result of differences in concentration of various anions and cations inside and outside the cell, which is further dependent upon the permeability properties of the external membrane, and the active transport of ions, particularly sodium and potassium, by the membrane. These various factors result in a high concentration of potassium, and of negatively charged, non-diffusible ions (proteins, etc) and, a low concentration of sodium and chloride ions, *inside* the cell, relative to their concentrations in the tissue fluid which bathes the cell externally. Calcium is also present within the cell. The resting potential can change in two distinct ways, giving rise to *graded potentials* or *action potentials* respectively. Graded potentials involve the membrane of *dendrites* and neuron *cell bodies*, and consist of fluctuating increases or decreases in the resting potential, i.e. their membranes are either relatively

[105] D. A. Sholl, *The Organisation of the Cerebral Cortex*, Methuen, London. 1956.

[106] J. T. Aitken and J. E. Bridger, *J. Anat.*, **95**, 1961.

[107] S. Gelfan, G. Kao and D. S. Ruchkin, *J. comp. Neurol.*, **139**, 1970.

[108] S. Gelfan and A. F. Rapisarda, *J. comp. Neurol.*, **125**, 1964.

[109] J. T. Eayrs, *Acta anat.*, **25**, 1955.

[110] B. Katz, *Nerve, Muscle, and Synapse*, McGraw-Hill, New York. 1966.

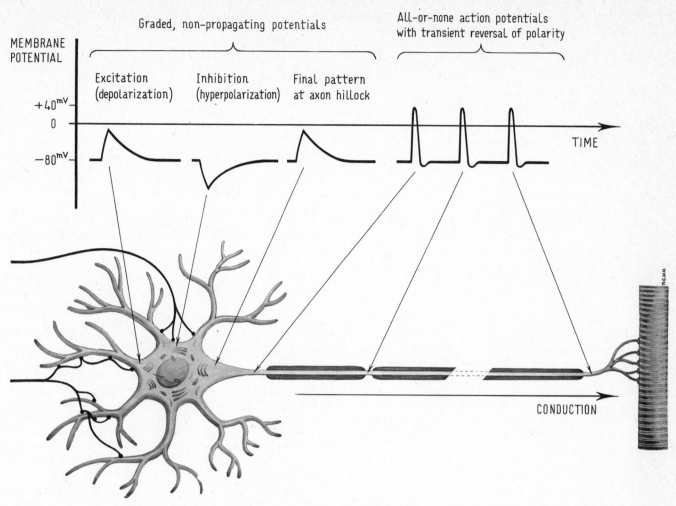

**7.16** A diagram showing the types of change in electrical potential which can be recorded across the cell membrane of a motor neuron at the points indicated by the arrows. Excitatory and inhibitory synapses on the surfaces of the dendrites and soma cause local graded changes of potential which summate at the axon hillock, and may initiate a series of all-or-none action potentials, which are conducted along the axon to the effector terminals.

*hyperpolarized* or *depolarized*. In contrast, the action potential involves a transient complete reversal of polarity across the membrane of *axons* (and also of some large dendrites which resemble axons in their structure).

**Graded potential variations** may be either *excitatory* or *inhibitory*. When excitatory, there occurs an increase in permeability of the membrane to sodium ions which therefore flow down their concentration gradient to enter the cell, and thereby progressively depolarize the membrane. The size and time course of the depolarization at a particular membrane locus, to which an effective stimulus has been applied, is related (logarithmically) to the stimulus strength. Furthermore, surrounding zones of membrane also suffer a depolarization, but with decreasing amplitude, at increasing distances from the initiating locus. Thus, the larger the initial depolarization, the greater the spread of effect to surrounding areas of membrane. Such a mechanism allows the *summation* of effect of multiple excitatory stimuli applied at numerous points over the receiving surface of the neuron. Inhibitory stimuli, thought to act by increasing the inflow of negatively charged chloride ions, therefore tend to increase the membrane potential (hyperpolarization), and thus they oppose or subtract from, the *total excitatory state* of the neuron.

**The action potential, nerve impulse** or **spike potential** in contrast, is characterized by a brief *reversal* of polarity caused by the sudden influx of sodium ions, followed by a return to the resting potential as potassium ions flow out; these processes take about 5 msecs in all. For any system, the amplitude and duration of successive

action potentials is identical, no matter how large the stimulus is above a certain *threshold value*, so the response is an *all-or-none* event. The wave of excitation associated with the action potential spreads away from the point of initiation, but, unlike the graded potential, its size and time course do not alter, so the wave sweeps rapidly over the membrane at a constant rate. The action potential is therefore said to be *propagated* and *non-decremental*. After a region of membrane has been stimulated, however, there is an irreducible *refractory period* during which another action potential cannot be elicited, thus fixing a maximum frequency of their formation. When a series of action potentials is generated, they are rapidly conducted along the neurite, maintaining their original frequency pattern precisely. This phenomenon is the basis of nervous communication, which is therefore said to be a *frequency-coded*.

The graded and action potentials are related to one another at specific points on the neuronal surface. For example, in a motor neuron, the graded potentials of the dendrites and soma sweep over the axon hillock to initiate action potentials at the *initial segment* of the axon. The greater the graded depolarization of the soma, the more frequent the action potentials, so that the *state of excitation* of the cell is reflected by the *frequency pattern* of the *volleys of action potentials* which flow along its axon.

When an action potential reaches the axon terminals, it causes the release of a discrete amount of *neurotransmitter substance* which further changes the excitability of the receiving cell, either another neuron, a muscle cell, or some other element. A closely grouped series of action potentials (*spike trains* or *volleys*) naturally causes a greater effect than single ones, since extracellular enzyme action, or other processes, limit the time during which the neurotransmitter can act.

Although the most common cell region for the change from graded to action potential to occur is the initial segment of the axon, in many peripheral receptors with an axon-like dendrite (for example cutaneous sensory neurons), it occurs in a region close to the sensory ending, often the first node of Ranvier, in myelinated fibres.

In amacrine cells (p. 1116) *all* their electrical activities may be of the graded type, and such cells are able to spread these changes in any direction depending on the point of stimulation. In cells with an axon, however, conduction occurs under physiological conditions in one direction only, that is, from the dendrites and cell body to the axon (*orthodromic conduction*); although when artificially stimulated at the periphery, axons can conduct in the opposite direction (*antidromic conduction*), and electrical changes then invade the cell body.

## SIGNIFICANCE OF NEURONAL MORPHOLOGY

Because of the mode of synaptic excitation and decremental conduction of the dendrites and perikarya, the shape of these structures and the distribution of excitatory and inhibitory synapses over their surfaces, undoubtedly play a vital part in determining the relation between the input and output of a neuron. This provides a cogent reason for analysing the geometry of neurons in as precise a manner as possible, in order to understand their role in different physiological processes.

## ULTRASTRUCTURE OF NEURONS

Since the pioneering studies of Palay and Palade,[111] and of de Robertis and Bennet,[112] much information on neuronal ultrastructure has been amassed (for example, see footnote reference[113]). Following the terminology of light microscopy, it is useful to distinguish between those regions of the nervous system consisting mainly of the cell bodies of neurons, or of regular arrays of their axons which constitute relatively discrete nuclear cell masses and fibre tracts respectively, and those parts made up of complex meshworks of axon terminals, dendrites and neuroglial processes which form the *neuropil* of the nervous system.[113] The different components of the neurons will now be considered in detail.

**The soma** consists of cytoplasm rich in granular and agranular endoplasmic reticulum (**7.**17, 18) with attached and free polyribosome clusters, often forming large aggregations; these are visible with the light microscope, by virtue of their constituent RNA, as basophilic *Nissl* or *chromatin bodies* or *granules*.[114] These are more obvious in highly active cells, such as the motor neurons of the anterior grey column of the spinal cord, where *stacks* of granular endoplasmic reticulum occur (**7.**18).

The *nucleus* is usually large, rounded and quite pale, that is, euchromatic, with one or more prominent *nucleoli*. All of these features are typical of cells actively engaged in protein synthesis, as too is the presence of numerous mitochondria as a source of energy, available also for other cellular activities. *Lysosomes* are another prominent cell component, as are also stacks of agranular cytomembranes

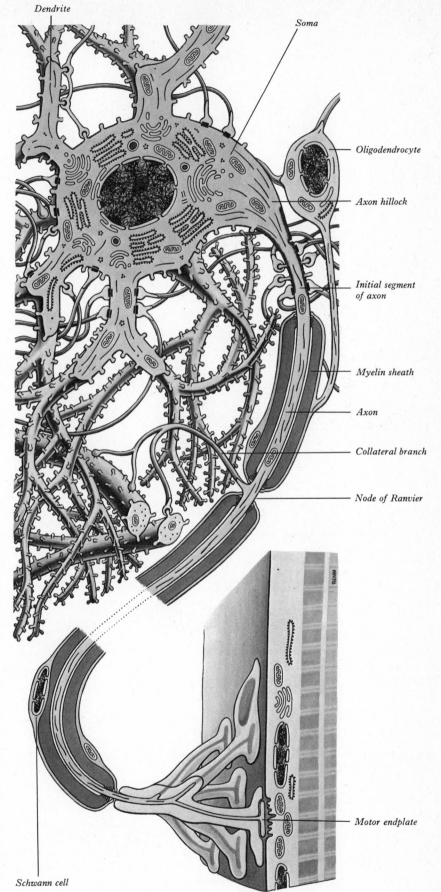

*Dendrite*

*Soma*

*Oligodendrocyte*

*Axon hillock*

*Initial segment of axon*

*Myelin sheath*

*Axon*

*Collateral branch*

*Node of Ranvier*

*Motor endplate*

*Schwann cell*

**7.**17  A schematic drawing of the ultrastructure of a motor neuron, showing part of its dendritic field (above left); the dendrites are studded with spines which are contacted by different types of synaptic terminal. The cytoplasm of the neuronal soma contains stacks of rough endoplasmic reticulum, and other organelles. See text for a detailed description.

[111] S. L. Palay and G. E. Palade, *J. biophys. biochem. Cytol.*, **1**, 1955.

[112] E. De Robertis and H. S. P. Bennett, *J. biophys. biochem. Cytol.*, **1**, 1955.

[113] A. Peters, S. L. Palay and H. de F. Webster, *The Fine Structure of the Nervous System*, Harper and Row, New York. 1970.

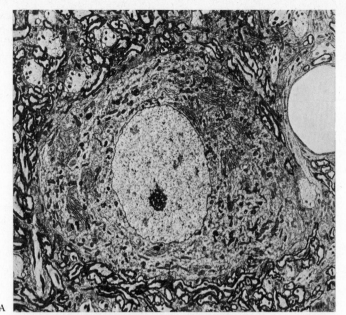

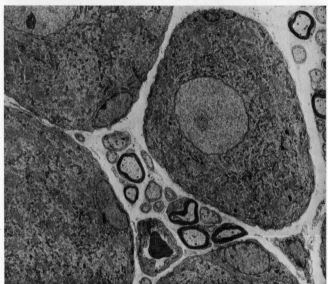

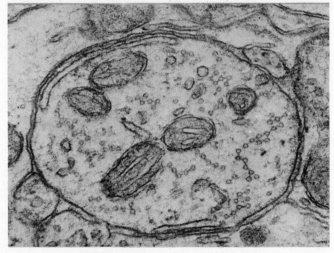

7.18 A–C   Electron micrographs of neuronal perikarya of the rat. A Typical ventral grey column multipolar neuron placed amongst numerous profiles of dendrites and axons, including myelinated nerve fibres. Note the prominent nucleolus, and in the cytoplasm the clusters of rough endoplasmic reticulum. B A section through the somata of a number of unipolar spinal ganglionic neurons, associated with which are small flattened capsular (satellite) cells. Myelinated and non-myelinated nerve fibres and a capillary are also present. C An electron micrograph of a transverse section through the initial segment of an axon, showing the rows of linked microtubules which characterize this region. (Specimens 7.18 A–C kindly provided by Dr. A. R. Lieberman of University College, London.)

comprising the *Golgi complex* which often form several distinct groups in different parts of the cell body. *Microfilaments* and *microtubules* are present in abundance, bundles of the former corresponding to the 'neurofibrils' of light microscopists. Microtubules and microfilaments extend into and throughout the lengths of **dendrites** and **axons**, the relative proportion of these two components varying with the type of neuron and the type of cell process involved. In general, dendrites are richer in microtubules than are axons, which may be almost completely filled with microfilaments; both microtubules and microfilaments appear to be continuous from the cell body to the tips of its neurites, and although bundles of them diverge at points of neurite branching, individual tubules and filaments do not branch.

*Centrioles*, formerly believed to be absent from mature neurons, have been described in every neuronal type so far investigated, and may be associated with the generation or maintenance of the microtubular apparatus. In some neurons, centrioles with cilium-like projections from the cell surface have been reported; although cilia appear to be common on the surface of neuroblasts, they have also been found in mature cells; their significance, except at some special sensory terminals, is obscure.

Various other inclusions are also commonly present in the cytoplasm of neurons. *Pigment granules* of various types characterize certain parts of the brain;[114] the substantia nigra (p. 882), for example, has a neuromelanin, whose presence is probably related to the catecholamine-synthesizing ability of these neurons, these neurotransmitters being closely related chemically to the pigment. In the locus coeruleus, likewise, a similar pigment, rich in copper, gives a bluish colour to the neurons. Other neurons are unusually rich in certain metals, zinc for example in the hippocampus, and iron in the oculomotor nucleus. These metals may be part of the prosthetic groups of various special enzymes. As neurons age, all of them tend to accumulate granules of a yellowish pigment termed *lipofuscin* (senility pigment), which becomes particularly prominent in the cells of the spinal ganglia.

**The dendrites** share many features of the cell body, containing microtubules, microfilaments, mitochondria, and, to a lesser extent, ribosomes and agranular endoplasmic reticulum (7.18, 20). **Axons** are similar, except that normally they do not contain ribosomes. The agranular endoplasmic reticulum in the neurites often takes the form of perforated transverse septa, or longitudinally orientated tubules and spherical vesicles. Various types of vesicle are also found clustered close to the points of neurotransmission to other cells (*vide infra*, p. 775).

As already mentioned, several of the features of neurons can be interpreted as indicating a high level of protein synthesis, prompting the question, for what purpose is this protein required? Maintenance and repair of cytoplasmic proteins are activities in which all living cells engage, and in view of the relatively huge volume of cytoplasm in the cell body and extensive neurites of many neurons, it is perhaps not surprising that the rate of protein synthesis is also high. However, a sizable proportion of the protein synthesized may also be involved in the elaboration of the transmitter materials released at nerve endings, and also in various cellular activities associated with the reception of stimuli at dendritic and cell body surfaces. Cholinesterase, for example, is present at the surface of many neurons, which are also rich in other enzymes associated with the active transport of ions, such as sodium and potassium stimulated ATP-ase.

Although the machinery of protein synthesis, that is, RNA and ribosomes, is found throughout the cell body

[114] H. Barden, *J. Neuropath. exp. Neurol.*, **28**, 1969.

and in the dendrites, these materials are usually absent from axons. This raises the question of how transmitter substances and other materials are transported to the extremities of the neuron.

## AXOPLASMIC FLOW

It has for some time been appreciated that the cytoplasm of nerve cells, like that of other cells, is in continual motion; in tissue culture streaming movements of particulate matter and vesicles along axons in both directions can be observed. A considerable body of evidence from several sources now shows that a similar movement occurs in the axons of living neurons, resulting in the net transport of materials along axons from the cell body to the terminals, with some lesser movement also in the other direction.[115] Experiments which involve following the progress of radioactive substances (for example, from the retina along the visual pathway), and other investigations involving the ligature and subsequent structural analysis of central tracts and peripheral nerves,[116] have shown that *two types of transport* can be detected, one slow and the other relatively fast. The first type is a *bulk flow of axoplasm* including mitochondria, lysosomes and vesicles at a rate of about 1–3 mm a day, constituting the *slow transport*; the second, *rapid transport*, carries selected proteins and other materials at the rate of about 100 mm a day, and in the neurosecretory pathway of the hypothalamohypophyseal tract (p. 908), at the maximum recorded speed of 2,800 mm a day. This rapid flow can be eliminated by treating the nerve trunk locally with colchicine, indicating that microtubules are associated with the phenomenon (see also p. 909). It has also been shown ultrastructurally, in lampreys, that vesicles with side projections line up along the outside margins of microtubules, suggesting that they may be transported along axons by shearing forces generated between the projections and the microtubules. Other investigators have pointed out the presence of cross-connexions between adjacent microtubules, and proposed them as a tentative basis for wave-like oscillations, which possibly generate a motile force for streaming movements of the cytoplasm.

Whatever the mechanism, several problems arise. For example, what happens to the materials transported to the periphery—do they pass out of the neuron, and if so, into what tissue compartment? Ligature experiments show that there is a build-up of vesicles on both sides of the ligature, so that any mechanism must account for *bidirectional movement* of cytoplasmic organelles. Many unsolved questions remain to be answered in this field.

## Morphology of Synapses

The concept that neural pathways are interrupted at specific junctional points, was derived first from the physiological observation that there is an irreducible delay period inherent in reflex responses to sensory stimuli, and that neural conduction occurs only in certain directions.[117, 118] When it was established histologically that the central nervous system consisted of large numbers of individual neurons, rather than a continuous syncytial network, it became possible to attempt the localization of the junctional zones or synapses morphologically. Studies with the silver impregnation methods of Golgi (*vide supra*, p. 767) showed various structural specializations at axon terminals in the central nervous system, and other methods demonstrated rather similar peripheral endings in muscles (7.19, 20, 26). Later studies with the electron microscope, correlated with a considerable body of physiological and pharmacological knowledge, have helped to establish the morphological basis of synapses, and their molecular organization. Since synapses conduct only in one direction as a rule, some type of asymmetry might be expected in their structure; and, being regions of apposition between adjacent neurons, they may involve the junction of almost any parts of the two neuronal surfaces. The most common type of synaptic junction (7.19, 20) is that between an axon and a dendrite or a soma, the afferent fibre being expanded to form a small bulb or *bouton*; this may either be the terminal expansion of an axonal branch (*bouton terminal*), or it may be one of a series of expansions which form a row of bead-like endings, each of which makes synaptic contact (*bouton de passage*, see 7.19). Such boutons may synapse with: (1) *dendritic spines* or with the *flat surface* of a *dendrite*; (2) the *spines* or *flat surface* of the *soma*; (3) the *initial segment* of an *axon*; (4) the *boutons* of other *axons*. The patterns of axon termination in different populations of neurons vary considerably; a single axon may synapse with only one neuron, for example the climbing fibres ending on cerebellar Purkinje cells (p. 866), or more commonly, with a number of cells, the parallel fibres of the cerebellum being an extreme instance of this type (p. 867). An axon may synapse primarily with the dendritic tree or it may enwrap and arborize around the soma. Afferent axons of different origins may synapse only with certain parts of the neuron: for example, in the pyramidal cells of the visual cortex, optic radiation afferents synapse chiefly with the basal segments of the apical dendrite. (See also the account of the differential distribution of afferent terminals on the pyramidal cells of the cornu ammonis on p. 941.)

In *synaptic glomeruli* groups of axons make contact with the dendrites of one or more neurons in localized regions encapsulated by neuroglial cells (7.21); often complex interactions take place which will be further described below (p. 776).

## SYNAPTIC SPINES

Thorn-like extensions of dendrites and other parts of the neuron surface (7.15, 17) are termed *spines* or *gemmules*; they form the receptive points of contact with many of the incoming boutons, and may take several forms. Most frequently they are slender extensions (7.15) not more than about 2 $\mu$m long, with one or more expansions at their free ends, but they can also be short and stubby, branched, and bulbous. Their fine morphology and distribution will be described later (p. 775).

## ULTRASTRUCTURE OF SYNAPSES

Ultrastructurally, synapses can be defined as regions of structural specialization between two or more neurons, which possess some type of asymmetrical organization. They can be classified in various ways, for example by the type of neuronal processes involved and the direction of transmission. Thus synapses may be *axodendritic* (most common), *axosomatic* (also quite common), and less commonly, *axoaxonic, dendrosomatic, dendroaxonic, dendrodentritic*, and *somatodendritic. Somatosomatic* synapses have also been observed in lower vertebrates.

Axodendritic and axosomatic synapses are found in all regions of the central nervous system and in autonomic

[115] P. A. Weiss, in: *The Neurosciences Second Study Program*, eds, F. O. Schmitt, G. C. Quarton, T. Melnechuk and G. Adelman, Rockefeller University Press, New York. 1970.
[116] K. Kapeller and D. Mayor, *Proc. R. Soc.*, B, **167**, 1967.
[117] C. S. Sherrington, *The Integrative Action of the Nervous System*, Yale University Press, New Haven, 1947.
[118] J. C. Eccles, *The Physiology of Synapses*, Springer-Verlag, Berlin. 1964.

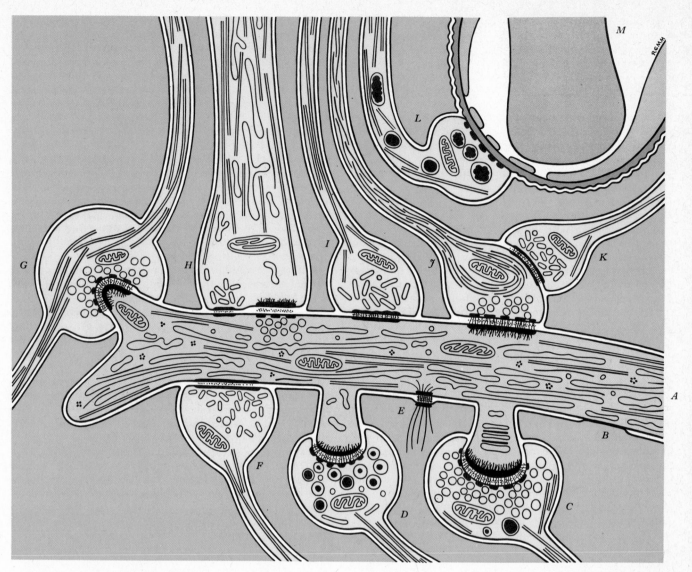

**7**.19 A scheme of the ultrastructural morphology of synapses, showing various junctional structures, grouped around a dendrite (A). The tight junction (B) and the desmosome (E) are without synaptic significance. Excitatory synaptic boutons are shown (C, G) containing small spherical translucent vesicles. D: a bouton with dense-cored, catecholamine-containing vesicles; F: an inhibitory synapse containing small flattened vesicles; H: a reciprocal synaptic structure between two dendritic profiles, inhibitory towards dendrite A and excitatory in the opposite direction; I: an inhibitory synapse containing large flattened vesicles. J and K: two serial synapses; J is excitatory to the dendrite; K is inhibitory to J. L: a neurosecretory ending adjacent to a vascular channel (M), surrounded by a fenestrated endothelium. All the boutons in this diagram are of the terminal type, except G which is a bouton de passage.

ganglia. Axoaxonic synapses occur between the boutons of two axon terminals (p. 750) and also between axon terminals and the initial segments of other axons (**7**.9, 20). The other types of synapse appear to be restricted to regions of complex interaction between the larger neurons of sensory pathways and microneurons.

For clarity, the **axodendritic arrangement**[100, 119, 120] will first be described in some detail (**7**.19, 20). Each synapse involves the apposition of a *presynaptic bouton* or *synaptic bag* with a postsynaptic process from which it is separated by a *synaptic cleft*. On both sides of this cleft there are zones of dense cytoplasm, usually broken on the presynaptic side into several groups, and on the postsynaptic side often extended into a filamentous meshwork, the *subsynaptic web*. The cleft shows indications of fine transverse filaments and contains polysaccharides. The presynaptic expansion is typified by numerous small membranous *synaptic vesicles* clustered in groups against the edge of the synaptic cleft and often, in a particular sectional profile, filling the whole bouton; mitochondria, membranous sacs and occasional lysosomes are also present. In some sites, the neurofilaments of the afferent axon enter the bouton and form a loop which takes a

variety of forms visible under the light microscope with silver stains. On the postsynaptic side there are often membranous structures such as the parallel cisternae (with intervening electron dense plates),—the *spine apparatus* of mammalian cortical dendritic spines. Glial cell processes commonly enwrap these various structures, but they do not extend into the synaptic cleft. The synaptic surface of the bouton is flat where it ends on the smooth surface of a dendrite or soma, but where postsynaptic spines are involved it may be highly curved to enwrap the spine or several spines belonging to adjacent neurons (**7**.19, 20). In some situations the dendrite surface itself forms a large spike, which interdigitates with the surface of the bouton. Conversely, dendritic expansions may be invaginated by one or more axonal terminals.

## FUNCTIONAL CLASSIFICATION OF SYNAPSES

Since we know that synapses may be either inhibitory or excitatory and that different transmitters are released in

[119] E. G. Gray, *J. Anat.*, **93**, 1959.
[120] E. G. Gray, *Prog. Brain Res.*, **31**, 1969.

774

their locality, it is important to look for corresponding structural differences between synapses. These can be classed morphologically on the basis of the shape of their synaptic vesicles and the arrangement of their pre- and post-synaptic cytoplasmic densities, into a number of distinct types. Thus, synapses which are rich in *catecholamines* (noradrenalin, adrenalin, dopamine), contain small (40–60 nm) *dense-cored vesicles* (7.20), similar to those of chromaffin cells in the adrenal medulla,[100] and their action in some sites is inhibitory, whilst in others it is excitatory. In contrast, *neurosecretory endings* such as those of the posterior pituitary contain relatively huge (50–200 nm) dense-cored vesicles of an irregular shape (7.20). Of the other types of central synapse, it was first recognized by Gray[121] in osmium-fixed material that two classes could be distinguished—a *type I* in which the zone of sub-synaptic dense cytoplasm is much thicker than that on the presynaptic side, and a *type II* in which the two zones are more symmetrical but thinner (7.19). The widths of the synaptic clefts are also different, being about 30 nm in type I synapses against 20 nm in type II synapses. With the advent of aldehyde perfusion as a method of fixation, these two types of synapse were found to be associated with two distinct classes of synaptic vesicles, type I endings containing small spherical vesicles about 50 nm in diameter, and type II boutons showing a variety of flattened forms (7.20). These are often known as 'S' (*spherical*) and 'F' (*flattened*) types of synaptic endings respectively.[122] Where the electrophysiology was known, as in the cerebellum, *type I synapses* could be correlated with *excitation* and *type II endings* with *inhibition*.[123] Recent reports, however, indicate that the situation is more complicated than this simple classification implies, since it is possible to distinguish between large ($25 \times 60$ nm) and small ($15 \times 40$ nm) flattened vesicles,[124] and also between discoidal and cigar-shaped forms.[125] Irregular (*pleomorphic*) shapes are also reported. Other studies have shown that in fresh specimens all vesicles may be spherical, but that some flatten on exposure to the buffers used in the preparative procedures. Different synaptic endings also show *mixed populations* of flat and spherical vesicles of varying proportions, depending upon the osmotic strength of the fixative. Although these various appearances are undoubtedly artefactual, they nevertheless point to real differences in the chemistry of the synapses.

The junction between the retinal receptors and bipolar neurons is also marked by a synapse-like structure, differing from the usual pattern in that the vesicles are clustered around an internal cytoplasmic rodlet rather than being situated at the margin of the synaptic cleft.[100]

## NEUROCHEMICAL TRANSMISSION

Transmission at all of the synapses described above is *neurochemical*, involving the release of *transmitters* associated with, or contained within, the synaptic vesicles, into the synaptic cleft. Here, the transmitter causes changes in potential at the postsynaptic surface, tending to depolarize it in the case of excitatory synapses, or to hyperpolarize the membrane in inhibitory ones.

Synaptic bags (*'synaptosomes'*)[126] can be separated by cell fractionation techniques from brain homogenates, and further subfractionated into various components. Where acetylcholine is the transmitter, enzymes capable of synthesizing this substance from its precursor, choline, are present in synaptosomes, and the transmitter is stored in association with the synaptic vesicles. Catecholamines have been demonstrated in the same way in synaptosomes, and are associated with the presence of dense-cored vesicles (*vide infra*, p. 791); further evidence of the catecholamine nature of such synapses comes from various studies of regions of the nervous system known to be rich in these substances, by autoradiographic methods and fluorescence microscopy (*see* p. 777). Glycine has also been demonstrated autoradiographically at type I ('F') synapses, and could be the transmitter in this species of ending.[127]

Detailed studies of the fine structure of synapses have shown the presence of a triangular grid of cytoplasmic densities on the deep aspect of the presynaptic surface (7.19) in type I endings,[128] which may have the function of guiding mobile synaptic vesicles to the edge of the cleft so that they momentarily fuse with the presynaptic membrane, thus releasing the stored transmitter into that gap; subsequently the vesicles may return to the interior of the synaptic bag for recharging with transmitter. It should be noted that the membranes of the synaptic vesicles and that of the cell surface are chemically different. The cue for transmitter release is the depolarization of the presynaptic membrane by the arrival of a nerve impulse, and the consequent release of calcium ions in the cytoplasm of the terminal.

## ELECTRICAL SYNAPSES

Although in mammals chemical transmission is more usual, in chick embryos and in lower vertebrates, and in several groups of invertebrates, electrically acting synapses are present in certain motor pathways where speed or synchrony of action is important.[129] Examples are the spoon-endings in the chick ciliary ganglion, club-endings on the giant Mauthner cells of the medulla in bony fishes, electromotor synapses in electrogenic fishes, and the giant fibre 'escape' systems of crayfish and earthworms. In structure and physiology, these synapses are essentially the same as the electrical junctions in cardiac muscle (p. 6), and non-striated muscle (p. 488), and are much more rapid than chemical synapses. Some of the invertebrate types can operate equally well in either direction, though usually the transmission is unidirectional.

## ORGANIZATION OF SYNAPTIC GROUPS

The way in which synaptic endings affect other neurons is partly dependent on their detailed arrangement on the cell surface, and their interrelations with other synapses. At *serial synapses* (7.19, 20), synaptic boutons end on other boutons, to affect their ability to respond to an invading volley of nerve impulses; this could be the basis of *presynaptic inhibition* observed physiologically in the spinal cord, although of course it could also be responsible for *presynaptic facilitation*, depending upon the types of synapse involved. In *reciprocal synapses* (7.19) found in the olfactory bulb and in the lateral geniculate body, transmission between two processes can occur in either direction by way of staggered synaptic zones placed on each side of the synaptic cleft. Commonly the zones appear to be excitatory in one direction and inhibitory in the other; they are believed to be the basis of lateral inhibition, at least at the first of these sites.[130]

[121] E. G. Gray, *J. Anat.*, **95**, 1961.
[122] D. Bodian, *J. Cell Biol.*, **44**, 1970.
[123] K. Uchizono, *Nature, Lond.*, **207**, 1965.
[124] A. J. Pinching and T. P. S. Powell, *J. Cell Sci.*, **9**, 1971.
[125] M. E. Dennison, *J. Cell Sci.*, **8**, 1971.
[126] V. P. Whittaker, in: *Handbook of Neurochemistry*, ed. A. Lajtha, vol. II, Plenum Press, New York. 1969.
[127] A. I. Matus and M. E. Dennison, *Brain Res.*, **32**, 1971.
[128] K. Pfenninger, C. Sandri, K. Akert and C. H. Eugster, *Brain Res.*, **12**, 1969.
[129] S. K. Malhotra, *Prog. Biophys. mol. Biol.*, **20**, 1970.
[130] W. Rall, G. M. Shepherd, T. S. Reese and M. W. Brightman, *Expl Neurol.*, **14**, 1966.

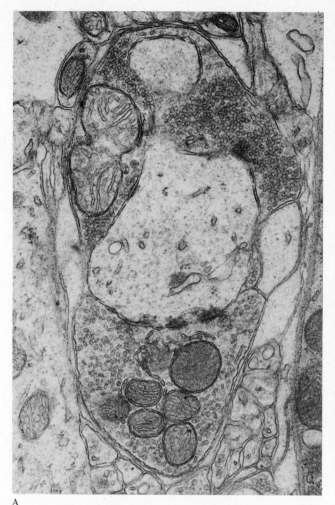

A

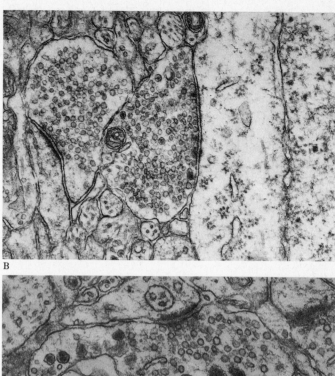

B

C

**7.20 A–C** Electron micrographs demonstrating various types of synapse. A This shows a pale cross-section of a dendrite upon which end two synaptic boutons. One of them (above) contains round vesicles, and the other (below) contains flattened vesicles of the small type. A number of pre- and post-synaptic thickenings mark the specialized zones of contact.

B Two types of synaptic structures are shown; one of them (left), a type I synapse between an axon terminal containing round vesicles, and a dendritic spine, the other (right), a type II synapse between an axon terminal containing pleomorphic vesicles, and the surface of a neuronal soma. C A type I synapse containing both small, round, clear vesicles, and also large dense-cored vesicles of the neurosecretory type.

In **synaptic glomeruli** (7.20, 21) several boutons may synapse with dendrites, and with each other, in localized regions of the neuropil which are usually encapsulated by layers of glial cells.[131] Sometimes, where microneurons are involved, the synaptic relationships are quite complex, involving both excitatory and inhibitory interactions between many cell processes. In **synaptic** or **neuropil cartridges**, a local region of a dendrite is enclosed partially by a glial sheath to isolate a cylindrical zone of synaptic endings on both spines and on the smooth dendritic surface between spines (7.19). Glial cells may also be so situated as to isolate or allow juxtaposition between various groups of interacting cells in various ways which may be of some physiological importance.[131] Although much is known about the arrangement of synapses in limited areas of the nervous system, much remains to be learnt about the disposition of different types of synapse on the surfaces of neurons. It has been suggested, for example, that inhibitory synapses might be particularly effective in blocking excitation if situated on the flat surfaces of the stems of dendrites, and on the soma and initial segment of the axon, where they could block excitation caused by other types of endings occurring on the spines of dendrites or other more peripheral positions, an example being the terminals of the basket cell axon which synapse with the 'pre-axon' of the Purkinje cell (p. 867).

## DEVELOPMENT AND PLASTICITY OF SYNAPSES

When first formed embryonically, synapses are recognizable by inconspicuous zones of density on each side of the synaptic cleft, and they only gradually mature into their fully differentiated structure.[132] Similar profiles are often seen in postnatal nervous systems, prompting the suggestion that synapses may be labile structures capable of being recruited for transmission, and perhaps dispersing when redundant. A change such as this is implicit in some theories of memory, which require synapses to be subject to modification according to the frequency of their use, thus establishing *preferential conduction pathways* in the brain. Unfortunately, what little evidence is available from training experiments, and from artificial stimulation, either does not support this hypothesis, or is equivocal. Neurophysiological recording of cortical neurons, however, suggests that synapses may become less easy to excite with repeated use, and they may change size. However, perhaps it is not necessary to postulate structural changes on this scale, since an increase of molecular receptor sites on the

[131] J. Szentágothai, in: *The Neurosciences. Second Study Program*, eds. F. O. Schmitt, G. C. Quarton, T. Melnechuk and G. Adelman, Rockefeller University Press, New York. 1970.
[132] D. Bodian, in: *The Neurosciences. Second Study Program*, eds. F. O. Schmitt, G. C. Quarton, T. Melnechuk and G. Adelman, Rockefeller University Press, New York. 1970.

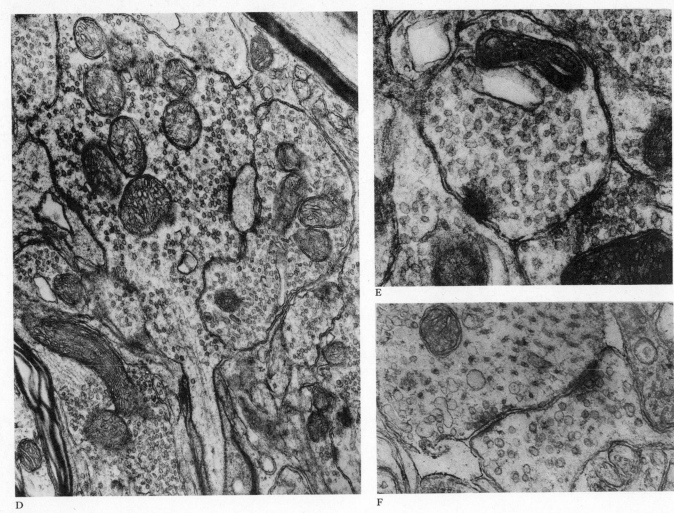

D

E

F

7.20 D–F   Electron micrographs of complex arrangements of synapses. D This shows a large terminal bouton of an optic nerve afferent fibre, which is making contact with a number of postsynaptic processes, in the dorsal lateral geniculate nucleus of the rat. One of the postsynaptic processes (right), also receives a synaptic contact from a bouton containing flattened vesicles. E Three neuronal processes in serial contact. On the lower right, a process, containing round vesicles, synapses with a second process (centre) containing flattened vesicles; in turn the latter makes contact with a third process (lower left): specimen from the dorsal lateral geniculate nucleus of the rat. F This demonstrates reciprocal synapses between two neuronal processes in the olfactory bulb of the rat. (7.20 A, D and E provided by Dr. A. R. Lieberman of University College, London.)

postsynaptic membrane, for example, would have the same effect as a change in the size of the presynaptic *bouton*. It is interesting that a somewhat controversial body of evidence has accumulated, suggesting that long-term memory formation is associated with increased protein synthesis; any change in the proteins associated with the synapse, even of receptor proteins, might require such an increase (*vide infra*).

## NEUROTRANSMITTERS

Up to the present time two major classes of transmitter substance, which have been authenticated as such and extensively examined, are *acetylcholine* and the catecholamines, *noradrenalin (norepinephrine)*, *adrenalin (epinephrine)* and *dopamine*.[133] The physiological effects of these vary considerably from one site to another and are beyond the scope of the present account. However, their common characteristics are that they are released from nerve endings when a nerve impulse arrives, and that they affect the resting potential of the cells which they influence, either to raise or lower it, for only a limited period of time. With acetylcholine, this temporal restriction is achieved by enzymic destruction of transmitter in the synaptic cleft, and the enzyme *acetylcholinesterase* can be demonstrated by various means, including cytochemical localization, in that region.[134] With the catecholamines, as with other

possible transmitters (*vide infra*), the transmitter is taken back into the nerve ending, to be restored for subsequent use, so terminating its extracellular action.

The mechanism of action of neurotransmitters is not yet fully understood, and most of our knowledge comes from investigations of peripheral motor endings. In the cholinergic endings in muscle, the subsynaptic sarcolemma of the muscle cells bears special *receptor molecules*, probably proteins, which bind the transmitter strongly, and presumably initiate the changes in the membrane which alter its permeability to ions. A similar, though more complex mechanism exists with the catecholamines (p. 775).

The distribution of particular neurotransmitters within the brain has been studied with a variety of methods, including pharmacological, radioactive tracer methods, fluorescence microscopy with respect to the catecholamines, cytochemical localization of cholinesterase, and so on. Acetylcholine is known to be present in the initial part of the Renshaw loop (p. 828), for example, and catecholamines are important in the reticular system of the brain stem and spinal cord, in the hypothalamus, corpus striatum, and substantia nigra, and other sites.

[133] L. S. Goodman and A. Gilman (eds.), *The Pharmacological Basis of Therapeutics*, 4th ed., Macmillan, London. 1970.
[134] P. R. Lewis and C. D. Shute, *J. Cell Sci.*, **1**, 1966.

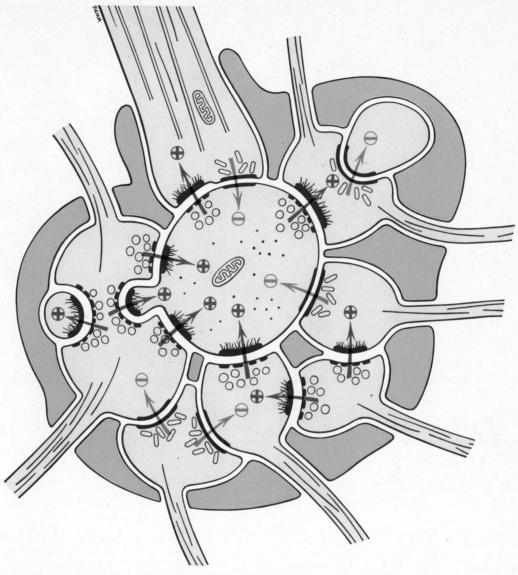

**7.21 A** and **B** Specialized multiple groups of synaptic contacts. **A** A synaptic glomerulus, showing various arrangements of synapses grouped around a centrally placed terminal dendritic expansion, seen in cross-section. Both excitatory (+) and inhibitory (−) synapses are shown; the direction of transmission is indicated by arrows (red for excitation, blue for inhibition). A glial capsule surrounds the whole complex.

The recognition of the aminergic status of neurons in the substantia nigra forms the basis of the treatment of Parkinsonian tremor with L-dopa, a precursor of dopamine, the synthesis of which is faulty in this condition (*see* p. 978).

Although a few neurotransmitters have been identified, many of the synapses of the central nervous system appear to operate by means of other transmitters of unknown chemistry. Many substances which can be extracted from the nervous system are known to have profound pharmacological effects at synapses, but have not so far satisfied the classical pharmacological criteria for neurotransmitters. Some of these agents are present in relatively large concentration in specific parts of the brain, and are known to be synthesized and metabolized locally. Among these materials are the amino acids glycine, gamma-aminobutyric acid (GABA), glutamic acid, aspartic acid, and serotonin (5-hydroxytryptamine).[147] Some of these may be precursors or breakdown products of transmitters, rather than actual transmitters themselves; however, some of them have been localized in synaptic endings, and are taken up from extracellular media in the same manner as catecholamines.

Morphological and pharmacological evidence points to a multiplicity of transmitters within the central nervous system; why so many are needed is not clear, but obviously much remains to be learnt about the physiology of central synapses which will have a direct bearing upon concepts of nervous organization. One simplifying concept, first formulated by Dale,[135] is that each neuron synthesizes only one transmitter substance, which is then released at all of its axon terminals including those of its collaterals. This concept has been upheld in many peripheral and central locations, although in the latter it is perhaps at variance with the occasional observation of mixed populations of synaptic vesicles within boutons.

## Neuroglia

In addition to neurons, several varieties of non-excitable cells are present in the nervous system,[136] forming a major component in its total composition (**7.22, 23**). In the central nervous system these are the *glial cell types* in the parenchyma of the brain and spinal cord, and the *ependymal cells* lining their internal cavities. In the ganglia

[135] H. H. Dale, W. W. Feldberg and M. Vogt, *J. Physiol., Lond.*, **86**, 1936.
[136] E. de Robertis and R. Carrera, *Prog. Brain Res.*, **15**, 1965.

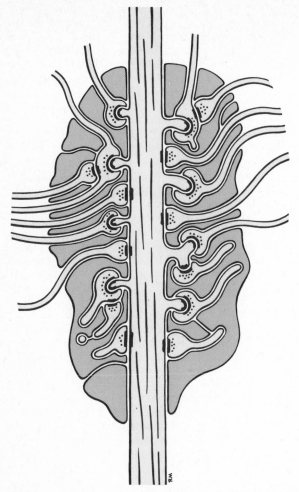

B A synaptic cartridge, with synapses grouped around a segment of a dendrite, and enclosed within a glial capsule (green).

like extensions. These cells can be further divided into star-like *protoplasmic astrocytes* with broad symmetrically spreading processes, confined to the grey matter, and *fibrous astrocytes* situated chiefly in the white matter, with asymmetrically spreading processes ramifying amongst the nerve fibres. The cytoplasmic processes of astrocytes carry fine, foliate extensions which partly engulf and separate neurons and their neurites, and often end in plate-like expansions on blood vessels, ependyma (*vide infra*), and on the pial surface of the central nervous system. Ultrastructurally, the cells are typified by a somewhat dense nucleus with an irregular outline (7.23), a cytoplasm which is rich in glycogen, lysosomes (corresponding to the *granules* or *gliosomes* of earlier light microscopy), Golgi complexes, and microfilaments extending throughout the cell processes.[138] Desmosomes and gap junctions (*see* pp. 5–6) form special contact zones between individual astrocytes, and sometimes between astrocytes and neurons. Cells with these features may take a number of different forms, and it appears likely, on the basis of isotopic labelling studies, that astrocytes, which are able to divide in mature animals, pass after mitosis through a series of structural transformations before finally disintegrating. In areas of brain injury they proliferate (gliosis), and also act as phagocytes to clear cellular débris.

**Oligodendrocytes** (7.22, 23), as their name implies, have fewer cell processes, and are present in two distinct areas, namely *intrafascicular* cells in myelinated tracts, and *perineuronal* oligodendrocytes where their processes come into apposition with neuronal surfaces. Some of the leaf-like expansions of the intrafascicular cells appear to be continuous with the myelin sheaths of central nerve fibres, a finding confirmed by electron microscopy.[139] A single oligodendrocyte may connect with the sheaths of more than one fibre. Ultrastructurally, these cells are characterized by a rounded nucleus and a cytoplasm rich in mitochondria, microtubules and glycogen. As with astrocytes, there is a spectrum of appearances, ranging from cells with relatively large euchromatic nuclei and a pale cytoplasm to ones with heterochromatic nuclei and a dense cytoplasm. Tritium labelling, again, shows that oligodendrocytes can proliferate in normal mature animals, and that they pass through stages of maturation and degeneration.

**Pituicytes** of the neurohypophysis are similar to astrocytes in some respects, except that their processes end mostly on the endothelial cells of vascular sinuses.

**Müller** cells of the retina (p. 1113) also have many features in common with astrocytes, and are of a similar origin.

**Bergmann glial cells** of the cerebellum (p. 866) have a special structure; their cell bodies and nuclei are situated in a row some distance below the pial surface. A single apical process passes superficially and then branches into terminal pial expansions. In many respects they have the appearance of a rather primitive glial cell type.

**Ependymal cells** are arranged as an epithelial layer one cell thick which lines the ventricles of the brain and the central canal of the spinal cord.[136] The cells vary from squamous to columnar according to their locality. At the surface they are in contact with each other by gap junctions and occasional desmosomes, and their free faces bear numerous microvilli and cilia which are often motile, their movements contributing to the flow of cerebrospinal fluid. Ultrastructurally,[140] the nucleus is rather

of the spinal nerve roots and autonomic nervous system, are the *capsular cells* which surround the cell bodies in those masses, and peripherally, the *Schwann cells* ensheathing the axons (*see* p. 287), terminal *lemmal cells* surrounding sensory capsules, *teloglial cells* ensheathing motor terminals, and the *supporting cells* of the sensory epithelia. Although the precise roles of the various cell types is not yet clear, their importance in the activity of the nervous system is becoming more and more obvious. One barrier to study has been their small size and variable appearance as seen with the special staining methods necessary to demonstrate them with light microscopy. Combined electron and light microscopic studies have helped to clarify some of these details, and a picture is gradually emerging, at least of their morphology.

## NEUROGLIAL CELL TYPES

In the central nervous system the chief non-nervous cells are the glial cell types (7.22, 23). These vary in numbers and type from one part of the nervous system to another, but two basic classes can be distinguished by their size and embryonic origin, namely the *macroglia*, relatively large cells derived from the neural plate, and the smaller *microglia*,[137] stemming from the mesodermal tissues surrounding the nervous system, which they enter at a relatively later stage of development.[138]

The *macroglia* (7.22, 23) comprises two cell types, the *astrocytes* (*astroglial cells*) and the *oligodendrocytes* (*oligodendroglial cells*).

**Astrocytes** possess small cell bodies (the nucleus is about 8μm in diameter in man) with ramifying dendrite-

[137] P. del Rio Hortega, *Bull. Soc. Sci. méd. biol.*, Montpellier, **5**, 1924.
[138] S. Mori and C. P. Leblond, *J. comp. Neurol.*, **139**, 1970.
[139] R. P. Bunge, *Physiol. Rev.*, **48**, 1968.
[140] M. W. Brightman and S. L. Palay, *J. Cell Biol.*, **19**, 1963.

heterochromatic, with an indented outline; the cytoplasm is rich in mitochondria, lysosomes, microtubules and microfilaments (7.22, 23). Secretion bodies are also sometimes present. In embryonic nervous systems, and in lower vertebrates, ependymal cells possess one or more long, radially orientated, processes which may branch and give off short side extensions, and are termed *tanycytes*, *ependymal astrocytes*, or *ependymoglial cells*. Later, in most, but not all, regions of mammalian brains, the basal process is resorbed.

*The functions of glial and ependymal cells* appear to be numerous although not fully explored:

7.22 A schema showing the types of non-neuronal cells in the central nervous system. The ependymal and glial cells are shown in green. The ependyma includes examples of ciliated and non-ciliated cells, and one tanycyte, with a centrally directed basal process. Two astrocytes are shown abutting on a neuronal soma and dendrites; one (above) also contacts a capillary, the other (below) expands on the pial surface. An oligodendrocyte (middle right) provide myelin sheaths for two axons. Two flattened microglial cells, one adjacent to a capillary (middle right), and the other within the neuropil at the top left, are also illustrated.

(1) Undoubtedly they act mechanically as a supporting component of the nervous system, and their microfilaments, microtubules, and surface contact zones fit them for this task. (2) They act as insulators, separating neurons and their processes from each other, or grouping interacting regions together. Electrical studies of glial cells in leeches, where they are particularly large, show that they can act in this way, and further that they lack the ability to conduct surface depolarizations for any distance.[141] (3) They can act defensively by phagocytosis of foreign material or cell débris, and can provide a means of limited repair to form glial scar tissue, or to fill the gaps left by degenerated neurons. (4) They have essential metabolic functions in regulating the biochemical environment of neurons (*see* p. 769), probably providing nutrients and regulating acid-base levels, amongst other actions. They may well provide transport channels between the local vasculature and the neuropil. Such a function has been recognized to be of great importance in maintaining the metabolism of cell processes which may extend for relatively enormous distances from the sites of nuclear control.[142] (5) Oligodendrocytes form and maintain the myelin sheaths of the larger neuronal processes of the central nervous system, in a manner similar to that of the Schwann cell in the periphery.[139] (6) Ependymal and related cells are associated with secretion into, and uptake and transport from, the cerebrospinal fluid; these functions have been explored in regions associated with the hypophysis cerebri where they are involved in transport of hormone-controlling factors in the median eminence and hypophysial stalk. (7) We can speculate that macroglial cells may play an important part in determining levels of physiological activity in the neuronal populations which they infiltrate. Although there is no evidence that glial cells supply ions to neurons during their activity, alterations in the metabolism of glial cells must have profound effect on the ionic environment of neurons and therefore on their patterns of excitability. Such alterations may be involved experimentally where anions such as chloride, applied topically to the brain surface, cause spreading electrical changes, the *spreading depression of Leao* (p. 965); it is conceivable that various metabolic changes within the brain may effect changes of electrical behaviour in its various parts by this means, either as a normal biological mechanism, or as a pathological one. Pathological disturbances of glial function may equally result in profound disturbances of neuronal function.

## Microglia

The microglial cells (7.22) are the smallest of the glial elements, and have flattened outlines, with fine, rather short, dendritic processes inserted between neurons, or applied to the external surfaces of capillaries. Ultrastructurally,[138] the cells contain rather dense, flattened, or indented, nuclei and, beside the usual organelles, large numbers of lysosomes. These features are identical with those of connective tissue macrophages, which indeed they are thought to be. Their phagocytic activities in combating infection and removing débris support this view.

## ORIGINS OF NEUROGLIA AND EPENDYMA

Early schemes of cellular differentiation in the neural tube such as that of His envisaged germinal cells giving rise, simultaneously, to *neuroblasts* and to glial stem cells or *spongioblasts*, which differentiate further into glioblasts and ependymo-glial cells. The glioblasts further differentiate

[141] J. G. Nicholls and S. W. Kuffler, *J. Neurophysiol.*, **27**, 1964.
[142] H. Hydén, in: *The Neurosciences, a Study Program*, eds. G. C. Quarton, T. Melnechuk and F. O. Schmitt, Rockefeller University Press, N.Y. 1967.

into astrocytes and oligodendrocytes and the ependymoglial cells into mature ependymal elements (p. 981). With the coming of autoradiographic methods of analysis, this scheme was modified in the sequence of events (*vide infra*), the germinal (matrix) cells *first* giving rise to neuroblasts, and *later* to the other cell elements (p. 792). As the matrix cell of later stages can only form non-nervous elements, it corresponds in principle to the spongioblast. However, it has been established that astrocytes and oligodendrocytes are also able to multiply once they have reached their position in the parenchyma of the nervous system (p. 792), even in mature animals.

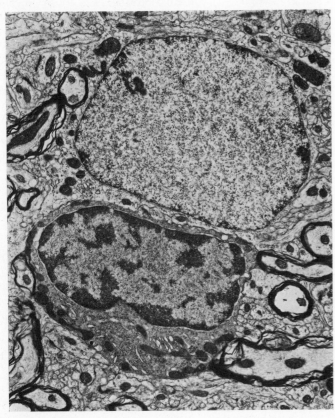

**7.23** An electron micrograph of two neuroglial cells situated amongst myelinated and non-myelinated nerve fibres, in the rat thalamus. An oligodendrocyte containing numerous mitochondria, a well-developed endoplasmic reticulum, and an indented nucleus is shown below; a larger astrocyte with a vesicular nucleus and scanty cytoplasm, is demonstrated above. (Kindly provided by Dr. A. R. Lieberman of University College; London.)

Ultrastructurally, the maturation of the glial and ependymal cells is marked by a gradual increase of intracellular membranes, to which ribosomes become attached, an increasing density of the nucleus and eventually the laying down of characteristic organelles such as filaments and microtubules.[161] These events accompany the cell migration and the contacting of the neuronal and vascular structures with which they establish their particular functional relationships. Microglia migrate in from the meninges, along the blood vessels, during embryonic development; they also appear able to divide in postnatal life.

## THE BLOOD-BRAIN BARRIER

In early investigations of the brain it was noticed that certain dyes, when injected into the circulatory system, failed to stain the parenchyma of the brain, although they passed easily into non-nervous tissues. Many subsequent studies confirmed that access from the circulation to the extracellular space of the central nervous system is severely limited for many substances, as though a physiological barrier existed at this junction. The precise nature of this '*blood-brain barrier*' has been the subject of much debate in view of its importance to drug therapy of nervous disorders, anaesthesia, and so on.[143] It is possible that because such an apparently small extracellular space exists in the brain (see, however, p. 993), the fluid in the gaps between its cells soon becomes equilibrated with materials diffusing from capillaries. Accordingly, more could only diffuse in when the cells begin to take the material up intracellularly, thus accounting for the selective nature of the barrier. However, many materials when injected into the *ventricles* can enter the brain with ease, indicating that the barrier is probably present at the level of the capillary. Recent experiments with peroxidase as an ultrastructural colloidal tracer[144] show that diffusion can occur quite freely in the interstices between the cells of the central nervous system. The tracer passes from the ventricles, through the ependymal layer, and across the nervous tissues to reach the pial surface. Diffusion is, however, stopped at the endothelial lining of capillaries, and it appears that central nervous capillaries are unusually impermeable to large molecules. It is probable then, that the vascular endothelium is a major element in the blood-brain barrier, but it is also possible that other metabolic factors may play a part in its ability to discriminate between different substances.

## EXTRACELLULAR SPACE IN THE BRAIN

When considering the movements of water and solutes in any tissue it is convenient to think of the system in terms of a number of physiological barriers which create a series of physiological compartments, namely the capillary bed, the lymphatic drainage, the intracellular space and the extracellular space.[143] The central nervous system lacks an intrinsic lymphatic drainage and the position is therefore simplified. At one time it was considered that large extracellular spaces were present between the cell processes, on the basis of light microscopy; but fine structural studies soon showed that the central nervous parenchyma consists of a complex three-dimensional meshwork of neurons and their processes, glial cells and capillaries, all apparently tightly packed with no more than a 20 nm gap between their surfaces. However, studies with physiological dilution methods, and electrical resistance recordings, indicated that the extracellular space should be much higher than that calculated from fine structural observations, that is about 20 per cent rather than 5 per cent. Later investigations partly resolved this problem, since it was found that in anoxic conditions the cells take up extracellular fluid and swell to fill all possible gaps, and that processing of tissues for electron microscopy can result in large changes in the spaces between cells.[145] It is probable, therefore, that the extracellular space of central nervous tissue is larger than the minimal value of about 5 per cent, but by how much is not clear.

## Study of Peripheral Nerve Fibres

As in the central nervous tracts, two types of nerve fibre are present in the peripheral nervous system, namely myelinated and non-myelinated fibres. Peripherally, however, they are ensheathed by the *cells of Schwann* instead

[143] H. Davson, *Physiology of the Cerebrospinal Fluid*, Churchill, London. 1970.
[144] M. W. Brightman and T. S. Reese, *J. Cell Biol.*, **40**, 1969.
[145] S. M. Sumi, *J. Ultrastruct. Res.*, **29**, 1969.

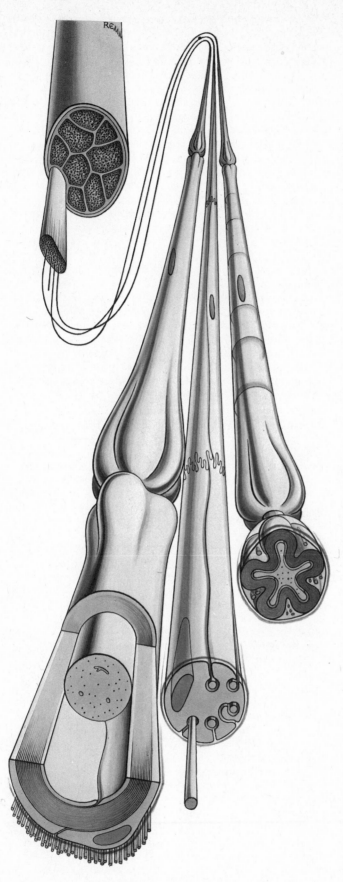

of the central oligodendrocytes. Both central and peripheral nerve fibres present a number of difficulties to the neurohistologist, either because of their small size in the case of unmyelinated fibres, or because the sheaths of myelinated fibres are badly disrupted by the lipid solvents employed for histological preparation. A number of special methods have been devised to overcome these problems; with myelin sheaths these are based chiefly on means of fixing and staining the myelin either in teased material which demonstrates individual fibres, or in blocks of tissue which can be later processed and sectioned in the usual way. The osmium-based methods are particularly valuable in this respect, either used as osmium tetroxide in aqueous solution, or with chromate and haematoxylin solutions, both methods fixing and staining the sheaths simultaneously. Other methods include the use of frozen sections stained with lipid-soluble dyes, examination of material prepared by any of these methods by polarization, phase or interference microscopy, and observation of freshly teased or living nerves *in situ* by various means including incident light techniques. The extension of time-lapse cinemicrography, and videotape recording techniques in conjunction with closed-circuit television, to this field of investigation have aided the analysis of living nerve fibres.[146] The various means of demonstrating central neurons already described (p. 767), have also been valuable in demonstrating peripheral nerve fibres including non-myelinated ones; as with other parts of the nervous system, electron microscopy has contributed greatly to our understanding of peripheral nerve structure.

## Structure of the Peripheral Nervous System

The peripheral nervous system comprises the cerebrospinal and autonomic systems of nerves, and their associated ganglia containing nerve cell somata, together with the cellular and connective tissue elements which ensheath them. All these structures, of course, lie peripheral to the pial envelope which covers the central nervous system, through which the central and peripheral nerve fibres are continuous at many points, but the histology of the two contrasts in a number of ways, and that of the peripheral structures will now be considered in some detail (7.24, 25, 26, 27, 28).

**The sensory ganglia** of the dorsal spinal nerve roots (7.25), and the corresponding ones on the trunks of the trigeminal, facial, glossopharyngeal and vagal cranial nerves, are ensheathed by periganglionic connective tissue which is similar to perineurium in composition (p. 994). The neurons are *unipolar*, possessing spherical or ovoid cell somata of varying size, which are aggregated in groups, interspersed with fasciculi of myelinated and non-myelinated nerve fibres. The fine structure of neuronal cytoplasm is described elsewhere (p. 771) and will not be pursued further here, but it should be noted that a single non-myelinated neurite (sometimes termed a 'dendro-axonal' process) leaves each cell soma. It often follows a highly convoluted course near the parent soma before bifurcating at a T-junction to become continuous with the central and peripheral processes of the sensory nerve fibre.[147] In the case of myelinated fibres, such a junction occurs at a node of Ranvier (p. 790). The peripheral process terminates in a sensory ending and since it

7.24A This diagram shows some structural features of peripheral nerve fibres. A nerve trunk (top left) is cut away to expose a single fasciculus, from which three fibres are indicated in detail. These include two myelinated axons, one on each side of a group of non-myelinated axons enclosed within a Schwann cell sheath. The myelinated fibre on the left has been cut away at various points to demonstrate the relationship between the axon, the Schwann cell, and its sheath of myelin.

[146] P. L. Williams and S. M. Hall, *J. Anat.*, **107**, 1970; **108**, 1971; **109**, 1971.

[147] A. S. Dogiel, *Der Bau der Spinalganglien des Menschen und der Saugethiere*, Fischer, Jena. 1908.

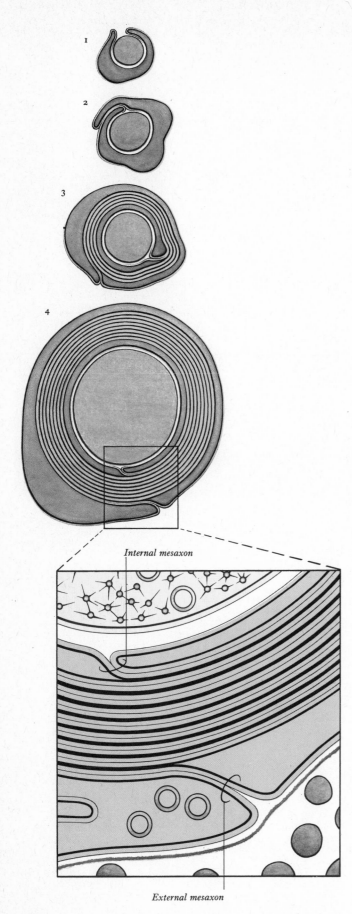

*Internal mesaxon*

*External mesaxon*

**7.24**B A diagram showing the development and organization of the myelin sheath of a peripheral nerve fibre. In stages 1–4 myelin formed by a Schwann cell (blue) progressively envelops the growing axon (yellow), to form the final pattern of spirally disposed myelin lamellae: see enlarged detail at the base of the diagram. Compare with **7.25**F and G, and consult text for further details.

conducts towards the cell body it is functionally an *elongated dendrite*, but it possesses all the morphological and physiological characteristics of a *peripheral axon* and, following common usage, will be so termed in this account. Each unipolar cell body is closely enveloped by a *nucleated capsule* consisting of flattened, epithelium-like *capsular cells*, also variously termed *amphicytes* or *satellite cells*. (It should be noted that the name satellite cell is used in a number of different ways. Some authors use the term for small rounded extracapsular ganglionic cells, others include ganglionic capsular cells and Schwann cells, and yet others include all non-neuronal cells both central and peripheral which are perineuronal in position. Further, the name is also applied to cells associated with the surfaces of striated muscle fibres—p. 481.) The cytoplasm of the capsular cells in many ways resembles that of Schwann cells (*vide infra*), and their deep surfaces are irregular, interdigitating with reciprocal irregularities on the surface of the subjacent nerve cell body. The layer of capsular cells is continuous with a layer of similar cells which encloses the convoluted part (*initial glomerulus*) of the dendro-axonal process, and this, in turn, is continuous with the Schwann cell layer of the peripheral and central processes of the nerve fibre. Outside these cell layers lies a delicate vascular connective tissue which is continuous with the endoneurium of the peripheral nerve and nerve root.

Sensory ganglionic neurons are not confined to the discrete ganglia of the cerebrospinal nerves, but either singly or in small groups, they often occupy 'heterotopic' positions either peripheral to the ganglia in the nerve trunks and their branches, or central to the ganglia between the fasciculi of the dorsal spinal nerve roots.

**The autonomic ganglia** have a different structure, since their cell bodies are multipolar with dendritic trees which receive synapses from incoming preganglionic visceral motor fibres, and sections show a mixed neuropil of afferent and efferent fibres, dendrites, synapses and cell bodies[148] (**7.25**). Satellite or capsular cells perform the role of neuroglia among the neuronal structures. Autonomic ganglia are found in the paravertebral sympathetic chains, near the roots of the great visceral arteries in the abdomen, and near or embedded within the walls of various viscera. Autonomic ganglion cells may also be highly modified, as in the case of the chromaffin cells of the adrenal medulla in which the axon is absent.

**The nerve trunks** and their principal branches are composed of roughly parallel bundles of nerve fibres comprising the efferent and afferent axons, their ensheathing Schwann cells, which in some cases elaborate *myelin sheaths*, surrounded by connective tissue sheaths at different levels of organization. The fibres are grouped together within the trunk in a number of *fasciculi* (**7.24**) each of which may contain from relatively few to many hundreds of nerve fibres. The size, number and pattern of the fasciculi vary greatly in different nerves and at different points along the length of a nerve. The number of fasciculi increases and their size decreases some distance before there is macroscopic evidence of *branching* of a nerve trunk. Similarly, where the nerve is subjected to considerable increases of pressure, as when passing deep to a fibrous retinaculum, the fasciculi are again increased in number and reduced in size; further, their volume of associated connective tissue and their vascularity also increases. Consequently, the nerve shows a pink, fusiform dilatation of contour at this point, which is sometimes termed a *pseudoganglion* or *gangliform enlargement*.

A dense irregular connective tissue sheath, the *epineurium*, surrounds the whole trunk, and a similar but less

[148] S. Ramon y Cajal, *Textura del Sistema Nervioso del Hombre y de los Vertebrados*, vol. I, Moya, Madrid. 1900.

fibrous *perineurium* encloses each fasciculus, within which the spaces between nerve fibres are penetrated by a loose delicate connective tissue network, the *endoneurium*. These connective tissue sheaths serve as convenient planes of access for the vasculature of peripheral nerves, the capillary bed and associated lymphatics running in the main parallel to the nerve fibres in the endoneurial spaces, but short oblique cross-connexions pass between them.

The epineurium is a collagenous adventitial coat with little regular organization;[149] the perineurium in contrast has a regular structure of highly flattened laminae of fibroblasts alternating with fine collagenous sheets running in various directions within the sheath (7.25). Macrophages are also present. The fibroblasts, which are surrounded by dense intercellular material, form junctional complexes with each other, and it appears from tracer experiments that these limit the diffusion of large molecules across the sheath.[150] The fibroblasts also show numerous pinocytotic vesicles, an indication of active transport mechanisms. Thus the sheath not only plays a mechanical and defensive role but also isolates the enclosed nerve fibres, to some extent, from the outside environment.

## THE CLASSIFICATION OF PERIPHERAL NERVE FIBRES

On the basis of total fibre diameter (i.e. the axon as well as its myelin sheath), and the rate of impulse conduction, the fibres in mixed peripheral nerves have been classified into three major classes, designated A, B and C.[151] Fibres in class A are the largest, consisting of various categories of myelinated somatic afferent and efferent fibres (7.25). Class B comprises the myelinated preganglionic fibres of the autonomic nervous system, and class C, non-myelinated autonomic and sensory fibres.

### A Fibres

These can be further subdivided and it has been found useful to create separate terminologies for sensory and motor components.

**The afferent (sensory) fibres in class A** are divided into groups I, II and III.

*Group I* fibres are large in diameter (up to 20 μm) and conduct at speeds of up to 100 m/sec. They include the primary sensory fibres from muscle spindles (subgroup Ia) and from tendon organs (subgroup Ib).

*Group II* includes cutaneous afferent fibres from various mechanoreceptors such as touch and Pacinian corpuscles, receptors associated with larger, 'guard' hair follicles, and fibres from the secondary endings on the intrafusal muscle fibres of muscle spindles. The diameters of group II fibres range from 5 to 15 μm, and their conduction velocities from 20 to 90 m/sec.

*Group III* fibres innervate follicle receptors associated with finer hair or 'down', sensory endings in the walls of some blood vessels, and a variety of pain receptors (nociceptors) in many tissues of the body. Their diameters range from 1 to 7 μm, and their conduction speeds from 12 to 30 m/sec.

**The efferent (motor) fibres in class A** are divided into three groups designated α, β and γ.

The α fibres innervate extrafusal muscle only, being about 17 μm in diameter, and conducting at 50–100 m/sec. The fibres to 'fast twitch' muscle are slightly larger and faster conducting than those to 'slow' muscle.

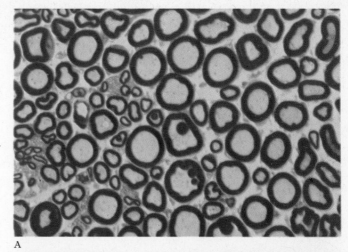

A

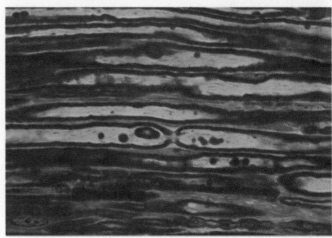

B

7.25 A Transverse section of part of a mixed peripheral nerve from a mouse, showing a wide range of diameters of myelinated nerve fibres. Myelin: dark blue; axoplasm: pale blue, embedded in which are slightly darker blue dots, the axonal mitochondria. Note particularly the wide range of axon diameters; the smaller axons possess thinner myelin sheaths. The fibre with a particularly thick, double-contoured myelin sheath (bottom left) is sectioned through an incisure of Schmidt-Lanterman. The large fibres with more complex profiles (centre and bottom) are sectioned near the commencement of paranodal bulbs. On the left, between the myelinated fibres, groups of non-myelinated axons, enclosed by Schwann cells (medium blue) are just visible. A 1 μm epoxy resin section, stained with osmium tetroxide solution, and toluidine blue, photographed using oil immersion optics.

B A longitudinal section of material prepared in a similar manner to that in 7.25 A. Note particularly the fibre just below the centre of the field which is sectioned through a node of Ranvier. As the internodal myelin sheath approaches the node, its diameter increases to a maximum (the paranodal bulb) and the myelin sheath then curves sharply inwards, to terminate at the limits of the 'nodal gap', The myelin profiles, apparently lying free within the paranodal bulbs, are demonstrated to be paranodal shelves of myelin, when serial sections are examined (compare with 7.25 H). Note also the constriction of the nodal axon; long, narrow axonal mitochondria are also visible.

C A transverse section through the centre of a node of Ranvier, with numerous finger-like processes of adjacent Schwann cells converging towards the nodal axolemma. Many microtubules and microfilaments are visible within the axoplasm (centre).

D A longitudinal section of a part of a myelinated nerve fibre of the mouse, including an incisure of Schmidt-Lanterman; this appears as oblique zones in the myelin sheath on both sides of the fibre. Consult text for structural details.

E A transverse section of an immature peripheral nerve of a rat, taken one week after birth, showing the profiles of numerous axons. Some of the latter are non-myelinated and, either singly or in groups, are invaginated into the surfaces of cytoplasmic processes of adjacent Schwann cells. Other axons are in the process of myelination. Note the Schwann cell nucleus (lower centre) to one side of a myelin sheath, and the ultrastructure of the Schwann cell cytoplasm at this stage of development.

[149] P. K. Thomas, *J. Anat.*, **97**, 1963.
[150] J. D. Waggener and J. Beggs, *J. Neuropath. exp. Neurol.*, **26**, 1967.
[151] J. Erlanger and H. S. Gasser, *Electrical Signs of Nervous Activity*, Univ. Penna. Press, Philadelphia. 1937.

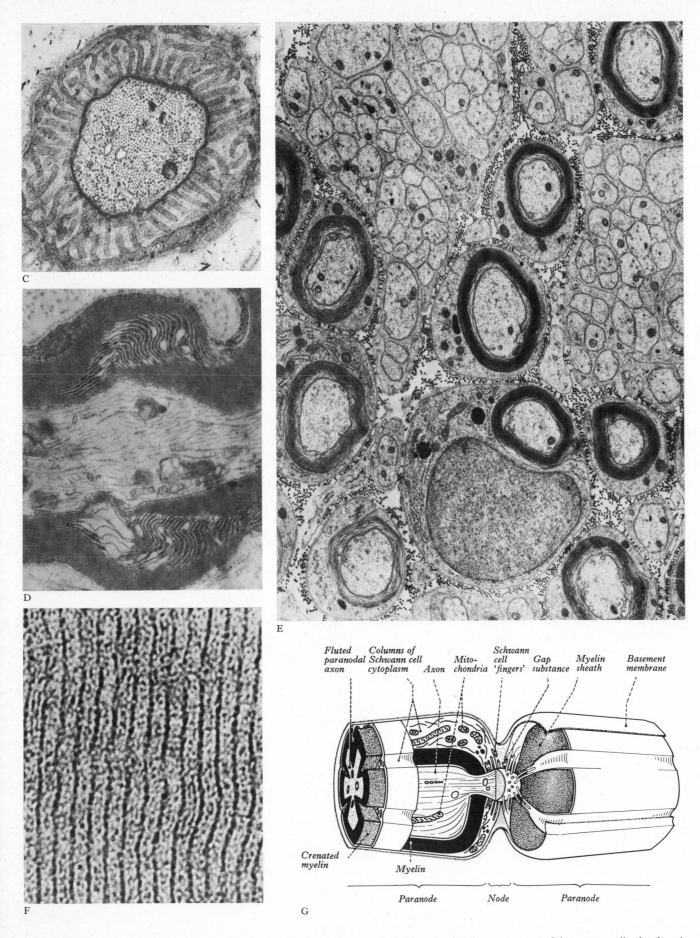

C

D

E

F

G

*Fluted paranodal axon*  *Columns of Schwann cell cytoplasm*  *Axon*  *Mito-chondria*  *Schwann cell 'fingers'*  *Gap substance*  *Myelin sheath*  *Basement membrane*

*Crenated myelin*

*Myelin*

*Paranode*    *Node*    *Paranode*

F   A high-power electron micrograph of part of a myelin sheath in section, showing dense period lines (the apposition of the cytoplasmic aspects of the cell membranes), alternating with less dense intraperiod lines (the apposition of the external aspect of the Schwann cell membranes). The preparative techniques used has caused the intraperiod line to split into two distinct lines in some areas.

G   A diagram showing the arrangement of the axon, myelin sheath and Schwann cell cytoplasm at the node of Ranvier and in the paranodal bulbs. (Supplied by P. L. Williams and D. N. Landon. Preparations **7.25** A–E kindly supplied by Dr. Susan Standring of Guy's Hospital, London.)

785

The $\beta$ fibres are few in number, and each appears to give a collateral branch to a muscle spindle, before the main branch continues to end on a 'slow twitch' extrafusal muscle fibre (p. 480).

The $\gamma$ fibres are probably exclusively fusimotor, and 'fast' and 'slow' ($\gamma1$ and $\gamma2$) fibres have been recognized, the latter being somewhat narrower and possessing thinner sheaths.[152] Gamma fibres are from 2 to 10 $\mu$m in diameter and conduct at velocities of 10–45 m/sec.

### B Fibres

The preganglionic autonomic B fibres lie in the diameter range of 3 $\mu$m or less and have conduction velocities of 3–15 m/sec.

### C Fibres

These are non-myelinated nerve fibres with diameters ranging from 0·2 $\mu$m to about 1·5 $\mu$m and conduction velocities of only 0·3–1·6 m/sec. Such fibres include autonomic efferents which are postganglionic in position, and both visceral and somatic sensory fibres, many of which are 'pain' fibres serving all the tissues of the body except the interior of the central nervous system. The smallest C fibres are found in the fila of the olfactory nerves.

Whilst such general forms of classification have proved of great assistance in neurophysiology, it must be emphasized that caution should be exercised before assuming that a single structural parameter, such as total fibre diameter, measured at one point along a nerve trunk, adequately categorizes the nerve fibre population along the length of a nerve (see also below).

## CONDUCTION IN PERIPHERAL NERVES

When a nerve trunk is stimulated, the *sum* of the action potentials in its many different nerve fibres, the *compound action potential*, can be recorded with extracellular electrodes. Since these potential variations travel at different speeds along different fibres, and since large fibres create larger electrochemical fluxes than small ones, a compound action potential recorded at a distance from the point of stimulation has a complex form, with at least four successive waves of different amplitude and velocity. These are known as the $\alpha$, $\beta$, $\gamma$ and $\delta$ waves. Just as each nerve trunk has its own characteristic spectrum of nerve fibres types, so the precise wave pattern is also distinctive. In the past, the fibre types have been classified by their conduction velocities, but it is now recognized that fibres of different physiological roles may have similar conduction velocities so that a more complex terminology taking into account size, conduction velocity and functional connexions has emerged (*vide supra*).

It is becoming clear that there are a series of factors which govern the conduction velocity of nerve fibres. In non-myelinated fibres, the action potential sweeps continuously over the axolemma as ionic eddy currents (electrotonus) which progressively excite neighbouring areas of membrane. The rate of spread is proportional to the cross-sectional area of the axon.[153] In myelinated fibres, however, the presence of an insulating layer of myelin prevents the membrane from being excited at any point except the nodes of Ranvier, but once an action potential is initiated at one node, the resultant ionic eddy currents spread to excite the next node and others in sequence. Since the longitudinal flow of ions in tissue fluid and axoplasm is much more rapid than a continuous electronic spread along the axonal membrane, much higher conduction velocities are possible by this mechanism, which is known as *saltatory conduction* or *saltation*.[154]

During excitation at a node of Ranvier, there is initially an increased permeability of the short, exposed, segment of nodal axolemma to sodium ions, which therefore flow down their concentration gradients to enter the nodal axon. Consequently, longitudinal ionic currents are generated which flow along the *internodal axon* to leave at the next node, the circuit being completed by longitudinal ionic currents in the reverse direction in the endoneural tissue fluid. When the outflowing current density at the *second node* rises to a critical *threshold level*, its

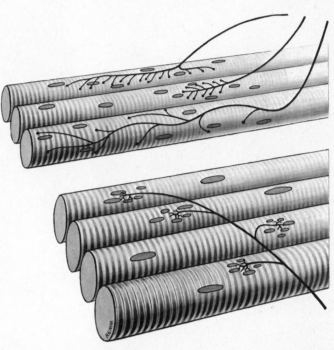

7.26 A   Diagram showing some types of innervation of striated muscle, including the 'en plaque' terminals of $\alpha$ efferents (below), and the more widely spread 'trail' and 'en grappe' endings of $\gamma$ efferents (above). (Intrafusal fibres shown relatively enlarged for clarity.)

depolarizing effect is sufficient to initiate similar permeability changes in the nodal axolemma, and the whole process is repeated, with excitation of the third and subsequent nodes. However, myelin is an imperfect insulator and, as a result, the longitudinal currents are not completely confined to the axoplasm and external tissue fluid. Some radial leak of current occurs between the axoplasm and tissue fluid, with a resulting loss of efficiency. The details of these relationships will not be pursued here, but it may be noted that for a given total fibre diameter, maximum efficiency is achieved when the diameter of the axon and the thickness of its myelin sheath are such that the *ratio* of axon diameter to total fibre diameter is 0·6. Only the largest mammalian myelinated nerve fibres reach this ratio during growth.

Despite the general usefulness of the classification of nerve fibres described above, based in part upon total nerve fibre diameter variations, it should be emphasized that other dimensions are importantly involved in determining the conduction characteristics of a myelinated nerve fibre. As just mentioned, these include the *diameter* of the *axon* and the *relative thickness* of its *myelin sheath*; in addition, the *internodal distance* between successive nodes of Ranvier, and the *area, characteristics*

[152] I. A. Boyd and M. R. Davey, *Composition of Peripheral Nerves*, Livingstone, Edinburgh. 1968.
[153] A. L. Hodgkin, *The Conduction of the Nervous Impulse*, Thomas, Springfield, Ill. 1964.
[154] R. Stämpfli, *Physiol. Rev.*, **34**, 1954.

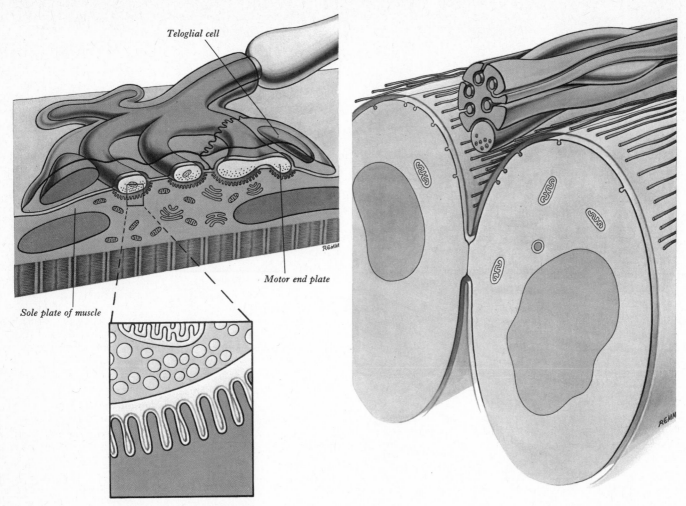

Teloglial cell

Motor end plate

Sole plate of muscle

B   A diagram of the detailed structure of an 'en plaque' neuromuscular junction. An enlarged portion of the terminal is shown below; note the folding of the sarcolemma to form subsynaptic gutters, the disposition of the basal lamina, and the synaptic vesicles within the axon terminal.

C   A diagram of an autonomic neuromuscular junction between a group of non-myelinated axons (above) and smooth muscle cells (below). The Schwann cell (blue) is reflected at intervals to expose enlargements of the axons (yellow) which contain synaptic vesicles.

and *microenvironment* of the *nodal axolemma* are important. These structural parameters vary between species, between different functional categories of fibre, and at different points along the length of individual fibres and their branches.[162]

## SCHWANN CELLS

Of neural crest origin, the cells of Schwann are the chief non-excitable cells of the peripheral nervous system, enfolding and enwrapping axons over most of their surfaces. Morphologically, Schwann cells vary with the type of fibre, but generally the nucleus is rather heterochromatic and ellipsoidal in shape, and the cytoplasm is rich in mitochondria, microtubules and microfilaments, in addition to prominent lysosomes, and a well-developed rough endoplasmic reticulum. A basement membrane is present at the external surface except where this lies adjacent to a nerve cell process.

Circumstantial evidence points to a close physiological relationship between Schwann cells and neurons. Embryonic growth of nerve cell processes, and regrowth of axons after local injury, only occur in the presence of Schwann cells, and in tissue culture, growth of the two occur simultaneously. The exact nature of the relationship is not clear: as with certain glial cells of the central nervous system, the sheaths which Schwann cells form around neurites limit the flow of ions occurring during electrical activity of the nerve fibre, or they affect its distribution in other ways. It has also been suggested that

in view of the large cytoplasmic volume and surface area of many neurons, which possess but a single diploid nucleus, and the exceptionally long distances through which metabolites must flow from the cell body to the more remote parts of their processes, Schwann cells may perform local nutritive and energy-supplying roles in maintaining the ensheathed nerve cell processes.[155] In myelinated fibres the Schwann cells also allow more rapid rates of conduction and a reduced energy consumption in fibres of relatively small diameter.

Apart from structural observations of, for example, the large numbers of mitochondria in Schwann cells at nodes of Ranvier in myelinated fibres (*vide infra*, p. 788), the evidence for this relationship is not complete and further critical experiments are needed to settle the problem. In addition to these metabolic functions, Schwann cells also provide mechanical support to nerve fibres and are capable of phagocytosis of cellular débris.

All of the larger axons of the nervous system of mammals are enwrapped in *myelin sheaths* and are termed *myelinated* or *medullated* fibres. The fatty composition of the myelin is responsible for the glistening whiteness of the peripheral nerve trunks and of the white matter centrally. Axons less than about $0.5–1.0$ $\mu$m in diameter generally lack these sheaths and are therefore termed *non-myelinated*, *non-medullated* or *grey* fibres. These two types of fibre have great physiological significance and will be described in some detail.

[155] D. N. Landon and P. L. Williams, *Nature, Lond.*, **199**, 1963.

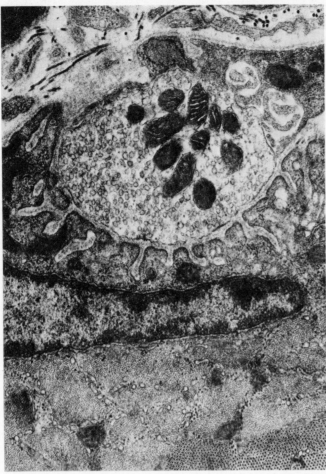

**7.27** An electron micrograph of a neuromuscular junction in striated muscle, showing part of a motor endplate containing synaptic vesicles (above). The latter is situated in a groove in the sarcolemma; this is further convoluted to form the subsynaptic gutters of the sole plate (below). (Kindly provided by Dr. D. N. Landon, Neurobiological Unit, National Hospital for Nervous Diseases, London.)

## NON-MYELINATED FIBRES

These comprise the smaller axons of the central nervous system, post-ganglionic axons of the autonomic nervous system, and several types of fine sensory fibres such as some of those responsible for signalling pain (but see also below and pp. 797, 833), the olfactory nerve axons, and others. Structurally these axons are engulfed either singly or in small bundles into longitudinal invaginations of a series of Schwann cells[113, 156] which therefore separate them from the endoneurial space (**7.27**). The original line of invagination during development of non-myelinated axons which are deeply embedded in Schwann cells is marked by a *mesaxon* consisting of a double layer of the Schwann cell plasma membrane, the external surfaces of which are parallel but separated by a gap of 15–20 nm. Deeply, the two layers separate to enclose the axon from which they are again separated by a *periaxonal space* of similar dimensions; superficially the mesaxonal layers separate to become continuous with the general outer plasma membrane of the Schwann cell. The endoneurial tissue fluid has access to that in the periaxonal space by way of the gap between the two layers of the mesaxon. Although narrow, these intercellular spaces are of sufficient dimensions to allow the mobility of ions necessary for the continuous electrotonic current fluxes which characterize non-myelinated fibre conduction.

Where synaptic or motor transmission occurs, the Schwann cell is reflected back from the axonal surface to expose the active regions. The terminal branches of mye-

linated fibres where they taper, are also provided with Schwann cell sheaths of a similar nature.

## MYELINATED FIBRES

Myelinated fibres form the bulk of the elements of the somatic nervous system. To understand the structure of the myelin sheath it is convenient to describe its development in the newborn. The formation of myelin begins some while before birth in many tracts and nerve trunks although it is not completed until a considerable time later. The pattern of myelination varies in its timing in different mammalian groups and in different parts of the same nervous system.

In the peripheral nervous system axons grow out from the central and ganglionic cell bodies along with Schwann cells which initially multiply as the nerve grows in length, but later they cease dividing and increase only in size. At first, all axons are non-myelinated, but later a flap-like extension of the Schwann cell cytoplasm begins to spiral around the neurite, with the bulk of the cytoplasm and nucleus remaining outside the spirals (**7.27, 28**). As development proceeds, more and more turns are made, and the spirals become transformed into compacted layers of cell membrane.[157] In electron micrographs, the myelin sheath, when mature, is seen as a laminated structure with regular dense *period lines* (representing the plane of apposition between the internal surfaces of the plasma membrane) alternating with less conspicuous *intraperiod lines*, representing appositions between the external surfaces of the plasma membrane spiral (**7.27**). Suitable osmotic treatment which causes the swelling of the sheath causes the intraperiod line to split, showing that the external surfaces are not fused to form a specialized junctional zone, but are apparently able to move on one another.[158] On the inside and outside of the myelin sheath is a delicate zone of Schwann cell cytoplasm which, in many parts of the internode in mature fibres, is only about 20–30 nm thick. The internal layer is covered deeply by the inner plasma membrane of the Schwann cell which adjoins the 15–20 nm wide *periaxonal space*, and which is continuous through an *internal mesaxon* with the deepest lamella of myelin. Similarly an *external mesaxon* connects the outermost myelin lamella with the superficial part of the plasma membrane of the Schwann cell. Larger accumulations of Schwann cell cytoplasm are found in the external layer related to the grooves in the paranodal myelin sheath, in the perinuclear region, where the nucleus dimples the external aspect of the myelin sheath near the mid-point of the cell, and also on the internal and external aspects of the Schmidt-Lanterman incisures (*vide infra*, p. 790). These cytoplasmic regions often contain mitochondria, lysosomes and a variety of vesicles and granules. The inner and outer zones of cytoplasm are also connected with each other by helical channels containing granular cytoplasm and microtubules at the nodes of Ranvier and Schimdt-Lanterman incisures (*vide infra*). The outer plasma membrane of the Schwann cell and its adjacent basement membrane correspond to the neurolemma of light microscopists.

When the lipids are removed from the myelin sheath chemically, as in the processing of histological material for wax embedding, without prior fixation and stabilization of the lipid components, a network of proteinaceous filaments, termed *neurokeratin*, is seen by light microscopy, but this has not yet been confirmed by other means.

[156] J. Ochoa and W. G. P. Mair, *Acta. Neuropath.*, **13**, 1969 *a* and *b*; and J. Ochoa, *J. Anat.*, **108**, 1971.
[157] J. D. Robertson, *J. biophys. biochem. Cytol.*, **1**, 1955.
[158] L. M. Napolitano and T. J. Scallen, *Anat. Rec.*, **163**, 1969.

## CHEMICAL COMPOSITION OF MYELIN

Myelin sheaths can be isolated by cell fractionation procedures and chemically characterized as a bulk material, *myelin*. In composition, myelin is similar to plasma membranes of other cells such as erythrocytes in being constituted of lipids and proteins, but is distinctive in the proportions of the various chemical components which are grouped in these categories.[159] In addition to the usual lipids—cholesterol, lecithin and the phospho-inositides—it is particularly rich in the characteristic glycolipid known as galactocerebroside; conversely, myelin contains less protein than is usual for cell membranes, but the proteins which are present include distinctive *basic proteins*. The latter are particularly strong allergens in experimentally-induced allergic encephalitis and possibly in other allergic disorders. In addition, myelin contains up to 30 per cent of bound water.

## FORMATION AND GROWTH OF MYELIN

Although the geometry of myelin is now understood in some detail, exactly how it is laid down during myelination is still debatable. Early models, supported by tissue growth.[139] Other possibilities are the interstitial deposition of myelin within the lamellae of the sheath, or ingrowth of the spiral by slipping of the turns on one another, new myelin being formed externally.[161] Alternatively, it was suggested that the enclosed axon may rotate to wind myelin upon itself; recent reports that myelin in different internodes of the same fibre have different directions of spiralization would appear to rule this possibility out, however.[161] Whilst perhaps excessive ingenuity has been expended in devising models which may explain 'spiralization' of the myelin sheath, much less attention has been paid to the other dimensional changes which are occurring. Thus, whilst the myelin sheath increases in *thickness* from the initial few lamellae to one containing perhaps 300, in a large mature peripheral fibre, the *axon* also increases in *diameter* from about 1 to 15 μm, and each internodal segment increases in length from about 150 μm to perhaps 1,500 μm.[162] After the onset of myelination, no further multiplication of Schwann cells occurs and each elongates in proportion to the overall growth in length of the part of the body in which the nerve lies.[163] Clearly, much remains to be learnt about the initiation, mechanisms, and cessation of myelination and the continued maintenance of the mature sheath.

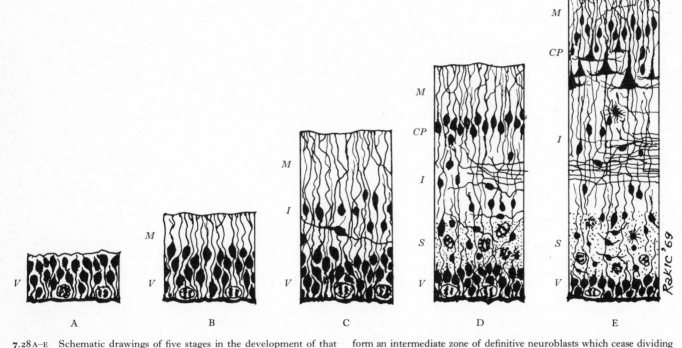

**7.28 A–E** Schematic drawings of five stages in the development of that part of the neural tube destined to form cerebral cortex, emphasizing a recently proposed revision of the terminology relating to the genesis and migration of cells. Abbreviations: V—ventricular zone; M—marginal zone; I—intermediate zone; S—subventricular zone; CP—cortical plate. A The early ventricular zone consisting of the pseudostratified columnar epithelial layer of 'ventricular cells' which undergo periodic proliferative cycles, during which the cell nuclei advance towards, and retreat from, the ventricular surface. This zone, and the 'elevator movement' of nuclei, correspond approximately to the matrix cell layer and its subdivisions, described by Fujita (*see* p. 127). B The nucleated ventricular zone is now distinguishable from the cytoplasmic non-nuclear parts of the cells which form the marginal zone. C Some cell progeny have now migrated to form an intermediate zone of definitive neuroblasts which cease dividing and commence differentiation. D Some cells of the intermediate zone, and others migrating through it from deeper zones, accumulate to form a more superficial early cortical plate of neuroblasts. A subventricular zone of round proliferative cells, with no elevator movement of their nuclei, is now distinguishable. Afferent axons from elsewhere in the nervous system invade the intermediate zone. E The progressive differentiation of the various types of neuron which characterize the area of cortex under consideration now occurs, and to these are added further generations of neuroblasts and glioblasts from deeper zones. (From: Boulder Committee, *Anat. Rec.*, **166**, 1970. By courtesy of Dr. R. L. Sidman and the Wistar Press.)

culture observations, involved the formation of a loop of Schwann cell cytoplasm around the enclosed axon, and the subsequent migration of the perinuclear region of the cell around it in a spiral manner.[160] In the central nervous system at least, such a mechanism appears to be ruled out since a single oligodendrocyte can simultaneously form myelin sheaths around several separate axons which would be impossible by the above method of

In late fetal and early postnatal development, myelination does not occur simultaneously in all parts of the nervous system, different nerves and tracts having their

[159] L. C. Mokrash, *Neurosciences Res. Prog. Bull.*, **9**, 1971.
[160] B. B. Geren, *Expl Cell Res.*, **7**, 1954.
[161] H. de F. Webster, *J. Cell Biol.*, **48**, 1971.
[162] P. L. Williams and C. P. Wendell-Smith, *J. Anat.*, **109**, 1971.
[163] A. D. Vizoso and J. Z. Young, *J. Anat.*, **82**, 1948.

own particular myelination characteristics which can be related to the functional maturity of various functional pathways.[156] Amongst other factors which are largely unknown, the onset of myelination is associated with the growth in diameter of the non-myelinated axons, and in those animals which have been investigated, the critical point appears to be reached when the axon is about 1·0 $\mu$m in diameter, although some larger nonmyelinated fibres are sometimes found[164] (and many fibres < 1 $\mu$m in diameter possess myelin sheaths). Once begun, myelination continues at a steady rate with the growth of the axon until this stops, so that there is a predictable mathematical relationship between axon diameter and sheath thickness. The exact numerical value of this relationship varies with the type of fibre and its distance from the cell body of the neuron.[162]

## THE NODE OF RANVIER

At the junction between adjacent Schwann cells or oligodendrocytes of myelinated nerve fibres is a gap where the axolemma is exposed, termed the node of Ranvier[165] (7.24, 25). These gaps are placed at regular intervals, the myelinated segments between being known as *internodes*. The distance between nodes varies directly with the diameter of the fibre from about 150 to 1,500 $\mu$m.[166] When fibres branch, they do so at nodes.

In peripheral nerves, the myelin sheaths on both sides of each node are usually expanded into *paranodal bulbs* (7.24) which often show an asymmetry related to the growth patterns of the surrounding topographical region. The surfaces of the bulbs and of the underlying axolemma are fluted as they approach the node, and numerous Schwann cell mitochondria are present in the external cytoplasm-filled grooves so formed.[155, 167] The axon itself also narrows considerably at the node. Where each myelin lamella terminates, it contacts the paranodal axolemma as an expanded loop (7.25) in which are situated spirally orientated microtubules and dense cytoplasm. The external paranodal cytoplasm of the Schwann cell sends a number of finger-like processes which curve towards, and their tips abut on, the otherwise naked axolemma of the node[155] (7.24). The fingers are numerous and form a regular hexagonal array in large fibres, but are few and irregular in small ones. The depression formed at the node by the narrowing of the axon at this point is filled between the nodal fingers with an acidic mucosubstance (*gap substance*)[168] which may form a reservoir of ions, or a selective barrier to their flow in the conduction of nerve impulses (*vide supra*, p. 786). The narrowing of the nodal axon probably increases the transmembrane current density and hence the efficiency of nodal excitation.

Central nodes have been less extensively investigated, but appear to be of a more simple construction, with few nodal fingers, and small or absent paranodal bulbs.[169]

## INCISURES OF SCHMIDT-LANTERMAN

Originally described as cytological features, the clefts or incisures of Schmidt-Lanterman were subsequently long regarded as artefacts of preparation. Ultrastructural and *in vivo* observations have restored them as characteristic features of central and peripheral myelinated fibres.[170] The incisures are fairly regular oblique discontinuities in the close packing of the myelin lamellae (7.27), forming funnel-shaped zones of cytoplasm spiralling between the internal and external layers of Schwann cell cytoplasm. Thus, at the incisure, the major dense line separates to enclose a helical band of granular Schwann cell cytoplasm, bearing one or more microtubules which follow this spiral

pathway, microfilaments, and occasionally other organelles. The dense cytoplasm is modified in places, where it is similar to that found in the zonula adherens of epithelial and other cells, forming an oblique row or *stack* of '*desmosomoid*' attachments at one or more points near the external surface of the incisure. The intraperiod line also splits at the incisure to create an extracellular space interconnecting the periaxonal and endoneurial spaces.

The incisures possibly provide conduction channels for metabolites into the depths of the myelin sheath and to the subadjacent axon; they have been claimed to be importantly involved in the initial stages of Wallerian degeneration[171] and focal demyelination.

The *classical view* of Wallerian degeneration was that the first week after crush or section of a peripheral nerve was largely a period of *morphological disruption* of the part of the nerve distal to the injury, but it was also a period of *biochemical stability*. The morphological disturbances included the formation of myelin *ovoids* containing 'digestion chambers' with disruption of the axon. Only in the second week was there considered to be any biochemical change, and this consisted principally of the degradation of phospholipid in the sheath with the liberation of cholesterol esters.

More recently, *in vivo* examination of nerves undergoing Wallerian degeneration, has shown that the time scale of events is considerably faster. The initial morphological changes include retraction of the paranodal myelin sheath, wide dilation of the incisures of Schmidt-Lanterman, with the subsequent collapse and rounding off of the myelin to form ovoids at these points. These changes start within minutes in zones near the lesion, and occur progressively over the next 36–48 hours in more distal parts of the nerve. Further, it has been shown that there is an increase in the concentration of hydrolytic enzymes within 12 hours of injury, which is associated with a loss of trypsin-digestible *basic protein* from the sheath which can be demonstrated as a loss of *trypanophilia* in histological sections.

Electron microscopically the changes associated with Wallerian degeneration have been described as an accumulation of membrane-bound bodies in the axoplasm proximal and distal to the site of injury. Distally, there follows a degradation of the axoplasmic organelles, and at the previous sites of dilated incisures, there is a collapse of the previously compact myelin lamellae, with alterations in their radial structural repeat distances. Within 4 days, lipid droplets accumulate around the degrading myelin within the Schwann cell cytoplasm, and these are then extruded into the endoneurial space, where they are subsequently phagocytosed by invading haematogenous macrophages. The early increase in acid phosphatase activity has been correlated with the appearance of numerous lysozomes within the Schwann cell cytoplasm at this time.

As degradation of the myelin proceeds, the Schwann cells begin to proliferate rapidly; in some nerves which contain many large diameter myelinated fibres, the total number of nuclei per transverse section of the nerve rises to about 16 times that of a normal nerve, by the end of the third week of degeneration. These proliferating Schwann cells become aligned in parallel longitudinal chains within

[164] M. A. Matthews, *Anat. Rec.*, **161**, 1968.
[165] A. Hess and J. Z. Young, *Proc. R. Soc. B.*, **140**, 1952.
[166] R. Kashef, *The Node of Ranvier*, Ph.D. Thesis, Univ. of London. 1966.
[167] C.-H. Berthold, *Acta Soc. Med. upsal.*, **73**, suppl. **9**, 1968.
[168] D. N. Landon and O. K. Langley, *J. Anat.*, **108**, 1971.
[169] A. Peters, *Q. J exp. Physiol.*, **51**, 1966.
[170] S. M. Hall and P. L. Williams, *J. Cell Sci.*, **6**, 1970.
[171] P. L. Williams and S. M. Hall, *J. Anat.*, **109**, 1971.

the persistent basement membrane, where they are of great importance in any subsequent regenerative phenomena which may ensue (p. 793).

## Peripheral Endings of Effector Neurons

Of the various types of effector endings, the most intensively studied are those which innervate muscles, and particularly those of skeletal muscle, which are quite distinct from the efferent nerve endings in smooth muscle. All such endings, termed *neuromuscular* or *myoneural junctions*, are, however, similar in being specialized regions of the neuronal cytoplasm from which neurotransmitters are released on to the surface of an adjacent muscle cell, causing a change in its electrical state. Because of the similarity between these junctions and synapses, and the relative ease with which neurophysiological studies can be carried out at the former, much general knowledge of neurotransmission stems from ultrastructural, physiological, biochemical and pharmacological analysis of neuromuscular junctions rather than synapses.

### NEUROMUSCULAR JUNCTIONS IN SKELETAL MUSCLE

The general structure of these has been outlined elsewhere (p. 482) and will be described only briefly here. Essentially, the terminals consist of end branches of somatic motor fibres, each of which innervates from a few to many hundreds of muscle fibres, depending upon the precision of muscle control. The structural specialization of the motor terminal varies with the type of muscle innervated. Two major types of ending have been recognized, the 'en plaque' terminals on fast twitch, 'phasic', skeletal muscle, and the 'en grappe' terminals on slow twitch, 'tonic', skeletal fibres. In the former type each terminal branch of the axon ends midway along a muscle fibre in a discoidal expansion, the *motor end plate* (7.26, 27). In the latter, the axon gives numerous subsidiary branches which form a cluster of small expansions which may extend for some distance along the muscle fibre (7.26). Both types of ending are characterized by a specialized region of the muscle fibre surface, the *sole plate*, in which a number of muscle fibre nuclei are grouped in a mass of granular sarcoplasm, and ultrastructurally, by the presence in the muscle of numerous mitochondria and the folding of the sarcolemma into a series of parallel grooves or gutters into which the external basement membrane fits (7.26, 27). The terminal expansion of the efferent fibre is separated by a gap of about 30–40 nm from this complex *subneural apparatus*, and contains mitochondria and large numbers of clear spherical vesicles similar to those of presynaptic boutons, which are clustered against the membrane throughout the zone of apposition. Ensheathing the motor terminal are Schwann cells sometimes termed *teloglia*, but these never project into the synaptic cleft. It is interesting that en plaque and en grappe endings differ in that the sarcolemmal gutters are deeper and the presynaptic vesicles more numerous in the former.[172]

Physiological and pharmacological studies[173] have shown that the neuromuscular junctions with skeletal muscle fibres are *cholinergic*, that is, they act by the release of *acetylcholine* from the nerve terminal on to the specialized surface of the underlying sarcolemma, and this changes its ionic permeability. The resulting depolarization of the sarcolemma, if sufficiently intense, initiates an action potential which is propagated over the surface of the muscle fibre and results in its contraction (p. 482). As with synapses, the quantity of neurotransmitter released depends upon the number of nerve impulses arriving at the motor terminal, and since the transmitter is inactivated at a constant rate by the enzyme *acetylcholinesterase*, the amount present at a particular time is dependent upon its *rate* of release, which in turn reflects the *frequency* of arrival of action potentials along the nerve fibre. In this way the contraction of a muscle is controlled by the frequency of firing of its efferent nerves. Even in quiescent muscle fibres, small sporadic depolarizations have been detected (*miniature end-plate potentials*), which are too small to cause contraction. When recorded electrophysiologically, their amplitudes cluster at a series of preferential levels, indicating that multiples of small *quanta* of transmitter are occasionally released in the resting stage; calculations suggest that the amount of transmitter necessary to cause these unitary changes probably occupies the volume of a single synaptic vesicle.[173]

Acetylcholinesterase can be demonstrated cytochemically in the myoneural cleft, and experiments with the specialized motor endings in the electric organ of the electric rayfish *Torpedo* show the enzyme to be located in the sarcolemma close to its site of action. Activity of the neurotransmitter can be blocked by *curare* and its derivatives, and by the sea-snake venom substance *bungarotoxin*, all of which bind irreversibly with the receptor molecules, so causing paralysis at the neuromuscular junction.[174] If the activity of the enzyme acetylcholinesterase is inhibited with *eserine* (*physostigmine*) or other poisons, transmitter action is cumulative and the muscle responds with a tetanic spasm. The neuromuscular junction is also partially blocked by high concentrations of lactic acid, and this is responsible for some types of muscle fatigue after prolonged exercise during which lactic acid accumulates.[174]

### AUTONOMIC MOTOR ENDINGS

Unlike those in skeletal muscle, autonomic nerve endings are not closely applied to the smooth muscle cells but end at variable distances from their surfaces.[100, 175] Non-myelinated autonomic axons branch to give many tapering, varicose collaterals (7.26, 27). At zones where transmission occurs, clusters of ultramicroscopic vesicles are present within the axoplasm, and the Schwann cell which closely enwraps the axon elsewhere, is retracted at this point so that the axon lies in a shallow groove, thus forming a free diffusion path between the axon and the muscle cells. In *sympathetic nerves* the vesicles are usually of the *dense-cored* catecholamine-containing type (p. 775), and these can be correlated with the characteristic fluorescence of catecholamines using light microscopy, when preparations which have been fixed in formalin vapour are viewed with ultraviolet illumination.[176]

Generally, *noradrenalin* is the transmitter at sympathetic postganglionic endings, and *adrenalin* is present chiefly in the *chromaffin cells* of the adrenal medulla. It is possible to distinguish ultramicroscopically between the synaptic vesicles which contain the two types of catecholamine by using the appropriate fixatives. Catecholamines can be released experimentally with various drugs, such as *reserpine*, and this constitutes a valuable research tool, in addition to its clinical usefulness.

At *parasympathetic* endings, clear spherical vesicles, similar to those in the motor end plates of skeletal muscle,

[172] H. A. Padykula, and G. F. Gauthier, *J. Cell Biol.*, **46**, 1970.
[173] B. Katz and R. Miledi, *Proc. R. Soc. B*, **161**, 1965.
[174] R. Miledi, P. Molinoff and L. T. Potter, *Nature, Lond.*, **229**, 1971.
[175] K. C. Richardson, *J. Anat.*, **96**, 1962.
[176] B. Falck and C. Owman, *Acta Univ. lund*, Sect. II, **7**, 1965.

are present. Several lines of evidence indicate that these are *cholinergic* in nature; similar terminals are also found in the neighbourhood of sympathetic endings, and it has been suggested that in addition to their action on non-nervous tissues, cholinergic endings may cause the release of catecholamines from sympathetic endings.[177]

The precise pattern of axonal branching in autonomic efferents is closely related to the nature of the controls which they exert;[178] in visceral smooth muscle, with a slow widespread action, the branching may be extensive, a single neuron innervating a large number of muscle cells. With quick-acting muscle which has a greater precision of control, such as that in the iris, the innervation is more localized, with much less branching of the axons. In addition to smooth muscle, many other tissues are innervated by autonomic efferents, including glands, myoepithelial cells, and adipose tissue. Many physiological actions depend upon autonomic control of the cardiovascular system whereby the activities of the tissues are in part regulated by varying the perfusion of blood through them.

## The Natural History of Neurons

The structure of mature neurons considered in the previous paragraphs covers only a limited aspect of the total biology of these cells. Their mature structure must be considered in the context of the development, maturation, reactions to morphogenetic and pathological influences, senescence, and final death of these cells.

### ORIGIN AND DEVELOPMENT OF NEURONS

Neurons originate from two main embryonic areas. Central nervous neurons stem from the neural plate and tube, whilst those of the cerebrospinal and autonomic ganglia arise from the neural crest (p. 130). The neural plate also gives rise to the ependymal and macroglial cells, whilst the neural crest gives origin to the Schwann cells of the peripheral nervous system, and to the chromaffin cells of the suprarenal medulla.

The development of the cells of the central nervous system has attracted much attention since the first detailed descriptions by His (p. 127), and many conceptual schemes have been advanced to explain the complex series of changes involved. Recently many of the difficulties of interpretation have been resolved by the use of autoradiographic methods which demonstrate the origin and subsequent fate of the various cell types involved in the development of the nervous system.

In the central nervous system, the earliest observers considered the wall of the neural tube to be divided into ependymal, mantle and marginal zones (p. 127). This was later modified to include the concept of a matrix cell layer (p. 127). Recently,[179] however, the latter has been further amplified into a fourfold division of the wall of the early neural tube into *ventricular, subventricular, intermediate* and *marginal* zones (7.27).

As described previously, the neural plate and early neural tube consists of a single layer of pluripotent epithelial stem cells which give rise to all the cell types of the central nervous system except the microglia. The nuclei of these stem cells are situated near the ventricular surface in the *ventricular zone* of the tube, with an anuclear cytoplasmic marginal zone consisting of the laterally extending 'tails' of the cells. As these cells undergo mitotic division they change shape, contracting during the act of mitosis so that the nucleus moves first towards, and then subsequently away from the ventricular surface

within the ventricular zone. Since the mitoses do not occur synchronously the nuclei appear at varying levels on histological section. Later, some of the progeny of these cell divisions cease mitosis permanently, and move deep to the ventricular zone to form an *intermediate* (mantle) *zone* where they differentiate into neuroblasts. Others, however, form a *sub-ventricular zone* between the ventricular and intermediate zones, where they continue to multiply, giving rise to further generations of neuroblasts and, later, glioblasts. Both of these cell types subsequently migrate into the intermediate and marginal zones. However, in particular brain regions (e.g. the cerebellar cortex), some of these mitotic subventricular stem cells migrate across the wall of the neural tube to assume a sub-pial position, where they establish a new zone of cell division and differentiation. Many of the cells formed remain in this sub-surface position, but others migrate, yet again, through the developing nervous tissue to their various deeply-placed definitive positions where final differentiation into neurons and macroglia occurs.

During the genesis of these various cell types, neuroblasts are the first to be formed, followed later by glioblasts. The timing of these events differs in the various parts of the central nervous system and also varies between species. The majority of neuroblasts are formed before birth in mammals, although a number of examples of postnatal neurogenesis are also known, namely, the granule cells of the cerebellar cortex, olfactory bulb, and hippocampus. In contrast gliogenesis continues after birth both near the ventricular surface and at other more deeply placed regions.

Autoradiographic studies have shown that particular classes of neurons develop at specific times. Usually large neurons differentiate before small ones; however, the subsequent pattern of migration appears to be independent of the time of initial formation. For example, the cerebellar Purkinje cells form before the main body of granule cells which arise at the sub-pial zone and later migrate towards the ventricle through the zone of maturing larger neurons. Other studies have shown that neurons can migrate for considerable distances through populations of maturing, relatively static cells, before arriving at their final destination. It is considered that the early migration of neurons is determined by intrinsic factors, or factors in their immediate vicinity, since at this stage they have no afferent connexions which might determine their paths of migration. Later, however, the final form of their neurites, cell volume, and indeed the continuance of the cell itself, often depends upon the establishment of the correct patterns of connexion with other neurons.

### STRUCTURE OF DEVELOPING NEURONS

Initially the neuroblast is a round or spindle-shaped cell the cytoplasm of which bears a prominent Golgi apparatus, many lysosomes, glycogen deposits and numerous unattached ribosomes.[180] As maturation proceeds the cell sends fine cytoplasmic processes (neurites) into the surrounding regions. The latter are rich in microfilaments and microtubules, and centrioles frequently occur at

[177] J. H. Burn, in: *Adrenergic Neurotransmission*, Ciba Foundation Study Group 33, eds. G. E. W. Wolstenholme and M. O'Connor, Churchill, London. 1968.

[178] G. Burnstock, in: *Smooth Muscle*, eds. E. Bulbring, A. F. Brading, A. W. Jones and T. Tomita, Arnold, London. 1970.

[179] R. L. Sidman, in: *The Neurosciences Second Study Program*, eds. F. O. Schmitt, G. C. Quarton, T. Melnechuk and G. Adelman, Rockefeller University Press, New York. 1970.

[180] V. M. Tennyson, in: *Developmental Neurobiology*, ed. H. Himwich, Thomas, Springfield. 1969.

the bases of the neurites where microtubules are being formed (p. 10). Internally, further maturation is marked by the development of the membranes of the endoplasmic reticulum, and the proliferation of attached ribosomes and mitochondria; glycogen is progressively reduced in maturing cells. With development one of the neurites becomes differentiated as the axon, whilst the other cell processes extend to establish the early dendritic tree. The growth of axons has been extensively studied, particularly in tissue culture; the rate of longitudinal growth is initially quite rapid—up to 1 mm per day. The tip of growing axons and dendrites is marked by a bulbous enlargement, the *growth cone*, which is rich in microfilaments (p. 772) and membranous vesicles, with small surface filopodia growing out in an 'exploratory' manner into the surrounding intercellular spaces.[181] Thus, like many other morphogenetic processes, axonal growth appears to depend upon the presence of microfilaments (*see* p. 10). Recent observations, however, suggest an alternative view of the structure of the growth cone, in which the advancing tip is formed by a 'glial' or Schwann cell, the axon tip following in train (p. 787).

The direction taken by a growing axon appears to be governed in part by mechanical factors such as the micellar architecture of neighbouring intercellular matrix, or the presence of other axons and Schwann cells along which further generations of axons grow to form bundles, and hence central nerve fibre tracts, or peripheral nerve trunks. The final direction and termination of axons, however, appear to be related to the overall fundamental plan of the nervous system, and much evidence is available to indicate that their growth patterns are determined by embryonic chemical concentration gradients, 'field effects', the chemical recognition of the surfaces of other cells, and so forth (*vide infra*). Experimental work, particularly on lower vertebrates, in which it is possible to graft or manipulate parts of the embryonic nervous system such as the visual pathway from the retina to the optic tectum, indicates that axons are able to establish precise relationships with various target regions of the brain in spite of mechanical interference, as though they are guided both by their relationship to surrounding axons, and also by a chemical recognition in their areas of termination. Similar considerations apply to the motor innervation of skeletal muscle. The mechanisms whereby such specific connexions are established are as yet unknown in detail, but may involve the sensing of metabolites such as 'nerve growth factor' produced by the target tissues, and the recognition of particular cells by the composition of their surfaces, impulse firing characteristics, and so on (but see also p. 131). There is also evidence[182] that if during embryonic development, the axon fails to establish the correct contacts, its parent perikaryon atrophies and finally disintegrates; such mechanisms may explain the close numerical relationship between the number of neurons in a given motor pool, and the number of muscle cells which it innervates.[180]

The final growth of the dendritic tree is also influenced by its pattern of afferent connexions, and if deprived of these experimentally, the dendrites fail to develop fully. Various metabolic factors are also known to affect the final branching pattern of dendrites; for example, thyroid deficiency in perinatal rats results in cerebral cortical neurons which are smaller and have less profuse branching of their dendrites than those of control animals. This is probably analogous to the mental retardation of cretinism.[109]

Once established, however, the dendritic tree in broad outline appears to be remarkably stable, and partial deafferentation affects only the detailed organization of dendritic spines or similar surface projections. If, however, cells lose their afferent connexions completely, atrophy and degeneration of much of the dendritic tree, and even of the whole neuron may ensue, although different regions appear to vary in the quantitative nature of such responses (anterograde transneuronal degeneration —*see* p. 759). Thus, as development proceeds there is a gradual loss of plasticity so that soon after birth the neuron is a stable structure with a reduced rate of growth. After this two main types of alteration occur. The first follows physical or chemical trauma to any part of the neuron, the second involves the ill-understood changes which accompany the establishment of temporary or permanent memory traces.

Reaction of neurons to physical trauma has been studied most extensively in motor neurons with peripheral axons, which are convenient of access, but also centrally where their axons form well-defined tracts, and incidentally the latter provides the basis for the various degenerative techniques for exploring neuronal connectivity (*see* p. 759). When an axon is crushed or severed, changes occur on both sides of the lesion.[183] Distally, the axon initially swells, and subsequently breaks up into a series of membrane-bound spheres; the process begins near the point of damage and progresses distally. These *anterograde* changes, which also involve the axon terminals, continue to total degeneration and removal of the cytoplasmic débris (see also p. 760). Proximally, a similar series of changes may occur close to the point of injury, followed by a number of sequential (*retrograde*) changes in the cell body.[184] The latter are firstly directed towards the removal of much of the original protein-synthesizing apparatus by autophagic lysosomal action. There is first a rise in cytoplasmic RNA which is associated in part with the increased synthesis of lysosomal acid phosphatase; this is followed by a dispersion of the large Nissl granules with a loss of affinity for stains in the cytoplasm (*chromatolysis*), reflecting a reduction of cytoplasmic RNA. Subsequently, this is followed by the formation of new protein-synthesizing organelles which produce distinctive proteins, many of which are destined for the regrowth of the axon. This is further indicated by the movement of the nucleoli to the periphery of the nucleus, and the restoration of polysome clusters in the cytoplasm, and the consequent return of stain affinity in the cytoplasm when prepared with Nissl's technique for light microscopy.

Where regrowth of the axon is possible, as in the peripheral nervous system, the presence of an intact endoneurial sheath near to and beyond the region of injury, is important if the axon is to re-establish satisfactory contact with its previous end-organ, or a closely adjacent one. The degeneration of the myelin sheath which occurs distal to the point of injury has already been mentioned (p. 768), and this is accompanied by mitotic proliferation of the Schwann cells, their progeny filling the space inside the basal lamina of the old endoneurial tube.[185] Further, where a gap is present between the severed ends of the nerve, proliferating Schwann cells emerge from the stumps (mainly the distal stump) and form a series of nucleated cellular cords (the *bands of Bungner*) which bridge the interval. These may persist for a long time, even in the absence of satisfactory nerve regeneration. The proximal part of the axon develops a terminal swelling from the surface of which many small axonal sprouts develop which grow into the surrounding tissues. The

[181] V. M. Tennyson, *J. Cell Biol.*, **44**, 1970.
[182] A. Hughes, *Aspects of Neural Ontogeny*, Academic Press, N.Y. 1968.
[183] W. J. H. Nauta and S. O. E. Ebesson, (eds.), *Contemporary Research Methods in Neuroanatomy*, Springer-Verlag, N.Y. 1970.
[184] B. G. Cragg, *Brain Res.*, **23**, 1970.
[185] H. de F. Webster, *Prog. Brain Res.*, **13**, 1964.

majority of these are ultimately abortive, but the successful one enters the proximal end of the endoneurial tube and grows distally in close contact with the surfaces of its contained Schwann cells. A process of *contact guidance* (p. 62) is involved between the growing tip of the axon and the Schwann cell surfaces in the endoneurial tube and, when present, those which form Bungner's bands. When the axon tip has reached and successfully reinnervated an end-organ, the surrounding Schwann cells commence to synthesize myelin sheaths, including typical junctional nodes of Ranvier and internodal Schmidt-Lanterman incisures. However, if regeneration is occurring in a mature animal in which general growth of the body and limbs has virtually ceased, there is no increase in the lengths of the internodal segments of myelin which remain uniformly short (often about 200 $\mu$m). Before full *functional regeneration* can occur, however, a considerable period of growth of both axonal diameter and myelin sheath thickness is necessary. When a high proportion of effective peripheral connexions have been established, the nerve fibre population eventually recovers a virtually normal nerve fibre diameter spectrum, but this does not occur with a lack of appropriate peripheral connexions or if the onset of regeneration is long delayed. Regeneration of central axons does not normally occur in mammals, perhaps because of the absence of definite endoneurial tubes, and the disorganized proliferation of macroglial cells which follows central nervous injury.

A second series of changes occur in nerve cells throughout the life of the individual. In addition to the normal turnover and replacement of the cytoplasm and surface of the neuron which occurs continuously, there are the constantly changing patterns of afferent nerve fibre activity, circulating hormone levels and other factors which are important to changes in neuronal behaviour in different parts of the brain. In the normal individual, cyclic or intermittent processes such as those involved in feeding, reproduction, aggression and so on, are obviously connected with such alterations of activity. It may be envisaged that changes in the chemical micro-environment of the cell can alter its electrical firing pattern in a probabilistic manner and thus change the characteristic responses of whole cell populations. More subtle changes are probably involved at the biochemical level so that the neuron modulates its responses (and structure) with reference to its previous history. This is a probable basis of certain aspects of memory formation which have received much attention in recent years. Changes in RNA content and composition have been reported to accompany the learning of conditioned responses, and claims have been made that experimental inhibition of protein synthesis also specifically inhibits certain types of memory formation.[186] Despite the interest of such findings, it is by no means clear what relevance they have to learning processes in the intact nervous system.

Finally, more drastic changes may occur; it is known that during fetal development many neurons degenerate and die. This process continues into post-natal life so that in senescence it has been estimated that up to 20 per cent of the original population of neurons is lost. In the embryo the loss of neurons can be seen as a process of 'thinning out' those which fail to establish proper functional connexions.[187] In post-natal life the loss of neurons is not so easily understood; it has been suggested that it may be a similar process, perhaps related to the stabilization of behaviour patterns formed during the early years. Certainly, with increasing age, the logical efficiency of the nervous system and its reaction speeds deteriorate, and it seems probable that this is related in some way to the loss of neurons, although whether as a direct result is unknown.

## TROPHIC INFLUENCE OF NEURONS

In addition to the functions of neurons in conduction and transmission, they have other important functions in the integration of the body during development, and in the continued post-natal maintenance of other tissues. Of course, nervous tissue is not unique in this respect since most tissues influence the metabolism of surrounding cell masses in some fashion, but the effects of nervous tissue are perhaps more dramatic and far reaching than elsewhere.

The most obvious relationship of this kind is the mutual dependence of motor neurons and the muscles which they innervate. If, during the course of development, a nerve fails to connect with a muscle, the nerve degenerates and likewise, if a muscle is denervated the muscle degenerates. If, however, the innervation of a slow (red) and a fast (white) skeletal muscle, each of which has distinct metabolic and physiological properties, is exchanged, the muscles change their structure and properties in accordance with the innervation, showing that the nerve determines the type of muscle and not vice versa. Trophic influences are best known in lower vertebrates, however, which are capable of regenerating whole limb structures after amputation, but only if the nerves to the limb are not destroyed.[188] In higher vertebrates, also, the trophic influences of axonal growth on dendritic trees is well known (p. 793), and it seems likely that many phenomena of sensory cell development, such as the specificity of gustatory sensory cells in the tongue, are under direct trophic influence from the afferent nerves.

It is interesting that in many invertebrates, also, regeneration of metameric segments is under direct neurosecretory control, and it has been suggested that the nervous system may have originated in the ancestral metazoans chiefly as a system for coordinating the regeneration and development of the body as a whole. Seen in this light, the neurosecretory activity of the hypothalamohypophyseal neurons may be a primitive survival from the distant past, other neurons being a subsequent specialization for more rapid types of communication.

## Sensory Receptors

As has already been stated, the manner in which an organism reacts to changes in its environment depends upon the presence of suitable sensory receptors which can monitor various parameters important to its survival. Although in unicellular organisms the whole cell may be able to detect mechanical deformation, changes of temperature, osmotic pressure, concentrations of various chemicals, light, and so on, in more elaborate animals individual cells have become differentiated to sense such changes with great acuity, different cells being responsive to their own particular range of physico-chemical variables. Such cells are termed sensory receptors; they take various forms in the animal kingdom, but in mammals there is, with minor exceptions, a common pattern which will be outlined below.

Structurally, sense organs take one of three basic forms, depending upon the relationship of the nervous system to the sensory surface. In **neuroepithelial receptors** the sensory cell is itself a neuron of which the perikaryon

[186] S. H. Barondes, *Int. Rev. Neurobiol.*, **12**, 1969.
[187] M. C. Prestige, in: *The Neurosciences Second Study Program*, ed. F. O. Schmitt, G. C. Quarton, T. Melnechuk and G. Adelman, Rockefeller University Press, New York. 1970.
[188] V. Hamburger, *Dev. Biol.*, suppl. **2**, 1968.

is peripherally situated near the sensory surface and the axon extends back into the central nervous system to connect with second order neurons. The only known example of this type of receptor in mammals is the sensory cell of the olfactory epithelium, although in many invertebrate groups it is the chief type of sensory receptor and must be regarded as phylogenetically primitive. A second arrangement is for the sensory cell to be a modified epithelial cell, an **epithelial receptor**, derived from the non-nervous tissue at the sensory surface and innervated by the peripheral process of a primary sensory neuron, the cell body of which is situated close to the central nervous system. Activity in this type of receptor involves the passage of excitation from the sensory cell across a synaptic gap; examples are gustatory and cochlear auditory receptors. It is known that in gustatory sensory receptors there is a high turnover of individual cells which are constantly being renewed from the pool of surrounding epithelial cells, a phenomenon which may also occur in other sensory systems of this general type. Visual receptors are in many ways similar in their organization, since they are formed from the lining of the ventricle of the fetal brain; but no cell replacement occurs. Thirdly, a neuronal receptor is itself a primary sensory neuron with a perikaryon situated in a craniospinal ganglion and a long peripheral process, the ending of which constitutes the actual sensory terminal. All cutaneous sensors and many proprioceptors are thought to be of this type, although the sensory terminals may in some cases be encapsulated or lie in association with specialized mesodermal or ectodermal elements which form an integral part of the sensory apparatus; however, it appears that these non-neuronal elements are not themselves excitable but rather create the right environment for the excitation of the neuronal dendrite.

## RECEPTOR RESPONSES

The various events occurring between the presentation of a stimulus and the signalling of this to the central nervous system have been extensively studied,[189] but are not yet entirely understood. It is convenient to divide these processes into a number of stages: initially there is the presentation of an effective stimulus, then its transduction at the receptor surface into a graded change of electrical potential (*generator potential*), and the initiation of an all-or-none action potential which passes to the central nervous system. All of these processes may occur within the confines of the receptor where this is a neuron, or some of them may take place partly in the receptor and partly in the dendrite of the neuron innervating it in the case of epithelial receptors.

The nature of the transduction process varies, of course, with the modality of the stimulus, and involves a change in the permeability to certain ions in the receptor membrane, usually to cause a depolarization (or in retinal cells, a hyperpolarization).

How a stimulus causes such a change is not yet known in any sensory cell. In mechanoreceptors it may involve a physical deformation in membrane structure; in chemoreceptors the action may correspond to that postulated for the action of acetylcholine at the neuromuscular junction (p. 482). Visual receptors appear to be rather similar to chemoreceptors except that chemical changes occur within the cell as a result of illumination and so presumably act on the *internal* aspect of its membrane. Osmoreceptors may be similar to mechanoreceptors except that they react to mechanical deformation of their cell surface resulting from osmotic inflow or outflow of water with respect to the cytoplasm.

It is interesting that in certain fishes a quite distinct type of transduction occurs in electroreceptors which are capable of sensing changes in the electric fields set up in the external medium by their own bioelectric processes, or by those of other fishes.[190] So far a similar sensory mechanism has not been reported in tetrapods.

The quantitative responses of sensory endings to stimuli vary greatly and give additional flexibility to the design of sensory systems. Although an increase in the level of excitation with increase of stimulus strength is a common pattern (the 'on' response), some receptors respond instead to a decrease in stimulus strength (the 'off' response). Even when not stimulated, receptors show varying degrees of spontaneous activity, sometimes of a high level, against the background of which an increase or decrease in activity occurs with changing levels of stimulus strength.

When a steady stimulus is presented, there is, in most receptors, an initial burst of activity followed by a gradual slowing or *adaptation* to the steady level of the stimulus. The rate of this adaptation is an important physiological factor; *rapidly adapting* endings give accurate estimates of *changes* in stimulus strength, whereas *slowly adapting* receptors are often found in situations where static stimuli such as those associated with position sense are involved. The stimulus strength necessary to elicit a response in a receptor (i.e. its *threshold level*) varies considerably. Such high and low threshold responses give added information on stimulus strength.

## GENERAL CLASSIFICATION OF RECEPTORS

Receptors can be classified in various ways, for example, by the particular energy forms or '*modalities*' to which they are especially sensitive. We can therefore group them into *mechanoreceptors* which are particularly responsive to mechanical disturbances (touch, pressure, sound waves, etc.), *chemoreceptors* sensitive to chemical changes, *photoreceptors* responsive to electromagnetic waves in the visual frequency range, *thermoreceptors* which sense changes in temperature, *osmoreceptors* which react to changes in osmotic pressures (in contrast to chemoreceptors which are activated by specific chemical groups in their environment).

Another type of classification divides receptors on the basis of their distribution and role in sensory activities of the body, into three main groups, namely, *exteroceptors*, *proprioceptors* and *interoceptors*. Exteroceptors and proprioceptors are the receptor end organs of the somatic afferent components of the nervous system and the interoceptors constitute the receptor end organs of the visceral afferent components.

**Exteroceptors** respond to stimuli from the external environment and are placed at or close to the surface of the body;[191] they can be divided into the *general* or *cutaneous sense organs* and the *special sense organs*. The general sense organs include the non-encapsulated and encapsulated terminals in the skin and around hairs; the special sense organs are the olfactory, visual, acoustic and taste receptors which will be described elsewhere (p. 1083).

**Proprioceptors** respond to stimuli arising in the deeper tissues particularly in the locomotor system. They are concerned with movement, position and pressure, and include the neurotendinous organs of Golgi, the neuromuscular spindles, deeply placed Pacinian corpuscles and perhaps other endings such as those of joints, and the

---

[189] R. Granit, *Receptors and Sensory Perception*, Yale University Press, New Haven. 1962.

[190] H. W. Lissmann and K. E. Machin, *J. exp. Biol.*, **35**, 1958.

[191] D. Sinclair, *Cutaneous Sensation*, Oxford University Press, London. 1967.

vestibular receptors in the membranous labyrinth. The proprioceptors are stimulated by the activity of the muscles, movements of joints and changes in the position of the body as a whole or its various parts, and are essential to the coordination of muscles, the grading of muscular contraction and the maintenance of its equilibrium.

**Interoceptors** include the receptor end organs in the walls of the viscera and blood vessels (see also p. 1081), where a variety of fibre terminations and end-organs including naked nerve endings, loops and encapsulated

The nerve terminals in the viscera are not, in general, responsive to the same stimuli which act on the exteroceptors placed at the surface of the body and with certain exceptions do not respond to localized mechanical and thermal stimuli. However, tension produced by over-stretching or excessive muscular contraction, often gives rise to visceral pain, particularly in pathological conditions, which is frequently poorly localized and of the deep-seated variety.

Amongst the interoceptors are included various vascular

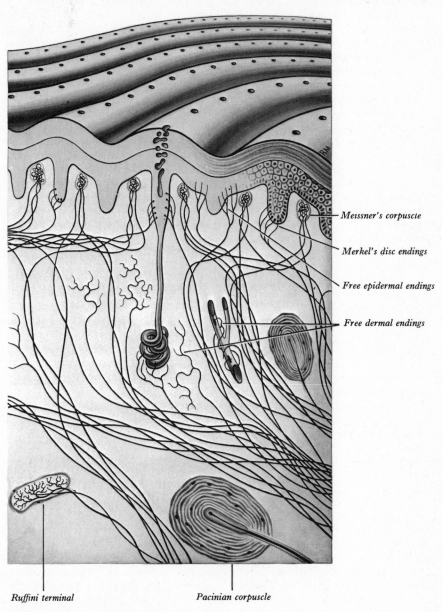

*Meissner's corpuscle*

*Merkel's disc endings*

*Free epidermal endings*

*Free dermal endings*

*Ruffini terminal*          *Pacinian corpuscle*

**7.29 A** Schematic illustration of some of the principal sensory endings of thick (hairless) skin and associated structures, including various types of encapsulated and 'free' endings, of the epidermis, dermis and subcutaneous connective tissue.

terminals, has been described. Nerve terminals are found in all layers of the visceral walls including the lining epithelium and they are numerous in the adventitia of blood vessels, although the nature of many of these endings is open to doubt. Lamellated corpuscles have been described in the heart, adventitia of blood vessels, pancreas and mesenteries; free terminal arborizations are also present in many situations including the endocardium, loose connective tissue, the endomysium of all types of muscle, and connective tissue generally.

chemoreceptors and baroceptors (pressure receptors) the activity of which is important in the regulation of blood flow and pressure in the whole cardiovascular system, the control of respiration and other important aspects of homeostasis.

It should be pointed out that this scheme of classification is in many cases arbitrary, since many types of end organ are present in all three classes, and also their activities may be closely linked in the central nervous system. For convenience, therefore, the sensory terminals will be classified in the following description on the basis of their structural characteristics.

## STRUCTURAL CLASSIFICATION OF SENSORY ENDINGS

In addition to the foregoing division of receptors into broad functional categories, the general receptors have been grouped on morphological grounds (7.29, 30, 31, 32). How much functional significance can be attached to some

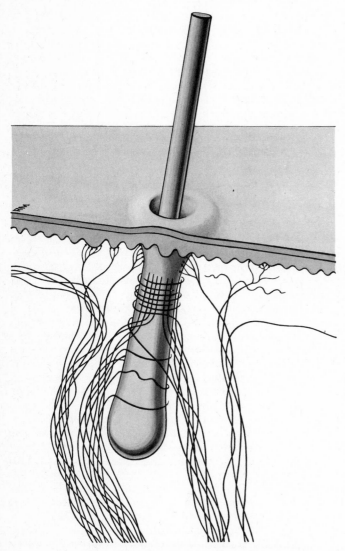

**7.29 B** The innervation of a hair follicle; fine and coarse axons terminate around the intermediate and superficial regions, some branching in a circular direction, and others pursuing a longitudinal course.

differences in detail in such a structural classification is debatable. Complicating factors include changes in receptor ending morphology associated with ageing, regeneration, local topography and also species differences. The terminology is further confused, as there is no general agreement on the structural definition of many types of sensory ending. Accordingly, the scheme which will be outlined below is not exhaustive. Some receptor endings are limited to a particular tissue or combination of tissues; others are present in many situations in the body. Generally, however, we may distinguish between *free nerve endings* which form plexuses or are otherwise spread freely without any particular association with other cell types, and *corpuscular endings* where specialized non-nervous cells are present at or near the sensory surface.

Such specialised non-sensory cells are, of course, additional to the Schwann cells which normally ensheath both types of sensory terminal except in the few instances mentioned below, although the two types may have a common origin.

## FREE NERVE ENDINGS

Sensory nerve fibre endings which branch repeatedly to form plexuses or terminate with fewer branches (7.30), occur in many different sites of the body. Such free nerve endings are found in all types of connective tissue including the dermis, fascia, ligaments, tendons, sheaths of blood vessels, meninges, joint capsules, periosteum, perichondrium, Haversian systems of bone, and the endomysial spaces of all types of muscle. They also innervate the epithelium of the integument, cornea, buccal cavity, and the alimentary tract with its associated glands, although in the latter examples they are devoid of Schwann cell sheaths; they are enveloped instead by the cells of the epithelium and are not truly 'free' endings.[192]

The afferent fibres from free terminals are both myelinated and non-myelinated, but are always of small diameter and low conduction speeds, being of the group III sensory afferent type. Where the fibre is myelinated, the terminal arborizations are non-myelinated and it is possible that they are devoid of Schwann cell sheaths altogether at their tips.

The functional significance of these endings is not yet clear; electrical recordings from their afferent fibres show that such fine terminals subserve a number of different modalities, but it cannot yet be settled if there are functionally specific endings amongst this type. The stimulus thresholds tend to be higher than those of larger fibres, and this may be related to their close functional relationship to the signalling of pain, since only very strong and potentially traumatic stimuli will cause a high level of activity in these fibres; indeed they are often referred to as 'pain fibres'. This terminology is, however, perhaps misleading since it appears that pain is experienced as a result of an imbalance in the differential activity of both small and large afferent fibres; where the small fibre activity predominates the sensation is pain or itch, whereas if the proportions are reversed the sensation is non-painful and may signal other stimuli (see also p. 833). Some authorities, therefore, prefer to regard the small diameter afferent fibre system as constantly monitoring the fluctuating 'general state' of the body tissues rather than constituting a system of specific 'pain afferents'.

## NERVE ENDINGS IN RELATION TO HAIR

Each hair follicle is innervated from the deep dermal cutaneous plexus of nerves by myelinated fibres; their number and size is related to the size of the hair follicle.[192] The fibres approach the hair follicle from different directions to reach it just below the duct of the sebaceous gland where they divide into branches which run parallel to the hair in the outer coat of the follicle (7.29). Some of these fibres pass into the middle of the outer coat where they give rise to naked axon filaments encircling the hair and terminating as free nerve endings amongst the collagen bundles. Others pass into the hyaline layer between the outer and inner coats and, after losing their myelin sheaths, break up into fine filaments which terminate amongst the cells of the outer root sheath. It has been shown that some of these endings instead of being 'free',

[192] N. Cauna, in: *Touch, Heat and Pain*, Ciba Foundation Symposium, eds. A. V. S. de Reuck and J. Knight, Churchill, London. 1966.

end in expansions in association with the outer root sheath with which are associated tactile discs of the Merkel type (*vide infra*). In some mammals at least three arrangements of sensory endings can be distinguished, namely those surrounding 'guard' hairs, 'down' hairs, and specialized patches of raised epithelium associated with hairs termed *tylotrich pads*. Each of these types has a specific pattern of electrical activity associated with mechanoreception; guard hair roots are surrounded by a highly branched network of endings (basket endings), the receptors being of the rapidly adapting type, and their fibres rapidly conducting (group II). Tylotrich endings have a similar response but their fibres conduct even more rapidly. Down hairs are innervated by more slowly conducting (group III) fibres.

## CORPUSCULAR NERVE ENDINGS

These are special end organs or encapsulated nerve endings which exhibit great variety in size and shape, but have one feature in common, that is, the termination of the nerve is enveloped by a capsule. Included in this group are the tactile and the lamellated corpuscles together with the neurotendinous endings and neuromuscular spindles, all of which are well defined morphological entities. Many other types of nerve endings have been described, such as bulbous corpuscles, articular corpuscles, genital corpuscles, tactile discs, Ruffini end organs and Golgi-Mazzoni endings, but there is considerable confusion as to their nature and function, contributed to by several factors, for example, technical difficulties, species and regional variations and age changes. (See **7**.29, 30, 31, 32.)

**The tactile corpuscles** (of Meissner) are found in the papillae of the skin of all parts of the hand and foot, in the front of the forearm and lips, palpebral conjunctiva and the mucous membrane of the tip of the tongue. They are found mainly in glabrous skin. Mature corpuscles are cylindrical in shape, orientated with their long axes perpendicular to the deep surface of the epidermis and about 80 $\mu$m long and 30 $\mu$m broad. The corpuscle consists of a capsule and a central core. The capsule is only loosely attached to the core of the corpuscle and is absent at the extremities. Light microscopists have maintained that the capsule consists of fine elastic fibres orientated along the long axis of the corpuscle and interspersed with fibrocytes and possibly other cell types. It has been claimed that the elastic fibres anchor the corpuscle to the epidermis.[193] Electron microscopy of tactile corpuscles in the monkey and other animals shows the capsule to be continuous with the perineurium of the nerves supplying the corpuscle and to consist of a variable number of lamellae of greatly flattened cells with their associated basement membranes. Between successive lamellae there is a substantial amount of collagen but no elastic fibres have been identified. Extensions of the capsule, often only one lamella in thickness, may form complete or incomplete septa dividing the corpuscle into lobules, particularly at the epidermal extremity. The core of the corpuscle consists of cells and nerve fibres. At the epidermal end the cells are described as disc-like, lightly staining, transversely disposed and about 2–4 $\mu$m thick and 30–40 $\mu$m in diameter; these cells are claimed to be epidermal in origin. At the opposite end of the core the cells are irregular in shape with small oval or round nuclei devoid of nucleoli and with deeply staining chromatin. These are believed to be Schwann cells. In addition to Schwann cells, electron microscopy reveals occasional fibroblasts and collagen fibres, disposed in bundles or singly and mainly orientated parallel to the nerve fibres; the flattened apical cells have been studied in electron micrographs (**7**.31E). Each tactile corpuscle is supplied by a few heavily myelinated nerve fibres derived from the deep corial plexus and possibly also by additional nonmyelinated fibres which are branches of myelinated fibres in the deep corial plexus. Within the corpuscle the nerve fibres ramify profusely and decrease in size; large numbers of both myelinated and nonmyelinated branches are visible in ultrathin sections, the former being most numerous at the deep extremity of the corpuscle and the latter constituting the majority at the epidermal extremity (**7**.31E) and in the smaller lobules. In all cases the nerve fibres are associated with Schwann cells or their processes and no naked axons are seen. Some of the unmyelinated fibres in the core of the corpuscle are less than 0·1 $\mu$m in diameter. The cytoplasm of the unmyelinated fibres may contain small vesicles but no special significance can be attached to them.

Tactile corpuscles develop just before or just after birth. There is a reduction of about 80 per cent in their numbers between birth and old age when the number of nerves supplying each corpuscle is also reduced and the nerve endings are confined to the deep end of the core.

**The lamellated corpuscles** (of Pacini) have been described in the subcutaneous tissue of the palmar aspects of the hand and plantar aspect of the foot and digits, in the genital organs of both sexes, the arm, neck, nipple, periostea, interosseous membranes of the forearm and leg, near joints and in the mesentery and pancreas of the cat. The corpuscles are oval in the fetus and oval, spherical or even irregularly coiled in the adult. They are up to 2 mm in length and 100–500 $\mu$m across, the larger ones being visible to the naked eye. Each corpuscle consists of a capsule, an intermediate growth zone and a central core containing the nerve terminal. The capsule comprises about 30 concentrically arranged lamellae of flattened cells each about 0·2 $\mu$m thick. The neighbouring cells overlap at their edges and successive lamellae are separated by intervals containing some amorphous material and collagen fibres. The latter tend to be disposed circularly and to be closely applied to the surfaces of the lamellae, in particular to their outer surfaces. The amount of collagen increases with age. The intermediate zone is a cellular layer between the capsule and core. Occasional mitoses are seen in this zone and with growth of the corpuscle the cells are incorporated either into the capsule or the core, and the intermediate zone is not a conspicuous feature of the mature corpuscle. The core of the corpuscle consists of about 60 bilaterally arranged, closely packed lamellae, placed on both sides of the central nerve terminal and separated by two longitudinally running clefts. Nucleated cell bodies are situated in the outermost part of the core, at its junction with the intermediate zone. From these cells there arise cylindrical cytoplasmic arms which infold into the longitudinal clefts. Here they give rise to flattened sheet-like processes which pass to one or both sides to form the core lamellae and interdigitate with processes from other cytoplasmic arms. Adjacent lamellae do not arise from the same arm.

Each corpuscle is supplied by one or, rarely, two thick myelinated nerve fibres derived directly from peripheral nerves without the intervention of the corial plexus. The fibre first loses its myelin sheath and at its junction with the core the Schwann cell sheath terminates. The naked axon traverses the length of the central axis core, usually without division or branching and terminates in an expanded end bulb. It is in contact with the innermost core lamellae and is oval in transverse section, with the longer axis in the plane of the longitudinal clefts between the core lamellae. It contains numerous large mitochondria, the

[193] T. A. Quilliam, in: *Touch, Heat and Pain*, eds. A. V. S. de Reuck and J. Knight, Ciba Foundation Symposium, Churchill, London. 1966.

more superficial of which are usually arranged radially in palisade fashion beneath the axolemma. Minute vesicles of about 5 nm diameter are also present; these tend to be aggregated opposite the longitudinal clefts. The cells comprising both the capsule and core lamellae are believed to be modified fibroblasts and appear to be distinct from Schwann cells.[194] Butyryl cholinesterase has been demonstrated in the core of the lamellated corpuscle. Lamellated corpuscles are said to be closely associated with glomerular arteriovenous anastomoses and to derive their blood supply from the capillaries accompanying the nerve fibre to the capsule at the site of entry. A condensation of the surrounding fibrous tissue forms an external capsule to the whole corpuscle.

Lamellated corpuscles commence to develop in the third month of fetal life; the nerve terminal becomes surrounded by capsular lamellae which continue to be laid down into adult life, thus increasing the size of the corpuscle.[195]

Lamellated corpuscles are believed to possess considerably turgidity due to fluid pressure between the capsular lamellae. They are generally accepted to be pressure receptors and effective stimuli probably include vibration.[196]

**The bulbous corpuscles** (of Krause) have been found in the papillae and adjoining part of the corium of hairless skin, mucocutaneous junctions and the mucous membranes supplied by somatic nerves. They have also been described in the skin of the forearm, salivary glands, walls of blood vessels, in the epineurium of nerve trunks and on the nerve endings in relation to hairs; the exact identity of the organs described in these various structures is, however, often difficult to ascertain on account of the scanty and diverse information available as to the structure of bulbous corpuscles. They are variable in form and appearance but in man are spheroidal in shape and about 50 $\mu$m in diameter. They consist of a capsule which shows signs of lamellation and is thought to be composed of endoneurium lined by the Schwann cells of the contained nerve fibre. The nerve fibre enlarges as it enters the capsule and is invested by its Schwann cells. It may be branched, coiled or run a relatively straight course before terminating in a club-shaped fashion. Cholinesterase is present in bulbous corpuscles, mainly in the capsule. In the pig these corpuscles begin to develop just before birth and reach a maximum concentration in early life, thereafter diminishing in number. Many authorities have questioned the status of the bulbous corpuscles and regard them as resulting from decay and regeneration of the distal ends of nerve fibres which are obstructed in their peripheral growth and devoid of a capsule or function as receptor organs, or as fibres which have been diverted from the epidermis when this tissue has become saturated with nerve terminals. There is evidence that cyclic degenerative and regenerative changes occur in nerve bundles, preterminal axons and terminal arborizations in the skin, cornea, carotid body and elsewhere, possibly to meet changing structural and functional conditions. It has been suggested that some of the more variable endings, such as bulbous corpuscles, represent stages in this cycle rather than specialized nerve endings.

**The tactile menisci** (of Merkel) have been described in the hairless skin and hair follicles of man and are characteristic of the epidermis of the snout of the pig.[197] Light microscopists describe them as shallow cup-shaped discs, in close contact with a single enlarged epithelial cell, the *tactile cell*, and associated, usually in groups, with nerve terminals in the stratum spinosum of the epidermis or the cells of the outer root sheath of the hair.[198] Lipid caps occur at the junctions of the discs and tactile cells. With the electron microscope the tactile cell is distinguishable,

in the opossum, as more electron lucid than adjacent epithelial cells; its nucleus is lobulated and the cytoplasm contains a prominent Golgi apparatus and secretory granules. Desmosomes occur between it and adjacent epithelial cells. It is closely related over a wide expanse with nerve filaments in the epidermis which contain an accumulation of mitochondria and lipids in this location. Few filaments terminate in proximity to the cell.[199]

**Articular corpuscles** have been variously described in fibrous joint capsules as structurally resembling bulbous corpuscles or lamellated corpuscles (see below for further description). *Genital corpuscles* are probably similar to bulbous corpuscles and have been described in the glans penis and clitoris.

**Golgi-Mazzoni endings** have been identified in the corium of the conjunctiva, external genitals, connective tissue of tendon and epimysium of muscles. They have been described as separate morphological entities but may be variants of the bulbous corpuscle. **Ruffini endings** are highly branches, spray-like end-organs, found in association with special capsule-like cells in deep fibrous structures of the corium, joint capsules and other connective tissues. Typically, the terminal branches of an axon form loosely encapsulated knot-like corpuscles, arranged in groups.

*Accessory nerve fibres* morphologically similar to pain conducting fibres have been described in association with encapsulated endings.

**Neurotendinous endings of Golgi** (Golgi tendon organs) are chiefly found near the junctions of tendons and muscles. Each is about 500 $\mu$m long and 100 $\mu$m in diameter and consists of small bundles of tendon fibres enclosed in a delicate capsule. The tendon fibres (*intrafusal fasciculi*) are less compact than those elsewhere in the tendon, the collagen fibres are smaller and the associated tendon cells are larger and more numerous. Like many other endings, such as lamellated and tactile corpuscles and neuromuscular spindles, the capsule consists of concentric sheets of cytoplasm, each about 100–300 nm thick, belonging to capsular cells. Within each layer the capsular cells are closely opposed and successive layers are separated by intervals of varying width containing basal laminae. Numerous minute flask-like invaginations of the plasma membranes (*caveolae intracellulares*) suggest that the capsular cells may be concerned with the maintenance of the internal environment of the ending. Outside the capsule is a thin layer of collagen fibres. One or more heavily myelinated group Ib-nerve fibres pierce the capsule and divide in a spray-like manner. The ramifications, which may lose their Schwann cell sheaths, terminate in leaf- or clasp-like enlargements, rich in small vesicles and mitochondria, which are wrapped around the tendon fasciculi with the basal lamina or Schwann cell cytoplasm intervening.

The endings are highly active when tendons are stretched either actively or passively, and initiate myotactic reflexes which inhibit the development of excessive tensions during muscular contraction. Structural and physiological evidence indicates that these sensory endings may be deformed by the surrounding collagen fibres which tend to lie more parallel and closer together as tension develops in the tendon.[200]

[194] D. C. Pease and T. A. Quilliam, *J. biophys. Biochem. Cytol.*, **3**, 1957.
[195] N. Cauna and G. Mannan, *J. Anat.*, **93**, 1959.
[196] J. A. B. Gray and M. Sato, *J. Physiol., Lond.*, **122**, 1953.
[197] M. R. Miller, H. J. Ralston and M. Kasahara, *Am. J. Anat.*, **102**, 1958.
[198] G. Weddell, E. Palmer and W. Pallie, *Biol. Rev.*, **30**, 1955.
[199] B. L. Munger, *J. Cell Biol.*, **26**, 1965.
[200] W. T. Catton, *Physiol. Rev.*, **50**, 1970.

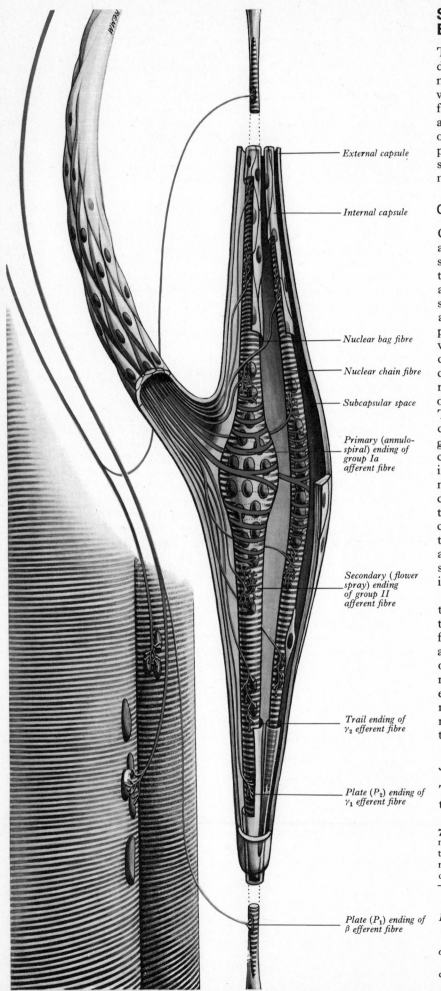

External capsule

Internal capsule

Nuclear bag fibre

Nuclear chain fibre

Subcapsular space

Primary (annulo-spiral) ending of group Ia afferent fibre

Secondary (flower spray) ending of group II afferent fibre

Trail ending of $\gamma_2$ efferent fibre

Plate ($P_2$) ending of $\gamma_1$ efferent fibre

Plate ($P_1$) ending of $\beta$ efferent fibre

## Special Configurations of Sensory Endings

The different varieties of sensory endings have now been discussed individually. Physiologically, however, it is necessary to consider *arrays* of several types of ending, which act in concert, to provide information about the forces and influences acting at a particular locality, to be analysed together in the central nervous system. Although our knowledge of such multiple patterns is as yet only partial, at least three situations have been explored in some detail. These are cutaneous and joint receptors, and neuromuscular spindles.

### CUTANEOUS RECEPTORS

Cutaneous sense organs have been generally considered to act as peripheral analysers which respond to stimuli in a specific and preferential manner,[191, 192, 200] so that each of the modalities of cutaneous sensation, pain, touch, cold and heat, is subserved by a specific end organ. It has been suggested that tactile corpuscles and the nerve endings around hair follicles respond to touch, the bulbous corpuscles to cold, the Ruffini type of receptor organ to warmth and the free nerve endings in the epidermis and dermis to pain. The lamellated corpuscles are sensitive to deformation.[201] It has, however, been shown that the modalities of sensation can be detected in areas wherein only free nerve endings and those around hair exist.[202] Touch, heat, cold and pain can be appreciated in the cornea, where only free nerve endings exist.[203] It is suggested that the appreciation of the different modalities of cutaneous sensation depends more on the pattern of the impulses arriving at the sensory cortex, including their number and spatial and temporal arrangements.[204] In the central nervous system the nerve fibres concerned with the transmission of impulses to the thalamus and cerebral cortex run in discrete tracts. The fibres in these tracts and their terminations in the thalamus and cortex appear to be arranged somatotopically, that is, they are arranged spatially, according to the topographical source of the impulses which they transmit.

Observations during the recovery of cutaneous sensation after nerve section has suggested that there are two types of sensibility, the *epicritic* and the *protopathic*, the former being of a fine discriminative type and the latter of a cruder variety.[205] This can be explained by the existence of two separate sensory systems regenerating at different rates but this is no longer regarded as valid. A more recent explanation is that the changes occurring during the recovery of cutaneous sensation are associated with the reformation of interweaving corial nerve plexuses, but this is by no means certain.[206]

### JOINT RECEPTORS

The arrays of sensory endings placed within and around the articular capsules of synovial joints are of great impor-

7.30 A   Schematic three-dimensional reconstruction of a mammalian neuromuscular spindle, showing nuclear bag and nuclear chain fibres; these are innervated by the sensory annulo-spiral and flower-spray terminals (blue) and by the γ and β fusimotor terminals (red). For further details consult text.

[201] E. D. Adrian and K. Umrath, *J. Physiol., Lond.*, **68**, 1929.
[202] E. Hagan, H. Knoche, D. C. Sinclair and G. Weddell, *Proc. R. Soc. B.*, **141**, 1953.
[203] P. P. Lele and G. Weddell, *Brain*, **79**, 1956.
[204] W. E. Le Gros Clark, *The Anatomical Patterns as the Essential Basis of Sensory Discrimination*, Clarendon Press, Oxford. **1947**.
[205] H. Head and W. H. R. Rivers, *Studies in Neurology*, **Froude**, London, **1920**.
[206] G. Weddell, *J. Anat.*, **75**, 1941.

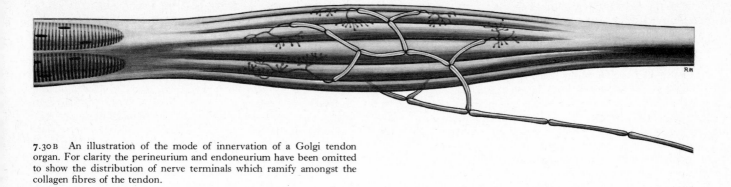

7.30 B   An illustration of the mode of innervation of a Golgi tendon organ. For clarity the perineurium and endoneurium have been omitted to show the distribution of nerve terminals which ramify amongst the collagen fibres of the tendon.

tance in providing information about the position, movements and stresses acting on these structures.[207] Both structural and physiological studies have shown that there are at least four classes of receptor terminals present, the proportion of each varying with the topographical position of the joint. Three of these classes comprise encapsulated endings and the fourth free terminal arborizations. Wyke[207] has named these terminals types I to IV, and this classification will be followed here.

**Type I endings** are encapsulated spray terminals of the Ruffini type (*vide supra*) present in the superficial layers of the fibrous capsule in small clusters, supplied by myelinated afferent fibres of the group II category. Physiologically they are slow-adapting receptors, giving conscious awareness of joint position and joint movement, responding, it is thought, to patterns of stress in the articular capsule. This type of ending is particularly common in articulations such as the hip joint, where static positional sense is of importance in the control of posture.

**Type II endings** are lamellated (Paciniform) receptors, similar to, but smaller than, Pacinian receptors found elsewhere in connective tissue. They are present in small groups throughout the joint capsule but particularly in the deeper layers and also, in the temperomandibular joint, in the posterior articular fat pads. They are rapidly-adapting, low-threshold receptor endings, highly sensitive to movement and to pressure change, responding to joint movement and transient stresses in the capsule. They are supplied by group II myelinated afferent fibres; but they are not considered to be associated with conscious awareness of joint sensation.

**Type III endings** are identical to Golgi tendon organs in structure and physiology (p. 799), being present in the specialized ligaments of joints, though not in their capsules. They are high-threshold, slow-adapting receptors which apparently serve to prevent excessive stresses being developed at joints by the reflex inhibition of the adjacent muscular activity. Their innervation is from the large myelinated group I b afferent nerve fibres.

**Type IV endings** are free, unencapsulated terminals of group III myelinated fibres which ramify within the capsule, the adjacent fat pads, and around blood vessels particularly of the synovial layer. These are also high-threshold, slow-adapting endings which are thought to sense excessive joint movements and also provide a basis for the signalling of joint pain.

## MUSCLE SPINDLES

The *muscle* or *neuromuscular spindles* form an important sensory element in the control of muscle contraction, and as might be expected from the complicated nature of this control, the detailed structure and behaviour of spindles are also complex and not entirely understood. The precise anatomy of spindles varies greatly in submammalian species, so the present account will apply only to mammals.[209, 210, 211]

Basically, each spindle consists of a few, small, specialized *intrafusal muscle fibres*, which are innervated by both sensory and motor nerve endings. This complex is surrounded in the equatorial region of the interfusal fibres by an expanded *spindle capsule* formed of connective tissue, divisible into an *outer sheath* of flattened fibroblasts, and collagen similar to those of the perineurium (p. 784), and elements of an *inner axial sheath* (of Sherrington) which form delicate tubes around the individual intrafusal muscle fibres. The space between the outer and inner sheaths is occupied by lymph which is rich in hyaluronic acid, and is in continuity with the lymphatic system of the surrounding tissues.

The intrafusal fibres number from six to fourteen, varying from one muscle to another, and also with species. Two distinct types of fibre are present in most mammalian spindles, the *nuclear bag* and *nuclear chain fibres*, distinguishable by the arrangement of nuclei within the sarcoplasm in the equatorial region of the spindle. In nuclear bag fibres the equatorial nuclei are gathered together in a cluster to give a slight expansion of the fibre profile, whereas in the nuclear chain type the nuclei form a single longitudinal row in the centre of the fibre. The nuclear bag fibres are greater in diameter and much longer, extending beyond the capsule to attach to the endomysium of the surrounding extrafusal muscle fibres; the nuclear chain fibres are attached at their poles to the capsule or to the sheaths of the nuclear bag fibres.

The contractile apparatus of the intrafusal fibres is similar to that of extrafusal ones except that the zone of myofibrils is rather thin at the equator where they ensheath the nuclei. Ultrastructurally, the nuclear bag fibres are similar to 'slow' extrafusal fibres of amphibians, lacking the M lines, possessing little sarcoplasmic reticulum, but containing abundant mitochondria and oxidative enzymes: nuclear chain fibres are more like immature 'fast' twitch muscles of mammals, containing M lines, well-formed sarcoplasmic reticulum and T-tube elements, fewer mitochondria and lower oxidative enzyme levels. Nuclear bag fibres, when stimulated, contract more slowly than the nuclear chain type, supporting the ultrastructural findings. **Sensory innervation** of muscle spindles is of two types, both of which are the nonmyelinated terminal branches of two distinct classes of myelinated

[207] B. D. Wyke, *Ann. R. Coll. Surg.*, **41**, 1967.
[208] R. B. Godwin-Austen, *J. Physiol., Lond.*, **202**, 1967.
[209] R. E. M. Bowden, *Ann. R. Coll. Surg.*, **38**, 1966.
[210] P. C. B. Matthews, in: *Scientific Basis of Medicine Annual Review*, 1971, ed. I. Gilliland and J. Francis, Athlone Press, London. 1971.
[211] D. N. Landon, in: *Control and Innervation of Skeletal Muscle*, ed. B. L. Andrew, Thompson, Dundee. 1966.

somatic sensory nerve fibres. The *primary or annulo-spiral* endings are placed centrally at the equator, and form spiral and sometimes annular terminals enwrapping the nuclear bag or chain portions of the intrafusal muscle fibre. A single large myelinated sensory fibre (group Ia), branches to provide the innervations of a number of intrafusal fibres in this way. Ultrastructurally, each terminal runs in a deep groove in the sacrolemma beneath the basement membrane, and it contains numerous mitochondria, vesicles, microfilaments, microtubules, and a pervading flocculent material. The *secondary or flower-spray* endings, which are largely confined to nuclear chain fibres, are branched terminals of slightly narrower myelinated group II afferents; these endings are beaded in appearance and spread in a narrow band on both sides of the primary endings near the equator. These beads, ultrastructurally, are expansions similar in content to the primary endings, and they lie in close apposition to the sarcolemma, although not in grooves.

## Motor Endings in Muscle Spindles

Three types of motor terminals have been distinguished, two being the endings of $\gamma$-efferents and one of a $\beta$-efferent nerve fibre. The first two comprise the *trail endings* nearest to the equatorial region, ramifying to form unspecialized cholinergic motor terminals with no obvious end plate or sole, and further pole-wards the P2 ending, with a typical 'en plaque' end plate and sole. At the extreme ends of nuclear bag fibres is the P1 ending, likewise forming a typical 'en grappe' end plate (p. 482),

whose efferent nerve fibre arises as a collateral branch of a myelinated $\beta$-efferent fibre supplying the extrafusal slow twitch muscle in the neighbourhood of the spindle. These motor endings are able to cause contraction of intrafusal myofibrils.

The activities of the spindle appear to provide information on the length of the extrafusal muscle, its velocity of contraction, and changes in velocity, and it is thought that these modalities are related to the different behaviours of the two types of intrafusal fibres when stretched, either actively by their motor endings, or passively by stretching of the extrafusal muscle surrounding them. It is probable that because of the composition of sarcoplasm in the equatorial nuclear zone of the intrafusal fibres a passive stretch causes greater elongation in that region than in the fibres on each side where the myofibrils are more numerous, causing the response to deformation in the primary sensory endings to be different from that of the secondary endings which are placed further pole-wards. The equatorial region of nuclear bag fibres will also stretch more than that of the nuclear chain types because of the lower viscosity of the former, giving differential responses from the two. From physiological studies it is thought that *nuclear bag fibres* may be largely concerned with *position* and *velocity sense* of a rapidly adapting nature (their *dynamic response*), and the *nuclear chain fibres* with static, slow adapting ones (the *static response*). The fusimotor fibre can adjust the length of the intrafusal fibre, and therefore the activity of its sensory fibres by causing the polar regions to contract. This can compensate for

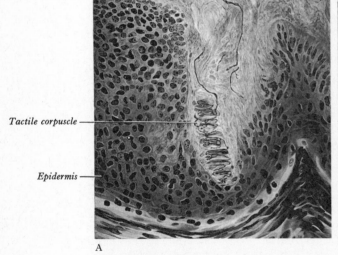

Tactile corpuscle —

Epidermis —

A

B

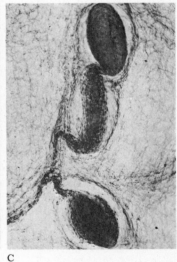

C

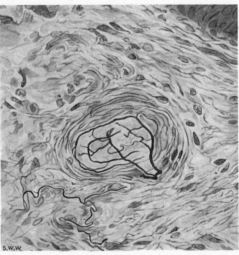

D

7.31 A–F  Specialized sensory end organs. A Tactile corpuscle of Meissner in human skin. (Gros-Bielschowsky technique, about × 250.) B Bulbous corpuscle from human anal canal. (Gros-Bielschowsky and haematoxylin, about × 480, material kindly supplied by Prof. M. J. T. FitzGerald, University College, Galway.) C Whole mount of developing Pacinian corpuscles in feline mesentery (Gros-Bielschowsky technique, about × 120, specimens A and C kindly provided by Prof. N. Cauna, University of Pittsburgh.) D Transverse section of mature feline Pacinian corpuscle; the blood vessels are filled with coloured gelatin. E Ultrastructure, near the apex, of a tactile corpuscle of Meissner in vertical section, showing flattened lemmal cells arranged horizontally, with their nuclei to the right of the field. The sectional profiles of the terminal nerve fibres, appearing between the lemmal cells, contain numerous dense mitochondria. (Magnification about × 5000.) F Ultrastructure of terminal nerve fibres in close association with a hair follicle in the auricle of a rat. Note, above, part of the nucleus and cytoplasm of a keratocyte; the plasma membrane adjoins a well-defined basal lamina, and presents a series of hemidesmosomes. The two nerve fibres contain numerous mitochondria and are enveloped by Schwann cell processes. Surrounding the latter are basal laminae, reticulin fibres (above) and collagen fibres (below). Magnification × 35,000. (E and F respectively from Ciba Foundation Symposium on *Touch, Heat and Pain*, 1966, and *J. comp. Neurol.*, **136**, 1969, by kind permission of Prof. N. Cauna and the publishers, J. & A. Churchill and the Wistar Press.)

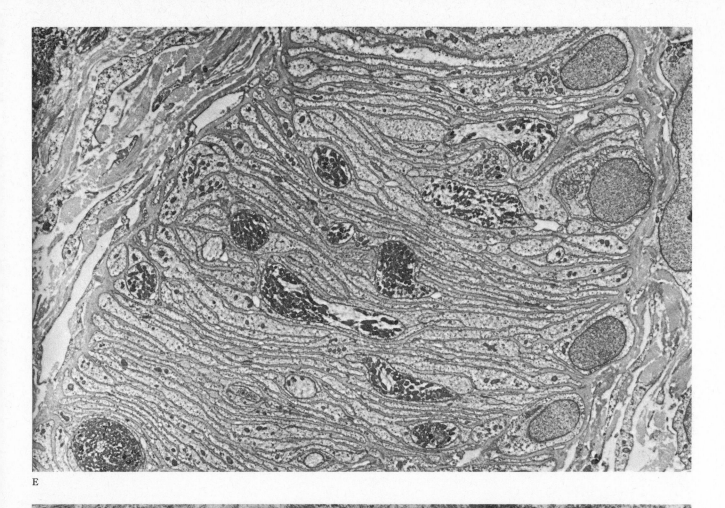

E

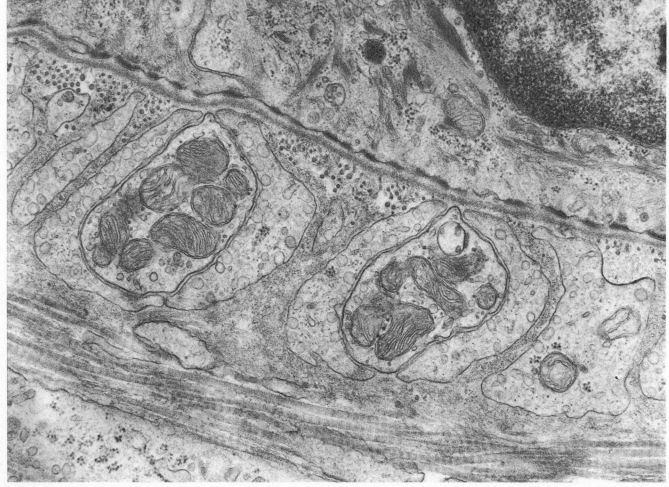

F

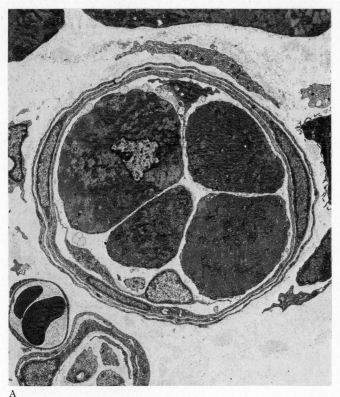

A

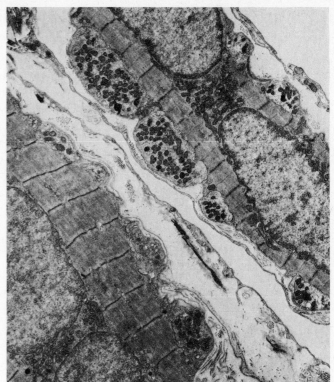

B

**7.**32 A and B    A    An electron micrograph of a neuromuscular spindle of a rat, in transverse section, showing the capsule, capsular space and four intrafusal muscle fibres, one with a centrally positioned nucleus. B    An electron micrograph of a longitudinal section through two intrafusal muscle fibres from a neuromuscular spindle of a rat. Note the primary (annulo-spiral) afferent nerve fibre endings cut in cross-section as they

spiral around the equatorial region of a nuclear chain fibre (top right) and of a nuclear bag fibre (lower left). Note also the large numbers of mitochondria present in the sensory fibres. See text for further description. A and B were kindly provided by Dr. D. N. Landon, National Hospital for Nervous Diseases, London.

shortening of the extrafusal fibres during normal muscle activity, or, as was formerly suggested, could be the normal means of causing extrafusal fibres to contract, these being stimulated by the intrafusal muscle. It is envisaged that $\gamma$-efferent fibres, by causing contraction in the intrafusal fibres, could stimulate the sensory endings, which would then initiate contraction in the extrafusal muscle by reflex excitation of $\alpha$-*motor* neurons.[212, 213] More recent evidence, however, indicates that activity in $\alpha$-motor neurons may, in some cases of voluntary movement, precede that in $\gamma$-

motor neurons during muscle contraction, so that the spindle probably monitors the *extent* of muscle contraction allowing *comparisons* to be made between *intended* and *actual movements*.[210] It should be noted that spindles do not appear to be involved in the conscious appreciation of limb position which is mediated by tendon, ligament and articular nerve endings (p. 801).

[212] R. Granit, *The Basis of Motor Control*, Academic Press, N.Y. 1970.
[213] I. A. Boyd, *Phil. Trans. R. Soc. Ser. B*, **245**, 1962.

# MAJOR DIVISIONS OF THE NERVOUS SYSTEM

Although in essence a continuum, the nervous system may be divided for convenience of study into a number of parts, regions, or sub-systems. The *encephalon* or brain (**7.**33) and the *medulla spinalis* or spinal cord together form the *central nervous system*. Extended from this in pairs are twelve cranial and thirty-one spinal nerves, constituting a *peripheral nervous system*. This itself includes not only all the ramifications of these nerves, which mediate *somatic sensory* and *motor* functions, but also the entire complex of *visceral* or *splanchnic* nerves, connected to the central nervous system through the somatic channels, thus forming a *peripheral autonomic nervous system*. This ·division into central and peripheral parts of the nervous system is basically justifiable, for the latter consists of relatively simple conductors connecting the peripherally situated receptor and effector organs to each other through the complex intermediation of the brain and spinal cord. Though the latter also contains certain further extensions of the long afferent and efferent pathways deployed through the peripheral nerves, the particular significance of the

whole central nervous system resides in extremely complex networks of interconnected neurons in which arise the appropriate patterns of response to the stimuli of both the external and the internal environment. This same highly intricate area of intermediation, between incoming patterns of afferent information and the emergence of suitable arrays of 'commands' to the effectors, is also the domain in which learning, memory and consciousness are intrinsic, each to a degree dependent upon the level of development of the central apparatus. Indeed, the elaboration of these activities, which clearly has increased along the lines of evolution, and especially along that leading ultimately to the human animal, is equally clearly related to a vastly increased population of central interneurons, rather than to changes in the peripheral afferent and efferent conductors. Nevertheless, the essential continuity and interdependence of all parts of the nervous system should never be overlooked.

The elements of which the nervous system is composed have already been described (p. 766). Whereas the peripheral nerves largely consist, except in their somatic and autonomic ganglia, of parallel and unconnected fibres, the central nervous system contains not only the terminations or beginnings of these peripheral axons but also very large numbers of nerve cells, together with their dendritic processes, the ramifications and synapses of which make up the greater part of the volume of the brain and spinal cord. Both parts of the nervous system also contain, of course, considerable amounts of either connective tissue and Schwann cells or neuroglia, and numerous blood vessels. The central nerve fibres and cells are distributed in an organized manner, and one or the other frequently predominates in particular regions. The somata of neurons are usually (but not always) gathered together into masses, which are called *nuclei* and sometimes *ganglia*; since they are devoid of any covering of myelin they appear darker to the unaided eye than do collections of nerve fibres, except where the latter are nonmyelinated. This difference is accentuated by fixation, and with alcohol treatment nerve cell aggregations appear somewhat grey and myelinated nerve fibres almost white, giving rise to the crude but useful terms 'grey' and 'white matter' or substance, although their colours are more nearly buff and cream in material fixed by the more commonplace formalin technique. It is not to be supposed that 'grey matter' contains no myelinated fibres; a large proportion of central axons are myelinated, and since every group of nerve cells will contain at least their own fibres, the grey or buff colour is merely due to the relatively low proportion of myelin. Similarly, tracts of myelinated nerve fibres, identified by the unaided eye as 'white matter', may nevertheless contain small numbers of nerve cells, and where the fibres are largely or entirely non-myelinated the colour will be 'grey'. With these provisos the two terms are usefully employed in the grosser descriptive topography of the central nervous system.

**The spinal cord** occupies approximately the cranial two-thirds of the vertebral canal, and it is arbitrarily considered to be continuous with the lowest part of the brain, the medulla oblongata, just below the level of the foramen magnum. The first pair of spinal nerves emerge from the spinal cord immediately caudal to this. The walls of the cord are thick, the cavity of the central nervous system being here reduced to an almost microscopic *central canal*, extending nearly the full length of the cord.

**The encephalon** or brain (**7.**33), which is wholly within the cranial cavity, is itself described as consisting of a number of regions, which are of considerable morphological and functional significance. These are—in ascending order from the spinal cord—the **rhombencephalon** or hindbrain, the **mesencephalon** or midbrain, and the **prosencephalon** or forebrain. The rhombencephalon includes the **myelencephalon** or medulla oblongata, the **metencephalon** or pons, and the **cerebellum**. The prosencephalon is also subdivided into the **diencephalon** ('between brain'), which is the central connecting part of the forebrain, corresponding approximately to the thalamus and hypothalamus, and the **telencephalon**, which comprises the two so-called cerebral 'hemispheres' or cerebrum. The midbrain, pons, and medulla oblongata are collectively termed the *brainstem*, connecting the forebrain and spinal cord. The relation of these divisions of the brain to each other will be appreciated more clearly if their development is considered (p. 132). The pattern of fore-, mid-, and hind-brain is not only an expression of ontogenetic growth in the individual, it is also phylogenetic, inasmuch as it represents the basic central nervous hierarchy of vertebrates. These three successive levels are sometimes regarded as the 'segments' of the brain, and in extension of this idea the telencephalic part of the forebrain, the cerebrum, and particularly the

cerebral cortex and its connexions, is described as 'supra-segmental', a term also applied to the cerebellum. Both are phylogenetically later outgrowths upon the basically elongated form of the primitive vertebrate brain.

The *medulla oblongata* is the most caudal part of the brainstem. It is immediately above the basilar region of the occipital bone, and is continuous with the pons above and the spinal medulla below. The *pons* is also related to the basi-occiput and to the dorsum sellae of the sphenoid bone. It is markedly greater in transverse and antero-posterior dimensions than the medulla, from which it is easily distinguished by the large lamina of transverse nerve fibres protruding from its ventral aspect. The *cerebellum*, consisting of paired lateral parts, or *hemispheres*, united by

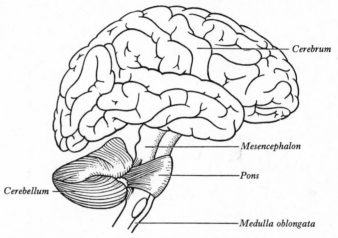

*Cerebrum*

*Mesencephalon*

*Pons*

*Cerebellum*

*Medulla oblongata*

**7.**33   Semi-diagrammatic scheme of the main divisions of the brain.

a median *vermis*, is dorsal to the pons and medulla, occupying most of the posterior cranial fossa. Ventrally it is continuous with the midbrain, pons, and medulla. The cavity of the rhombencephalon or hindbrain is expanded as the *fourth ventricle*, which occupies the dorsal parts of both the pons and the cranial half of the medulla, being continuous with a fine canal in the caudal part of the medulla, and through this with the central canal of the spinal cord. The fourth ventricle contracts at its cranial end into a narrow channel in the mesencephalon, somewhat inappropriately termed the *cerebral aqueduct*. The *midbrain* is a relatively short part of the brainstem and somewhat constricted in comparison with the pons. The *diencephalon*, which is almost completely embedded in the cerebrum and thus largely hidden from surface view, contains a narrow, vertical *third ventricle*, which communicates caudally with the aqueduct.

The *cerebrum* is the most cranial or rostral part of the brain, and it accounts in mankind for much the major fraction of its volume. It occupies the anterior and middle cranial fossae and is directly related to almost the whole concavity of the vault of the skull. It is described as consisting of two large convoluted *cerebral hemispheres*. In fact, the halves of the cerebrum are *not* hemispherical; together they do form roughly a hemisphere, and perhaps the term was originally used in the singular, but the plural usage, however unsuitable as regards shape, is customary. Each hemisphere is roughly equal to a quarter of a sphere in shape and contains a large, crescentic *lateral ventricle*, continuous medially with the third ventricle in the diencephalon. Each hemisphere has an external layer of grey matter, the *cerebral cortex*, and a central core of white matter, or *medullary substance*, in which are several large masses of grey matter, the *basal ganglia* or *nuclei*.

As already mentioned, the *peripheral nervous system* contains a somatic component, the *cerebrospinal nervous system*, and a visceral component, the *autonomic nervous system*. In the former the efferent nerve fibres pass directly from their cells of origin in the central nervous system to the effector organs, muscles. The efferent autonomic fibres, however, do not do so, but terminate in ganglia outside the central nervous system, where they form synapses with neurons whose axons pass onwards to innervate non-striated muscle and glandular tissue. Autonomic efferent pathways thus consist of two orders of neurons termed, for obvious reasons, *preganglionic* and *postganglionic*. The arrangement of afferent fibres is, on the other hand, similar in both cerebrospinal and autonomic systems.

The autonomic nervous system consists of *sympathetic* and *parasympathetic* divisions. Preganglionic sympathetic efferent fibres issue from a region of the spinal cord limited to the segments between the first thoracic and second or sometimes third lumbar levels. Preganglionic parasympathetic efferent fibres emerge from the central nervous system only in certain cranial nerves (oculomotor, facial, glossopharyngeal, vagus, and accessory) and in the second, third and fourth sacral spinal nerves. These two groups of autonomic efferents are therefore usually designated the *thoracolumbar* (sympathetic) and *craniosacral* (parasympathetic) *outflows*. A detailed description of the autonomic system appears on p. 1065.

# THE CENTRAL NERVOUS SYSTEM

## THE SPINAL MEDULLA OR CORD

The spinal cord (medulla spinalis) is the elongated, approximately cylindrical part of the central nervous system which occupies most of the vertebral canal. Its average length in the European male is 45 cm and its weight about 30 gm. It extends from the level of the cranial border of the atlas to the caudal border of the first or cranial border of the second lumbar vertebra. This level of termination is, of course, subject to variation, showing also some correlation with the length of the trunk, especially in females.[214] The cord's termination may be as

high as the lower third of the twelfth thoracic vertebra or as low as the disc between the second and third lumbar vertebrae. The position of the termination is elevated slightly by flexion of the vertebral column. The spinal cord is enclosed in three membranes or *meninges*; these are, from without inwards, the *dura*, *arachnoid*, and *pia maters*, which are separated from each other by *subdural* and *subarachnoid spaces*, the former being merely potential, the latter being occupied by the cerebrospinal fluid (p. 991). Continuous cranially with the medulla oblongata, the spinal cord narrows caudally to a sharp tip, the *conus medullaris*. From the apex of this the *filum terminale*, a fine connective tissue filament, descends to the dorsum of the first coccygeal segment (7.34).

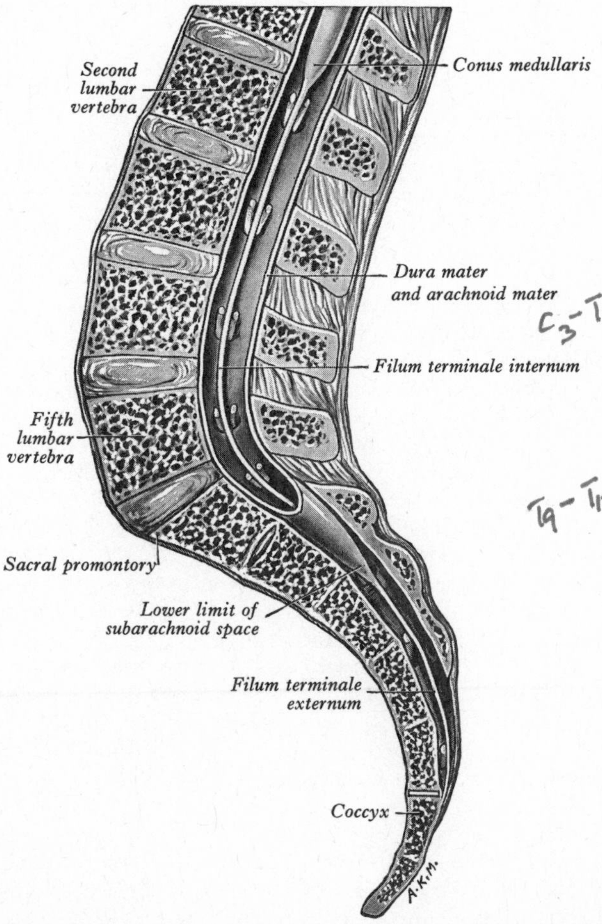

In *transverse width* the spinal cord varies from level to level. It shows a general tapering from cranial to caudal extremities, but this is obscured to some extent by enlargements at cervical and lumbar levels. Moreover, it is not cylindrical, being greater in its transverse dimension at all levels, and especially so in its cervical segments.

The *cervical enlargement* is the more pronounced and corresponds to the large spinal nerves supplying the upper limbs. Hence it extends from the third cervical to the second thoracic segment, its maximum circumference (about 38 mm) being in the sixth cervical. (A spinal cord segment is the region of attachment of one pair of spinal nerves.)

The *lumbar enlargement* similarly corresponds in level to the segmental innervation of the lower limbs, beginning at the first lumbar segment and extending to the third sacral, the equivalent vertebral levels being ninth to twelfth thoracic. Its greatest circumference (about 35 mm) is level with the lower part of the twelfth thoracic vertebra, beyond which it rapidly dwindles into the conus medullaris.

*Fissures* and *sulci* mark the external surface of the spinal cord through most of its length. An anterior median fissure and a posterior median sulcus and septum almost completely divide the cord into symmetrical right and left halves, joined across the midline by a commissural band of nervous tissue, in which is the central canal (7.35, 36).

The *anterior median fissure*, traversing the whole length of the ventral surface of the spinal cord, has an average depth of 3 mm, being deeper than this at more caudal levels. It contains a reticulum of pia mater, and immediately dorsal to it is a lamina of nerve fibres, the *anterior*

Second lumbar vertebra

Conus medullaris

Dura mater and arachnoid mater

Filum terminale internum

Fifth lumbar vertebra

Sacral promontory

Lower limit of subarachnoid space

Filum terminale externum

Coccyx

**7.34** Median sagittal section of the lumbosacral part of the vertebral column to show the conus medullaris and filum terminale. The section has opened up the subarachnoid space as far as the first sacral vertebra. Note the difference in levels between the inferior limits of the spinal cord and its meninges.

806

[214] I. Jit and J. Charnalia, *J. Anat. Soc. India*, **8**, 1959.

# SPINAL MEDULLA OR CORD

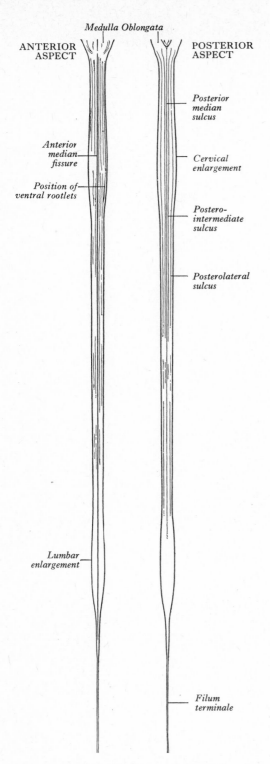

Medulla Oblongata

ANTERIOR
ASPECT

POSTERIOR
ASPECT

Posterior
median
sulcus

Anterior
median
fissure

Cervical
enlargement

Position of
ventral rootlets

Postero-
intermediate
sulcus

Posterolateral
sulcus

Lumbar
enlargement

Filum
terminale

**7.35A**   Diagram to show the main features of the spinal cord.

**7.35B**   The brain and spinal cord with attached spinal nerve roots and dorsal root ganglia, photographed from the dorsal aspect. Note the relative sizes of the cerebral and cerebellar hemispheres, and the fusiform cervical and lumbar enlargements of the spinal cord. The median longitudinal fissure between the hemispheres which contains the falx cerebri and falx cerebelli is visible, together with the horizontal cleft between cerebrum and cerebellum which receives the tentorium cerebelli. Contrast the irregular pattern and dimensions of the cerebral gyri and sulci with the more regular, largely transverse pattern of the smaller cerebellar folia, and their intervening fissures. Note also the changing obliquity of the spinal nerve roots in their craniocaudal progression, the stouter roots attached to the limb enlargements and the formation of the cauda equina and filum terminale. The cauda is undisturbed on the right, and has been fanned out on the left to facilitate identification of its individual components. (Dissection by Dr M. C. E. Hutchinson, Department of Anatomy, Guy's Hospital Medical School.)

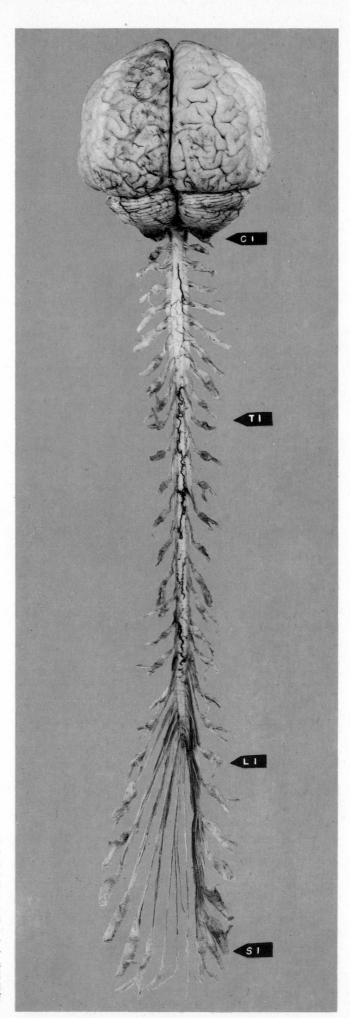

*white commissure.* Perforating branches of the spinal vessels pass from the fissure into the commissure to supply the central region of the spinal cord.

The *posterior median sulcus* is much shallower, and from it a *posterior median septum* of neuroglia penetrates somewhat more than half way into the substance of the cord, reaching almost to the central canal. The septum varies in its anteroposterior extent from 4 to 6 mm, diminishing caudally as the canal becomes more dorsal in position and the cord itself contracts.

A *posterolateral sulcus* exists on each side of and a short distance from the posterior median sulcus, and along it the dorsal spinal nerve roots enter the cord. The white substance of the cord between the posterior median and posterolateral sulci on each side is the *posterior funiculus.* Through the cervical and upper thoracic segments the surface of this funiculus presents a further longitudinal furrow, the *postero-intermediate sulcus,* which marks the position of a septum extending into the posterior funiculus and dividing it into two large tracts of fibres, the *fasciculus gracilis,* which is medial, and the *fasciculus cuneatus* which is lateral.

The region of the spinal cord between the posterolateral sulcus and anterior median fissure is the *anterolateral funiculus,* and this is further subdivided into *anterior* and *lateral funiculi* by the issuing anterior roots of the spinal nerves. The anterior funiculus lies medial to (and includes) the zone of emergence of the ventral roots, whilst the lateral funiculus lies between the roots and the posterolateral sulcus (**7.**36, 38). In the upper cervical segments a series of nerve roots emerges through the lateral funiculus on each side to form the spinal part of the accessory nerve by their union, which ascends in the vertebral canal lateral to the spinal cord to enter the posterior cranial fossa through the foramen magnum (**7.**59). It is composed of fibres which supply the sternocleidomastoid and trapezius muscles.

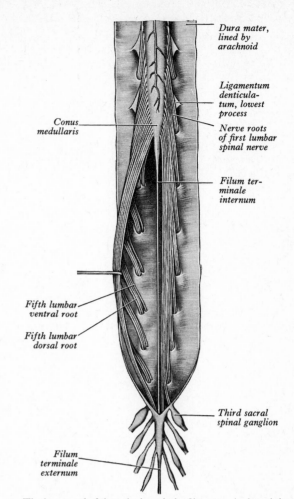

**7.**37   The lower end of the spinal cord, the filum terminale and the cauda equina exposed from behind. The dura mater and the arachnoid have been opened and spread out.

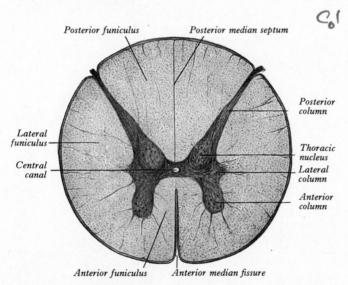

**7.**36   Typical transverse section of the spinal cord at a mid-thoracic level. Magnification about ×8.

The *filum terminale* (**7.**34, 37), a fine filament of connective tissue about 20 cm long, descends from the apex of the conus medullaris. Its cranial 15 cm, the *filum terminale internum,* is surrounded by tubular extensions of the dural and arachnoid meninges and reaches as far as the lower border of the second sacral vertebra. Beyond this its final 5 cm, the *filum terminale externum,* is closely united with the investing sheath of dura mater, descending to an attachment to the dorsum of the first coccygeal

vertebral segment. The filum, consisting mainly of fibrous tissue, is continuous at its cranial end with the pia mater of the spinal cord; adherent to the upper part of its surface are a few strands of nerve fibres which probably represent the roots of rudimentary second and third coccygeal spinal nerves. The central canal of the cord is also continued into the filum terminale for 5 or 6 mm. A particularly roomy part of the subarachnoid space surrounds the internal stretch of the filum; it is the site of election for spinal (lumbar) puncture.

Continuous with the cord at intervals along it are the paired dorsal and ventral roots of the spinal nerves (**7.**38). These cross the subarachnoid space, traverse the dura mater separately, and then unite in or close to their intervertebral foramina to form the spinal nerves. Since the spinal cord is markedly shorter than the vertebral column, the more caudal spinal roots descend for varying distances around and beyond the cord to reach their corresponding foramina; and in so doing they form, largely caudal to the apex of the cord, a divergent sheaf of spinal roots, the *cauda equina,* gathered around the filum terminale in the spinal theca.

The *ventral spinal roots* consist of efferent somatic and, at certain levels, visceral (sympathetic) nerve fibres, the axons of which are emerging from their sources in the spinal cord. The *dorsal spinal roots* are characterized by ovoid swellings, the *spinal ganglia,* one on each root just proximal to its junction with a corresponding ventral root in its intervertebral foramen. Each dorsal root fans out into six to eight rootlets which enter the cord in a vertical series along the posterolateral sulcus. The dorsal roots are generally regarded as consisting entirely of afferent nerve

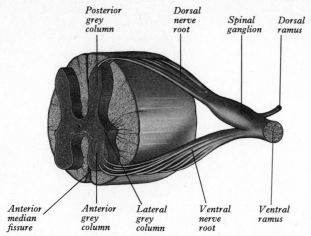

**7.38** Diagram of a spinal cord segment showing mode of formation of a typical spinal nerve, and the gross relationships of the grey and white matter.

fibres derived from unipolar nerve cells in the spinal root ganglia, but it has been suggested that a small number of them (3 per cent) are efferent,[215] and that autonomic vasodilator fibres may issue in dorsal roots (p. 1068). These views have not received wide support. Each ganglion nerve cell has a single very short process which almost immediately divides into a medial process entering the spinal cord through the dorsal root and a lateral one which passes peripherally to some form of sensory end organ. The central process is morphologically an axon, whereas the lateral or peripheral extension is derived from a dendrite. The region of the spinal cord associated with a given pair of spinal nerves is described as a *spinal segment*, but there is no clear indication of segmentation apart from this.

## Internal Structure of the Spinal Cord

The internal structure of the spinal cord may be considered from several different but complementary points of view. Ignoring for the present the all-pervading supply and support tissues, blood vessels and neuroglia, the arrangement of the nerve cells and their processes can be studied by a variety of means, including dissection and unaided observation of sections, by light and electron microscopy, and by experimental techniques, and, of course by combinations of these. The first method reveals little more than the general layout of nerve fibres and cells; microscopy provides much more detailed information of cell types and fibre calibres and of their intimate disposition in the substance of the cord. While both light and electron microscopy have contributed greatly to knowledge of the interconnexions between neuronal elements, the potential of these techniques can only be fully exploited in conjunction with experimental manœuvres, such as degeneration and microelectrode methods. We shall therefore consider spinal organization in a series of steps: (*a*) the large-scale arrangement of the grey and white matter, (*b*) the distribution of nerve cells in the grey matter, (*c*) the white substance and the deployment of tracts of fibres in it, and (*d*) the more detailed organization of the spinal neurons.

### GENERAL ARRANGEMENT OF GREY AND WHITE MATTER

The grey matter of the spinal cord is central in situation and has the form of a fluted column throughout, except where this pattern is modified at its continuation into the medulla oblongata and in its tapered caudal extremity, the

conus medullaris. In transverse sections (7.39) this column consists of symmetrical right and left comma-shaped masses connected by a transverse *grey commissure*, the whole somewhat resembling a letter H. The commissure is traversed by the central canal, which may be just visible to unaided vision. Each of the lateral crescentic masses has a concavity directed laterally and can be regarded as having *anterior* and *posterior* parts or *columns* relative to the grey commissure. At some levels a small *lateral column* projects from the intermediate region of the concavity. In transverse sections of the spinal cord these various columns appear as more or less pointed projections and are hence commonly called 'horns'. This picturesque nomenclature is misleading and unnecessary, and the elongated divisions of the grey matter will be referred to as columns in this account. The central grey matter is surrounded by the white matter of the cord, the latter consisting largely of nerve fibres, many of which are longitudinal in direction and are therefore grouped appropriately into *funiculi* (little cords) or *white columns*. The general arrangement of these as dorsal, lateral and ventral funiculi has already been described above, and further details of the types and arrangements of nerve fibres in these white columns will be the concern of a subsequent section (p. 817 *et seq.*).

**The anterior or ventral grey column** projects ventrally and somewhat laterally with respect to the grey commissure. It is comparatively short and broad and does not reach the surface of the spinal cord, being separated from this by the lateral part of the anterior funiculus (7.39). Its anterior and posterior limits are sometimes named its head and base—arbitrary terms of little value.

**The posterior or dorsal grey column** projects dorsolaterally, and in contrast to the anterior column it is transversely narrow and also extends almost to the surface near to the posterolateral sulcus, from which it is separated by a thin lamina of nerve fibres, the *dorsolateral tract* (p. 824). It also is considered to have a base, where it is continuous with the intermediate grey region, a constricted neck which expands into an oval or fusiform head, and an apex, which is capped by a mass of somewhat translucent nervous tissue, the *substantia gelatinosa*. This crescentic mass of small nerve cells and fibres is intimately concerned with the connexions of incoming afferent nerve fibres, further details of which appear later (p. 830).

**The lateral grey column** is a small, angular projection extending from the second thoracic to the first lumbar segment of the cord and does not appear at other levels.

The boundary between white and grey matter is in most places definite, but in the cervical region of the cord strands of grey matter invade the lateral funiculus from the base of the dorsal grey column; these strands are separated by interlacing groups of nerve fibres, and this gives the arrangement the appearance of a loosely interwoven net, whence its name, the *reticular formation*, or formatio reticularis. Similar regions appear, in a less developed form, at more caudal spinal levels; and more recently reticular formations have been identified in the brainstem, in connexion with which physiological investigations have led to the concept of an extensive *reticular system*, of great functional importance, widely deployed throughout the neuraxis. See pp. 888–890 for details.

The respective positions of the main masses of white and grey matter are what might be expected in simple terms of peripheral conductors and longitudinally arranged spinal tracts of fibres, but this general structure is also an expression of the development of the cord (p. 127). The dimensions of the spinal cord and the relative

[215] J. Z. Young and S. Zuckermann, *J. Anat.*, **71**, 1936.

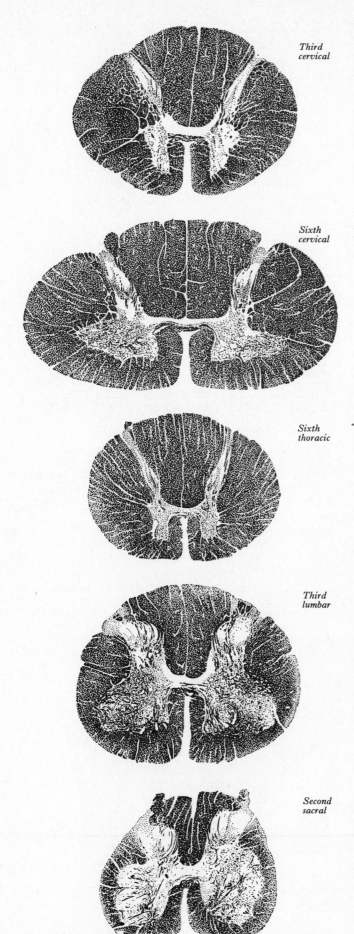

*Third cervical*

*Sixth cervical*

*Sixth thoracic*

*Third lumbar*

*Second sacral*

**7.39** Transverse sections through the spinal cord at representative levels. Magnification about × 5. Note changes in overall profile, and the relative changes in grey and white regions.

810

volumes of peripheral fibres and centrally aggregated nerve cells at different levels (7.39) can be explained by the amounts of muscle, skin and other tissues innervated by different segments, and by consideration of the fact that the fibres in the longitudinal tracts are on the whole inevitably more numerous as the cord is traced in a cranial direction. In the thoracic region the grey matter is absolutely and relatively small in volume, while the white substance shows a progressive increase in the ascending direction. In the cervical and lumbar enlargements the amount of grey matter, especially in the ventral columns, is much increased by the presence of large accumulations of nerve cells concerned in the innervation of the limbs; but, while the amount of nerve fibres at cervical levels is marked, in the lumbar enlargement and particularly the conus medullaris the white funiculi contain very many less fibres passing through these segments; 7.39 shows these details in several representative segments of the spinal cord, and it is obvious that various levels can easily be distinguished from each other. It is, however, more important to recognize the explanation of these differences in terms of the criteria noted above.

The **central canal** exists throughout the spinal cord and also extends into the caudal half of the medulla oblongata, opening out above this into the fourth ventricle (p. 878). In the caudal part of the conus medullaris it expands into a fusiform *terminal ventricle*, triangular in section with its base ventrally directed. It is about 8 to 10 mm in length, but tends towards obliteration above the age of forty years. At cervical and thoracic levels the canal is slighly ventral to the midpoint of the cord, central in the lumbar enlargement, and more dorsal in position in the conus medullaris. It extends for 5 or 6 mm into the filum terminale. During life it contains cerebrospinal fluid, and it is lined by a columnar, ciliated epithelium, the *ependyma*, which is encircled by a zone consisting principally of neuroglia but also containing a few nerve cells and fibres, the *substantia gelatinosa centralis*. This is traversed by processes spreading centrifugally from the basal aspects of the ependymal cells. The grey matter surrounding the central canal external to the gelatinous substance is the *grey commissure.* Ventral to the canal the commissure is thin, and further ventral still is a slender lamina of decussating nerve fibres, the *ventral white commissure* (p. 817). The grey commissure is traversed by two longitudinal veins (p. 840). The part of it dorsal to the canal is contiguous with the ventral edge of the posterior median septum; it is thinnest in the thoracic region of the cord and thickest in the conus medullaris; it is permeated by a variable number of transverse white myelinated nerve fibres which, collectively, are sometimes termed the *dorsal white commissure.*

## Internal Structure of the Grey Matter

Like other parts of the central nervous system the spinal grey matter (7.40) consists of a complex intermingling of nerve cells and their processes with neuroglia and blood vessels. The predominance of the somata of neurons in relation to their myelinated processes, which are also present, is responsible for the so-called grey appearance, as we have seen above. The neuroglia (p. 778) forms a most intricate lattice among the nerve cells and their neurites, being particularly condensed in the central gelatinous substance around the central canal. The processes of the nerve cells will be described in detail later in this section in connexion with the tracts of the spinal cord (p. 817) and with the organization of its interneuronal networks (p. 828); they include axons arriving from or departing to the fibre tracts of the white funiculi, the commencement of efferent and the termination of afferent

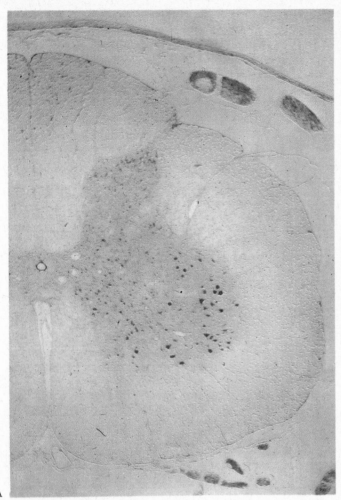

A

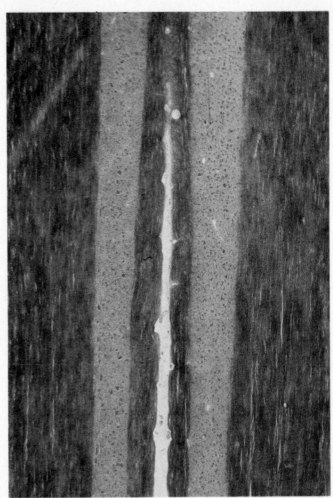

B

7.40 A and B  Transverse and longitudinal sections of spinal cord. A Transverse section of left half of human spinal cord at a mid-lumbar level. Note dorsal and ventral grey columns and commissural grey mass. The larger motor neurons in the ventral grey column are visibly grouped. For details see text. (Stained with cresyl fast violet.) B Longitudinal section of feline spinal cord showing the anterior median fissure, and anterior white columns, and lateral to these the ventral grey columns, in which motor neurons show some degree of grouping into longitudinal columns. (Material prepared by the late Prof. L. Laruelle and kindly supplied by Professor J. André-Balisaux, Institut Neurologique Belge, Brussels.)

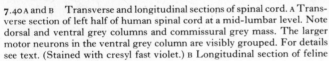

peripheral nerve fibres, together with collaterals from these sources and a most complex neuropil, the latter being composed of the innumerable neurites of nerve cells which are largely confined to the grey matter or at least to the spinal cord itself. Many cell processes cross the midline in the commissures, and the right and left halves of the cord, including its grey matter, are a functional continuum. The nerve cells in the grey substance are multipolar, varying much in size and other characteristics, and particularly in the length and morphology of their axons and dendrites. Many are Golgi types I and II nerve cells (p. 768), the axons of the former being long and passing out of the grey matter into the ventral spinal roots or the fibre tracts of the white matter. The axons and dendrites of the Golgi type II cells are largely confined to the neighbouring grey matter. Some neurons are *intrasegmental*, being deployed within the limits of a single segment; others spread through several segments, being *intersegmental* in distribution. Details of this kind will, however, be described later (p. 838). We shall here be concerned only with the mode of arrangement of the actual nerve cell bodies or somata in the different regions of the grey matter.

In many parts of the central nervous system nerve cells are gathered together in groups, often in large numbers; and this usually indicates involvement in some particular common function. In some instances a large group exhibits division into smaller subgroups sufficiently constant in occurrence in different individuals to justify description and the application of specific names. The existence of such constant patterns of nerve cell distribution inevitably suggests functional implications, though the influence of developmental or growth processes may be of even greater significance in many places. The nerve cells of the spinal grey matter are not distributed evenly or at random; they also occur in major and minor aggregations, some of which have obvious broad functional significance, while the meaning of others remains obscure or a subject of controversy. The following details of the cytoarchitecture of the spinal grey substance are described in the first place as purely topographical arrangements, and in doing this it is convenient to divide this account into sections dealing with the ventral and dorsal columns and with the intermediate region between them, including with the latter the lateral grey column. After this the functional interpretations of some of the subgroups in these columns will be considered in the light of the available evidence.

## NERVE CELL GROUPS OF THE ANTERIOR GREY COLUMNS

The nerve cells of the ventral columns vary greatly in size; most prominent are large multipolar elements exceeding 25 μm in average dimensions of their somata, and with axons emerging as the fibres of ventral roots which innervate striated skeletal muscles as α-efferents. Large numbers of smaller nerve cells, of the order of 15 to 25 μm, also occur

25 μm

15-25 μm.

811

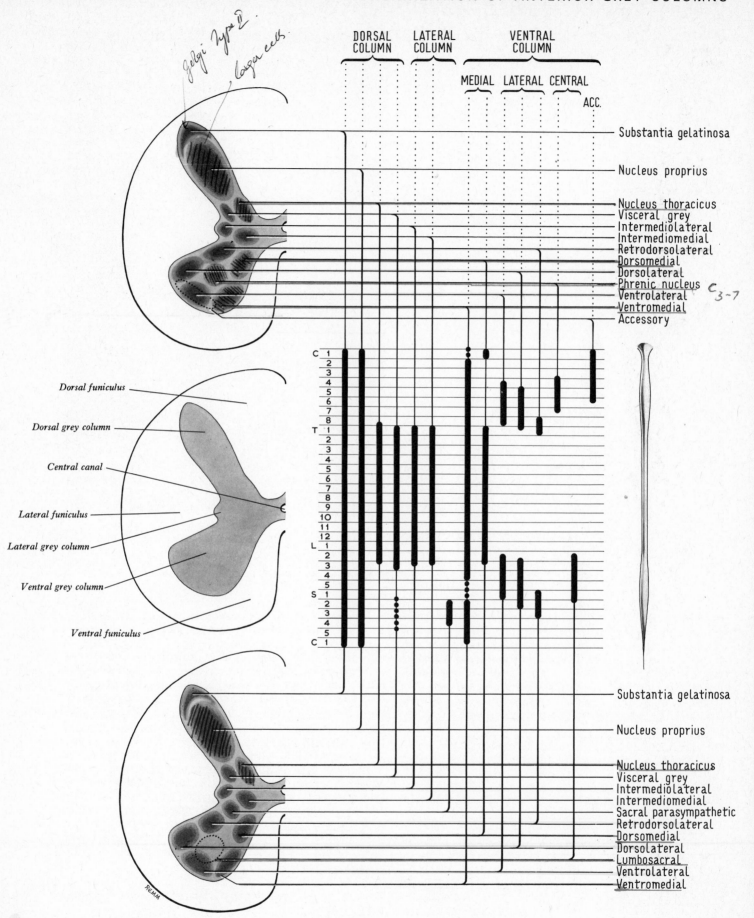

**7.41** The groups or nuclei of nerve cells in the grey columns of the human spinal cord as generally accepted. Relative positions of these columnar groups, as well as their extension through varying series of spinal segments, are as indicated. (Adapted from data in *Correlative Anatomy of the Nervous System*, by E. C. Crosby, T. Humphrey and E. W. Lauer, Macmillan, 1962, with the permission of the authors and publishers.)

and the axons of some of these are the γ-efferents which innervate the intrafusal muscle fibres of neuromuscular spindles. On the evidence of retrograde degeneration experiments and other considerations, not all the smaller nerve cells in this column produce such efferents, and most in fact are interneurons (see also p. 828).

As in other parts of the spinal grey matter, the ventral column cells are basically arranged in elongate groups, a number of separate longitudinal columns extending through characteristic series of segments in the cord. This arrangement is perhaps seen most easily in transverse sections (7.40 A) and is usually so studied; longitudinal sections are rarely described or depicted. In these, however, it is clear that these columns of nerve cells are themselves not uniformly continuous through the cord (7.40 B), but are clustered in small aggregations, which are too diminutive to bear any segmental significance.[216, 217] The basic division of the ventral grey region is into three columnar groups—*medial, central*, and *lateral*, but all of these exhibit further subdivision at certain spinal levels, usually into dorsal and ventral parts. Thus a considerable nomenclature has accumulated, and while there is a satisfactory measure of agreement regarding the organization of the ventral column into cell groups, some confusion persists in the naming of these. The terms employed here are derived from a recent authority widely consulted,[218] but as yet many of these terms are not officially established in *Nomina Anatomica*. As will be more easily appreciated from illustration 7.41, the **medial group** extends through most segments of the cord, being perhaps absent from the fifth lumbar and first sacral. Through all the thoracic and the upper three of four lumbar segments it is divided into subsidiary **ventromedial** and **dorsomedial groups**, and in segments cranial and caudal to this the medial group is represented only by its ventromedial moiety, except in the first cervical segment, where only the dorsomedial group is considered to exist.

The **central group** of the ventral grey column is the least extensive and is identifiable only in some cervical and lumbosacral segments. In the cervical cord, through the third to seventh segments, is a centrally situated columnar group termed the **phrenic nucleus**; there is abundant experimental and clinical evidence that these nerve cells innervate the diaphragm, probably constituting the least controversial individual motor pool in the entire spinal cord.[217, 219, 220] The **lumbosacral nucleus**, traversing the second lumbar to first sacral segments, is also central in the ventral column, the distribution of its axons being unknown. Nerve cells whose axons are considered to enter the spinal part of the accessory nerve form an irregularly shaped **accessory group**, in the upper five or six cervical segments, occupying the ventral border of the anterior grey column in an intermediate or central position. They are, however, lateral to the dorsomedial group in the first cervical segment; the ventral siting of this nucleus may be coupled with the absence of the lateral groups from the first three cervical segments (7.41).

The **lateral group** of the ventral column can be further divided into ventral, dorsal, and retrodorsal groups, all of which are largely confined to spinal segments innervating the limbs. Their individual extents are indicated in illustration 7.41, and the significance of their arrangements will be discussed below (p. 814).

## NERVE CELL GROUPS OF THE POSTERIOR GREY COLUMNS

The cell groups of the dorsal region of the spinal grey matter comprise two which extend through the whole length of the cord and two limited to the thoracic and upper lumbar segments.

The **substantia gelatinosa**, present at all levels, consists chiefly of small Golgi type II neurons with some larger nerve cells. The connexions of these with incoming fibres from dorsal roots and with spinothalamic tract fibres have long been accepted, but somewhat drastic review of this teaching in its details is occasioned by recent experimental work (pp. 830, 832). Also extending throughout the cord is a column of rather large cells, ventral to the gelatinous substance, the **dorsal funicular group** or nucleus proprius. As in the case of the anterior column, a thin lamina of nerve cells, distinguishable from those of the substantia gelatinosa by their larger size, is described by some authorities as a *marginal zone*, dorsal to the substantia (7.40, 41).

The **nucleus dorsalis** or *thoracicus* (of Clarke) occupies the basal region of the posterior grey column, immediately dorsal to the intermediate zone (but see also p. 828). At most levels it is close to the dorsal white funiculus and may project slightly into it. There are variable accounts of its extent, but in the human spinal cord it can usually be identified from the eighth cervical caudally to the third or fourth lumbar. Similarly situated groups of nerve cells have been described as occurring at cervical levels cranial to the nucleus dorsalis, and extensive prolongations in caudal levels of the cord appear to exist in some long-tailed monkeys.[221] But since these 'cervical' and 'sacral' nuclei consist of cells of considerably different characteristics, and have only been described in other mammals, it is premature to extrapolate such observations to the human spinal cord. The cells of the dorsal nucleus itself vary in size, most being comparatively large, especially in the lower thoracic and lumbar segments. Some of these cells send axons into the dorsal spinocerebellar tract (p. 822), some are interneurons.

Lateral to the nucleus dorsalis, and dorsal to the intermediolateral column (7.41), is a small region of nerve cells of medium size, extending throughout the same segments (approximately first thoracic to third lumbar) as the intermediate columns.[222] This columnar group is identifiable in the human cord, but its functional status is uncertain, though it has naturally been associated with the neighbouring autonomic nerve cells.

## NERVE CELL GROUPS OF THE INTERMEDIATE GREY MATTER

The intermediate region of the spinal grey matter (7.40, 41), which includes the lateral grey column, is composed of relatively small nerve cells, many with the features of autonomic preganglionic cells, which develop from elements in the embryonic cord at first dorsolateral to the central canal. Many of these migrate to a position lateral to it and at some little distance from it; these nerve cells constitute the **intermediolateral group**. An **intermediomedial column** is formed from nerve cells which remain nearer to the central canal. The intermediolateral group forms the projecting lateral grey column proper, and a large proportion of its cells send axons into the ventral spinal roots and via the white rami communicantes to reach the sympathetic trunk (p. 1068); preganglionic nerve fibres are similarly derived from some of the cells of the intermediomedial group (the remainder being interneurons). Both groups extend from the eighth cervical or

[216] L. Laruelle and M. Reumont, *Rev. Neurol.*, **44**, 1933.
[217] R. Warwick and G. A. G. Mitchell, *J. comp. Neurol.*, **105**, 1956.
[218] E. C. Crosby, T. Humphrey and E. W. Lauer, *Correlative Anatomy of the Nervous System*, Macmillan, New York. 1962.
[219] W. J. W. Sharrard, *J. Bone Jt. Surg.*, **37 B**, 1955.
[220] N. H. Keswani and W. H. Hollinshead, *Anat. Rec.*, **125**, 1956.
[221] H.-T. Chang, *J. comp. Neurol.*, **95**, 1951.
[222] D. Takahashi, *Arb. neurol. Inst. Univ. Wien*, **20**, 1913.

first thoracic segment as far as the second or third lumbar, thus corresponding approximately to the thoracolumbar outflow. In the second, third and fourth sacral segments a similar group of nerve cells, intermediate in position, is the source of the pelvic or sacral outflow of parasympathetic preganglionic nerve fibres (p. 1068). This **sacral parasympathetic grey column** is lateral to the central canal and substantia gelatinosa centralis, in the junctional zone between the bases of the anterior and posterior grey columns. It shows no division into medial and lateral parts, nor does it project from the intermediate grey zone like the thoracolumbar lateral grey column. The emergence of parasympathetic preganglionic nerve fibres from other segments of the cord has been described by some workers,[223, 224] their cells of origin being ascribed to the basal region of the dorsal grey column and perhaps to be associated with the intermediate grey zone. Such fibres were stated to issue from the cord in *dorsal* roots, to be vasodilator in function, and to form synapses with small multipolar nerve cells in corresponding dorsal spinal root ganglia.[225, 226] These interesting views have not, however, received general acceptance nor any substantial confirmation.

The foregoing description of the arrangement of nerve cells in the spinal cord, which is largely dependent upon the study of material specifically stained to show the *somata* of neurons rather than their processes, has of late been considerably amplified by a *laminar concept* of spinal grey matter organization, an account of which follows below (p. 827). This concept is more widely based upon the interconnexions of nerve cells, and its structural data have been correlated with the results of degeneration experiments to a much greater degree than in the case of the older mode of description outlined above, combining also more aptly with the observations of microelectrode studies. The laminar pattern of organization has thus helped to establish a more precise definition of spinal cord activities, but the two modes of description are not exclusive and, as will become apparent, the older scheme of columnar grouping of nerve cells is in most of its features adaptable into the newer laminar pattern. The latter does, nevertheless, involve some important modifications in regard to the structural relationships between the nerve cells of the dorsal grey column and the fibres of the dorsal roots and spinal tracts, and also involves more precise concepts of functional implications.

There is one aspect of the spatial relationships of nerve cells in the spinal grey matter which so far has scarcely been mentioned; this concerns the significance of cell grouping in the ventral grey columns in relation to individual muscles and movement, and to this attention must now be directed.

## THE FUNCTIONAL IMPLICATIONS OF ANTERIOR GREY COLUMN CELL GROUPS

Even in the earliest accounts of the columnar arrangement of nerve cells in the spinal cord—most of which were based on Nissl stained material studied only in transverse sections, and derived from a truly extraordinary miscellany of animals (including tadpoles, an ostrich, a gorilla, and occasionally man!)—a somatotopic interpretation of cell grouping in the ventral column was advanced with some confidence.[227] Thus, it was an early tenet of such speculations that the medial groups innervate axial musculature (supplied by posterior primary rami), the limbs being innervated from the lateral groups. This attractive hypothesis, originally based entirely on structural data, has in fact been confirmed to some degree by subsequent experimental work, as will appear below. The criticism has been made that few of the investigators in this field

have observed the grouping of ventral grey column cells in longitudinal sections, and that the errors which may arise in tracing elongated aggregations of cells through transverse series of sections probably account for at least some of the disagreements and variations between the topographical results of many earlier workers. Obviously an agreed pattern of cell groups, free at least from major discrepancies, is a necessary prelude to any attempts to assess how far such grouping might represent, for example, the neurons innervating an individual muscle. Considerable agreement in this regard is apparent in the most recent work on this problem, particularly among observers who have examined the distribution of ventral grey column cell groups in fetal material, where it is agreed that the groups are more discrete and hence more easily identified.[228, 229] It is also of importance to note that results of this kind were markedly similar in cat and human material, though only one human fetus was examined. On the other hand, the degree of motor cell grouping in the ventral column is much less developed in amphibians and reptiles, or even mammals such as the bat and mole, all of which possess a fairly complex forelimb musculature, than in the whale, in which the same muscle system is much simplified.[230] It must be added that these comparative observations are of limited value, having been carried out on a somewhat heterogeneous collection of vertebrates, usually in extremely small series and often single animals, with little reference to taxonomic relationships. Moreover, little new information appears to have been recorded during the last two decades and certainly no major series of observations.

These difficulties must be mentioned in some detail to introduce some element of caution into further consideration of the functional interpretations of the motor neuron groups which undoubtedly occur in the ventral grey column, and not to deny the existence of such patterns. Pattern is always significant, and a topographical pattern certainly exists in the ventral column. The question in the present context is—What is the physiological meaning of cell grouping in this region? That it concerns the innervation of skeletal muscles seems inescapable, and it would appear a relatively simple, if tedious, undertaking to cut the nerves supplying individual muscles and to observe the distribution of the resultant retrograde degeneration in the motor neurons of the ventral columns. Few experimental studies of this kind have in fact been carried out— at least, on an extensive scale—and since they have involved the use of different species of animal and sometimes different levels of the spinal cord, they provide only limited checks upon each other. In an investigation of the lumbosacral region of the cord in cats, in which various peripheral nerves were divided in the hind limb[231], the affected groups of nerve cells were all in the lateral part of the anterior column, and the cells innervating the more distal muscles in the limb were dorsal to the 'motor columns' for proximal muscles. In general terms these findings corroborated the speculations of earlier topographical observers, and limited experimental confirmation, also in the cat, has been recorded with regard to the

[223] K. Kuré, G. Saégusa, K. Kawaguchi and K. Shiraishi, *Q. Jl exp. Physiol.*, **20**, 1930.

[224] D. Sheehan, *Anat. Rec.*, **55**, 1933.

[225] F. Kiss, *J. Anat.*, **66**, 1932.

[226] K. Kuré, S. Murakami and S. Okinaka, *Z. Zellforsch. mikrosk. Anat.*, **22**, 1934.

[227] H. C. Elliott, *Am. J. Anat.*, **70**, 1942.

[228] G. J. Romanes, *J. Anat.*, **75**, 1941.

[229] H. C. Elliott, *Am. J. Anat.*, **72**, 1943.

[230] G. J. Romanes, in: *The Spinal Cord*, ed. G. E. Wolstenholme, Ciba Foundation Symposium, Churchill, London. 1953.

[231] G. J. Romanes, *J. comp. Neurol.*, **94**, 1951.

anterolateral group of leg muscles.[232] In the former investigation it was concluded that the cell groups identifiable topographically were not usually individual *motor pools*, but more often (but not always) represented a somatotopic grouping of the motor nerve cells innervating muscles involved together in some *common effect on a joint*.

Another investigator has interpreted his experimental results in monkeys as indicating that the ventral column cell groups can be accounted for not only on the above basis, but also and equally well in terms of peripheral nerves, limb segments, and muscles grouped on a morphological or developmental basis.[233] In this investigation the effects of division of dorsal and ventral primary rami of

THE INNERVATION OF THE LOWER LIMB MUSCLES

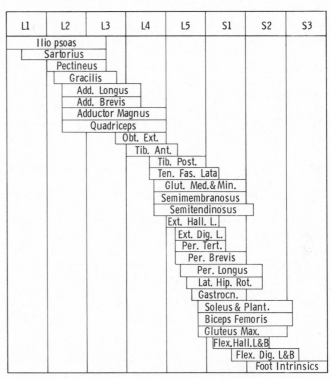

| L1 | L2 | L3 | L4 | L5 | S1 | S2 | S3 |
|---|---|---|---|---|---|---|---|
| Ilio psoas | | | | | | | |
| Sartorius | | | | | | | |
| | Pectineus | | | | | | |
| | Gracilis | | | | | | |
| | Add. Longus | | | | | | |
| | Add. Brevis | | | | | | |
| | Adductor Magnus | | | | | | |
| | Quadriceps | | | | | | |
| | | Obt. Ext. | | | | | |
| | | Tib. Ant. | | | | | |
| | | | Tib. Post. | | | | |
| | | | Ten. Fas. Lata | | | | |
| | | | Glut. Med.& Min. | | | | |
| | | | Semimembranosus | | | | |
| | | | Semitendinosus | | | | |
| | | | Ext. Hall. L. | | | | |
| | | | | Ext. Dig. L. | | | |
| | | | | Per. Tert. | | | |
| | | | | Per. Brevis | | | |
| | | | | Per. Longus | | | |
| | | | | Lat. Hip. Rot. | | | |
| | | | | Gastrocn. | | | |
| | | | | | Soleus & Plant. | | |
| | | | | | Biceps Femoris | | |
| | | | | | Gluteus Max. | | |
| | | | | | Flex.Hall.L&B | | |
| | | | | | | Flex. Dig. L&B | |
| | | | | | | Foot Intrinsics | |

**7.42 B** The segmental arrangement of the innervation of the lower limb muscles. (According to W. J. W. Sharrard, *Ann. R. Coll. Surg.*, **35**, 1964.)

spinal nerves were studied both in the segments innervating limbs and at thoracic levels; and this led to a denial of the differentiation of the ventral grey column into medial and lateral groups in thoracic segments. Even in the limb enlargements of the cord, where both groups were admitted to be present, both appeared to be sources of fibres entering dorsal and ventral rami, a direct confutation of the classical view assigning the innervation of axial and limb musculature respectively to the medial and lateral groups.[234] The same worker, in a later communication, re-emphasized his view that the concept of columnar organization of the ventral grey region had become so ingrained as to be a serious source of error in functional interpretation of this part of the spinal cord. While this is perhaps an extreme view, it does at least underline the unsatisfactory state of knowledge in these matters, which require a wider re-investigation in primate animals, a formidable undertaking. More precise and reliable description of the motor neuron groups in the ventral grey column might, of course, prove to be of rather limited interest in functional interpretation, though it would clearly be of some value when applied in clinical situations involving spinal lesions in mankind. In this connexion it is interesting to note that the effects of poliomyelitis on

Left figure labels:
L₁
Erector spinae
Psoas

L₂
Femoral adductors
Quadriceps extensor
Sartorius

L₃

L₄
Tibialis posterior
Tibialis anterior
Femoral flexors
Tensor fasciae latae
Femoral abductors

L₅
Long digital extensors
Gastrocnemius and Soleus
Peronei

S₁
Intrinsic foot muscles
Long digital flexors
Gluteus maximus
Lateral femoral rotators

S₂

S₃
Perineal muscles

R.E.M.M.

**7.42 A** Diagram of the approximate location in the transverse plane, and in longitudinal extent, of the nerve cell groups innervating muscles, chiefly in the leg, in the lumbosacral segments of the human spinal cord. (Based on clinicopathological studies of poliomyelitis, by W. J. W. Sharrard, *J. Bone Jt Surg.*, 1955).

[232] K. Balthasar, *Arch. Psychiat. NervenKrankh.*, **188**, 1952.

[233] J. M. Sprague, *Am. J. Anat.*, **82**, 1948.

[234] O. Kaiser, *Die Funktionen der Ganglionzellen des Halsmarkes*, Nijhoff, Haag. 1891.

motor neurons in the ventral column have been correlated be several clinical observers with the distribution of the resultant paralysis. The most detailed report of this kind[235, 236] is of special interest, being not only concerned with human conditions but also a confirmation to a considerable extent of some of the experimental findings in cats referred to above (7.42). It is much to be hoped that further data will be forthcoming from such clinico-pathological correlation.

To summarize, it must be admitted that, despite a copious literature reporting a large number of topographical studies and a much smaller succession of experimental investigations, very considerable uncertainties remain to be clarified. That the topographical arrangement of the nerve cells of the ventral grey columns is basically columnar is well established, but many points of imprecision require further study; and perhaps the columnar mode of organization—to some extent inevitable in an elongated structure such as the spinal cord, has been somewhat over emphasized. Somatotopic organization with respect to muscles, either in individual representation or in functional groupings, appears to be confirmed in general terms; but the evidence is against the occurrence of discrete motor pools for individual muscles, of which few have been satisfactorily demonstrated. Overlapping of the nerve cell groups of associated muscles seems to be a commoner pattern of functional organization. It may be added that most of the workers in this field of study and experiment have apparently allowed their concentration upon the somata of neurons to divert consideration too far from the dendritic regions between them, which in simple ratio occupy a much greater volume in the spinal grey matter. It is to this aspect of spinal organization that we shall return after consideration of the 'white matter' in the next section.

## Nerve Fibre Tracts of the Spinal Cord

The 'white matter' of the spinal cord consists of nerve fibres, neuroglia and blood vessels. It surrounds the fluted column of grey matter and its whiteness is, of course, due to the large proportion of myelinated nerve fibres. Its arrangement into anterior, lateral and posterior funiculi has already been described (7.36). Its constituent fibres vary much in calibre, large numbers being small and non-myelinated. Some tracts are characterized by fibres of a small diameter, for example the dorsolateral tract, the fasciculus gracilis and the central part of the lateral funiculus. The nerve fibres in the fasciculus cuneatus, anterior funiculus, and the peripheral zone of the lateral funiculus all contain many large diameter fibres. Most regions of the white substance of the spinal cord contain a considerable *spectrum of fibre diameters*, extending from I $\mu$m or less up to about 10 $\mu$m. Fibres with a diameter of 3 $\mu$m or less predominate, and those at the upper end of the spectrum (a few of which may exceed 10 $\mu$m) form only a small fraction of the total. Detailed studies of the distribution of fibres of differing diameter in the human spinal cord have been few,[237, 238] but it has been claimed that many tracts can be identified on this basis alone. The proportion of fibres of particular diameters has been estimated in a few instances,[239] but in general precise data of this kind are lacking. In any case, delineation of tracts by such observations in transverse sections of normal material can only be regarded as valid when confirmed by the results of experimentation. Most of the available information regarding the tracts of the spinal cord is derived from the results of controlled selective damage of fibres in the cord itself, in experimental animals, but the effects of damage to dorsal nerve roots and of lesions

placed in the brainstem, cerebellum and cerebrum have also provided much information. In all such experiments retrograde degeneration indicates the nerve cells from which particular fibres proceed, while anterograde terminal degeneration provides the evidence for their sites of termination. Suitable staining to reveal Wallerian degeneration of the fibres at intermediate levels demonstrates the position of a tract and the degree to which its fibres are compacted together, dispersed, or overlapped with others. It must be emphasized at once that, while certain tracts are relatively discrete and most are located regularly in definable parts of the funiculi, reciprocal overlapping at least of their fringes is usual (*vide infra*). This accounts in part for the variation in their extent, as seen in diagrams of transverse sections of the cord according to different authorities; in all such diagrams arbitrary boundaries must necessarily be set to delineate the supposed limits of tracts. This is especially true in regard to the human spinal cord; deliberate experimentation is here impossible, and the only data available are the results of disease and injury, neither of which produce the selective and clear-cut kind of lesions possible in animal experimentation. The results of such investigations, particularly when derived from experiments on other primates, can be regarded as likely to be closely similar to the human arrangements; but it would obviously be unwise to accept them as being identical. The evidence collected from examination of the human spinal cord for degenerating nerve fibres resulting from disease or injury does in general support the presumption that the layout of tracts in the human primate is very much the same as in others. The amount of information accumulated from this source is surprisingly large, though usually less precise; it was in fact the principal source of information at first (p. 764), and a very large number of reports of this kind are scattered through neurological literature.[240]

The very predominance of data derived from clinical sources has produced a curious vicious circle in associating an observed grouping or *syndrome* of sensory and motor disturbances with injury to or disease in particular regions of the spinal cord—the exact extent of the latter being not invariably assessed with precision. Because some tracts are undeniably concentrated in certain parts of the white funiculi, their delineation has become artificially crystallized. The fringe overlap mentioned above may be quite extensive; some tracts are in fact almost completely mingled, and others are merely a concept, rather than a circumscribed reality, their fibres being scattered far and wide. Experimental observations, pursued in parallel with clinical deductions, have now far outstripped the latter in their recognition of the intermingling of spinal tracts, whose supposed discrete nature is still widely accepted in clinical practice, but can become an impediment rather than an aid to accurate diagnosis.

The account of spinal tracts which follows is primarily concerned with their arrangement in the human spinal cord, but inevitably reference to findings in animal experimentation must be made at many points where adequate clinicopathological or other data based on human material are not available. In the succeeding section (p. 825), dealing with the finer details of neuronal organization and activity in the spinal cord, evidence derived from animals other than man predominates, but

[235] W. J. W. Sharrard, *J. Bone Jt. Surg.*, **37 B**, 1955.
[236] W. J. W. Sharrard, in: *British Surgical Progress*, 1956.
[237] G. Häggqvist, *Z. Zellforsch. mikrosk. Anat.*, **39**, 1936.
[238] S. P. Giok, *Localization of Fibre Systems within the White Matter of the Medulla Oblongata and the Cervical Cord in Man*, Ijdo N.V., Leiden. 1956.
[239] J. Szentágothai-Schimert, *Z. Anat. EntwGesch.*, **111**, 1941.
[240] P. W. Nathan and M. C. Smith, *Brain*, **78** and **82**, 1955 and 1959.

it is improbable that the deductions from this are not largely applicable to the human spinal cord.

As a convenient simplification, the nerve fibres in the white matter of the spinal cord may be assigned to five groups: (a) afferent fibres from the cells in the dorsal root ganglia which have entered by the dorsal roots and extend for longer or shorter distances in the cord; (b) long ascending fibres, derived from nerve cells in the cord and conducting afferent impulses to supraspinal levels; (c) long descending fibres from supraspinal sources which synapse with cord cells; (d) fibres effecting intrasegmental and intersegmental connexions; and (e) fibres from the motor neurons in the ventral and lateral grey columns which issue in the ventral spinal nerve roots.

analysis of tracts in the cat and monkey, and a critical review of some of the difficulties in their determination, see footnote references [241], [242], [243]. The general positioning of the major tracts is illustrated in a simplified form in 7.43 and in greater detail at two spinal levels in 7.44 A and B. Some features are further summarized in 7.47 A and B.

## TRACTS IN THE ANTERIOR FUNICULUS

### 1. Descending Tracts

(a) The **anterior corticospinal tract** is usually small, but varies in size inversely with the lateral corticospinal tract. It lies alongside the anterior median fissure. It is present in the upper part of the spinal cord, gradually diminishing

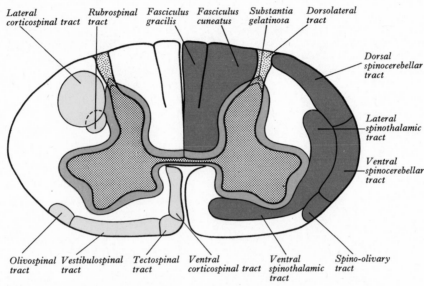

7.43   Simplified diagram of the main tracts of the spinal cord. The ascending tracts are shown in red on the right side of the figure; the descending tracts are shown in yellow on the left side; the 'intersegmental' tracts are shown in orange on both sides.

Fibres in all these categories except the last form the *longitudinal tracts* of the spinal cord. Arrangements are not, however, as simple as this. Examination of the cord in different planes reveals that many fibres proceed for considerable distances in oblique and even horizontal directions, particularly when crossing the midline, as many do in the grey and white commissures. Many of these are *decussating* fibres, that is to say they are crossing to the opposite side of the cord to continue to some more distant point. Many others are *commissural*, being intrasegmental connexions which link nerve cells in the grey columns on one side of the cord to cells on the other. Moreover, some of the longitudinal tracts are polysynaptic, that is, composed of a train of neurons. Most, if not all, of the fibres entering by the dorsal root divide into ascending and descending branches which both give off a series of collateral branches extending into the grey matter. In the latter the number of nerve cells which either send axons into the ventral roots or into the tracts in the white funiculi is a mere fraction of the total, the majority being interneurons (p. 829).

In the following account of the spinal tracts an arbitrary order has been adopted, those in the anterior, lateral and posterior funiculi being described in that order; in each region the descending, ascending and intersegmental tracts are successively considered. This is done primarily to present a relatively orderly topographical picture of the arrangement of tracts which is useful in the context of medical diagnosis, and in phylogenetic studies. However, tracts vary somewhat in their relative positions at different levels in the cord, and in different species. For a detailed

in size as it descends; it cannot be traced below the middle of the thoracic region. The origin and termination of its constituent fibres are considered with those of the lateral corticospinal tract (p. 820). This tract is found only in primates, its precise significance is unknown; it is subject to much variation;[244] it may be absent or it may, very rarely, contain all the corticospinal fibres. Usually it is composed of about 10–30 per cent of them. Its variations have been said to accord with its late phylogenetic and ontogenetic development.[245]

(b) The **vestibulospinal tract**, which is principally derived from both the large and small cells of the lateral vestibular nucleus (p. 852), descends along the periphery of the anterior funiculus; its fibres end around cells in the anterior grey column. This tract is uncrossed and brings the anterior column cells under control of the vestibular nuclei of the same side, serving as an efferent pathway for equilibratory control. The most medially situated fibres of the vestibulospinal tract have, however, been described as starting from cells in the medial and perhaps also the lateral and inferior vestibular nuclei,[246] though the most recent work suggests that only the medial

[241] W. J. C. Verhaart, *Acta anat.*, **18**, 1953 and **20**, 1954.
[242] G. T. van Beusekom, *Fibre analysis of the anterior and lateral funiculi of the cord in the cat*, Thesis, Leiden. 1955.
[243] W. J. C. Verhaart and G. T. van Beusekom, *Acta psychiat. neurol. scand.*, **33**, 1958.
[244] R. Nyberg-Hansen and E. Rinvik, *Acta neurol. scand.*, **39**, 1963.
[245] T. Humphrey, *Proc. 2nd Internat. Meeting of Neurobiologists*, Elsevier, Amsterdam. 1960.
[246] A. T. Rasmussen, *J. comp. Neurol.*, **54**, 1932.

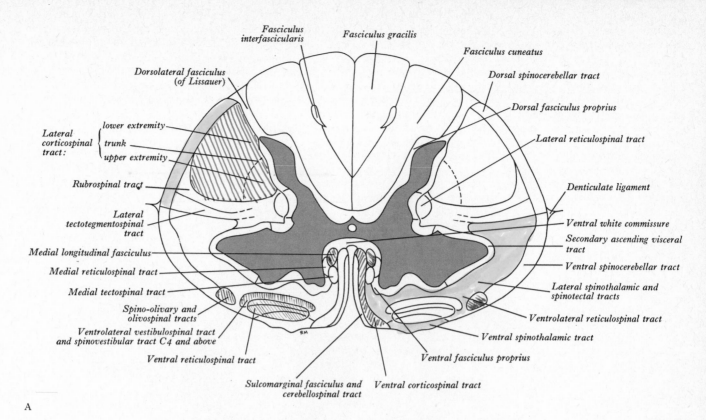

Fasciculus interfascicularis

Fasciculus gracilis

Fasciculus cuneatus

Dorsolateral fasciculus (of Lissauer)

Dorsal spinocerebellar tract

Dorsal fasciculus proprius

Lateral corticospinal tract:
- lower extremity
- trunk
- upper extremity

Lateral reticulospinal tract

Rubrospinal tract

Lateral tectotegmentospinal tract

Denticulate ligament

Medial longitudinal fasciculus

Ventral white commissure

Secondary ascending visceral tract

Medial reticulospinal tract

Ventral spinocerebellar tract

Medial tectospinal tract

Lateral spinothalamic and spinotectal tracts

Spino-olivary and olivospinal tracts

Ventrolateral reticulospinal tract

Ventrolateral vestibulospinal tract and spinovestibular tract C4 and above

Ventral spinothalamic tract

Ventral reticulospinal tract

Ventral fasciculus proprius

Sulcomarginal fasciculus and cerebellospinal tract

Ventral corticospinal tract

A

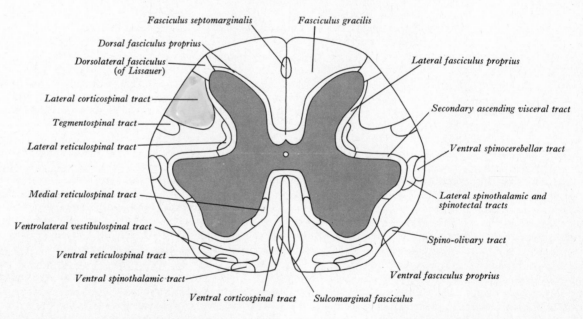

Fasciculus septomarginalis

Fasciculus gracilis

Dorsal fasciculus proprius

Dorsolateral fasciculus (of Lissauer)

Lateral fasciculus proprius

Lateral corticospinal tract

Secondary ascending visceral tract

Tegmentospinal tract

Ventral spinocerebellar tract

Lateral reticulospinal tract

Medial reticulospinal tract

Lateral spinothalamic and spinotectal tracts

Ventrolateral vestibulospinal tract

Spino-olivary tract

Ventral reticulospinal tract

Ventral spinothalamic tract

Ventral fasciculus proprius

Ventral corticospinal tract

Sulcomarginal fasciculus

B

**7.44**A and B   Diagrams of the approximate relative positions of nerve fibre tracts of the human spinal cord at midcervical (A) and lumbar (B) levels. (Adapted from *Correlative Anatomy of the Nervous System*, by E. C. Crosby, T. Humphrey and E. W. Lauer, Macmillan, 1962.)

nucleus is a source.[247] These fibres, which pursue a different course in the medulla oblongata, descending in the medial longitudinal fasciculus (p. 885), constitute the *medial vestibulospinal tract*. This tract is partly crossed and probably does not reach lumbar segments of the cord, and may therefore be concerned with the upper extremity and neck alone. In the white funiculus it is dorsal to the tectospinal tract and immediately adjacent to the anterior median fissure (7.43, 44) in the position of the so-called *sulcomarginal fasciculus*. The remainder of the vestibulospinal fibres, (i.e. the majority, which are uncrossed and descend from the lateral nucleus) may hence be regarded as a *lateral vestibulospinal tract*, which extends to all levels in the cord. The fibres of both tracts terminate in the medial part of the anterior grey column (laminae VII and VIII, *see* p. 828), and they influence both α and γ motor neurons through interneurons;[248] but there is physiological evidence that some fibres end monosynaptically on motor neurons. Both tracts have been widely regarded as uncrossed, but, as we have seen, decussating fibres have been described in the medial tract. There is some degree of somatotopic representation in the lateral vestibular nucleus (p. 861).

(c) The **tectospinal tract** is adjacent to the ventral rim

[247] O. Pompeiano and A. Brodal, *Archs ital. Biol.*, **95**, 1957.
[248] B. E. Gernandt, M. Iranyi and R. B. Livingston, *Expl Neurol.*, **1**, 1959.

of the anterior median fissure. Its fibres arise in the superior colliculus of the opposite side (p. 887) and end by forming synapses with cells in the anterior grey column, especially in the cervical segments of the cord. These fibres influence motor neurons through interneurons,[249] their terminations being probably in laminae VI–VIII (p. 828). The contralateral origin of this tract now seems well established; suggestions of a bilateral origin from the superior colliculi may have arisen through confusion with the *lateral tectotegmentospinal tract* of some authors. When the latter is recognized, the tectospinal fibres which descend in the anterior funiculus are often termed the *medial tectospinal tract*. For further discussion of the tectospinal systems *see* pp. 821 and 887.

(*d*) **Reticulospinal fibres** are also widely scattered through the anterior funiculus, chiefly in its medial part. They arise from the nerve cells of the ipsilateral pontine reticular nuclei (p. 890), but some may decussate shortly before their spinal terminations.[250] They descend throughout the cord in the anterior funiculus and probably end by synapses with interneurons in the medial part of the ventral grey column (laminae VII and VIII,[251] p. 828), through which they possibly exert a facilitatory effect on motor neurons. This tract is commonly known as the *medial* (pontine) *reticulospinal tract*, its origin in the pons corresponding in level to the 'facilitatory area' of many physiologists. (Contrast the lateral reticulospinal tract— p. 821.) These details are entirely derived from observations in non-human tissues; for a discussion of the reticulospinal tracts in man see footnote references[252, 253].

(*e*) The **interstitiospinal tract** has its origin in the interstitial nucleus (p. 885) and its fibres descend without crossing into the medial longitudinal fasciculus (p. 885), and thence into its spinal continuation, the ipsilateral fasciculus proprius (anterior intersegmental tract). In the cat the tract is claimed to be traceable to sacral levels,[254] but no such details are available for the human spinal cord, although the tract as an entity has long been recognized.[255]

(*f*) The **solitariospinal tract** (of Cajal[256]) is a small group of descending fibres which may originate in the neurons of the caudal part of the solitary nucleus (p. 846); it has been best documented in the cat,[257] and has been equated with part of the medial reticulospinal tract by another authority.[258] It was named by Cajal and may be involved in visceral reflexes involving the oesophagus and stomach.

## 2. Ascending Tracts

The **anterior spinothalamic tract** is in fact continuous with the lateral tract of the same name, but may be considered to be the part of this complex in the anterior funiculus, medial to the fibres of the ventral nerve roots and dorsal to the vestibulospinal tract (7.43), which it overlaps, as it does all its neighbours. It has been claimed, largely on clinical evidence, that it is chiefly concerned with crude tactile and with pressure sensibility (but this does not wholly accord with recent physiological investigations— pp. 833, 896). The precise locations of the nerve cells of origin of this tract have not been identified; they have usually been described as 'secondary neurons' situated in the dorsal grey column which receive direct synapses from the axons which enter via the dorsal roots from the primary sensory neurons in the dorsal root ganglia. Since the investigations of Cajal it has been known that some neurons in all regions of the grey matter (dorsal and ventral columns, and the intermediate zone) have axons which cross the midline and ascend in the anterolateral white funiculus, whilst more recently investigators using the Golgi technique have claimed that these are particularly concentrated in spinal cord laminae IV–VII. Whilst many of these may well contribute to the spinothalamic

tracts, such evidence is not conclusive, since it is impossible to follow the axons to their destination. Similarly, studies of the retrograde responses in spinal cord cell somata after cordotomy at a higher level, or after placing lesions in the brainstem or diencephalon, are equally inconclusive because other pathways in addition to the spinothalamic tracts will inevitably have been damaged. Physiological experiments have thrown some light on this matter in the cat and the rat.[368] Electrical stimulation of the region where the medial lemniscus and spinothalamic systems enter the thalamus was accompanied by intracellular recording of antidromic responses from the various grey matter laminae in the cord. Responsive cell somata were identified in laminae V and VI, and this provides some confirmation of the origin of the spinothalamic tracts; but it should be noted that with the limited sampling inherent in such a technique, responding cells in other laminae may well have been missed. Further, it is by no means certain that all spinothalamic fibres are the axons of 'secondary neurons'; in some cases one or more interneurons may be interposed between the primary dorsal root afferents concerned and the spinothalamic tract neuron.

The evidence from cordotomies in man and from other sources suggests that most of the fibres cross the cord, probably within a single segment above their origin, the decussation being in the anterior white commissure. Although physiological studies (p. 833) suggest some spatial separation of neuronal elements concerned with different combinations of the sensory modalities associated with the spinothalamic tracts in the dorsal grey column, the arrangement of the ascending fibres in these tracts is also upon a somatotopic basis.[259, 260] Fibres crossing at any particular level join the medial aspect of those already ascending on the contralateral side of the cord, so that both tracts are segmentally laminated (7.45), fibres originating in lower segments, and therefore of greater total length, being most superficial. In addition a slight spiral twist is evident, the more superficial fibres being progressively more dorsal in position as the tracts ascend the cord. This arrangement is continued through the medulla and pons to the nucleus ventralis posterior lateralis of the thalamus (p. 896). Intermingling with the anterior spinothalamic fibres are not only descending *reticulospinal fibres*, already mentioned, but also numbers of ascending *spinoreticular fibres*. It is possible that the spinothalamic fibres give off collaterals to the brainstem reticular nuclei, but it is now considered that the majority of their afferents form separate spinoreticular pathways, some of which are probably polysynaptic in nature. As in the case of other ascending tracts, there is definite physiological evidence that the spinal cells of origin of the spinothalamic tracts, or their associated interneurons, may be inhibited by fibres descending from nerve cells in the sensory and motor parts of the cerebral cortex, in the anterior cerebellar lobe, and certain regions of the brainstem reticular formation; but the spinal distribution and

[249] J. Szentágothai, *J. Neurophysiol.*, **11**, 1948.
[250] A. Torvik and A. Brodal, *Anat. Rec.*, **128**, 1957.
[251] R. Nyberg-Hansen, *J. comp. Neurol.*, **124**, 1965.
[252] P. W. Nathan and M. C. Smith, *Brain*, **78**, 1955
[253] A. Brodal, *The Reticular Formation of the Brain*, Oliver and Boyd, Edinburgh. 1957.
[254] R. Nyberg-Hansen, *Ergebn. Anat. EntwGesch.*, **39**, 1966.
[255] L. J. J. Muskens, *Brain*, **36**, 1914.
[256] S. R. y Cajal, *Histologie du système nerveux de l'homme et des vertébrés*, Maloine, Paris. 1909.
[257] A. Torvik, *J. Anat.*, **91**, 1957.
[258] E. C. Crosby, T. Humphrey and E. W. Lauer, *Correlative Anatomy of the Nervous System*, Macmillan, N.Y. 1962.
[259] P. W. Nathan, *J. Neurol. Neurosurg. Psychiat.*, **26**, 1963.
[260] F. Morin, H. G. Schwartz and J. L. O'Leary, *Acta psychiat. neurol. scand.*, **26**, 1951.

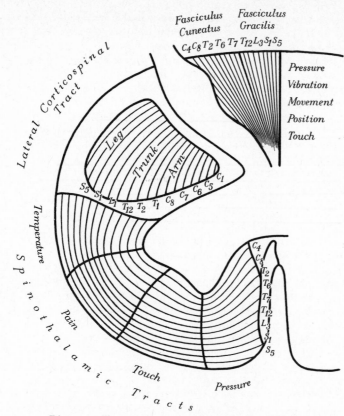

**7.45** Diagram to illustrate the segmental organization of the fibres in the posterior funiculus, the lateral corticospinal tract and the lateral and anterior spinothalamic tracts. The probable cross-sectional areas of these tracts are enlarged to provide adequate space. (After Dr. O. Foerster, by kind permission of Springer-Verlag, Berlin.)

sites of termination of these inhibitory fibres have not yet been clarified. Consult reference [261] for details. Finally, mention should be made of a small *spinovestibular tract* which is intermingled with the vestibulospinal system, and which conveys both exteroceptive and cutaneous information to the vestibular nuclei. This tract may be confined to cervical levels of the cord; the degree of crossing of its fibres is uncertain, but they are thought to terminate in restricted regions of the lateral and descending vestibular nuclei. The cells of origin of the tract probably correspond to those of the spinocerebellar system.

### 3. Intersegmental Tracts

The remaining fibres of the anterior funiculus constitute the **anterior intersegmental tract**. It consists of intersegmental fibres, some of which have crossed from the opposite side. Intermingled with them are believed to be reticulospinal and descending autonomic fibres. The tract is continuous above with the medial longitudinal bundle. Although it is perhaps preferable to combine together all the intersegmental or propriospinal fibres in the anterior funiculus under one term, a number of separate entities have been described in this region by the classical neuroanatomists of the past, as in the case of the propriospinal tracts elsewhere in the cord,[262] and the finer details of distribution of such fibres will be briefly considered with the dorsolateral tract (p. 824).

### TRACTS IN THE LATERAL FUNICULUS

### 1. Descending Tracts

(a) The **lateral corticospinal tract** extends throughout nearly the whole length of the spinal cord. It gradually diminishes in size as it descends, and it ends about the level of the third or fourth sacral segment. On transverse

section it occupies an oval area in front of the posterior grey column and medial to the posterior spinocerebellar tract (7.44); in the lumbar and sacral regions, where the posterior spinocerebellar tract is absent, the lateral corticospinal tract reaches the surface of the spinal cord. The anterior and lateral corticospinal tracts are widely accepted as important motor pathways in the spinal cord, but in recent years physiological experiments have focused attention on other important functional associations of these pathways (pp. 833, 836). They contain about a million fibres of varying diameter, 70 per cent of which are myelinated. About 90 per cent of the fibres have a diameter of 1–4 $\mu$m, about 9 per cent are from 5 to 10 $\mu$m and less than 2 per cent range from 11 to 22 $\mu$m. However, it should be noted that here, as at many other points in the nervous system, these figures and particularly those concerning the small-diameter fibres, may well need substantial revision in the future, when systematic quantitative studies using the electron microscope have been carried out. Many of the fibres arise from cells in the motor area (area 4 of Brodmann) of the frontal lobe; the thicker fibres (11–22 $\mu$m in diameter) are believed, from cell and fibre counts, to be the axons of the giant pyramidal cells of Betz (pp. 949, 954). Some fibres come from other layers in area 4, but experimental evidence shows that at least two-thirds of the corticospinal fibres arise elsewhere. A number start from other cortical areas in the frontal and parietal lobes, especially areas 3, 1, 2 and 6 of Brodmann. However, the origin of about 50 per cent only of the total number of fibres can be thus explained.[263] All the fibres descend through the internal capsule of the cerebrum, traverse the cerebral peduncle and pons and enter the pyramids of the medulla oblongata. In the lower part of the medulla oblongata a variable number, usually about two-thirds, cross the median plane and turn caudally in the lateral funiculus of the spinal cord as the lateral corticospinal tract, while the remainder do not cross but are continued into the same side of the spinal cord, where they form the anterior corticospinal tract. The lateral corticospinal tract also contains some fibres which are derived from the cerebral hemisphere of the same side (*uncrossed lateral corticospinal fibres*).[264]

The corticospinal tracts, anterior and lateral, thus defined, have commonly been described as the *pyramidal* pathway, a usage which is likely to persist. It is true that they consist of the fibres which pass through the pyramids of the medulla oblongata (p. 841), but the same expression is sometimes also made to include *corticobulbar* fibres which diverge cranial to this level to terminate in association with the motor nuclei of the cranial nerves (p. 283). But the chief objection to the continued use of the term 'pyramidal' lies elsewhere. The corticospinal tracts have a single distinction, in that they descend without interruption from cerebral cortex to a termination in the spinal grey matter; and in this they have become contrasted with a group of other descending tracts, such as the rubrospinal and vestibulospinal and others, the fibres of which form intermediate synapses with nerve cells in the cerebrum and brainstem, and which have been collectively labelled as 'extrapyramidal'. The functional distinction between these so-called 'systems' is rapidly becoming blurred, and clinical concepts based upon them are in process of gradual dissolution. The more recent revelation of the reticular system (p. 888) has added further confusion, because in both structural and functional details

[261] D. Carpenter, A. Lundberg and U. Norrsell, *Acta physiol. scand.*, **59**, 1963.
[262] P. W. Nathan and M. C. Smith, *Brain*, **82**, 1959.
[263] A. M. Lassek, *The Pyramidal Tract*, Thomas, Springfield, Ill. 1954.
[264] J. F. Fulton and D. Sheenan, *J. Anat.*, **69**, 1935.

it overlaps much of the 'extrapyramidal' system. The latter concept is probably to be regarded as obsolescent, and for this reason the term 'pyramidal' is perhaps also better avoided.

Throughout its course in the cerebrum and brainstem, with the possible exception of the pons, somatotopic arrangement of its fibres has been established, chiefly as a result of clinical observations in man (7.45). The details of this arrangement will be described in the appropriate sections below. Whether the same kind of distribution obtains in the medullary pyramids and spinal cord is a matter of controversy,[265, 266] but in the cord the longer fibres are said to be most superficial, the shorter ones being internal to them. The majority of the corticospinal fibres, in both ventral and lateral tracts, probably terminate in synapses with interneurons situated in the basal part of the dorsal grey column and spreading ventrally from this through the intermediate zone into the ventral grey column (laminae IV–VII, see p. 836).[267, 268, 269] In these experimental investigations, mostly in cats, no corticospinal fibres were traced as far as motor neurons; but monosynaptic connexions of this kind have been described in monkeys,[270] and it is presumed that such findings indicate similar arrangements in the human spinal cord, perhaps in greater numbers. Nevertheless, it appears certain that the majority of corticospinal fibres, which influence motor neurons innervating skeletal muscle, do so through polysynaptic chains of interneurons. Physiological evidence suggests that this influence is facilitatory with regard to flexors and inhibitory in the case of extensors—the reverse of the effects mediated by the lateral vestibulospinal tract (p. 818). Both α and γ motor neurons are influenced by corticospinal fibres. There is some evidence that corticospinal fibres from the precentral or motor cortex terminate in a more ventral position than those from the postcentral or sensory area;[271] and a considerable number of them (perhaps up to one quarter in some cases) reach their termination without crossing the midline. The influence of corticospinal fibre activity on the transmission of sensory information has been mentioned elsewhere (p. 833, 836).

*Ascending spinopontine* and *spinocortical fibres* have been described in both the anterior and the lateral corticospinal tracts in the cat[272] and in man,[273] derived from all levels of the spinal cord, but especially from cervical segments. They may be concerned in the transmission of cutaneous afferent information.[274] These circumstances add further confusion to the traditional concepts of 'pyramidal' and 'extrapyramidal' systems.

(*b*) The **rubrospinal tract** is composed of nerve fibres of variable diameter which descend from large and small cells in the red nucleus; immediately caudal to this they decussate, and in the lateral funiculus they form a relatively compact band ventral to the lateral corticospinal tract (7.43, 44). Similar fibres have been said to be derived from other nerve cells in the tegmentum of the midbrain caudal to the red nucleus, constituting a *tegmentospinal tract* associated with the ventral border of the rubrospinal tract.[275] The latter was first established in the cat, in which animal it has been most extensively studied; but it is also well authenticated in the macaque monkey, and in both these species it descends through the whole cord to lumbosacral levels. It is important to note that fibres from the smaller nerve cells of the red nucleus reach the most caudal segments of the cord. Because an erroneous view was at one time current that only the largest cells in the nucleus (p. 884) were the source of such long fibres, and since there are few large cells in the human red nucleus, a persuasion has gradually developed that the rubrospinal tract is negligible in man, an opinion doubtless aided by the dearth of information from clinical

observation.[276] Since the tract is well attested in the monkey and chimpanzee, it may exist in mankind; and although the details stated here apply to other mammals, it is wiser to maintain an open verdict as regards the human condition.

In their origins from the red nucleus the rubrospinal fibres show, in the cat,[277] a somatotopic arrangement on a dorsoventral plan, the shortest fibres arising in the most dorsal cells and proceeding to cervical levels in the cord to influence, presumably, the muscles of the neck and upper limb—probably through intermediary neurons. The axons of the most ventral rubral nerve cells are considered to be concerned with the movements of the lower limbs. Some of the fibres leave the tract in the brainstem to influence the motor neurons of cranial nerves, possibly through interneurons in the reticular formation, and some of these *rubrobulbar* axons may reach the ipsilateral inferior olivary nucleus.[278]

The distribution of the terminals of the rubrospinal fibres is similar to that of the corticospinal tract, largely to laminae V–VII (7.47 B), except that the rubrospinal terminals do not extend quite so far ventrally, none reaching the motor neurons. This spatial overlap of the terminals of the two tracts suggests a close interaction of their effects on the motor neurons through a common interneuron pool. It is worthy of note here (see also p. 884) that the red nucleus receives afferent fibres not only from the cerebellum but also from the cerebral cortex, including the 'motor' cortex (area 4) and other areas which are concerned in the origins of the corticospinal pathway. This corticorubral projection displays a somatotopic arrangement in the cat[279] and in primates[280] similar in its details to the corticospinal pathway. Both tracts appear to exercise somewhat similar effects on the spinal motor neurons, such as facilitation of those concerned with flexor musculature; and it is therefore probably misleading to separate them, either in physiological or clinical thinking, as 'pyramidal' and 'extrapyramidal'. However, it would be premature to formulate a revised outlook upon these tracts and their functioning *in man*, despite the highly suggestive data available from investigations in other primates.

It is appropriate to mention here that the cells of origin of the *tegmentospinal fibres* mentioned above are thought to receive the synaptic terminals of *tectotegmental fibres* from the superior colliculi of both sides. Further, some direct tectospinal fibres from both colliculi may accompany the tegmentospinal fibres. This complex of descending fibres (which are closely associated topographically with the rubrospinal system) are accordingly often grouped as the *lateral tectotegmentospinal tract*.

(*c*) The **lateral reticulospinal tract** is usually described as medial to the rubro- and cortico-spinal fibres,

[265] O. Foerster, in: *Handbuch der Neurologie*, ed. Bumke and Foerster, vol. 6, Springer-Verlag, Berlin. 1936.

[266] J. W. Barnard and C. N. Woolsey, *J. comp. Neurol.*, **105**, 1956.

[267] E. C. Hoff and H. E. Hoff, *Brain*, **57**, 1934.

[268] W. W. Chambers and C.-N. Liu, *J. comp. Neurol.*, **108**, 1957.

[269] R. Nyberg-Hansen, *Expl Brain Res.*, **7**, 1969.

[270] C.-N. Liu and W. W. Chambers, *J. comp. Neurol.*, **123**, 1964.

[271] M. E. Scheibel and A. B. Scheibel, *Brain Res.*, **2**, 1966.

[272] F. Walberg and A. Brodal, *J. comp. Neurol.*, **99**, 1953.

[273] P. W. Nathan and M. C. Smith, *J. Neurol. Neurosurg. Psychiat.*, **18**, 1955.

[274] A. Brodal and F. Walberg, *A.M.A. Archs Neurol. Psychiat.*, **68**, 1952.

[275] R. T. Woodburne, E. C. Crosby and R. E. McCotter, *J. comp. Neurol.*, **85**, 1946.

[276] P. W. Nathan and M. C. Smith, *Brain*, **78**, 1955.

[277] O. Pompeiano and A. Brodal, *J. comp. Neurol.*, **108**, 1957.

[278] F. Walberg, D. Bowsher and A. Brodal, *J. comp. Neurol.*, **110**, 1958.

[279] M. Mabuchi and T. Kusama, *Brain Res.*, **2**, 1966.

[280] H. G. J. M. Kuypers and D. G. Lawrence, *Brain Res.*, **4**, 1967.

but its constituent fibres are to some degree dispersed among those of the neighbouring tracts. This description applies to experimental animals, for although there is little doubt that reticulospinal pathways exist in the human spinal cord, there is as yet little direct evidence of this. The lateral reticulospinal tract differs in several characteristics, anatomical and physiological, from the medial tract (p. 819). Its axons are largely derived from large nerve cells in the medullary zone of the brainstem reticular formation (nucleus reticularis gigantocellularis), but also from smaller cells, this origin according with the varying diameters of the reticulospinal fibres. In contrast with the pontine reticulospinal fibres in the anterior funiculus, the lateral tract is largely crossed, but some fibres also remain on their side of origin. Each half of the medullary reticular formation hence exerts a distinctly bilateral effect on the spinal cord. The terminals of the lateral, like the medial reticulospinal tract, form synapses with interneurons in the intermediate grey region and the medial zone of the anterior grey column, but they are more dorsal in position[281] (chiefly lamina VII), though some may reach motor neurons (lamina IX). These details apply chiefly to the cat, and in the same study it was established that reticulospinal fibres descend to all levels of the cord, contrary to earlier views.[282] The medullary origin of the lateral reticulospinal tract approximates in extent to the brainstem 'inhibitory area', and this again contrasts with the facilitatory effect of the medial tract. In addition to these motor influences, which extend to both α and γ neurons in the activities of the medial and lateral tracts, the reticulospinal axons may also modify the transmission of afferent impulses. (See also 7.47 B and p. 838).

(d) **Descending autonomic fibres**, mediating both direct and crossed connexions between brainstem visceral 'centres' and the preganglionic nerve cells of the spinal cord, must obviously exist, as is attested by an abundance of physiological evidence. Nevertheless, accurate knowledge of their positions and terminations in the spinal cord is exiguous and conflicting. That such fibres are predominantly in the lateral funiculus is generally agreed, but it is likely that a smaller number also descend in the anterior funiculus. The failure of experimental efforts to define any compact groups of degenerating nerve fibres in the spinal cord as a result of hypothalamic or brainstem lesions has naturally led to the concept that descending autonomic connexions are diffusely dispersed through the cord. But individual investigations have associated them with the lateral corticospinal, reticulospinal and intersegmental tracts, and have also assigned some of them to a superficial position in the lateral funiculus.[283] The descending pathways are considered to consist for the most part of small-diameter fibres, probably arranged in polysynaptic chains. Since lesions which were supposed to interrupt reticulospinal fibres have been associated with disturbances of visceral function, such as vasomotor and sudomotor control,[284] it is probable that some of these fibres are to be regarded as autonomic. Vasomotor changes can be elicited by stimulation of the precentral area of the cerebral cortex, and there is thus a possibility that some of the corticospinal fibres are autonomic in function. In sum the evidence, much of it negative in character, suggests that the descending autonomic fibres are dispersed through much of the anterolateral region of the cord; hence lesions in any part of this are likely to be associated with disturbance of visceral control.

(e) The **olivospinal tract** (of Helweg) is described in considerable detail in most textbooks, and these descriptions are markedly uniform in assigning it to a small triangular area, as seen in transverse spinal sections, immediately lateral to the most lateral of the issuing ventral root fibres. It is said to be confined to upper cervical segments,

and to contain fibres which end in the ventral grey column, and also fibres which form an ascending *spino-olivary tract* (*see* p. 824).[285] The olivospinal tract was identified in the human spinal cord, but there appears to be no experimental evidence that its axons are in fact derived from the nerve cells of the inferior olivary nucleus.[61] Because of this uncertainty it has been suggested that the tract be named *bulbospinal*, but this merely displaces the uncertainty elsewhere. These conflicting views serve to emphasize the need of further evidence in this matter.

## 2. Ascending Tracts

(a) The **posterior spinocerebellar tract** is a flattened band situated at the periphery of the posterior region of the lateral funiculus; medially it is in contact with the lateral corticospinal tract; dorsally, with the dorsolateral tract. It begins about the level of the second or third lumbar nerve, increases in size as it ascends, and finally passes into the cerebellum through the inferior cerebellar peduncle. Its fibres are the axons of the cells of the ipsilateral thoracic nucleus. This nucleus receives *afferent* impulses from two sources. (1) Many of the long ascending fibres of the posterior funiculus give off collaterals which form synaptic connexions with the cells of the thoracic nucleus. (2) Terminals of the intermediate ascending fibres of the posterior column may behave in the same way, especially in the thoracic segments of the spinal cord. It is uncertain which of these two sources preponderates in the formation of the posterior spinocerebellar tract.

(b) The **anterior spinocerebellar tract**, as seen on transverse section, is a crescentic, flattened tract which occupies the periphery of the lateral funiculus, in front of the area occupied by the posterior spinocerebellar tract. The precise origin of its constituent fibres cannot be regarded as settled, but they are usually said to be derived from the large cells of the posterior grey column. They are therefore secondary neurons on the spinocerebellar pathway. The primary neurons concerned are probably similar to those described above in connexion with the posterior spinocerebellar tract, but the ascending axons of the secondary neurons are mostly derived from the opposite side of the spinal cord, only a small proportion ascending on the ipsilateral side.[286] Recent experimental evidence indicates that the 'secondary neurons' are in fact sited dorsolaterally in the ventral grey column.[287] The tract commences in the upper lumbar region and extends upwards to cranial pontine levels, where it turns to descend dorsally in the superior cerebellar peduncle to reach the cerebellum.

The fibres in the spinocerebellar tracts have a laminated arrangement, with those carrying impulses from the lower limb being placed most superficially.[288, 289] They convey to the cerebellum both exteroceptive and proprioceptive impulses arising in receptors of the skin and locomotor apparatus which are essential for the adjustments of muscle and for synergic control during the performance of voluntary movements. As already stated (p. 813), the thoracic nucleus diminishes in size as it is traced upwards, and does not extend cranial to the first thoracic or last cervical segments. It would appear, therefore, that the posterior

[281] R. Nyberg-Hansen, *Expl Neurol.*, **124**, 1965.
[282] A. Torvik and A. Brodal, *Anat. Rec.*, **128**, 1957.
[283] D. M. Enoch and F. W. L. Kerr, *Archs Neurol. Psychiat., Chicago*, **16**, 1967.
[284] D. A. Johnson, G. M. Roth and W. M. Craig, *J. Neurosurg.*, **9**, 1952.
[285] J. Jansen and A. Brodal, *Aspects of Cerebellar Anatomy*, Grundt Tanum, Oslo. 1954.
[286] J. Jansen and A. Brodal, *Aspects of Cerebellar Anatomy*, Grundt Tanum, Oslo. 1954.
[287] H. Ha and C.-N. Liu, *J. comp. Neurol.*, **133**, 1968.
[288] R. E. Yoss, *J. comp. Neurol.*, **97, 99**, 1952/3.
[289] M. C. Smith, *J. comp. Neurol.*, **108**, 1957.

spinocerebellar tracts are concerned chiefly with the trunk and lower limbs, and evidence has been adduced[290] to show that the corresponding proprioceptive impulses from the upper limbs travel by the posterior external arcuate fibres which originate in the accessory cuneate nucleus in the medulla oblongata (p. 845), forming a *cuneocerebellar tract*. In addition to the classical spinocerebellar pathways there is considerable evidence for at least two indirect projections, interrupted by synapses in the inferior olivary and lateral reticular nuclei of the medulla, both of which have been shown to project to the cerebellum, receiving their afferents respectively from the dorsal funiculi and the spinothalamic tracts. Consult reference [61] for further details and discussion.

It has long been established that the spinocerebellar tracts convey proprioceptive information; more recently physiological evidence has demonstrated that the posterior, or dorsal, tract also mediates impulses from touch and pressure endings. Both tracts display a marked somatotopic termination in the cerebellum in experimental animals, including monkeys, and in man, a topic which will be considered in greater detail later (p. 863). The posterior spinocerebellar tract ends in an area of cerebellar cortex concerned with the hind limb, while its associated cuneocerebellar tract reaches a fore-limb area. The anterior spinocerebellar fibres end in the hind-limb area only; but recent physiological evidence[291, 292] indicates the existence of ascending fibres functionally associated with the anterior spinocerebellar tract and serving tendon stretch receptors in fore-limb muscles; this has been tentatively named the *rostral spinocerebellar tract*.

Some of the neuron somata which contribute to the spinocerebellar tracts have been studied using intracellular recording techniques. Some receive the termination of only one type of exteroceptive or proprioceptive afferent, whilst others show a convergence and interaction of different types of afferent upon single cells. Their impulse transmission characteristics are modified by activity in tracts which descend from the brainstem.

(c) The **lateral spinothalamic tract**, which lies medial to the anterior spinocerebellar tract in the lateral funiculus of the spinal cord, is an exteroceptive pathway conveying information concerned with pain and thermal variations from the opposite side. As mentioned above (p. 819) it is continuous with the anterior spinothalamic tract, and on clinical evidence appears to differ chiefly in the localization of the different 'modalities' of sensory inflow mediated, the anterior tract being concerned with tactile and deep pressure mechanoreception. However, it should be noted that the simple zonal, 'modality-specific' pattern of fibres implied in this view contrasts sharply with the great variation in physiological responses of the cell types investigated in the grey matter laminae IV–VII, some of which probably give rise to spinothalamic fibres. As we shall see (pp. 833, 834), these variations include marked differences in the size, characteristics, specificity and somatotopic mapping of the receptive fields of the different cells, and in the degree of convergence of different functional types of primary afferent fibre on to single interneurons. In view of this, it seems likely that some, at least, of the spinothalamic fibres transmit complex patterns of information, and the assumption that they are all modality specific is certainly an oversimplification. (Reference is made to the possible role of the substantia gelatinosa in the pain pathway on p. 833.)

The somatotopic lamination of the anterior spinothalamic tract is also evident in the lateral. This arrangement is of considerable practical importance to the neurosurgeon, and it is maintained throughout the passage of the lateral tract through the medulla oblongata and the pons. In the midbrain, however, the fibres from the lower limbs extend dorsally, and in this part of their course it is possible for the surgeon to divide the pain and temperature fibres from the upper limb and trunk without injury to the corresponding fibres of the lower limb.[293]

Although it is generally accepted that the lateral spinothalamic tract is the predominant pathway for somatic pain and thermal sensibilities, it has not infrequently been suggested that an alternative pathway may exist and is provided by a series of intersegmental fibres with their neuronal bodies situated in the grey matter of the spinal cord (p. 890). In addition, the spinotectal tract has been regarded by others[294] as an alternative pathway for painful and thermal sensibility.

It is convenient to add at this juncture a brief reference to a so-called *spinocervical tract* and an associated *spinocervico-thalamic system* of connexions. The *lateral cervical nucleus*, though small in man, is an accepted entity and is situated in the lateral funiculus lateral to the dorsal grey column in the upper two cervical segments of the cord. The tract is said to contain fibres derived from nerve cells in the thoracic nucleus (Clarke's column), and from cells in the dorsal and ventral grey columns among those giving rise to axons of the spinocerebellar tracts. It extends upwards from lumbosacral levels. The further projection from the lateral cervical nucleus was at first considered to enter the cerebellum, but the most recent anatomical and physiological studies indicate that the axons from the cells in this nucleus ascend with the medial lemniscus to the nucleus ventralis posterior lateralis of the contralateral thalamus, that they mediate tactile and pressure modalities of sensation (and perhaps also joint sensibility), and are hence for the present to be associated with the spinothalamic system.[295, 296] Interestingly, a column of nerve cells, considered to be identical with the lateral cervical nucleus has been described in the rat as extending throughout the spinal cord.[297]

Little definite information is available concerning the pathway followed by impulses arising in connexion with painful pathological conditions of viscera. It has been clearly shown that the first neuron fibres travel in the splanchnic nerves, and it seems certain that they enter the spinal cord via white rami communicantes and dorsal spinal roots. Whatever pathway they follow in the spinal cord they are all interrupted by the operation of bilateral cordotomy of the lateral funiculi carried out at the level of the first thoracic segment,[298] and on this account it has been suggested that they travel in the lateral spinothalamic tract. The reader should note that, although hitherto defined as being formed by the union of the lateral and anterior spinothalamic tracts, the spinal lemniscus may now be defined more accurately as the brainstem continuation of the lateral spinothalamic tract alone.

Owing to the fact that the fibres which form the lateral spinothalamic tract cross at once, decussating with the corresponding fibres of the opposite side, lesions affecting the commissural area, such as occur in the disease, *syringomyelia*, produce a bilateral loss of pain and thermal sensibilities for the areas represented in the particular segments involved.

[290] A. Ferraro and S. E. Barrera, *Archs Neurol. Psychiat.*, Chicago, **33**, 1935.
[291] O. Oscarsson and N. Uddenberg, *Acta physiol. scand.*, **62**, 1964.
[292] O. Oscarsson, *Physiol. Rev.*, **45**, 1965.
[293] A. Earl Walker, *Archs Neurol. Psychiat.*, Chicago, **48**, 1942.
[294] A. Earl Walker, *Res. Publs Ass. Res. nerv. ment. Dis.*, **23**, 1943.
[295] F. Morin and J. V. Catalano, *J. comp. Neurol.*, **103**, 1955.
[296] H. Ha and C.-N. Liu, *J. comp. Neurol.*, **127**, 1966.
[297] D. G. Gwyn and H. A. Waldron, *Brain Res.*, **10**, 1968.
[298] O. R. Hyndman and J. Wolkin, *Archs Neurol. Psychiat.*, Chicago, **50**, 1943.

(*d*) The **spinotectal tract** is medial to the anterior spino-cerebellar tract and anterior to the lateral spinothalamic tract, the three tracts being intimately related throughout their ascending course in the spinal cord and brainstem. Its constituent fibres arise in the deep grey matter laminae of the opposite side and soon cross the median plane to reach the lateral funiculus. The tract is most easily identified at cervical levels. Its fibres ascend to the mid-brain where they terminate in the superior colliculus of the tectum. They provide an ascending pathway for spino-visual reflexes. In this connection it is to be remembered that the superior colliculi constitute a reflex centre in the visual path and are not concerned with the transmission of visual impulses to the cerebral cortex. Afferent impulses passing up the spinotectal tract result in movements of the head and eyes towards the source of stimulation.

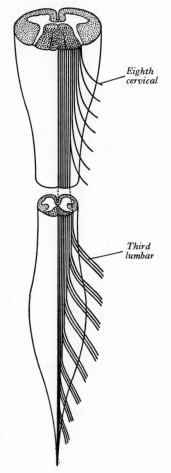

*Eighth cervical*

*Third lumbar*

7.46 Diagram showing the lamination of the fibres in the posterior funiculus. The spinal cord is viewed from the dorsal aspect. The drawing shows that the posterior funiculus is formed by the long ascending fibres of the dorsal roots and that the sacral fibres lie next the median plane, the lumbar to their lateral side, the thoracic more laterally, and the cervical most lateral of all.

However, some fibres of the tract pass onwards to the ventral thalamus, and are considered to mediate cutaneous pain and perhaps other modalities.

(*e*) The **dorsolateral tract** (of Lissauer) is a small strand of fine myelinated and non-myelinated fibres situated between the tip of the posterior grey column and the sur-face of the spinal cord, close to the dorsal roots. It is formed in part by fibres of the lateral bundle of the dorsal roots which bifurcate into ascending and descending branches. The ascending branches travel one or two seg-ments in the tract; they give collaterals to and terminate around cells in the posterior grey column (pp. 830, 832).

Although the dorsolateral tract is present throughout the cord, no fibres travel more than a few segments in it, and it is hence more appropriate to regard it as a *fasciculus*. This is all the more desirable in view of the experimental confirmation,[299, 300, 301] of an old suggestion[302] that the tract contains many propriospinal fibres, the contribu-tion from entering dorsal root fibres amounting to no more than 25 per cent of the total at any particular level.[300] (It is interesting to note that Flechsig's suggestion con-siderably predated Lissauer's descriptions in 1886.) Many of the propriospinal fibres are axons of the small neurons of the substantia gelatinosa (laminae II and III, *see* p. 830).

(*f*) **Spinoreticular fibres** have been described in the lateral funiculus as a result of experiments in the cat;[303] these are intermingled with spinothalamic fibres and hence do not form a discrete identifiable tract. The majority of these ascending fibres do not cross, but there appears to be a generalized and bilateral projection to nuclei at all levels of the brainstem reticular formation, though particularly to those at pontine and medullary levels. The existence of such spinoreticular connexions has also been demonstrated in the human brainstem.[304]

(*g*) The **spino-olivary tract** is described as arising from neurons in the deeper laminae of the spinal grey matter, the axons of which cross the midline and then ascend near the surface of the cord at the junction of the anterior and lateral white funiculi, to terminate in specific 'spinal' regions of the dorsal and medial accessory olivary nuclei.[305] The tract conveys information derived from cutaneous as well as proprioceptive receptors—both muscle and tendon organs.[306] A functionally similar pathway which constitutes a *dorsal spino-olivary system* has been sug-gested on physiological grounds as ascending with the dorsal white funiculi and then relaying in the dorsal column nuclei before projecting on to the accessory olivary nuclei.[307] Interest in these pathways has heightened in company with the increased awareness of the impor-tance of the olivocerebellar system of climbing fibres with their specific localized excitatory effects on the cerebellar Purkinje cells (pp. 860, 869).

### 3. Intersegmental Tracts

The **lateral intersegmental tract** constitutes the re-mainder of the lateral funiculus, separated ventrally from the anterior intersegmental tract by the emerging fibres of the ventral nerve roots. It consists of intersegmental fibres, some of which have passed from the opposite side of the spinal cord and, probably, reticulospinal and descending autonomic fibres.

## TRACTS IN THE POSTERIOR FUNICULUS

### 1. Ascending Tracts

This funiculus comprises two large ascending tracts, the fasciculi gracilis and cuneatus, which are separated from each other by the postero-intermediate septum.

The **fasciculus gracilis** commences at the caudal limit of the spinal cord and is composed mainly of the long ascending branches of the medial bundle of fibres of the

[299] L. J. Poirier and C. Bertrand, *J. comp. Neurol.*, **102**, 1955.
[300] K. M. Earle, *J. comp. Neurol.*, **96**, 1952.
[301] J. Szentágothai, *J. comp. Neurol.*, **122**, 1964.
[302] P. Flechsig, *Die Leitungsbahnen im Gehirn und Rückenmark des Menschen, auf Grund entwicklungsgtschichtlicher Untersuchungen.* Engel-mann, Leipzig. 1876.
[303] A. Brodal, *J. comp. Neurol.*, **91**, 1949.
[304] W. R. Mehler, in: *Basic Research in Paraplegia*, ed. J. D. French and R. W. Porter, Thomas, Springfield, Ill. 1962.
[305] N. Mizuno, *J. comp. Neurol.*, **127**, 1966.
[306] G. Grant and O. Oscarsson, *Expl Brain Res.*, **1**, 1966.
[307] O. Oscarsson, *Brain Res.*, **5**, 1967.

dorsal nerve roots. They run upwards in the posterior funiculus, and as the tract ascends it receives accessions from each dorsal root. The fibres which enter in the coccygeal and lower sacral regions are thrust medially by the fibres which enter at higher levels. The fasciculus gracilis, which contains fibres derived from the lower thoracic, lumbar, sacral and coccygeal segments, occupies the medial part of the posterior funiculus in the upper part of the spinal cord (7.45). The **fasciculus cuneatus** commences in the mid-thoracic region and derives its fibres from the dorsal roots of the upper thoracic and cervical nerves and, in consequence, is situated lateral to the fasciculus gracilis (7.45, 46).

Both fasciculi are heavily myelinated, and the fibres are larger in the fasciculus cuneatus than they are in the fasciculus gracilis. Both fasciculi contain the central processes from cells in the spinal ganglia, i.e. receptor or *primary afferent* neurons, and these pass without interruption or decussation to the medulla oblongata, where they end in the *gracile* and *cuneate nuclei*, in which the second neurons of this pathway begin. The majority of the fibres of the second neurons sweep ventrally round the central grey matter (7.61) as the *internal arcuate fibres*, and take part in the decussation of the lemnisci. Thereafter, as the *medial lemnisci*, they ascend on each side to the ventral nucleus of the thalamus (p. 896) and are there relayed to the cortex of the post-central gyrus (areas 3, 1 and 2). Some of the second neurons form *posterior external arcuate fibres* (p. 845) which pass to the cerebellum.

These two tracts, which occupy nearly the whole of the posterior funiculus, convey proprioceptive sensibility, including vibration and pressure and some elements of exteroceptive tactile sensibility. The fibres concerned all pass up to the medulla oblongata in the ipsilateral posterior funiculi, together with the fibres which convey sensations of posture and of movements, both active and passive. It should also be noted, however, that during their passage in the cord a number of the long ascending dorsal column fibres give rise to a series of collateral branches which enter the dorsal column of spinal grey matter.

The laminar somatotopic pattern of the gracile and cuneate tracts has been shown to be more intricate than the segmental arrangement described above; there is also a segregation of fibres on the basis of modality, those conducting impulses from hair receptors being most superficial, followed by fibres mediating tactile and vibratory sensibility in successively deeper layers.[308] Physiological experimentation has also indicated that the somatotopic arrangement is carried through to the nuclei gracilis and cuneatus, and that these contain numerous interneurons; unit recording in the nuclei shows a high specificity in fibres arriving along the two tracts. Stimuli immediately outside the receptive field from which a single unit can be activated may show an inhibitory effect. There is evidence of a projection of descending fibres from the pre- and post-central cerebral cortex which travel in the corticospinal projection and exert facilitatory and inhibitory influences on the interneurons of the gracile and cuneate nuclei. It is to such modulating effects that the highly discriminative nature of activity in the dorsal funicular pathways is probably due, and these tracts, like others, can no longer be regarded as a simple through route for sensory information. (For further discussion see p. 834).

## 2. Descending Tracts

A somewhat confusing number of small tracts of descending fibres have been described in the dorsal funiculi by a variety of observers, who worked chiefly in the late nineteenth century and based their accounts on pathological appearances in human spinal cords. Thus, extending through cervical and upper thoracic levels, in the medial part of the cuneate tract, is the *comma tract* (of Schultze), also known as the *semilunar tract* or, more recently, the *interfascicular fasciculus*. In lower thoracic segments a thin superficial strand of fibres has been described, but this is almost certainly the cranial end of the *septomarginal tract*, which is ascribed to a deeper situation bordering the posterior median septum. The so-called 'oval field of Flechsig' and the 'triangular field of Gombault and Philippe' are also merely different levels of the septo-marginal tract, which appears to alter its shape and position remarkably as it descends in the cord from lower thoracic segments. It is tempting to assume that the interfascicular fasciculus and septomarginal tract are also continuous, but this remains a matter of doubt. They are reputed to differ in one respect; the former is said to consist only of the descending branches of entering dorsal root fibres, whereas the septomarginal tract is considered to contain also large numbers of intersegmental connexions. It must be emphasized that almost all the literature concerning these descending dorsal column fibres is based on clinical observation, experimental evidence being scant. For an exhaustive review see reference [309].

## 3. Intersegmental Tracts

Occupying the anterior or deepest part of the posterior funiculus is a small strand of fibres named the **posterior intersegmental tract**. It is somewhat crescentic on transverse section, and is just posterior to the grey commissure (7.43, 44); it is best marked in the lumbar region, but can be traced into the thoracic and cervical regions. Its fibres, which are intersegmental, are derived from the cells of the posterior grey column; they divide into ascending and descending branches which re-enter and ramify in the grey matter.

# Further Aspects of Spinal Cord Organization

The more traditional and somewhat simplified account of spinal cord organization given in the preceding pages has been considerably expanded, complemented, and in a number of respects modified, in recent years following the intensive application by many investigators of both the classical and newer methods of neuroanatomy and neurophysiology.[310, 311, 312] Their researches include more detailed comparative studies in a wide array of vertebrates, alternative schemes for the classification of the spinal cord grey matter based upon cytoarchitectonics, and more precise analyses of the dendritic patterns and axonal arborizations using modified Golgi techniques. The more recent degeneration techniques have added considerably to our knowledge of the sites of termination of dorsal spinal nerve root afferent fibres and their collaterals, the siting of terminals of fibre systems which descend from supraspinal levels, and some approach has been made to unravel the exceedingly complex intrinsic organization of the cord by placing minute focal lesions within the grey matter and following subsequent degenerative events in neighbouring regions. Many of these neuroanatomical investigations, based upon light microscopical techniques, have been improved progressively by the

[308] N. Uddenberg, *Expl Brain Res.*, **4**, 1968.
[309] P. W. Nathan and M. C. Smith, *Brain*, **82**, 1959.
[310] J. C. Eccles and J. P. Schadé, *Prog. Brain Res.*, **11**, 1964.
[311] J. C. Eccles and J. P. Schadé, *Prog. Brain Res.*, **12**, 1964.
[312] K. Lissák (ed.), *Results in Neuroanatomy, Neurochemistry, Neuropharmacology, and Neurophysiology*, Akadémiai Kiadó, Budapest. 1967.

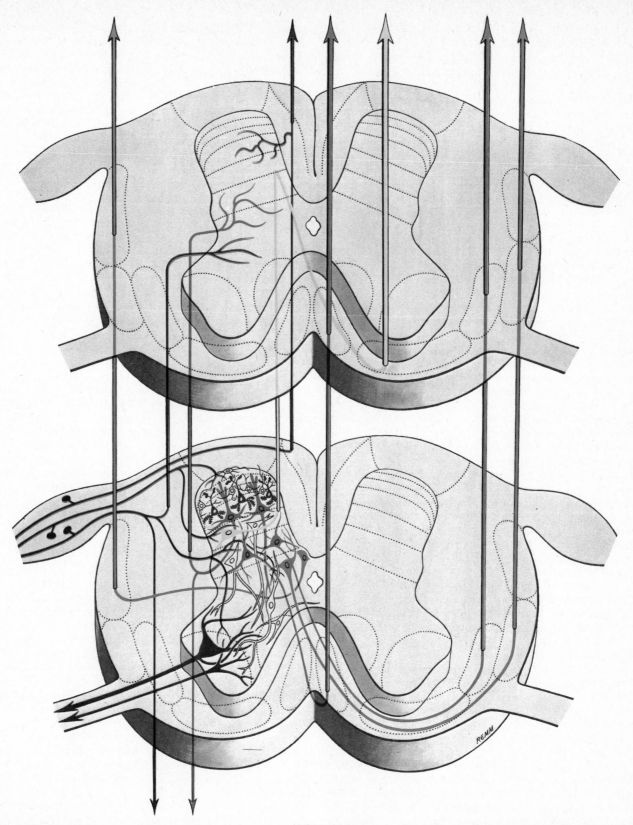

**7.47 A** Scheme of some of the major ascending tract systems of the spinal cord and some features of grey matter organization. Within the grey matter the dotted lines show the laminar pattern, within the white matter they are an approximate guide to the topography of the tracts. Attempts have been made to indicate in a simplified manner the overlapping of dendritic fields described in the text. An alpha and a gamma motor neuron (grey) are included, together with some of the structural features of the substantia gelatinosa which are described and illustrated more fully in 7.49. Some of the small substantia gelatinosa neurons are uncoloured, as are some interneurons in the deeper laminae. The larger substantia gelatinosa neurons are solid black. Large lamina IV cells, and associated ascending and descending intersegmental fibres are green. Primary sensory afferent fibres, including a fibre in the fasciculus gracilis, are purple. Spinotectal fibre—orange; anterior spinothalamic fibre—yellow; lateral spinothalamic fibre—magenta; and dorsal and ventral spinocerebellar fibres—blue.

application of quantitative histological methods, whilst in some regions detailed ultrastructural studies of the synaptic arrangements have provided new data.

This intensified interest in cord morphology has greatly assisted, and equally been assisted by, parallel studies in neurophysiology. In particular, the electrophysiological analyses of the dorsal and ventral spinal nerve root fibres under different conditions, recordings from different points within the grey matter, and unit recordings made with microelectrodes which have impaled single neuron somata, can with some success be correlated with the anatomical findings. As a result, whilst some of the classical views have been substantiated, others have needed a drastic revision and new concepts have been proposed.

## LAMINAR ARCHITECTURE

For many years the *general outline* of the grey matter of the spinal cord as seen in transverse section provided a basis for a terminology used by morphologists and experimentalists alike. In this manner, as we have seen elsewhere (p. 809), dorsal, lateral and ventral columns were recognized. The ventral column was considered to consist of a 'base' and a ventrolateral 'head', whilst the dorsal column was dignified with an 'apex', 'head', 'neck' and 'base' proceeding from dorsal to ventral. Between these, a rather imprecisely defined intermediate zone was recognized, whilst more easily defined subdivisions included the substantia gelatinosa, the thoracic nucleus (Clarke's column) and the various subgroupings of large motor neurons which, in considerable variety, characterize a part of the ventral column (p. 811). Whilst much valuable pioneering work was carried out using this scheme, the increasing volume of experimental analysis, both structural and functional, has revealed a relative lack of precision, proving a hindrance and prompting further attempts to classify cord structure.[313, 314, 315] The most widely adopted scheme stemmed initially from extensive studies using thick as well as the more usual thin sections, stained by the method of Nissl for cell somata, of newborn, young and adult specimens of the feline spinal cord. Based upon observations on the size, shape, packing density, and cytological features of the neurons in different regions of the grey matter, nine *cell layers* or *laminae* have been distinguished which are roughly parallel with the dorsal and ventral surfaces of the grey matter, and which extend throughout the length of the cord, together with a region surrounding the central canal. As an example, the disposition of the laminae as seen in a transverse section through the fifth lumbar segment of the cord is shown in illustration **7.48** A. Briefly the constitution of the cell layers is as follows:

**Lamina I** is an extremely thin layer with an ill-defined boundary adjoining the white matter (within which outlying cell groups occur). It presents a reticular appearance because of the presence of many coarse and fine nerve fibre bundles. It contains small, intermediate and fairly large neuron somata, many being spindle-shaped. Alternative names proposed are *lamina marginalis* or the *layer of Waldeyer*[316] (who recognized a similar zone in 1888).

**Lamina II** consists of tightly-packed small cells crossed, especially medially, by numerous fibre bundles which enter from the dorsal funiculus. An outer (dorsal) zone, which appears darkly stained because of its high density of the smallest cells, stands in contrast to an inner (ventral) pale zone.

**Lamina III** consists of neuron somata which are in general larger, more variable in shape and less closely packed than those in lamina II.

**Lamina IV**, thicker than the preceding layers, is a loosely packed, heterogeneous zone permeated by many fibres. The cell somata vary greatly in size and shape, from small and round, through intermediate and triangular, to very large star-shaped profiles.

Laminae I–IV correspond to the general term *head* of the dorsal column of previous workers. Lamina II (and some workers consider in addition part or all of lamina III) correspond to the *substantia gelatinosa* of earlier accounts, whilst the imprecisely defined *nucleus proprius* of the dorsal column roughly corresponds to some of the cell constituents of laminae III and IV.

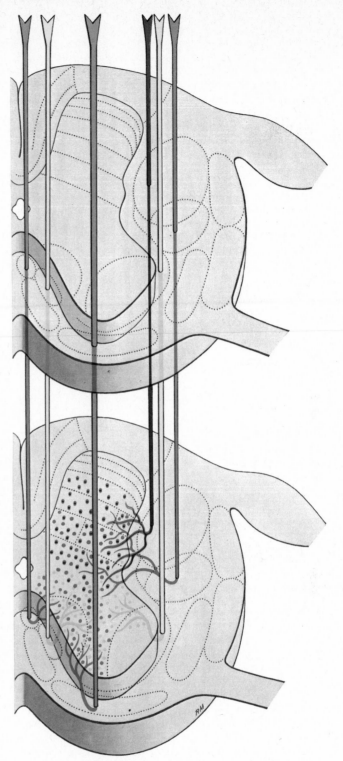

**7.47** B A scheme of some of the major descending tract systems of the spinal cord including their overlapping zones of termination in the grey matter. The significance of the dotted lines is the same as for **7.47** A. Corticospinal tract—mauve; rubrospinal tract—magenta; reticulospinal tracts—yellow; vestibulospinal tracts—blue.

**Lamina V**, a thick layer which includes the *neck* of the dorsal column, is divisible into a lateral one-third and a medial two-thirds. Both have a mixed population of cell somata, but the former contains a large number of prominent well-stained cells interlaced by numerous

[313] B. Rexed, *J. comp. Neurol.*, **96**, 1952.
[314] B. Rexed, *J. comp. Neurol.*, **100**, 1954.
[315] B. Rexed, *Prog. Brain Res.*, **11**, 1964.
[316] H. Waldeyer, *Das Gorilla—Rückenmark*, Akademie der Wissenschaften, Berlin. 1888.

bundles of nerve fibres running transversely, dorsoventrally and longitudinally—hence the restricted use of the term 'formatio reticularis' for this region, particularly well seen in the cervical region, and recognized for over a century.[317] (It should be noted, however, that in modern neurology the term *reticular formation* is used much more widely—p. 888.)

**Lamina VI**, most easily recognized in the limb enlargements, particularly of young animals, consists of a medial one-third of small tightly-packed cells and a lateral two-thirds which possesses larger triangular or star-shaped cells, more loosely packed. Accordingly, in lamina VI the medial zone stains more heavily than the lateral zone, in contrast to lamina V where the converse applies. Lamina VI corresponds roughly to the topographical *base* of the dorsal column.

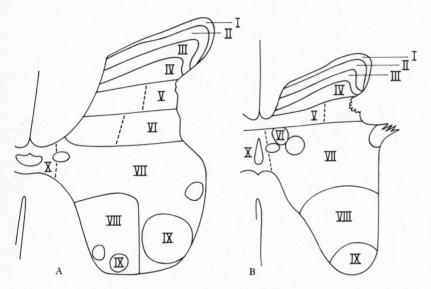

7.48 A and B The pattern of lamination proposed by B. Rexed (*Progress in Brain Research*, Vol. II) for the spinal cord grey matter of the cat, viewed in transverse section. A the fifth lumbar segment. B the third thoracic segment. (With the permission of the author and the Elsevier Publishing Company.)

Laminae VII–IX present a variety of complex forms in the limb enlargements (7.48 A), and to assist understanding the simpler arrangement found at thoracic levels is included for comparison (7.48 B).

**Lamina VII**—this corresponds to much of the *intermediate grey column* or *zone* of previous authors. Within its confines it includes the prominent cells of the *thoracic nucleus* (Clarke's column) and the *intermediomedial* and *intermediolateral cell columns* at appropriate levels in the spinal cord—these have been detailed elsewhere (p. 813). The remaining large areas of lamina VII (i.e. between these cell columns and, in the limb enlargements, extending ventrally between lamina VIII and the constituent groups of IX) consist of a rather homogeneous population of medium-sized triangular or star-shaped cell somata.

**Lamina VIII** spans the base of the thoracic ventral column, but in the limb enlargements it is restricted to its medial aspect. It consists of a heterogeneous mixture of cell sizes and shapes from small to moderately large.

**Lamina IX** comprises the complex array of cell columns (p. 811) which include the very large somata of the α motor neurons, and numerous smaller cells. The smaller cells include motor neurons which give rise to the small-diameter efferent fibres (γ efferents) to the muscle spindles, and numerous interneurons some of

which may be the inhibitory Renshaw cells (*vide infra*). The location of the γ motor neurons was long in doubt, but studies of the retrograde changes in the cell somata following section of peripheral nerves[318] and intracellular recording with microelectrodes[319] have demonstrated that these cells are dispersed between the α motor neurons within the motor cell columns. The precise location and morphology of the Renshaw cells, however, is still rather uncertain. Intracellular microelectrode recordings have indicated the presence of inhibitory interneurons in the ventral extension of cell lamina VII, where it is insinuated between laminae VIII and IX.[320] Studies of this region with Golgi technique[321] has failed to demonstrate typical Golgi type II neurons (with profuse, short, local arborizations of their axons)—the cell type long assumed to be the basis of Renshaw loop inhibition. Nevertheless, another view has been expressed, namely that neurons with longer axons are not incompatible with such an inhibitory function, and further, that the ventral extension of lamina VII receives the greatest density of initial collateral branches from the axons of the α motor neurons (and which are assumed to synapse with the Renshaw cells).[322]

The remaining area of grey matter **(lamina X)** surrounds the central canal, and consists of the *dorsal* and *ventral grey commissures* and the *substantia gelatinosa centralis.*

## FURTHER ASPECTS OF SPINAL LAMINAR ARCHITECTURE

It must be emphasized that the preceding description is the barest outline of the proposed scheme of classification and for further details the extensive original papers quoted should be consulted.

It should also be noted that the scheme only applies in full to the spinal cord of the *cat* and no comparably detailed study has yet been carried out on the spinal cord of man or any other primate. Nevertheless, the same general principles of laminar organization (with doubtless considerable variation in detail) are considered to apply to the spinal cords of all higher mammals.[323] The originator of the scheme proposed the following tentative functional analysis of the laminar pattern (although a number of his conclusions have been revised by subsequent workers—see below).

Laminae I–IV were considered the main receiving areas for the cutaneous exteroceptive primary afferent fibre terminals and collateral branches. (For further details of this sensory input, see below.) From this region are initiated many complex polysynaptic reflex paths, both ipsilateral and contralateral, and both intrasegmental and intersegmental. It was also considered that from this region arise many of the long ascending tracts to higher centres (but see below for further discussion and alternative points of view).

Laminae V and VI were thought to receive most of the terminals from proprioceptive primary afferents and also profuse connexions from corticospinal fibres descending from the motor and sensory regions of the cerebral cortex, and descending systems from other sub-cortical centres.

[317] O. Deiters, *Untersuchungen über Gehirn und Rückenmark des Menschen und der Säugethiere*, Vieweg, Braunschweig. 1865.
[318] R. Nyberg-Hansen, *Expl Neurol.*, **13**, 1965.
[319] J. C. Eccles, R. M. Eccles, I. Iggo and A. Lundberg, *Acta physiol. scand.*, **50**, 1960.
[320] W. D. Willis and J. C. Willis, *Archs ital. Biol.*, **104**, 1966.
[321] M. E. Scheibel and A. B. Scheibel, *Archs ital. Biol.*, **104**, 1966.
[322] J. Szentágothai, in: *Recent Advances in Clinical Neurophysiology, Electroenceph. clin. Neurophysiol.*, suppl. 25 (ed. L. Widén), Elsevier, Amsterdam. 1967.
[323] B. Rexed, *Prog. Brain Res.*, **11**, 1964.

Accordingly, these laminae were regarded as being of great importance in the detailed regulation of movement patterns.

Lamina VII in its lateral part has extensive ascending and descending connexions with midbrain centres and the cerebellum (e.g. via spinocerebellar, spinotectal, spinoreticular, tectospinal, reticulospinal and rubrospinal tracts, and is hence of importance in the regulation of posture and movement. The medial part of lamina VII has a wealth of propriospinal reflex connexions with neighbouring regions of grey matter and adjacent segments concerned both with movement patterns and autonomic functions (p. 907). As we have seen, the ventral extension of lamina VII may be in part occupied by inhibitory interneurons (Renshaw cells—pp. 751, 828).[324, 325]

Lamina VIII again consists of a mass of propriospinal interneurons receiving terminals from adjacent laminae, profuse commissural terminals from the contralateral lamina VIII, and descending pathway terminals from interstitiospinal, reticulospinal, and vestibulospinal tracts, and the medial longitudinal fasciculus. Their axons influence both contralateral and ipsilateral motor neuron pools, perhaps directly, but more probably by an excitatory action on the small motor neurons which supply $\gamma$-efferent fibres to the muscle spindles.

Lamina IX consists of an admixture of $\alpha$ and $\gamma$ motor neurons and also many interneurons.

The large $\alpha$ *motor neurons* supply the motor end plates of the extrafusal muscle fibres in the *motor units* of striated muscle (p. 482). They vary in size and physiological recording techniques have demonstrated two varieties, *tonic* and *phasic* $\alpha$ neurons.[326] The former have a lower rate of impulse firing, a lower conduction velocity in their axons, and are assumed to be dimensionally smaller. Attempts have also been made to correlate these varieties with different structural and functional types of striated muscle fibre, e.g. *slow* and *fast* muscle—see p. 480. However, as yet there is no histological means of differentiating these types of $\alpha$ motor neuron. Additionally, some of the large motor neurons (sometimes termed $\beta$ *motor neurons*) have been considered to supply both extrafusal and intrafusal muscle fibres.

Similarly, there are at least two physiologically distinct types of $\gamma$ *motor neuron*, the axons of which (fusimotor fibres) innervate the intrafusal fibres of the muscle spindles. It has been shown that the 'static' and 'dynamic' responses of muscle spindles (p. 802) are subject to separate control mechanisms mediated by *static* and *dynamic fusimotor fibres* which are distributed to *nuclear chain* and *nuclear bag* intrafusal fibres respectively. However, again it has proved impossible to differentiate the types of $\gamma$ motor neuron somata histologically, although two types of neuromuscular junction—*plate endings* and *trail endings*—have been recognized, as have two varieties of $\gamma$-efferent myelinated nerve fibre ($\gamma$ *1* and $\gamma$ *2*) in peripheral nerves to muscle.[327] How closely these varieties can be correlated has been disputed.

## THE GEOMETRY OF SPINAL NEURONS

Since the unrivalled pioneering investigations of Cajal[328], which foreshadowed so much of what was to follow and, indeed, remain today a primary source of information, there has gradually accumulated a volume of increasingly precise data on the form of spinal neurons. As we have seen, much has been learned from a study of the sizes, shapes, distribution, packing density and cytological characteristics of *cell somata* following staining by the Nissl technique or one of its modifications. However, as has been emphasized, such techniques provide only

limited information and they must be supplemented by alternative techniques which allow analyses, preferably in quantitative terms, of the patterns of dendritic ramifications, and of the courses, arborizations and sites of termination of axons and their collateral branches. Furthermore, degenerative techniques are necessary for a precise determination of their connexions with other cells.

Excellent examples of such quantitative approaches may be found in footnote references [329, 330] in which the lumbosacral regions of the spinal cord of the cat were studied. Whilst the results cannot be examined in detail here, they contained the following kind of information. In the ventral zone of the ventral column of one complete spinal segment (lumbar 6) there was a total neuron population of about 7,000; of these 700 were considered to be the small cells from which the $\gamma$-efferent fibres to the muscle spindles originated; of the larger cells 3,276 were propriospinal (interneurons), 126 were classified as 'spinal border' cells, whilst 2,898 were $\alpha$ motor neurons. Thus, in this region about half the cells were interneurons and half motor neurons; if the whole ventral column is assessed, the ratio is about 7 interneurons to 1 motor neuron, and if the intermediate zone and base of the dorsal column are included also, the ratio rises to about 13 to 1. Neuron packing density was estimated and was highest in the intermediate zone of grey matter (7 cells per 100 $\mu$m cube of tissue) and lowest in the ventral column (1–2 cells per 100 $\mu$m cube). The *total* surface area of individual cell somata and associated dendrites ranged from 11,000 to 97,000 $\mu$m$^2$, whereas the surface area of the *cell somata* alone ranged up to 25,000 $\mu$m$^2$; the number of stem dendrites varied up to a maximum of 13, whilst *dendritic* surface area ranged up to about 76,000 $\mu$m$^2$. In this study the dendrite surfaces formed up to 80 per cent of the total receptive surface of the neuron, dendrites sometimes extending as far as 1,000 $\mu$m from the parent soma, in which cases the terminal dendrites passed into the adjacent white matter, as much as 50 per cent of the estimated receptor surface of the neuron being more than 300 $\mu$m from the parent cell body. The latter figure is particularly interesting, since many types of neuron have very wide arborizations of their dendritic trees; but neurophysiological evidence[331] has cast doubt on the possible effectiveness of synapses situated at distances greater than 300 $\mu$m from the soma; their functional role still remains to be determined. In the second series of investigations cited[330] estimates were provided of the percentage of grey matter occupied by cell somata and their surface areas, and the percentage occupied by dendrites and their surface areas. A mean value of 7,500 $\mu$m$^3$ was estimated for the volume of the soma of an interneuron, and 29,000 $\mu$m$^3$ for the soma of a motor neuron. The surface area of the 'average' cell body ranged from $4·4$ to $5·9 \times 10^3$ $\mu$m$^2$ and that of the 'average' dendritic tree from 59 to $73 \times 10^3$ $\mu$m$^2$ in different specimens.

Other investigations[332, 333] have also been concerned with the complex dendritic patterns of ventral column motor neurons and of interneurons located in adjacent

[324] B. Renshaw, *J. Neurophysiol.*, **4**, 1941.

[325] B. Renshaw, *J. Neurophysiol.*, **9**, 1946.

[326] R. Granit, H. D. Henatsch and G. Steg, *Acta physiol. scand.*, **37**, 1956.

[327] I. A. Boyd, *Phil. Trans. R. Soc. Ser. B*, **245**, 1962.

[328] S. Ramón y Cajal, *Histologie du système nerveux de l'homme et des vertébrés*, Vol. 1, Maloine, Paris. 1909.

[329] J. T. Aitken and J. E. Bridger, *J. Anat.*, **95**, 1961.

[330] J. P. Schadé, *Prog. Brain Res.*, **11**, 1964.

[331] J. C. Eccles, *The Physiology of the Nerve Cell*, Johns Hopkins Press, Baltimore. 1957.

[332] G. J. Romanes, *Prog. Brain Res.*, **11**, 1964.

[333] J. M. Sprague and H. Ha, *Prog. Brain Res.*, **11**, 1964.

cell laminae. Emphasis is placed upon the wide arborization of the dendrites of the motor neurons, seen to best advantage when both transverse and particularly longitudinal sections are examined. Not only do the dendrites of adjacent cells interlace horizontally in complicated patterns, but they also spread even more widely, overlapping the territories of other motor neuron cell columns; some penetrate adjacent cell laminae (VII and VIII), inter-weaving with their dendrites and cell somata, whilst still others pass quite deeply into the superjacent white matter, weaving between the longitudinal myelinated nerve fibres and terminating at varying depths (sometimes

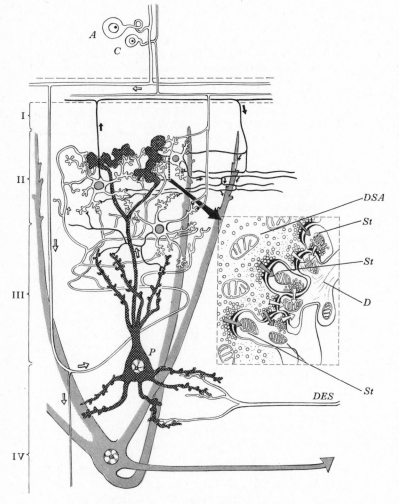

**7.49** Diagram of the arrangement of neurons and their interconnexions in a longitudinal section through the dorsal grey column of the spinal cord, which includes the substantia gelatinosa and adjacent neuronal laminae (Roman numerals I–IV). Inset (right) shows synaptic detail of the area indicated. Two primary sensory afferent fibres are shown: a cutaneous afferent of large calibre (A), and a small calibre non-myelinated afferent (C). Small substantia gelatinosa interneurons are in white with black outline; their axons are single black lines. A pyramidal cell with dendrites and spines, and a recurrent axon expanding into synaptic complexes is shown in black with white dots. A large multipolar neuron of lamina IV with long radial dendrites and initial axon is in cross-hatch. DES—axon descending from a supraspinal source. Arrows on main diagram show presumed direction of impulse conduction. Note (1) the different sites of synaptic termination of primary afferents A and C, (2) the axonal pattern and terminals of substantia gelatinosa interneurons, and (3) the synaptic complexes formed between the recurrent axon expansions of the pyramidal cell, the small gelatinosa interneuron dendrites, and the primary sensory axon terminals. See inset for details: DSA—pyramidal cell axon terminal; D—dendrite of gelatinosa interneuron; St—primary afferent fibre axon terminal; white arrows—axodendritic synapses; cross-hatched arrows—axoaxonic synapses. Consult text for a discussion of the 'gate' theory and structural details. (By courtesy of Professor J. Szentágothai and *Experimental Brain Research*.)

one-third to one-half the thickness of the white matter is traversed).[332] Even more prominent is the longitudinal spread of dendritic branches from α motor neurons which occurs within their cell column of origin, and which may overlap the territories of many hundreds of neighbouring motor neurons. Again, these observations raise the question of the functional role of axodendritic synapses far removed from the cell soma. Clearly, the causal mechanisms responsible for the relatively circumscribed grouping of motor neuron *somata* into cell columns contrasts sharply with those related to the development of interlacing *dendritic fields*. The significance of the latter is by no means clear but attempts have been made to interpret the patterns of overlap in terms of the geometry of the terminals of primary afferent fibres from muscle nerves, and those of the interneurons in the adjacent cell laminae, both of which spread longitudinally for distances of three or four spinal cord segments (for details consult footnote references [333, 334]).

A further detailed study of the dendritic fields in spinal cord grey matter has recently been published[335] whilst particular regions which have been the subject of intensive study include the *thoracic nucleus* (Clarke's column)[336, 337] and the *substantia gelatinosa*.[338, 339]

The general arrangement of neurons in the **substantia gelatinosa** is as follows. The neurons of the thin lamina I usually possess large dendritic networks which spread tangentially across the dorsal aspect of the dorsal grey column, where they interdigitate with the deepest fibres of the dorsolateral (Lissauer's) tract and some of the dorsal nerve root afferents; their axons ramify in the subjacent laminae. The small neurons of lamina II and the somewhat larger ones of lamina III have predominantly radially disposed dendrites (i.e. they occur in longitudinal 'sheets' which are perpendicular to the surface of the dorsal column); possibly a few of their axons may pass ventrally to the deeper laminae but the vast majority remain within the substantia gelatinosa (*vide infra*). These fine axons ramify immediately, either after ascending or descending a short distance within lamina II or after passing briefly into the dorsolateral tract and then returning to either lamina II or III. Between the radial dendrites of the small cells are two other principal components also radially disposed—the terminal parts of the long dendrites of the larger, more deeply situated cells of lamina IV and the terminal branches of many primary afferent cutaneous dorsal nerve root fibres. The small-diameter non-myelinated afferents approach the substantia gelatinosa from its dorsal aspect and their terminal branches point ventrally, whilst the larger diameter afferents curve around the substantia and approach it from its ventral aspect, their terminals point dorsally.

Recently another detailed study of the substantia gelatinosa has been carried out, based upon the Golgi technique and ultrastructural methods, combined with either dorsal root transection or chronic surgical isolation of the dorsal grey column. The morphology of the neurons in laminae II and III were studied, and particular reference was made to a larger pyramidal type of neuron sited at the junctional zone between laminae III and IV. The latter possess recurrent axons which pass into lamina II, where they expand to form the core of large *glomerular*

[334] P. Sterling and H. G. J. M. Kuypers, *Brain Res.*, **4**, 1967.

[335] M. A. Scheibel and A. B. Scheibel, *Brain Res.*, **9**, 1968.

[336] J. Szentágothai and A. Albert, *Acta morph. Acad. Sci. hung.*, **5**, 1955.

[337] C. C. Böhme, *The Fine Structure of Clark's Nucleus of the Spinal Cord*, Thesis, University of Pennsylvania, 1962.

[338] J. Szentágothai, *J. comp. Neurol.*, **122**, 1964.

[339] H. J. Ralston, *Z. Zellforsch. mikrosk. Anat.*, **67**, 1965.

*synaptic complexes*. These glomeruli contain axodendritic synapses between the pyramidal cell axons and the dendrites of the small gelatinosa cells, and axoaxonic contacts between the pyramidal cell axons and the terminals of primary dorsal root afferent fibres. The principal structural features of these synapses, together with some synaptic details of the input from primary dorsal root afferents, the axonal ramifications and terminals of the small gelatinosa neurons, the main output channel via lamina IV neurons, and terminals of fibres descending from supraspinal sources, are summarized in illustration **7.49** which is taken from footnote reference [340]; this should be consulted for further details. Consideration of the possible functional significance of this arrangement is given in subsequent paragraphs.

## THE SITES OF TERMINATION OF DORSAL ROOT AFFERENT FIBRES

The mode of formation, general topography, and division into a lateral fine-fibred and a medial coarse-fibred bundle of a dorsal spinal nerve root have been described elsewhere (p. 824), Consideration has also been given to the manner in which these fibres divide into ascending and descending branches, each of which gives rise to a series of collateral branches which approach the grey matter of the dorsal column at various levels over a substantial length of the cord, the longest ascending branches of the medial division proceeding as far as the gracile and cuneate nuclei in the medulla. In the present section, the zones of termination of these dorsal root fibres in the various regions of the spinal grey matter are discussed.

There have been two principal approaches to this problem: anatomical and neurophysiological. In the former, the fields of termination of fibres at different levels have been followed by application of the techniques of Glees and Nauta after severance of individual dorsal roots and the elapse of appropriate time intervals to allow terminal degeneration to occur. In the latter, the focal electrical potentials generated in the spinal grey matter have been explored by using microelectrodes to record the results of stimulation of muscle and cutaneous nerves and dorsal nerve roots.

In relation to degeneration studies a number of points should be noted. Extensive and informative studies of dorsal root terminals[341, 342] have been carried out on the spinal cord of the *cat* (although similar general principles probably apply to all higher mammals, *details* cannot be applied without reserve to the spinal cord of man). The authors relate their findings to the laminar architecture of the grey matter described previously (p. 827), and include a critical review of the limitations and advantages of the Nauta technique. It is pointed out that the degenerating terminals seen are only those in association with cell somata and dendrite trunks, whereas the branches of the dendrites of many neurons radiate widely from the cell (p. 830). Since the dendrites are encrusted with synaptic contacts throughout their length,[343-348] numbering some thousands in large neurons, and since these are not revealed by the degeneration techniques mentioned, it is essential to correlate such studies with others carried out using the Golgi techniques.

The fields of termination of fibres examined after section of the sixth right lumbar dorsal spinal nerve root in the cat is shown at three levels (spinal cord segments, lumbar 5, 6 and 7) in illustration **7.**50 A, B, C. These findings are briefly summarized as follows.

All the large calibred fibres of the dorsal funiculus (excepting some of the medially placed ones) have collaterals which pass through the medial two-thirds of laminae I, II and III, many curving around the medial aspect of these laminae and these form a dense plexus of degenerating fibres of passage (in transit to other regions) and degenerating terminals around the majority of the cells in the broad lamina IV. Many of the fibres of passage recurve to approach the substantia gelatinosa from its ventral aspect, into which they pass, forming numerous degenerating terminals between the radially disposed dendrites of the small cells of laminae II and III and the terminal segments of the long dorsally directed dendrites from lamina IV.

Degeneration occurs in the fine fibres of the dorsolateral tract for distances of three segments both cranial and caudal to the level of the severed root, and from these, collaterals pass directly into laminae I, II and III, in all of which they form degenerating terminals.

From lamina IV many larger fibres pass to the medial zones of V and VI (a region containing commissural interneurons), whilst many others form a rich mass of degenerating terminals in the central zone of laminae V and VI. From this central concentration 'fingers' of degenerating terminals radiate through laminae VII and VIII and, running with them, are fibres of passage which then converge upon the various motor neuron pools and their associated interneurons, which constitute lamina IX. It has been demonstrated[341] that degenerating synaptic terminals from dorsal root afferents terminate both on the cell somata and the dendritic surfaces of the large multipolar motor neurons where they are interspersed between the numerous terminals derived from interneurons in other laminae and at other levels in the cord. In the cat such monosynaptic terminals of dorsal root afferents on motor neurons were found to extend for two segments cranial and caudal to the severed root, whereas terminals on interneurons in other laminae were also identified one or two segments even more cranial or caudal to this. Similar extensive studies have also been carried out on the spinal cord of the rhesus monkey.[349, 350] In a number of respects the findings correspond with those in the cat, but a number of differences in detail have also emerged, but will not be discussed here; the interested reader should consult the footnote references quoted.

In recent years there have been numerous attempts to correlate the architectural features of the spinal cord grey matter derived from Nissl, Golgi, and degeneration techniques, of the kind detailed in the preceding pages, with more critical analyses of the sites of origin and termination of the tract systems in the white matter, with the exceedingly complex array of propriospinal interneurons, and with electrophysiological studies of their functional activities. In relation to the latter a voluminous literature has accumulated which lies outside the scope of the present volume. Only a few points can be mentioned briefly and superficially here, and further details may be sought in the readily available review articles and original publications in this field, for example [351, 352]

[340] M. Réthelyi and J. Szentágothai, *Expl Brain Res.*, **7**, 1969.

[341] J. M. Sprague, *Proc. R. Soc. B.*, **149**, 1958.

[342] J. M. Sprague and H. Ha, *Prog. Brain Res.*, **11**, 1964.

[343] J. Armstrong, K. C. Richardson and J. Z. Young, *Stain Technol.*, **31**, 1956.

[344] R. W. G. Wyckoff and J. Z. Young, *Proc. R. Soc. B.*, **144**, 1956.

[345] G. L. Rasmussen, in: *New Research Techniques of Neuroanatomy*, W. F. Windle (ed.), Thomas, Springfield. 1957.

[346] J. Z. Young, *Electroenceph. clin. Neurophysiol.*, suppl. **10**, 1958.

[347] L. Illis, *Brain*, **87**, 1964.

[348] S. Gelfan and A. F. Rapisarda, *J. comp. Neurol.*, **123**, 1964.

[349] J. E. Shriver, B. M. Stein and M. B. Carpenter, *Am. J. Anat.*, **123**, 1968.

[350] M. B. Carpenter, B. M. Stein and J. E. Shriver, *Am. J. Anat.*, **123**, 1968.

[351] J. C. Eccles, *The Physiology of the Nerve Cell*, Johns Hopkins Press, Baltimore. 1957.

[352] J. C. Eccles and J. P. Schadé (eds.), *Prog. Brain Res.*, **12**, 1964.

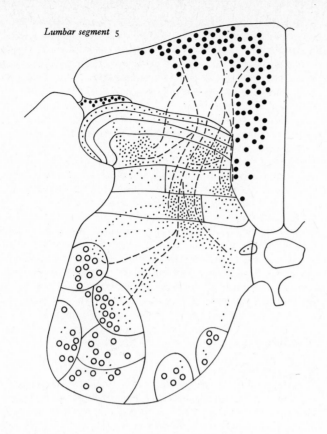

*Lumbar segment 5*

A

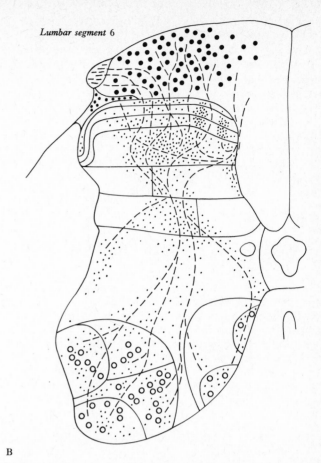

*Lumbar segment 6*

B

7.50 A–C The pattern of degeneration of nerve fibres and their terminals, demonstrated with the Nauta-Laidlaw technique in the ipsilateral half of the spinal cord at various segmental levels, five days after surgical division of the *sixth* lumbar dorsal spinal nerve root of the cat. A the fifth lumbar segment; B the sixth lumbar segment; and C the seventh lumbar segment. The large dots indicate degeneration of fibres in the dorsal funiculus; intermediate dots—degenerating fibres in the dorso-lateral tract of Lissauer; fine dots—degenerating nerve terminals;

## SOME NEUROPHYSIOLOGICAL CORRELATES

In addition to providing a most convenient site in which to study the sequence of cytological changes which follow the severance of their axons (p. 759), the large multipolar neurons of the motor columns in lamina IX of the spinal cord formed the basis for Sherrington's classical study of the characteristics of reflex responses.[353] During this emerged the first clear evidence of *integrative* activities occurring at the contact points between neurons, and the foundations for the concepts of opposing *excitatory* and *inhibitory* action were laid. Subsequently the large size and position of the somata of these cells enabled investigators to impale them with microelectrodes. The additional fact that they can be caused to fire volleys of nerve impulses (or to be inhibited from so doing) *orthodromically* by the stimulation of appropriate peripheral nerves or dorsal nerve roots, and that they can be invaded *antidromically* by stimulation of ventral nerve roots was of great assistance to experimentalists. These means have made possible detailed analyses of the electrical and ionic events which occur at synapses during the generation of *excitatory* and *inhibitory postsynaptic potentials*. Similarly, the early recognition of inhibitory interneurons[324, 325] (Renshaw cells—p.828), in the neighbourhood of the large motor neurons, has led to an increasing volume of enquiry into *lateral* and *feedback* inhibitory phenomena, not only in the spinal cord but at many other cell stations throughout the nervous system.

Since 1940 much evidence has accumulated concerning another form of inhibitory action, namely *presynaptic inhibition*, in which spinal neurons have, again, provided a major experimental source (for reviews see footnote reference [354]). In presynaptic inhibition the synaptic terminals (A) which impinge upon a neuron (B) are themselves subjected to the action of synaptic terminals (C) from an inhibitory interneuron, i.e. there exist axoaxonic synapses. When the inhibitory terminals (C) are active they are held to cause a relative depolarization of terminals (A), thus reducing the effectiveness of the latter in causing a postsynaptic change in neuron (B). Usually two or more interneurons are interposed on a presynaptic inhibitory pathway. Further, in common with postsynaptic excitatory and inhibitory phenomena, presynaptic inhibition may be mediated by fibre system terminals which have descended from supraspinal sources.

Once thought to be uncommon, *presynaptic inhibitory effects* have now been demonstrated in relation to all varieties of primary afferent fibre terminals. In this manner the flow of sensory information into the nervous system does not simply and directly reflect environmental changes; it is continually readjusted and modified at the first synapse depending upon local conditions in the grey matter. A particularly interesting and intensively investigated site at which presynaptic effects occur is the substantia gelatinosa (laminae II and III).[355–359] The anatomy of this region has been described elsewhere (pp. 813, 830) and it has been proposed as a mechanism whereby

[353] C. S. Sherrington, *The Integrative Action of the Nervous System*, Scribner, New York. 1906.

[354] J. C. Eccles, *Prog. Brain Res.*, **12**, 1964.

[355] P. D. Wall, *J. Physiol., Lond.*, **172**, 1964.

[356] L. M. Mendell and P. D. Wall, *J. Physiol., Lond.*, **172**, 1964.

[357] R. Melzack and P. D. Wall, *Science, N.Y.*, **150**, 1965.

[358] L. M. Mendell, *Expl Neurol.*, **16**, 1966.

[359] L. Heimer and P. D. Wall, *Expl Brain Res.*, **6**, 1968.

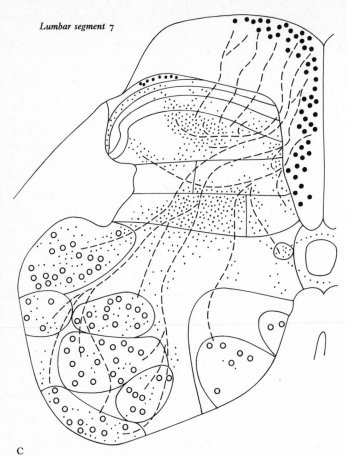

*Lumbar segment 7*

C

dashed lines—degenerating fibres of passage. (From J. M. Sprague and H. Ha, *Progress in Brain Research*, Vol. II, with the permission of the authors and the Elsevier Publishing Company.)

inflowing impulses from cutaneous afferents are subjected to a *tonic control mechanism* involving relative levels of depolarization and hyperpolarization of the primary afferent fibre terminals. The effect is thought to be mediated by the small and pyramidal cells of the substantia gelatinosa, but the precise synaptic mechanisms at work are still the subject of much research.[360] An interesting theory concerning the possible mode of operation of this system, in providing a 'gate' in relation to the inflow of impulses along pain and other afferent pathways, is summarized in 7.51, based on data in footnote reference [357], which should be consulted for further details. Briefly, it is proposed that large-diameter afferents (e.g. from hairs and touch corpuscles) are excitatory to both small gelatinosa interneurons (SG) and to the larger neurons (T-cells) of the deeper lamina IV (from which, directly or indirectly, spinothalamic fibres arise). In contrast, small-diameter and non-myelinated afferents are excitatory to the T cells but inhibitory to the SG cells, whilst the axons of the latter, it is proposed, can exert presynaptic inhibition upon the terminals of all afferents which synapse with the T-cells. Within such a system, a low level of activity in the small-diameter afferents inhibits the SG cells, which therefore cannot inhibit the T-cells, and thus the gate to the lamina IV T-cells is open and will transmit intermittent small volleys of impulses from the large fibres. A prolonged high-frequency volley of impulses in the large-diameter afferents, however, will be transmitted to lamina IV T-cells initially, but this soon ceases as activity in the SG cells closes the gate. Conversely, a persistent high level of activity in the small-calibre afferents will open the gate wide resulting in a massive bombardment of the lamina IV cells. The latter include

some high threshold cells which are only activated by such an intense bombardment, and it is thought that onward transmission from these cells over the lateral spinothalamic tract will be appreciated as pain in supraspinal centres. In this concept, therefore, pain results from the imbalance between varieties of inflowing impulses which occurs when there is a disproportionately large traffic along the small-diameter afferents. The latter, perhaps, are not to be regarded as 'specific pain afferents' but as the fibre system which continually monitors the *state of the tissues* innervated.

Other varieties of electrophysiological investigation have involved the exploration of the spinal grey matter with microelectrodes during the stimulation of muscle and cutaneous nerves,[361, 362] and during the 'natural' stimulation of peripheral receptors.[363, 364] The focal extracellular potentials evoked by such means correspond well with certain specific regions of the grey matter laminae and with the areas of termination of dorsal root afferent fibres determined by degeneration techniques. For further details the references quoted should be consulted.

## UNIT RECORDING WITH INTRACELLULAR MICROELECTRODES

Physiological recordings made with microelectrodes inserted into individual cell somata deep within the spinal cord grey matter have, in recent years, provided much information, often of an unexpected nature, which has necessitated a radical reappraisal of many widely held views. Excellent examples of this experimental approach are a series of investigations of the activities of cells in spinal laminae IV–VI during natural forms of skin stimulation, passive limb movements, stimulation of cutaneous, muscle and visceral nerves in various combinations, and on occasion, sumultaneous stimulation of various fibre tracts which descend from supraspinal sources (or after the removal of such influences).[365, 366, 367]

In the earlier experiments[365] it was confirmed that a *functional lamination* exists which corresponds in large measure to that proposed on cytoarchitectonic grounds (p. 827). It was demonstrated that cells in all three laminae would respond to cutaneous stimulation, whereas movement only elicited a response in lamina VI. Cells in lamina IV possessed small receptive fields and responded as if many different types of specific cutaneous afferents *converged* upon an *individual cell* (e.g. it responded to hair movement, touch, skin cooling, etc.). Lamina V cells responded as if many cells of lamina IV converged upon each of them; they possessed much larger and more diffuse receptive fields. Response to movement was limited to cells in lamina VI, but many of the latter responded to both passive movement and cutaneous stimulation. Simultaneous stimulation of corticospinal fibres affected cells in all three laminae, sometimes facilitating and sometimes inhibiting their responses. It was also demonstrated that activity of certain brainstem centres inhibited cutaneous stimulation responses but enhanced responses to movement and could even *switch the 'modality'* of lamina VI cells from cutaneous to pro-

[360] M. Réthelyi and J. Szentágothai, *Expl Brain Res.*, 7, 1969.
[361] J. C. Eccles, P. Fatt, S. Landgren and G. J. Winsbury, *J. Physiol., Lond.*, **125**, 1954.
[362] J. S. Coombs, D. R. Curtis and S. Landgren, *J. Neurophysiol.*, **19**, 1956.
[363] G. M. Kolmodin, *Acta physiol. scand.*, **40**, suppl. **139**, 1957.
[364] G. M. Kolmodin and C. R. Skoglund, *Acta physiol. scand.*, **50**, 1960.
[365] P. D. Wall, *J. Physiol., Lond.*, **188**, 1967.
[366] B. Pomeranz, P. D. Wall and W. V. Weber, *J. Physiol., Lond.*, **199**, 1968.
[367] P. D. Wall, *Brain*, **93**, 1970.

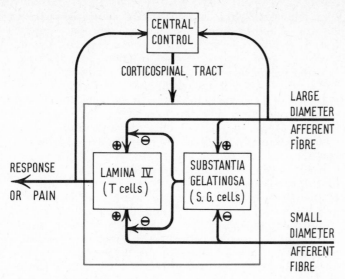

7.51  The sensory 'gate' mechanism which has been proposed by R. Melzack and P. D. Wall for the mode of operation of the dorsal laminae of grey matter of the spinal cord. See text for a discussion of the effects of an imbalance in the sensory inflow along the large and small diameter afferent fibres. (From an illustration in *Science*, Vol. 150, with the permission of the authors and publishers. Copyright, 1965, American Association for the Advancement of Science.)

prioceptive. In later investigations[366] in which cutaneous, muscle, and visceral nerves were stimulated, the findings were expanded and refined. Particular emphasis was placed upon lamina V in which *fine myelinated afferents* from the *three* sources converged on *individual cells* and interacted in various ways. They possessed very large, non-discriminative receptive fields and it was proposed that in some way they signalled information concerning the general 'state' of the various tissues. These results will not be examined in detail here, but they are well summarized in a subsequent publication[367] in which the characteristics of the spinal cord cells in laminae IV–VI are compared with those of the dorsal column nuclei (nucleus gracilis and nucleus cuneatus). The former are now considered to provide an important source of the crossed spinothalamic tract,[368] which is, as we have seen (p. 819), one of the principal ascending sensory pathways, whilst the latter receive the terminals of the fasciculi gracilis et cuneatus, the second major ascending sensory pathway. Their respective roles have long been a subject of controversy and a comparison emphasizes some important features of sensory physiology.

## COMPARISON OF THE DORSAL COLUMN–MEDIAL LEMNISCUS AND THE SPINOTHALAMIC TRACT PATHWAYS

It is instructive to compare the size of the receptive fields, the degree of anatomical localization (somatotopical mapping), the maintenance of specificity of channels or the convergence and interaction among them, and the forms of control of transmission of impulses in the two systems.

**The cells of the dorsal column nuclei**[369, 370] receive the synaptic terminals of the long, ascending, uncrossed, primary afferent fibres of the fasciculus gracilis and cuneatus (p. 824) which carry information concerning deformation of the skin, movement of hairs, joint movement, and rhythmical vibration of the tissues. In the cat, the fibres from hair receptors are superficial, whilst touch and vibration receptors are more deeply placed. The somatotopical localization of fibres in the dorsal white columns has already been described (p. 825) and further

consideration of the structure and connexions of the dorsal column nuclei will be considered with the medulla oblongata (p. 844).

Unit recording with microelectrodes implanted in the cells of the dorsal column nuclei has shown that their *receptive fields* for touch (that is the skin area from which a response can be elicited) vary in size in different regions, but are generally small (and smallest in the digits). Some receptive fields have an *excitatory centre* and an *inhibitory surround*; thus a stimulus applied just outside the excitatory receptive area will inhibit the cell in question. The cells of the nuclei are spatially organized into an accurate somatotopic map of the periphery (in accord with the similar localization in the dorsal columns). *Specificity* in the cells is high, each responds to *only one type* of afferent fibre stimulation; thus a cell may respond to hair movement alone, or to joint movement, or to an applied sinusoidal vibration, but never to two of these. Indeed, a number of fibres converge upon a single cell but they are always of the same functional type.

The transmission of impulses from the dorsal columns to the medial lemniscus are subjected to a variety of control mechanisms.[371, 372] Concomitant activity in neighbouring dorsal column fibres may result in presynaptic inhibition by depolarization of the presynaptic terminals of one of them. Stimulation of the sensorimotor cortex also modulates the transmission of impulses by both pre- and post-synaptic inhibitory mechanisms, and sometimes by facilitation. These descending influences are mediated by the corticospinal tract. Modulation of transmission also follows reticular formation stimulation.

Clearly, the dorsal column nuclei are not simple 'relay nuclei' as was long supposed. They have been described[367] as having the characteristics of 'a private and highly reliable telephone system in which afferent information is separated in channels which are discrete both for spatial origin and stimulus specificity of afferent fibres'. These features contrast strongly with those of the cells of origin of the spinothalamic tracts.

**The cells in laminae IV–VI of the spinal cord** have very different receptive fields. Those of lamina IV have small fields and there is a high degree of somatotopic localization of the cells, whereas those of lamina V have extremely large diffuse fields, and respond to a wide range of stimulus strengths. *Specificity* of separate channels as it exists in the dorsal column nuclei is absent in the laminae of the cord. *Convergence of different functional types* of afferent fibre on to the *same cell* is the rule in the cord, the convergence varying with the lamina. Lamina IV cells receive large cutaneous afferents, lamina V cells receive fine afferents from skin, muscle, and splanchnic nerves in various combinations, whilst lamina VI cells receive large muscle and cutaneous afferents. The converging synaptic terminals from different sources result in an interaction between excitatory and inhibitory states, which summate to determine the output from the cell. The control of impulse transmission is modulated in a variety of ways. Firstly, the cutaneous afferents are probably influenced by the tonic regulating mechanism of the substantia gelatinosa described previously. In addition, impulse transmission is greatly influenced by a variety of descending tracts from the sensorimotor cortex and brainstem centres (*vide supra*). The degree of control varies from

[368] P. N. Dilly, P. D. Wall and K. E. Webster, *Expl Neurol.*, **21**, 1968.

[369] V. B. Mountcastle, *Medical Physiology*, 12th ed., Mosby, St. Louis. 1968.

[370] A. C. Norton, U.C.L.A. *Brain Information Service, Updated Review Project—Cutaneous Sensory Pathways: Dorsal Column—Medial Lemniscus System*, University of California Press, Berkeley. 1968.

[371] S. J. Jabbur and A. L. Towe, *J. Neurophysiol.*, **24**, 1961.

[372] P. Andersen, J. C. Eccles, R. F. Schmidt and T. Yokota, *J. Neurophysiol.*, **27**, 1964.

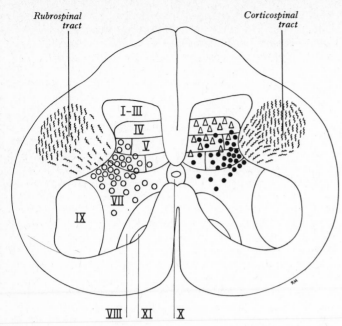

*Rubrospinal tract*

*Corticospinal tract*

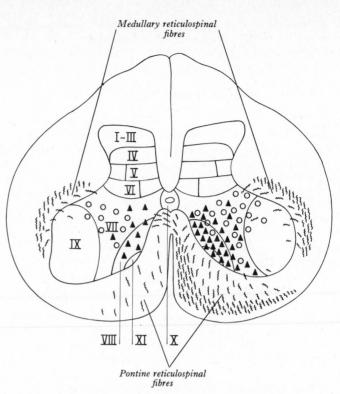

*Medullary reticulospinal fibres*

*Pontine reticulospinal fibres*

**7.**52 A–C  The spinal terminations of various descending tracts of the spinal cord determined experimentally in the cat, and referred to the laminar pattern of the grey matter which is described elsewhere in the present section. (Redrawn from *Neurological Anatomy* by A. Brodal, Oxford University Press, 1969, by courtesy of the author and publishers).

A  Terminations of corticospinal fibres from 'motor' areas of the cerebral cortex—black dots; corticospinal fibres from 'sensory' areas of cerebral cortex—white triangles; rubrospinal fibres—white dots.

C  Terminations of reticulospinal fibres; those originating in the medulla oblongata—white dots—are in general more dorsally placed than those originating in the pons—black triangles.

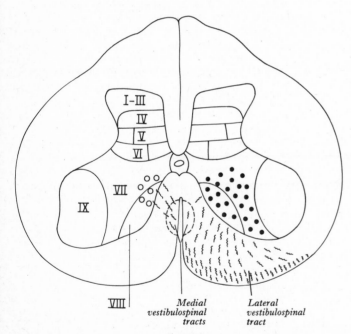

*Medial vestibulospinal tracts*

*Lateral vestibulospinal tract*

B  Terminations of vestibulospinal fibres; those from the lateral vestibulospinal tract—black dots; those from the medial vestibulospinal tract are shown on the opposite side of the cord as white dots.

section can in fact discriminate for weight, texture, two-point stimulation, vibration and position. It is proposed that environmental stimuli may be classified into two types: those which are 'passively impressed on an animal' and those that 'must be actively explored by motor movement or sequential analysis before they can be successfully discriminated'. Reception of the former is considered the role of the spinothalamic system, whilst that of the dorsal column system is to initiate and programme an exploration of a source of stimulation, and to carry the resultant flow of information. Further evidences in this field, perhaps derived from intracellular microelectrodes carried by freely moving animals—a technique currently being developed—will be awaited with great interest.

## THE SPINAL TERMINATIONS OF DESCENDING TRACTS FROM SUPRASPINAL SOURCES

In recent years degeneration techniques such as that of Nauta have added considerably to our knowledge of the sites of termination within the spinal cord grey matter of many of the principal descending fibre tract systems.[373–381] The majority of these investigations, again, involve the spinal cord of the cat and occasionally primates other than man. The results, which may well embody general principles applying to many higher mammals, must not, however, be extrapolated in detail directly to the situation in the human cord. Some of the principal results are summarized in illustration **7.**52 A, B and C based upon the above

simple changes in excitability of the cells in lamina IV to a complete reversal of modality in lamina VI.

The roles of the two major sensory pathways—dorsal column and spinothalamic tract—have aroused considerable controversy. The classical view[369] holds that the dorsal column is the *essential discriminatory pathway* and that in its absence a mechanical stimulus is recognized as having occurred, but that it is impossible to specify it exactly as to location, intensity and shape. This view has recently been strongly challenged[367] and it is pointed out that experimental animals with a complete dorsal column

[373] R. Nyberg-Hansen, *J. comp. Neurol.*, **122**, 1964.
[374] R. Nyberg-Hansen, *Expl Neurol.*, **9**, 1964b.
[375] R. Nyberg-Hansen, *J. comp. Neurol.*, **124**, 1965.
[376] R. Nyberg-Hansen, *Ergebn. Anat. EntwGesch.*, **39**, 1966.
[377] R. Nyberg-Hansen, *Archs ital. Biol.*, **104**, 1966.
[378] R. Nyberg-Hansen, *Expl Brain Res.*, **7**, 1969.
[379] R. Nyberg-Hansen and A. Brodal, *J. comp. Neurol.*, **120**, 1963; *J. Anat.*, **98**, 1964.
[380] R. Nyberg-Hansen and T. Mascitti, *J. comp. Neurol.*, **122**, 1964.
[381] A. Brodal, *Neurological Anatomy*, Oxford University Press, London. 1969.

references, in which the distributions of the terminals are related to the laminar architecture of the grey matter. The following salient points, some of which have already received brief mention with the human tracts, may be noted.

**The corticospinal tract** fibres in the cat terminate almost exclusively on interneurons in laminae IV–VII. Perhaps all such fibres terminate in this manner, but because of the very extensive ramifications of the dendrites of the multipolar motor neurons of lamina IX, some of which penetrate lamina VII, the presence of a few axodendritic contacts with motor neurons cannot be entirely excluded. Further experiments demonstrated that the corticospinal fibres which arise from 'sensory' cortical regions terminate chiefly in laminae IV and V, whereas those from 'motor' regions end in V–VII with the greatest concentration in the lateral part of lamina VI. Thus, although some overlap occurs, the two types of corticospinal fibre (from different cortical regions) are fairly distinct in their areas of termination. These findings are of particular interest in relation to the increasing volume of evidence concerning the corticospinal (pyramidal) tract as one of the principal supraspinal systems that *modulate the inflow of sensory information*. As we have seen, the latter may be mediated either by presynaptic inhibition of the terminals of the primary afferent fibres, or by postsynaptic inhibition or facilitation of the second (or subsequent) neurons in the afferent pathway. It should also be pointed out, however, that in contrast to the cat there is both anatomical[382–384] and physiological[385–387] evidence that in monkeys a small proportion of corticospinal fibres end monosynaptically on large α motor neurons. Much less is known with precision about the synaptic terminals in man; the majority undoubtedly end upon interneurons, but some evidence[388] again indicates a small population of fibres ending directly on motor neurons.

Briefly, it may again be mentioned that recent physiological studies[389] in the cat indicate that the corticospinal tract influences both α and γ motor neurons, and that in both cases the effect is mediated via interneurons. In general there is an excitatory effect on motor neurons which supply flexor musculature and an inhibitory one to those supplying extensor musculature.

**The rubrospinal tract** fibres in the cat arise from both the large and small celled parts of the contralateral red nucleus, which shows evidences of some degree of somatotopic organization. Degeneration studies after stereotactic lesions of the nucleus indicate that the tract descends throughout the cord to lumbosacral levels and that its terminals end upon interneurons in spinal cord laminae V–VII. Its zones of termination correspond rather closely with those of the corticospinal fibres which arise in 'motor' regions of the cerebral cortex. Again there are physiological evidences that activity of the rubrospinal projection influences both α and γ motor neurons, via interneurons, facilitating flexor groups and inhibiting extensor ones. Since in some experimental animals a somatotopically organized *corticorubral projection* of fibres has been demonstrated from the sensorimotor cortex, some authors have stressed the presence of dual pathways from the cortex to the cord, one a *direct corticospinal projection*, the other an *indirect corticorubrospinal projection*. Both have similar terminations in the cord and many physiological attributes in common. Little precise knowledge is available, as we have seen, concerning the origin, localization, termination and functional significance of the rubrospinal system in man. Although often stated to be rudimentary and of little significance, clear evidence for such a view is lacking.

**The vestibulospinal tracts**, medial and lateral, have also been quite intensively investigated in experimental animals, but are much less well understood in man. As stated previously, the lateral vestibulospinal tract originates from both large and small cells of the *lateral vestibular nucleus* of the same side, descends in the anterolateral white column throughout the cord, its fibres terminating at successive levels largely in laminae VII and VIII, only a trivial number of terminals entering lamina IX. The medial vestibulospinal tract arises mainly from the medial vestibular nuclei of both sides. The fibres run in company at brainstem levels with other components of the medial longitudinal fasciculi and then descend, perhaps to midthoracic levels only, on both sides of the anterior median fissure of the cord. They, too, terminate in a more restricted zone which includes parts of laminae VII and VIII. Activation of the main lateral vestibulospinal tract results in excitation of extensor motor neurons and inhibition of flexor motor neurons. The excitation is a direct monosynaptic effect and it must be concluded that the terminals of the vestibulospinal fibres make synaptic contact with the extensive dendrites of some of the motor neurons that penetrate laminae VII and VIII. Gamma motor neurons are also considered to be facilitated whilst the inhibitory effect to the flexors is presumably mediated by inhibitory interneurons of the laminae in which the fibres terminate.

**The reticulospinal tracts** have been notoriously difficult to evaluate in the spinal cord of man and, again, much more precise information is available in the cat, from studies using the Nissl method for studying the acute retrograde responses in cell somata after spinal cord section, and also the Nauta technique for anterograde terminal degeneration after the placing of stereotactic lesions in the brainstem. Both pontine and medullary reticulospinal fibres from one side of the brainstem apparently pass to *both sides* of the cord, but the pontine fibres are much more densely concentrated on the ipsilateral side, whereas the medullary fibres also send a substantial population to the contralateral side. The spinal cord course of the two differs, the medullary fibres are claimed to pass in the lateral funiculi whilst the pontine fibres are concentrated ventromedially. Their zones of termination are summarized in **7.52**C. Briefly it may be mentioned that similar experiments indicate that the **tectospinal tract** from the contralateral superior colliculus and the **interstitiospinal tract**, which arises mainly in the ipsilateral interstitial nucleus of Cajal in the cranial midbrain, both terminate in spinal cord laminae VI–VIII. The latter and the reticular formation will be further discussed in subsequent sections.

## SUMMARY OF SPINAL CORD ORGANIZATION

It has been proposed[390] that in broad outline it is convenient to consider the grey matter of the spinal cord as composed of a *central core* with paired *dorsal* and *ventral appendages*, each with some distinctive characteristics (**7.53**). (The unfamiliar terms core and appendage are retained in this summary since they do not correspond

[382] E. C. Hoff and H. E. Hoff, *Brain*, **57**, 1934.
[383] H. G. J. M. Kuypers, *Brain*, **83**, 1960.
[384] C.-N. Liu and W. W. Chambers, *J. comp. Neurol.*, **123**, 1964.
[385] C. G. Bernhard, E. Bohm and I. Petersen, *Acta physiol. scand.*, **29**, 1953.
[386] J. B. Preston and D. G. Whitlock, *J. Neurophysiol.*, **24**, 1961.
[387] S. Landgren, C. G. Phillips and R. Porter, *J. Physiol., Lond.*, **161**, 1962.
[388] H. G. J. M. Kuypers, *Brain*, **81**, 1958.
[389] R. Corazza, E. Fadiga and P. L. Parmeggiani, *Archs ital. Biol.*, **101**, 1963.
[390] J. Szentágothai, in: *Recent Development of Neurobiology in Hungary*, Vol. I ed. K. Lissak, Akadémiae Kiadó, Budapest, 1967.

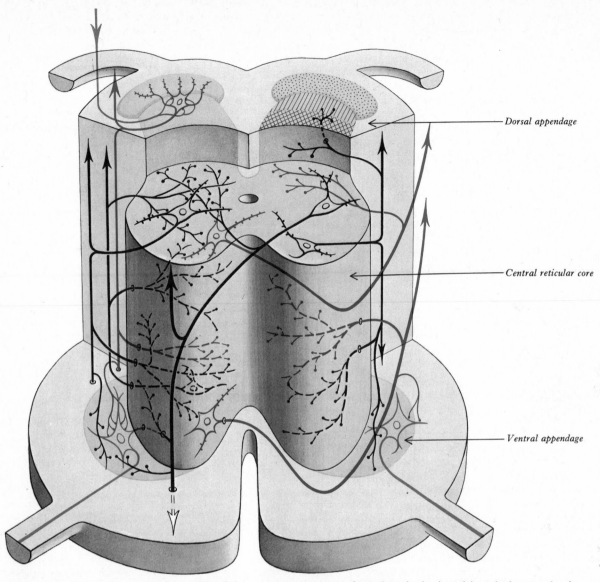

**7.53** A highly simplified stereodiagram illustrating the concept of the spinal cord as consisting of a central 'reticular core' of grey matter, with related dorsal and ventral 'appendages' of grey matter. Many structural features are omitted, and only a few examples, relevant to the concept, are included. A dorsal column neuron, and others, more ventrally placed, which give rise to descending, long ascending, and local collateral branches, are shown in blue. Varieties of interneuron are in black. Two motor neurons are shown in red; also in red is a single example of a fibre descending from a supraspinal source. See text for a more detailed description; see also **7.47**A and B for the origin of the tracts, and **7.49** for the fine structure of the substantia gelatinosa. (Redrawn from J. Szentágothai in: *Recent Development of Neurobiology in Hungary*, I. K. Lissák (ed.). By courtesy of the author and publishers, Akadémiai Kiadó, Budapest, 1967.)

precisely with the dorsal and ventral grey columns of topographical neuroanatomy.)

The core, with our present methods of investigation, appears to present a diffuse, non-discriminative, reticular type of organization, within which there is both a great divergence and convergence of information paths; the majority of its interneurons interconnect with many hundreds, perhaps thousands of other core interneurons distributed over a substantial length of the cord. In contrast the dorsal and ventral appendages have a greater degree of precise discriminative organization in terms of somatotopic mapping and various orders of functional localization. To give precise topographical limits to core and appendages is probably an intellectual abstraction and is certainly impossible at the present rudimentary state of our knowledge; indeed, the concept itself will undoubtedly need much revision (and perhaps lose much of its relevance) as knowledge and understanding increase. Roughly the central core is considered to encompass the interneurons of laminae VII and VIII (i.e. the intermediate zone of previous workers and the areas between the motor neuron columns). However, it may well be that many of the interneurons of the deeper laminae of the dorsal column and those within the motor cell columns should also be included under the concept of a reticular core. The ventral appendage corresponds to the cell columns of lamina IX whilst the dorsal appendage includes laminae I–VI.

**The dorsal appendage** is, as we have seen (pp. 813, 830), the principal receiving zone of the various exteroceptive, proprioceptive and interoceptive dorsal nerve root afferent fibres. The dorsally situated laminae (I–IV) are the main cutaneous afferent receiving areas, lamina V receives small-diameter afferents from skin, muscle and viscera, whilst lamina VI receives proprioceptive and some cutaneous afferents. It should be emphasized, however, that relatively few investigations have as yet been carried out; the functional boundaries are certainly not as clear-cut as the above description suggests, and undoubtedly a great variety of further functional 'types' of interneuron with many other grades and subtleties of interaction between them remain to be discovered.

Further, it is inherent in the technique of intracellular microelectrode recording that because of their situation, size and morphology, some cells can be investigated with relative ease, others with difficulty, and a large (and indeterminate) number are beyond our current technical reach; for these reasons a bias in our view of cord dynamics is inevitable.

Nevertheless, it is becoming clear from the existing recordings that the dorsal appendage cells abstract information about the internal and external environment in many different forms. Cells and cell groups in different regions show great variety in their degree of somatotopic mapping, the size and response characteristics of their receptive fields, in their specificity or in the degree of convergence and interaction of different types of afferent channel upon a single cell. A brief comparison between the behaviour of the cells in the dorsal appendage of the cord with those in the dorsal column nuclei of the medulla oblongata has been given elsewhere (p. 834). Clearly, the simple view of spinal cord cells as providing merely relays in a series of invariant, discrete, 'unimodality' channels which transmit an elementary punctate view of the environment, either ventrally to motor neurons or cranially to brain centres, as they are often presented in neurological textbooks, must now be firmly rejected. A series of complex transformations of the patterns of inflowing information have already occurred within the dorsal appendage. The outflow along the axons of the dorsal appendage neurons passes to many destinations, either directly to motor neuron columns in the ventral appendage, indirectly via more ventrally situated laminae including the exceedingly complex arrangements of interneurons in the reticular core, on both sides of the cord and cranial and caudal to the level of the input in question. Long axoned cells of both the dorsal appendage and the reticular core contribute to the long ascending tracts, which reach a multiplicity of centres in the brainstem.

Further, transmission of impulses to and beyond the dorsal appendage cells may be modified in various ways by mutual interaction and the operation of controlling mechanisms. Mention has already been made (p. 833) of the facilitatory and inhibitory effects which may follow simultaneous activity in different categories of afferent fibre which converge on the same cell, and of the postulated tonic modulating system of the substantia gelatinosa, which affects the inflow of impulses from cutaneous afferents. In addition, much evidence is now accumulating which demonstrates that impulse transmission in all the laminae of the dorsal appendage (as in the remainder of the spinal cord grey matter) are strongly influenced by fibre systems which descend from supraspinal sources such as the sensorimotor cortex and the reticular formation of the brainstem; such effects may be mediated by either pre- or post-synaptic contacts and be either facilitatory or inhibitory depending upon the site and the circumstances. The biological significance of these mechanisms which control sensory input channels are still far from clear; they may be concerned with eliminating redundancy, reducing confusion by excessive bombardment of central networks, or be linked to 'states of readiness' of central mechanisms, or to the temporary 'preoccupation' of such centres with more immediately significant transformations. The subject is under intense and continuing analysis. It is increasingly clear, however, that the majority of fibre tract systems that descend from the brain and influence motor patterns of behaviour, do so by modifying the state and impulse transmission characteristics of interneurons in the deeply placed laminae of grey matter and much less frequently by influencing the motor neurons directly.

**The reticular core** interneurons form an exceedingly complex network in which each cell receives inputs from and transmits to large numbers of others. The core receives an input from the axonal terminals of some cells of the dorsal appendage, from proprioceptive dorsal root afferent fibres, and from some of the long descending tract systems. Because of the wealth of interneuronal connexions in this region, analysis has proved of the greatest difficulty, but the earlier view that it almost approaches a *random nerve network* in form is receding with the extensive application of the newer methods of analysis. The latter include the placing of minute stereotactic lesions within the core and observing subsequent degenerative phenomena, intracellular recording, and elegant researches on thousands of specimens using the Golgi technique (for an extensive review of this field consult the collection of essays in footnote reference [391]). One type of organization that has emerged concerns the quantitative analysis of connectivity or 'transmitting power' of different types of interneuron and some of the descending tract systems. Details cannot be given here, but briefly some axonal terminals pursue an extremely long course through the grey matter giving off perhaps only two or three synaptic end bulbs to each of the many hundreds of interneurons encountered in transit. Others concentrate large numbers of terminals on one or a small group of neurons. Thus, diffuse or *'non-discriminative'* connexions have been contrasted with *'discriminative'* ones. Further, it has been shown that contrary to earlier opinion many proprioceptive afferents have terminals in the core that are strictly 'segmentally' localized to narrow transverse 'sheets' of grey matter (in contrast to the dorsal appendage cutaneous afferents which terminate in extensive narrow longitudinal sheets). It is largely through such complex interneuronal aggregates that inflowing sensory information interacts with that descending from higher centres to set in train the endless variety of locomotor responses; and although our understanding of them is still in its infancy, the continued application of modern powerful methods offers a considerable prospect of further success in this region.

**The ventral appendage** as described elsewhere (pp. 811, 814, 828) consists of a columnar organization of the cell somata of α and γ motor neurons and again neighbouring interneurons. Attention was also directed to the physiological evidence for 'tonic' and 'phasic' types of α cell related to different varieties of striated muscle fibre, and to the existence of different types of γ cell whereby the 'static' and 'dynamic' responses of the muscle spindles are under independent central control mechanisms. Unfortunately, the detailed synaptology of these different cell types is uncertain. Further, it was shown that whilst a considerable degree of somatotopic localization exists in the ventral columns, its detailed arrangement and significance also remain to be determined.

The principal synaptic connexions of the *motor neurons* are derived from: (1) direct monosynaptic terminals from proprioceptive dorsal root afferents within the same or neighbouring spinal cord segments; (2) terminals from collateral branches of the axons of dorsal appendage interneurons; (3) terminals from interneurons of the reticular core which are of high density and 'discriminative' when derived from the same spinal segment, and diffuse or 'non-discriminative' when derived from neighbouring segments; (4) a few direct monosynaptic terminals from the vestibulospinal and (in various primates including man) the corticospinal tracts, although in the main these tracts end on interneurons.

How these various channels which converge on the

[391] M. A. B. Brazier (ed.), *The Interneuron*, University of California Press, Berkeley and Los Angeles. 1969.

motor neurons interact to produce integrated motor behaviour is still far from clear. However, a few generalizations can be made. The principal descending pathways can be grouped into those which are predominantly excitatory to flexor musculature and inhibitory to extensors (the corticospinal, rubrospinal and medullary reticulospinal tracts) and those which have the converse effect (the vestibulospinal and pontine reticulospinal pathways). However, this simple view of the broad dualistic action of certain descending tracts does little justice to the large volume of detailed investigation that has been reported on the complex modifications of reflex activities by descending systems; but, as yet, it has proved difficult to fit these into an overall behavioural picture.

Secondly, there are two distinct pathways by which a muscle may be thrown into a state of contraction (or relaxation); the first or α *pathway* involves an immediate and direct change in the excitatory level of the α motor neurons innervating the motor units. It is considered that such a mechanism operates only infrequently and that is when a sudden forceful response is appropriate. In the majority of instances a γ *pathway* is operative in which the sequence appears to be—activity in local interneurons, followed by activity (or inhibition) of the γ efferents to the muscle spindles, which in turn via the local muscle servo-loop mechanism (p. 802) causes an appropriate change in the tonic and phasic α motor neurons. The detailed mechanism whereby this so-called α-γ *linkage* is maintained or broken under different conditions is still under investigation.[392] It should also be noted, however, that some recent researches have indicated that during voluntary actions, initiating activity in the α system may be more frequent than was previously recognized (*see* p. 804).

*Applied Anatomy.* In injury to the spinal cord the segmental level of the interference may be determined accurately from clinical data and the application of accurate anatomical knowledge.

Complete division of the spinal cord above the fifth cervical segment causes death by respiratory failure resulting from paralysis of the phrenic and intercostal nerves. Lesions between $C_5$ and $T_1$ produce paralysis in all four limbs (quadriplegia); the degree of paralysis in the upper limb varies with the site of the lesions. At the fifth segment the upper limb paralysis will be complete; at the sixth the arms adopt a position of abduction and lateral rotation, with the elbows flexed and the forearms supinated due to the unopposed activity of the deltoids, spinati, rhomboids, bicipites and brachiales, which are supplied by the fifth cervical nerve. In cervical lesions at progressively lower levels the innervation of correspondingly more muscles of the upper limb is retained. Lesions of the first thoracic segment result in paralysis of the small muscles of the hand together with interference with sympathetic outflow, resulting in contraction of the pupil, recession of the eyeball, narrowing of the palpebral fissure and absence of sweating on the face and neck (Horner's syndrome). Sensation will be retained in areas deriving their innervation from segments above the site of the lesions. In particular, cutaneous sensation will be retained in the neck and chest down to the second intercostal space, because this area is innervated by the supraclavicular nerves ($C_2$ and $C_4$).

In the thoracic region, division of the spinal cord results in paralysis of the trunk below the segmental level of the lesion and of both lower limbs (paraplegia).

The first sacral neural segment is opposite the junction of the thoracic and lumbar vertebrae and injury, which commonly occurs here, results in paralysis of the urinary bladder and rectum and of the muscles supplied by the sacral segments. Cutaneous sensibility is lost in the 'saddle' area in the perineum and buttocks, back of the thigh, leg and sole of the foot. The lumbar nerve roots which pass distally to join the cauda equina at this level may be divided and then the result is complete paralysis of both lower limbs. Lesions below the first lumbar vertebra may divide or damage the nerves of the cauda equina, but severe nerve damage is uncommon and is usually confined to the nerve root at the level of the bony injury.

Neurological symptoms may also arise from interference with the blood supply of the spinal cord, particularly in the lower thoracic and upper lumbar regions.

## The Vertebral Levels of Spinal Cord Segments

Clinically it is important to know the position of the spinal segments relative to the vertebrae. In the cervical region the tip of the spine of a particular vertebra corresponds to the level of the succeeding cord segment (i.e., the sixth cervical spine is opposite the seventh cord segment); in the upper thoracic region the apex of a vertebral spine corresponds to two segments lower in number (i.e., the fourth spine is level with the sixth segment); in the lower thoracic region there is a difference of three segments (i.e., the tenth thoracic spine is level with the first lumbar segment). The eleventh thoracic spine overlies the third lumbar segment and the twelfth thoracic spine is opposite the first sacral segment. In the newborn child, on the other hand, the spinal cord extends to the upper border of the third lumbar vertebra.

## Blood Vessels of the Spinal Cord

Blood reaches the spinal cord along the spinal branches of the vertebral, deep cervical, intercostal and lumbar arteries which, with the anterior and posterior spinal arteries, contribute to the formation of longitudinal anastomotic channels along the cord[393] (*see* pp. 641 and 658). The spinal branches gives rise to anterior and posterior radicular arteries which approach the spinal cord along the ventral and dorsal nerve roots. Most of the anterior radicular arteries are small and terminate within the ventral nerve roots or in the plexus in the pia around the cord. A small but variable number (usually four to nine), mainly situated in the lower cervical, lower thoracic and upper lumbar regions, are larger than the remainder and in addition reach the anterior median sulcus of the spinal cord, where they divide into slender ascending and large descending branches. These branches anastomose with one another and with the anterior spinal arteries above to form a single, or in places paired, longitudinal vessel of uneven calibre along the anterior median sulcus. Frequently one of these anterior radicular arteries is considerably larger than the remainder and is often termed the *arteria radicularis magna*. Its exact position varies, but it arises from one of the intersegmental branches of the descending aorta in the lower thoracic or upper lumbar vertebral levels. In two-thirds of cases it arises on the left-hand side. Reaching the spinal cord, this vessel sends one branch to join the anterior spinal artery below and another to anastomose with the division of the posterior spinal artery lying in front of the dorsal roots. The arteria radicularis magna may be responsible for most of the blood supply of the lower two-thirds of the spinal cord.

From the anterior spinal artery central branches pass into the anterior median fissure. Here each one passes either to the right or left to supply the anterior grey

---

[392] R. Granit, *The Basis of Motor Control*, Academic Press, London and New York. 1970.

[393] L. A. Gillilan, in: *Correlative Anatomy of the Nervous System*, by E. C. Crosby, T. Humphrey and E. W. Lauer, Macmillan, N.Y. 1962.

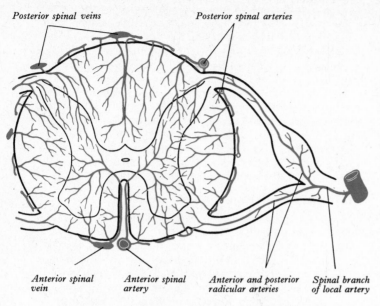

*Posterior spinal veins*  *Posterior spinal arteries*

*Anterior spinal vein*  *Anterior spinal artery*  *Anterior and posterior radicular arteries*  *Spinal branch of local artery*

**7.54**  Diagram of the intrinsic blood vessels of the spinal cord.

anastomotic ramus from the descending branch of the arteria radicularis magna.

The central branches of the anterior spinal artery are responsible for the supply of as much as two-thirds of the cross-sectional area of the spinal cord. The remainder of the posterior grey columns, posterior white columns and the peripheral parts of the lateral and anterior white columns are supplied by numerous small radially directed vessels derived from the posterior spinal arteries and from the vessels forming the plexus in the pia mater.[394, 395] In a detailed microangiographic investigation of the human spinal cord at cervical levels[396] there were from 1 to 6 anterior, and 0 to 8 posterior radicular spinal arteries. Each centimetre of the anterior spinal artery gave rise to 5 to 8 central branches. No anastomoses were observed within the cord itself. Overlapping of the territories of the central spinal arteries was confirmed, and similar overlapping in the longitudinal direction was emphasized..

The veins of the spinal cord drain into six tortuous, often plexiform and longitudinal channels, one along the anterior median fissure and a second along the posterior median sulcus and the others, often incomplete, situated on each side, one pair just behind and the other in front of the line of attachment of the ventral and dorsal nerve roots. These six vessels communicate freely with one another and above with the veins of the cerebellum and the cranial venous sinuses. The veins accompanying the anterior spinal artery receive sizeable venules from the central grey matter, while much of the blood draining the periphery of the spinal cord enters the veins of the pia mater. Further details of these veins are found on p. 702.

[394] L. A. Gillilan, *J. comp. Neurol.*, **110**, 1958.
[395] J. B. D. Torr, *The Blood Supply of the Human Cord*, M.D. Thesis, University of Manchester. 1957.
[396] I. M. Turnbull, A. Brieg and O. Hassler, *J. Neurosurg.*, **24**, 1966.

column, base of the posterior grey column, including the dorsal nucleus, and the adjacent white matter (7.54).

Each posterior spinal artery gives rise to a pair of longitudinally running channels which anastomose frequently, one lying in front of, the other behind the attachment of the dorsal roots. These longitudinal channels are reinforced at intervals by posterior radicular arteries, which are variable both in number and size but are more numerous than the anterior radicular arteries. In addition the vessel in front of the dorsal nerve roots receives an

# THE RHOMBENCEPHALON OR HINDBRAIN

The rhombencephalon comprises the medulla oblongata, pons and cerebellum; its cavity is the fourth ventricle. The medulla oblongata and pons are traversed by fibre tracts which interconnect these and other parts of the central nervous system and contain, amongst others, collections of nerve cells which constitute the nuclei of several of the cranial nerves. The following cranial nerves have their superficial origins from the pons and medulla oblongata: trigeminal, abducent, facial, vestibulocochlear, glossopharyngeal, vagus, cranial roots of the accessory, and hypoglossal. Scattered among the nuclei and tracts is the *reticular formation* (p. 888) which consists of intermingled grey and white matter and also nuclei of nerve cells concerned with the control of the heart, the respiratory apparatus and the alimentary tract.

# THE MEDULLA OBLONGATA

**The medulla oblongata** extends from the lower margin of the pons to a transverse plane passing above the first pair of cervical nerves; this plane corresponds with the upper border of the atlas behind, and the middle of the dens of the axis in front; at this level the medulla oblongata is continuous with the spinal cord. However, it must be emphasized that the plane of junction is arbitrary; the internal structure of the spinal cord changes *gradually* to that of the medulla oblongata. The anterior surface of the medulla oblongata is separated from the basilar part of the occipital bone and the upper part of the dens by the membranes of the brain and the occipito-axial ligaments. Posteriorly it is received into the notch between the hemispheres of the cerebellum, and the upper portion of this surface forms the lower part of the floor of the fourth ventricle.

The medulla oblongata is somewhat piriform in shape (7.55, 56), its broad extremity being directed upwards to merge with the pons, while its narrow lower end is continuous with the spinal cord. It measures about 3 cm longitudinally, 2 cm transversely at its widest part, and 1·25 cm anteroposteriorly. The central canal of the spinal cord is prolonged into its lower half, and then expands as the cavity of the fourth ventricle; the medulla oblongata may therefore be divided into a lower, *closed part* containing the central canal, and an upper, *open part* corresponding with the lower half of the fourth ventricle. Its anterior and posterior surfaces are marked by median fissures.

**The anterior median fissure** contains a short fold of pia mater, and extends along the entire length of the medulla oblongata; below, it is continuous with the anterior median fissure of the spinal cord; above, it ends at the lower border of the pons in a small triangular expansion termed the *foramen caecum*. Its lower part is interrupted by bundles of fibres which cross obliquely from one side to the other, the *decussation of the pyramids*. Some fibres, the *anterior external arcuate fibres*, emerge from the fissure above this decussation and curve laterally over the surface of the medulla oblongata.

**The posterior median sulcus** is a narrow groove which exists only in the closed part of the medulla oblongata; it is continuous below with the posterior median sulcus of the spinal cord, but becomes rapidly shallower at cranial levels, and ends about the middle of the medulla oblongata, where the central canal expands into the cavity of the fourth ventricle.

Many of the cranial nerves emerge from or enter the substance of the medulla oblongata, and they appear at the surface in line with the roots of spinal nerves. The fibres of the hypoglossal nerve correspond in position with ventral spinal roots and emerge in linear series from a furrow termed the *anterolateral sulcus*. Similarly, the accessory, vagus, and glossopharyngeal nerves are in line with dorsal spinal roots (p. 808) and enter or leave through the bottom of a sulcus named the *posterolateral sulcus*. Advantage is taken of this arrangement to subdivide each half of the medulla oblongata into anterior, middle and posterior regions. Although these three regions appear to be directly continuous with the corresponding funiculi of the spinal cord, they do not contain precisely the same nerve fibres, since some of the fasciculi of the spinal cord end or begin in the medulla oblongata, while others alter their course in passing through it.

**The anterior region** of the medulla oblongata (7.55, 56) lies between the anterior median fissure and the anterolateral sulcus, forming an elongated surface elevation which is named, somewhat inappropriately, the *pyramid*. Its upper end is slightly constricted and between it and the pons the fibres of the abducent nerve emerge; below, it tapers into the anterior funiculus of the spinal cord, with which it is superficially continuous.

The two pyramids contain descending fibres which pass from the cerebral cortex to the spinal cord. When traced downwards, approximately 70–90 per cent of these fibres leave the pyramids in successive bundles, and decussate in the anterior median fissure, forming what is termed the *decussation of the pyramids*. Having crossed the median plane, they pass down in the posterior part of the lateral funiculus of the spinal cord as the lateral corticospinal tract. The remaining fibres—i.e. those in the lateral part of the pyramid—do not cross the median plane; some descend as the anterior corticospinal tract (7.57) into the anterior funiculus of the same side of the spinal cord while others incline backwards and laterally to join the lateral corticospinal tract of the same side (p. 820). The corticospinal tracts display a clear segregation of their descending fibres upon a topographical basis at almost all levels; and in the medullary pyramids this arrangement is similar to that which exists at cranial levels, the most lateral fibres being concerned with the innervation of the legs, the most medial with the arms and neck. How far the same pattern is carried on into the ventral corticospinal tracts or through the decussating corticospinal fibres is not fully clarified, but a similar somatotopic sorting of fibres is usually described in the lateral corticospinal tracts as they extend into the spinal cord.

**The lateral region** of the medulla oblongata (7.58) is limited in front by the anterolateral sulcus and the roots of the hypoglossal nerve, and behind by the posterolateral sulcus and the roots of the accessory, vagus and glossopharyngeal nerves. Its upper part consists of a prominent oval mass which is named the *olive*, while its lower part

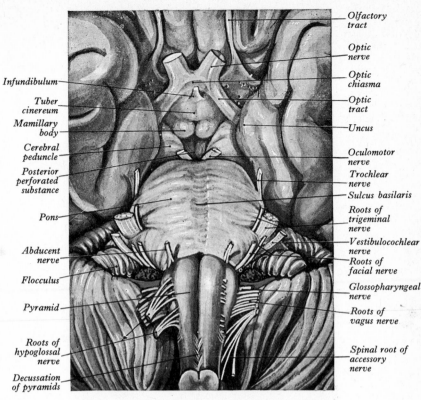

Olfactory tract
Optic nerve
Optic chiasma
Optic tract
Uncus
Oculomotor nerve
Trochlear nerve
Sulcus basilaris
Roots of trigeminal nerve
Vestibulocochlear nerve
Roots of facial nerve
Glossopharyngeal nerve
Roots of vagus nerve
Spinal root of accessory nerve

Infundibulum
Tuber cinereum
Mamillary body
Cerebral peduncle
Posterior perforated substance
Pons
Abducent nerve
Flocculus
Pyramid
Roots of hypoglossal nerve
Decussation of pyramids

**7.55** The ventral aspect of the brainstem and the interpeduncular fossa. The wall of the lateral recess of the fourth ventricle is shown in blue, and the choroid plexus, which protrudes through the foramen of the lateral recess into the subarachnoid space, is coloured crimson. Note that the lateral recess covers the medial part of the flocculus and is itself partially obscured by the root of the glossopharyngeal nerve.

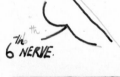

6$^{th}$ NERVE.

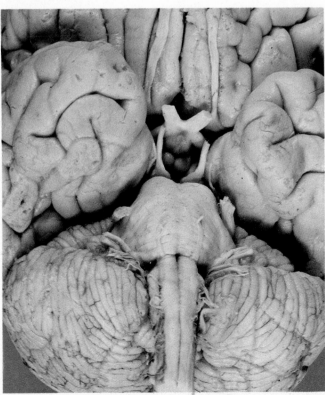

**7.56** The ventral aspect of the brainstem, interpeduncular fossa and adjacent parts of the cerebellar and cerebral hemispheres. For identification of the various structures, compare with **7.55**. (Dissection by Dr. E. L. Rees, Department of Anatomy, Guy's Hospital Medical School.)

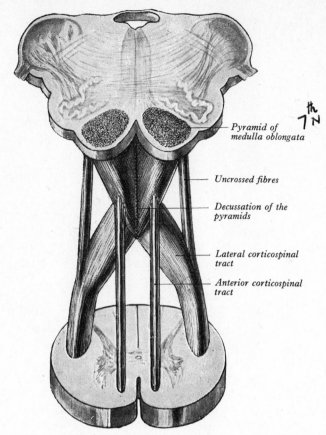

Pyramid of
medulla oblongata

Uncrossed fibres

Decussation of the
pyramids

Lateral corticospinal
tract

Anterior corticospinal
tract

**7.57**  Schematic dissection to show the decussation of the pyramids.

is of the same width as the lateral funiculus of the spinal cord, and appears on the surface to be a direct continuation of it. Only a portion of the lateral funiculus of the spinal cord is continued upwards into this region, because the lateral corticospinal tract is derived mainly from the contralateral pyramid, and most of the fibres of the posterior spinocerebellar tract leave the funiculus to enter the inferior cerebellar peduncle in the posterior region of the medulla. The lateral intersegmental tract and the anterior spinocerebellar tract are continued upwards in the lateral region of the medulla oblongata.

**The olive** is a smooth, oval elevation between the anterolateral and posterolateral sulci and lateral to the pyramid. It is caused by an underlying group of nerve cells forming the *inferior olivary nucleus* (p. 847). It is lateral to the pyramid, separated by the anterolateral sulcus and the fibres of the hypoglossal nerve. It is about 1·25 cm long, and dorsolateral to its cranial end there is a slight depression at the lower border of the pons in which the roots of the facial nerve appear. The anterior external arcuate fibres emerge from the anterior median fissure, and wind backwards across the pyramid and the olive to enter the inferior cerebellar peduncle (7.67).

**The posterior region** of the medulla oblongata (7.58 A, B; 59) lies behind the posterolateral sulcus and the roots of the accessory, vagus and glossopharyngeal nerves, and, like the lateral region, is divisible into caudal and cranial levels.

The *caudal part*, limited behind by the posterior median sulcus, consists of the upward continuation of the *fasciculus gracilis* and the *fasciculus cuneatus* of the spinal cord. The fasciculus gracilis flanks the posterior median sulcus, and is separated from the fasciculus cuneatus by the cranial continuation of the postero-intermediate sulcus and septum of the cervical spinal cord (p. 808). These two fasciculi are at first vertical; but at the caudal end of the fourth ventricle they diverge from the median plane, and each presents an elongated swelling. The swelling on the fasciculus gracilis is the *gracile tubercle*, and is produced by the upper end of a subjacent nucleus of grey matter termed the **nucleus gracilis**; that on the fasciculus cuneatus is termed the *cuneate tubercle*, and is caused similarly by the **nucleus cuneatus**. Most of the fibres of these two fasciculi end by forming synapses with the cells in their respective nuclei. A third elevation, the *tuberculum cinereum*, can sometimes be recognized in the caudal part of the posterior region of the medulla (7.58). It is located between the fasciculus cuneatus and the roots of the accessory nerve, and is narrow below but wider above. It is produced by a nucleus which is continuous below with the substantia gelatinosa, and in which the fibres of the spinal tract of the trigeminal nerve

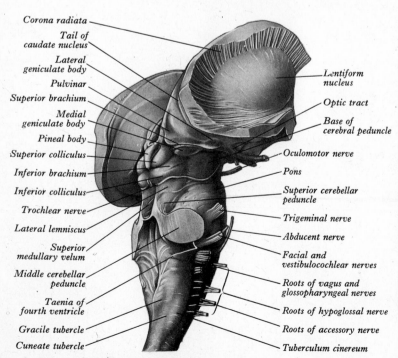

Corona radiata

Tail of
caudate nucleus

Lateral
geniculate body

Pulvinar

Superior brachium

Medial
geniculate body

Pineal body

Superior colliculus

Inferior brachium

Inferior colliculus

Trochlear nerve

Lateral lemniscus

Superior
medullary velum

Middle cerebellar
peduncle

Taenia of
fourth ventricle

Gracile tubercle

Cuneate tubercle

Lentiform
nucleus

Optic tract

Base of
cerebral peduncle

Oculomotor nerve

Pons

Superior cerebellar
peduncle

Trigeminal nerve

Abducent nerve

Facial and
vestibulocochlear nerves

Roots of vagus and
glossopharyngeal nerves

Roots of hypoglossal nerve

Roots of accessory nerve

Tuberculum cinereum

**7.58 A**  The brainstem, posterolateral aspect.

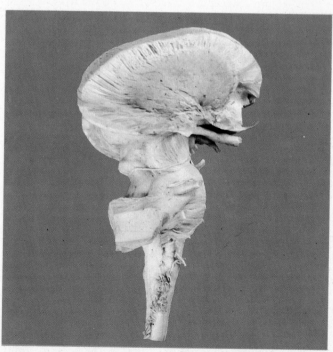

**7.58 B**  The right lateral aspect of the brainstem, lentiform nucleus and corona radiata. For identifications compare with 7.58 A. (Dissection by Dr. E. L. Rees, Dept. of Anatomy, Guy's Hospital Medical School.)

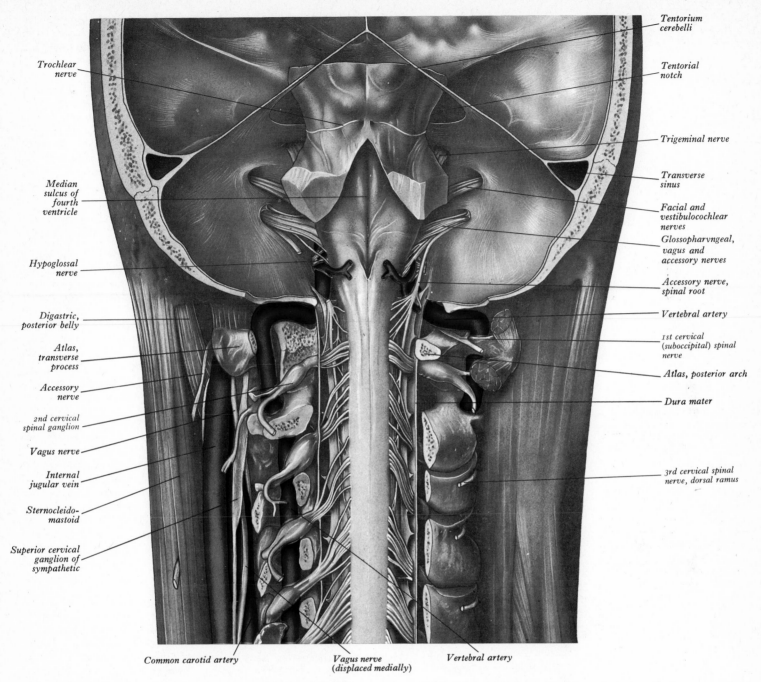

Trochlear nerve

Median sulcus of fourth ventricle

Hypoglossal nerve

Digastric, posterior belly

Atlas, transverse process

Accessory nerve

2nd cervical spinal ganglion

Vagus nerve

Internal jugular vein

Sternocleido-mastoid

Superior cervical ganglion of sympathetic

Tentorium cerebelli

Tentorial notch

Trigeminal nerve

Transverse sinus

Facial and vestibulocochlear nerves

Glossopharyngeal, vagus and accessory nerves

Accessory nerve, spinal root

Vertebral artery

1st cervical (suboccipital) spinal nerve

Atlas, posterior arch

Dura mater

3rd cervical spinal nerve, dorsal ramus

Common carotid artery

Vagus nerve (displaced medially)

Vertebral artery

7.59  Dissection exposing the brainstem and upper five cervical spinal segments after removal of large portions of the occipital and parietal bones and the cerebellum together with the roof of the fourth ventricle. On the left the foramina transversaria of the atlas and the third, fourth and fifth cervical vertebrae have been opened to expose the vertebral artery. On the right the posterior arch of the atlas and the laminae of the succeeding cervical vertebrae have been removed.

end; these fibres separate the nucleus from the surface of the medulla oblongata (p. 855). For further details of this region, including the obex and the taeniae of the fourth ventricle, see p. 878.

The *cranial part* of the posterior region of the medulla oblongata is occupied by the *inferior cerebellar peduncle*, a thick rounded ridge situated between the lower part of the fourth ventricle and the roots of the glossopharyngeal and vagus nerves. The two inferior cerebellar peduncles incline away from the dorsolateral aspect of the medulla oblongata towards the cerebellum. As they ascend, they diverge from each other, and form the lower parts of the lateral boundaries of the fourth ventricle; higher up, they are directed backwards, each passing into the corresponding cerebellar hemisphere. Near their entrance into the cerebellum they are crossed by several strands of fibres, the *striae medullares*, which run to the median sulcus of the

floor, or anterior wall, of the fourth ventricle (7.88, 90). The inferior cerebellar peduncle is not the upward continuation of the fasciculus gracilis and fasciculus cuneatus, although it appears to be so, for the fibres of these fasciculi end in the gracile, cuneate and accessory cuneate nuclei. The composition of the inferior cerebellar peduncle is described on p. 860.

## INTERNAL STRUCTURE OF THE MEDULLA OBLONGATA

The internal structure of the medulla oblongata, like that of other parts of the brainstem, has been studied chiefly in transverse sections by a combination of histological and experimental methods, three-dimensional reconstructions also being largely based upon serial transverse sections. It is hence customary and convenient to reconstruct such

843

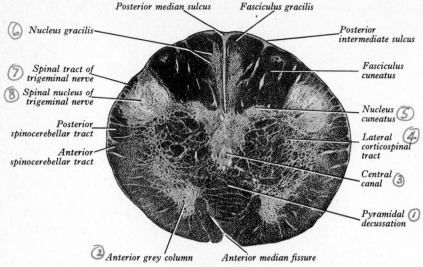

7.60 Transverse section through the medulla oblongata at the level of the pyramidal decussation. Weigert Pal preparation. Magnification ×7.

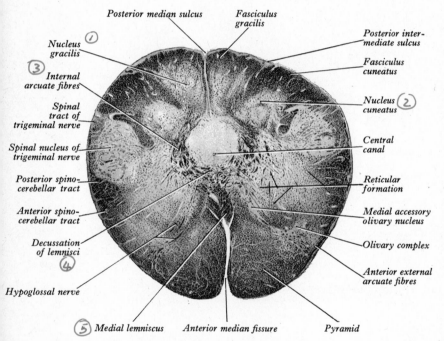

7.61 Transverse section through the medulla oblongata at the level of the decussation of the lemnisci. Weigert Pal preparation. Magnification *c.* ×6.

regions in description by reference to appearances in sample transverse sections at a variety of levels. In the account which follows, both of the medulla and other brainstem levels, this method will be employed, the medulla being considered at four successive levels, the first being the most caudal. The disposition of the principal brainstem nuclei is shown in profile in illustrations **7.62** and **7.64**, which should be consulted frequently when reading the subsequent sections.

(1) **A transverse section through the lowest part of the medulla oblongata** shows details very similar to those at the cranial end of the spinal cord, as would be expected (**7.60**). The posterior, lateral and anterior funiculi can be identified, and they contain the same nerve tracts. The grey matter shows two very striking alterations. The anterior grey column is separated from the central grey matter by the decussating corticospinal fibres, which are coursing backwards and laterally to reach the lateral

funiculus of the opposite side. In the upper part of the medulla oblongata the corticospinal fibres occupy the pyramid in its ventromedial portion, but in the lower part the majority of the corticospinal fibres cross the median plane, inclining backwards, as they do so (**7.57**), and decussating anterior to the central grey matter. The decussation takes place in an orderly manner with the fibres which terminate in the cervical segments of the spinal cord decussating first. This *decussation of the pyramids* is the most striking feature in sections of the medulla oblongata at this level. The actual proportion of the fibres which take part is subject to variation, but, as a rule, at least three-quarters do so and continue down the spinal cord in the lateral funiculus as the lateral corticospinal tract. Of the remaining fibres some retain their ventromedial position and descend in the anterior funiculus of the spinal cord as the anterior corticospinal tract; others descend with the crossed fibres in the lateral funiculus of the same side (**7.57**). As a result of this decussation the anterior intersegmental tract of the spinal cord is displaced nearer to the central grey matter, which also takes up a more dorsal position so that the central canal inclines backwards as it ascends. The continuity between the anterior grey column and the central grey matter, maintained throughout the whole length of the spinal cord, is severed. The detached anterior grey column rapidly diminishes in size as it ascends; it is subdivided into the *supraspinal nucleus*, the source of efferent fibres of the first cervical nerve, and the *spinal nucleus of the accessory nerve*, which lies dorsolaterally and gives origin to the upper fibres of the spinal part of that nerve. The supraspinal nucleus is continuous above with that of the hypoglossal nerve. The nucleus of the spinal part of the accessory nerve is continued into the upper five segments of the spinal cord where it lies in the dorsolateral part of the anterior grey column. Above it merges with the nucleus ambiguus (p. 848).

The outline of the posterior horn of the grey matter can still be made out, but it, too, has undergone some modification. A narrow, strip-like portion of grey matter appears in the middle of the fasciculus gracilis, continuous ventrally with the base of the posterior horn. This is the inferior end of the *nucleus gracilis*, which extends upwards as far as the caudal limit of the fourth ventricle and forms an elevation on the posterior surface of the medulla oblongata, already described as the gracile tubercle (p. 842). A second cuneiform projection from the base of the posterior horn, beginning at a slightly higher level, invades the ventral part of the fasciculus cuneatus, and constitutes the *nucleus cuneatus*.

The *substantia gelatinosa* is a prominent feature in the direct upward continuation of the apex of the posterior grey column of the spinal cord. Here this apex is continuous with the lower end of the *nucleus of the spinal tract of the trigeminal nerve*, and the fibres of the tract itself are interposed between the nucleus and the surface of the medulla oblongata (**7.60**). It is considered in detail on pp. 855 and 1029.

(2) **A transverse section just above the decussation of the pyramids** shows an accentuation of the differences already noted and the appearance of certain new elements (**7.61**).

The *nucleus gracilis* has increased in breadth and the fibres of its corresponding fasciculus are grouped together on its dorsal, medial and lateral surfaces; the *nucleus cuneatus* has undergone a similar change. At first both retain their continuity with the central grey matter, but this is lost at higher levels. The fibres of the fasciculus gracilis and cuneatus have ascended uncrossed through the spinal cord, and the majority terminate in their respective nuclei at different levels by forming synapses with their contained nerve cells. New fibres arise in the nuclei and constitute the second neurons on the pathway of tactile and proprioceptive sensibilities. These *internal arcuate fibres* emerge from the ventral aspects of the nuclei and, curving forwards and laterally at first round the central grey matter, they bend medially to reach the median plane, where they decussate with the corresponding fibres of the opposite side (7.61). Thereafter, they turn upwards and ascend on the opposite side close to the median raphe, constituting the *medial lemniscus*. The *decussation of the lemnisci* occurs in the area dorsal to the pyramids and in front of the central grey matter, which is in this way displaced still more dorsally towards the dorsal surface of the medulla oblongata. As the internal arcuate fibres sweep forwards they intervene between the spinal tract of the trigeminal nerve and the central grey matter. From the foregoing remarks it might appear that the gracile and cuneate nuclei are simply relay stations on a main sensory pathway widely regarded as the major route for impulses concerned with the more discriminative aspects of tactile and locomotor sensibility. During the last decade abundant anatomical and physiological evidence has led to a reappraisal of these views. It is clear that both nuclei contain interneurons[397] and that the nerve cells directly related to incoming afferents are chiefly concentrated at intermediate levels in them, especially in the case of tactile information.[398] The somatopic arrangement in the tracts is also evident in the nuclei, within which there is also a most specific distribution of terminals on the basis of sensory modalities, including hair displacement, light touch, pressure, vibration and joint movements. Receptive fields for individual fibres in these pathways have been intensively studied, indicating high degrees of specificity and inhibitory effects from adjoining fibres. The inhibitory and enhancing influences of cortical projections upon the gracile and cuneate cells have already been mentioned (p. 834). The precise functional significance of the gracile and cuneate tracts, including their projections, has recently become a topic of marked controversy, but it seems highly probable that the over-simplified account of them current in most general texts is no longer adequate.[399, 400] (See also pp. 834, 835.)

The *accessory cuneate nucleus* lies dorsolateral to the cuneate nucleus. It contains large cells similar to those of the thoracic nucleus of the spinal cord and gives origin to the *posterior external arcuate fibres* (p. 860); these enter the cerebellum through the ipsilateral inferior cerebellar peduncle. The accessory cuneate nucleus receives its afferents from the lateral fibres in the fasciculus cuneatus which are derived from the cervical segments. It provides a pathway, the *cuneocerebellar tract*, for proprioceptive impulses from the upper limb, destined for the cerebellum, which enter the spinal cord above the upper limit of the thoracic nucleus.[401]

The *nucleus of the spinal tract of the trigeminal nerve* (7.62) is at this level separated from the central grey matter by the internal arcuate fibres. It is separated from the lateral surface of the medulla oblongata only by the spinal tract of the trigeminal nerve, the fibres of which terminate in the nucleus, and by some of the fibres of the posterior spinocerebellar tract, which is beginning to incline dorsally to enter the inferior cerebellar peduncle (p. 860).

Two additional collections of grey matter occur at this level. One is dorsal to the lateral part of the pyramid, while the other is placed to its medial side and not far from the median plane. These are parts of the *medial accessory olivary nucleus* and will be considered together with the inferior olivary nucleus (p. 847).

The central grey matter, now occupying a position near the dorsal surface of the medulla oblongata, contains

three important nuclei. A prominent group of large motor nerve cells, interspersed with myelinated fibres, is situated in the ventromedial part of the central grey matter. This is the *nucleus of the hypoglossal nerve*. It extends upwards into the open part of the medulla oblongata, where it lies under the medial part of the trigonum hypoglossi in the floor of the fourth ventricle. Immediately adjacent to the hypoglossal nucleus are several other smaller groups of nerve cells collectively spoken of as the 'perihypoglossal' complex or 'perihypoglossal grey'. Neither term has more than topographical significance, for none

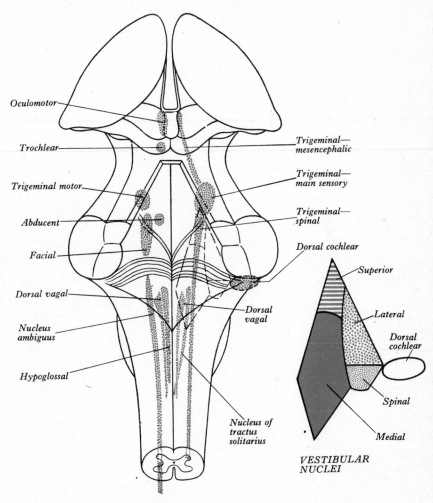

7.62 Surface projection of the nuclei of the cranial nerves on the dorsal aspect of the brainstem. Motor nuclei in red; sensory in blue. The vestibular nuclei are indicated in the main diagram by interrupted lines and are shown in detail in the small diagram. The olfactory and optic centres are not shown.

of them is known to be in any way connected with the hypoglossal nerve or its nucleus. Included in the complex are the nucleus intercalatus (of Staderini), the 'sublingual' nucleus (of Roller), the nucleus prepositus hypoglossi, and the nucleus paramedianus dorsalis (reticularis), all of which contain cells suggestive in their characteristics of reticular connexions, which have been definitely ascribed to the paramedian nucleus.[402] Gustatory and visceral afferent connexions have been attributed

[397] P. Andersen, J. C. Eccles, R. F. Schmidt and T. Yokota, *J. Neurophysiol.*, **27**, 1964.

[398] P. J. Hand, *J. comp. Neurol.*, **126**, 1966.

[399] V. B. Mountcastle, *Medical Physiology*, 12th ed., Mosby, St. Louis. 1968.

[400] P. D. Wall, *Brain*, **93**, 1970.

[401] A. Ferraro and G. E. Barrera, *J. comp. Neurol.*, **62**, 1935.

[402] A. Brodal, *The Reticular Formation of the Brainstem*, Oliver and Boyd, Edinburgh. 1957.

to the intercalated nucleus, but there is more convincing evidence that the perihypoglossal nuclei in general project to the cerebellum, at least in the cat[403] and the monkey.[404] A topographical representation of lingual musculature has been described in the hypoglossal nucleus (p. 1026).

Dorsolateral to the hypoglossal nucleus, there is a second group of cells, the *dorsal nucleus of the vagus*. It is a mixed nucleus, containing cells of at least two types. The larger cells give rise to the fine fibres which innervate non-striated muscle; the smaller spindle-shaped cells may possibly be concerned with visceral afferent impulses. On the other hand many authorities believe that all the vagal visceral afferent fibres terminate in the nucleus of the tractus solitarius (*vide infra*). At a higher level the dorsal nucleus of the vagus lies to the lateral side of the hypoglossal nucleus in the floor of the fourth ventricle and corresponds in position to the trigonum vagi.

with the dorsal vagal nucleus and nucleus ambiguus. There is evidence that the solitary nucleus projects to the upper levels of the spinal cord through a solitario-spinal tract (p. 819) both in man[408] and the cat.[409] The nucleus is considered to receive fibres from the spinal cord, cerebral cortex and cerebellum.[410] Nerve cells aggregated in a position ventrolateral to the nucleus of the solitary tract have sometimes been termed the *nucleus parasolitarius*.[411]

Numerous scattered islets of grey matter occur in the centre of the ventrolateral portion of the medulla oblongata. They occupy an area which is freely intersected by nerve fibres running in all directions and which is therefore termed the *reticular formation*. It is present at all levels of the medulla oblongata and extends upwards into the tegmentum of the pons and midbrain. There is no clear demarcation between the reticular formations in

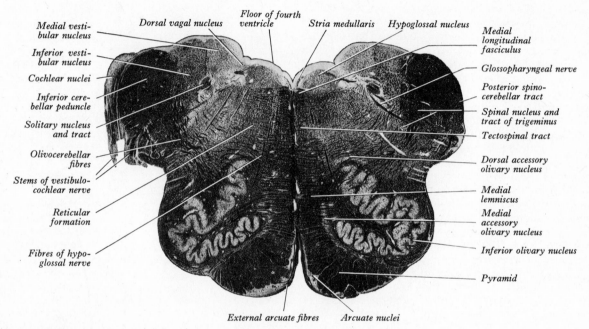

Medial vesti-bular nucleus — Dorsal vagal nucleus — Floor of fourth ventricle — Stria medullaris — Hypoglossal nucleus — Medial longitudinal fasciculus

Inferior vesti-bular nucleus — Glossopharyngeal nerve

Cochlear nuclei — Posterior spino-cerebellar tract

Inferior cere-bellar peduncle — Spinal nucleus and tract of trigeminus

Solitary nucleus and tract — Tectospinal tract

Olivocerebellar fibres — Dorsal accessory olivary nucleus

Stems of vestibulo-cochlear nerve — Medial lemniscus

Reticular formation — Medial accessory olivary nucleus

Inferior olivary nucleus

Fibres of hypo-glossal nerve — Pyramid

External arcuate fibres — Arcuate nuclei

**7.63** Transverse section through the medulla oblongata at mid-olivary level. Weigert Pal preparation. Magnification *c.* ×4·5.

A third group of cells lies dorsolateral to the dorsal nucleus of the vagus at this level. It is the *nucleus of the tractus solitarius* (**7.65**), and it is intimately related to a group of descending fibres which constitute the *tractus solitarius* itself. At the caudal end of the medulla, solitary and dorsal nuclei fuse dorsal to the central canal. As the nucleus of the tractus solitarius is traced upwards it comes to lie more deeply in the medulla oblongata, on the ventro-lateral aspect of the dorsal nucleus of the vagus, with which it is practically coextensive. The tractus solitarius receives afferent fibres from the facial, glossopharyngeal and vagus nerves, and they enter the nucleus in that order from above downwards, conveying to it gustatory sensibility from the mucous membrane of the tongue and palate (facial, glossopharyngeal and vagus), and, according to many authorities, visceral sensibility from the pharynx (glossopharyngeal and vagus) and from the oesophagus and the abdominal part of the alimentary canal (vagus). In this craniocaudal representation there is some degree of overlap.[405, 406] The nerve cells of the solitary nucleus are smaller than those of the dorsal vagal nucleus. It is presumed that their axons project to the thalamus and perhaps thence to the cerebral cortex, though experimental attempts to establish this in the cat have failed.[407] The same study demonstrated connexions

these various regions and they are considered collectively on p. 888.

The white matter has undergone an important re-arrangement above the corticospinal decussation. The *pyramids* contain corticospinal and corticonuclear fibres, the latter being distributed to the motor nuclei of the cranial nerves. They form two large bundles in the ventral part of the section, on each side of the anterior median fissure. Dorsally they are related to the accessory olivary nuclei and the decussation of the lemnisci.

The fibres of the *medial lemniscus* (p. 845), after emerging from the lemniscal decussation, turn upwards on each side in the form of a flattened tract, closely applied to the median raphe. In this position they ascend to the pons, increasing in number as additional fibres join

[403] A. Torvik and A. Brodal, *J. Neuropath exp. Neurol.*, **13**, 1954.

[404] W. R. Mehler, M. E. Feferman and W. J. H. Nauta, *Brain*, **83**, 1960.

[405] H. G. Schwartz, G. E. Roulhac, R. L. Lam and J. O'Leary, *J. comp. Neurol.*, **94**, 1951.

[406] F. W. L. Kerr, *Archs Neurol. Psychiat., Chicago*, **6**, 1962.

[407] D. K. Morest, *J. comp. Neurol.*, **130**, 1967.

[408] J. Collier and E. F. Buzzard, *Brain*, **26**, 1903.

[409] A. Torvik, *J. Anat.*, **91**, 1957.

[410] P. Angaut and A. Brodal, *Archs ital. Biol.*, **105**, 1967.

[411] E. C. Crosby, T. Humphrey and E. W. Lauer, *Correlative Anatomy of the Nervous System*, Macmillan, N.Y. 1962.

them from the upper levels of the decussation. Ventrally they are related to the pyramidal tract, and dorsally to the medial longitudinal bundle and the tectospinal tract. In the decussation the fibres undergo a rearrangement whereby those derived from the gracile nucleus come to lie ventral to those derived from the cuneate nucleus; at a higher level where the disposition of the medial lemniscus in the brainstem becomes altered (p. 883), the gracile fibres are lateral and the cuneate fibres medial. The fibres of the medial lemnisci at this level have been shown to

the large olivary nucleus, the arcuate nucleus and nuclei associated with two divisions of the vestibulocochlear, the glossopharyngeal, vagus and accessory nerves.

The *inferior olivary nucleus* is a large hollow mass of grey matter, with irregularly crenated walls and a longitudinal hilus placed on its medial side. It is surrounded by a capsule of myelinated fibres forming the *amiculum of the olive.* Situated dorsolateral to the pyramid, the nucleus corresponds to the surface elevation of the olive, but extends upwards almost to the pons. The olivary nucleus

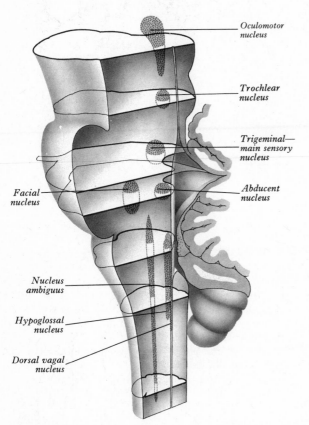

7.64 Diagram of motor nuclei of the cranial nerves. The sectional planes shown correspond to those depicted elsewhere in the text.

- Oculomotor nucleus
- Trochlear nucleus
- Trigeminal—main sensory nucleus
- Facial nucleus
- Abducent nucleus
- Nucleus ambiguus
- Hypoglossal nucleus
- Dorsal vagal nucleus

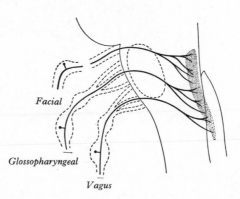

- Facial
- Glossopharyngeal
- Vagus

7.65 Diagram of afferent fibres of the facial, glossopharyngeal and vagus nerves, conveying gustatory impulses to the nucleus of the tractus solitarius.

display in the monkey[412] and chimpanzee[413] a laminar somatotopic arrangement on a segmental basis.

The *medial longitudinal fasciculus* forms a small compact tract of nerve fibres, situated close to the median plane and ventral to the hypoglossal nucleus. Below, it is continuous with the anterior intersegmental tract of the spinal cord, but at this medullary level it is displaced dorsally by the decussations of the pyramids and lemnisci. It is continued upwards through the pons and the midbrain in the same position relative to the central grey matter and the median plane, and therefore comes into intimate relationship throughout its course with the somatic efferent column of the grey matter. The constituent fibres of the tract run relatively short courses within it, for they are derived from a variety of sources, which are detailed on p. 885.

The spinocerebellar, spinotectal, vestibulospinal, rubrospinal and lateral spinothalamic (spinal lemniscal) tracts are all in the anterolateral area, limited dorsally by the nucleus of the spinal trigeminal tract and ventrally by the pyramid.

(3) **A transverse section at the level of the caudal limit of the fourth ventricle** (7.63), shows a number of new elements, together with most of those already described at a lower level. The total amount of grey matter shows a distinct increase owing to the presence of

consists of small cells, a large number of their axons forming the *olivocerebellar tract.* These axons emerge from the hilus or through the adjacent wall and run medially, intersecting the fibres of the medial lemniscus (7.63, 66). They cross the median plane and sweep dorsal to or traverse the olivary nucleus of the opposite side, intersecting the lateral spinothalamic tract, rubrospinal tract and nucleus of the spinal tract of the trigeminal nerve to enter the inferior cerebellar peduncle, by which they are conveyed to the cerebellum. Afferent connexions to the nucleus can be divided into ascending and descending fibres. The ascending fibres, mainly crossed, reach the nucleus from all levels of the spinal cord travelling in one or, possibly, two *spino-olivary tracts.* Some ascending connexions also reach the inferior olivary complex via the dorsal white columns.[414] The descending fibres arise from the cortex of the cerebrum, thalamus, basal nuclei, red nucleus and central grey matter of the midbrain.[415] Some of these are said to travel in a bundle called the *central tegmental fasciculus.*[416]

The *medial accessory olivary nucleus* is a curved lamina of grey matter which is found at this level. The concavity of the curve is directed laterally and the nucleus is interposed between the medial lemniscus and the pyramid, on the one hand, and the medial and ventral aspects of the inferior olivary nucleus on the other.

The *dorsal accessory olivary nucleus* is a second lamina of grey matter, placed dorsal to the medial part of the inferior olivary nucleus.

Both the inferior and the accessory olivary nuclei are intimately associated with the cerebellum. Phylogenetically, the accessory olivary nuclei are older than the inferior nucleus, and they send their fibres to the palaeocerebellum (p. 860). The inferior olivary nucleus occurs

[412] A. Ferraro and S. E. Barrera, *J. comp. Neurol.,* **64**, 1936.
[413] A. E. Walker, *Proc. K. ned. Akad. Wet.,* **40**, 1937.
[414] P. J. Hand and C.-N. Liu, *Anat. Rec.,* **154**, 1966.
[415] F. Walberg, *J. comp. Neurol.,* **114**, 1960.
[416] J. Jansen and A. Brodal, *Aspects of Cerebellar Anatomy,* Grundt Tanum, Oslo. 1950.

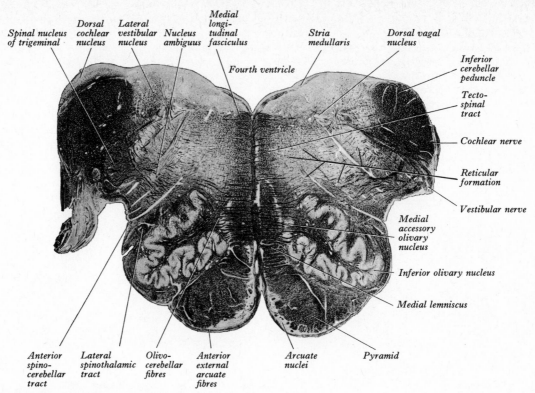

*Spinal nucleus of trigeminal*  *Dorsal cochlear nucleus*  *Lateral vestibular nucleus*  *Nucleus ambiguus*  *Medial longitudinal fasciculus*  *Stria medullaris*  *Dorsal vagal nucleus*

*Fourth ventricle*

*Inferior cerebellar peduncle*
*Tecto-spinal tract*
*Cochlear nerve*
*Reticular formation*
*Vestibular nerve*
*Medial accessory olivary nucleus*
*Inferior olivary nucleus*
*Medial lemniscus*

*Anterior spino-cerebellar tract*  *Lateral spinothalamic tract*  *Olivo-cerebellar fibres*  *Anterior external arcuate fibres*  *Arcuate nuclei*  *Pyramid*

**7.**66 Transverse section through the superior half of the medulla oblongata. Weigert Pal preparation. Magnification *c.* ×4·5.

only in mammals and, in the course of evolution, it has enlarged in a caudal direction. In all their connexions, whether with higher levels in the cerebral hemispheres, the spinal cord, or the cerebellum, the olivary nuclei show a marked and often highly specific organization upon a somatotopic basis. This is particularly so in the case of cerebellar connexions, which are considered in detail later (pp. 860, 863, 869).

The *arcuate nuclei* form curved, interrupted bands of grey matter which are closely applied to the anterior and medial aspects of the pyramids; they appear to be caudally displaced nuclei pontis.[417] They give origin to the anterior external arcuate fibres.

The central grey matter, which, at this level, is spread out over the floor of the ventricle, contains the *hypoglossal nucleus* and the *dorsal nucleus of the vagus*, the *nucleus of the tractus solitarius* lying ventrolateral to the last-named; lateral to these, and on the medial side of the inferior cerebellar peduncle, the lower part of the *inferior and medial nuclei of the vestibular nerve* may be recognized (p. 851). Between the hypoglossal nucleus and the dorsal nucleus of the vagus is the *nucleus intercalatus* (p. 845).

A small isolated group of large motor nerve cells, termed the *nucleus ambiguus*, is placed deeply in the reticular formation. It extends upwards as far as the upper limit of the dorsal nucleus of the vagus. The fibres which emerge from its upper end join the glossopharyngeal nerve, and those which emerge at a lower level join the fila of the vagus and cranial part of the accessory nerves. Inferiorly it is continuous with the spinal nucleus of the accessory nerve (p. 844). It consists of large motor neurons, the fibres of which are distributed to striated muscle of branchial origin (p. 1027). These first pass dorsally and medially for a short distance and then curve laterally to join the emerging fila of the cranial portion of the accessory, the vagus and glossopharyngeal nerves. Histologically, the nucleus ambiguus can be divided into several groups of cells in man, as in other mammals; experimentally some degree of representation of the muscles innervated has been established[418] (p. 1028).

The nucleus gracilis and the nucleus cuneatus, now diminishing in size and irregular in outline, occupy the dorsolateral portion of the section, and ventral to them the *nucleus of the spinal tract of the trigeminal nerve* can be recognized without difficulty.

The *cochlear nuclei* may be observed on the surface of the inferior cerebellar peduncle (pp. 852, 853).

The white matter of the medulla oblongata shows little change at this level apart from the development of the inferior cerebellar peduncle on the lateral side of the fourth ventricle. The pyramid, the medial lemniscus, the tectospinal tract and the medial longitudinal bundle occupy the same relative positions as they did at a lower level. The fibres of the olivocerebellar tract, sweeping across the median plane and turning dorsally to join the inferior cerebellar peduncle, have already been described in connexion with the olivary nucleus (p. 847). The *anterior external arcuate fibres* have their cells of origin in the arcuate nuclei of both sides and, emerging from the anterior median fissure, they run laterally, backwards and upwards over the surface of the pyramid, the olive and the spinal tract of the trigeminal nerve. Reaching the posterior spinocerebellar tract, they ascend with it to enter the inferior cerebellar peduncle (**7.**67).

The emerging fila of the hypoglossal nerve leave the ventral aspect of its nucleus and run forwards through the reticular formation. Passing lateral to the medial lemniscus and medial to, or sometimes through the wall of, the olivary nucleus, they curve laterally to emerge from the anterolateral sulcus. A relatively small lesion in the ventral part of the medulla oblongata at this level may therefore involve both the corticospinal tract and the hypoglossal nerve, causing a characteristic crossed paralysis. The muscles of the tongue are paralysed on the same side as the lesion, but it is the limbs of the opposite side of the body that are affected, for the lesion is situated above the level of the pyramidal decussation.

[417] A. T. Rasmussen and W. T. Peyton, *J. comp. Neurol.*, **84**, 1946.
[418] A. M. Lawn, *J. comp. Neurol.*, **127**, 1966.

More dorsally, the reticular formation is traversed by the fibres of the vagus, travelling from their origin in the dorsal nucleus, the nucleus ambiguus and the nucleus of the tractus solitarius to the posterolateral sulcus, where they emerge.

The *spinal lemniscus* (p. 823), lies dorsal to the olivary nucleus and separated from the surface of the medulla oblongata by the anterior spinocerebellar and the spinotectal tracts. There is evidence from surgical procedures in man, and experiments in other animals,[419] that the fibres are arranged somatotopically; those conveying impulses from the lower limb are superficial, those from the upper limb deep and those from the trunk intermediate. As it ascends through the upper part of the medulla oblongata, the spinal lemniscus is closely related to the nucleus ambiguus, and a small lesion in the ventral part of the reticular formation may cause paralysis of the vocal fold and of the soft palate of the same side, but a loss of sensibility to pain and temperature on the opposite side of the body.

(4) **A transverse section of the most cranial part of the medulla oblongata** shows little change. The dorsal surface of the medulla oblongata here is relatively flat as compared with the preceding level and may show a few fibres of the stria medullaris just under this surface (p. 854). The inferior olivary nucleus occupies the same relative position, but the accessory olivary nuclei are broken up and diminishing (7.66).

The medial nucleus of the vestibular nerve has widened and lies on the lateral and dorsal sides of the dorsal vagal nucleus, which is now depressed below the floor of the rhomboid fossa. The inferior nucleus of the vestibular nerve intervenes between the medial nucleus and the inferior cerebellar peduncle. At the pontomedullary junction the *lateral vestibular nucleus* replaces the inferior nucleus and the lower parts of the cochlear nuclei are usually seen. (See p. 851 for details of the vestibular nuclei.)

The nucleus of the tractus solitarius, the nucleus of the spinal tract of the trigeminal nerve and the nucleus ambiguus show little alteration in position.

The arrangement of the white substance at this level shows no conspicuous alteration. The lateral spinothalamic tract, or spinal lemniscus, ascends dorsal to the olivary nucleus, its fibres retaining the somatotopical arrangement already described (p. 823). The *inferior cerebellar peduncle* has increased in size and forms a well-marked elevation on the dorsolateral aspect of the medulla oblongata. The extensive array of fibres, from many sources, which compose the peduncle are described on p. 860.

The disposition of the *medial lemniscus* (p. 848) alters in the upper part of the medulla oblongata. Its ventral region widens and becomes insinuated between the dorsal aspect of the pyramid and the narrowing cranial end of the olivary nucleus (7.71). At the same time its dorsal part recedes from the tectospinal tract and the medial longitudinal bundle. This alteration is continued

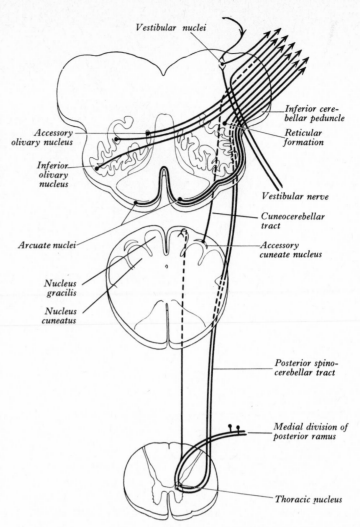

7.67 Diagram to show some of the afferent components of the inferior cerebellar peduncle; the efferent components have been omitted. See text for further details.

so that, as it enters the pons, the medial lemniscus is extended in a coronal plane (7.70) in the ventral part of the tegmentum (p. 855). The medial lemniscus comprises the projection fibres on the pathway for proprioceptive and tactile sensibility. It is believed that, in its course through the medulla oblongata, it is joined by the fibres of the anterior spinothalamic tract (p. 819). On entry into the pons, therefore, the medial lemniscus contains many of the proprioceptive, tactile and pressure fibres from the lower limb, the trunk and the upper limb of the *opposite* side and there are good grounds for believing that the lower limb fibres are placed most laterally and adjoin those from the upper limb, while those from the neck lie most medially.

[419] E. Gardner and H. M. Cuneo, *Archs Neurol. Psychiat., Chicago*, **53**, 1945.

# THE PONS

**The pons** is ventral to the cerebellum. Cranial to it is the midbrain. Inferiorly the pons is continuous with the medulla oblongata, but is demarcated from it in front and on each side by a transverse furrow in which the abducent, facial and vestibulocochlear nerves appear.

The *ventral* or *anterior surface* of the pons (7.55, 56) is prominent, being markedly convex from side to side, less

so from above downwards. It consists of transverse fibres arched like a bridge across the median plane, and converging on each side into a compact mass which forms the middle cerebellar peduncle. It adjoins the dorsum sellae of the sphenoid bone and the adjacent basilar part of the occipital bone, and is limited above and below by well-defined borders. The anterior surface of the pons is

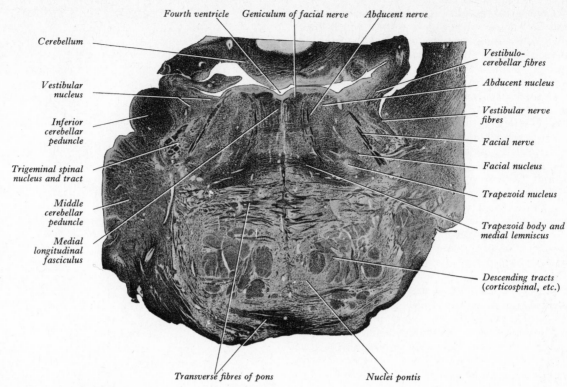

**7.68** Transverse section through the pons at the level of the facial colliculus. Weigert Pal preparation. Magnification *c.* × 3·5.

marked by the shallow median *sulcus basilaris*, which usually lodges the basilar artery; this sulcus is bounded on each side by an eminence caused by the descent of the corticospinal fibres through the substance of the pons. Lateral to these eminences, a little above the mid level of the pons, the trigeminal nerves make their exit, each consisting of a smaller, superomedial, motor root, and a larger, inferolateral, sensory root; vertical lines, drawn immediately lateral to the attachments of the trigeminal nerves, may be taken as arbitrary boundaries between the ventral surface of the pons and the middle cerebellar peduncles.

The *dorsal* or *posterior surface* of the pons is hidden by the cerebellum. It contributes to the upper half of the rhomboid fossa, with which it is described (p. 879).

Transverse sections through the pons show that it is divided into a dorsal region or *tegmentum* and a *ventral* (*basilar*) *part.* The tegmentum is the direct upward continuation of the medulla oblongata, excluding the pyramids. The ventral part contains bundles of longitudinal fibres, some of which are continued into the pyramids of the medulla oblongata, numbers of transverse fibres and scattered collections of grey matter which constitute the *nuclei pontis.* (It should be noted that the term 'pons' is commonly used in two senses: firstly, to denote the externally visible protuberance of the ventral part of the region and, secondly to designate both this and the tegmental part, i.e. the whole of the brainstem between medulla oblongata and mesencephalon.)

In mammals a correlation exists between the degree of development of the cerebral hemispheres, ventral part of the pons and cerebellum (neocerebellum, p. 858). The ventral part of the pons is not present in submammalian forms; it is present in marsupials and higher mammals and may be represented in the lowliest mammals, the monotremes.[420] As the mammalian scale is ascended, the ventral part increases in size *pari passu* with cerebrum and cerebellum.

## INTERNAL STRUCTURE OF THE PONS

**The ventral part of the pons** presents a similar arrangement of its grey and white matter at all levels. The longitudinal bundles (**7.71**) comprise the corticopontine, corticonuclear and corticospinal (motor) fibres, which are continued downwards from the crus cerebri (p. 882). As they enter the upper limit of the ventral part of the pons, they form a compact collection of fibres, but they rapidly become dispersed into numerous smaller bundles, separated from one another by the *nuclei pontis* and the transverse fibres of the pons. The *corticospinal fibres* descend through the whole length of the pons and enter the pyramids of the medulla oblongata, where they converge

**7.69** Diagram of central course of the fibres of the facial nerve, superior aspect, in a transverse section of the pons.

[420] A. A. Abbie, *Proc. R. Soc. B.*, **115**, 1934.

into compact tracts (p. 840). They are accompanied by *corticonuclear fibres*, some of which pass to the contralateral motor nuclei of the cranial nerves in the pons; the remainder continue into the medulla oblongata to end in a similar manner. Clinically there is evidence that the facial nucleus and certain other nuclei (p. 854) also receive ipsilateral corticonuclear fibres. The *corticopontine fibres*, which are derived from the cerebral cortex of the frontal, temporal, parietal and occipital lobes, terminate at different levels in the nuclei pontis (7.68). The axons of the cells of the nuclei pontis form the *transverse fibres of the pons* (pontocerebellar fibres), and constitute the middle cerebellar peduncle. The frontopontine fibres terminate in the nuclei pontis above the level of the emerging roots of the trigeminal nerve and are relayed to the opposite half of the cerebellum as the upper transverse fibres of the pons. A few of the pontocerebellar fibres do not cross the midline; they all end as mossy fibres of the cerebellar cortex (p. 869). Some degree of somatotopic organization is carried through this system of connexions. Axons from the tectum of the midbrain may also relay in the nuclei pontis,[421] as may in addition some from spinal levels.

The *nuclei pontis* comprise all the masses of nerve cells which are scattered throughout the ventral part of the pons. They are of various sizes and shapes. As already indicated, they constitute cell stations on the pathway from the cerebral cortex to the cerebellum. The cells of the nuclei pontis are derivatives of the rhombic lip which migrate ventrally and cranially.

the eighth nerve on the lateral side (but for an alternative view see p. 854). The afferent fibres to the nucleus have been claimed to traverse the whole length of the pons with the corticospinal fibres and leave them only in the medulla oblongata. They course obliquely backwards and upwards over the surface of the olive, to reach their destination, forming part of the *fasciculus circumolivaris pyramidis* (7.77).

The dorsal, tegmental part of the pons varies in its internal details at different levels, especially in regard to its cytoarchitecture. These differences can be adequately illustrated for general purposes by sections at two representative levels, one cranial, one caudal.

**A transverse section through the caudal part of the tegmentum** passing through the facial colliculus (7.68), contains the motor nuclei of the abducent and facial nerves, the nuclei of the vestibular and cochlear divisions of the eighth nerve, and certain isolated collections of grey matter which will be described below.

The *medial nucleus* of the vestibular nerve is continued upwards for a short distance into the tegmentum of the pons. The *lateral vestibular nucleus* lies between it and the inferior cerebellar peduncle.

The *vestibular nuclei* lie subjacent to the vestibular area in the rhomboid fossa (p. 879) and comprise the medial, lateral, inferior and superior. They receive fibres from the vestibular division of the vestibulocochlear nerve and send their axons to the cerebellum, medial longitudinal fasciculus, spinal cord and lateral lemniscus. The *medial vestibular nucleus* extends from the medulla oblongata at

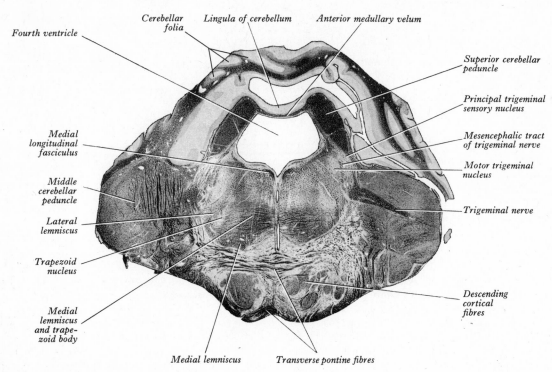

*Fourth ventricle*

*Cerebellar folia*

*Lingula of cerebellum*

*Anterior medullary velum*

*Superior cerebellar peduncle*

*Principal trigeminal sensory nucleus*

*Medial longitudinal fasciculus*

*Mesencephalic tract of trigeminal nerve*

*Motor trigeminal nucleus*

*Middle cerebellar peduncle*

*Lateral lemniscus*

*Trigeminal nerve*

*Trapezoid nucleus*

*Medial lemniscus and trapezoid body*

*Descending cortical fibres*

*Medial lemniscus*

*Transverse pontine fibres*

**7.70** Transverse section of the pons at the level of the trigeminal nerve. Weigert Pal preparation. Magnification *c.* ×2·5.

All the cells which migrate in this direction do not succeed in reaching the ventral part of the pons. Some of them remain, forming an oblique ridge across the dorsolateral aspect of the inferior cerebellar peduncle, and constitute the *nucleus of the circumolivary bundle* (corpus pontobulbare). It has been held that the fibres to which this discrete part of the nuclei pontis gives origin run vertically upwards on the surface between the emerging seventh nerve on the medial side, and its sensory root and

the level of the upper end of the olive into the lower part of the pons. As it ascends it broadens, so that the dorsal nucleus of the vagus becomes depressed below the floor of the fourth ventricle. It is crossed by the striae medullares, which separate it from the floor of the fourth ventricle. Caudally it is continuous with the nucleus intercalatus.

421 G. W. Pearce, in: *Structure and Function of the Cerebellar Cortex*, eds. D. B. Tower and J. P. Schadé, Elsevier, Amsterdam. 1960.

The *inferior vestibular nucleus* lies between the medial nucleus and the inferior cerebellar peduncle. It extends from the level of the cranial limit of the nucleus gracilis to the pontomedullary junction. It is interspersed by bundles of fibres from the descending part of the vestibular nerve and from the vestibulospinal tract. The *lateral vestibular nucleus* lies immediately cranial to the inferior nucleus and extends upwards almost to the level of the nucleus of the abducent nerve. It is composed of large multipolar cells. The cells of this nucleus give origin to the fibres of the vestibulospinal tract. The *superior vestibular nucleus* is small and lies above the medial and lateral nuclei.

The *fibres of the vestibular part of the vestibulocochlear nerve* can be seen entering the medulla oblongata between the inferior cerebellar peduncle and the spinal tract of the trigeminal nerve and are directed towards the vestibular area. After entering the brainstem, they separate into

and via the medial longitudinal fasciculus to the motor nuclei of the ocular muscles.

A number of minor groups of neurons in the vicinity of the named vestibular nuclei have been identified in experimental animals; only one of these, the *interstitial nucleus* of the vestibular nerve, is known to receive axons from it. The *nucleus parasolitarius* (p. 846) may be associated with the vestibular complex on the basis of afferent connexions from the fastigial nucleus of the cerebellum (p. 873). The total number of nerve cells in the vestibular nuclei much exceeds the complement of afferent fibres in the vestibular part of the eighth cranial nerve, and this is linked with the observation that vestibular afferents reach only limited regions of the vestibular nuclei, many of whose cells may be interneurons, many also being the sources of the varied projections mentioned above. There is considerable evidence of spatial representation of the vestibular

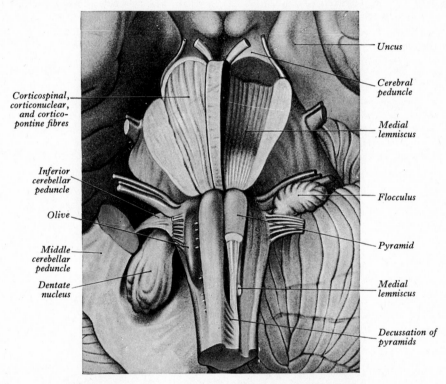

Corticospinal, corticonuclear, and cortico-pontine fibres

Inferior cerebellar peduncle

Olive

Middle cerebellar peduncle

Dentate nucleus

Uncus

Cerebral peduncle

Medial lemniscus

Flocculus

Pyramid

Medial lemniscus

Decussation of pyramids

**7.71** Ventral aspect of a dissection of the pons, the medulla oblongata and the right cerebellar hemisphere. In the pons and medulla, the dissec-tion is deeper on the left (right side of figure). Note the spiralling of the medial lemniscus and compare with **7.103**.

ascending and descending bundles and branches. The descending fibres terminate in the medial, lateral and inferior vestibular nuclei. They descend on the medial side of the inferior cerebellar peduncle and intermingle with the cells of the inferior nucleus. The ascending fibres pass either into the superior and medial nuclei and a few to the cerebellum. The fibres to the cerebellum pass superficially through the inferior cerebellar peduncle (in the juxtarestiform body) to terminate in the nucleus fastigii, the flocculonodular lobe and the uvula (p. 860). The vestibular nuclei not only project extensively to the cerebellum (p. 861), but also receive axons from parts of the cerebellar cortex and the fastigial nuclei (p. 861). Their projections to the spinal cord, through the vesti-bulospinal tract, have already been described (p. 817). Vestibular connexions also reach the cord through the medial longitudinal fasciculus (p. 818). Efferent axons are also projected to higher levels in the cerebrum, prob-ably mediating a bilateral cortical representation, but evidence for this is scanty. The vestibular complex sends fibres in addition to the pontine reticular nuclei (p. 890)

apparatus in the nuclei (p. 1016). For an appraisal of the large volume of experimental research in connection with the vestibular pathway see references [422, 423].

The *fibres of the cochlear division of the vestibulocochlear nerve* partially encircle the lateral surface of the inferior cerebellar peduncle to terminate in the *dorsal* and *ventral cochlear nuclei*, which project slightly from the surface of the peduncle. The *dorsal cochlear nucleus*, which forms the auditory tubercle (p. 879), is on the posterior aspect of the peduncle and is continuous medially with the vesti-bular area in the rhomboid fossa. The *ventral cochlear nucleus* is on the anterolateral side of the peduncle in the interval between the cochlear and vestibular fibres of the vestibulocochlear nerve. The two parts of the vestibulo-cochlear nerve and the cochlear nuclei are usually seen in sections at the pontomedullary junction.

[422] A. Brodal, O. Pompeiano and F. Walberg, *The Vestibular Nuclei and their Connexions, Anatomy and Functional Correlations*, Oliver and Boyd, Edinburgh. 1962.

[423] G. L. Rasmussen and W. F. Windle (eds.), *Neural Mechanisms of the Auditory and Vestibular Systems*, Thomas, Springfield, Ill. 1960.

**The ventral cochlear nucleus** is highly complex in its cytoarchitecture, consisting of many cell types, variously described as giant, large and small spherical, multipolar, granular, and so on, the variants being on the whole grouped in separate regions of the nucleus. [424, 425] (See also p. 1016.) Degeneration experiments demonstrate a marked degree of topographical order in the termination of cochlear nerve fibres in the nucleus, in that different parts of the spiral organ of the cochlea and differing frequencies of stimulation appear to be related to specific cells serially arrayed in the ventrocaudal part of the ventral nucleus. [426, 427] All the cochlear nerve fibres enter the nucleus, bifurcating as they do so into ascending branches, which terminate in the ventral nucleus, and descending branches traversing it to reach the dorsal cochlear nucleus (*vide infra*). The total number of cochlear nerve fibres has been estimated at about 25,000 in man, and since the ventral nucleus alone contains at least three times as many nerve cells as this in the cat, whose cochlear fibres are about half the human complement, it is clear that the cells in the cochlear nuclei greatly outnumber the fibres in the nerve. Thus, a mere fraction of the cochlear nerve cells receive terminals from the nerve, though it is said that each fibre forms connexions with several cells. [428] These terminals are limited to the ventral and caudal region of the ventral cochlear nucleus, some of whose neurons are probably local interneurons, the remainder being the sources of axons leaving the nucleus, as described below.

**The dorsal cochlear nucleus** is topographically almost continuous with the ventral nucleus, the two being separated by a thin stratum of nerve fibres. The dorsal nucleus also shows a complex organization, based upon a laminar pattern and containing a considerable spectrum of nerve cell types, including giant cells and other types like those in the ventral nucleus and also a fusiform or pyramidal type peculiar to it. Again, the terminals in the dorsal nucleus appear to be limited in their distribution, being derived, of course, from the descending branches of the cochlear nerve mentioned above. [429]

While details of the types of cells in the cochlear nuclei which project from them are not yet available, such axons are probably derived from several types, since a large proportion of the total number of cells have efferent axons, a few only being confined to the nuclei. These efferents all end at pontine levels in the superior olivary, trapezoid, and lateral lemniscal nuclei (*vide infra*), and they leave the cochlear nuclei by at least three routes. (1) The most ventral contingent of efferent fibres are also the most numerous, forming by their decussation the trapezoid body at the level of the pontomedullary junction (7.70). These axons ascend slightly as they approach the midline to decussate, but a minor number do not cross; they form connexions in the ipsilateral superior olivary nuclei. Those which decussate relay in the contralateral nuclei, and in both cases the next order of axons ascend in the corresponding lateral lemniscus. A few of the decussating fibres pass through the contralateral superior olive into the lateral lemniscus, where they relay in the lemniscal nuclei. (2) Some of the axons derived from ventral cochlear nucleus cells pass dorsally superficial to the descending spinal fibres of the trigeminal nerve and to the cerebellar fibres in the inferior peduncle, together with axons of the dorsal cochlear nucleus, which form the third group. These ventral cochlear fibres, which are smaller in calibre than those forming the trapezoid decussation, swerve ventromedially to cross the midline ventral to the medial longitudinal fasciculus as the *intermediate acoustic striae* (of Held[430]); their further progress is uncertain, but they probably pass cranially within the opposite lateral lemniscus. (3) The most dorsal group of cochlear projection fibres, derived from the dorsal cochlear nucleus, turn

medially around the dorsal aspect of the inferior cerebellar peduncle and continue towards the midline as the *dorsal acoustic striae* (of Monakow[431]). They are not to be confused with the striae medullares of the fourth ventricle (p. 854), to which they are ventral and thus more deeply situated. As the dorsal acoustic striae incline ventromedially they approach and cross the midline to reach and ascend in the opposite lateral lemniscus, in the nuclei of which they probably relay.

The *superior olivary complex of nuclei* is located laterally in the reticular formation at the level of the pontomedullary junction. Medial to the complex are the trapezoid nucleus and body, inferior to it the much larger inferior olivary group of nuclei (p. 847). The superior olive consists of a number of named nuclei and other small groups of nerve cells. [432] The *lateral superior olivary nucleus* (the S-shaped segment of the feline olivary complex) is relatively small in primates, including man. Medial to it is the *medial (accessory) superior olivary nucleus* (the para-olivary nucleus of Winkler), which is large in man. Medial again to this is the nucleus of the trapezoid body (*vide infra*). Dorsally situated in the complex is a *retro-olivary group* of nerve cells, reputed to be the origin of the efferent cochlear fibres described below. Interconnexions between the individual nuclei of the superior olivary complex have been described. Unit recording from the lateral nucleus in the cat[433] has established the existence of a tonotopical mode of organization, adjoining groups of nerve cells being related to ipsilateral cochlear fibres concerned with different but related acoustic frequencies. The medial superior olivary nucleus receives impulses from both cochlear spiral organs, and physiological evidence suggests that it forms part of a pathway concerned in auditory localization. Together with the trapezoid nuclei, the superior olivary groups are the main relay stations of the ventral and largest projection of the cochlear nuclei. Their complex connexions, as demonstrated in experimental animals, are not yet well authenticated in the human brainstem.

The *trapezoid nucleus* is sometimes described as consisting of two parts—a ventral component of cells scattered among the fascicles of the trapezoid body and a more compact dorsal nucleus located medial to the superior olivary complex. Although usually regarded as relay stations on the auditory pathway, the trapezoid nuclei in man remain in this regard an uncertain issue. Some of the axons of the trapezoid nuclei may enter the medial longitudinal fasciculus, ascending therein to terminate in the trigeminal and facial nuclei and also those of the motor nerves of the extraocular muscles. Such connexions could mediate reflexes involving the muscles in the middle ear (stapedius and tensor tympani) and the eye muscles.

The *nucleus of the lateral lemniscus* consists of small aggregations of nerve cells dispersed among the fibres of this fasciculus. Lateral and medial groups have been described. They receive bilateral afferent axons from both cochlear nuclei, and their efferents pass cranially into the midbrain through the lateral lemniscus; their further connexions will be considered later (pp. 886, 915).

[424] S. Ramon y Cajal, *Histologie du système nerveux, de l'homme et des vertébrés.*, Maloine, Paris. 1909.

[425] R. Lorente de Nó, *Laryngoscope, St Louis*, **43**, 1933.

[426] H. F. Schuknecht, in: *Neural Mechanisms of the Auditory and Vestibular Systems*, eds. G. L. Rasmussen and W. F. Windle, Thomas, Springfield. 1960.

[427] I. C. Whitfield, *The Auditory Pathway*, Arnold, London, 1960.

[428] F. H. Lewy and H. Kobrak, *Archs Neurol. Psychiat., Chicago*, **35**, 1936.

[429] K. K. Osen, *Acta otolar*, **67**, 1969.

[430] H. Held, *Arch. mikrosk. Anat. EntwMech.*, 1893.

[431] C. v. Monakow, *Gehirnpathologie*, 2nd ed., Hölder, Vienna. 1905.

[432] R. Irving and J. M. Harrison, *J. comp. Neurol.*, **130**, 1967.

[433] W. B. Warr, *Expl Neurol.*, **14**, 1966.

*Efferent cochlear nerve fibres* travel centrifugally in the cochlear nerves to innervate the spiral organ.[430, 434] Though comparatively few in number (about 500 in the cat), experiment suggests that they play an important part in hearing, perhaps being involved in both inhibitory and excitatory reflexes through the cochlear nuclei.[435] Lateral inhibition has also been demonstrated by the unit recording technique applied at the trapezoid level of the auditory pathway. The efferent cochlear fibres appear to be derived from retro-olivary cells in the superior olivary complex, fibres from each side proceeding to both cochleae—hence the term 'olivocochlear' fibres. No clear details of higher connexions in this regard are available.

The *striae medullares of the fourth ventricle*, as already stated above, are not formed of nerve fibres involved in the auditory pathway. There is considerable evidence on the contrary that they are part of an aberrant cerebropontocerebellar connexion, in which the arcuate nuclei (p. 848), pontobulbar body (p. 851), and the external arcuate fibres (p. 848) are all concerned. Some confusion exists among the accounts of various authorities, especially regarding the role of the pontobulbar body. The following description merely presents the consensus of these views, some of which appear to be more reliably established than others. Embryological evidence (p. 134) suggests that some of the nerve cells which migrate ventrally towards the pons from the rhombic lip to form the nuclei pontis largely fail to do so and remain near the fourth ventricle as the pontobulbar body or nucleus. Others migrate further and are scattered superficially over the ventral aspect of much of the extent of the medullary pyramids as the arcuate nuclei, a sizable congregation of them occurring immediately caudal to the pons. Both groups of cells are considered to receive corticopontine projections, those to the arcuate nuclei descending in the pyramids with the corticospinal fibres. Axons from the arcuate nuclei of both sides pass dorsally round the side of the medulla, cranial, superficial and caudal to the inferior olive as a thin stratum, fascicles of which are usually visible on the surface. All these fibres pass into the inferior cerebellar peduncle, being known collectively as *external arcuate fibres*. Some external arcuate fibres (so-called) follow an *internal* course, passing dorsally from the arcuate nuclei through the substance of the medulla close to the median raphe. Reaching the floor of the fourth ventricle, these fibres decussate and turn laterally subjacent to the ependymal lining of the ventricle, entering the cerebellum by the inferior peduncle. In this latter part of their course these fibres form the striae medullares; from their connexions they are also known as the *arcuatocerebellar tract*. There is some evidence that this ends in the flocculus.[436] Some of these fibres are said to end in the pontobulbar nucleus, but this may be a confusion with projection fibres of the nucleus. Some of the latter may travel ventrally forming part of a compact bundle, the *circumolivary fasciculus*, which skirts the caudal pole of the inferior olive, usually appearing as a surface feature of this part of the medulla. The fasciculus and the pontobulbar nucleus have been found absent in aplasia of the pons, an interesting confirmation of their affiliation with the pontocerebellar projection.[437] The efferent circumolivary fibres which pass ventrally join the arcuatocerebellar tract, with which they reach the striae medullares and enter the contralateral inferior cerebellar peduncle. However, as pointed out previously (p. 851) afferent fibres to the pontobulbar nucleus have also been considered to run in the circumolivary fasciculus, and the precise contribution of efferent and afferent fibres to the fasciculus cannot yet be regarded as settled.

**The nucleus of the abducent nerve** is in the central grey matter a short distance from the median plane, and in line with the nuclei of the third and fourth cranial nerves, above, and the hypoglossal nerve, below, thus forming a somatic motor column (p. 133). It is close to the medial longitudinal fasciculus, which is placed to its ventromedial side. In this way fibres from the vestibular and cochlear nuclei and the nuclei of other cranial nerves, especially the oculomotor communicate with the abducent, which also bears an intimate relation to the emerging fibres of the facial nerve (*vide infra*). The outgoing fibres of the sixth nerve pass ventrally downwards through the reticular formation, intersecting the trapezoid body and the medial lemniscus and traversing the basilar part of the pons to emerge at its lower border.

**The facial nucleus** lies in the ventrolateral part of the reticular formation of the pons, immediately behind the dorsal nucleus of the trapezoid body. Dorsal to it, and somewhat to its lateral side, is the spinal tract of the trigeminal nerve and its associated nucleus. The facial nucleus receives fibres from the corticonuclear tract of the opposite side, a smaller number from that of the same side (p. 884), and also fibres from the ipsilateral rubroreticular tract. Its large motor cells give origin to the fibres of the facial nerve. These fibres do not pass directly from their origin to the surface of the brainstem, but pursue a very remarkable course. At first they incline dorsally and medially towards the rhomboid fossa, passing below the abducent nucleus (7.69). They then course upwards on the medial side of this nucleus, coming into close relationship with the medial longitudinal fasciculus, through which the facial nerve may be brought into communication with the other cranial nerves. Finally, the fibres of the facial curve forwards and laterally around the upper pole of the abducent nucleus forming the *genu of the facial nerve* and pass forwards, laterally and downwards through the reticular formation. In the last part of their course to the surface they pass between their own nucleus medially and the nucleus of the spinal tract of the trigeminal nerve lateral to them.

The unusual behaviour of the emerging fibres of the facial nerve provides apparent evidence in favour of the theory of neurobiotaxis (p. 133). In the 10 mm human embryo the facial nucleus lies in the floor of the fourth ventricle, occupying the position of the branchial (special visceral) efferent column, and at this stage it is placed at a higher level than the abducent nucleus. As growth proceeds, the facial nucleus migrates at first caudally, dorsal to the sixth nucleus, and then ventrally to reach its adult position. As it migrates the axons to which its cells give rise elongate, and their subsequent course maps out the pathway along which the facial nucleus has travelled.

It must be remembered that the facial nucleus not only receives fibres from the corticonuclear tracts for volitional control, but also afferents from its own sensory root (through the nucleus of the tractus solitarius) and from the nucleus of the spinal tract of the trigeminal nerve. These latter sources of stimulation complete local reflex arcs, in every way similar to the segmental reflex arcs in the spinal cord. It is considered that to retain its proximity to the nucleus of the tractus solitarius and to the nucleus of the spinal tract of the trigeminal nerve that the facial nucleus migrates from its original position in the basal lamina.

The nucleus of the facial nerve is divided into several parts. The cells which give rise to the axons innervating

[434] G. L. Rasmussen, in: *Sensori-neural Hearing Processes and Disorders*, ed. A. B. Graham, Little, Brown & Co., Boston. 1967.

[435] J. T. Allanson and I. C. Whitfield, *Third London Symposium on Information Theory*, Butterworth, London. 1955.

[436] J. Szentágothai, *Acta Morph. (Budapest)*, **2**, 1955.

[437] R. v. Baumgarten and L. Aranda Coddou, *Acta neurol. lat. amer.*, **5**, 1959.

the muscles in the scalp and upper part of the face are placed towards the dorsal part of the nucleus and are believed to receive corticonuclear fibres from both sides.[438, 439] The subgroups of neurons which form the nucleus may represent discrete motor pools (p. 1011).

**The salivatory nucleus** is near to the rostral end of the dorsal nucleus of the vagus, just above the junction of the medulla oblongata and pons.[440] It is in close relation to the caudal end of the nucleus of the facial nerve. It is customary to divide it into *superior and inferior salivatory nuclei* which send their secretomotor fibres to the salivary and, perhaps, the lacrimal glands through the facial and glossopharyngeal nerves respectively (p. 1067).

**The nucleus of the spinal tract of the trigeminal nerve** is continued up through the lower part of the pons, the fibres of the tract still being closely applied to the lateral aspect of the nucleus. It is placed ventral to the lateral vestibular nucleus and is intersected by the fibres of the vestibular nerve destined for that nucleus. The inferior cerebellar peduncle lies to its lateral side below, but inclines dorsally as it ascends to the cerebellum, and the spinal tract of the trigeminal nerve and its nucleus are subsequently related laterally to the middle cerebellar peduncle. Above, the nucleus becomes continuous with the superior sensory nucleus of the trigeminal. The spinal 'tract' is unfortunately named, for it does not consist of fibres originating in the central nervous system but of the descending axons of the trigeminal nerve derived from nerve cells in the trigeminal ganglion. From these fibres collaterals and terminals enter the spinal nucleus, which is continuous at its caudal end with the substantia gelatinosa of the dorsal grey column in the spinal cord (p. 1001). Cranially it merges with the main sensory nucleus of the nerve. It is mainly concerned with the mediation of pain and thermal sensibilities in the trigeminal area. There is a well-established topographic organization within the nucleus. (For further details see p.1002).

In addition to tracts already studied at a lower level the white matter of the lower part of the tegmental region of the pons contains the trapezoid body, the lateral lemniscus and the emerging fibres of the sixth and seventh cranial nerves, which are new elements not present in the upper part of the medulla oblongata.

The *medial lemniscus* occupies the ventral part of the tegmentum. Its outline, on transverse section, is a flattened oval, extending laterally from the median raphe (7.68). The vertically running fibres of the medial lemniscus are intersected by the horizontal fibres of the trapezoid body. Laterally they are related to the *lateral spinothalamic tract* and to the *trigeminal lemniscus*. The fibres of the latter are derived from the cells of the nucleus of the spinal tract of the trigeminal nerve of the opposite side, and convey painful and thermal impressions from the skin of the face, the mucous membranes of the conjunctiva, tongue, mouth, nose, etc. The lemnisci are now arranged as a transverse band composed, from the medial to the lateral side, of the medial and trigeminal lemnisci, lateral spinothalamic tract and lateral lemniscus.

The *trapezoid body* is formed by fibres derived from the cochlear nuclei (mainly the ventral) and from the nuclei of the corpus trapezoideum. They run transversely and rostrally in the ventral part of the tegmentum, and, having intersected or passed ventral to the vertical fibres of the medial lemniscus, they cross the median raphe, decussating with the corresponding fibres of the opposite side. Before they reach the emerging fibres of the facial nerve the fibres of the trapezoid body turn upwards to form the *lateral lemniscus*, which is the ascending auditory pathway.

The course of the outgoing fibres from the nuclei of the abducent and facial cranial nerves has already been examined.

The *medial longitudinal fasciculus* is sited close to the midline, immediately ventral to the floor of the fourth ventricle. It is closely related to the nucleus of the abducent nerve and to the emerging fibres of the facial nerve, as they ascend on the medial side of that nucleus. The proximity of the fasciculus suggests that it may receive fibres from and transmit fibres to both structures (p. 885). As it lies in the lower part of the pons, the medial longitudinal fasciculus receives fibres from the vestibular nuclei and possibly from the dorsal nucleus of the trapezoid body (p. 853), through the peduncle of that nucleus. These contributions from the eighth nerve form the greater part of the fasciculus (p. 885) which is the main 'intersegmental' tract in the brainstem, particularly concerned with interactions between the nuclei innervating the ocular muscles, and between these and the vestibular system.

**A transverse section at a cranial level in the tegmentum** of the pons contains new elements in connexion with the trigeminal nerve (7.70), but otherwise shows no very notable alteration.

**The motor nucleus of the trigeminal nerve** lies in the reticular formation of the pons, deep to the lateral part of the floor of the fourth ventricle in line with the fibres of the trigeminal nerve traversing the ventral part of the pons (7.70).

**The principal (superior) sensory nucleus of the trigeminal nerve** lies on the lateral side of the motor nucleus, intervening between it and the middle cerebellar peduncle, and is continuous below with the nucleus of the spinal tract. The second neuron fibres from the principal sensory nucleus cross the median plane and ascend with the medial lemniscus to the thalamus (p. 1029).

The *nucleus of the lateral lemniscus* is a small collection of cells placed on the medial aspect of the tract in the cranial part of the pons. It receives synaptic terminals from some fibres of the lateral lemniscus; some of its efferent fibres enter the medial longitudinal bundle, whilst others return to the lemniscus. It is to be associated, as a relay station, with the nucleus of the trapezoid body.

The white matter of the tegmentum at this level is marked by the absence of the trapezoid body, which is now replaced by the lateral lemnisci, and the invasion of its dorsolateral part by the superior cerebellar peduncles.

The *medial lemniscus* (7.71) occupies a position in the ventral part of the tegmentum, but it has moved laterally a short distance from the median raphe. Here it is joined medially by the projection fibres from the principal sensory nucleus of the trigeminal nerve, which convey proprioceptive, tactile and pressure impulses from the receptive area covered by it. More laterally it is related dorsally to the trigeminal lemniscus and lateral spinothalamic tract, conveying pain and thermal impulses, and to the lateral lemniscus and its nucleus. As the lateral lemniscus ascends, it passes dorsally and lies close to the surface. It will be seen subsequently to send its fibres into the inferior colliculus and the medial geniculate body. The *medial longitudinal fasciculus* retains its paramedian position.

The *superior cerebellar peduncle* is formed by a large collection of fibres which take origin in the dentate nucleus of the cerebellum (p. 873), and pass upwards and forwards to enter the lateral part of the roof of the fourth ventricle. As it ascends in this position it inclines forwards and medially and enters the dorsolateral part of the tegmentum. The *anterior spinocerebellar tract* is intimately associated with the foregoing. It has already been traced up through the medulla oblongata, where it lies dorsal to

[438] J. W. Papez, *J. comp. Neurol.*, **43**, 1927.
[439] C. van Buskirk, *J. comp. Neurol.*, **82**, 1945.
[440] P. R. Lewis and C. C. Shute, *Nature, Lond.*, **183**, 1959.

the olivary nucleus and separated from the surface only by the anterior external arcuate fibres. In the lower part of the pons it inclines dorsally between the sensory nucleus of the trigeminal nerve and the middle cerebellar peduncle until it reaches the lateral aspect of the superior

peduncle. Its fibres then descend dorsally in a curve to enter the cerebellum.

The *reticular formation* is continued through all levels of the pons and is described in further details on p. 888.

# THE CEREBELLUM

The cerebellum, the largest part of the hindbrain, lies behind the pons and medulla oblongata, and its median portion is separated from these structures by the cavity of the fourth ventricle. It lies in the posterior cranial fossa and is covered by the tentorium cerebelli (p. 986). It is somewhat ovoid in form, but constricted in its median part, and flattened from above downwards, its greatest diameter being from side to side. Its average weight in the male is about 150 grams. In the adult the proportion between the cerebellum and cerebrum is about 1 to 8, in the infant about 1 to 20.

## GENERAL FORM OF THE CEREBELLUM

The cerebellum consists of two *cerebellar hemispheres* joined by a narrow median strip, the *vermis*. On the *superior surface*, however, there is no deep grooving in the parasagittal planes, so that the surface of the superior vermis, which is raised into a slight median ridge, is directly continuous with the hemisphere on each side (7.72). Anteriorly the superior vermis projects beyond the free margin of the tentorium cerebelli, and from there it slopes downwards and backwards, related above to the straight sinus. The upper surface of each hemisphere is in contact with the tentorium cerebelli, and slopes downwards and laterally from the superior surface of the vermis.

*Superior vermis*

*Horizontal fissure*

*Anterior lobe*

*Fissura prima*

*Postlunate fissure*

*Middle lobe*

*Posterior cerebellar notch*

**7.72**   Superior aspect of the cerebellum to show major fissures and lobes. Compare with **7.74**.

It is bounded, in front, by an anterolateral margin, which corresponds to the attachment of the tentorium cerebelli to the superior border of the petrous part of the temporal bone, and behind, by a curved posterior margin, which abuts against the transverse sinus as it lies in the attached margin of the tentorium cerebelli.

On the *inferior surface* the cerebellar hemispheres are separated from each other by a deep hollow, which is

termed the *vallecula* (7.75). The inferior surface of the hemisphere is irregularly convex and lies in contact with the posterior surface of the petrous part of the temporal bone, the sigmoid sinus, the mastoid part of the temporal bone and the lower part of the squamous portion of the occipital bone. The inferior surface of the vermis projects into the floor of the vallecula and is limited on each side by the *sulcus valleculae*.

*Anteriorly* the cerebellum presents a wide, shallow *anterior cerebellar notch*, which lodges the pons and the upper part of the medulla oblongata, but these portions of the brainstem are separated from it by the fourth ventricle. In the floor of the anterior cerebellar notch the peduncles pass into the white centre of the cerebellum.

*Posteriorly* the hemispheres are separated from each other by the posterior cerebellar notch, which is a deep and narrow interval containing the falx cerebelli of the dura mater.

## SURFACE TOPOGRAPHY OF THE CEREBELLUM

The surface of the cerebellum is everywhere marked by closely set transverse and somewhat curved fissures which give it a laminated appearance and separate its constituent *folia*. Some of the fissures are deeper than others and divide the organ into several lobules. The most conspicuous of these fissures is the *horizontal fissure*. This extends around the lateral and posterior borders of each cerebellar hemisphere from the middle cerebellar peduncle in front to the posterior cerebellar notch behind; it marks the junction of the superior and inferior surfaces of the cerebellum.

**Superior surface** (7.72, 85). The most conspicuous fissure on the superior surface is the *fissura prima*. This is somewhat V-shaped with its apex directed dorsally, and cutting into the superior surface of the vermis at the junction of its anterior two-thirds with the posterior third. The lines of the fissure are directed anterolaterally around the superior surfaces of the cerebellar hemispheres to meet the horizontal fissures close to their anterior ends.

The superior surface of the vermis is divided by short, deep fissures into the *lingula, central lobule, culmen, declive* and *folium vermis* in that anteroposterior order. Each of these divisions, excepting the lingula, is continuous laterally with the adjoining lobule of the cerebellar hemispheres (7.73, 85). The fissura prima cuts the superior surface of the vermis between the culmen and declive.

The lingula consists of a single lamella which presents four or five poorly marked folia on its surface; its white matter is directly continuous with that of the superior medullary velum. The lingula is separated from the central lobule by the *postlingual fissure*. The central lobule is continuous laterally with the *alae of the central lobule*. These are limited behind by the *postcentral fissure*. Between this fissure and the fissura prima lies the culmen medially and the *quadrangular lobule* laterally.

The superior surface of the cerebellar hemispheres and vermis behind the fissura prima is divided by the curved *postlunate fissure* into an anterior portion which consists of the declive with its lateral extensions, the *lobuli simplices* and a posterior portion, the folium vermis with the adjoining parts of the cerebellar hemisphere termed the *superior semilunar lobules* which are limited behind by the horizontal fissures.

**Inferior surface** (**7.**75, 85). This includes the inferior surface of the vermis and the inferior aspect of each cerebellar hemisphere. The inferior vermis is divided into four smaller portions named from behind forwards the tuber vermis, pyramid, uvula and nodule. The tuber vermis is continuous laterally with the *inferior semilunar nodules*. These parts are bounded, behind, by the horizontal fissure and, in front, by the *prepyramidal fissure*. The *pyramid* is separated from the *uvula* by the *post-pyramidal fissure* or *fissura secunda* and is continuous laterally with the *biventral lobule* on the inferior surface of each hemisphere. In front of the uvula and separated from it by the median portion of the *posterolateral sulcus* is the nodule (**7.**73, 75).

On the inferior aspect of the cerebellar hemisphere, anterior to the biventral lobule, is a deep fissure, the *retrotonsillar*, which passes laterally from the sulcus valleculae opposite the fissura secunda and then curves forwards to gain the anterior part of the inferior surface of the hemisphere. Together with the anterior part of the sulcus valleculae it bounds a circumscribed portion of the cerebellum, termed the *tonsil*, which is connected to the uvula across the floor of the sulcus valleculae by a strip of cortex, termed the *furrowed band* (**7.**75). Superiorly the tonsil lies in intimate relation with the inferior surface of the inferior medullary velum.

The *nodule* is the most anterior part of the inferior surface of the vermis. Behind, it is separated from the uvula by the posterolateral sulcus, and on each side it is connected to the flocculus and the white core of the hemisphere by the inferior medullary velum. Its anterosuperior aspect is directed towards the fourth ventricle. Anteriorly it is covered with grey matter and crossed by two or three

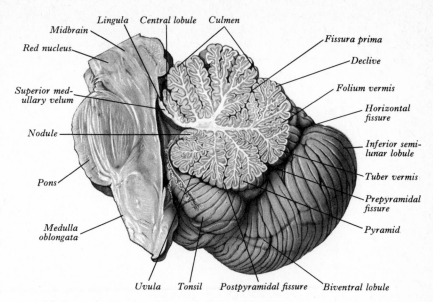

**7.**73 Median sagittal section of the cerebellum and brainstem.

white core would be exposed, were it not directly continuous with the nervous layer of the inferior medullary velum.

The *flocculus* is a small, partially detached portion of the cerebellum which lies immediately below the vestibulocochlear nerve as it enters the brainstem, and is crossed anteriorly by the fila of the glossopharyngeal and vagus nerves as they pass laterally to reach the jugular foramen. It is somewhat oval in outline, with a crenated margin, and from its medial end a narrow band of white fibres emerges, which constitutes the *peduncle* of the flocculus; it is covered anteriorly by the lateral recess of the fourth ventricle and the part of the choroid plexus

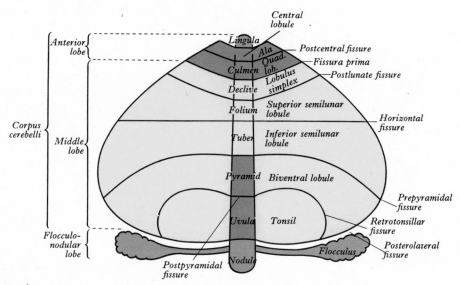

**7.**74 Diagram to show the morphological and functional subdivisions of the cerebellum. *Blue*: archicerebellum. *Green*: paleocerebellum. *Yellow*: neocerebellum. See also illustration **7.**85 for further details.

shallow fissures. In this situation it is separated from the ventricular cavity by a double layer of pia mater and its contained choroid plexus, and the ventricular ependyma (**7.**89). Posteriorly the grey matter is deficient, and the white matter is on the surface covered only with a layer of neuroglia and the ependyma (**7.**89). The lateral aspect of the nodule is free anteriorly and is covered with grey matter; posteriorly, it presents a narrow strip, where its

which projects from the aperture of the recess (**7.**55). The peduncle contains both afferent and efferent fibres. At the lateral angle of the floor of the fourth ventricle it divides into dorsal and ventral parts. Through the dorsal part the flocculus establishes connexions with the nodule and the uvula. The ventral part passes medially and turns upwards close to the lateral border of the pontine part of the floor of the ventricle. Many of these fibres are afferent

857

and are derived from the vestibular nuclei and also, according to some authorities, from the medial accessory olivary nucleus, but others are efferent to the vestibular nuclei and some appear to ascend to a higher level.

## THE LOBES OF THE CEREBELLUM

The cerebellum can be divided into two fundamental parts termed the flocculonodular lobe and the corpus cerebelli, the latter comprising an anterior and middle lobe (7.74, 85A). These subdivisions possess functional as well as morphological and embryological significance. The *flocculonodular lobe* consists of both flocculi, their peduncles and the nodule. The *corpus cerebelli* comprises the remainder of the cerebellum and is separated from the flocculonodular lobe by the posterolateral fissure, which is the first to appear on the cerebellum both in phylogeny and ontogeny. The corpus cerebelli is subdivided by the fissura prima into anterior and middle lobes. The *anterior lobe* lies in front of the fissure and comprises the lingula, central lobule, culmen, alae of the central lobules and quadrangular lobules. The remainder of the corpus cerebelli is termed the *middle lobe* and comprises the declive, folium vermis, tuber vermis, pyramid, uvula, lobuli simplices, biventral lobules, semilunar lobules and tonsils.

Certain sectors of the cerebellum are phylogenetically older than the rest. The flocculonodular lobe, which is predominantly *vestibular* in its connexions, together with the lingula, which receives spinocerebellar in addition to vestibular connexions, constitute the oldest part of the cerebellum, the *archicerebellum*. The anterior lobe, excluding the lingula, but together with the pyramid and uvula of the middle lobe, is phylogenetically the next part

the neocerebellum intervenes between the anterior and flocculonodular lobes (7.74, 7.85 A).

**The superior medullary velum** is a thin lamina of white substance, which stretches between the superior cerebellar peduncles (brachia conjunctiva), and with them forms the roof of the cranial part of the fourth ventricle; its deep surface is covered with the ventricular ependyma. The velum is narrow anterosuperiorly, where it extends into the interval between the inferior colliculi, and broader posteroinferiorly, where it is continuous with the white substance of the superior part of the vermis. The folia of the lingula are prolonged on to the dorsal surface of its lower half, and a median ridge, termed the *frenulum veli*, descends upon its superior part from between the inferior colliculi. The trochlear nerves emerge at the sides of the frenulum (7.87).

**The inferior medullary vela** are two thin, somewhat crescentic, sheets placed one on each side of the nodule. Each consists of a thin layer of white matter and neuroglia, surfaced over internally by the ventricular ependyma, and externally by the pia mater. Its internal surface forms the lower wall of the lateral dorsal recess of the fourth ventricle (p. 878); its external surface is related to the superior aspect of the tonsil. Its convex peripheral margin is continuous with the white core of the cerebellum and with the sides of the pyramid, uvula and nodule; its anterior (sometimes inferior) border is free (7.87) and from it the ventricular ependyma is prolonged downwards in close apposition with the pia mater to form the thin part of the roof of the ventricle and to reach the taeniae. At its anterolateral corner the velum is continuous with the dorsal part of the peduncle of the flocculus, from which most, if not all, of its nerve fibres are derived (7.75).

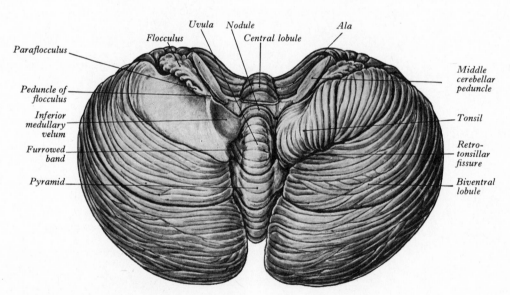

**7.75** Inferior aspect of the cerebellum. The tonsil and the adjoining part of the biventral lobule of the right side have been removed.

to appear and is predominantly *spinocerebellar* in its connexions, constituting the *paleocerebellum*. At this stage in phylogeny, this newly acquired lobe separates the archicerebellum into two parts, the lingula in front and the flocculonodular lobe behind. With the evolution of the neopallium in the mammal, there is a further expansion of the cerebellum with the addition of the middle lobe, excepting the pyramid and uvula. This addition constitutes the *neocerebellum* and is predominantly *corticopontocerebellar* in its connexions. Like the paleocerebellum,

## DEVELOPMENT OF THE CEREBELLUM

For the early stages of cerebellar development see p. 134. Early in the third month the cerebellum is represented by a mass which stretches across the roof of the cranial part of the hindbrain vesicle, becoming bilobed like an hour-glass. Its narrow median part is destined to form the vermis, and its enlarged extremities develop into the hemispheres. As growth proceeds a number of transverse grooves appear on the dorsal aspect of the cerebellar rudiment, and give rise to the numerous fissures which characterize the surface of the cerebellum (**7**.75, 76).

The lateral parts of the *posterolateral fissure* appear before any of the others and demarcate the most caudal portions from the rest of the cerebellar rudiment, enabling the flocculi to be identified. The right and left parts of this fissure extend medially and meet in the median plane, where they demarcate the nodule. The flocculonodular lobes can now be recognized and constitute the most caudal part of the cerebellum at this stage; but, owing to the growth of the adjoining areas, they come to occupy the anterior part of the inferior surface in the adult. They are formed in close proximity to the line of attachment of the epithelial roof, i.e. to the rhombic lip (p. 135).

At the end of the third month a transverse furrow appears on the cranial slope of the cerebellar rudiment, and deepens to form the *fissura prima*, which cuts into the vermis and both hemispheres, separating off the most cranial region of the rudiment to form the anterior lobe.

About the same time two short transverse grooves appear on the inferior surface of the vermis behind the postnodular fissure. The first of these is the *fissura secunda*, which demarcates the uvula, and the second is the *prepyramidal fissure*, which demarcates the pyramid (**7**.76). The whole cerebellum grows in a dorsal direction, and the caudal, or inferior, aspects of the hemispheres undergo much greater enlargement than the inferior surface of the vermis, which therefore becomes buried at the bottom of a deep hollow—the *vallecula*. While these changes are taking place numerous additional fissures develop, but they have little morphological significance. The most extensive of them forms the *horizontal fissure*.

In many mammals a portion of the hemisphere im-

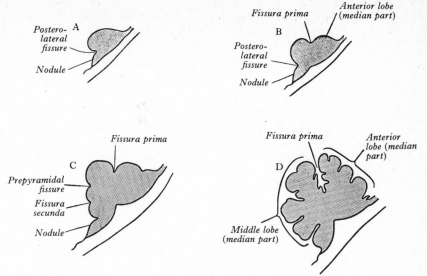

**7**.76 Median sagittal sections through the developing cerebellum at four successive stages.

mediately cranial to the flocculus becomes demarcated, and in some it forms a very prominent part of the cerebellum. Owing to its relation to the flocculus, it is termed the *paraflocculus*, but the relationship is purely topographical, and, in contradistinction to the flocculus, the paraflocculus derives its afferent connexions mainly, if not entirely, from the cerebral cortex. It is uncertain whether any homologue of the paraflocculus exists in the human cerebellum, or whether it is represented by some small patches of grey matter which are found not infrequently on the inferior surface of the middle cerebellar peduncle.

## INTERNAL STRUCTURE OF THE CEREBELLUM

The cerebellum exhibits a profound difference in structure from the spinal cord, the medulla oblongata and the pons, for the grey and white matter of which it is comprised are arranged in the opposite manner. The grey matter or cortex covers the whole surface of the cerebellum, dipping in to line the various fissures which cross its surface. Certain aggregations of grey matter are found in its interior, but that does not in any way alter the prominence of the peripheral distribution of the grey matter and the central arrangement of the white matter. In this way the cerebellum resembles the cerebrum, and it is this modification of the disposition of the grey matter which has rendered possible the enormous degree of expansion which these two parts of the nervous system have undergone during the process of evolution.

### The White Matter of the Cerebellum

The white matter forms a central core, which is much thicker in the lateral parts than it is in the median area, where it forms a flattened strip connecting the enlarged lateral portions with each other. From its surfaces a series of nearly parallel plates or laminae project towards the surface, and these give off secondary laminae, usually more or less at right angles to the primary laminae. In turn the secondary laminae may give off still shorter laminae, all of which are covered with grey matter. When a section is made through the cerebellum parallel with the median plane it divides the primary laminae at right angles, and

the cut surface presents a characteristic branched appearance which is termed the *arbor vitae* (**7**.73).

The white matter consists of (1) fibrae propriae, (2) projection fibres, and (3) the myelinated axons of the Purkinje cells (*vide infra*).

**The fibrae propriae** or intrinsic fibres, as their name suggests, do not leave the cerebellum, but interconnect different regions of the organ. The *association fibres* connect

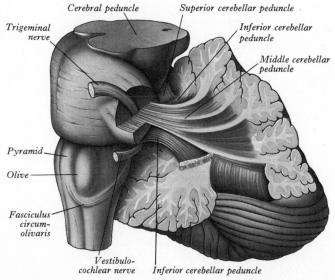

**7**.77 Dissection (by the late Dr. E. B. Jamieson) of the left cerebellar hemisphere and its peduncles.

adjacent or more distant folia of the cerebellar cortex, including those of the vermis. They do not cross the midline and the majority are relatively short bundles. Their detailed anatomy has not been extensively investigated (but see also p. 867). Numerous *commissural fibres* interconnect the two hemispheres; many are grouped into an *anterosuperior commissure*. A *postero-inferior commissure* also exists and crosses the midline near the fastigial nuclei (*vide infra*). In addition to interhemispheric cortical connexions, and running with them, are *decussating* spinocerebellar and cerebellovestibular fibres.

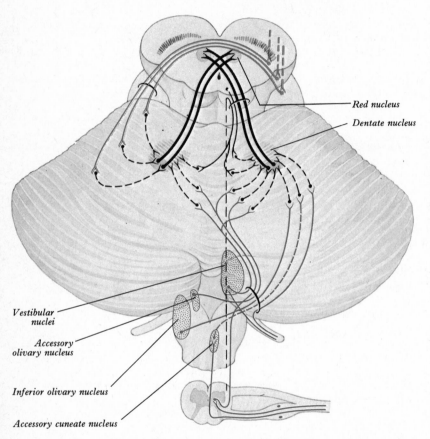

Red nucleus

Dentate nucleus

Vestibular nuclei

Accessory olivary nucleus

Inferior olivary nucleus

Accessory cuneate nucleus

**7.78** A simplified diagram of the connexions of the cerebellum showing some components of the peduncles—inferior (blue), middle (magenta) and superior (black). The important cerebellothalamic fibres and other efferent systems, have been omitted.

**The projection fibres** connect the cerebellum with other parts of the brain and spinal cord. They are grouped together into three large bundles or *peduncles* (**7.77**) on each side and these issue from the anterior cerebellar notch. The superior peduncles connect the cerebellum to the midbrain, the middle peduncles to the pons, and the inferior peduncles to the medulla oblongata. Some of these connexions are shown in a highly simplified manner in **7.78**.

## THE INFERIOR CEREBELLAR PEDUNCLE

The inferior cerebellar peduncle is a thick bundle of white fibres, both entering and leaving the cerebellum from many sources and to many destinations. As described elsewhere (p. 843) it is formed on the dorsolateral aspect of the superior half of the medulla oblongata. The two peduncles diverge as they continue to ascend, but upon reaching the anterior cerebellar notch, each bends sharply posteromedially to enter into its respective hemisphere. As it bends and curves backwards it is insinuated between

the middle peduncle on its lateral aspect and the superior peduncle medially. Some authorities consider it convenient to divide the inferior peduncle, for descriptive purposes, into a small medially placed strand, the *juxtarestiform body*, and a large lateral bundle, the *restiform body*. The relation of the oblique *pontobulbar body* to the dorsolateral aspect of the peduncle has already been mentioned (p. 851).

*The tracts entering the cerebellum* through the inferior peduncle stem from a variety of sources in the spinal cord and medulla. They include the olivocerebellar, parolivocerebellar, vestibulocerebellar, reticulocerebellar, posterior spinocerebellar, cuneocerebellar and trigeminocerebellar tracts, together with the anterior external arcuate fibres and other arcuatocerebellar fibres (the striae medullares). The tracts *leaving* the cerebellum through the inferior peduncle include the cerebello-olivary, cerebellovestibular and cerebelloreticular pathways, with minor bundles of cerebellospinal and cerebellonuclear fibres.

(1) **The posterior spinocerebellar tract**, as we have seen (p. 822), originates from cells in the thoracic nucleus of the same side, shows a somatotopic lamination of its fibres, and conveys a variety of types of information from both cutaneous exteroceptors and proprioceptors from the hind limb and lower trunk. Some fibres are 'modality specific' whilst others carry information converging from more than one source; the transmission along both types of fibre may be modulated by activity in descending tracts from the brainstem. The dorsal spinocerebellar fibres terminate in the 'hind-limb' regions of the cerebellar cortex (*vide infra*) which includes the vermis of the anterior lobe (central lobule, culmen and some of the declive) together with the neighbouring parts of their adjacent lobules, whilst other fibres end in the pyramid and uvula.

(2) **The cuneocerebellar tract** (posterior external arcuate fibres) passes from the cells of the external (accessory) cuneate nucleus to gain the anterior and posterior regions of the vermis of the same side. This tract and its nucleus of origin are somatotopically organized, and are functionally similar to the posterior spinocerebellar tract, but in relation to the fore limb and upper trunk. The anterior and posterior areas of the cerebellar cortex which receive spinal afferents, and the localization of afferent terminals within these areas, are illustrated in **7.85** A, B.

(3) **The olivocerebellar tract** is composed of the axons of neurons in the inferior olivary nucleus, whilst (4) **the parolivocerebellar tracts** originate from the dorsal and medial accessory olivary nuclei. It had long been suspected that a close correspondence existed between points on the surface of the inferior olive and ones on the cortex of the contralateral cerebellar hemisphere. Subsequent studies of human cases with degenerative disease, and both physiological and anatomical experimentation in animals, have confirmed this. Further, it has been shown that a remarkably precise point-to-point interconnexion exists between all points of the olivary complex of nuclei and the opposite hemisphere. Broadly, a dorsoventral and a mediolateral correspondence exists with the inferior olive projecting to the larger and more lateral parts of the hemisphere, whilst the accessory olives project to the vermal and paravermal regions. Illustration **7.85** E is a simplified summary of these findings based largely on clinical cases (for further details see footnote references [61,441]). Whilst the olivocerebellar fibres largely cross the midline, some authorities have described a few fascicles which terminate ipsilaterally. The olivocerebellar fibres

[441] J. Jansen and A. Brodal (eds.), *Aspects of Cerebellar Anatomy*, Grundt Tanum, Oslo. 1954.

end in the cortex as *climbing fibres* which have, in recent years, been recognized as of great functional significance—they are discussed further below. In association with this it should be emphasized that afferents converge upon the olivary nuclei both from the spinal cord, the cerebral cortex and other subcortical centres. The spino-olivary tracts already described (p.,822) convey cutaneous and proprioceptive afferents to the accessory olivary nuclei, which in turn project largely on to the 'spinal regions' of the contralateral cerebellar hemisphere completing a *spino-olivocerebellar* system. Cortico-olivary fibres descend largely from motor regions of the cerebral cortex and terminate in localized areas of the inferior and accessory olivary nuclei,[442] completing a *cortico-olivocerebellar pathway*. Additionally, other subcortical nuclei, including the corpus striatum, red nucleus and brainstem reticular formation, all project on to restricted regions of the olivary complex and may thus differentially affect cerebellar cortical activity.

Not all olivocerebellar fibres, however, terminate as climbing fibres in the cortex—some end in the contralateral fastigial, emboliform, globose and dentate intracerebellar nuclei, and the projections are to some degree somatotopically organized. These various nuclei will be further discussed below.

(5) **The reticulocerebellar tract** arises mainly from both large and small cells of the *lateral reticular nucleus* of the medulla, but other *perihypoglossal* and *paramedian* reticular nuclei also contribute—p. 845. The reticulocerebellar fibres end in the 'spinal' regions of the cerebellar vermis mentioned above.

It should be noted at this point that various indirect channels to the cerebellum thus exist through the intermediary of the medullary reticular nuclei, because of the convergence on them of spinoreticular, vestibuloreticular and corticoreticular pathways which are described elsewhere in this section.

(6) **The vestibulocerebellar tract** is in the main composed of primary afferent (root) fibres of the vestibular part of the vestibulocochlear nerve, but some secondary fibres stem from cells of the medial and inferior vestibular nuclei. The fibres terminate ipsilaterally in the cortex of the archicerebellum, principally in the flocculus and nodule, but a small number are considered to end also in the uvula and lingula. Other vestibulocerebellar fibres are distributed to the fastigial nuclei of both sides. It is held[443] that the primary vestibulocerebellar fibres are mainly those with sensory endings in the ampullae of the semicircular ducts. In contrast, the nuclei of origin of the secondary fibres are the sites of termination of the rather small spinovestibular tract (p. 820). The vestibulocerebellar fibres occupy part of the juxtarestiform body (*see* p. 860).

The remaining pathways which enter the cerebellum through its inferior peduncle are less well understood.

(7) **The anterior external arcuate fibres** arise from arcuate nuclei of both sides and, together with some superficial reticulocerebellar fibres, course over the surface of the inferior peduncle to enter the cerebellum. As stated above, the arcuate nuclei are possibly homologous with the pontine nuclei, and accordingly, the anterior external arcuate fibres form part of a *cortico-arcuatocerebellar* pathway, but the cerebellar termination and significance of the latter is unclear.

(8) **The striae medullares**, encountered previously, (p. 854) are also thought to originate in the arcuate nuclei; they partially decussate and pass to the flocculus. They are sometimes termed the *arcuatofloccular tract* (fibres of Piccolomini) and are probably to be grouped with the anterior external arcuate fibres, and those derived from the pontobulbar body (p. 851).

(9) **Trigeminocerebellar fibres** both crossed and uncrossed, are known to enter the cerebellum from the superior sensory and descending (spinal) nuclei of the trigeminal nerve. Their distribution, and the status of other nucleocerebellar tracts which have been described are uncertain in the human cerebellum.

*The tracts leaving the cerebellum* in the inferior peduncle include:

(10) **Cerebello-olivary fibres**, as yet of uncertain origin, which leave in the inferior peduncle to terminate on cells of the inferior olivary nucleus.

(11) **Cerebellovestibular fibres**, which issue from the ipsilateral flocculus, nodule, and fastigial nucleus (and to some extent the opposite fastigial nucleus). They run with other constituents of the juxtarestiform body to reach the four vestibular nuclei, in which they terminate. Other cerebellovestibular fibres are the axons of Purkinje cells in the anterior and posterior regions of the vermis which do not synapse in the intracerebellar nuclei, but pass directly to the lateral vestibular nucleus. The anterior vermian projection shows a somatotopic localization which corresponds with that of the origin of the lateral vestibulospinal tract (p. 818). Further vermian projections pass to the fastigial nucleus, and thence to the lateral vestibular nucleus in the fastigiovestibular tract—again these pathways are somatotopically organized.[444]

(12) **Cerebelloreticular fibres**, which start in both, but mainly the contralateral, fastigial nuclei. They pursue an indirect course, partially decussating and then proceeding as the *hook bundle of Russell*, which curves around the cerebellar end of the superior peduncle before joining the inferior peduncle. In the main these fascicles are distributed to the pontine and medullary reticular formation. Accordingly, different functional zones of the nucleus fastigii (*vide infra*) and *fastigiovestibular* and *fastigiobulbar* tracts have been recognized. However, the two tracts are partially admixed in both the direct juxtarestiform body pathway and in the less direct hook bundle described above. Some observers believe that a proportion of the hook bundle fibres pass through the medulla oblongata to enter the anterior funiculus of the spinal cord as a *cerebellospinal tract*. The evidences with regard to the latter, and those concerning direct *cerebellonuclear tracts* to brainstem motor nuclei remain meagre and unconvincing.

## THE MIDDLE CEREBELLAR PEDUNCLE

The middle cerebellar peduncle (brachium pontis) is more massive than the superior and inferior peduncles, and passes lateral to them as it continues from the dorsolateral region of the pons, curving dorsally and then radiating to become continuous with the laminae of white matter within the cerebellar hemisphere (7.77). It is composed almost exclusively of the axons from the second neurons on the extensive *corticopontocerebellar pathway*. These neurons constitute the nuclei pontis which are scattered throughout the substance of the ventral (basilar) part of the pons. The fibres arising from the nuclei in one half of the pons almost all cross the midline, traversing the opposite middle peduncle to reach the cortex of the contralateral hemisphere. However, much of the vermis probably receives pontocerebellar fibres from both sides of the pons, whilst the lingula, some small regions of the anterior lobe and the flocculonodular lobe receive no pontocerebellar projection.

[442] A. Sousa-Pinto and A. Brodal, *Expl Brain Res.*, **8**, 1969.
[443] B. M. Stein and M. B. Carpenter, *Am. J. Anat.*, **120**, 1967.
[444] A. Brodal, O. Pompeiano and F. Walberg, *The Vestibular Nuclei and their Connections*, Oliver and Boyd, Edinburgh. 1962.

THE SUPERIOR CEREBELLAR PEDUNCLE

The fibres of each middle peduncle are arranged in three fasciculi, superior, inferior and deep. The *superior fasciculus* is derived from the upper transverse fibres of the pons; it is directed backwards and laterally superficial to the other two fasciculi, and is distributed mainly to the lobules on the inferior surface of the cerebellar hemisphere, and to the parts of the superior surface adjoining the posterior and lateral margins. The *inferior fasciculus* is formed by the lowest transverse fibres of the pons; it passes inferomedial to the superior fasciculus and is continued downwards and backwards more or less parallel with it, to be distributed to the folia on the under surface close to the vermis. The *deep fasciculus* comprises most of the deep transverse fibres of the pons. It is at first covered by the superior and inferior fasciculi, but crossing obliquely it appears on the medial side of the superior, from which it receives a bundle; its fibres spread out and pass to the upper anterior cerebellar folia. The fibres of this fasciculus cover those of the inferior peduncle.

Despite a number of investigations the precise distribution of pontocerebellar fibres from different regions of the pons in terms of the localization of their cerebellar terminals has not yet been satisfactorily explored. In general, the most lateral and also the most medial pontine nuclei project to the vermis, whilst the intermediate ones project to the contralateral hemisphere.

The pontine nuclei receive the terminals of corticopontine fibres which arise from many, perhaps all, parts of the cortex of the ipsilateral cerebral hemisphere, and they also receive collateral branches from some of the descending corticospinal fibres. While the origin of corticopontine fibres is undoubtedly extensive, the quantitative contribution from different cortical regions, and any precise somatotopic pattern of the projection from the different cerebral lobes on to specific groups of pontine nuclei, cannot yet be regarded as established in primates, including man. However, experimental investigations demonstrate that a fairly precise somatotopic pattern of corticopontine fibres extends from the sensorimotor cortical regions in the cat.[445, 446] Similarly, isolated reports of *spinopontine* and *tectopontine* fibre systems in the cat have, as yet, received no definite confirmation in primate brains, although they may well be present.

## THE SUPERIOR CEREBELLAR PEDUNCLE

The superior cerebellar peduncles (**7.77, 90**) emerge from the cranial part of the anterior cerebellar notch and are hidden from view by the anterior lobe of the cerebellum. When that structure is pulled aside they can be seen connected with one another by the superior medullary velum, and ascending in the lateral part of the roof of the fourth ventricle to disappear just caudal to the inferior colliculus.

A number of fibres *enter* the cerebellum through the superior peduncle (*vide infra*), but the great majority of the fibres which constitute the strand are *leaving* the cerebellum, and take origin for the most part in the cells of the nucleus dentatus. They emerge from the hilus of this nucleus and, having been joined by efferent fibres from the emboliform, globose and fastigial nuclei, they pass upwards, forwards and medially, covered over at first by the medial fibres of the inferior and the deep fibres of the middle peduncle. As they ascend in the roof of the fourth ventricle the fibres gradually incline anteriorly and sink into the tegmental region of the midbrain medial to the lateral lemniscus. They then sweep medially and the majority of the fibres decussate with the corresponding contralateral fibres. However, a proportion do not decussate and accordingly, considering the contribution from both peduncles, there is now, on both sides of the midline, a small uncrossed component and a much larger

crossed component of the superior cerebellar peduncles. Both the crossed and uncrossed components now separate into ascending and descending bundles. Each of these will be considered briefly, but it must be emphasized that the *crossed ascending* bundle is by far the most prominent, and is often the only one referred to in elementary accounts.

**The uncrossed component** of the superior cerebellar peduncle which arises in part from the fastigial nucleus, is mainly distributed to the brainstem reticular formation. Ascending fibres terminate in the reticular nuclei of the midbrain tegmentum and the grey matter surrounding the aqueduct of the midbrain, whilst the descending fibres reach reticular nuclei of the pons and medulla.

**The crossed descending fibres** of the superior cerebellar peduncle are distributed mainly to the inferior and accessory olivary nuclei and neighbouring reticular formation. Some authorities describe additional fascicles which pass into the spinal cord and others which run in company with the medial longitudinal fasciculus to the motor nuclei of the nerves supplying the extrinsic eye muscles.

**The crossed ascending fibres** of the superior cerebellar peduncle are quantitatively the major outflow from the cerebellum. They arise from the neurons of the dentate, globose and emboliform nuclei (p. 873) and form the *cerebellorubral* and *dentatothalamic tracts*. **The cerebellorubral fibres** are principally axons from the globose and emboliform nuclei (of the opposite side) and they terminate on the cells of the red nucleus which lies in the midbrain tegmentum (p. 884). On the basis of animal experimentation, a somatotopic localization of the cells in the globose and emboliform nuclei and in the issuing cerebellorubral tract, which corresponds with that in the red nucleus and rubrospinal tract, has been described.

**The dentatothalamic fibres**, having issued from the cells of the opposite dentate nucleus and crossed the midline, now by-pass the red nucleus and terminate in synaptic relationship with the neurons of the nucleus ventralis intermedius (lateralis) and, to a lesser degree, the nucleus ventralis anterior of the thalamus (*see* p. 898). From these thalamic centres fibres radiate to end in the 'motor' regions of the cerebral cortex. In this manner large areas of the cortex of the cerebellar hemispheres, through their connexions with the dentate nucleus, and then via the dentothalamic tract and the thalamocortical radiation, are able to influence the activities of the motor areas of the cerebral cortex.

In addition, some authors have described fibres in the crossed ascending component of the superior peduncle which terminate in other thalamic nuclei, including the nucleus centromedianus, the reticular nucleus, the nuclei ventralis posterior and lateralis posterior, and also in a variety of nuclei in the subthalamus and hypothalamus.[447, 448, 449, 450]

Fibre systems which *enter* the cerebellum through the superior cerebellar peduncle include the anterior spinocerebellar and tectocerebellar tracts.

The origin and constitution of the **anterior spinocerebellar tract** was considered previously (p. 822). As this superficial laminated tract ascends the cord it consists of some fibres which originated on the same side, but a majority which crossed from neurons on the opposite side of the cord. It continues to ascend superficially in the brainstem and then curves posteriorly along

[445] P. Brodal, *Expl Brain Res.*, **5**, 1968.
[446] P. Brodal, *Archs ital. Biol.*, **106**, 1968.
[447] R. Hassler, *Dt. Z. Nervenheilk.*, **163**, 1950.
[448] D. Cohen, W. W. Chambers and J. M. Sprague, *J. comp. Neurol.*, **109**, 1958.
[449] K. Nimi, N. Fujiwara, T. Takimoto and S. Matsugi, *Tokushima J. exp. Med.*, **8**, 1962.
[450] R. S. Snider, *Prog. Brain Res.*, **25**, 1967.

the lateral aspect of the superior peduncle to enter the cerebellum, within which many of the fibres which crossed the midline in the cord recross in the inferior cerebellar commissure to regain their side of origin. The fibres terminate in the 'hind-limb' receiving areas of the anterior and posterior vermian and paravermian regions of the cerebellar cortex (7.85 A, B). As mentioned previously, the existence of a **rostral spinocerebellar tract** which is the fore-limb counterpart of the anterior spinocerebellar tract, has been recognized by physiological recording techniques in experimental animals. Its anatomical verification, and the demonstration of its existence in the primate brain, including that of man, is still awaited.

**The tectocerebellar tracts** descend from the tectum of the midbrain to the cerebellum through the neural substance of the superior medullary velum close to the midline. They probably arise from the inferior and superior colliculi of both sides, and their fibres terminate in the intermediate vermal and paravermal regions of the cerebellar cortex, including the posterior part of the anterior lobe, the declive and lobulus simplex, the folium, tuber and pyramid (7.85 D). The precise origin and constitution of these tracts await further analysis. While it is widely assumed that they convey both auditory and visual information directly to the cerebellum, alternative routes have been proposed; these include *tectopontocerebellar* and *occipitopontocerebellar* pathways.

## A Summary of Cerebellar Connexions

The foregoing account of the cerebellar peduncles and their contained tracts is rendered particularly lengthy, complex, and the overall pattern somewhat obscured, by the multiple nature of the topographic pathways involved and the plethora of tract names. In the following paragraphs some details of the topography of the peduncles and tracts will be ignored, and certain groupings of connexions emphasized, which would otherwise perhaps be less apparent.

### THE CEREBELLAR INPUT

The input to the cerebellum may be direct or indirect. Fibres passing into the cerebellum *directly* without intervening synapses, to terminate predominantly in the cerebellar cortex, stem from neuron groups in the spinal cord, medulla oblongata, pons and midbrain. All other tracts which influence cerebellar activity do so *indirectly* by converging on one or more of the direct sources just mentioned.

**The main direct cerebellar inputs** are: (1) from the spinal cord via the various spinocerebellar pathways (including functionally the cuneocerebellar tract); (2) from the olivary, reticular, vestibular and arcuate nuclear complexes of the medulla oblongata; (3) from the pontine nuclei in the ventral part of the pons; and (4) from the tectum of the midbrain via the tectocerebellar tract. These are detailed in previous pages.

Reference has already been made to a useful approximate subdivision of the cerebellar cortex on phylogenetic and ontogenetic grounds into archicerebellum, paleocerebellum and neocerebellum (*see* 7.85 A). Ignoring for our present purposes minor inconsistencies and some degree of overlap, the *archicerebellum* or 'vestibulocerebellum' receives principally vestibular connexions; the *paleocerebellum* or 'spinocerebellum' receives direct terminals from the spinal cord, the medullary reticular formation and the accessory olivary nuclei; the *neocerebellum* receives, laterally in the large hemispheres of the middle lobe, the massive *pontocerebellar* connexions

and those from the inferior olive, whilst nearer the median plane, in its vermian and paravermian regions, it receives *tectocerebellar* connexions. (Perhaps to correspond to the rather imprecise but useful terms 'vestibulocerebellum' and 'spinocerebellum', the addition of 'pontocerebellum' and 'tectocerebellum' would seem appropriate.) This crude parcellation of the cerebellar cortex into the receiving areas for the main groups of *direct* afferent inputs, despite some overlap, can aid further discussion of the complexities added when indirect pathways are included, and it has also proved useful in clinicopathological description (*vide infra*).

**The indirect routes** by which cerebellar cortical activity can be modified must, as pointed out above, necessarily involve the convergence of pathways on to the direct pathways just summarized. In particular, other routes from the spinal cord, various subcortical nuclei and the extensive projections from the cerebral cortex must be considered.

In addition to the array of direct spinocerebellar pathways previously described, it will be recalled that both the accessory olivary nuclei and the medullary reticular formation also project to the spinocerebellum, and it is interesting that both the latter receive spinal cord projections through the spino-olivary and spinoreticular tracts. Further, circumscribed regions of the vestibular nuclei and the tectum both receive spinal connexions through the spinovestibular and spinotectal tracts, although the degree to which information flowing into the cerebellum along the vestibulocerebellar and tectocerebellar tracts is modified by influences from the spinal cord remains uncertain. Nevertheless, it is clear that information from the cord may reach the cerebellum in many different orders of complexity. The direct spinocerebellar pathways convey relatively elementary forms of information; single fibres may carry impulse patterns which follow stimulation of a single type of cutaneous or proprioceptive peripheral receptor, whilst others may carry patterns derived from the convergence and interaction of fibres from two or more types of peripheral receptor—even here, however, impulse transmission at the first synapse in the pathway may be modulated by activity in descending pathways such as the corticospinal. In the indirect spinal pathways there are presumably mechanisms for the further integration of impulses from the cord with those flowing along the other pathways which converge on the medullary reticular formation, accessory olivary nuclei, etc., before transmission into the cerebellum.

Similar considerations apply to the numerous routes by which the cerebral neocortex may modify cerebellar cortical activity. As we have seen, the most massive is the corticopontocerebellar pathway with which many observers would link a cortico-arcuatocerebellar pathway. In addition it must be remembered that other cell stations from which axons reach the cerebellar cortex are also in receipt of connexions from the cerebral cortex. Thus, there are corticotectal, corticoreticular, and cortico-olivary tracts; and as mentioned above, even the cells of origin of the spinocerebellar tracts are influenced by descending corticospinal fibres. Accordingly, it will be appreciated that cerebral cortical activity may well influence the information flow into the cerebellum along most of the pathways that enter the organ.

However, the various brainstem centres which project to the cerebellum are not homogeneous systems with respect to their connexions; on the contrary, there is much evidence that, for example, the olivary complex is not only somatotopically organized in relation to its projections to the cerebellar cortex, but varies much in its different parts in terms of their afferent connexions. Thus, some parts may be largely concerned with particular through routes, e.g.

the spino-olivocerebellar pathway; other regions may provide sites for the *pre-integration* of the information flow along various afferent channels which converge on the olivary nuclei. The latter include some of the afferents from the spinal cord and cerebral cortex just mentioned, and others from the corpus striatum, the red nucleus and the brainstem reticular formation.

Without elaborating further here, it is clear that for a fuller understanding of cerebellar mechanisms, much more needs to be known about all the forms in which information is presented to the cerebellar cortex. The relatively simple direct spinocerebellar and vestibulo-cerebellar pathways have already been analysed quite extensively, but the significance of the cerebral cortical control systems, and the degree to which complex transformations occur by pre-integration in the various brainstem centres remain obscure, but are the subject of much current research.

### THE CEREBELLAR OUTPUT

The output from the cerebellum commences with the axons of the Purkinje cells of the cerebellar cortex and involves the four intracerebellar nuclei (fastigial, globose, emboliform and dentate), on both sides of the midline. Both the Purkinje cells and the nuclei will be further detailed in subsequent sections, but for our present purposes it must be stated that the vast majority of the Purkinje cell axons converge upon and synapse with the neurons of the nuclei just mentioned; the axons of the latter form the main outflow tracts from the cerebellum. However, some of the Purkinje cells situated in the cortex of the flocculonodular lobe and others in the anterior and posterior parts of the vermis send axons which by-pass the intracerebellar nuclei, to extend directly to their destinations outside the cerebellum.

The most obvious effects of cerebellar dysfunction are disturbances in patterns of muscle contraction, and it is instructive to consider the cerebellar outflow in relation to the regions known to be intimately concerned, at least in part, with locomotor control. Whilst a few cerebello-spinal and cerebellonuclear fascicles have occasionally been mentioned in the research literature, it seems that direct cerebellar connexions to motor neuron pools in either the spinal cord or brainstem are either non-existent, or so sparse as to be of little functional significance. In contrast, all the major motor control regions of the brainstem and cerebrum receive, directly or indirectly, profuse connexions from the cerebellum. These include the vestibular nuclear complex, the brainstem reticular formation, the red nucleus, the tectum, and, via the thalamus, the corpus striatum and motor regions of the cerebral cortex. From these nuclei arise all the main descending pathways, corticospinal, tectospinal, vestibulospinal, rubrospinal, reticulospinal, etc. by which—usually through the intermediary of local interneurons—the patterns of activity in the α and γ motor neurons are varied. These pathways will not be further detailed here, but it is evident that for a comprehensive view of cerebellar control to emerge, it will be necessary to consider the control which is exerted at all these levels simultaneously. Further, despite the prominence of *locomotor* sequelae in states of deranged cerebellar function, there may well be many other activities in which the cerebral and cerebellar cortices cooperate and which are not revealed by current methods of investigation. Certainly a number of aspects of *autonomic* regulatory functions may be modified in cases of cerebellar disease or after experimental stimulation or ablation. There is also an increasing weight of evidence that the cerebellum may play a role in modifying the electrical activity of the sensory areas of the cerebral

cortex; and through its connexions with the reticular formation and thalamus it may modulate transmission in *ascending* sensory pathways.[451]

## The Grey Matter of the Cerebellum

The cerebellar grey matter is distributed in two locations —as an extensive surface coat, the cerebellar cortex, and as independent masses deep within the substance of the organ, the intracerebellar nuclei.

### THE CEREBELLAR CORTEX

The surface grey matter of the cerebellar cortex is, as we have seen (p. 856), folded by a large number of predominantly transverse but somewhat curved fissures. The latter are closely arranged, approximately parallel, and vary considerably in depth, dividing the organ into a series of lobes, lobules and folia. These subdivisions correspond to the primary, secondary, tertiary and sometimes quaternary laminae of the central cerebellar white matter. The smallest terminal laminae and their curved caps of grey matter constitute individual *cerebellar folia* (7.73, 84). So deeply grooved is the surface of the cerebellum, that if 'unfolded' the anteroposterior length of the cortex would be more than one metre, while its transverse dimension is only one-seventh of this at its maximum. Throughout its whole extent the cerebellar cortex shows a virtually uniform microscopic structure. Local differences which are so characteristic of the cerebral cortex do not occur in the cerebellum, so that it is impossible to distinguish between sections taken from different areas. Not only is the cerebellar cortex of man homogeneous structurally in all regions, but also a similar structure obtains throughout the mammalia and with only minor differences throughout the vertebrates.

The cerebellar cortex shows a high degree of geometric order, many of its elements being precisely arranged with respect to the surface and to the longitudinal and transverse axes of individual folia (7.79). It consists of: (*a*) the terminations of fibres entering the cortex ('climbing' and 'mossy' fibres); (*b*) five varieties of neuron—granule cells, outer stellate cells, basket cells, inner stellate (Golgi) cells, and finally, the Purkinje cells, whose axons leave the cerebellar cortex; (*c*) specialized neuroglial cells and blood vessels.

The cortex of the cerebellum consists of two main strata, external *molecular* and internal *granular layers*. Some authorities consider that a third *Purkinje cell layer* should be distinguished which is intermediate in position, but in this account it is treated as the deepest part of the molecular layer. In the following paragraphs the constituents of each layer are listed and briefly summarized, and subsequently individual features are treated in greater detail. Nevertheless, the detailed researches on the anatomy and physiology of the cerebellar cortex are now so numerous and contain such a wealth of data, that all cannot be treated in depth here. For further details and extensive bibliographies the interested reader should consult footnote references [452–456].

In brief, the exceedingly numerous granule cells of the

[451] R. S. Snider, *Prog. Brain Res.*, **25**, 1967.
[452] R. S. Dow, *Biol. Rev.*, **17**, 1942.
[453] J. Jansen and A. Brodal (eds.), *Aspects of Cerebellar Anatomy*, Grundt Tanum, Oslo. 1954.
[454] R. S. Dow and G. Moruzzi, *The Physiology and Pathology of the Cerebellum*, University of Minnesota Press, Minneapolis. 1958.
[455] J. C. Eccles, M. Ito and J. Szentágothai, *The Cerebellum as a Neuronal Machine*, Springer-Verlag, Berlin, N.Y. 1967.
[456] C. A. Fox and R. S. Snider (eds.), *Prog. Brain Res.*, **25**, 1967.

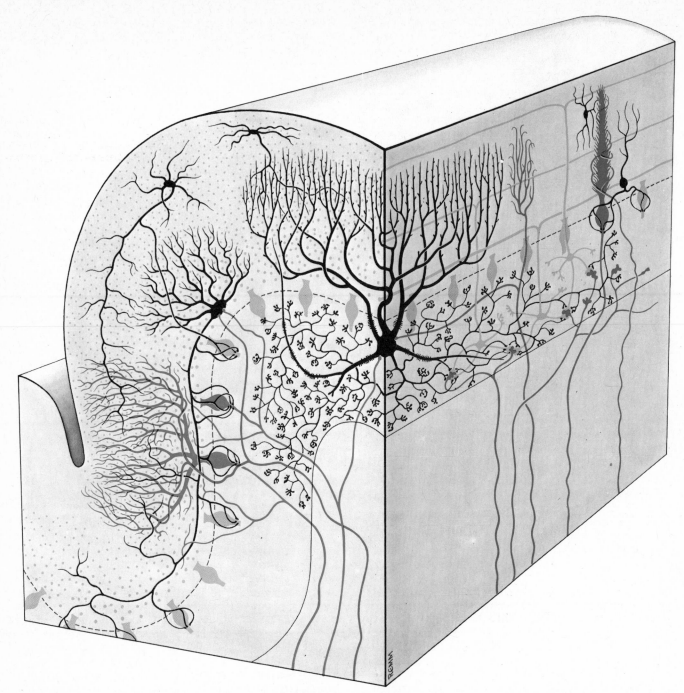

**7.79**  The general organization of the cerebellar cortex: a single cerebellar folium has been sectioned vertically, both in its longitudinal axis
(right part of the diagram) and transversely (on the left). Note: (1)
Purkinje cells (red); (2) inhibitory interneurons (black) including outer
stellate, basket and Golgi cells; (3) granule cells and their ascending
axons which bifurcate into longitudinally disposed horizontal fibres
(yellow); (4) climbing fibres and mossy afferents (blue). Note also the
synaptic glomeruli formed between the terminals of the mossy afferent
fibres, the complex dendrite tips of the granule cells, and the ramifications of the Golgi cell axon. (Redrawn from: *The Cerebellum as a Neuronal
Machine* by J. C. Eccles, M. Ito and J. Szentágothai. With the permission
of the authors and the publishers Springer, 1967.)

inner layer are one of the two principal *input* stations of the
cerebellar cortex, since they receive the synaptic terminals
of the mossy afferents (i.e. *all* the fibre systems converging
on the cerebellar cortex other than the olivocerebellar
fibres). The large Purkinje cells form the *output* channel
from the cerebellar cortex, most of their axons converging
upon the deeply placed intracerebral nuclei, from which
the various outflow tracts leave the cerebellum for the
numerous destinations described in the previous pages.

   The dendritic trees of the Purkinje cells receive synaptic
terminals from the profuse array of *parallel fibres* derived
from the granule cell axons, and from the *climbing fibre*
input to the cortex derived from the olivocerebellar
tract. The remaining neurons, i.e. outer stellate cells,
basket cells and Golgi cells, are essentially *inhibitory*

*interneurons*, which interconnect the various elements in
the cerebellar cortex in complex geometrical patterns
(*vide infra*).

   In broad outline, therefore, the cerebellar cortex
receives *two lines of input*, the climbing olivocerebellar
fibres which synapse directly with the Purkinje cells, and
the mossy fibres which do so through the intermediary of
numerous granule cells and their parallel-fibred axon
terminals. Both are excitatory to the Purkinje cells but are
completely contrasting, as we shall see, in their structural
arrangement and presumed modes of operation. The
outgoing axons of the Purkinje cells are inhibitory to the
cells of the intracerebral nuclei, which in turn modify
the activities of all the major motor control centres of the
brainstem and cerebrum. Purkinje cell activity is further

complicated by the operation of complex surrounding 'shells' of inhibitory interneurons.

## THE LAYERS OF THE CEREBELLAR CORTEX

**The molecular layer** is some 300–400 μm in thickness and consists of a rather sparse population of different types of neuron, numerous dendritic arborizations, non-myelinated axons and neuroglial cell processes. In conventional histological preparations it appears rather featureless, hence its name, in contrast to the immense tightly-packed nuclear population of the granular layer. The molecular layer contains (7.79):

(1) In its deepest part a single layer of the flask-shaped cell somata of Purkinje cells which are flattened in the transverse axis of the folium, and appear narrow when the folium is sectioned longitudinally.

(2) The rich dendritic trees of the Purkinje cells which reach towards the surface of the cortex and are also flattened in the transverse plane of the folium.

(3) Recurrent collaterals from Purkinje cell axons.

(4) The dendritic trees of the Golgi cells whose somata occupy the outer granular zone; these dendritic trees also reach towards the surface of the cortex, but are not flattened, and they span the territories of a number of Purkinje cells both transversely and longitudinally.

(5) The cell somata, dendrites and axonal branches of the outer stellate cells which are superficially placed.

(6) The cell somata, dendrites and axonal branches of the more deeply placed basket cells.

(7) The axonal terminals of the more deeply placed granule cells which pass radially into the molecular layer, where each divides into two branches which proceed in opposite directions in the longitudinal axis of the folium, giving, with others, the parallel fibre bundles which intersect with the various dendritic trees just mentioned.

(8) The terminals of the olivocerebellar climbing fibres, which ascend from the deeper parts of the hemisphere through the granular layer to become closely applied to the surfaces of the Purkinje cell dendrites in the molecular layer.

(9) The radially disposed branches of large neuroglial cells which are sited in the granular layer; these branches surround or intervene between the foregoing neuronal elements, except at points of synaptic contact, and at the surface of the cortex form conical expansions which meet neighbouring ones to make an external limiting membrane for the cerebellar cortex.

The general disposition of these different elements is summarized in illustration 7.79.

**The granular layer** of the cerebellar cortex (7.79) varies in thickness, being about 100 μm deep in the furrows and 400–500 μm at the apex of the folia. It contains an almost unbelievably large population of 'micro-neurons', the *granule cells*, which are about $2.4 \times 10^6$ per cubic millimetre for the cerebellar cortex of the monkey and $3–7 \times 10^6$ per cubic millimetre in the human cortex.[457, 458] In summary the granular layer consists of:

(1) The cell somata of the granule cells just mentioned and the initial parts of their axons which ascend to the molecular layer to form the parallel fibres.

(2) The dendritic extensions of the granule cells, with their claw-like terminal expansions.

(3) The branching terminals of the mossy afferent fibres to the cerebellar cortex.

(4) The climbing fibres passing through to the molecular layer.

(5) The cell somata, basal dendrites and the profuse and complex axonal arborization of the Golgi cells.

(6) The cerebellar *glomeruli* which are synaptic complexes involving four types of neurite; the mossy fibre

terminal establishes synaptic contacts with both granule cell and Golgi cell dendrites, whilst the granule cell dendrites also receive synaptic contacts from Golgi cell axon terminals (p. 869).

(7) The cell bodies of the large neuroglial cells mentioned above.

The cells and synaptic contacts of the cerebellar cortex will now be described in greater detail.

## THE PURKINJE CELL

As mentioned above the Purkinje neurons are a highly differentiated type of cell, with a specific geometry, and throughout the vertebrates are characteristically found in the cerebellar cortex and in no other part of the nervous system.

Their flattened cell bodies are flask-shaped when viewed in a transverse section across a folium and appear as a vertical narrow strip in longitudinal section. They are arranged in a single stratum in the deepest part of the molecular layer of the cortex (7.79), immediately adjacent to the granular layer; individual Purkinje cells are separated by about 50 μm transversely and 50–100 μm longitudinally. Their cell bodies have a vertical diameter of 50–70 μm and a transverse diameter of 30–35 μm.

One, sometimes two large, smooth primary dendrites arise from the 'neck' of the flask, that is, the superficial pole of the cell, but its precise pattern of branching varies with the position of the cell. In the depths of the furrows between folia the primary dendrite branches almost immediately into two large smooth stems which recede from each other at nearly 180° in the transverse plane of the folium, and from these a remarkably rich arborization of second, third and subsequent order sub-branches arise and pass towards the surface of the cortex. Near the apex of a folium the primary dendrite passes superficially for some distance before branching at a more acute angle. In both cases, however, the branches of the dendritic tree are confined to a narrow 'sheet' of tissue which lies precisely in the transverse plane of the folium. The Purkinje cells are rather more tightly packed together at the apices of the folia than in the depths of the fissures, and this, together with the variations in dendrite branching, have been interpreted as Cartesian transformations which correspond to the convexities and concavities of the surface, consequent upon the 'folding' of the tissue planes which occurs during development.

The primary dendrite and its first and second order branches have smooth surfaces, as noted above, but the third order branches and subsequent ramuli are densely covered over much of their surfaces by short, thick *dendritic spines* which form synaptic contacts with the parallel fibres derived from the granule cell axons (*vide infra*). The terminal *spiny branchlets* of the dendritic tree carry about 45 spines on each 10 μm of their length, and it has been computed[457] that on average each Purkinje cell carries about 180,000 spines on the whole of its dendritic tree—this is further discussed below.

The base of the cell body of a Purkinje cell, which lies near the granular layer, gives origin to the axon, which passes through the granular layer into the subjacent white matter. The initial 30 μm or so of the process, however, is narrow, non-myelinated, has ultrastructural features which correspond with those of the soma rather than the true axon, and its surfaces make specialized synaptic contacts with basket cell axon terminals. For these reasons some authorities prefer to call this initial region the *preaxon*; beyond this point it suddenly increases in dia-

[457] C. A. Fox and J. W. Barnard, *J. Anat.*, **91**, 1957.
[458] V. Braitenberg and R. P. Atwood, *J. comp. Neurol.*, **109**, 1958.

meter, acquires a myelin sheath and gives rise to a number of collateral branches. The principal part of the axon continues through the white matter and eventually breaks up into a basket-work of terminals which form synapses with cells of one of the intracerebellar nuclei, but a small proportion of the axons by-pass these nuclei and pass directly to the vestibular nuclei of the brainstem (p. 861). The collateral branches of the Purkinje axon interweave to form supra- and infra-ganglionic plexuses internal and external to the level of the Purkinje cells. Their termination is still rather an open question, but any significant number of these recurrent collaterals ending upon neighbouring Purkinje cells seems doubtful. The majority probably pass to make synaptic contacts with the dendrites of basket and Golgi cells in the same, neighbouring and even quite distant folia, and may well form the so-called cortical association fibres, the significance of which has long remained obscure.

*Synaptic contacts are made with Purkinje cells* (7.80) by: (1) the parallel fibre bundles of the granule cell axons, which synapse with the dendritic spines of the Purkinje cell; (2) the climbing fibres from the olivocerebellar system; one climbing fibre is largely restricted to a single Purkinje cell and its numerous branches follow the subdivisions of the Purkinje dendrites and establish hundreds, perhaps thousands of synaptic contacts with the nonspiny (i.e. smooth interspine) areas of the spiny branchlets; (3) synaptic terminals from the outer stellate cells on the smooth surfaces of the large primary and secondary dendrites; (4) synaptic contacts from collaterals of basket cells, which end interspersed between those of the stellate cells; (5) complex 'beard-like' terminals of the basket cell axons which surround the Purkinje cell preaxon described above. These various contacts are summarized in 7.80.

The ultrastructure of the Purkinje cell has been well studied;[459, 460, 461] it contains all the elements common to neurons (p. 771) and particular emphasis has been placed upon distinctive arrays of compressed lamellar systems of membranes which assist microscopic identification. They will not be further detailed here. Other than at points of synaptic contact with other neuronal processes, all parts of the cell surface are clothed with the processes of Bergmann glial cells.

## THE GRANULE CELL

The varying thickness of the granular layer and its immense population of granule cells (up to 7,000,000 per cubic millimetre in man) has been mentioned above. Each granule cell has a spherical nucleus of only 5–8 $\mu$m diameter with a mere veil of cytoplasm 0.5–1.0 $\mu$m thick containing a few small mitochondria, ribosomes and a diminutive Golgi complex. From the deep aspect of the granule cell pass usually 3–5 dendrites (occasionally 1–7), and each dendrite is some 10–30 $\mu$m in length and often remains single, but sometimes branches before breaking up into claw-like terminal expansions. The latter receive the synaptic terminals of the mossy fibre input and the other components adjoining them to form the *cerebellar glomeruli*, which occupy the small clear crevices between the granule cells, seen when they are examined with conventional light microscope techniques.

The small-diameter axon of each granule cell passes from its superficial aspect into the molecular layer and then dichotomises at a T-junction, the branches diverging parallel to the long axis of the cerebellar folium. The total length of the two branches is 2–3 mm, and together with those of other granule cells, they form the system of *parallel fibres* (7.79, 80). Near the point of bifurcation the parallel fibres are smooth, but throughout much of their course they develop intermittent fusiform dilatations of

outline, and then near their termination a series of short hook-like or club-like surface projections. The dilatations and projections are sites of synaptic contact between the parallel fibre and the numerous types of dendrite in the molecular layer. Some quantitative aspects of these connexions will be mentioned below, but by far the most numerous are those with the dendritic spines of the Purkinje cells, less frequent are those with the spines of Golgi cell dendrites, and with the dendrites of the outer stellate and basket neurons. It may be noted that quantitative histological studies suggest that 200,000–300,000 parallel fibres cross, and probably synapse with, the dendrites of a *single* Purkinje cell.

## THE BASKET NEURONS

These neurons are of stellate form and occupy the deeper half of the molecular layer of the cerebellar cortex. Their dendritic trees have no special geometry in their details of branching, but again, like the Purkinje cells, their dendrites are confined to thin 'sheets' of tissue which lie strictly in the transverse plane of the cerebellar folia. The dendritic surfaces carry rather sparse, irregular, long, thin dendritic spines which make synaptic contact with the parallel fibres that intersect the dendritic tree at right angles. The cell body is also densely beset with axosomatic synapses, derived it is thought from climbing fibre collaterals and from recurrent collaterals of the Purkinje cell axons.

The basket cell axons course in the deeper part of the molecular layer just superficial to the layer of Purkinje cells, and again, the principal axon passes in the transverse plane of the folium. It continues for a distance of about 1 mm, covering the territories of about 10–12 Purkinje cells in its course. From the second Purkinje cell onwards, descending collateral branches pass towards the cell somata of the Purkinje cells, where they interweave with collaterals from other basket cells, forming the pericellular networks of fibres from which the cells derive their name. Side branches pass from each descending collateral and from the main axon, and pass longitudinally in the folium to reach an additional 3–6 rows of Purkinje cells on both sides of the main axon. Accordingly, 100–200 Purkinje cells may be reached by the synaptic terminals of a single basket cell. The general cell body surfaces of Purkinje neurons are devoid of synaptic contacts and those derived from the descending collaterals of the basket cell axons are clustered in a complex fashion around the point of origin and throughout the length of the preaxon mentioned above (7.80). The basket cell axons also give rise to a much less profuse system of ascending collateral branches which probably synapse with the smooth bases of the Purkinje cell dendrites.

Thus, the basket cells provide a unique synaptic system. Activity in a longitudinal bundle of parallel fibres will activate a longitudinal row of basket cells whose dendrites are intersected by the bundle. Because the basket cell axons pass transversely in the folium, they will therefore exert a powerful synaptic action on the origins of axons from Purkinje cells which lie in longitudinal strips on both sides of the parallel fibre bundle (see also below).

## THE OUTER STELLATE NEURONS

Smaller than the basket cells, the outer stellate neurons are scattered through the superficial half of the molecular

[459] R. M. Herndon, *J. Cell Biol.*, **18**, 1963.
[460] J. Hámori and J. Szentágothai, *Acta biol. Hung.*, **15**, 1965 and *Expl Brain Res.*, **1**, 1966; **2**, 1966.
[461] C. Léránth and J. Hamori, *Acta biol. Acad. Sci. hung.*, **21**, 1970.

header at top right

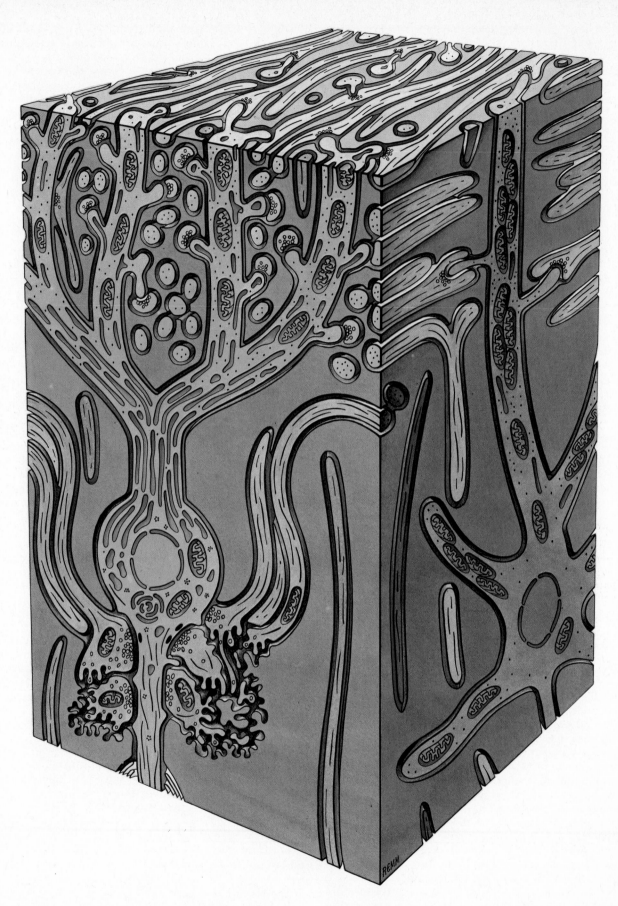

**7.80**  Detailed cytoarchitecture of part of the cerebellar cortex which includes the layer of Purkinje cell somata and the zones immediately superficial and deep to this. The vertical block face to the right is in the longitudinal axis of the cerebellar folium; the vertical face to the left is in the transverse plane of the folium; the upper face is tangential with respect to the convex summit of the folium. The cell details are shown in the following colours: red—the soma of the Purkinje cell, its 'preaxon' passing from the lower pole, and its apical stem dendrite with its first-order branches bearing dendritic spines. Blue—climbing fibres. Orange/ yellow—horizontal fibres derived from the bifurcation of the ascending axons of granule cells. Mauve—Golgi cell soma, dendrites with spines and initial segment of its axon. Pale brown—the descending basket cell axons forming complex synapses on the preaxon of the Purkinje cell. Green—areas occupied by glial cell processes. Note the synapses between the horizontal axons and the dendritic spines of the Purkinje cell and Golgi cell. (Compounded and redrawn from information and illustrations in: *The Cerebellum as a Neuronal Machine* by J. C. Eccles, M. Ito and J. Szentágothai.)

layer of the cerebellar cortex. Their dendritic trees, although smaller than those of basket cells, are similar in their general form, possession of spines and their transversal disposition in the folium. Again, they are intersected at right angles by bundles of parallel fibres, with which their spines and interspine smooth areas establish synaptic contacts. The origin of the sparse axosomatic synapses which have been seen on these cells is uncertain.

The smallest stellate neurons have profuse local axonal arborizations, which terminate on Purkinje cell dendritic spines, whilst the longer axons of the larger stellate cells again pass transversely in the folium to similar destinations on more distant Purkinje cells. The deepest and largest stellate neurons are similar but possess a number of descending collaterals which accompany those of the typical basket cells.

## THE GOLGI NEURONS

These are the largest neurons of a stellate form in the cerebellar cortex and they occupy the superficial zone of the granular layer, immediately below the Purkinje cell bodies. A series of large dendrites radiate from every aspect of the cell, but many eventually curve to enter the molecular layer, within which they arborize, their course within the latter being predominantly at right angles to the surface of the cortex. Their dendritic trees are not compressed into the transverse plane of the folium, and they appear much the same in both transverse and longitudinal folial section. In both these planes they overlap the territories of three Purkinje cells. Thus, the whole dendritic tree of a Golgi cell approaches, but does not overlap appreciably, those of adjacent Golgi cells, and each is intermingled, within the molecular layer, with the dendritic fields of about ten Purkinje cells. Some of the Golgi dendrites, however, do not enter the molecular layer, but divide within the granular layer and make a contribution to the cerebellar synaptic glomeruli (*vide infra*).

The Golgi cell axon arises from the deep aspects of the cell soma or from the base of one of its deeper dendrites, and immediately breaks up into a profuse arborization which permeates the full thickness of the granular layer, occupying a volume of tissue which corresponds on a deeper plane, to that of its dendritic tree in the molecular layer, i.e. does not overlap that of adjacent Golgi cells.

The main synaptic input to the Golgi neuron is from the parallel fibres of the molecular layer which synapse with the rather sparse spines on its dendrites. The axonal terminals of the Golgi cell take part in the formation of the cerebellar synaptic glomeruli.

In relation to the Golgi cells, therefore, the cerebellar cortex may be thought of as consisting of a series of tissue units, each roughly hexagonal in surface view, which abut on each other but do not overlap. Within each unit are about 10 Purkinje cell territories and deep to these an enormous population of granule cells and synaptic glomeruli.

## INPUTS TO THE CEREBELLAR CORTEX

As we have seen elsewhere, there are two lines of input to the cerebellar cortex, namely, the climbing fibres and the mossy afferents (7.79).

**The climbing fibres**, although recognized and illustrated by Cajal, their origin was for long in doubt and only recently has it been established that many are olivocerebellar fibres. The precise point-for-point correlation between the olivary complex of nuclei and the cerebellar cortex has already been mentioned (p. 860).

Each climbing fibre passes straight without branching through the white matter and the granular layer to become attached to a single Purkinje cell. It then divides repeatedly and its terminal arborization is closely applied to the surfaces of the branching Purkinje cell dendrites throughout much of their length, making large numbers of synaptic contacts with the smooth areas of dendrites between the dendritic spines.

A few collateral branches leave the climbing fibre and some of these descend to synapse with the cell somata and dendrites of Golgi neurons, whilst others make synaptic contacts with neighbouring basket or outer stellate cells. Physiological studies have now established that both mossy and climbing fibres are excitatory in their effects. Thus, climbing fibres are able to exert a powerful, localized, excitatory effect upon single Purkinje cells and also a much weaker effect upon the different varieties of interneuron in its neighbourhood.

**The mossy afferent fibres** are now widely considered to include all the afferent systems other than those of the olivocerebellar tract described above. They also are excitatory in their effects, but in all other respects they contrast markedly with the sharply localized climbing fibre input.

As each mossy fibre traverses the white matter of the cerebellum it gives off a series of collateral branches which diverge to a number of adjacent folia, and within each folium the branch runs through the central lamina of white matter, again giving off numerous sub-branches to the granular layer on both aspects of the folium. Each sub-branch then enters the granular layer and divides yet again into two or three terminal branchlets which expand into a group of grape-like synaptic terminals, or mossy fibre *rosettes*, each of which occupies the centre of a cerebellar *glomerulus* or islet.

**The cerebellar glomeruli** are complex synaptic arrangements involving a central mossy fibre rosette, the dendrites of a number of granule cells, the synaptic terminals of Golgi cell axons; in addition, certain glomeruli are also invaded by a Golgi cell dendrite. Each glomerulus is roughly spherical or ovoid, about 20 $\mu$m in its greatest dimension, and the ratio of glomeruli to granule cells is about 1 to 5.

All synaptic contacts in the glomerulus are of the axodendritic type. The central rosette establishes contact with the internal surfaces of a surrounding leash of up to 20 granule cell dendrites and, when present, with the spine-studded surface of a Golgi cell dendrite. The terminals of the Golgi cell axons establish synaptic contact with the lateral or external surfaces of a number of the granule cell dendrites. These arrangements are most easily appreciated by reference to a diagram (7.81).

The mossy fibre terminals are excitatory and can thus excite the granule cell dendrites and, if included, a Golgi cell dendrite. Conversely, the Golgi cell, which is an inhibitory interneuron, can inhibit the granule cell through its axodendritic contacts.

## SOME QUANTITATIVE ASPECTS OF CEREBELLAR CORTICAL STRUCTURE

Because of its regularly repetitive geometry, the cerebellar cortex has been much studied using quantitative neurohistological methods.[455, 457, 462, 463] A few prominent features only can be mentioned here. In its different zones, it shows extremes in terms of neuronal population, in the convergence, divergence and one-to-one relationship of transmission paths, and in the complex geometries of its inhibitory interneuronal pathways.

[462] C. A. Fox, D. E. Hillman, K. A. Siegesmund and C. R. Dutta, *Prog. Brain Res.*, **25**, 1967.
[463] V. Braitenberg, *Prog. Brain Res.*, **25**, 1967.

A vertical column of cerebellar cortex 1 mm in cross-sectional area, taken at the summit of a folium in the human cerebellum, contains roughly 500 Purkinje cells, 600 basket cells, 50 Golgi cells and perhaps 3,000,000 granule cells, with some 600,000 synaptic glomeruli.

On the input side each climbing fibre synapses with *only one* Purkinje cell (but through its collaterals with an undetermined number of neighbouring interneurons). In contrast a single mossy afferent fibre shows an enormous divergence—it may make synaptic contact with 400 or more granule cells within a single folium, and if its branches to neighbouring folia are included, the number probably rises to several thousand. Conversely, each granule cell probably receives synaptic contacts from 4 to 5 different mossy fibre terminals.

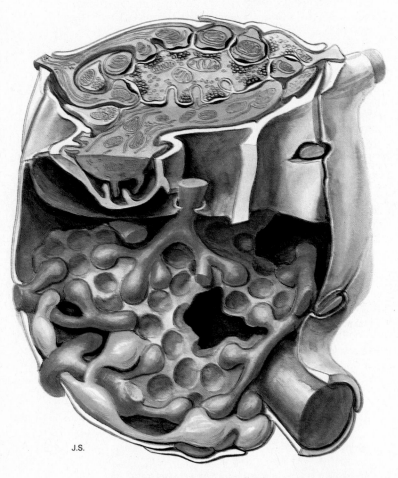

7.81  A stereodiagram illustrating the structure of a cerebellar synaptic glomerulus. *Blue:* mossy afferent fibre rosette. *Red:* granule cell dendrites. *Yellow:* terminals of Golgi cell axon. *Green:* Golgi cell dendrite. *Grey:* neuroglial capsule. Note that the essential synaptic contacts are axodendritic between: mossy afferent fibres and granule cell dendrites; mossy afferents and Golgi cell dendrites; Golgi cell axons and granule cell dendrites. (From: *The Cerebellum as a Neuronal Machine,* by J. C. Eccles, H. Ito and J. Szentágothai, by courtesy of the authors, and the publishers, Springer, 1967.)

The ascending axons of the granule cells, as we have seen, bifurcate to form parallel fibres which run longitudinally in the molecular layer and enter into synaptic contact with the various dendritic trees in their paths, i.e. those of Purkinje cells, Golgi cells, basket cells and outer stellate cells. The total length of the parallel fibre from a single granule cell axon is about 2–3 mm and in its path it makes a synaptic contact with 300–450 Purkinje cells. Thus the divergence from a single mossy afferent fibre through the intermediary of granule cells is to perhaps hundreds of thousands of Purkinje cells. The uncertainty

in the latter calculation stems from our lack of knowledge concerning the degree of overlap in parallel fibre territories. Finally, there is an enormous convergence of paths on to individual Purkinje cells, the dendritic tree of each cell receiving up to 200,000 synaptic contacts from different parallel fibres.

## MECHANISMS OF THE CEREBELLAR CORTEX

The large volume of structural research on the cerebellum ranging from comparative morphology, developmental analysis, and gross connectivity studies, to the quantitative cytology, cell geometry and synaptic relationships pursued by ultrastructural techniques, has been paralleled by an equally impressive volume of neurophysiological research (for example footnote references [452, 454, 455, 464–470]). The increasing interdependence of these approaches has led to the postulation of a number of elementary mechanisms which probably interlock during the normal functioning of the cerebellar cortex; only some brief comments indicating these kinds of approach will be included here.

It is clear, as repeated in previous sections, that the cerebellar cortex has two highly distinctive lines of input—the climbing and the mossy fibres—and only one line of output, the axons of the Purkinje cells (7.82). Both the climbing fibres and the mossy fibres ultimately convey information to the cerebellar cortex derived, at least in part, from similar sources, namely the exteroceptors and proprioceptors, the brainstem reticular formation and the cerebral cortex (see previous paragraphs). Further, both input channels are excitatory in their effects; but the climbing fibre exerts a one-to-one, powerful, all-or-none excitation on individual Purkinje cells, whilst each mossy afferent diffuses its excitatory effect through hundreds of excitatory granule neurons to thousands of Purkinje cells. The Purkinje cells are exclusively inhibitory in their action and their outflowing axons exert varying inhibitory patterns upon the intracerebellar and vestibular nuclei.

The remaining cells of the cerebellar cortex—basket, outer stellate and Golgi cells—each with its distinctive cell geometry, input and output, all function as inhibitory interneurons, the particular shape, site and kind of inhibitory effect varying with the cell type in question.

Whatever means of neurophysiological recording is employed, and whatever type of tissue preparation used, from the cerebellar cortex of the unanaesthetized animal to the chronically isolated slab of cortex, most of the cellular elements show a low level of 'background' impulse discharge even under conditions of minimal sensory input. Some researchers have used the term 'spontaneous' for this type of activity, but whether it represents an intrinsic characteristic of the individual neurons and their assemblies remains unclear; nevertheless, it is upon such a background that the more dramatic and orderly responses to specific patterns of input occur.

It has been suggested[471] that the climbing fibres and their terminal synapses, which are largely concentrated on individual Purkinje cells, do not provide an integrative

[464] R. S. Dow, *J. Physiol., Lond.,* **94**, 1938; *J. Neurophysiol.,* **2**, 1939; **12**, 1949.

[465] J. C. Eccles, *Perspect. Biol. Med.,* **8**, 1965.

[466] J. C. Eccles, R. Llinas and K. Sasaki, *Nature, Lond.,* **203**, 1964; *Expl Brain Res.,* **1**, 1966a, b, c; *J. Physiol., Lond.,* **182**, 1966a, b, c.

[467] J. C. Eccles, K. Sasaki and P. Strata, *Expl Brain Res.,* **2**, 1966; **3**, 1967a, b.

[468] M. Ito and M. Yoshida, *Expl Brain Res.,* **2**, 1966.

[469] M. Ito, M. Yoshida and K. Obata, *Experientia,* **20**, 1964.

[470] R. S. Snider, *Prog. Brain Res.,* **25**, 1967.

[471] J. Szentágothai, in: *Recent Development of Neurobiology in Hungary* Vol. I, ed. K. Lissák, Akadémiai Kiádo, Budapest. 1967.

mechanism, and it is presumed that for the climbing fibres their information flow has been *pre-integrated* from the various channels which converge and synapse with the cells of the olivary nuclear complexes. Further, it is suggested that the important *integrative units* of the cerebellar cortex involve the mossy afferent input, granule cells, parallel fibres, Purkinje cells and the varieties of interneuron. Some of their possible elementary interactions are summarized in **7**.82, 83.

It may be imagined that activity in some of the mossy afferents has excited a small locus of granule cells with resultant activity in a narrow bundle of parallel fibres in the molecular layer of the cortex. The bundle of active parallel fibres, about 3 mm in length, courses longitudinally within the folium and exerts an excitatory effect upon the dendritic fields in its path, i.e. those of Purkinje, Golgi, basket and outer stellate cells. If the bundle is very narrow, or its activity of a low order, none of these cells will respond. However, as the size of the bundle increases until it roughly corresponds to the width of the Purkinje cell dendritic fields, excitatory responses follow in a row of Purkinje cells and also in the related basket and outer stellate cells. Under these conditions the Golgi neurons do not respond, because only a small proportion of their much larger dendritic fields are receiving an input from the parallel fibre bundle. The net result, therefore, is that a single row of Purkinje cells about 3 mm long and parallel to the long axis of the folium respond with volleys of impulses along their axons. Because of the transverse disposition of the basket and outer stellate cell axons and their terminals, simultaneous activation of these inhibitory interneurons by the bundle results in longitudinal strips of cortex containing inhibited Purkinje cells which flank the active row on both sides. It is considered that with the continual fluctuations of activity in the mossy fibre input, the essential response of the cerebellar cortex is one of a constantly changing pattern of innumerable 'unit rows' of excited Purkinje cells flanked by inhibitory zones. The latter provide a process of neural sharpening by which the more active bundles of parallel fibres are selected from the general background of cortical activity. Should the active bundle of parallel fibres become too wide (i.e. much greater than the width of a single Purkinje cell row), another mechanism comes into play mediated by the Golgi cells. If sufficiently wide, the parallel fibres excite the Golgi cells via their dendrites and these, in turn, cause a reduction in the mossy fibre input via the granule cells by means of their inhibitory synaptic terminals on the granule cell dendrites in the synaptic glomeruli (p. 869). Hence, the principal function of the Golgi neurons appears to be in providing a 'choke' whereby excessive broadening of the active bundle of parallel fibres is prevented.

It is upon this incessantly changing pattern of excited, inhibited or relatively quiescent rows of Purkinje cells, that the sharply localized excitatory effect of the climbing fibres is exerted, the resultant effect upon any individual Purkinje cell depending upon the strength of the climbing fibre stimulus and the state of the Purkinje cell upon its receipt. By mechanisms such as these, fluctuating inhibitory patterns are transmitted by the Purkinje cells to the intracerebellar nuclei, and thence to the motor control centres in the cerebrum and brainstem.

There are, of course, many other orders of complexity in the intracortical circuits of the cerebellum. These include the added complication of the effects of Purkinje cell and climbing fibre collateral branches on the various inhibitory interneurons, the problems posed by the presence of Golgi cell dendrites in the synaptic glomeruli, and differential 'on' and 'off' responses in the different categories of interneuron. Further interesting mathematical analyses of the structural arrangements in the cerebellum have led to proposals concerning its possible mode of operation as an accurate timing device or *biological clock*, which incorporates critical *delay paths* in its design; these may be important in controlling the correct temporal sequence of events in, for example, rapid 'voluntary' movements.[472] These will not be pursued further here, but perhaps enough has been said to indicate the general lines along which our knowledge of the *higher integrative units* of the cerebellar cortex is increasing. Despite such increases in understanding, they still fall far short of a comprehensive view of how the cerebellum as a whole integrates its total complex inflow of information, and utilizes it to regulate the overall locomotor patterns of the complete organism.

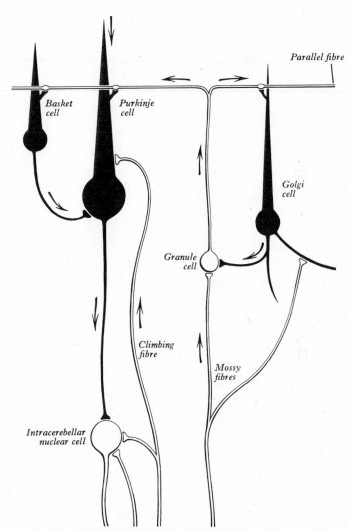

**7**.82 An analysis of the essential circuitry and synaptic contacts between the climbing and mossy afferent fibres, the main neuronal elements of the cerebellar cortex, and the neurons of the intracerebellar nuclei, based upon cytological and microelectrode studies. Excitatory cells, neurites and terminals are white surrounded by a black line; inhibitory elements are solid black. By courtesy of Professor J. C. Eccles.

## THE INTRACEREBELLAR NUCLEI

Four independent accumulations of grey matter are embedded in the white matter of the cerebellum of man on each side of the midline. These are the *intracerebellar nuclei*, sometimes also rather imprecisely termed the 'roof' nuclei because of the close relationship of some of them to the roof of the fourth ventricle.

[472] V. Braitenberg, *Prog. Brain Res.*, **25**, 1967.

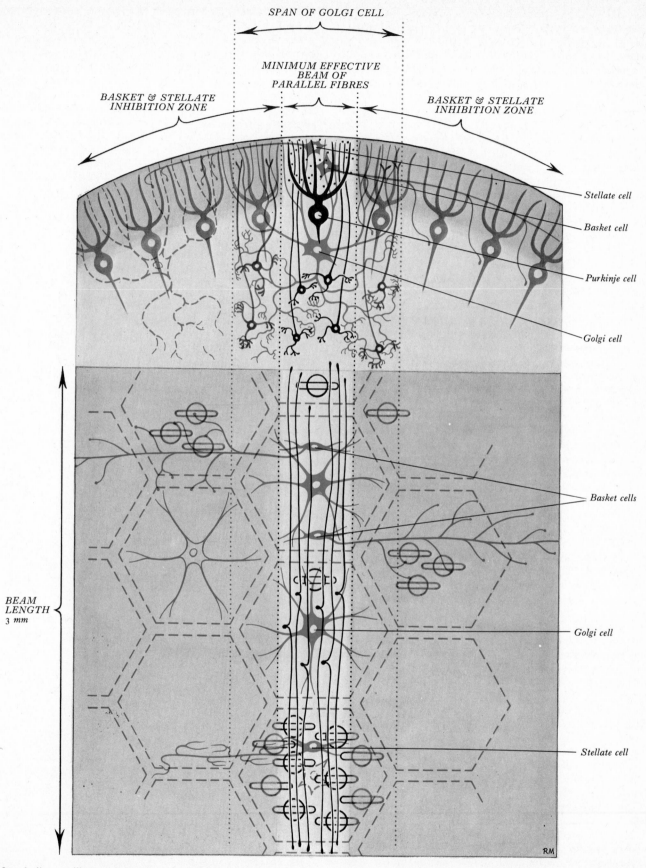

SPAN OF GOLGI CELL

MINIMUM EFFECTIVE
BEAM OF
PARALLEL FIBRES

BASKET & STELLATE
INHIBITION ZONE

BASKET & STELLATE
INHIBITION ZONE

Stellate cell

Basket cell

Purkinje cell

Golgi cell

Basket cells

BEAM
LENGTH
3 mm

Golgi cell

Stellate cell

**7.83** A diagram illustrating the concept of the complex neuronal integrative units of the cerebellar cortex. The neurons and their processes are shown in a transverse section of a cerebellar folium (above) and in surface view (below). Neurons in full colour (black, red or blue) or in full coloured outline, are in a state of excitation. Neurons in grey or interrupted outlines are inactive. *Full black or grey, black or grey outlines:* Purkinje cells, granule cells and their parallel fibre bundles; *blue:* basket and stellate cells; *red:* Golgi cells. The white longitudinal strip indicates activation of a locus of granule cells, their bundle of parallel fibres, and the associated longitudinal row of Purkinje cells. Simultaneous activation of the basket and stellate inhibitory interneurons by the parallel fibre bundle causes zones of lateral inhibition (grey shading) to flank the activated strip. These zones of inhibited Purkinje cells are in reality about ten rows wide—only four rows are illustrated here (grey profiles). If the active bundle of parallel fibres reaches a critical width, inhibitory Golgi interneurons become active, and reduce or stop mossy fibre input in the cerebellar glomeruli. The inhibitory territories of the Golgi cells are indicated by the array of red hexagons. See text for further description. (Redrawn from J. Szentágothai in: *Recent Development of Neurobiology in Hungary,* I. K. Lissák (ed.). By courtesy of the author and publishers, Akadémiai Kiadó, Budapest, 1967.)

Most laterally placed and the largest is the nucleus dentatus, on the medial aspect of which are the smaller nucleus emboliformis and nucleus globosus, whilst nearest the midline lies the nucleus fastigii. In most mammals, however, only three nuclei are recognized—a nucleus lateralis corresponding in part to the nucleus dentatus, a nucleus interpositus which corresponds largely to the globose and emboliform nuclei of man, and finally a nucleus medialis which corresponds to the nucleus fastigii. However, the precise homologies of the nucleus interpositus have been the subject of some debate.[473]

The nucleus fastigii is phylogenetically the oldest and is largely associated with the archicerebellum (vestibulo-cerebellum); the globose and emboliform nuclei are more recent and associated with the paleocerebellum (spino-cerebellum), whilst the nucleus dentatus is the most recent and is associated with the neocerebellum (ponto-cerebellum). These associations are, however, approximate only, and are further discussed below.

**The nucleus dentatus** (7.84) is situated a little to the medial side of the centre of the white matter of the hemisphere. It consists of an irregularly folded grey lamina containing white matter centrally, the fibres of which are derived in large measure from the axonal processes of the cell somata in the grey lamina. The grey lamina is deficient anteromedially and through this so-called 'hilus' of the nucleus the white fibres stream to form a large part of the superior cerebellar peduncle (p. 862). **The nucleus emboliformis** lies close to the medial side of the nucleus dentatus and partially covers its hilus, whilst the **nucleus globosus** is still more medially placed and despite its name is elongated anteroposteriorly. **The nucleus fastigii** is larger than the latter and is situated close to the median plane in the anterior part of the superior vermis.

The most prominent cells of the cerebellar nuclei are fairly typical large multipolar neurons possessing rather simple, stellate but irregular dendritic arborizations, the numbers of dendrites increasing from the fastigial to the dentate nucleus. However, the dendritic trees of adjacent neurons overlap considerably in the fastigial nucleus and are much more distinct, having their own territories, in the dentate nucleus. These large multipolar neurons give rise to axons which make one or two characteristic loops before leaving the nuclei to form the **cerebellar outflow tracts** in the superior and inferior cerebellar peduncles for the various destinations in the brainstem detailed in the previous pages. During the looped part of their course the axons give off a number of recurrent collateral branches which terminate locally in the nuclei of origin. The intracerebellar nuclei also contain numerous small neurons, some of which are probably local Golgi type II interneurons, whilst others contribute to the peduncles. (Experimentally some of the small cells show retrograde chromatolytic changes after section of the peduncles.[474, 475])

**The afferent connexions** to the cells of the intracerebellar nuclei are from both cerebellar and extracerebellar sources. Primarily they receive both axodendritic and axosomatic synapses from the terminals of Purkinje cell axons. The latter enter the nuclei and each axon branches to form pericellular nests around a number of neurons, whilst conversely, each pericellular nest receives contributions from the branches of more than one Purkinje cell axon, i.e. there is both an element of divergence and of convergence in the construction of the nucleus.

It is now widely held that the Purkinje cells are exclusively inhibitory in their action and this fact has focused attention on other afferents, many of which are presumably excitatory to the intracerebellar nuclei. Fibres have been described as reaching these nuclei from the red nucleus, i.e. rubrocerebellar fibres,[476] and also collateral branches from the spinocerebellar, pontocerebellar, olivocerebellar and reticulocerebellar tracts.[477] The outflow of information through the cerebellar peduncles, therefore, is thought to stem from an integration within the intracerebellar nuclei of the patterns of excitation delivered from these various extracerebellar sources with the inhibitory patterns delivered by Purkinje cell axons, and modified by the action of local interneurons.

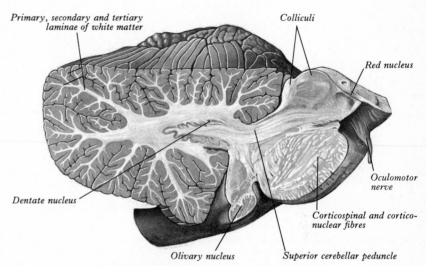

Primary, secondary and tertiary laminae of white matter

Colliculi

Red nucleus

Dentate nucleus

Oculomotor nerve

Olivary nucleus

Corticospinal and cortico-nuclear fibres

Superior cerebellar peduncle

7.84 Oblique vertical section through the right cerebellar hemisphere and right half of the brainstem.

## STRUCTURAL AND FUNCTIONAL LOCALIZATION IN THE CEREBELLUM

Since the cerebellar cortex shows an identical microscopic structure and microcircuitry in all parts of the cerebellum, it may be assumed—and physiological investigations support this—that its operational characteristics in terms of this local circuitry is also identical in all regions. In this sense, therefore, a functional localization does not exist within the cerebellar cortex *itself* as it does, for example, in the different laminae of grey matter in the spinal cord.

Structural and functional localization in the cerebellum is thus a reflection of the manner in which functionally dissimilar afferent tracts end preferentially in different regions of this homogeneous cortex. Equally, it is a reflexion of how the different areas of cortex project to particular intracerebellar nuclei, and therefore influence different brainstem centres. A vast number of investigations have been directed towards the problem of cerebellar localization and the foundations have been laid by comparative morphological, developmental and gross connectivity studies.[441, 478−482] These were supplemented by more detailed analyses of connectivity patterns using degeneration techniques in experimental animals.[61]

[473] J. Jansen and A. Brodal (eds.), *Aspects of Cerebellar Anatomy*, Grundt Tanum, Oslo. 1954.
[474] J. Jansen and J. K. S. Jansen, *J. comp. Neurol.*, **102**, 1955.
[475] S. Flood and J. Jansen, *Acta anat.*, **63**, 1966.
[476] J. Courville and A. Brodal, *J. comp. Neurol.*, **126**, 1966.
[477] J. C. Eccles, M. Ito and J. Szentágothai, *The Cerebellum as a Neuronal Machine*, Springer-Verlag, Berlin, N.Y. 1967.
[478] G. E. Smith, *J. Anat.* **36**, 1902; **37**, 1903.
[479] H. A. Riley, *Archs Neurol. Psychiat.*, Chicago, **24**, 1930.
[480] O. Larsell, *Archs Neurol. Psychiat.*, Chicago, **31**, 1934; **38**, 1937.
[481] O. Larsell, *J. comp. Neurol.*, **87**, 1947; **89**, 1948; **97**, 1952; **99**, 1953.
[482] R. Nieuwenhuys, *Prog. Brain Res.*, **25**, 1967.

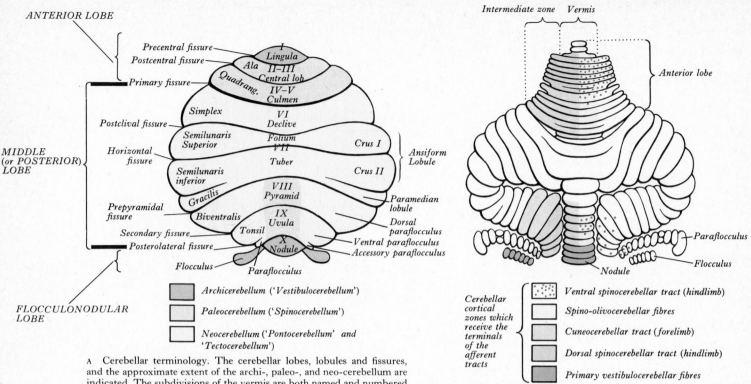

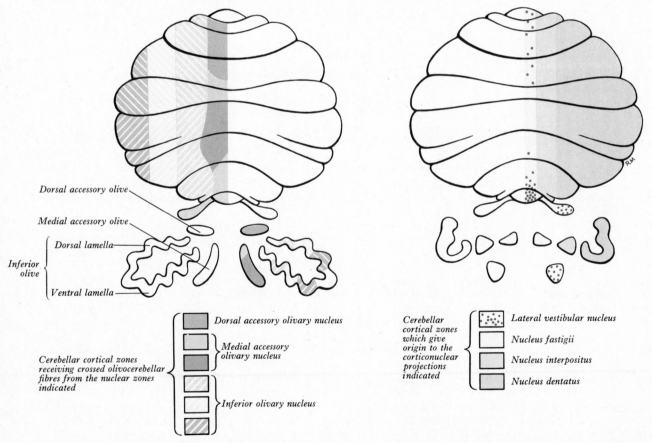

A   Cerebellar terminology. The cerebellar lobes, lobules and fissures, and the approximate extent of the archi-, paleo-, and neo-cerebellum are indicated. The subdivisions of the vermis are both named and numbered (after Larsell). On the left are terms widely used in human neuroanatomy; on the right are additional terms often used in general mammalian neuroanatomy.

B   The cerebellar cortical areas of termination of the afferent tracts indicated, derived from experimental studies.

E   An analysis of the topical organization of the cortical zones of the cerebellum which receive crossed olivocerebellar (climbing) fibres from the different parts of the inferior olivary complex of nuclei.

F   An analysis of the topically organized projections of cerebellar cortical Purkinje cell axons on to the lateral vestibular nucleus, and the intracerebellar nuclei.

**7.85** A–H   This series of diagrams is to illustrate certain features of the localization of structure and function in the cerebellum. G is a median sagittal section of the feline cerebellum; in all the remaining diagrams it is assumed that the cerebellum has been flattened and viewed from the dorsal aspect, so that its whole cranio-caudal extent can be seen. A, E and F are approximate outlines of the human cerebellum; B, C, D and H are of the feline cerebellum. Detailed descriptions of the information in these diagrams are in the text, and in the footnote references quoted.

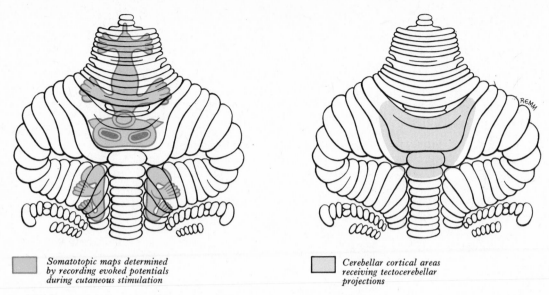

| | |
|---|---|
| ▨ Somatotopic maps determined by recording evoked potentials during cutaneous stimulation | ▨ Cerebellar cortical areas receiving tectocerebellar projections |

C  The somatotopic arrangement of the evoked potentials recorded from the cerebellar cortex during cutaneous stimulation.

D  The cerebellar cortical areas receiving tectocerebellar projections.

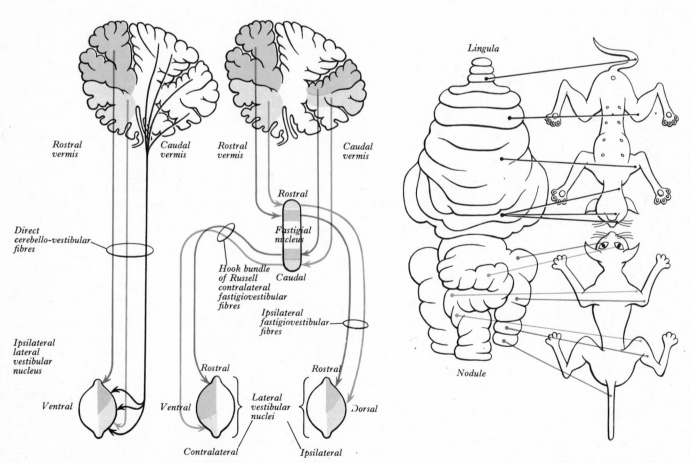

G  The arrangement of direct cerebello-vestibular and indirect cerebello-fastigio-vestibular projections from the cerebellar vermis of the cat.

H  The somatotopic pattern of movements elicited in different parts of the body during stimulation of the cerebellar cortex in the decerebrate cat.

(Illustrations B, F and G were redrawn and modified from *Neurological Anatomy*, 1969, by courtesy of the author Professor A. Brodal and the publishers, Oxford University Press; C, D and H were redrawn and modified from *Publications of the Association for Research in Nervous and Mental Disease*, **30**, 1952, by courtesy of the authors Professor R. Snider (C and D) and of Professors J. L. Hampson, C. R. Harrison and C. N. Woolsey (H), and the publishers, The Williams and Wilkins Company, Baltimore, U.S.A.)

Neurophysiological studies of the changes in electrical potential evoked by the 'natural' or 'artificial' stimulation of peripheral receptors including the special sense organs, peripheral nerves, and different regions of the cerebrum brainstem and spinal cord, have been carried out. [483, 484, 485, 486] The type of recordings have varied from rather crude monitoring of the surface of the exposed cerebellum, through recording of focal potentials by electrodes inserted into the cerebellar tissues, to unit recording with intracellular microelectrodes. Stimulation of the exposed cerebellar cortex in animals has been used to determine whether discrete movements are elicited, and which cerebellar regions influence movements that have been initiated reflexly or by stimulation of the cerebral cortex. Another extensive field of research has involved the study of the behavioural effects of selective cerebellar ablation in experimental animals and the effects of cerebellar disease in man. For details of these important fields the interested reader should consult the articles quoted, some of which are devoted exclusively to these topics. A few examples only can be mentioned and illustrated here; further, since the various experiments have been carried out on a range of mammals, and because their considerable variations in cerebellar morphology cannot be treated here, the illustrations are referred to simplified plans of the cerebellum, and the areas indicated may well vary considerably between species and in mankind.

Reference has already been made to the primary division of the cerebellum into archicerebellum, paleocerebellum and neocerebellum, and how these correspond approximately, with some degree of overlap, to the major patterns of afferent cerebellar connexions summarized in the terms 'vestibulocerebellum', 'spinocerebellum' and 'pontocerebellum' (7.85 A), the latter including the 'tectocerebellum'.

Experimental determinations, in the cat, of the areas of termination of the primary vestibulocerebellar fibres, and of the spinocerebellar, cuneocerebellar and spinoolivocerebellar tracts are illustrated in 7.85 B. The double areas of distribution of these various spinal tracts to separate anterior and posterior, vermal and paravermal zones should be noted. These areas make up the spinocerebellum noted above, and within them a general somatotopic separation of hind-limb and fore-limb regions is shown. The primary vestibular fibres are shown ending mainly in the flocculus, nodule and part of the uvula.

Illustration 7.85 C shows the somatotopic map of the cerebellar cortex produced by recording the evoked potentials during stimulation of cutaneous receptors distributed over the body surface, based on the findings of Snider.[487, 488] There is a marked correspondence between this and diagram 7.85 B, which was based upon neuroanatomical degeneration techniques. Again, the anterior and posterior parts of the spinocerebellum are evident, but in this case the responses to stimulation of the face are also included. It is seen that the different regions of the body are represented in reverse order in the anterior and posterior receiving areas; further, in the anterior area the representation is ipsilateral, whereas in the posterior area it is bilateral. As would be expected, a rather similar map is produced on stimulation of proprioceptive endings, and therefore need not be reproduced here.

In illustration 7.85 D is shown the area from which responses are recorded during visual and auditory stimulation, and also during stimulation of the occipital areas of the cerebral cortex. The visual and auditory areas are virtually coincident and include the central regions of the vermis and their adjacent paravermal zones, overlapping the face area of the anterior spinocerebellum

determined by tactile stimulation. How far these visual and auditory responses are due to direct tectocerebellar pathways, or to the involvement of other less direct pathways is uncertain (p. 863).

Repeated reference has been made in the previous pages to the strict point-to-point correlation that exists between the nuclei of the olivary complex and the opposite cerebellar cortex—the general correspondence of zones is illustrated in a simplified form in 7.85 E.

The foregoing examples of cerebellar localization are based upon the differential distribution of afferent tracts to the cerebellar cortex, and broadly, the main receiving areas are arranged as a sequence of *transverse* strips which proceed from the (morphologically) anterior to posterior ends of the cerebellum. Equally clear evidences exist for a localization based upon the different destinations of Purkinje cell axons which leave the cerebellar cortex, but this is a *longitudinal* form of organization.[441, 489–492]

It will be recalled that the majority of the Purkinje cell axons terminate in the intracerebellar nuclei, but some by-pass the latter and pass directly to the lateral vestibular nucleus. The main features of the corticonuclear projections in the cerebellum are summarized in illustration 7.85 F. It is seen that direct cerebellovestibular fibres pass to the vestibular complex from the flocculus, nodule and much of the remainder of the vermis, but particularly from its anterior and posterior regions. The projections to the intracerebellar nuclei show an orderly longitudinal arrangement, and on both sides of the midline the cerebellar cortex is considered to be divided into *medial*, *intermediate*, and *lateral* zones. The fibres which leave the medial zone (vermis) converge upon the nucleus fastigii and their cranio-caudal sequence is preserved during this convergence and in their termination in the nucleus. The intermediate zone (a longitudinal paravermian strip) projects to the nucleus globosus and nucleus emboliformis, whilst the lateral zone (the cerebellar hemisphere) projects to the nucleus dentatus. In each case the orderly cranio-caudal sequence of the cortical origin of the axons is preserved through to their terminations in the nuclei. The vast majority of these corticonuclear projections are ipsilateral, but the fastigial nuclei receive some axons from the vermian cortex on both sides of the midline.

Recalling the main cerebellar outflow tracts and their nuclei of origin (pp. 862, 873), it will thus be appreciated that the vermis principally exerts a control over the vestibular nuclei and the brainstem reticular formation. The intermediate paravermian cortex controls the red nucleus and midbrain tegmentum, whilst the cerebellar hemisphere, through the nucleus dentatus and thalamus, mainly influences activity in the corpus striatum and cerebral cortex.

Interestingly, some parts of these outflow pathways have also been shown to be somatotopically organized. These include the direct and indirect vermal projections

[483] R. S. Snider, *J. comp. Neurol.*, **64**, 1936; **72**, 1940; *Anat. Rec.*, **91**, 1945; *Archs Neurol. Psychiat., Chicago*, **64**, 1950.

[484] R. S. Snider and E. Eldred, *J. comp. Neurol.*, **95**, 1951; *J. Neurophysiol.*, **15**, 1952.

[485] R. S. Snider and A. Stowell, *Fedn Proc. Fedn. Am. Socs exp. Biol.*, **1**, 1942; *J. Neurophysiol.*, **7**, 1944.

[486] R. S. Dow and G. Moruzzi, *The Physiology and Pathology of the Cerebellum*, University of Minnesota Press, Minneapolis. 1958.

[487] R. S. Snider, *Res. Publs Ass. Res. nerv. ment. Dis.*, **30**, 1952.

[488] J. L. Hampson, C. R. Harrison and C. N. Woolsey, *Res. Publs Ass. Res. nerv. ment. Dis.*, **30**, 1952.

[489] R. P. Eager, *J. comp. Neurol.*, **120**, 1963; **126**, 1966.

[490] D. C. Goodman, R. E. Hallett and R. B. Welch, *J. comp. Neurol.*, **121**, 1963.

[491] J. Voogd, *The Cerebellum of the Cat. Structure and Fibre Connexions*, Van Gorcum and Co., N. V., Assen. 1964.

[492] A. K. Korneliussen, *J. Hirnforsch*, **9**, 1967; **10**, 1968.

to the lateral vestibular nucleus[493] (7.85 G), and the intermediate projections to the red nucleus;[494] this correlates well with the organization of the lateral vestibular and red nuclei themselves, and also that of the lateral vestibulospinal and rubrospinal tracts. Further, a similar localization has been shown in the nucleus ventralis lateralis of the thalamus which receives the dentato-thalamic projections, and itself projects to the motor regions of the cerebral cortex.[495]

It should be emphasized at this point that the foregoing descriptions are based upon a range of experimental animals, but it is most likely that the general principles will apply to the cerebellum of man. Similarly, in experimental animals, interesting physiological parallels have been demonstrated. Cerebellar stimulation at different points often modifies movements which are being generated by simultaneous reflex or cerebral cortical stimulation, whilst cerebellar stimulation in the decerebrate animal elicits discrete movements (7.85 H). Again, anterior and posterior areas which correspond to the spinocerebellum have been shown to display a somatotopic order in respect to such movement patterns.[496] The anterior area when stimulated gives ipsilateral responses whereas the posterior area gives bilateral responses.

Such investigations, combined with the effects of ablation,[497] suggest that the vermis controls the posture, tone, locomotion and equilibrium of the *whole body*, whilst the intermediate zone controls the posture and discrete movements of the *ipsilateral limbs*. The lateral zone is much less well understood.

## CEREBELLAR FUNCTION AND DYSFUNCTION

There have been innumerable reports on the behavioural effects of cerebellar disease in man and on those of selective or total cerebellar ablations in experimental animals. Only the briefest mention can be made here and the interested reader should consult the excellent reviews which are readily available.[498–502]

In essence, the cerebellum receives an informational input from cutaneous receptors, proprioceptors, the eyes, ears, brainstem reticular formation and cerebral cortex, which is integrated and then discharged to the motor controlling centres of the cerebrum and brainstem. Its normal functioning is necessary for smooth, coordinated, effective locomotor responses to occur.

Without reference to particular cerebellar regions the more obvious effects of cerebellar dysfunction may include: (*a*) disturbances in equilibrium of the whole body; (*b*) disturbances in muscle 'tone' or their resistance to stretch, tendon reflexes and ability to stabilize joint positions; (*c*) incoordination of movements (*ataxia*) due to irregularities in the timing of onset, rate and force of contraction of synergistic muscle groups.

*Disequilibrium* in man is manifest by a tendency to fall forwards, backwards or laterally when standing, and by an unsteady staggering gait; it may be accompanied by sensations of spinning, nausea, etc.

There is usually a 'softness' in the affected muscle bellies on palpation, diminished tendon reflexes, and the muscles tire easily (*asthenia*). The lowering of joint control may progress to pendular swinging of a dependent limb segment after displacement, or to the condition of 'flail joints'.

*Muscular incoordination* is the essential feature of most varieties of cerebellar dysfunction. It may affect different regions of the body and to varying degrees; for this reason a variety of symptoms may occur, and a wide array of clinical tests have been devised to demonstrate its presence. Briefly, the term *asynergia* is often used to denote the diminished capacity for smooth, cooperative,

sequential action between a series of muscle groups. A complex movement may be carried out as a sequence of irregular disjointed episodes—*decomposition of movements*. There may develop an inability to carry out rapid movements which alternate in direction, e.g. supination and pronation of the forearm and hand, *dysdiadochokinesis*; control of the range of movement may be lost with either 'undershoot' or 'overshoot'—*dysmetria*. Disturbances of locomotion with a *staggering gait* and a tendency to fall, and—particularly with closed eyes—deviations from the intended direction of progression, are common. Similarly, the inability to point with the finger in a particular direction—*past pointing*—or to trace a specified course with either finger or heel may be present. *Tremor* is usually absent when the arm and hand are at rest, but a coarse transverse *intention tremor* may appear, which intensifies as the movement nears completion; tremor may also affect movements of the head or trunk. Muscular incoordination may lead to characteristic *defects of speech*, with a slowness of onset, slurring, jerky intermittent sound production which sometimes is intensified and has an explosive nature—so-called *scanning speech*. A *cerebellar nystagmus* may be present; there is an inability to fixate an object with the eyes, resulting in a repetitive conjugate drift of the visual axes away from the object, followed by a rapid return. The nystagmus is sometimes *positional*, i.e. more pronounced when the body adopts particular postures, or it may be *directional*, i.e. increasing when the subject attempts to gaze in a particular direction.

Attempts to correlate particular groups of clinical signs and symptoms of cerebellar disease in man with the different regions of the organ involved, or with the results of animal experimentation, have met with only partial success.

In the *flocculonodular syndrome*, with damage to the nodule, uvula and flocculus, both in man and experimental animals, the principal features are loss of equilibratory control of the whole body, swaying when standing, staggering when attempting to walk, and a tendency to fall, usually backwards. A positional nystagmus is often present. These effects are attributable in general to the upset of integration between the vestibular nuclei and the *vestibulocerebellum*.

In experimental animals *ablation* of the vermis of the anterior lobe increases the tendon reflexes and the rigidity already present in a decerebrate preparation, whereas vermian *stimulation* reduces the rigidity. The opposite responses occur with ablation or stimulation of the paravermian parts of the anterior lobe. Further, these effects are somatotopically organized; but, so far, corresponding results, which may stem from involvement of the anterior spinocerebellum, have not been clearly demonstrated in man.

The majority of cases of human cerebellar disease may be classified as *neocerebellar*, with involvement of one or both cerebellar hemispheres or their outflow tracts. In

[493] A. Brodal, O. Pompeiano and F. Walberg, *The Vestibular Nuclei and their Connexions. Anatomy and Functional Correlations*, Oliver and Boyd, Edinburgh. 1962.

[494] J. Courville, *Expl Brain Res.*, **2**, 1966.

[495] A. E. Walker, *J. comp. Neurol.*, **60**, 1934.

[496] J. L. Hampson, C. R. Harrison and C. N. Woolsey, *Res. Publs Ass. Res. nerv. ment. Dis.*, **30**, 1952.

[497] W. W. Chambers and J. M. Sprague, *J. comp. Neurol.*, **103**, 1955; *Archs Neurol. Psychiat., Chicago*, **74**, 1955.

[498] G. Holmes, *Brain*, **62**, 1939.

[499] B. D. Wyke, *Med. J. Aust.*, **2**, 1947.

[500] J. R. Brown, *J. Am. med. Ass.*, **141**, 1949.

[501] R. S. Dow and G. Moruzzi, *The Physiology and Pathology of the Cerebellum*. University of Minnesota Press, Minneapolis. 1958.

[502] R. S. Dow, in: *Handbook of Clinical Neurology*, Vol. 2, eds. P. J. Vinken and G. W. Bruyn, North Holland Publishing Co., Amsterdam. 1969.

unilateral disease, if sufficiently extensive, the various manifestations of hypotonia and incoordination listed above appear on the *same side* as the lesion, but gross intention tremor and staggering gait only supervene if the dentate nucleus or superior cerebellar peduncle are involved. It should be emphasized that relatively small cortical cerebellar lesions cause little obvious effect, and even quite extensive disease, although causing a transient derangement of function, is followed by rapid and marked improvement in locomotor control. The mechanism of this *cerebellar compensation* remains obscure.

Finally, as mentioned above, despite the prominence of *locomotor* effects in states of cerebellar dysfunction, it is probable that the cerebellum is less obviously, but importantly, involved in other central nervous activities such as *autonomic homeostasis* and the *modulation of transmission* along sensory input channels.

## The Fourth Ventricle

The fourth ventricle (7.86, 89, 90) is a somewhat tent-shaped space situated ventral to the cerebellum, and dorsal to the pons and cranial half of the medulla. Developmentally considered, it consists of three parts: a *superior* belonging to the isthmus rhombencephali (p. 133), an *intermediate*, to the metencephalon, and an *inferior*, to the myelencephalon. It is lined with ependyma, and its inferior limit is continuous with the central canal

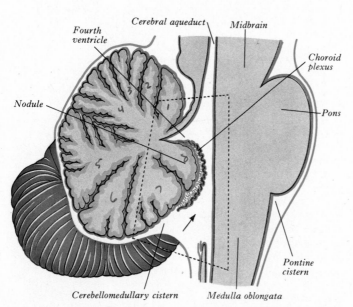

7.86   Sagittal section through the brainstem and the cerebellum close to the median plane. The black arrow is placed in the median aperture of the fourth ventricle. The area enclosed by the interrupted lines is shown enlarged in 7.89. *Blue*: arachnoid mater. *Red*: pia mater. *Green*: ependyma.

of the medulla oblongata; cranially, it is continuous with the cerebral aqueduct, which connects it to the cavity of the third ventricle. From its middle level a narrow, curved pouch, named the *lateral recess*, is prolonged on each side between the inferior cerebellar peduncle and the peduncle of the flocculus, reaching as far as the medial part of the flocculus itself. The recess is crossed anteriorly by the fila of the glossopharyngeal and vagus nerves and its lateral extremity is open, allowing a portion of the choroid plexus of the fourth ventricle to protrude into the subarachnoid space (7.55). In the median plane the cavity extends dorsally into the white core of the

cerebellum, forming a *median dorsal recess* (7.86) cranial to the nodule; and on each side a *lateral dorsal recess* extends still further dorsally (7.143), lying cranial to the inferior medullary velum and caudal to the cerebellar nuclei, from which it is separated by a thin layer of white matter.

The fourth ventricle possesses lateral boundaries, a roof or dorsal wall, and a diamond-shaped ventral floor, the rhomboid fossa.

**Lateral boundaries.** The caudal part of each lateral boundary is constituted by the gracile and cuneate tubercles, the fasciculus cuneatus, and the inferior cerebellar peduncle, the cranial part, by the superior cerebellar peduncle.

**The roof or dorsal wall** (7.87). This extends backwards into the median and lateral dorsal recesses. The cranial portion of the roof is simple, and is formed by the superior cerebellar peduncles and the superior medullary velum. The *superior cerebellar peduncles* (p. 862), on emerging from the central white matter of the cerebellum, pass cranially and ventrally, forming at first the lateral boundaries of the upper part of the ventricle; on approaching the inferior colliculi, they converge, and their medial margins overlap the ventricle and form part of its roof. The *superior medullary velum* (p. 858) fills the angular interval between the superior cerebellar peduncles, and is continuous dorsally with the central white core of the cerebellum; it is covered on its dorsal surface by the lingula of the superior vermis (7.89).

The *caudal part* of the roof is more complicated. Over most of its extent it consists of an exceedingly thin sheet, entirely devoid of nervous tissue and formed by the ventricular ependyma and the pia mater of the tela choroidea of the fourth ventricle, which covers it posteriorly (7.89). Caudally, the continuity of the sheet is broken by a gap, termed the *median aperture* (7.87), through which the cavity of the ventricle communicates freely with the subarachnoid space. The *tela choroidea of the fourth ventricle* is a double layer of pia mater which occupies the interval between the cerebellum and the lower part of the roof of the ventricle. Its posterior layer provides a covering of pia mater for the inferior vermis and, after reaching the nodule, is reflected ventrally and caudally in immediate contact with the ependyma. In the tela choroidea are highly vascular fringes forming the choroid plexus of the fourth ventricle. On each side, the layer of the tela choroidea in contact with the ependyma of the caudal part of the roof reaches the inferolateral border of the ventricular floor, which is marked by a narrow, white ridge, termed the *taenia*; the two taeniae are continuous below with a small, curved margin, the *obex*, which covers the inferior angle of the ventricle and is covered by ependyma on both aspects (7.89). Cranially, these taeniae pass laterally and horizontally along the inferior borders of the lateral recesses.

**The openings in the roof.** In the caudal part of the roof of the fourth ventricle are three openings, one median and two lateral. The *median aperture* is a large opening, situated caudal to the nodule (7.87); it varies considerably in its extent, and its irregular cranial border is drawn dorsally towards the inferior surface of the vermis in a somewhat funnel-shaped manner to face the cerebello-medullary cistern (7.89). The *lateral apertures* are situated at the ends of the lateral recesses and are partly occupied by parts of the choroid plexus, which protrude into the subarachnoid space (7.55). The ependyma and pia mater are continuous at the margins of these openings. Through these openings alone the ventricular cavity communicates with the subarachnoid space. Occasionally one of the lateral recesses may fail to open into the subarachnoid space, but the median aperture is constantly present.

**The choroid plexuses.** Two highly vascular fringe-like processes of the tela choroidea contain the choroid plexuses of the fourth ventricle; they invaginate the caudal part of the roof of the ventricle and are everywhere covered by ependyma, which is modified to form a true secretory epithelium.[503] Each consists of a vertical and a horizontal region. The former consists of two longitudinal fringes adjacent to the median plane, fusing at the cranial margin of the median aperture and frequently prolonged beyond this margin on to the ventral aspect of the vermis to which they adhere.[504] The horizontal portion projects into the fourth ventricle, passes into the lateral recess and emerges through the lateral aperture still covered by ependyma. The entire structure presents the form of the letter T, the vertical limb of which, however, is double.

**The rhomboid fossa** (7.90). The floor of the fourth ventricle is rhomboidal in shape; it is formed by the posterior surface of both the pons and the cranial, open part of the medulla oblongata. It is covered by a layer of grey matter continuous with that surrounding the central canal of the medulla oblongata and spinal cord; superficial to this there is a thin lamina of neuroglia covered with ependyma. The floor consists of three parts, superior, intermediate and inferior. The *superior* part is triangular in shape and limited laterally by the superior cerebellar peduncles; its cranial apex is directly continuous with the wall of the cerebral aqueduct; its base is represented by an imaginary line at the level of the cranial ends of two small depressions, named the *superior foveae*. The *intermediate* part extends from this level to that of the horizontal sections of the taeniae of the ventricle and is prolonged into the lateral recesses. The *inferior* part is triangular, and its caudally directed apex is continuous with the wall of the central canal of the closed part of the medulla oblongata.

The rhomboid fossa is divided into symmetrical halves by a *median sulcus*, which reaches from its upper to its lower apex and is deeper below than above. On each side of this sulcus there is an elevation, the *medial eminence*, bounded laterally by a sulcus, the *sulcus limitans*. In the superior part of the floor the medial eminence has a width equal to that of the corresponding half of the floor, but opposite the superior fovea it forms an elongated swelling, the *facial colliculus*, which overlies the nucleus of the abducent nerve, and is in part produced by the ascending section of the root of the facial nerve. In the inferior part of the floor the medial eminence forms a triangular area, termed the *hypoglossal triangle* or *trigonum hypoglossi*. When examined closely with a lens the hypoglossal triangle is seen to consist of medial and lateral areas separated by a series of oblique furrows; the medial area corresponds with the cranial part of the nucleus of the hypoglossal nerve, the lateral with the *nucleus intercalatus*.

The *sulcus limitans* forms the lateral boundary of the medial eminence. Its superior part corresponds with the lateral limit of the floor and presents a bluish-grey area, named the *locus coeruleus*, which owes its colour to a patch of deeply pigmented nerve cells termed the *substantia ferruginea*. The *nucleus coeruleus* corresponds to some extent with the locus of the same name in the floor of the fourth ventricle, but it ascends cranially beyond this as far as the caudal end of the mesencephalic trigeminal nucleus; it may even overlap the latter, appearing in the same sections in the most caudal level of the midbrain. Its cells are of medium size and some contain a melanin pigment, especially so in the human midbrain, and it is this which is responsible for the colour of the locus coeruleus.[505] At pontine levels it spreads into the reticular formation, and is regarded as a reticular element by some observers.[506] Its connexions are not fully known, but include afferents from the trigeminal nuclei and possibly

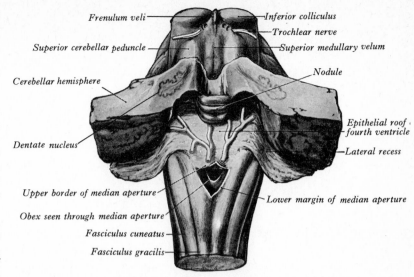

7.87 Dorsal aspect of the roof and the lateral recesses of the fourth ventricle, exposed by removal of parts of the cerebellum.

from neighbouring reticular nuclei; its efferents have been traced to the ipsilateral reticular formation in the region of the inferior olivary nuclei. The fine structure of its cells and synapses has been the subject of a recent study.[507] It may be associated with the pontine 'pneumotaxic centre'; further associations with a pontine centre concerned with active sleep states have also been suggested. At the level of the facial colliculus the sulcus

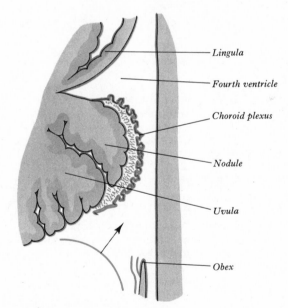

7.88 An enlargement of the part of 7.86 which is enclosed by an interrupted line. *Blue*: arachnoid mater. *Red*: pia mater. *Green*: ependyma. The black arrow traverses the median aperture of the roof of the fourth ventricle.

limitans widens into an angular depression, termed the *superior fovea*, and in the inferior part of the floor presents a distinct dimple termed the *inferior fovea*. Lateral to the foveae there is a rounded elevation named the *vestibular area*, which extends into the lateral recess, where it forms the *auditory tubercle* produced by the underlying dorsal

[503] W. E. Le G. Clark, *The Tissues of the Body*, 6th ed., Clarendon Press, Oxford. 1971.
[504] W. Hewitt, *J. Anat.*, **94**, 1960.
[505] J. M. Foley and D. Baxter, *J. Neuropath. exp. Neurol.*, **17**, 1958.
[506] G. V. Russell, *Tex. Rep. Biol. Med.*, **13**, 1955.
[507] N. Shimizu and K. Imamoto, *Archs histol. jap.*, **31**, 1970.

cochlear nucleus and cochlear part of the vestibulocochlear nerve (p. 852). Winding round the inferior cerebellar peduncle, and crossing the vestibular area and the medial eminence to pass deeply at the median sulcus, are a

cells of moderate size. The inferior part of the floor of the fourth ventricle towards its apex, presents the appearance of a pen nib, and is hence called the *calamus scriptorius.*

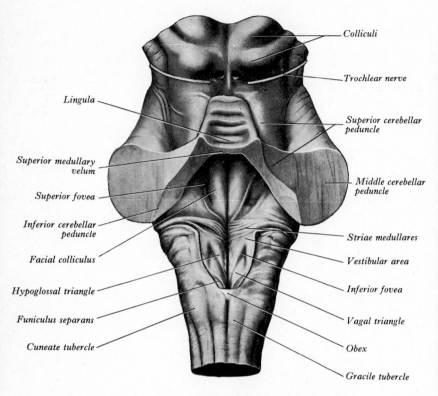

Colliculi

Trochlear nerve

Lingula

Superior cerebellar peduncle

Superior medullary velum

Superior fovea

Middle cerebellar peduncle

Inferior cerebellar peduncle

Facial colliculus

Striae medullares

Vestibular area

Hypoglossal triangle

Inferior fovea

Funiculus separans

Vagal triangle

Cuneate tubercle

Obex

Gracile tubercle

**7.**89   The rhomboid fossa, or 'floor' of the fourth ventricle.

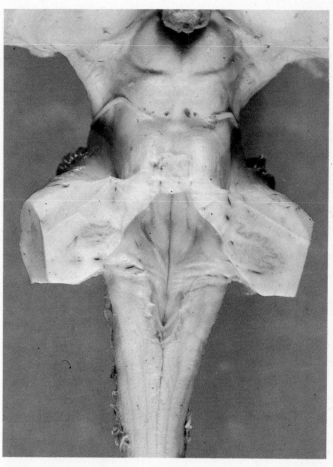

number of white strands termed the *striae medullares* (*see* p. 854). Caudal to the inferior fovea, and between the hypoglossal triangle and lower part of the vestibular area, a triangular dark field, the *vagal triangle or trigonum vagi,* overlies the dorsal nucleus of the vagus nerve (p. 1019). The lower part of the vagal triangle is crossed by a narrow translucent ridge, named the *funiculus separans,* and between this funiculus and the gracile tubercle is a small tongue-shaped area, termed the *area postrema.* On section it is seen that the funiculus separans is formed by a strip of thickened ependyma, and the area postrema by loose, highly vascular, neuroglial tissue containing nerve

**7.**90   A dorsal view of the brainstem including the floor of the rhomboid fossa—for identification of structures compare with **7.**89. In addition to the structures shown in the latter, note: (1) the crenated outlines of the right and left dentate nuclei in the sectioned surface of the cerebellar white matter opposite the widest part of the rhomboid fossa; (2) the midline pineal body cranial to the superior colliculi; (3) the midline third ventricle cranial to the pineal; (4) the rounded pulvinar of the dorsal thalami which encroach on the uppermost part of the photograph; (5) the right and left habenular trigones immediately lateral to the base of the pineal; and (6) the medial geniculate bodies, lateral to the superior colliculi. (Dissection by Dr. E. L. Rees, Department of Anatomy, Guy's Hospital Medical School.)

# THE MESENCEPHALON OR MIDBRAIN

The mesencephalon or midbrain is derived from the intermediate of the three primary cerebral vesicles. In the course of its development in man and in its phylogenetic history it retains a much simpler form than either the forebrain or the hindbrain. In lower vertebrates the leading feature of the midbrain is the development in its roof plate of higher visual (p. 887), and, later, higher auditory centres. In the mammals these become reflex centres and their original function as 'higher' or sensory centres becomes transferred to the cerebral cortex. As this change, telencephalization, increases, the midbrain is traversed by an increasing number of axons subserving cortico-spinal and spino-cortical pathways. Midbrain mechanisms also contribute extensively to the reticular system (p. 888).

## EXTERNAL FEATURES

The midbrain lies athwart the hiatus in the tentorium cerebelli and connects pons and cerebellum with the forebrain. It is the shortest segment of the brainstem, being not more than 2 cm in length. On each side it is related to the parahippocampal gyrus, which hides its lateral aspect from view when the inferior surface of the brain is examined. Its long axis inclines ventrally as it ascends.

The midbrain can for description be divided into right and left halves, the *cerebral peduncles,* each of which is further subdivided into a ventral part, the *crus cerebri,* and a dorsal *tegmental part,* by a lamina of pigmented grey matter, the *substantia nigra.* The two crura are separate, whereas the tegmental parts are united. The tegmentum is traversed by the *cerebral aqueduct*, which connects the third and fourth ventricles. The region of the tegmentum dorsal to the cerebral aqueduct is called the *tectum* and comprises the *colliculi* which consist of four rounded elevations, symmetrically arranged in superior and inferior pairs; these contain visual and auditory reflex centres respectively.

The *crura cerebri* are two white, superficially corrugated structures which emerge from the cerebral hemisphere, one on each side of the median plane. They converge as they descend and meet where they enter the pons; here they form the posterior boundaries of the *interpeduncular fossa* (p. 904). The surface of the posterior part of the interpeduncular fossa is formed by a greyish area, the *posterior perforated substance* (p. 904), through which pass the central branches of the posterior cerebral artery.

The ventral surface of each crus is crossed close to the

inferior colliculus, the rest passing into the brachium of the inferior colliculus.

The *colliculi* (*corpora quadrigemina*) (7.97) are four rounded eminences, situated cranial to the superior medullary velum, and caudal to the pineal gland and posterior commissure, the whole region inclining ventrally as it ascends. They are inferior to the splenium of the corpus callosum, and are partly overlapped on each side by the pulvinar of the thalamus. The colliculi are arranged in pairs (superior and inferior), and are separated from one another by a cruciform sulcus. The vertical part of this sulcus expands superiorly to form a slight depression in which the *pineal body* (7.97) lies. From the inferior end of the vertical sulcus a white ridge, the *frenulum veli*, is prolonged caudally to the superior medullary velum; at the sides of this ridge the trochlear nerves emerge, pass ventrally on the lateral aspects of the cerebral peduncles and traverse the interpeduncular cistern to reach the

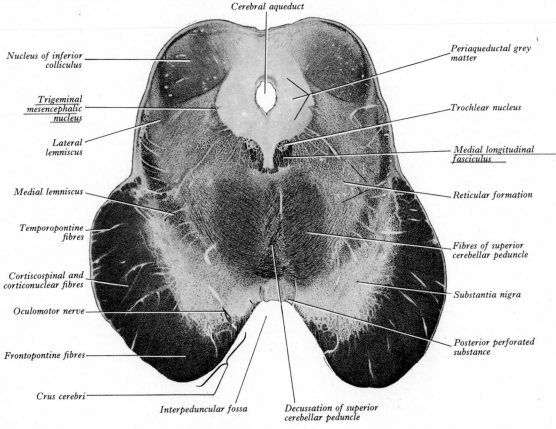

Cerebral aqueduct

Nucleus of inferior colliculus

Trigeminal mesencephalic nucleus

Lateral lemniscus

Medial lemniscus

Temporopontine fibres

Cortiscospinal and corticonuclear fibres

Oculomotor nerve

Frontopontine fibres

Crus cerebri

Interpeduncular fossa

Decussation of superior cerebellar peduncle

Periaqueductal grey matter

Trochlear nucleus

Medial longitudinal fasciculus

Reticular formation

Fibres of superior cerebellar peduncle

Substantia nigra

Posterior perforated substance

**7.91**  Transverse section of midbrain through the inferior colliculi. Weigert Pal preparation. Magnification *c.* ×4·1.

pons, from medial to lateral, by the superior cerebellar and posterior cerebral arteries; near to the point of entry of the crus into the cerebral hemisphere, the optic tract winds backwards around it. Over the surface of the crus, also close to the pons, a thin white band, the *taenia pontis*, is frequently seen as it enters the cerebellum between the middle and superior peduncles.

The medial surface of each crus bears a longitudinal groove, the *medial sulcus*, from which the roots of the oculomotor nerve emerge (7.92). The lateral surface of each peduncle is in relation with the parahippocampal gyrus of the cerebral hemisphere and is crossed in a ventral direction by the trochlear nerve (7.97). This surface is marked by a longitudinal groove, the *lateral sulcus*; the fibres of the lateral lemniscus come to the surface in this sulcus, and then turn dorsally, some to enter the

posterior end of the cavernous sinus. The *superior colliculi* are larger and darker in colour than the inferior, and constitute centres for visual reflexes (p. 887). The *inferior colliculi*, though smaller, are somewhat more prominent than the superior and are associated with the auditory pathway (p. 886). The difference in colour is due to the greater accumulation of nerve cells near the surface of the superior colliculus (p. 887).

From the lateral aspect of each colliculus a ridge, termed the *brachium*, ascends in a ventrolateral direction. The *brachium of the superior colliculus* passes inferior to the pulvinar. It partly overlaps the medial geniculate body and is partly continued into the lateral geniculate body (p. 915), and partly into the optic tract. It conducts fibres from the retina and from the optic radiation to the superior colliculus. The *brachium of the inferior colliculus*

ascends ventrally from the inferior colliculus; it conveys fibres from the lateral lemniscus and the inferior colliculus to the medial geniculate body.

## INTERNAL STRUCTURE OF THE MIDBRAIN

On transverse section, each cerebral peduncle is seen to consist of a dorsal and a ventral part, separated by a deeply pigmented lamina of grey matter, termed the *substantia nigra* (7.91, 92). The dorsal part is named the *tegmentum*; the ventral, the *crus cerebri*. The crura are separated from each other, but the tegmental parts are continuous with one another across the midline, and the term *tegmentum* usually implies the bilateral mass between both nigral masses and the tectum. The latter is the part dorsal to the cerebral aqueduct and contains the colliculi.

The crus cerebri is semilunar on transverse section, and consists of corticospinal, corticonuclear, and corticopontine fibres (7.91). The *corticospinal* and *corticonuclear* fibres occupy the middle two-thirds of the crus; they descend through the pons and medulla oblongata, where the corticonuclear fibres end in the nuclei of the motor cranial nerves, mainly of the opposite side; the corticospinal fibres are continued into the pyramid of the medulla oblongata. The corticopontine fibres arise in the cerebral cortex and terminate in the nuclei pontis, where they are relayed mainly to the opposite cerebellar hemisphere.

A band of fibres, named the *tractus peduncularis transversus*, is sometimes seen emerging from the optic tract on the lateral aspect of the cerebral peduncle; it passes round the ventral surface of the peduncle about midway between the pons and the optic tract, and disappears by entering the interpeduncular fossa behind and lateral to the corpus mamillare, where it terminates in a small *nucleus of the transverse peduncular tract* which lies medial to the substantia nigra. The tract is a constant structure in many lower mammals, but is only identifiable in 30 per cent of human brains. Since it undergoes atrophy after enucleation of the eyeballs, it may be considered as being associated with the visual pathway; the nucleus projects to the oculomotor nuclei in some mammals.[508] (But see also p. 914).

**The substantia nigra** is a lamina of grey matter containing numerous, deeply pigmented, multipolar nerve cells and extending throughout the whole length of the midbrain. Owing to its pigmentation it can readily be recognized with the naked eye in transverse or coronal sections (7.98) through the midbrain. The functional significance of the pigment is obscure; it increases with age, is greater in amount in primates, maximal in man,[509] and is even present in albinos.

The substantia nigra is semilunar on transverse section, its concavity being directed towards the tegmentum; from its convex surface, processes extend between the

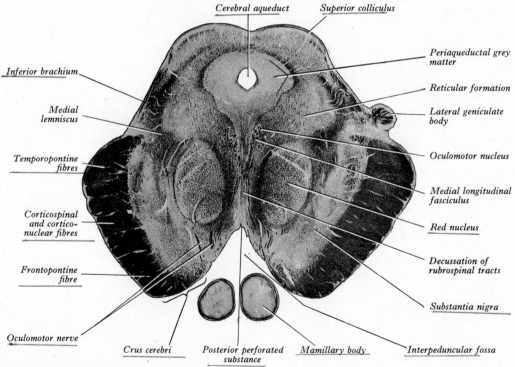

Cerebral aqueduct    Superior colliculus

Inferior brachium

Medial lemniscus

Temporopontine fibres

Corticospinal and cortico-nuclear fibres

Frontopontine fibre

Oculomotor nerve

Crus cerebri    Posterior perforated substance    Mamillary body

Periaqueductal grey matter

Reticular formation

Lateral geniculate body

Oculomotor nucleus

Medial longitudinal fasciculus

Red nucleus

Decussation of rubrospinal tracts

Substantia nigra

Interpeduncular fossa

**7.92** Transverse section of the midbrain through the superior colliculi. Weigert Pal preparation. Magnification *c.* × 3.

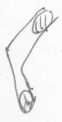

They are subdivided into two main groups: (*a*) *frontopontine* and (*b*) *temporopontine*. (*a*) The frontopontine fibres arise in the frontal lobe, principally areas 6 and 4 of Brodmann, traverse the anterior limb of the internal capsule, and occupy the medial sixth of the crus cerebri. (*b*) The temporopontine fibres arise in the temporal lobe, traverse the posterior limb of the internal capsule and occupy the lateral sixth of the crus cerebri; they end in the nuclei of the pons. *Parieto-* and *occipito-pontine* fibres are also described in the crus cerebri. They are medial to the temporopontine fibres.

fibres of the crus cerebri. Thicker medially than laterally, it reaches from the medial to the lateral sulcus, and extends from the upper surface of the pons to the subthalamic region; its medial part is traversed by the fibres of the oculomotor nerve as they stream forwards to reach the oculomotor sulcus. It is divided into a dorsal *compact* part containing medium-sized cells, many of which are pigmented, and a ventral *reticular* part intermingled with

[508] L. A. Gillilan, *J. comp. Neurol.*, **74**, 1941.
[509] D. Marsden, *J. Anat.*, **95**, 1961.

fibres of the crus cerebri and containing fewer cells, only some of which contain a small amount of pigment. The reticular part extends into the subthalamic region, where it is considered to be continuous with the globus pallidus, which it resembles structurally; both nuclei contain iron in unusual amounts. In vertebrates below mammals a well-developed pars lateralis is present; this is recognizable but almost insignificant in man.[510] It has nevertheless been shown to project to the tectum in primates.[511]

The substantia nigra is connected with the cerebral cortex, spinal cord, hypothalamus and basal nuclei. Corticonigral fibres arise from the precentral and, probably, the postcentral gyri and terminate on cells in the reticular region, but they are few in number, many being fibres of passage to the red nucleus and reticular formation. Collaterals from fibres in the sensory tracts ascending from the spinal cord are also said to terminate in the substantia. Fibres from the mamillary peduncle and subthalamic nucleus have also been traced on to its cells. The connexions with the basal nuclei are efferent nigrostriatal fibres which pass to the caudate nucleus, putamen and possibly also the globus pallidus; afferent strionigral fibres also exist. Efferent fibres also pass into the tegmentum of the midbrain, probably to terminate on cells of the reticular formation, whence impulses arising in the substantia nigra are relayed to anterior column cells of the spinal cord. The nigrotegmental projection was observed to be a major efferent connexion in cats.[512] Lesions in the medial part of the substantia, also in cats,[513] suggest that some fibres pass to the ventral thalamus; nigrocortical connexions have been described in the same experimental animal.[514]

For further discussion of the aminergic nigrostriate pathway and its relationship to Parkinsonism see p. 978.

**The tegmentum of the midbrain** presents appearances which differ according to the level of the section examined. Caudally, it is directly continuous with the tegmentum of the pons and contains the same fibre tracts.

At the level of the inferior colliculi, the grey matter is restricted to the immediate environs of the cerebral aqueduct, to the scattered collections in the reticular formation (7.91) and to the tectum, which is described separately (p. 886).

The *nucleus of the trochlear (fourth cranial) nerve* lies in the ventral region of the central grey matter, close to the midline. It occupies a position homologous with the abducent and hypoglossal nuclei at lower brainstem levels. Closely related throughout to the medial longitudinal fasciculus, which is on its ventral aspect, the nucleus extends through the caudal half of the midbrain, and it is just caudal to the oculomotor nucleus. In some primates the nuclei are merged and only distinguishable by the arrangement of their cells, which are also smaller in the trochlear nucleus. Its *outgoing fibres* pass laterally and dorsally round the central grey matter. Descending dorsally on the medial side of the mesencephalic nucleus of the trigeminal nerve, they reach the cranial end of the superior medullary velum, wherein they decussate to emerge at the lateral side of the frenulum veli (7.90). A few fibres probably do not decussate. The trochlear nerve fibres emerge dorsally and largely decussate in all vertebrates. It has been suggested that the nerve originally supplied the muscles of the pineal eye, which would account for its dorsal course. Embryological evidence[515] and phylogenetic data support a more dorsal origin of this nucleus.

The *mesencephalic nucleus of the trigeminal nerve* is in the lateral part of the central grey matter. It extends from the cranial end of the main sensory nucleus of the trigeminal nerve in the pons to the level of the superior colliculus in the midbrain. It is accompanied by a tract composed of the peripheral and central branches of the axons of its cells. The large ovoid nerve cells of this nucleus are unipolar and resemble those of sensory ganglia. They occur in many small groups each containing only a few cells; these groups extend as curved laminae on each side, in the lateral margins of the periaqueductal grey matter. For connexions of this nucleus see pp. 1002, 1029.

Apart from these nuclei the tegmentum at this level contains large numbers of scattered nerve cells, most of which are included in the reticular formation (p. 888).

The *white matter* at this level of the midbrain contains all the tracts which have already been mentioned in the tegmentum of the pons, and it is characterized by the great decussation of the fibres of the superior cerebellar peduncles.

The *superior cerebellar peduncle*, which has already been described (p. 860), enters the dorsolateral part of the tegmentum and passes ventromedially round the central grey matter to reach the median raphe, where the majority of its fibres form with their fellows the *decussation of the superior cerebellar peduncles*. Having crossed the median plane, the fibres separate into ascending and descending bundles. Some of the *ascending* fibres and branches terminate in and give collaterals to the red nucleus, which they encapsulate and penetrate. Numerous others are continued cranially to end in the nucleus ventralis lateralis of the thalamus. Some of the fibres, however, are uncrossed, and branches are believed to end in the periaqueductal grey matter and reticular formation of the midbrain, in the interstitial nucleus (of Cajal) and the nucleus of the posterior commissure (sometimes, perhaps mistakenly,[516] called the nucleus of Darkschewitsch). The latter is considered to send efferent fibres to the medial longitudinal fasciculus and posterior commissure, the significance of which is uncertain. The *descending* branches end in the reticular formation of the pons and medulla oblongata, the olivary complex, and possibly the motor nuclei of certain cranial nerves (see also pp. 862, 864).

The *medial longitudinal fasciculus* retains its intimate relationship to the somatic efferent column, and therefore lies dorsal to the decussating fibres of the superior cerebellar peduncles.

The *medial, trigeminal* and *lateral lemnisci* and *lateral spinothalamic tract* (spinal lemniscus) form a curved band lying dorsal to the lateral part of the substantia nigra. At this level some of the fibres of the lateral lemniscus terminate in the nucleus of the inferior colliculus around which they form a capsule. These fibres synapse with cells in the inferior colliculus. Accompanied by fibres from cells in the inferior colliculus, the remaining fibres of the lateral lemniscus enter the brachium of the inferior colliculus, which commences at this level, and conducts them to the medial geniculate body. Some of these fibres give collaterals which also synapse with cells in the inferior colliculus.

Cranially, on a level with the superior colliculus, the tegmentum is strikingly modified by the appearance of a large nucleus, which extends upwards into the subthalamic region and is termed the *red nucleus,*

The *central grey matter* surrounds the aqueduct and

[510] A. C. Huber and E. C. Crosby, *J. comp. Neurol.*, **57**, 1933.
[511] R. T. Woodburne, E. C. Crosby and R. McCotter, *J. comp. Neurol.*, **85**, 1946.
[512] A. Afifi and W. W. Kaelber, *Expl Neurol.*, **11**, 1965.
[513] A. L. Marcós, *Anales Anatomia*, **18**, 1969.
[514] P. M. Negro, *Anales Anatomia*, **18**, 1969.
[515] A. A. Pearson, *J. comp. Neurol.*, **78**, 1943.
[516] W. R. Ingram and S. W. Ranson, *J. nerv. ment. Dis.*, **81**, 1953.

contains in its ventromedial part the *nucleus of the oculo-motor nerve*. This elongated nucleus is closely related on its ventrolateral aspect to the medial longitudinal fasciculus; inferiorly it extends to the trochlear nucleus (**7.**91). The nucleus of the oculomotor nerve is divisible into a number of cell groups which can be correlated with the motor distribution of the nerve. They include a visceral efferent accessory oculomotor nucleus, the Edinger-Westphal nucleus, dorsal to the main nucleus (and are all described on p. 999).

**The red nucleus (nucleus ruber)** is an ovoid mass of nerve cells with a pinkish tinge, about 5 mm in diameter, situated dorsomedial to the substantia nigra (**7.**92). The colour is most apparent in freshly sectioned, unfixed mid-brains, and is due to the presence of an iron-containing pigment which occurs in many, but not all, of the cells in the nucleus. These are mostly multipolar and of varying sizes, rather large and small categories being predominant. The proportions and distribution of these types differ in various mammalian groups; in primates, including man, the *magnocellular* element is relatively decreased, with a reciprocal augmentation of the *parvocellular* complement of cells. These small multipolar cells occur in all parts of the nucleus, but in man the large cells are restricted to the caudal part of the nucleus. Cranially, the boundary of the red nucleus is poorly demarcated from other cell groups, where it fades into the reticular formation and the caudal pole of the interstitial nucleus.[517] Some division of the red nucleus into caudal *compact* and rostral *diffuse* architectonic regions has been described, and the whole mass is traversed and encapsulated by fascicles of nerve fibres, including many of the fibres emerging from the oculomotor nucleus (**7.**92). These bundles impart a reticular appearance to the nucleus. Its magnocellular element is regarded as phylogenetically the older, which accords with the predominance of the parvocellular part especially in man, but also in other primates.

The *afferent connexions* of the red nucleus are complex and numerous, and only those for which the evidence is strong will be described here. Of these, some have been established only in experimental animals and are uncertain in man. An uncrossed corticorubral projection from the 'motor cortex' is demonstrable in the cat (from the anterior sigmoid gyrus); in the same animal an area anterior to the medial part of the precentral gyrus (p. 957), which is termed the 'supplementary motor area' in the feline cerebrum, projects bilaterally upon the red nuclei. A somatotopic arrangement of these corticorubral fibres and their terminations in the nucleus has been demonstrated; this conforms with the localization of the cells of origin of the rubrospinal tract (*vide infra*). There are also bilateral connexions, probably in both directions, with the superior colliculi. The red nucleus also receives nerve fibres from the contralateral nucleus interpositus in the cat; this corresponds to the nuclei globosus and emboli-formis of the human cerebellum. Afferents are also derived from the contralateral dentate nucleus. All these cerebellar connexions, and perhaps others (p. 862), pass through the superior cerebellar peduncle. They are said to display some degree of somatotopic organization. Connexions from other sources have been reported—from the globus pallidus, subthalamic and hypothalamic nuclei, substantia nigra, and spinal cord—but these are only putative in regard to the human red nucleus. (Some of the connexions of the red nucleus are outlined in **7.**93.)

The main *efferent outflow* of axons is into the **rubro-spinal tract** (p. 821), which is derived from both the large and small cells in the nucleus in other mammals, and probably also in mankind. As mentioned elsewhere (p. 821), this tract is currently dismissed as unimportant in man by many authorities, clinical and academic, who state that it

is derived only from the magnocellular neurons in the nucleus, and that even their axons do not travel far down the spinal cord. The evidence for this negative view is exiguous; all the studies carried out on the tract in other mammals, chiefly the cat and monkey, indicate that it reaches lumbosacral levels. The tract and its nuclear origins are somatotopically localized, the axons ending at cervical levels being from cells segregated in the dorso-

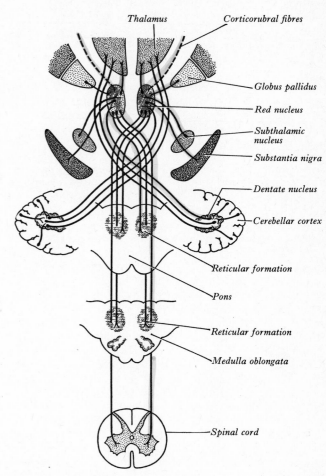

**7.**93 Simplified diagram of the principal connexions of the red nucleus.

medial region of the nucleus, those for lumbosacral segments in its ventrolateral part, and those with a destination in the thoracic cord are in an intermediate position. This mode of organization has been confirmed by recording antidromic impulses arriving in the nucleus as a result of stimulation of different levels of the tract. Some of the efferent axons terminate in the brainstem, as a *rubrobulbar tract*, which projects upon the motor nuclei of the tri-geminal and facial nerves. Fibres are also claimed to pass to the inferior olive, and the nuclei of the oculomotor, trochlear and abducent nerves; in the cat *rubrocerebellar* connexions to the dentate nucleus have been described.[518] A projection to the ventrolateral thalamic nuclei from the caudal third of the red nucleus has been described.

As it descends, the rubrospinal tract decussates at once in the ventral decussation of the tegmentum, ventral to the decussation of the tectospinal tracts, and then passes caudally, ventral to the decussation of the superior cerebellar peduncles, and continues through the reticular formation of the pons and medulla to reach the spinal cord. Since its spinal terminals are distributed to almost

---

[517] H. A. Davenport and S. W. Ranson, *Archs Neurol. Psychiat., Chicago*, **24**, 1930.
[518] J. Courville and A. Brodal, *J. comp. Neurol.*, **126**, 1966.

Labels on figure 7.93:
Thalamus
Corticorubral fibres
Globus pallidus
Red nucleus
Subthalamic nucleus
Substantia nigra
Dentate nucleus
Cerebellar cortex
Reticular formation
Pons
Reticular formation
Medulla oblongata
Spinal cord

the same laminae of grey matter in the cord as those of the corticospinal tract, the cortico-rubro-spinal projection can be regarded as a kind of indirect corticospinal pathway (p. 821).

Closely associated with the rubrospinal fibres are *tegmentospinal* fibres which arise in the tegmental reticular formation lateral and caudal to the red nucleus. These are probably to be grouped with the other (medullary and pontine) reticulospinal tracts (p. 836).

The *tectospinal* and the *tectobulbar tracts* also take origin at this level. Their fibres arise in the grey matter of the superior colliculi and sweep ventrally round the central grey matter to decussate with one another in the median raphe ventral to the oculomotor nucleus and the medial longitudinal bundle, forming the *dorsal part of the tegmental decussations*. Emerging from this the tectospinal tract descends on the ventral aspect of the medial longitudinal fasciculus until the decussation of the medial lemniscus in the medulla oblongata. Thereafter it diverges ventrolaterally and in the spinal cord it lies in the anterior column adjacent to the ventral end of the anterior median fissure. The tectobulbar tract is mainly composed of crossed fibres and descends close to the tectospinal tract. It ends in the pontine nuclei and motor nuclei of the cranial nerves, particularly those concerned with the innervation of the orbital muscles. It serves as a pathway for reflex movements of the eyes in response to visual stimuli. (See also references to the lateral tectotegmento-spinal tract, p. 821.)

**The medial longitudinal fasciculus** (7.94) is a heavily myelinated composite tract lying on the ventrolateral aspect of the oculomotor nucleus. At this level its fibres are more spread out than they are at lower levels in the brainstem, but the intimate relationship to the efferent nuclei is retained. The fasciculus extends cranially to the *interstitial nucleus* (of Cajal)—a collection of cells situated in the lateral wall of the third ventricle immediately above the cranial end of the cerebral aqueduct—which contributes fibres to it. As has already been seen, the medial longitudinal fasciculus retains its position relative to the central grey matter throughout the midbrain, pons and cranial part of the medulla oblongata. It is displaced ventrally by the successive decussations of the medial lemnisci and the lateral corticospinal tracts, and becomes continuous with the anterior intersegmental fasciculus of the spinal cord.

The intimate relationship which the fasciculus bears successively to the nuclei of the oculomotor, trochlear and abducent nerves, to the emerging fibres of the facial, the fibres from the dorsal cochlear nucleus in the floor of the fourth ventricle and the nucleus of the hypoglossal nerve, renders it a very convenient pathway for the passage of fibres from one nucleus to another in the brainstem. Its continuity with the anterior intersegmental tract of the spinal cord provides a route for connexions from these nuclei to the cervical anterior grey column cells, principally those innervating neck musculature. The harmonious cooperation obviously existing between the facial and hypoglossal nerves in movements of the lips and tongue in speech is frequently attributed to connexions between their nuclei conveyed by the medial longitudinal fasciculus. It is, however, doubtful whether it is the medial longitudinal fasciculus which provides the pathway for these connexions. It has long been established that the most substantial contributions to the fasciculus are made by the vestibular nuclei, and that its chief function is to ensure the coordinate movements of the eyes and head in response to stimulation of the vestibulocochlear nerve. Lesions of the fasciculus are associated with partial ophthalmoplegia. Fibres from the vestibular nuclei, both of the same and of the opposite side, join the fasciculus,

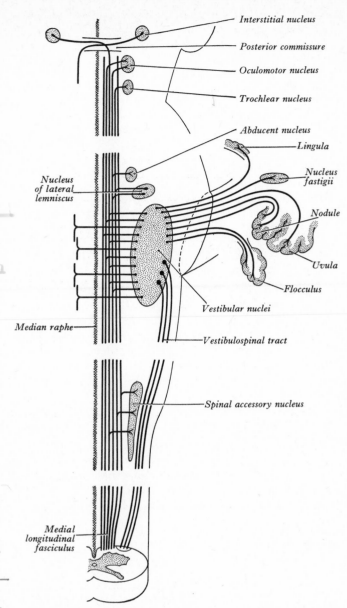

7.94 Simplified diagram of the components of the *medial longitudinal fasciculus* and of the distribution of its fibres to cranial nerve nuclei.

where they ascend, descend or divide into ascending and descending branches.[519] These vestibular fibres send collaterals to, or they may end in, the nuclei of the third, fourth, fifth and sixth cranial nerves and the spinal nucleus of the eleventh nerve (7.94). All four vestibular nuclei contribute ascending fibres to the fasciculus, those from the superior nucleus remaining uncrossed,[520] the others crossing in part. Some of these fibres, as stated, pass to the nuclei of the nerves of the eye muscles, some pass further to reach the interstitial nucleus and the nucleus of the posterior commissure, through which a proportion decussate before ending in these two nuclei.[521] Descending axons, from the medial vestibular nuclei, perhaps joined by some from the lateral and inferior nuclei, partially decussate and pass to the spinal cord, in the fasciculus, as the *medial vestibulospinal tract*[522] (pp. 818, 836). In addition, fibres join the fasciculus from the dorsal nucleus of the trapezoid body, the nucleus of the lateral lemniscus

[519] A. R. Buchanan, *J. comp. Neurol.*, **67**, 1937.
[520] R. E. McMasters, A. H. Weiss and M. B. Carpenter, *Am. J. Anat.*, **118**, 1966.
[521] S. Matano, *J. Hirnforsch.*, **12**, 1970.
[522] A. Brodal, O. Pompeiano and F. Walberg, *The Vestibular Nuclei and their Connexions*, Oliver and Boyd, Edinburgh. 1962.

and the nucleus of the posterior commissure. It is probable, therefore, that the cochlear as well as the vestibular nerve is capable of influencing the movements of the eyes and head through the fasciculus. Some fibres conveying vestibular impulses may ascend in the fasciculus to the thalamus.

A number of other longitudinal nerve fibre systems have been described in the midbrain, some of which extend through much of the entire brainstem. It is not possible to detail all of these here, but two in particular must be mentioned. **The dorsal longitudinal fasciculus** runs in the central grey matter of the midbrain, pons and part of the medulla, in a position ventrolateral to the aqueduct. It is a pathway for descending and ascending connexions, largely uncrossed, between the hypothalamic region and a number of cell groups in the brainstem, including the accessory nuclei (Edinger-Westphal) of the oculomotor complex, the superior colliculus, nucleus ambiguus, the salivatory nuclei, and the facial, solitary and hypoglossal nuclei.[523]

**The central tegmental fasciculus**, already mentioned as a feature of the medulla oblongata (p. 847), is more ventral in the midbrain, being at first lateral to the medial longitudinal fasciculus and dorsolateral to the red nucleus and the decussation of the superior cerebellar peduncles. As it descends through the pons and into the medulla it swerves further laterally to end in the inferior olivary complex of the same side.[524] Although few of its fibres are derived from the thalamus, it is sometimes called the thalamo-olivary tract. Most of its descending fibres are said to proceed from nerve cells in the central grey zone surrounding the cerebral aqueduct at the level of the superior colliculus, but fibres from the basal ganglia and red nucleus also travel in it. Through the red nucleus, ansa lenticularis (p. 904) and the lenticular nucleus, the central tegmental fasciculus mediates a pathway from the motor cortex via these structures to the inferior olivary nucleus. For a further discussion of olivary connexions see pp. 847, 860. The fasiculus ends in the medulla.

**The brachium of the inferior colliculus** forms a rounded strand on the lateral aspect of the upper part of the midbrain (7.107). Its fibres are derived from the inferior colliculus and from the lateral lemniscus and ascend to reach the medial geniculate body. In their course they separate the dorsolateral fibres of the medial lemniscus from the surface.

## THE TECTUM OF THE MIDBRAIN

Although the tectal part of the midbrain exhibits dorsal swellings from the earliest vertebrate stages, its full differentiation into superior and inferior pairs of colliculi (corpora quadrigemina) appears only in the mammals (7.90). Even in the first mammals, the prototherian monotremes, only a single pair of elevations, the *optic lobes* (corpora bigemina), can be distinguished. The optic lobes are highly developed in fishes, being actually larger than the olfactory lobes in Osteichthyes. It is interesting to note that at this and later levels of vertebrate evolution the olfactory lobes are in volume the major development of the forebrain. With the emergence of the cerebral hemisphere, i.e. a forebrain development with more than olfactory connexions, the optic lobes become relatively smaller, but remain substantial structures in amphibians, reptiles and birds. Their connexions and functions show a progressive cranial shift from reptiles through to mammals, a process called *telencephalization*. In this process the dominant position of the optic lobes, which in earlier vertebrates are probably concerned with all sensory modalities other than olfactory, shows a gradual diminu-

tion. This may be coupled with a decrease in the complexity of cytoarchitectonic organization in the optic lobes which is considered to reach its acme in primates, whose highly developed cerebrum has taken over much of the activity of the primitive tectum. The differentiation of the optic lobes into superior and inferior colliculi appears in the eutherian mammals, the inferior being perhaps a derivative of the optic lobes. Though it has been usual to link the superior colliculi with visual and the inferior pair with auditory behaviour, to accept this as an exclusive interpretation is likely to mislead; the superior colliculi in particular appear to be concerned in other ascending afferent pathways from cutaneous receptors and perhaps in auditory connexions. The inferior colliculi are certainly interconnected with the superior; it will nevertheless be more convenient to consider them separately.

**Each inferior colliculus** consists internally of a central main nucleus, ovoid in form, derived embryologically from the periaqueductal grey matter, with which it preserves some degree of continuity. This nucleus is surrounded by a laminar zone of nerve fibres, many of which are from the lateral lemniscus (p. 853) and terminate in the nucleus. Small and medium-sized nerve cells, many being stellate or multipolar, predominate in the nucleus, and some of these are scattered in the nerve fibres surrounding it, particularly on its lateral and medial aspects. These are sometimes regarded as constituting a separate nuclear entity, and they almost certainly have a different origin, being continuous through scattered cells with the superficial lamina of the superior colliculus. The two inferior colliculi are connected by a substantial commissure, which contains not only axons derived from their own cells but also lateral lemniscal fibres passing across the midline to end in the contralateral colliculus. The chief afferent pathway to the colliculi is the lateral lemniscus, whose origins have been described elsewhere (p. 853); similarly, its major contingent of efferent fibres passes through the inferior brachium to the medial geniculate body, a largely ipsilateral projection, though a crossed connexion, through the intercollicular commissure, may exist.[525] The lemniscal fibres relay only in the main collicular nucleus.[526] Some of them pass through without relay to reach the medial geniculate body, and similarly some of the colliculogeniculate fibres do not actually relay in the body, but pass on with those which do into the auditory radiation (p. 1017) to reach the auditory cortex (area 42). As in other sensory pathways there is a descending projection from the same cortical area to the inferior colliculus via the medial geniculate body, through which some may pass without relay. This descending pathway may produce effects at various levels, from the medial geniculate body onwards; it is likely that it links with efferent cochlear fibres, through the superior olivary and cochlear nuclei, as previously noted (p. 854). A tonotopical projection of the lateral lemnisci on the inferior colliculi has been described in cats; it is likely that some similar orderly arrangement extends throughout these auditory connexions, ascending and descending (see Auditory Cortex, p. 963 and reference[427]).

Projection pathways from the inferior colliculi to the brainstem and spinal cord appear to pass first to the superior colliculi, through which connexions with the tectospinal and tectotegmental tracts are effected.[527] These collicular projections are relatively small, and it is possible that the customary view of the inferior colliculi as reflex centres for auditory responses may require modification.

[523] E. C. Crosby and R. T. Woodburne, *J. comp. Neurol.*, **94**, 1951.
[524] J. Bebin, *J. comp. Neurol.*, **105**, 1956.
[525] H. W. Ades, *J. Neurophysiol.*, **7**, 1944.
[526] J. M. Goldberg and R. Y. Moore, *J. comp. Neurol.*, **129**, 1967.
[527] R. Y. Moore and J. M. Goldberg, *Expl Neurol.*, **14**, 1966.

There is, however, considerable evidence that they are concerned in the ability to localize the source of sounds.[528]

**The superior colliculus**, unlike the inferior, which reaches full development only in the mammals, is generally regarded as much simplified in the higher vertebrates, and particularly so in the primates. In man, however, it still exhibits much of the complex laminar organization of earlier forms. At least six laminae have been described in the human colliculus and considerably more intricate arrangements in some other mammals.[529] In this pattern of organization the superior colliculus closely resembles the cerebellar and cerebral cortex which, indeed, it surpasses in complexity in lower vertebrates. This resemblance has prompted the view that the optic lobes, from which the superior colliculi are derived, were the first suprasegmental development of the vertebrate brain which mediates as a summating or integrating mechanism on a much wider basis than the term optic lobe indicates. Such considerations are worthy of attention, if only as a corrective to the widely current teaching that the superior colliculus is exclusively concerned with visual activities.

The laminae of the human colliculus have been variously named, and official terms for them are not yet established. From the exterior inwards strata zonale, cinereum, opticum and lemnisci are recognized, the stratum lemnisci itself being divisible into strata griseum medium, album medium, griseum profundum and album profundum. These seven layers have also been termed zonal, superficial grey, optic, intermediate grey, deep grey, deep white and periventricular strata.[530] The two systems of description do not completely accord, but as a generalization the layers may be considered to be alternately composed of nerve cells or their fibres and dendrites, though some admixture occurs. For example, the most external, the *zonal layer*, consists chiefly of medullated and non-medullated nerve fibres derived from the occipital cortex (areas 17, 18 and 19—*see* p. 960), and arriving as the *external corticotectal tract*; but among these fibres are a few small cells, typically horizontal in arrangement. The next layer, the *superficial grey layer* (stratum cinereum) consists of numerous small multipolar interneurons, with which the cortical fibres in part form synapses, the whole mass forming a cap-shaped lamina, thicker at its centre, over the deeper layers. The *optic layer* consists partly of the fibres of the optic tract which reach the colliculus, a much diminished afferent element in higher primates; as they terminate, these fibres invade neighbouring layers with numerous collateral branches. The optic layer also contains nerve cells, some being large multipolar in type; efferent fibres to the retina are said to start in this layer in man[531] and other mammals. The remaining four layers are sometimes considered together as the stratum lemnisci, but will be briefly outlined here as separate strata. The next two, the *intermediate grey* and *white layers*, are collectively the main reception zone of the colliculus. As the names indicate these layers consist of nerve cells of various sizes intermixed with numerous axons and dendrites. Its main afferent source is the medial corticotectal pathway from the occipital cortex (area 18) and possibly preoccipital cortex (area 7); these areas are concerned with following movements of the eyes (p. 960). These layers also receive afferents from the spinal cord through spinotectal and spinothalamic routes, and probably from the inferior colliculus. Finally, the *deep grey* and *deep white* layers appear most deeply situated, immediately adjacent to the periaqueductal grey substance, again containing a mixture of cell types, with dendrites extending peripherally as far as the optic layer and axons forming many of the efferent connexions of the colliculus.

The superior colliculus thus receives afferents from a wide area,[532, 533] including fibres from the retina, spinal cord, inferior colliculus and occipital cortex, the first three conveying visual, tactile, and probably thermal, pain and auditory impulses, the cortical projection acting as a 'command' and possibly modulating pathway. Its efferents pass out to the retina and to a wide array of brainstem and spinal nerve cell groups. Thus, *tecto-oculomotor* fibres may run to nuclei of the ocular muscles, *tectospinal* fibres (p. 818) travel caudally to the cervical segments of the spinal cord, *tectotegmental* projections reach various reticular masses in the tegmentum, passing also to the substantia nigra, red nucleus and probably as far as the spinal cord. *Tectopontine* fibres, which probably descend in the tectospinal tract, terminate in the dorsolateral part of the pontine nuclei, whence a relay carries this path into the cerebellum (p. 863). All these descending fibres decussate, mostly in the dorsal tegmental decussation, but also to a lesser extent through a commissure which unites the two superior colliculi. For a review of these connexions see reference [534].

The relative paucity of the retinal projection to the superior colliculus in primates throws doubt upon the validity of the commonly accepted view of it as an important centre for visual reflexes, though it certainly has this function in many other mammals. But while the projection of the retinal quadrants on the superior colliculi in cats and rodents has been established with a satisfactory measure of agreement, both by degenerative and stimulation techniques, attempts to extend such experiments to monkeys have been much less successful, probably because of the great reduction in the retinocollicular projection in primates. Clinical evidence merely suggests that a similar pattern of organization may exist in man, this pattern being an association of the craniomedial half of each colliculus with the inferior retinal quadrants and the caudolateral with the superior quadrants. Even the connexions to the eye muscle motor nuclei, which are held to accord with the collicular somatotopic pattern, have been put in doubt by experiments on cats, though it is suggested that these may be merely interrupted by a relay in the pretectal area. For the moment these matters must remain *sub judice*.

Much attention has been focused upon behavioural observations in experimental animals subjected to various types of damage to subcortical parts of the visual pathway in recent times.[535] In addition the visual projection on the optic tectum has been mapped and compared by electrophysiological techniques in a wide series of lower vertebrates from fish to mammals. In general a similar pattern of retinal representation exists in the widely different groups examined, the chief difference in mammals being the degree of ipsilateral projection. This accords with the findings with respect to the movements elicited by stimulation of different parts of the tectum. For example, central collicular stimulation produces a contralateral movement of the head, natural in character, in the cat.[536] A considerable array of similar responses, identical with those occurring in the intact animal, have been observed

[528] R. B. Masterton, J. A. Jane and I. T. Diamond, *J. Neurophysiol.*, **30**, 1967.

[529] S. R. y Cajal, *Histologie du système nerveux, de l'homme et des vertébrés.*, Maloine, Paris. 1909–11.

[530] E. C. Crosby, T. Humphrey and E. W. Lauer, *Correlative Anatomy of the Nervous System*, Macmillan. New York. 1962.

[531] J. R. Wolter and L. Liss, *Albrecht v. Graefes Arch. Ophthal.*, **158**, 1956.

[532] J. M. Sprague, *Anat. Rec.*, **145**, 1963.

[533] T. H. Meikle and J. M. Sprague, *Int. Rev. Neurobiol.*, **6**, 1964.

[534] J. Altman and M. B. Carpenter, *J. comp. Neurol.*, **116**, 1961.

[535] D. Ingle and G. E. Schneider (eds.), *Subcortical Visual Systems*, Karger, Basel. 1969.

[536] W. R. Hess, M. Brügger and V. M. Bucher, *Mschr. Psychiat. Neurol.*, **111**, 1946.

in a number of experimental species, involving eyes, ears, head, trunk and limbs, suggesting that the superior colliculus is concerned in complex integrations between vision and widespread bodily activity.[537] In view of the bilateral representation of the retinae in the colliculi the results of various brain splitting experiments are of special interest. Division of the tegmentum, for example, leads in cats to profound changes in visual behaviour, not so much in reflex responses as in the ability of the animal to interpret its visual environment and to adapt to it.[538] Responses to threatening stimuli are permanently abolished, and the ability to locate edges and follow them is also lost. Similar results have been observed in the monkey. These results have something in common with the split brain syndrome in human patients (p. 967).

**The pretectal nucleus** is a somewhat indistinctly demarcated mass of nerve cells in the pretectal area, at the junction of the mesencephalon and diencephalon. It extends from a position dorsolateral to the posterior commissure towards the superior colliculus, with which it is in part continuous. It receives fibres through the superior brachium from the occipital and preoccipital cortex and from the lateral root of the optic tract (p. 914).[539] Its efferent fibres pass to both accessory oculomotor nuclei (of Edinger-Westphal).[540] Those which decussate pass ventral to the aqueduct or through the posterior commissure. By the autonomic outflow from these nuclei, with a relay in the ciliary ganglia (p. 999), the sphincter muscles of the iris in both eyes are made to contract in response to impulses from either (7.108). This light reflex appears to be the only activity mediated by the pretectal nucleus, but some of its efferent axons are said to enter the tecto-bulbar and tectospinal tracts. The significance of the descending cortical projection is not yet established.

**The cerebral aqueduct** is a narrow canal, about 15 mm long, connecting the third with the fourth ventricle. (Since it is in the midbrain, and certainly does not conduct fluid *to* the cerebrum, it is misnamed.) Its form, as seen in transverse sections, varies at different levels, being T-shaped below, triangular above, and oval in the middle, at which level it is slightly dilated.[541] It is lined with ependyma which is surrounded by a layer of grey matter named the *central grey*; the latter is continuous below with the grey matter in the floor of the fourth ventricle, and above with that of the third ventricle. Remains of the sulcus limitans, apparent on each lateral wall in embryonic development, may persist. Dorsally the aqueduct is partly separated from the grey matter of the colliculi by the fibres of the stratum lemnisci; ventral to it are the medial longitudinal bundles, and the reticular formation of the midbrain. Scattered throughout the central grey matter are numerous nerve cells of various sizes, interlaced by a network of fine fibres. Besides these scattered cells it contains three groups, which constitute the nucleus of the mesencephalic tract of the trigeminal nerve and the nuclei of the oculomotor and trochlear nerves.

---

[537] K. P. Schaefer and H. Schneider, *Arch. Psychait. NervKrankh.*, **211**, 1968.

[538] T. J. Voneida, *Anat. Rec.*, **151**, 1965.

[539] H. Kuhlenbeck and R. N. Miller, *J. comp. Neurol.*, **91**, 1949.

[540] S. W. Ranson and H. W. Magoun, *Archs Neurol. Psychiat.*, Chicago, **30**, 1933.

[541] G. Flyger and U. Hjelmquist, *Anat. Rec.*, **127**, 1959.

# THE RETICULAR FORMATION

It has long been recognized that scattered amongst the more conspicuous fibre bundles and nuclei of the brainstem are extensive fields of intermingled grey and white matter collectively termed the **reticular formation**. Throughout the present section of this volume there are numerous references, some brief and some in greater detail, to the supposed distribution, connexions and possible functions of various parts of this 'system'. When appropriate, reference should be made to these accounts, and to the detailed reviews which have appeared.[542–553] What follows here is a brief summary of some of the main points.

## GENERAL CONSIDERATIONS

A strict scientific definition of the criteria to be used when designating a particular region of the nervous system as 'reticular' or not has proved impossible to achieve. Simple inspection of sections of the vertebrate nervous system prepared by conventional neuroanatomical methods, however, allows some measure of distinction. Many areas consist of either predominantly grey or white matter (p. 753) and their contained neurons or fibre bundles have definite and recognizable quantitative cytological variations which are polarized with respect to the three principal planes of the body. Thus, many regions of white matter contain fibre bundles with a characteristic fibre diameter spectrum, and a definable direction, either longitudinal, transverse, oblique or curved, which carries them between a series of more or less well-defined origins and destinations. Similarly, many areas of grey matter contain populations of neurons with their somata, axon collaterals, dendritic trees and synapses organized into fairly precise three-dimensional arrays. These constitute the main nuclei, cortical formations and fibre tracts of the nervous system. Obvious examples are the well-defined cell columns or laminae in the dorsal and ventral appendages of the spinal cord (p. 837) and their homologues in the brainstem, many other brainstem, diencephalic and telencephalic nuclei, the cerebral and cerebellar cortices, the tectum, and the named tracts of white matter throughout the nervous system, the majority of which are described individually in the present section. Between these geometrically organized *non-reticular* nuclei and tracts are found areas where the grey and white matter is admixed, the fibre bundles interlace in many directions, and the

[542] G. Moruzzi and H. W. Magoun, *Electroenceph. clin. Neurophysiol.*, **1**, 1949.

[543] H. Meessen and J. Olszewski, *A Cytoarchitectonic Atlas of the Rhombencephalon of the Rabbit*, Karger, Basel. 1949.

[544] J. Olszewski, in: *Brain Mechanisms and Consciousness*, eds. E. D. Adrian, F. Bremer and H. H. Jasper, Blackwell, Oxford. 1954.

[545] J. Olszewski and D. Baxter, *Cytoarchitecture of the Human Brain Stem*, Karger, Basel. 1954.

[546] A. Brodal, *The Reticular Formation of the Brain Stem. Anatomical Aspects and Functional Correlations*, Oliver and Boyd, Edinburgh. 1957.

[547] E. Ramón-Moliner and W. J. H. Nauta, *J. comp. Neurol.*, **126**, 1966.

[548] E. Taber, *J. comp. Neurol.*, **116**, 1961.

[549] F. Valverde, *J. comp. Neurol.*, **116, 117, 119**, 1961a and b, 1962.

[550] H. Jasper, L. D. Proctor, R. S. Knighton and R. T. Costello (eds). *Reticular Formation of the Brain.* Henry Ford Hospital International Symposium. Little, Brown & Co., Boston. 1958.

[551] G. A. Horridge, *Interneurons*, Freeman, London and San Francisco. 1968.

[552] M. A. B. Brazier (ed.), *The Interneuron*, University of California Press, Berkeley and Los Angeles. 1969.

[553] M. E. Scheibel and A. B. Scheibel in: *The Neurosciences, A Second Study Program*, eds. F. O. Schmitt, G. C. Quarton, T. Melnechuk and G. Adelman, Rockefeller University Press, N.Y. 1970.

scattered neurons have diffuse, ill-defined patterns of connectivity (*vide infra*); these constitute the *reticular regions of the nervous system*. However, although many authorities agree concerning the geometric organization and non-reticular nature of the majority of the main nuclei and tracts, the status of a number of regions remains unclarified, and the following points should be noted.

The structural extremes of a mathematically precise, repeating geometric organization on the one hand, and a truly random nerve network on the other, are abstractions which do not exist in nervous systems. Even the highly regular cerebellar cortex shows considerable quantitative variation in different regions when examined critically (p. 866), and the most 'reticular' parts of the nervous system show some distinctive structural features. Thus, a graded range of levels of structural organization exists and, inevitably, those with a more diffuse structure prove the more difficult to investigate. For this reason, coupled with the fact that detailed knowledge of the quantitative aspects of neuronal morphology and connexions is still in its infancy, many authorities have expressed divergent views about which regions of the nervous system should be embraced by the term *the reticular formation*. Most are agreed about the inclusion of certain deeply placed areas of the medulla, pons and midbrain (*vide infra*), and some would restrict the use of the term to these regions. The status of other cell groups in these parts of the nervous system such as the olivary complex, the parvocellular part of the red nucleus, the pars reticularis of the substantia nigra, the nucleus of the posterior commissure, the interstitial nucleus, the intracerebellar nuclei and others, is uncertain, being included by some and excluded by others. Further disagreement reigns concerning the inclusion of the central regions of grey matter of the spinal cord which have been termed a 'reticular core' by some investigators (p. 838), and whether the non-specific nuclei of the thalamus (p. 898) and certain hypothalamic nuclei should be included. These terminological debates merely serve to emphasize the undesirable nature of rigidly categorizing some centres as reticular or non-reticular, and the need for further researches, in the light of which the necessity for such crude parcellations of the nervous system will gradually recede.

No attempt will be made in the present account to draw precise boundaries between such areas, but it should be appreciated that *all* levels of the neuraxis, including the spinal cord, brainstem and diencephalon, have regions with a relatively high level of ordered structure, which are interlocked both structurally and functionally with neighbouring reticular regions where the organization is much more diffuse.

The more obviously reticular regions of the nervous system are often regarded as phylogenetically ancient, representing the 'random nerve network' of early ancestors, upon which background, during subsequent evolution, the more circumscribed, highly organized, discriminative parts of the nervous system have appeared. But, as pointed out elsewhere (p. 752), even the most primitive known nervous systems possess both diffuse and more highly organized regions, which cooperate in their responses to different environmental stimuli. It is perhaps preferable to regard both these elements as evolving together, each providing indispensable and interdependent contributions to the total response patterns of the organism.

## THE RETICULAR PARTS OF THE NERVOUS SYSTEM

In general terms, the reticular parts of the nervous system consist of: (1) deeply placed, rather poorly defined groups of neurons and fibres with diffuse patterns of connexions; (2) the conduction paths through these regions are difficult and often impossible to define anatomically, but physiological evidence indicates that they are complex and often *polysynaptic*; (3) both *ascending* and *descending* components can be recognized; (4) stimulation of a locus on one side often elicits responses both on the ipsilateral and the contralateral side, i.e. both the ascending and descending systems contain *crossed* and *uncrossed* elements; (5) they mediate both *somatic* and *visceral* functions.

Whilst the earlier investigators discerned little structural variation in different regions, and simply dubbed all regions other than the specific named nuclei and tracts as reticular; more recently, a series of critical studies have shown that zonal variations in structure are present in these reticular regions. These include differences in cell size, number, packing density, cytochemistry, and in some measure, differences in their connexions. On this basis a series of *reticular nuclei* have been named in a variety of animals, but their borders are often indistinct, and some variation exists between species. These details cannot be reviewed here and for them the references quoted should be consulted.

Studies with the Golgi technique have shown that in the brainstem few of the reticular neurons are of the classical Golgi type II with short axons which branch locally. The majority have wide arborizations of their dendritic trees which spread mainly at right angles to the long axis of the brainstem. This manner of dendritic branching is sometimes termed *isodendritic*, and the area covered by the dendrites of a single reticular neuron is large—sometimes almost 50 per cent of the transverse sectional profile of that half of the brainstem in which the neuron lies. Consequently, there is a great degree of overlap of the dendritic fields of adjacent reticular neurons, and they are intersected at right angles by huge numbers of longitudinally running nerve fibres with which many synaptic contacts are established. The axons of reticular neurons take a longitudinal course, either ascending, descending, or bifurcating to pass in both directions. They traverse considerable lengths of the brainstem and give off a series of collateral branches many of which pass at right angles to re-enter the reticular fields, whilst others pass to neighbouring 'specific' centres. Some of the caudally directed axons pass into the spinal cord, whilst cranially directed ones may reach a number of the diencephalic nuclei. In addition, there are numerous afferent inputs from other regions of the nervous system (*vide infra*). Clearly, there are massive opportunities for convergence and divergence of information paths in such a system. The reticular neurons are either excitatory or inhibitory, the proportion varying in different regions, and are either cholinergic or aminergic (containing 5-hydroxytryptamine, dopamine, or various catecholamines), and again the proportions vary in different sites.

Of the various topographical regions often included in the reticular formation, the following are described elsewhere in this volume: the reticular core of the spinal cord (pp. 809, 838), the non-specific nuclei of the thalamus (p. 898), some of the hypothalamic nuclei (p. 905), and a number of structures in the sections devoted to the brainstem. Numerous references are also made to connexions of the reticular areas in the descriptions of the cerebellum, corpus striatum and subdivisions of the diencephalon.

Some only of the more prominent named brainstem reticular nuclei can be mentioned here. In the medulla, the reticular formation is often divided into *lateral* and *medial* regions on each side of the emerging roots of the hypoglossal nerve, in which grey and white matter predominate respectively. In the lateral part, the largest collection of prominent reticular neurons constitutes the *lateral reticular nucleus*, which is dorsolateral to the olivary nuclear complex. Dorsomedial to the olivary complex is the *inferior medial reticular nucleus*, which is closely associated with the central tegmental fasciculus. Near the midline are scattered groups of neurons interspersed with many bundles of fine decussating fibres, which collectively form the *nucleus of the raphe*, whilst a number of *parahypoglossal nuclei* are often also included in the medullary reticular formation. Extending cranially, near the midline, from the medulla to central pontine levels, is a narrow darkly staining column of cells which constitutes the *inferior central tegmental reticular nucleus* of the pons. More prominent pontine reticular aggregations lie somewhat laterally in the intermediate and lateral parts of the tegmentum—caudal to the motor nucleus of the trigeminal nerve is the *caudal pontine reticular nucleus* which continues cranially into the *oral pontine reticular nucleus*. In the midbrain, as stated above, many authorities regard parts of the red nucleus, substantia nigra, and the interstitial and posterior commissural nuclei, as reticular. In addition, throughout the whole extent of the dorsolateral part of the midbrain tegmentum, and extending towards the cerebral aqueduct, are a number of neuronal aggregates which are included in the reticular formation. Useful collective terms for these are the *deep tegmental reticular nuclei* and the *nuclei of the periaqueductal grey matter*. The numerous subdivisions and terminologies proposed for these regions will not be pursued here.

## CONNEXIONS OF THE RETICULAR FORMATION

The majority of these have been described elsewhere in the present section and will only be listed here.

**Afferent projections** reach the reticular formation from: (1) the spinal cord via the *spinoreticular pathways*, and also via *collateral branches* of the *long ascending tracts*, although the latter may not be as profuse as was thought previously; (2) collateral branches from some primary, and many secondary, afferent neurons associated with the *cranial nerves*, including the central *vestibular and acoustic* pathways; (3) the *cerebellum* via the various *cerebelloreticular pathways* described previously; (4) indirectly from the *visual* and *acoustic* pathways, and other afferent channels, via *tectoreticular fibres*; (5) from various *thalamic*, *subthalamic* and *hypothalamic nuclei*, which are further detailed elsewhere; (6) from the *corpus striatum*, both directly and indirectly through its complex of outflow paths; (7) direct *corticoreticular fibres* from the *sensorimotor regions* of the cerebral cortex, with smaller contributions from other cortical areas; an unknown proportion of such fibres are collaterals of other corticofugal systems such as the corticospinal tract; (8) from various parts of the *limbic system*, including the *septal areas*, the *amygdaloid nuclei* and the *hippocampus* through a variety of descending pathways.

Thus, many different afferent pathways converge upon the reticular formation, and although there is some evidence for a degree of zonal localization in the levels of termination of diverse afferents, there is also abundant evidence for much overlap and convergence of different channels. Unit recording with intracellular microelectrodes has provided much information that supports this view. Single units have been studied in experimental animals during multimodal forms of stimulation of cutaneous receptors and proprioceptors in many parts of the body, and during stimulation of a wide variety of peripheral nerves, the special sense organs, and diverse parts of the central nervous system including the spinal cord, the cerebral and cerebellar cortices, the hippo-campus, corpus striatum, etc. For example, units are found which respond solely to nociceptive stimuli applied to different body regions; others respond to a wide range of cutaneous stimuli, again from extensive bilateral receptive fields; yet others respond to stimulation of many different regions of the cerebral cortex, and so forth. Further, individual units can be identified which respond to the stimulation of a number of different types of afferent channel, e.g. visual, acoustic, cortical, cerebellar, etc. These different afferent channels also interact in various ways, some with mutual enhancement, others with mutual inhibition. Although the different levels of the reticular formation are not all equivalent in terms of their input and output, there is still a high degree of convergence of afferent channels, and a profusion of interconnexion between its neurons. The question of how such a bewilderingly complex and fluctuating array of information channels is used to direct cooperative responses, remains one of the central and most intractable problems in neurology.[554]

**The efferent connexions** of the reticular formation are: (1) to the autonomic and locomotor control centres, and interneuronal pools of the *spinal cord* via the *reticulospinal tracts*; (2) by short descending pathways to similar centres in the *brainstem*; (3) to the *cerebellum*; (4) to the *red nucleus, substantia nigra* and *tectum* of the midbrain; (5) to numerous nuclei in the *subthalamus, thalamus* and *hypothalamus*; (6) indirectly, through radiations of the latter diencephalic nuclei, to the corpus striatum and to the cerebral cortex, including most regions of the neocortex and many areas of the limbic system.

In short, therefore, the reticular formation receives convergent information channels from all the principal parts of the nervous system and, in turn, it projects directly or indirectly back to all these regions. Functional studies with implanted microelectrodes, and following focal stimulation or ablation of the system, also support the view that it is essentially involved in all the major functional activities of the nervous system, although the detailed manner of its operation remains unknown. Thus, the reticular formation is intimately concerned with:

(1) **Locomotor control**, not only through its direct reticulospinal projections to lower motor centres, but indirectly, by influencing the activities of the cerebellum, red nucleus, substantia nigra, subthalamic centres, the corpus striatum and the cerebral cortex.

(2) **Long and short term homeostasis** through its descending pathways to lower autonomic centres, and its ascending pathways conveying *visceral* and *somatic* information to the hypothalamus and limbic system (*see* pp. 909, 943). It is considered to include subsidiary brainstem centres related to cardiovascular, respiratory and gastrointestinal control mechanisms, and also the diffuse, bilateral, ascending, nociceptive ('slow pain') pathways.

(3) The rhythms of different **sleep** and **waking** **states**. It is thus part of the hierarchical system of *hypnogenic zones* found at different levels throughout the brainstem. The latter is considered to be in balance with the *ascending activating system*, mediated by various reticulo-diencephalic connexions and their radiations to the cerebral cortex (p. 898), which are responsible for the *arousal reaction*, or *desynchronization* of the electrical responses of the cerebral cortex.

[554] W. L. Klimer, W. S. McCulloch, J. Blum, E. Craighill and D. Peterson, in: *The Mind, Biological Approaches to its Functions*, W. C. Corning and M. Balaban (eds.), Interscience Publishers, N.Y. 1968.

# THE PROSENCEPHALON OR FOREBRAIN

The prosencephalon or forebrain develops from the most cranial of the three midline primary cerebral vesicles (p. 132). This *forebrain vesicle* and its contained cavity, the future *third ventricle*, is soon divisible into a caudal *diencephalon* and a cranial *telecephalon*. From the side walls of the latter right and left diverticula form and develop into the cerebral hemispheres. Each hemisphere contains a lateral ventricle, and the sites of evagination are marked by the interventricular foramina, through which the lateral ventricles communicate with each other and with the cavity of the third ventricle. (Survey photographs of the cerebrum in sagittal and coronal section are shown in **7**.95, 96, 110.)

Thus, the *diencephalon* corresponds in large measure to the third ventricle and the structures which bound it, whilst the telencephalon consists of a midline *telencephalon medium* or *impar* containing the cranial extension of the third ventricle, and the massive *bilateral telencephalic cerebral hemispheres* each containing a lateral ventricle. (For the development of these regions *see* p. 138.)

# THE DIENCEPHALON OR "INTERBRAIN"

As stated, the cavity of the diencephalon forms the greater part of the median slit-like third ventricle, which narrows caudally to continue into the aqueduct of the midbrain, while cranially it extends into the telencephalon medium (*vide supra* and p. 904).

More precise topographic limits for the diencephalon are: caudally—a plane which includes the posterior commissure and the caudal margins of the mamillary bodies; cranially—a plane which passes from the interventricular foramina through the posterosuperior border of the midline part of the optic chiasma. Cranial to the latter plane are the structures comprising the telencephalon medium. It should be emphasized, however, that while the boundaries just described have some measure of developmental and phylogenetic significance, in terms of the functional anatomy of the brain they are merely arbitrary descriptive aids, since many systems cross the boundaries into adjacent areas.

Thus, the diencephalon is a midline structure with symmetrical right and left halves. Traversing each lateral wall of the third ventricle is a *hypothalamic sulcus* of variable prominence, which extends from the cerebral aqueduct to the interventricular foramen (p. 919). The line of the sulcus is used to divide each lateral half of the diencephalon into a *pars dorsalis* and a *pars ventralis diencephali*.

The pars dorsalis diencephali consists on each side of: (1) the dorsal thalamus, (2) the metathalamus, and (3) the epithalamus; whilst the pars ventralis diencephali includes (1) the hypothalamus, and (2) the ventral thalamus.

Briefly, above the hypothalamic sulcus most of each side wall of the third ventricle is formed by a large egg-shaped mass of grey matter and associated laminae of white matter which together constitute the *dorsal thalamus*. The unqualified term *thalamus* is used by the majority of neuroanatomists as synonymous with dorsal thalamus and will frequently be used in this manner in the following account. As described in greater detail below, the thalamus can be divided into a series of major *parts*, and each of these can be subdivided into several *nuclei*. Inferior to the caudal end of the thalamus, and partly continuous with it, are two further swellings—the *medial* and *lateral geniculate bodies*—which overlie nuclei of the same names, and which together constitute the *metathalamus*. The roof of the diencephalon is largely formed by a layer of ependyma which is continuous with that lining the remainder of the third ventricle. Throughout most of its extent this ependyma is in close apposition with the overlying vascular pia mater, with no nervous tissue intervening. However, in the caudal part of the roof and in the adjoining lateral walls of the diencephalon, are the habenular nuclei and their commissure, the epiphysis cerebri or pineal body, and the posterior commissure. Together these constitute the *epithalamus*.

Some neuroanatomists include the whole of the pars ventralis diencephali in an 'anatomical' definition of the hypothalamus, but this includes regions which are quite dissimilar functionally, and, accordingly, a more restricted

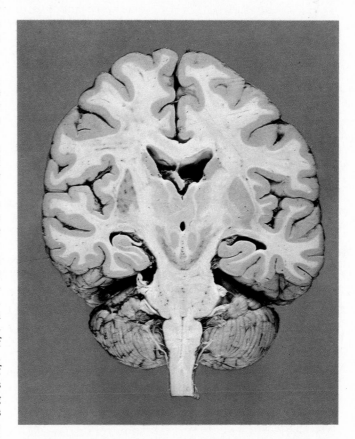

**7**.95    The dorsal half of a brain sectioned in an oblique coronal plane which passes through the cerebral hemispheres, diencephalon, midbrain, pons and medulla oblongata, to show the general disposition of main structures, many of which are labelled on **7**.98. Note: (1) the complex folding of the cerebral cortical gyri and sulci of the frontoparietal, insular and temporal regions; (2) the sectioned surfaces of the corpus callosum, septum pellucidum, body of the fornix, the corona radiata, internal capsule, ventral pons and medulla oblongata; in the latter, part of the decussation of the corticospinal tracts is visible. Note also: (3) the body and inferior horn of the lateral ventricle; (4) the lentiform and caudate nuclei, and the dorsal thalami which are fused across the midline. This illustration includes features referred to at many points in the text which are too numerous to include in a caption; these should be studied as appropriate. (Dissection by Dr. E. L. Rees.)

definition is preferred in this account. The *hypothalamus* extends from the lamina terminalis to a vertical plane immediately caudal to the mamillary bodies, and dorso-ventrally from the hypothalamic sulcus to include the structures in the side wall and floor of the third ventricle. The latter include the mamillary bodies themselves, the tuber cinereum and infundibulum, and nervous tissue adjacent to the optic chiasma (7.104). Cranially, the preoptic region, which lies adjacent to the lamina terminalis and is therefore strictly a telencephalic structure, is for functional reasons usually included in descriptions of the hypothalamus.

The remaining zones of the pars ventralis diencephali are situated in part lateral to the hypothalamus, as a thin sheet immediately ventral to the dorsal thalamus, and as a thick zone which merges caudally with the tegmentum of the midbrain. Collectively these zones constitute the *ventral thalamus* or *subthalamus*. The region includes the cranial extensions of the red nucleus and substantia nigra, the prominent subthalamic nucleus, the prerubral field, the zona incerta, and their associated complexes of nuclei and fibre tracts.

## The Thalamus

The thalami (7.95, 96, 97, 98) are two large ovoid masses of grey matter, situated one on each side of the third ventricle and reaching for some distance caudal to that cavity. Each thalamus is about 4 cm long, and has two ends and four surfaces.

The *anterior end* is narrow; it lies close to the median plane and forms the posterior boundary of the interventricular foramen.

The expanded *posterior end*, the *pulvinar*, is directed dorsally and laterally and overhangs the superior colliculus and its brachium. On the inferior aspect of its lateral part the lateral geniculate body (p. 915) forms a small, oval elevation. Inferiorly, the pulvinar is separated from the medial geniculate body (p. 915) by the brachium of the superior colliculus.

The *superior surface* (7.97) is free, slightly convex, and covered by a layer of white matter, termed the *stratum zonale*. It is separated laterally from the ventricular surface of the caudate nucleus by a white band, termed the *stria terminalis*, and by the thalamostriate vein (p. 985). It is separated medially from the medial surface by the reflection of the ependyma of the third ventricle to form its roof. This reflection is termed the *taenia thalami*. The superior surface is divided into a lateral and a medial part. The lateral part forms a portion of the floor of the lateral ventricle. It is covered with the epithelium of that cavity, and is partly hidden by the vascular fringe of the choroid plexus (7.98). The medial part of this surface is covered with the tela choroidea of the third ventricle, by which it is separated from the body of the fornix which grooves the surface. Between the lateral edge of the fornix and the upper surface of the thalamus the lateral margin of the tela choroidea with its contained plexus is invaginated into the ventricle through the choroidal fissure (7.157). In front, the superior surface is separated from the medial surface by a narrow, raised ridge from which the epithelial lining of the third ventricle is reflected to the under surface of the tela choroidea. This ridge covers a small bundle of white fibres, named the *stria medullaris thalami* (p. 901). Posteriorly it turns medially to form the anterior boundary of the *trigonum habenulae* (7.97), from which the superior surface of the thalamus is separated by the *sulcus habenulae*.

The *inferior surface* rests upon and is continuous with the cranial prolongation of the tegmentum (*subthalamus*).

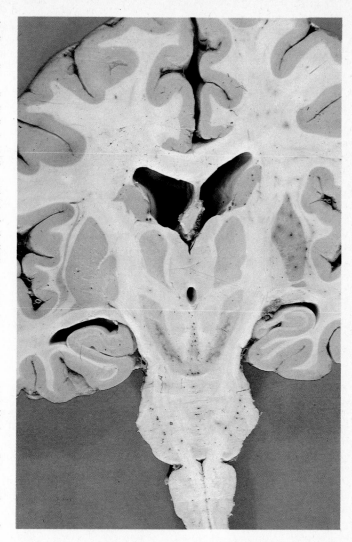

7.96 The central area of the ventral part of the oblique coronal section of the brain shown in 7.95, photographed at higher magnification to show some structural features in greater detail; compare with 7.98 for appropriate labelling. Note in particular: (1) the anterior, medial and lateral parts of the dorsal thalamus, separated by the internal medullary laminae; (2) the relation of the caudate nucleus to the anterior and inferior horns of the lateral ventricle; (3) the lentiform nucleus, divided into an external putamen and an internal globus pallidus; the latter again divided into internal and external parts; (4) the internal capsule, external capsule, claustrum, extreme capsule and insular cortex; (5) the profiles of the sectioned subthalamic and red nuclei and substantia nigra; (6) the hippocampus projecting into the floor of the inferior horn of the lateral ventricle. Other structural features on this section are referred to at many points throughout the text. Compare also with 7.152. (Dissection by Dr. E. L. Rees.)

In front of this it rests on that part of the hypothalamus lying in the lateral wall of the third ventricle.

The *medial surface* (8.195) is the superior part of the lateral wall of the third ventricle; it is usually connected to the corresponding surface of the opposite thalamus by a flattened grey band, named the *interthalamic adhesion* (*connexus interthalamicus*). This band is posterior to the interventricular foramen, and averages about 1 cm in its anteroposterior diameter; it sometimes consists of two or even three parts, and occasionally is absent. It contains nerve cells and nerve fibres; some of the latter cross the median plane, but many of them pass towards the median plane and then curve laterally on the same side. This surface of the thalamus is limited below by a curved groove, often ill-defined, termed the *hypothalamic sulcus*. It curves antero-superiorly from the cranial end of the cerebral aqueduct to the floor of the interventricular foramen and is usually regarded as the cranial continuation of the sulcus limitans of the spinal cord and brainstem, but this view has been strongly challenged.[555]

On the *lateral surface* there is a thick band of white substance consisting of projection fibres, which form the posterior limb of the internal capsule and separate the thalamus from the lentiform nucleus of the corpus striatum (**7**.98).

## The Gross Structure and Parts of the Thalamus

The thalamus is chiefly of grey matter but its superior surface is clothed by a layer of white matter, the *stratum zonale* and its lateral surface by a similar layer, the *external medullary lamina*. Internally, the thalamic grey matter is incompletely divided by a vertical sheet of white matter, the *internal medullary lamina* which splits anterosuperiorly in a Y-shaped manner. Accordingly, the main mass of the thalamus is divided into three major *parts*—anterior, medial and lateral; the lateral part is further divided into dorsolateral and ventromedial *parts*. Each of these major parts of the thalamus contains a *group of thalamic nuclei* and, further, these large groups are separated by more restricted groups of nuclei which occur within the internal medullary lamina, and also flank the medial and lateral surfaces of the thalamus.

**The main nuclear groups** of the thalamus are therefore:

(1) The *anterior group*, which constitutes the anterior part of the thalamus.

(2) The *medial group*, which lies between the internal medullary lamina laterally, and approaches but does not reach, the ependymal lining of the third ventricle medially.

(3) The *lateral group*, which constitutes the dorsolateral moiety of the lateral part of the thalamus, and which expands posteriorly to form the pulvinar.

(4) The *ventral group*, which occupies the ventromedial moiety of the lateral part of the thalamus.

(5) The *intralaminar group*, embedded in the substance of the internal medullary lamina.

(6) The *nuclei of the midline*, which are small, interlaced with a periventricular system of fine nerve fibres and which constitute part of the periventricular grey matter separating the medial part of the thalamus from the ependyma of the third ventricle and in part forming the variable interthalamic adhesion (p. 892).

(7) The *reticular nucleus of the thalamus*, which is a long, thin, curved lamina of cells separating the external medullary lamina from the white matter of the posterior limb of the internal capsule.

The anterior and medial part of the thalamus, together with some of the smaller groups of nuclei, are often regarded as phylogenetically the older regions, and designated *paleothalamus* in contrast with the lateral part or *neothalamus*, which reaches its greatest development in anthropoid apes and man. However, such modifications have occurred in the 'older' parts of the thalamus during the course of evolution, and the structural and functional relationships of the various regions of the primate thalamus are so intermingled, that some authorities regard such a division as little more than a convenient aid to elementary teaching.

As we shall detail further below, many parts of the thalamus are connected via relatively well-defined fibre bundles with all the main subcortical parts of the nervous system—the brainstem and spinal cord, cerebellum, hypothalamus and corpus striatum. Further, many parts of the thalamus establish reciprocal connexions with many parts of the cerebral cortex, and classically these two-way radiations of fibres between thalamus and cortex are

grouped into four *peduncles* or *stalks of the thalamus*. Taken together, however, these peduncles form an almost continuous fan-like radiation from the ventral, superior, posterior and inferolateral margins of the thalamus to most regions of the cortex, and they form a substantial part of the internal capsule and corona radiata (**7**.99, 150B, and p. 973). The *anterior* or *frontal thalamic peduncle* interconnects the anterior and medial parts of the thalamus with much of the cortex of the frontal lobe of the cerebrum. The *superior peduncle* interconnects the ventral and lateral thalamic regions with the pre- and post-central gyri and the neighbouring parts of the frontal and parietal lobes. The *posterior peduncle* joins the occipital and posterior parietal cortex with the posterior parts of the lateral thalamus including the pulvinar and lateral geniculate body. Finally, the *inferior thalamic peduncle*, smaller than the others, interconnects the posterior thalamus and medial geniculate body with restricted regions of the temporal lobe cortex.

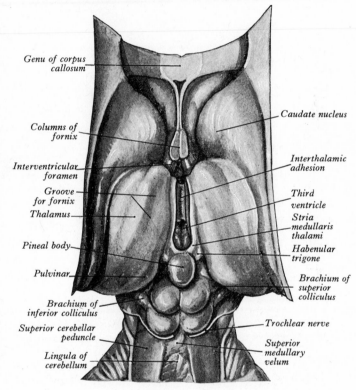

**7**.97 Dorsal aspect of the caudate nuclei, thalami, pineal body and tectum, revealed by removal of most of the corpus callosum, the body of the fornix, and of the tela choroidea.

## The Thalamic Nuclei and their Connexions

The nuclear groups of the thalamus outlined above have been intensively studied since the close of the nineteenth century in man and a number of other mammalian and submammalian forms. A number of these studies have been purely structural, concerning the cytoarchitectonics as revealed by the Nissl technique, or the general disposition of the white matter, whilst the Golgi method has given much information on the morphology of individual neurons and their processes. Many investigations of connectivity patterns have been carried out with the methods of Nauta and Marchi; the effects of selective stimulation

[555] J. F. Christ, in: *The Hypothalamus*, eds. W. Haymaker, E. Anderson and W. J. H. Nauta, Thomas, Springfield, Ill. 1969.

and ablation have been recorded; more recently, in as yet only restricted regions of the thalamus, there have been detailed ultrastructural studies of its synaptology, and unit recording with microelectrodes.

What emerges from these studies, which are far too numerous to review here, is that the thalamus is a region of immense structural complexity, composed of a large number of often interdependent, but functionally distinctive zones. Whilst substantial agreement has been reached concerning the broad parcellation of the thalamus into nuclear groups, and often individual nuclei, it is still

tionally. The general anatomy and thalamic termination of the more prominent long ascending pathways and those from neighbouring centres have been well established for a considerable period, but the finer details of their sites and modes of termination, and those of less substantial pathways are often uncertain and the source of much disagreement. Many thalamic nuclei show marked degenerative changes after experimental resection of regions of the cerebral cortex—hence the term *cortically dependent thalamic nuclei* for such centres. Again, some nuclei, whilst having local and intrinsic connexions, are

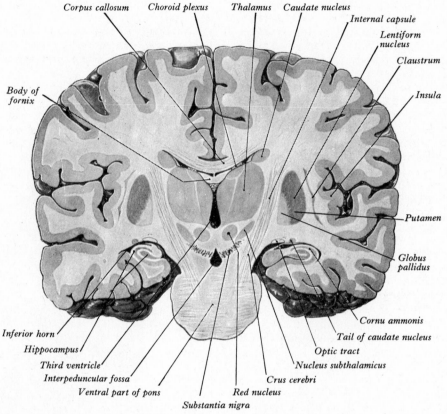

Corpus callosum — Choroid plexus — Thalamus — Caudate nucleus — Internal capsule — Lentiform nucleus — Claustrum — Insula — Body of fornix — Putamen — Globus pallidus — Cornu ammonis — Tail of caudate nucleus — Optic tract — Nucleus subthalamicus — Inferior horn — Hippocampus — Third ventricle — Interpeduncular fossa — Ventral part of pons — Red nucleus — Crus cerebri — Substantia nigra

7.98   Coronal section of the brain through the ventral part of the pons.

premature to assume that we possess a comprehensive picture of the structural and functional design of the organ. Difficulties of investigation stem from the large number of nuclear groups, some of them very small, which are closely packed together, their afferent and efferent fibre systems often passing through or near neighbouring nuclear territories. Accordingly, stereotactic lesions almost invariably affect unwanted regions in addition to the target area of the experiment. Similarly, retrograde degenerative changes are difficult to assess in the smaller thalamic neurons, and these are equally difficult to study with microelectrode techniques. Nevertheless, despite these problems of technique, a large volume of data has accumulated and the main nuclei of the thalamus and their best substantiated connexions will be summarized here (7.100, 101). For details and an introduction to extensive bibliographies the reader should consult footnote references [556–565].

In general terms a thalamic nucleus may establish connexions with: (1) other thalamic nuclei; (2) neighbouring subcortical masses of grey matter; (3) long ascending pathways from the brainstem and spinal cord; and (4) the cerebral cortex. The intrinsic connexions with other thalamic nuclei are the most difficult to analyse and thus are the least well understood both structurally and func-

predominantly in receipt of a discrete, often somatotopically organized input tract, and give rise to an equally well-organized projection to the cortex. These are often termed *relay nuclei* in contrast to *association nuclei* in which multiple subcortical connexions predominate. However, the former are not to be regarded as 'simple' relays since complex transformations of the flow of information are the rule in such centres. Further, based upon focal stimulation of the thalamus, together with recording from the cerebral cortex, thalamic nuclei have often been termed either *specific* or *non-specific*. In the former, a rapid,

[556] W. E. Le G. Clark, *J. Anat.*, **67**, 1933; **70**, 1936; **71**, 1937; *Brain*, **55**, 1932; **56**, 1933; *Lancet*, 1948.
[557] A. E. Walker, *The Primate Thalamus*, University of Chicago Press, Illinois. 1938.
[558] J. E. Toncray and N. J. S. Kreig, *J. comp. Neurol.*, **85**, 1946.
[559] J. G. Sheps, *J. comp. Neurol.*, **83**, 1945.
[560] A. Dekaban, *J. comp. Neurol.*, **99**, 1953.
[561] A. Dekaban, *J. comp. Neurol.*, **99**, 1953.
[561] H. Kuhlenbeck, *Confinia neurol.*, suppl., **14**, 1954.
[562] R. Hassler, in: *Introduction to Stereotaxis with an Atlas of the Human Brain*, eds. G. Schaltenbrand and P. Bailey, Grune and Stratton, N.Y. 1959.
[563] C. Amjone Marsan, *Archs ital. Biol.*, **103**, 1965.
[564] M. E. Scheibel and A. B. Scheibel, *Brain Res.*, **1**, 1966; **6**, 1967.
[565] D. P. Purpura and M. D. Yahr (eds.), *The Thalamus*, Columbia University Press, N.Y., London. 1966.

sharply localized, ipsilateral response is recorded, whilst with the latter the response is widespread, bilateral and occurs after a greater latency. With increasingly refined methods of investigation, however, many nuclei previously thought to have no connexion with the cerebral cortex are now shown to be 'cortically dependent', and the distinction between specific and non-specific nuclei is becoming less clear cut as a considerable measure of interaction between the two is becoming apparent.

## SYNAPTIC ORGANIZATION OF THALAMIC RELAY NUCLEI

Studies with the electron microscope have shown that the ultrastructural organization of the principal sensory 'relay' nuclei is extremely complex, and attempts to analyse synaptic relationships are in their infancy. A striking feature of all such nuclei so far studied is the *synaptic glomerulus*, a spherical, ovoid or more irregularly shaped tissue unit from 2 or 3 $\mu$m to 20 $\mu$m or more along one axis, consisting of closely packed axons and dendrites of different types, establishing with each other a large number and usually a considerable variety of synaptic relationships.[566] (See also p. 776 and 7.21.) These neural components, which include dendrites or dendritic appendages of the thalamic neurons together with axon terminals of different types, are encapsulated, and separated from the surrounding and generally more simply organized neuropil, by thin, sheet-like astrocyte processes. It is principally within synaptic glomeruli that the specific afferents terminate (for example, the axons of the optic nerve and tract in the lateral geniculate nucleus and those of the medial lemniscus in the nucleus ventralis posterior lateralis). Because of the synaptic interactions occurring within the environment of the glomeruli, each probably functions to some extent as an independent integrative unit whose output (to the cortically projecting thalamic neuron), following the arrival of an impulse in the specific afferent, is modified according to other variable factors, such as activity in the cortico-thalamic and other afferent systems and the extent of activity in neighbouring specific afferents and synaptic glomeruli.

One of the most interesting recent findings has been the discovery[567] in thalamic nuclei of *presynaptic dendrites* morphologically similar to conventional dendrites but containing, in addition to the usual organelles, clusters of synaptic vesicles and establishing synaptic contacts with other dendrites. Some cells with presynaptic dendrites may also have conventional axons; others may resemble the amacrine cells of the retina and olfactory bulb and bear only one type of 'dual-purpose' neurite. Recent ultrastructural analyses[568] have shown that the presynaptic dendrites eventually give rise to boutons, packed with distinctive disc-like synaptic vesicles. These dendritic boutons are very similar to axonal boutons, and constitute one of the principal classes of synaptic endings in the thalamic glomeruli. The significance of presynaptic dendrites in the information processing activities of thalamic nuclei is not yet understood.

## THE ANTERIOR GROUP OF NUCLEI

This group is divisible into three nuclei: *anterior dorsalis* (AD), *anterior medialis* (AM) and *anterior ventralis* (AV), the first being the least prominent. The anterior group of nuclei is interconnected with both the medial and lateral groups of thalamic nuclei, and possibly with the contralateral anterior group. It receives some fibres directly from the postcommissural fornix, and the substantial mamillothalamic tract from the mamillary nuclei of the same side, a few fascicles stemming from the oppo-

site side, and it also sends a small contingent of thalamo-mamillary fibres back to these nuclei. The main radiation from the anterior group are thalamocortical fibres to many parts of the gyrus cinguli (cortical areas 23, 24 and 32), and the anterior group also receives corticothalamic fibres from the same areas.

The anterior thalamic nuclei are thus a principal centre linking the activities of the hippocampus and hypothalamus with other thalamic nuclei and with extensive cortical areas which belong to the limbic system (p. 930). Stimulation or ablation of the mamillothalamic tract causes alterations in autonomic control and is presumably involved in complex homeostatic cycles involving visceral responses. A normally functioning hippocampus-fornix-mamillary body-thalamus-limbic cortex system is now widely considered necessary for the establishment of a *recent memory trace*. In Korsakow's syndrome, characterized by a memory loss for recent events, lesions in the mamillothalamic system are common.[569, 570] However, recent experiments in rats[571, 572] failed to show disturbances of recent memory following such lesions, and the interesting suggestion was made that the system is important in determining the balance between repetitive stereotyped behavioural responses and the initiation of 'novel' exploratory responses under different conditions of environmental stimulation.

## THE MEDIAL GROUP OF NUCLEI

This consists of the large *nucleus medialis dorsalis* (MD) and a series of smaller nuclei (*parafascicularis, submedius, paracentralis* and *centralis lateralis*)—the connexions and significance of the latter are uncertain in man and will not be pursued further here.

The *nucleus medialis dorsalis* presents a rostral magnocellular part and a caudolateral parvocellular part, and is considered to interconnect with virtually all the other groups of thalamic nuclei. It receives, in certain regions, fibre connexions from the amygdaloid complex of nuclei (p. 936) and the piriform cortex, and establishes two-way connexions, thalamostriate and striato-thalamic, with parts of the corpus striatum (p. 978), but the precise regions of the latter involved are still rather uncertain.

The most widely described connexions of the nucleus medialis dorsalis of the thalamus are with the hypothalamic nuclei and with the cerebral cortex of the frontal lobe. The two-way connexions with the hypothalamic nuclei are thought to run in the *periventricular system* of fibres, which are fine myelinated or nonmyelinated fibres and which pursue vertical or oblique courses immediately deep to the ependymal side wall of the third ventricle, where they are intermingled with patches of periventricular grey matter. Some of the periventricular pathways may be polysynaptic, and the system is often described as consisting of a cranio-caudal series of fascicles which connect different parts of the medial thalamus with the preoptic, tuberoinfundibular and mamillary parts of the hypothalamus respectively (p. 907). The most caudal fascicles continue into the *dorsal longitudinal fasciculus* of the periaqueductal grey matter of the midbrain. It should be noted, however, that not all investigators regard the

[566] J. Szentágothai, in: *The Neurosciences, Second Study Program,* eds. F. O. Schmitt, G. C. Quarton, T. Melnechuk and G. Adelman, Rockefeller University Press, New York, 1970.
[567] H. J. Ralston and M. N. Hernan, *Brain Res.*, **14**, 1969.
[568] A. R. Lieberman and K. E. Webster, *Brain Res.*, **42**, 1972.
[569] G. A. Talland, *Deranged Memory: A Psychonomic Study of the Amnesic Syndrome,* Academic Press, N.Y., 1965.
[570] J. Barbizet, *J. Neurol. Neurosurg. Psychiat.*, **26**, 1963.
[571] E. E. Krieckhaus, *Acta Biol. exp., Vars.*, **27**, 1967.
[572] E. E. Krieckhaus and D. Randall, *Brain*, **91**, 1968.

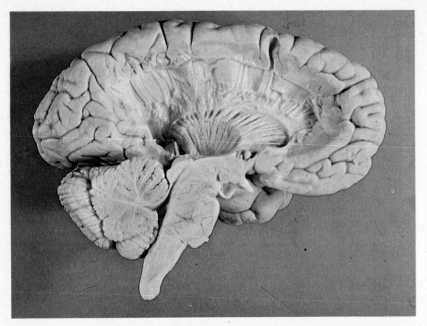

**7.99** After median sagittal section of the brain, the left cerebral hemisphere has been dissected from its *medial* aspect to display the fibre bundles of the corona radiata and internal capsule. This entailed the removal of the cingulate gyrus and subjacent white matter, much of the paramedian corpus callosum and fornix, the dorsal thalamus, and the head and body of the caudate nucleus. The oval depression previously occupied by the dorsal thalamus can clearly be seen within the curved depression left after removal of the caudate nucleus. (Dissection by Dr. Andrew Seal, Dept. of Anatomy, Guy's Hospital Medical School.)

existence of thalamohypothalamic connexions in the periventricular system as proven.[573, 574]

Profuse thalamocortical and corticothalamic connexions exist between the nucleus dorsalis medialis and almost the whole of the prefrontal cortex of the frontal lobe of the cerebral hemisphere which lies cranial to cortical areas 6 and 32 (p. 958). These radiations show an orderly topographic arrangement, specific regions of the nucleus connecting with specific cortical areas.

Clearly the medial part of the thalamus is a region of great functional significance, as evidenced by the wealth and complexity of its interconnexions; but equally it is impossible to attach simple functional labels to such a region of the nervous system. It probably provides mechanisms for the integration of a great variety of information channels, olfactory, visceral and somatic, by the convergence of multiple paths via the hypothalamus, amygdaloid complex, piriform cortex, corpus striatum and prefrontal cortex, and in turn has an output which can affect these and many other regions of the nervous system.

Stimulation of the dorsomedial thalamic nucleus in monkeys elicits movement patterns even after ablation of cortical motor areas, but the patterns disappear on ablation of the corpus striatum. Stimulation, disease or surgical ablation of the nucleus in man results in complex changes in motivational drive, the ability to solve problems and in the consciousness level, general 'personality' and subjective feeling states or 'affective tone' of the individual. The effects of ablation parallel in many ways the results of prefrontal lobotomy.

## THE VENTRAL GROUP OF NUCLEI

The ventral thalamic group form a craniocaudal sequence of three main nuclei: *ventralis anterior* (VA), *ventralis intermedius* (VI) and *ventralis posterior* (VP). (Many workers use the term ventralis lateralis (VL) rather than

the official term ventralis intermedius.) The *nucleus ventralis posterior* can be further subdivided into the important nuclei *ventralis posterior lateralis* (VPL) and *ventralis posterior medialis* (VPM), together with smaller and less well-understood nuclei which are inferior and oral in position.

The connexions of the main nuclei in this group include some intrinsic ones with adjacent thalamic nuclei such as the centrum medianum and pulvinar (*vide infra*), and also with neighbouring centres in the subthalamus and corpus striatum. However, by far the most prominent connexions of these nuclei are with the large ascending sensory systems, the medial, spinal and trigeminal lemnisci, and gustatory pathways, and also two-way links with the cerebral cortex. The origin, course and constitution of these ascending systems has already been described. The VPL receives the terminals of the medial and spinal lemnisci, whilst the VPM receives the trigeminal and gustatory pathways. (The cells receiving trigeminal terminals are sometimes called the *arcuate* or *semilunar nucleus*, whilst the gustatory fibres are sometimes held to end in an *accessory arcuate nucleus*.) Much research has been directed towards an understanding of the structural and functional localization and the types of interaction which occur during impulse transmission through these thalamic nuclei.

Briefly, there is an overall somatotopic pattern in the ascending pathways, in the nuclei themselves and in their connexions with the cerebral cortex. Both medial lemniscal and spinothalamic fibres from caudal body segments (i.e. from the nucleus gracilis in the case of medial lemniscal fibres) end in the lateral zone of the VPL, while fibres from successively more cranial body segments end in more medially placed zones in the nucleus. Still more medially placed is the VPM, which receives the trigeminothalamic fibres conducting information from the face and head, whilst most medial are the solitariothalamic gustatory fibres from the nucleus of the solitary tract. Other authors have emphasized that whilst such a lateromedial localization undoubtedly exists, the various tracts are not simply superimposed but end in different craniocaudal regions. The lateral spinothalamic tract has been described as ending in the caudal nuclear regions followed by the medial lemniscal and anterior spinothalamic fibres, while the trigeminothalamic fibres end in a craniomedial position.

The terminations of medial lemniscal and spinothalamic tract fibres show further contrasting features. The lemniscal fibres are wholly crossed, originating exclusively in the gracile and cuneate nuclei of the opposite side and their terminals are confined to the VPL. Whilst the majority of the spinothalamic fibres are also crossed, an appreciable number ascend on the same side and terminate in the ipsilateral thalamus. Further, although many spinothalamic terminals occur in the VPL, others proceed to a number of alternative destinations, including restricted parts of the medial geniculate nucleus, a small suprageniculate nucleus and various 'non-specific' thalamic nuclei—these are sometimes called the posterior (PO) group of terminals.[575] The latter may receive the terminals of high threshold spinal cord neurons which transmit nociceptive information (p. 833). Studies of the fine morphology of ascending tract terminals in the VPL have been carried out with the Golgi technique.[576] Spinothalamic and

[573] J. Szentágothai, B. Flerkó, B. Mess and B. Halász, *Hypothalamic Control of the Anterior Pituitary*, 2nd ed., Akadémiai Kiadó, Budapest. 1968.

[574] G. Raisman, *Br. med. Bull.*, **22**, 1966.

[575] G. F. Poggio and V. B. Mountcastle, *Bull. Johns Hopkins Hosp.*, **106**, 1960; *J. Neurophysiol.*, **26**, 1963.

[576] M. E. Scheibel and A. B. Scheibel, in: *The Thalamus*, eds. D. P. Purpura and M. D. Yahr, Columbia University Press, N.Y., London. 1966.

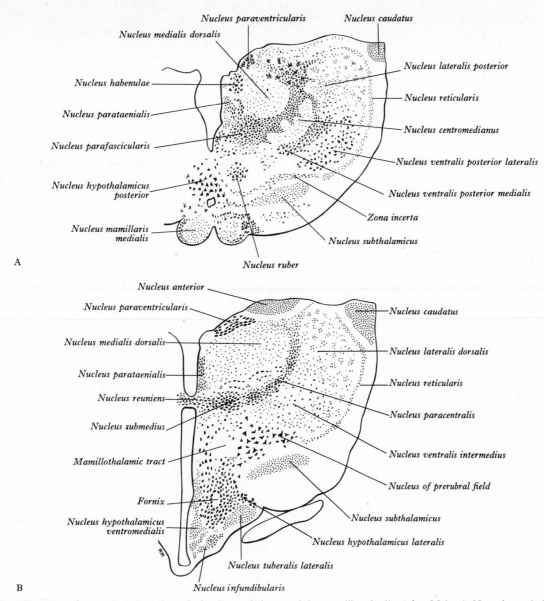

Nucleus paraventricularis
Nucleus caudatus
Nucleus medialis dorsalis
Nucleus lateralis posterior
Nucleus habenulae
Nucleus reticularis
Nucleus parataenialis
Nucleus centromedianus
Nucleus parafascicularis
Nucleus ventralis posterior lateralis
Nucleus ventralis posterior medialis
Nucleus hypothalamicus posterior
Zona incerta
Nucleus mamillaris medialis
Nucleus subthalamicus
A
Nucleus ruber

Nucleus anterior
Nucleus paraventricularis
Nucleus caudatus
Nucleus medialis dorsalis
Nucleus lateralis dorsalis
Nucleus parataenialis
Nucleus reticularis
Nucleus reuniens
Nucleus paracentralis
Nucleus submedius
Nucleus ventralis intermedius
Mamillothalamic tract
Nucleus of prerubral field
Fornix
Nucleus subthalamicus
Nucleus hypothalamicus ventromedialis
Nucleus hypothalamicus lateralis
Nucleus tuberalis lateralis
B
Nucleus infundibularis

7.100 A and B   Drawings of coronal sections through the diencephalon, stained with the method of Nissl to show the main nuclear aggregations of nerve cell somata. A   at the level of the tuber cinereum; B   at the level of the mamillary bodies (after Malone). Note the variations in cell size, shape and packing density, which characterize the nuclear masses of the dorsal thalamus, subthalamus and hypothalamus at these levels.

reticulothalamic terminals form diffuse interweaving networks, medial lemniscal fibres end as small cone-shaped bushy terminals arranged in regular laminae, whilst corticothalamic fibres have terminal arborizations confined to narrow disc-shaped 'sheets' of tissue which encompass the territories of many lemniscal fibres. Ultrastructural studies have demonstrated the presence of small local interneurons within the VPL, whilst others have started to explore the detailed synaptology of the nucleus [577, 578] (see p. 895). Unit recordings have been taken with microelectrodes inserted into cells of the VPL during medial lemniscal and spinothalamic tract activity in the monkey, by a number of investigators, and also in man, before the placing of stereotactic lesions in the thalamus for various types of locomotor disease. In the monkey, units responding to lemniscal activity retained many of the features described previously for the cells of the gracile and cuneate nuclei. The VPL cells were in this case highly specific for both the type of stimulus and the bodily site of origin. Units responded to contralateral stimulation which consisted of either mechanical distortion of the skin or hairs, or joint movement, or static joint position, or sinusoidal tissue vibration, but never to two of these varieties. Their receptive fields were small

and sharply localized, the smallest being recorded by stimulation of the terminal segments of the limbs. Units responding to spinothalamic tract activity in general showed rather larger receptive fields, and whilst some were 'modality specific' others showed interaction due to convergence of impulses from different types of stimulus pattern (p. 834). Impulse transmission in the VPL is now shown to be a most complicated series of events. Many of the units show the phenomenon of lateral inhibition or 'inhibitory surround' discussed previously (p. 751) which greatly enhances their discriminative value. Furthermore, transmission in the nucleus may be modulated by activity in descending corticothalamic fibres and in those which converge on the nucleus from other thalamic and extrathalamic sources. In this regard physiological studies have demonstrated that both presynaptic and postsynaptic inhibitory and facilitatory effects occur in the nucleus. [578, 579]

[577] T. Tömböl, *Brain Res.*, **3**, 1967.
[578] P. Andersen, J. C. Eccles and T. A. Sears, *J. Physiol., Lond.*, **174**, 1964.
[579] P. Andersen, C. McC. Brooks, J. C. Eccles and T. A. Sears, *J Physiol., Lond.*, **174**, 1964.

The recordings made in the nucleus ventralis posterior lateralis of the human thalamus, although necessarily more restricted in scope, substantially support the findings concerning somatotopic localization, and modality specificity of units demonstrated in the monkey. Furthermore, localized stimulation of the nucleus in conscious subjects evoked sharply circumscribed sensations described as 'tingling', 'numbness', etc. on the opposite side of the body.

The main thalamocortical radiations from the VPL and VPM proceed through the posterior limb of the internal capsule to the primary somatic sensory areas of the cerebral cortex—the postcentral gyrus which includes cortical areas 1, 2 and 3 (p. 958). Throughout this radiation the precise somatotopic organization of the nuclei of origin is preserved. The same cortical areas project corticothalamic fibres back to the nuclei. Unfortunately, the thalamic projections to the secondary somatic sensory areas cannot yet be regarded as settled.

*The nucleus ventralis intermedius* (VI, or nucleus ventralis lateralis, VL, of many authors) has been less extensively investigated. It establishes connexions with adjacent thalamic nuclei but its main sources of input are from the contralateral nucleus dentatus of the cerebellum via the dentatothalamic tract and rubrothalamic fibres of the ipsilateral red nucleus (pp. 862, 884). It also receives some fascicles from the globose and emboliform nuclei of the cerebellum and from the globus pallidus. These various afferents are constituents of the *thalamic fasciculus* (*see* p. 904).

The main projection from the VI is somatotopically arranged and passes through the internal capsule to reach the motor and premotor regions of the cerebral cortex (areas 4 and 6).

The *nucleus ventralis anterior* (VA) has a complex organization and has come into greater prominence in recent research, together with the nucleus ventralis intermedius, because of the therapeutic placing of destructive lesions in or near these nuclei in various types of locomotor disorder.

The nucleus ventralis anterior has numerous interconnexions with other thalamic nuclei, but in particular with the nucleus centromedianus (*vide infra*), the other intralaminar nuclei, the nuclei of the midline, and the reticular thalamic nucleus, i.e. all the so-called 'non-specific' thalamic nuclei. In addition the VA receives an input from the midbrain reticular formation and profuse connexions from the globus pallidus through the *thalamic fasciculus* (*see* p. 904), together with the most cranial of the dentatothalamic fibres of the superior cerebellar peduncle. Thalamocortical fibres radiate from the VA to the premotor cortex (area 6), to a lesser extent to the motor cortex (area 4), and fibres to restricted regions of the insular cortex have also been described. In turn corticothalamic fibres leave areas 6 and 4 and converge upon the VA. (For a detailed Golgi study of the nucleus see footnote reference [580].)

Thus, the VA is an important focal centre through which the corpus striatum, the ascending reticular formation and non-specific thalamic nuclei, and to a lesser degree the cerebellum, are able to exert a powerful effect on the activities of the motor and premotor cortices and probably on many other regions of the cortex as well. To what degree the information flowing in the various channels which converge on the VA is integrated, before onward transmission to the cortex, is not clear.

Views concerning the possible functional significance of the VA are rapidly changing. Some relationship to the motor control systems is evident—stimulation of the nucleus increases Parkinsonian rigidity and tremor, whilst ablation of the nucleus (often with, however, some

surrounding tissue) may be effective in reducing or abolishing the tremor. In experimental animals, stimulation of the caudate nucleus is followed by a reduced level of activity in both VL and VA and their related areas of cerebral cortex, and this is accompanied by a loss of learned behavioural responses. It should also be noted that stimulation of the VA causes desynchronization of the electroencephalogram, and increasingly the nucleus is regarded as an important link in the final stages of the 'ascending activating system' (see also p. 890).

## THE LATERAL GROUP OF NUCLEI

This group is commonly divided craniocaudally into three —the *nuclei lateralis dorsalis* (LD), *lateralis posterior* (LP), and most caudally the greatly expanded *pulvinar*, which occupies almost the whole of the caudal quarter of the thalamus. The pulvinar is a late phylogenetic development, only becoming prominent in the higher mammals and increasingly so in the primates, including mankind. It is sometimes divided into three or more subregions but these will not be considered separately here.

The three nuclei of the lateral group are all presumed to have interconnexions with other thalamic nuclei, but the details are not yet clear. Additionally, the pulvinar has been described as in receipt of connexions from the lateral geniculate nucleus, possibly the medial geniculate nucleus and amygdaloid complex, and some investigators have described direct projections from the optic tract, but the latter have not been substantiated. Whilst numerous connexions with such subcortical centres seem probable, further evidences must be awaited before definite conclusions are possible.

The best established connexions of the lateral group are two-way links with specific regions of the cerebral cortex, the LD with inferior parietal and posterior cingulate regions, LP with much of the parietal cortex behind the postcentral gyrus, whilst the pulvinar interconnects with wide areas of the parietal, occipital and temporal lobe cortices.

## THE 'NON-SPECIFIC' GROUPS OF THALAMIC NUCLEI

Since the recognition nearly a quarter of a century ago[581] that stimulation or ablation of different regions of the brainstem reticular formation was followed by widespread changes in the state of synchronization or desynchronization of electroencephalograms, attention has been focused upon possible cranially directed pathways from the reticular formation to the cerebral cortex. The suggestion soon followed that the brainstem reticular centres established profuse connexions with a series of thalamic nuclei from which proceeded a widespread *diffuse thalamocortical radiation* to virtually all parts of the cerebral cortex. Further, since stimulation of a number of these nuclei caused extensive, bilateral changes in cortical electrical activity, which were characterized by a slow onset and then a progressive build-up to a maximum, followed by fluctuations in level (recruitment)—the responses, and the nuclei themselves were called *non-specific*. It was widely assumed that the latter effects provided a background level of preparedness of the cortex which is necessary for the effective reception of the rapid, sharply localized ipsilateral, impulse patterns stemming from the larger *specific relay nuclei*, which have precise somatotopically organized thalamocortical and corticothalamic

[580] M. E. Scheibel and A. B. Scheibel, *Brain Res.*, 1, 1966.
[581] G. Moruzzi and H. W. Magoun, *Electroenceph. clin. Neurophysiol.*, 1, 1949.

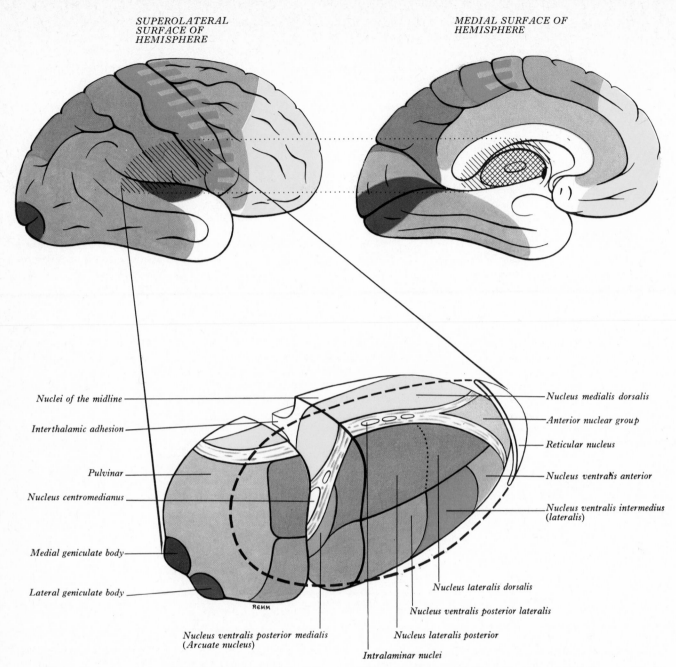

SUPEROLATERAL
SURFACE OF
HEMISPHERE

MEDIAL SURFACE OF
HEMISPHERE

Nuclei of the midline

Interthalamic adhesion

Pulvinar

Nucleus centromedianus

Medial geniculate body

Lateral geniculate body

REMM

Nucleus medialis dorsalis

Anterior nuclear group

Reticular nucleus

Nucleus ventralis anterior

Nucleus ventralis intermedius
(lateralis)

Nucleus lateralis dorsalis

Nucleus ventralis posterior lateralis

Nucleus lateralis posterior

Nucleus ventralis posterior medialis
(Arcuate nucleus)

Intralaminar nuclei

**7.101** The main nuclear masses of the dorsal thalamus (below) have been labelled and colour coded, and the same colours have been used to indicate the areas of cerebral neocortex interconnected with these nuclei. The lack of colour in the centromedian, intralaminar and reticular nuclei, and in restricted areas of the frontal and temporal lobes are *not* related to the colour code. The boundaries of the coloured cortical zones may well need revision in the future as experimental and pathological data accumulate.

connexions. A large research literature has accumulated around this subject and, whilst many of the general concepts remain valid today, it is increasingly evident that the reticulocortical pathways involved are multiple and much more complex than originally envisaged, some involving extrathalamic pathways through the ventral diencephalon. Further, there is such extensive interaction between specific and non-specific parts of the thalamus that whilst the terms retain a general usefulness, and are so widely used that they will be retained here, it must not be assumed that they imply a sharp, separable distinction between two aspects of thalamic organization and function.

The non-specific nuclear groups are usually considered to include the intralaminar nuclei, the nuclei of the midline, and the reticular nucleus of the thalamus.

### The Reticular Nucleus of the Thalamus

This is a thin curved sheet of cells situated between the white matter of the external medullary lamina and that of the posterior limb of the internal capsule. Accordingly, all the corticothalamic and thalamocortical fibres which run in the internal capsule pass through the territory of the nucleus.

The reticular nucleus has for long been regarded as an important final link in the diffuse thalamocortical radiation mentioned above, because of widespread effects on cortical activity which follow stimulation of the nucleus, and the nuclear degeneration which follows experimental resection of the cerebral cortex. However, more recent studies using the Golgi technique[579] have shown that the axons of the cells in this nucleus run *caudally*, giving off a series of collateral branches to many of the thalamic nuclei and the midbrain reticular formation. The whole of the cerebral cortex projects in an orderly manner on to the reticular nucleus of the thalamus,[582] and the degeneration which follows cortical resection is now thought to be

[582] J. B. Carman, W. M. Cowan and T. P. S. Powell, *J. Anat.*, **98**, 1964.

transneuronal and not retrograde in type.[583] Other afferents to the nucleus are from the brainstem reticular formation, and the globus pallidus. Thus, afferents converge on the reticular nucleus from these various sources and its output is mainly to other thalamic nuclei both specific and non-specific.

The intralaminar nuclei include a number of small aggregations of grey matter (the *nuclei paracentralis*, *centralis lateralis*, and *limitans*) and the much larger *nucleus centromedianus* (*vide infra*).

**The nuclei of the midline** form a complex and well-developed series in many mammals but are often poorly developed in man. Small but recognizable groups are sometimes to be found near the taenia thalami, the interthalamic adhesion when present, and others scattered in the periventricular wall. They will not be named and described individually here.

Because of their topography the non-specific nuclei are extremely difficult to investigate both anatomically and physiologically. In general, they are thought to receive the terminals of ascending fibres from the brainstem reticular formation, while some establish connexions with the corpus striatum, cerebellum, spinothalamic tracts, the hypothalamus, and many intrathalamic connexions with specific and non-specific nuclei on both sides of the midline. The most cranial of the non-specific nuclei project to the cerebral cortex including the phylogenetically older prepiriform and entorhinal cortices together with the parieto-occipital and frontal regions of the neocortex. Clearly, much remains to be learned about the arrangement connexions and significance of these nuclei.

**The nucleus centromedianus**, which is embedded in the white matter of the internal medullary lamina, only becomes a prominent structure in primates, and it is an easily recognized landmark in the human thalamus. Despite intensive investigation there has been much disagreement concerning its status and connexions.

However, the majority of investigators are now agreed that it is not connected with the cerebral cortex. A variety of ascending pathways have been described as ending partly in this nucleus; these include collaterals or terminals from a small proportion of the fibres of the spinal, medial and trigeminal lemnisci, ascending reticulothalamic fibres, and a contribution from the superior cerebellar peduncle. However, its main connexions are with parts of the corpus striatum, some of which are topically organized, and other profuse interconnexions with the remaining non-specific nuclei on both sides of the midline, and also with some 'specific' nuclei, particularly the nucleus ventralis anterior.

## SUMMARY

Clearly, the dorsal thalamus is a region of immense structural complexity and of outstanding functional significance, but despite a voluminous research literature we still possess only the most rudimentary concepts of its mode of functioning.

Most prominent is the large number of information channels which *converge* upon the thalamus where, through the profuse intrathalamic connexions, many are *integrated*, i.e. they interact, and the resulting information patterns, now of much greater range and complexity, *diverge* to many destinations. In this manner, the thalamus is importantly involved in the activities of *all* the major subregions of the central nervous system. Thus, all the main sensory systems (with the exception of the olfactory pathways), most regions of the cerebral cortex, the corpus striatum, cerebellum, hypothalamus, subthalamus and brainstem reticular formation all send fibre systems which converge on various nuclei of the thalamus and metathalamus, and in turn, most of these cortical and subcortical centres receive reciprocal connexions from the thalamus.

The thalamus is not essential for olfactory perception, which occurs in the primary and secondary olfactory cortical areas (p. 936), but higher order olfactory information, after integration with other channels, is transmitted to the thalamus from the amygdaloid complex, the piriform lobe, and the hippocampus via the mamillary body.

The specific relay nuclei, including the geniculate bodies, receive the various major sensory tracts where, often after interaction with other channels, somatotopically organized thalamocortical radiations pass to the different sensory receiving areas of the cerebral cortex. Reference has already been made to the complex transformations in the flow of information which occur during transmission through these nuclei. The latter include interaction between parallel and converging channels, pre- and post-synaptic facilitatory and inhibitory effects, the phenomenon of inhibitory 'surround' with neural sharpening, and the modulation of transmission which follows activity in the corticothalamic and other fibre systems which converge upon the nucleus in question. Some of the thalamocortical fibres preserve a high degree of specificity with respect to single modalities and their site of origin in the periphery, whilst others transmit more complex orders of information derived from the convergence of a number of channels. Ablation of the thalamocortical radiations to the somatosensory cortex results in a loss or diminution of the ability to localize a tactile stimulus, and an impairment of two-point discrimination, and the appreciation of texture, weight and shape of an object, and the assessment of the position or movement pattern of a bodily segment. Nevertheless, knowledge that contact with an object has occurred, and a rough, poorly localized awareness of pain-evoking and thermal stimuli, still occurs, provided the thalamic mechanisms are intact. Whilst it is clear that some form of pain appreciation can occur after loss of the cerebral cortex, the degree to which the cortex is involved in an intact nervous system has still not been solved.[584] Disease in the lateral or central thalamus is sometimes followed by sudden apparently 'spontaneous' attacks of an unexplained type of *thalamic pain*. Paradoxically, in addition to spinal, medullary, or mesencephalic tractotomy as surgical measures for the relief of pain, selective thalamotomy with ablation of either the nucleus ventralis posterior and surrounding regions, or of the intralaminar nuclei including the nucleus centromedianus, has sometimes been effective in pain relief. In summary, therefore, it appears that the VPL and VPM, the so-called PO group (including areas of the medial geniculate, suprageniculate and intralaminar nuclei), the nucleus centromedianus, and probably the nucleus dorsalis medialis, are all involved in pain appreciation, but how they cooperate in this activity remains unclear.

The rich interconnexions of the nucleus dorsalis medialis with the frontal cortex, hypothalamus, and other specific and non-specific thalamic nuclei has already been described. It is generally regarded as the principal centre for the complex integration of visceral and somatic functions. Through its hypothalamic connexions it is importantly involved in a wide array of autonomic and endocrine activities. It appears to be concerned with the emotional content, subjective feeling states, and identification of 'self'; as mentioned, ablation or disease in the nucleus causes changes in personality, drive, intellectual

[583] J. E. Rose, *Res. Publs Ass. Res. nerv. ment. Dis.*, **30**, 1952.
[584] D. Albe-Fessard and J. Delacour, *J. Psychol. norm. path.*, **65**, 1968.

performance, indifference to pain, emotional level etc., which are similar in some respects to those following ablation of the frontal cortex.

The anterior group of thalamic nuclei integrates the complex flow of information along the mamillothalamic tract derived from many visceral pathways and the hypothalamus, with that from other thalamic nuclei and from the cingulate cortex, and the group has reciprocal connexions with these centres. These circuits are important in complex homeostatic mechanisms and are possibly involved in the establishment of recent memory, and in determining the balance between 'repetitive and stereotyped', or 'novel and exploratory' forms of behaviour.

The non-specific nuclear groups establish profuse interconnexions with each other and with the specific thalamic nuclei of both sides. They receive an input from many of the sensory pathways, the cerebellum and corpus striatum, and through their diffuse cortical projections they exert a powerful effect upon the background activity levels in wide areas of the cerebral cortex—the *arousal reactions*. The latter particularly affect the parietal, orbital, cingulate and occipital association areas of the cortex, the most marked responses being in the prefrontal areas.

The nuclei ventralis anterior and lateralis are important cell stations where outflows from the corpus striatum and cerebellum interact with those from other thalamic nuclei, and then project on to the motor and premotor cortices. They are important in locomotor control, and it should be recalled that the nucleus ventralis anterior shows features common to both specific and non-specific nuclei.

Finally, it must be re-emphasized that the activities of most of the major regions of cerebral cortex are in some measure under thalamic influence, whilst information from the cortex converges on to the majority of the thalamic nuclei.

## The Epithalamus—Pineal Body and Habenula

The epithalamic structures, as stated previously, occupy the caudal roof of the diencephalon together with adjacent areas on the side walls of the third ventricle (7.95). They include the right and left *habenular nuclei*, each situated deep to the floor of a *habenular trigone*, and each receives the termination of a complex fibre bundle, the *stria medullaris thalami*. The epithalamus also includes the midline *pineal body* or epiphysis cerebri, and the *habenular* and *posterior commissures*, which cross the midline in the cranial and caudal laminae of the pineal stalk. The pineal body is described on p. 137.

The *trigonum habenulae* is, as its name suggests, a small triangular surface depression on each side, situated cranial to the superior colliculus and medial to the pulvinar of the thalamus from which it is separated by the *sulcus habenulae*. The trigone is bounded craniomedially by the caudal end of the ridge occupied by the stria medullaris thalami and by the pineal stalk.

**The habenular nucleus**, sometimes regarded as consisting of medial and lateral parts, is a station on some of the olfactory reflex pathways. A number of connexions have been described but their complete pattern is still uncertain. Many afferents to the nucleus run in the *stria medullaris thalami* which is formed near the anterior pole of the thalamus. These include connexions from the amygdaloid complex of nuclei via the stria terminalis (p. 937), and from the hippocampal formation via the fornix (p. 942). Other components of the stria are from the olfactory tubercle, anterior perforated substance, the

preoptic and septal areas and various hypothalamic nuclei. Direct tectohabenular fibres from the superior colliculi have been described.

The stria medullaris courses across the superior part of the medial surface of the thalamus, skirts the medial margin of the trigonum habenulae, and many of the fibres end in the ipsilateral nucleus habenulae. Others, however, cross the midline in the cranial leaflet of the pineal stalk, interlacing with their fellows to form the *habenular commissure*, so reaching the contralateral habenular nucleus. Some of the fibres which also follow this route are truly commissural and interconnect the amygdaloid complexes and the hippocampal cortices of the two sides; crossed tectohabenular fibres accompany them in the commissure.

Thus, although the habenulae are relatively small in man, they provide a nodal point for the integration of a considerable variety of olfactory, visceral and somatic afferent pathways.

The main outflow paths from the habenular nuclei pass to the interpeduncular nucleus, the nucleus medialis dorsalis of the thalamus, the tectum, and to the reticular formation of the midbrain tegmentum. The largest of these paths constitutes the *habenulopeduncular tract*—often known as the *fasciculus retroflexus* (of Meynert) (7.103). The latter courses cranioventrally, skirts the caudal zone of the nucleus medialis dorsalis of the thalamus, and then passes through the craniomedial part of the red nucleus to reach the interpeduncular nucleus from which fibres relay to the midbrain reticular formation. From these centres, descending fibres such as the tectotegmentospinal tracts and the dorsal longitudinal fasciculi ultimately connect with the autonomic preganglionic centres through which control of salivation, gastric and intestinal secretory activity and motility are effected, and others pass to the motor centres for the muscles concerned in mastication and swallowing. It should also be noted that ablation of the habenular complexes in experimental animals leads to extensive changes in metabolism, endocrine regulation and thermo-regulation.[585]

**The posterior commissure** is a complex fibre bundle which crosses the midline in the caudal lamina of the pineal stalk. Its size is relatively reduced in primates and its fibre constitution is imperfectly known in man. It acquires its myelin sheaths early, and some estimates of the number of fibres in different specimens of the commissure have been made.[586] Various nuclei are associated with the commissure—small groups scattered along its length and sometimes called the *interstitial nuclei of the posterior commissure*, accumulations in the periventricular grey matter which constitute *dorsal nuclei of the posterior commissure*, the *nucleus of Darkschewitsch* in the cranial part of the periaqueductal grey matter, and the *interstitial nucleus* (of Cajal) situated near the rostral end of the oculomotor nucleus and closely linked with the medial longitudinal fasciculus (p. 885). Fibres from all these nuclei, and continuations from the medial longitudinal fasciculus all cross the midline in the posterior commissure. Other centres which contribute fibres to the commissure include the posterior thalamic nuclei, the pretectal nuclei, the superior colliculi, and connexions between the tectum and habenular nuclei. The precise destinations and functional significances of many of these bundles in the human brain are incompletely understood and will not be discussed further here.

Caudal to the commissure, the ependymal cells lining the dorsal aspect of the cerebral aqueduct are specialized,

[585] J. Szentágothai, B. Flerkó, B. Mess and B. Halász, *Hypothalamic Control of the Anterior Pituitary*, Akadémiai Kiadó, Budapest. 1962.
[586] J. Tomasch and A. J. Malpass, *Anat. Rec.*, **130**, 1958.

being tall, columnar and ciliated, with a granular basophilic cytoplasm and characteristic histochemical reactions. This patch of cells, which are probably secretory, with their products passing into the cerebrospinal fluid, is sometimes termed the *subcommissural organ*.[587, 588]

## The Ventral Thalamus or Subthalamus

As mentioned previously, the pars ventralis diencephali, which lies caudoventral to the hypothalamic sulcus, may be divided on phylogenetic, ontogenetic and functional grounds into a *hypothalamus* and a *ventral thalamus* or *subthalamus*. The hypothalamus, which includes the structures forming the floor of the third ventricle as far caudally and including the mamillary bodies, together with the structures embedded in the cranioventral side wall of the ventricle, will be described in a later section. The remainder of the pars ventralis diencephali constitutes the subthalamus. It merges caudally with the tegmentum of the midbrain, and the cranial extensions of the substantia nigra and red nucleus project into the caudal subthalamus, whilst important fibre tracts ascend and descend between the two regions (7.103). Dorsally, the subthalamus adjoins the ventral nuclei of the dorsal thalamus, whilst craniomedially it is bounded by the various subdivisions of the hypothalamus (7.100). Ventrolaterally and directly laterally, the subthalamus is in contact with the expanding and rotating junctional zone where the cerebral peduncle merges into the internal capsule; and the latter separates the subthalamus from the medial aspect of the globus pallidus of the lentiform nucleus.

**The main aggregations of nerve cells** in the subthalamus are: (1) the cranial end of the red nucleus; (2) the cranial end of the substantia nigra; (3) the nucleus subthalamicus; (4) the zona incerta; (5) the nucleus of the prerubral or tegmental field; and (6) the entopeduncular nucleus or nucleus of the ansa lenticularis.

**The main tracts of nerve fibres** in the subthalamus are: (1) the cranial ends of the medial, spinal and trigeminal lemnisci and the solitariothalamic tract, as they approach their terminations in the thalamic nuclei; (2) the dentatothalamic tract from the opposite superior cerebellar peduncle accompanied by ipsilateral rubrothalamic fibres; (3) the fasciculus retroflexus; (4) the fasciculus lenticularis; (5) the fasciculus subthalamicus; (6) the ansa lenticularis; (7) the fibre aggregates of the prerubral field (the H field of Forel); (8) the continuation of the fasciculus lenticularis (in the $H_2$ field of Forel); and (9) the fasciculus thalamicus (the $H_1$ field of Forel).

The topographical neuroanatomy of the subthalamus is rather complex and is best understood by reference to three-dimensional models and closely graded series of coronal and parasagittal sections in the practical laboratory; a parallel study of the corpus striatum (p. 976) from which a number of the prominent subthalamic tracts are derived is also helpful. Illustration 7.102 may assist with the complicated terminology of the region, but the topography can only be appreciated in part from such a two-dimensional diagram.

As the cranial ends of the red nucleus and the substantia nigra pass into the caudal part of the subthalamus they gradually diminish in cross-sectional area to terminate a little caudal to the mamillary bodies. The changing relationship of the lemnisci to the red nucleus and substantia nigra as they ascend through the midbrain has already been described. The leminiscal fibres enter the subthalamus largely lateral to the red nucleus, and as they continue to ascend they pass on to the dorsal aspect of the nucleus to reach the inferior surface of the nucleus

ventralis posterior of the thalamus, in which the majority of their fibres terminate. Dentatothalamic and rubrothalamic fibres run in company with pallidothalamic fibres and form part of the thalamic fasciculus, which passes cranial to the termination of the lemnisci noted above to distribute largely to the nuclei ventralis intermedius and anterior of the thalamus (see pp. 898, 901, and below for further description).

**The nucleus subthalamicus** does not occur in submammalian forms, is small in most mammalian groups, and is prominent only in primates. In man the nucleus is an aggregation of medium to fairly large multipolar neurons and classically described as of the general shape of a biconvex lens when seen in coronal section. It lies in the caudal subthalamus, but extends into the junctional zone of subthalamus and midbrain tegmentum, where it lies dorsolateral to the cranial end of the substantia nigra and lateral to the cranial margin of the red nucleus. The subthalamic nucleus is closely related to the medial aspect of the internal capsule, which separates it from the globus pallidus of the corpus striatum. Medially, the subthalamic nucleus abuts on the hypothalamic region, whilst dorsally it is separated from the ventral nuclei of the thalamus by a thin strip of grey matter, the zona incerta, which is sandwiched between complex fibre bundles, the continuation of the fasciculus lenticularis, and the thalamic fasciculus (7.102, and see below).

The connexions of the nucleus subthalamicus are numerous, some being well established, whilst considerable uncertainty attaches to the remainder. The principal connexions are with the corpus striatum; two-way fibre systems pass by a number of routes between the globus pallidus and the subthalamic nucleus. Interconnexions with the putamen and caudate nucleus have also been described but are less well documented. The other connexions reported include ones with the opposite subthalamic nucleus and globus pallidus, and with the homolateral red nucleus, substantia nigra, the reticular formation of the midbrain tegmentum, the zona incerta and other small nuclei in the subthalamus, various hypothalamic and thalamic nuclei, and possibly with regions of the cerebral cortex.

The subthalamic nucleus is clearly an important site for the integration of a number of motor control centres, but particularly through its connexions with the corpus striatum and midbrain tegmentum. Relatively discrete lesions of one subthalamic nucleus in man result in the condition of *hemiballismus*, with uncontrollable, violent, torsional movements, choreiform in type, affecting the contralateral side of the body. The movements, which often continue for long periods, usually affect the proximal musculature of one or both limbs and may mimic throwing or kicking; but facial and trunk muscles may also be involved, though with a much lower incidence. Interestingly, unlike most of the other *dyskinesias*, hemiballismus can be reproduced in the experimental animal; in the monkey the condition follows surgical ablation of at least one-quarter of the subthalamic nucleus, provided the surrounding fibre systems associated with the globus pallidus are preserved intact. The hemiballismus so generated is unaffected by ablation of the rubrospinal, vestibulospinal and reticulospinal tracts, or area 6 of the cerebral cortex, but the condition *is* abolished by ablation of the globus pallidus or its outflow tracts, the nucleus ventralis anterior of the thalamus, area 4 of the cerebral cortex or the corticospinal tract. It is assumed, therefore, that the subthalamic nucleus exerts an inhibitory form of control on the globus pallidus, and therefore on its main outflow

[587] G. B. Wislocki and E. Leduc, *J. comp. Neurol.*, **97**, 1953.
[588] M. L. F. Keene and E. E. Hewer, *J. Anat.*, **69**, 1935.

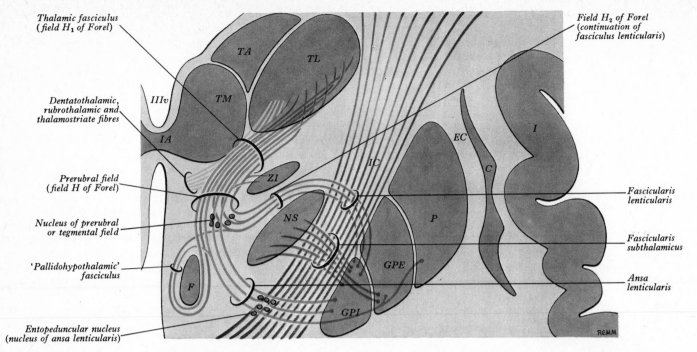

**7.102** A diagram of the nuclear masses of grey matter and fibre tract systems associated with, or closely related topographically to, parts of the dorsal thalamus, subthalamus and globus pallidus. The information presented is compounded from a series of closely spaced coronal sections through this region, attempts being made to include what are essentially three-dimensional structures in a two-dimensional diagram; it must be emphasized that all the structures shown would not appear on the same single coronal section. In addition to the features which are fully labelled, the significance of the letters is as follows: TM—medial nuclear group of thalamus; TA—anterior nuclear group of thalamus; TL—lateral nuclear group of thalamus; IA—interthalamic adhesion; ZI—zona incerta; F—column of fornix; NS—nucleus subthalamicus; IC—internal capsule; GPI and GPE—internal and external parts of globus pallidus; P—putamen; EC—external capsule; C—claustrum; and I—cortex of insula.

pathway via the thalamus to the motor cortex, the principal origin of the crossed corticospinal tract.[589–594]

**The zona incerta** is a thin lamina of grey matter interspersed with fine fibre bundles which extends throughout most of the diencephalon a little ventral to the thalamus but separated from it by the fibres of the thalamic fasciculus (*vide infra*). Laterally the zone is continuous with the reticular nucleus of the thalamus, whilst ventrally it is in apposition with fibres of the fasciculus lenticularis (*vide infra*). Functionally associated with the zona incerta are scattered groups of neurons along its caudomedial border which constitute the *nucleus of the prerubral* or *tegmental field*, and other groups interspersed between the fibre bundles of the ansa lenticularis (*vide infra*), which some authorities regard as 'detached' parts of the globus pallidus and which constitute the *entopeduncular nucleus*. These various cell groups are to be regarded in the main as stations on discharge pathways from the globus pallidus to the reticular formation in the tegmentun of the midbrain, some of the descending fibres running with the central tegmental fasciculus as far as the inferior olivary complex of nuclei (p. 847). Additionally, fibres descending from the cerebral cortex to terminate in the zona incerta have been described, and these various subthalamic nuclear masses probably also interconnect with the main subthalamic nucleus, the intralaminar and ventral nuclei of the thalamus, and with the red nucleus. Much remains to be learned concerning their functional significance.

In addition to the termination of the lemniscal systems and that of the dentatothalamic and rubrothalamic tracts (p. 898), the subthalamus is characterized by a series of bundles of white fibres, often interspersed with small groups of neurons. The fibre constitution of these bundles and their topography is complex, and a number of rather confusing and sometimes conflicting terminologies have been proposed. One approach, adopted here, is to consider the various bundles in relation to the main fibre systems which flow out of the corpus striatum (their relationships

to that organ are further discussed on p. 978). The various fibre bundles derived in part from the putamen, but predominantly from the globus pallidus, appear at the surfaces of the latter, from which they diverge medially in a fan-shaped radiation. The dorsal and intermediate fibres of the fan intersect with the fibres of the internal capsule, whilst the ventral fibres curve around the caudoventral border of the capsule. Earlier investigators[595] termed the whole radiation the ansa lenticularis and considered it to consist of dorsal, intermediate and ventral divisions. The term ansa lenticularis is, however, now restricted to the ventral division, the intermediate division is termed the fasciculus subthalamicus, whilst the dorsal division is termed the fasciculus lenticularis (see 7.102 for an outline of these relationships).

**The fasciculus lenticularis** consists of the dorsal bundle of pallidofugal fibres which pass through the internal capsule, intersecting with its fibres, from lateral to medial side. They then course medially, closely related to the medial aspect of the internal capsule, and partly intermingled with the dorsal aspect of the subthalamic nucleus and the ventral aspect of the zona incerta; in this part of its course the fasciculus traverses what is sometimes called the $H_2$ field of Forel. Having reached the medial border of the zona incerta, the fibres of the fasciculus lenticularis meet and intermingle with the fibres of the ansa lenticularis, with the scattered cell groups of the nucleus of the prerubral field, and also with bundles of dentatothalamic and rubrothalamic fibres. This zone of

[589] J. R. Whittier and F. A. Mettler, *J. comp. Neurol.*, **90**, 1949.
[590] M. B. Carpenter, *Archs Neurol. Psychiat., Chicago*, **63**, 1950.
[591] M. B. Carpenter and G. M. Britten, *J. Neurophysiol.*, **21**, 1958.
[592] M. B. Carpenter, J. W. Correll and A. Hinman, *J. Neurophysiol.*, **23**, 1960.
[593] M. B. Carpenter and C. S. Carpenter, *J. comp. Neurol.*, **95**, 1951.
[594] M. B. Carpenter, J. R. Whittier and F. A. Mettler, *J. comp. Neurol.*, **92**, 1950.
[595] C. v. Monakow, *Arch. Psychiat. NervKrankh.*, **12**, 1882.

merging of diverse fibre pathways and associated cell groups is variously called the *prerubral, tegmental,* or *H field of Forel.*

**The ansa lenticularis** has a complex origin from both parts of the globus pallidus, the putamen and possibly other neighbouring centres; its fibres partly relay in scattered cell groups along its course—the *entopeduncular nucleus.* The fibres of the ansa curve medially around the ventral border of the internal capsule and then continue to curve dorsomedially until they meet and become admixed with the other fibre systems mentioned above in the prerubral field. A number of the fibres in both the fasciculus and ansa lenticularis synapse with cells in the nucleus subthalamicus, the nucleus of the prerubral field and the zona incerta, whilst the remainder continue in

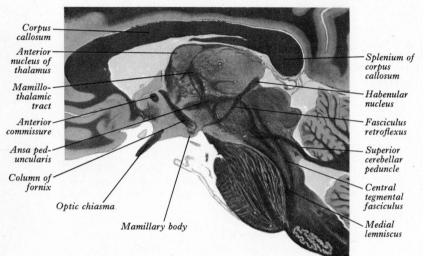

Corpus callosum
Anterior nucleus of thalamus
Mamillo-thalamic tract
Anterior commissure
Ansa peduncularis
Column of fornix
Optic chiasma
Mamillary body

Splenium of corpus callosum
Habenular nucleus
Fasciculus retroflexus
Superior cerebellar peduncle
Central tegmental fasciculus
Medial lemniscus

7.103 Parasagittal section of the brain passing through the right mamillary body, viewed from the left. Myelin stain. The fasciculus retroflexus is seen crossing the medial side of the red nucleus, which is surrounded by a capsule of white fibres derived chiefly from the superior peduncle. (After C. Foix and J. Nicolesco, *Anatomie cérébrale,* Paris. 1925.)

company with the other fibre bundles, and then loop laterally and cranially to reach a number of thalamic nuclei, particularly nuclei ventralis anterior, intermedius and centromedianus.

**The thalamic fasciculus** is the complex bundle of fibres which extends from the prerubral field, passing dorsal to, but also partly traversing, the zona incerta, and related dorsally to the ventral nuclear groups of the thalamus. It contains the continuation of the fasciculus and ansa lenticularis just described, dentatothalamic and rubrothalamic fibres, and, running in the opposite direction, bundles of thalamostriate fibres. Another name often used for the territory occupied by the thalamic fasciculus is the *H₁ field of Forel.*

**The 'pallidohypothalamic' fasciculus** is the name commonly given to a bundle of fibres which leaves the main pallidofugal system in the prerubral field and then pursues a curious course, curving ventromedially around the column of the fornix to approach the hypothalamus[596-598], where it was for long widely assumed to terminate in its dorsomedial nucleus. However, there is no conclusive evidence for a hypothalamic termination, and more recent experiments in the monkey[599] indicate that the bundle recurves yet again, passing laterally below the column of the fornix, and then dorsally to rejoin the main system of fibres in the H₁ field of Forel.

**The fasciculus subthalamicus** comprises the profuse two-way array of fibres which passes through the internal

capsule, interdigitating at right angles with its main fibre systems, to interconnect the nucleus subthalamicus with the globus pallidus, and to a lesser extent with the putamen.

Some of these connexions will be mentioned again in the description of the basal ganglia (p. 978).

## The Hypothalamus

The general position and extent of the hypothalamus has been considered previously (p. 891). In the present account it will be assumed to extend from the lamina terminalis to a vertical plane caudal to the mamillary bodies, and from the hypothalamic sulcus, to include the structures in the ventral side-wall and floor of the third ventricle. Strictly, the most cranial part of this region, the preoptic area, belongs to the telencephalon impar, but is included for functional reasons. *Lateral* to the hypothalamus lies the cranial part of the subthalamus, the internal capsule and the optic tract; *caudally* the hypothalamus abuts on the tegmental part of the subthalamus which is continuous caudally with the tegmentum of the midbrain; *dorsal* to the hypothalamus lie the various nuclei of the dorsal thalamus; *cranially* the optic chiasma, lamina terminalis and the anterior commissure separate the preoptic area from the precommissural septum, i.e. the continuation of the diagonal band of Broca into the paraterminal gyrus (p. 935), anterior to which lies the parolfactory gyrus. As mentioned previously, however, these topographical 'boundaries' are arbitrary, and functionally continuous systems cross many of them.

The structures which form the floor of the third ventricle extend to the free surface of the brain in the **interpeduncular fossa** (7.104) and consist, craniocaudally, of: (1) the optic chiasma; (2) the tuber cinereum with its eminences, and the stalk of the infundibulum; (3) the mamillary bodies; and (4) the posterior perforated substance which is not usually included in the hypothalamus, but is included here for convenience.

**The posterior perforated substance** is a small depressed area of grey matter which lies in the caudal part of the interval between the diverging crura cerebri. It is pierced by a number of small apertures which transmit the central branches of the posterior cerebral arteries. Deep to its floor lies the *interpeduncular nucleus,* a relatively small structure in man which is homologous with a much more extensive nuclear complex in submammalian forms. It receives the curiously looped terminals of the fibres of the fasciculus retroflexus (p. 901) of both sides, and establishes further connexions with the reticular formation of the midbrain tegmentum and with the mamillary bodies.

**The mamillary bodies** are a pair of smooth, hemispherical masses, each about the size of a small pea, placed side by side in the floor of the interpeduncular fossa just cranial to the posterior perforated substance. Each is enclosed by bundles of white fibres derived in large part from the column of the fornix; internally are a number of aggregations of grey matter; these and their connexions are described further below.

**The tuber cinereum** lies cranial to the mamillary bodies and caudal to the optic chiasma. It is, as its name suggests, a convex mass of grey matter when viewed from its inferior aspect, but it is not a completely smooth convexity, its surface presenting a series of eminences with intervening grooves which vary in their prominence. In

[596] P. Bard and D. Mck. Rioch, *Bull. Johns Hopkins Hosp.,* **60,** 1937.
[597] F. Vidal, *Archs Neurol. Psychiat., Chicago,* **44,** 1940.
[598] W. R. Ingram, *Res. Publs Ass. Res. nerv. ment. Dis.,* **20,** 1940.
[599] W. J. H. Nauta and W. R. Mehler, *Brain Res.,* **1,** 1966.

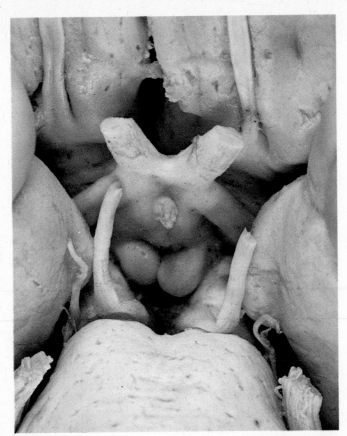

7.104 The interpeduncular fossa and surrounding structures. Note from above downwards: (1) the gyri recti of the frontal lobes, and the olfactory tracts, trigones and anterior perforated substances; (2) the optic nerves, chiasma and diverging optic tracts which disappear beneath the medial borders of the unci hippocampi; (3) the tuber cinereum with the attached superior part of the infundibular stem; (4) the mamillary bodies; (5) the deep recess between the mamillary bodies, the diverging crura cerebri and the cranial border of the pons, the floor of which is the posterior perforated substance; (6) on each side the prominent oculomotor nerves, more laterally the slender trochlear nerves, and bordering the pons, the thick trigeminal nerves are visible. (Dissection by Dr. E. L. Rees.)

the midline caudal to the optic chiasma, the hollow, conical *infundibulum* proceeds ventroinferiorly to become continuous with the solid expanded posterior lobe of the hypophysis cerebri (p. 1367). The tuber cinereum around the base of the infundibulum is raised to form a *median eminence* which, however, is superficially marked by a shallow tuberoinfundibular sulcus along their lines of junction. The tuber cinereum also presents a pair of *lateral eminences* and a midline *postinfundibular eminence*, whilst caudolaterally, on each side, a row of two or three minute hillocks project into the shallow groove between the tuber cinereum and the mamillary bodies.

## THE DIVISIONS AND NUCLEI OF THE HYPOTHALAMUS

Most regions of the hypothalamus contain populations of neurons which have been divided on the basis of phylogenetic, developmental, cytoarchitectonic, connectivity and histochemical studies into a number of nuclear aggregations, which have been given specific names, but some are much more clearly defined than others. A number of well-defined fibre tracts characterize parts of the hypothalamus, whilst the remaining regions are permeated by a complex series of interconnexions and more diffuse fibre arrays entering, leaving, passing through, or intrinsic to the region. Although the connexions of some of these fibres are fairly well established, others are known only

in outline. Further complications arise in the study of this small but immensely complex region of the brain; different authorities have, on occasion, used different criteria for its classification and their terminology does not always correspond. Only the major nuclear groups and principal connexions of the hypothalamus, followed by a brief outline of its main functional associations can be given here. For details, extended discussion and comprehensive bibliographies consult footnote references [600–604].

In general, the hypothalamus may be divided into a craniocaudal sequence of three zones—*supra-optic, infundibulotuberal* and *mamillary*. Similarly, a longitudinal division has been proposed into *lateral* and *medial zones* on each side. These are separated by the parasagittal plane, which include on each side the prominent fibre bundles of the column of the fornix, the mamillothalamic tract, and the fasciculus retroflexus. Some authorities prefer to subdivide the medial zone into a thin subependymal *periventricular zone*, and a thicker *intermediate* (or medial) *zone*.

Some of the main nuclear groups of the hypothalamus are illustrated in 7.105 and a more complete list is given below for reference purposes. Many of the latter are small and poorly localized, but despite this, some authorities even subdivide these into smaller aggregations. Each zone may be considered as a rough, craniocaudal sequence of nuclei, but some overlap occurs dorsoventrally, and the preoptic grey matter is common to all three zones.

**The periventricular zone** consists of: (1) part of the *preoptic* nucleus; (2) a small *suprachiasmatic* nucleus; (3) the large *paraventricular* nucleus; (4) the *infundibular* nucleus; and (5) the *posterior* nucleus of the hypothalamus. In general, these masses of grey matter are interspersed between the periventricular region of fibres (p. 895, 907) with which some of them are functionally associated. The most prominent nucleus of this zone, and the best understood in functional terms, is the paraventricular nucleus, which is further discussed below.

**The intermediate zone** (the medial zone of many authors) consists of: (1) part of the *preoptic* nucleus; (2) the *anterior* nucleus; (3) the *dorsomedial* nucleus; (4) the *ventromedial* nucleus; and (5) small *premamillary* nuclei.

**The lateral zone** consists of: (1) part of the *preoptic* nucleus; (2) the well-known *supra-optic* nucleus; (3) the extensive *lateral* nucleus; (4) the *tuberomamillary* nucleus; and (5) the *lateral tuberal* nuclei.

Finally, the mamillary body, with its main *medial* and *lateral mamillary* nuclei and a number of smaller associated aggregations of grey matter, may be considered as lying between the intermediate and lateral zones of the hypothalamus, although in fact they overlap both these zones.

A detailed description of the shapes, sizes, architectonics, and what is known of the connexions of these individual nuclei cannot be given in this volume, and for this, the references quoted should be consulted; but the following outstanding points may be noted. The preoptic, anterior, dorsomedial, and ventromedial nuclei and part of the posterior nucleus are mainly composed of small or medium-sized neurons and, in man, are rather poorly differentiated from their surroundings. Relatively large scattered neurons surrounded by small ones characterize the rest of the posterior nucleus and much of the lateral

[600] W. E. Le G. Clark, J. Beattie, G. Riddoch and N. M. Dott, *The Hypothalamus*, Oliver and Boyd, Edinburgh. 1938.
[601] E. Crosby and R. T. Woodburne, *Res. Publs Ass. Res. nerv. ment. Dis.*, **20**, 1940.
[602] G. W. Harris, *Neural Control of the Pituitary Gland*, Arnold, London. 1955.
[603] J. Szentágothai, B. Flerkó, B. Mess and B. Halász, *Hypothalamic Control of the Anterior Pituitary*, Akadémiai Kiadó, Budapest. 1962.
[604] W. Haymaker, E. Anderson and W. J. Nauta (eds.), *The Hypothalamus*, Thomas, Springfield, Illinois. 1969.

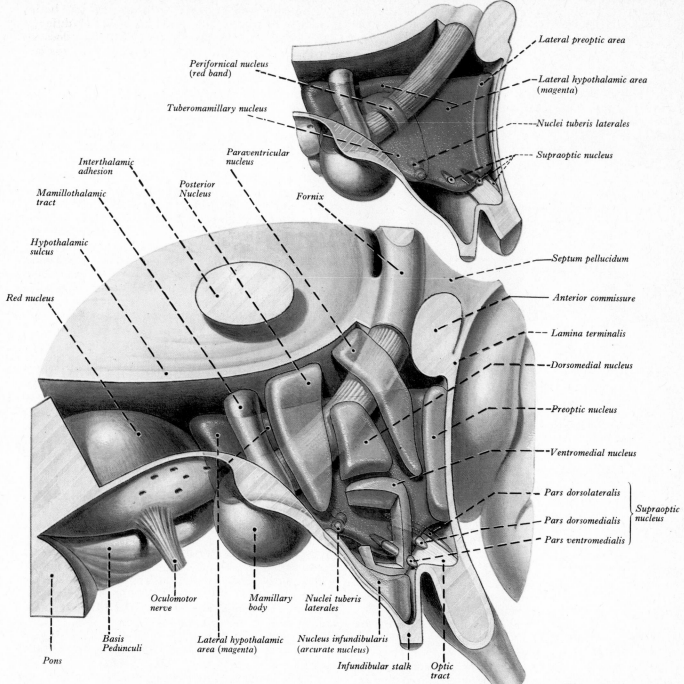

Perifornical nucleus (red band)

Tuberomamillary nucleus

Lateral preoptic area

Lateral hypothalamic area (magenta)

Nuclei tuberis laterales

Supraoptic nucleus

Interthalamic adhesion

Paraventricular nucleus

Posterior Nucleus

Mamillothalamic tract

Fornix

Hypothalamic sulcus

Red nucleus

Septum pellucidum

Anterior commissure

Lamina terminalis

Dorsomedial nucleus

Preoptic nucleus

Ventromedial nucleus

Pars dorsolateralis

Pars dorsomedialis

Pars ventromedialis

Supraoptic nucleus

Oculomotor nerve

Mamillary body

Nuclei tuberis laterales

Basis Pedunculi

Lateral hypothalamic area (magenta)

Nucleus infundibularis (arcuate nucleus)

Pons

Infundibular stalk

Optic tract

7.105 Schemata of the hypothalamic region of the left cerebral hemisphere from the medial aspect to display the major hypothalamic nuclei. In the upper diagram the medially placed nuclear groups have been removed, whilst in the lower diagram both lateral and medial groups are included. Lateral to the fornix and the mamillothalamic tract is the lateral hypothalamic region (magenta), in which the tuberomamillary nucleus is situated. Situated rostrally in this area is the lateral preoptic nucleus. Surrounding the fornix is the perifornical nucleus (red band), which joins the lateral hypothalamic area with the posterior hypothalamic nucleus. The medially situated nuclei (yellow) fill in much of the region between the mamillothalamic tract and the lamina terminalis, but also project caudal to the tract. The nuclei tuberis laterales (blue) are situated ventrally, largely in the lateral hypothalamic area. The supraoptic nucleus (green) consists of three parts. See text for further description. (From *The Hypothalamus*, by courtesy of the authors, W. J. H. Nauta and W. Haymaker, and the publishers, Charles C. Thomas, Springfield, Illinois, 1969.)

nucleus. The lateral tuberal nuclei, although small, are well defined, each being encapsulated by a dense meshwork of fine fibres, and each is located within one of the caudolateral surface hillocks between the tuber cinereum and mamillary body described above. The large size of the medial mamillary nucleus is characteristic of the human brain. The supraoptic nucleus, which covers the lateral part of the optic chaisma, and the large subependymal paraventricular nucleus are richly vascularized and they have certain distinguishing cytological features in common. They are composed in part of large, bipolar or multipolar neurons, which are sometimes multinucleate

and which, using Nissl's method, stain much more densely than the cells of surrounding nuclei. Their cytoplasm contains characteristic granules or droplets of neurosecretory material (p. 908).

## THE CONNEXIONS OF THE HYPOTHALAMUS

As mentioned previously, some hypothalamic connexions constitute fairly discrete fibre bundles, whilst others are diffuse, difficult to investigate, and hence often of uncertain origin and termination.

In broad outline, fibre systems *converging* on the hypothalamus include ascending visceral and somatic sensory pathways, olfactory pathways, and numerous tracts from the midbrain, diencephalon, 'limbic' structures, and from the neocortex. *Outflowing* paths from the hypothalamus return to many of these areas but, in particular, control paths reach the lower centres from which the *peripheral autonomic nervous system* originates; and it also controls the secretory cycles of the *hypophysis cerebri* and, through these activities, the *endocrine system* of the body.

More precisely, the different parts of the hypothalamus establish direct connexions with: (1) the tegmentum and periaqueductal grey matter of the midbrain; (2) subthalamic nuclei and indirectly with the globus pallidus; (3) thalamic nuclei; (4) the hippocampal formation; (5) the anterior olfactory areas; (6) the amygdaloid nuclear complex; (7) the septal areas; (8) the prefrontal cerebral cortex; (9) the hypophysis cerebri; and (10) possibly some direct fascicles from the retina, superior cerebellar peduncle and the globus pallidus. Some of the more important pathways will now be summarized.

### Afferent Connexions

The ascending sensory pathways to the hypothalamus include collateral branches of the lemniscal somatic afferent fibres, but in the main they are considered to be polysynaptic routes conveying visceral and gustatory information from the spinal cord and brainstem. They include the **mamillary peduncle** which is formed by the convergence of a number of fibre systems in the midbrain tegmentum to give a discrete bundle which ends in the mamillary body; ascending fibres run with the other components of the **dorsal longitudinal fasciculus** (*see* p. 886 and below) to reach the hypothalamus, and a number of smaller ascending pathways from the brainstem reticular formation have also been described.

Direct projections reach the hypothalamus from the subthalamic nucleus and zona incerta of the same and the opposite side, the latter crossing in the supraoptic decussations. Thalamohypothalamic connexions pass from the dorsomedial nucleus of the thalamus to many of the hypothalamic nuclei through the **periventricular system** of fibres previously described (p. 895) and probably also by traversing the medial part of the **inferior thalamic peduncle**.

A group of forebrain structures, many of which were originally regarded as mainly olfactory in their functional associations, have now been recognized as of much wider functional significance, and are often described together as the **limbic system** (p. 930). These structures include the hippocampal formation, amygdaloid and septal complexes, the piriform lobe and adjacent regions of neocortex which will be detailed further in subsequent sections. For our present purposes, however, it is necessary to state that the limbic structures give rise to a series of prominent pathways to the hypothalamus—the fornix, the stria terminalis, the medial forebrain bundle and the ventral amygdalofugal pathways.

**The fornix** is complex both in its topography and fibre constitution (p. 942), containing both commissural and projection fibres from a number of sources to a series of destinations. In the present context it is the main outflow from the neuronal laminae of the hippocampal formation, and as these fibres curve ventrally to approach the region of the anterior commissure they are joined by fascicles from the cingulate gyrus, possibly the indusium griseum, and many from the septal areas. As it continues ventrocaudally the fornix divides around the anterior commissure into pre- and post-commissural components. The precommissural fornix distributes in part to the preoptic regions of the hypothalamus, whilst during its descent the postcommissural (column) of the fornix gives offshoots to

the dorsal, lateral and periventricular regions of the hypothalamus before continuing to its main termination in the mamillary nuclei.

The amygdaloid complex of nuclei project on to the preoptic area and most of the hypothalamic nuclei cranial to the mamillary bodies. These amygdalohypothalamic fibres are conducted along two pathways—the complex curve fibre bundle called the *stria terminalis*, and also by a *ventral amygdalofugal route*. The latter consists of a diffuse array of fibres passing inferior to the lentiform nucleus through the anterior perforated substance to reach the hypothalamus. The amygdaloid complex and stria terminalis are further described below (p. 936).

**The medial forebrain bundle** is another complex fibre pathway which, although relatively reduced in the human brain, still constitutes the principal longitudinal fibre system of the hypothalamus (**7.123**). It contains both ascending and descending components. It interconnects the anterior olfactory, hypothalamic and midbrain tegmental centres, and it runs through the lateral zone of the hypothalamus, giving off and receiving numerous small fascicles throughout its course. Descending afferents to the hypothalamus running in the bundle include numerous *septohypothalamic fibres* from the septal areas (p. 937), *olfactohypothalamic fibres* from parts of the piriform cortex, and possibly *corticohypothalamic fibres* from the orbitofrontal cortex. Ascending visceral afferents reach the hypothalamus through the caudal part of the medial forebrain bundle. It should also be noted that descending fibres from the anterior terminations of the fornix and stria terminalis accompany the medial forebrain bundle and its branches. The details of some of these fibre systems have only been established in subprimate brains, but it is widely assumed that they also exist in the human brain.

**Corticohypothalamic fibres** project to the hypothalamus from wide areas of the prefrontal cortex by direct and indirect routes, but there has been much debate concerning the relative importance of the two pathways. The indirect fibres converge on the nucleus medialis dorsalis of the thalamus where they relay, and are then continued to the hypothalamus in the periventricular fibre system. In different experimental animals direct corticohypothalamic fibres have been variously described as ending in the lateral, dorsomedial, mamillary and posterior nuclei of the hypothalamus, but these have been denied by some authors. (For a detailed review of these and other hypothalamic connexions consult the article by Nauta and Haymaker in footnote reference [604].) Finally, as mentioned previously, some hypothalamic nuclei receive an input from the superior cerebellar peduncle, but direct projections from the retina which occur in submammalian forms, and direct projections from the globus pallidus cannot be regarded as proven in the primate brain.

### Efferent Connexions

In broad outline the connecting pathways from the hypothalamus include: (1) reciprocal paths to parts of the limbic system; (2) a series of descending polysynaptic paths to lower autonomic and motor centres; and (3) nervous and vascular links with the hypophysis cerebri.

The septal areas and the amygdaloid complex receive hypothalamic fibres which return along the pathways described above.

The prominent medial nucleus of the mamillary body gives rise to a large fibre bundle which ascends and, partly by branching of its individual fibres, diverges into two substantial tracts. The *mamillothalamic tract* (**7.117**) continues to ascend and terminates in all parts of the anterior nuclear group of the thalamus, where, after relay, massive projections radiate to the cingulate gyrus (pp. 895, 965).

The *mamillotegmental tract* curves caudally to enter the midbrain ventral to the medial longitudinal fasciculus and is distributed to tegmental nuclei of the reticular formation. Small bundles of *mamillosubthalamic fibres* pass to the prerubral field of the subthalamus, but their destination is uncertain. In addition to the mamillotegmental tract, descending fibres from the hypothalamus also reach the midbrain tegmentum in the *dorsal longitudinal fasciculus* and in the caudal extension of the *medial forebrain bundle*.

As mentioned above, the **connexions of the hypothalamus with the hypophysis cerebri** are by means of: (1) *nerve fibres* derived from various groups of hypothalamic neurons, which terminate at different levels throughout the median eminence, infundibulum, and *posterior lobe* of the hypophysis; and (2) a system of long and short *portal blood vessels* which interconnect plexuses of sinusoids in the median eminence and infundibulum with other plexuses in the *anterior lobe* of the hypophysis. The anatomy of these nervous and vascular channels is further considered with that of the hypophysis (p. 1371), but certain points must be emphasized here. The main glandular mass of the anterior lobe of the hypophysis receives no nerve supply, and virtually the whole of its blood supply is from the hypothalamohypophysial portal vessels. Direct observation in the living experimental animal has established that the direction of the blood flow in these vessels is from a series of complex sinusoidal tufts in the median eminence and infundibulum, through the portal vessels, to discharge into the blood sinusoids which run between the cords of glandular cells in the anterior lobe.

It is now widely accepted that a process of *neurosecretion* is involved both in the production and release of the posterior lobe hormones *oxytocin* and *vasopressin*, and also in the neurovascular mechanism whereby secretory activity in the various types of glandular cell in the anterior lobe is controlled. The hypothalamic centres containing neurons whose axons terminate in the infundibulum, or pass through it to terminate in the posterior lobe of the hypophysis, include the supraoptic, paraventricular, and infundibular nuclei, and part of the ventromedial nucleus.

**The supraoptic nucleus**, as mentioned above, is draped over the lateral part of the optic chiasma, and some authorities divide it into three or more subsidiary nuclei which are named according to their relationship to the chiasma. It is composed of a uniform population of large cells. **The paraventricular nucleus**, which causes a visible bulging of the ependyma into the third ventricle, extends from the hypothalamic sulcus and crosses the medial aspect of the column of the fornix, whilst its ventrolateral angle points towards the supraoptic nucleus. A number of its cells are large like those of the latter, but in addition there are many intermediate and small cells of varying shapes. **The infundibular nucleus** (often called the *arcuate nucleus*) occupies the median zone of the postinfundibular part of the tuber cinereum, and it extends into the median eminence and largely encircles the base of the infundibulum. However, it is deficient cranially where the infundibulum adjoins the midline part of the optic chiasma. No glial layer intervenes between the nucleus and the ependymal lining of the infundibular recess of the third ventricle. In contrast to the other nuclei just described, it is composed exclusively of numerous small cells, which appear round in coronal section and oval or fusiform in sagittal section.

Thus, the neurons which project into or through the infundibulum may be considered in two groups: *magnocellular*, including the large and intermediate cells of the paraventricular nucleus, and the large cells of the supraoptic nucleus, and *parvocellular*, which includes the small cells of the infundibular nucleus and possibly some in neighbouring nuclei. Whilst the magnocellular group is characterized by the presence of neurosecretory material (*vide infra*), it must be emphasized that both groups consist of true neurons. Each cell possesses a soma, dendrites and an axon with collateral branches, and these contain the usual neuronal organelles (p. 771). Furthermore, they receive axodendritic and axosomatic synapses from unknown sources, and their axons conduct volleys of nerve impulses. Their axonal terminals expand into end-bulbs which contain mitochondria and clear synaptic vesicles about 40–60 nm in diameter, and many of them are closely applied to the basement membranes of capillaries with no intervening neuroglia, in either the infundibulum or the posterior lobe. Whilst it is clear that important neural connexions exist which may influence the activities of these various nuclei—probably stemming from other hypothalamic nuclei and also from a number of the channels which converge upon the hypothalamus from other centres—their precise connexions have not yet been established. Equally, the significance of volleys of nerve impulses in these neurons, and the functional meaning of the presynaptic vesicles is by no means clear: no direct relationship to the process of neurosecretion has been demonstrated. (For further details see p. 1370.)

The terminology used in connexion with the neural pathways from the hypothalamus to the hypophysis has undergone several changes with increasing knowledge. This has resulted in an array of terms, some of which lack precision, and often different meanings attach to the same term when used by different authorities.

The term *supraopticohypophysial tract* was often used to denote *all* fibres which entered the infundibulum, whatever their origin or destination, but its use is now often restricted to those originating in the supraoptic and paraventricular nuclei. Since the nuclei are by no means equivalent in either their cytology or functional associations, some workers in the field prefer the more specific terms *supraopticohypophysial* and *paraventriculohypophysial tracts*. However, it must be realized that many of their fibres end in the infundibulum and do not reach the posterior lobe. The term *tuberohypophysial* or more precisely *tuberoinfundibular tract* is used to denote the fibres of the small neurons of the infundibular and possibly related nuclei, which end in the infundibulum.

The cells and axons of the magnocellular neurosecretory pathways from the supraoptic and paraventricular nuclei contain what were originally termed colloid droplets. These vary in size, are sometimes found between the cells and fibres, and they stain selectively with the chrome-alum haematoxylin stain of Gomori, when the fine axons and their branches are seen to contain a row of stained masses, each of which distends the axon, the whole appearance resembling a 'string of beads'. Irregularly distended nerve terminals containing large masses of neurosecretory material are termed *Herring bodies*. Ultrastructurally, the material consists of membrane-bound aggregations of dense granules, the whole mass varying from 200 to 300 nm in diameter. Much intensive research has been directed towards an understanding of neurosecretion, and the methods used include: studies on the effects of transection of the infundibulum; transplantation of the hypothesis; culture of neurohypophysial explants; autoradiography following the administration of labelled cysteine; subcellular fractionation and extraction followed by biological assay or chemical analysis; studies on the effects of dehydration, hydration, various drugs and stressful situations; chemical or electrical stimulation and ablation of focal points in the hypothalamus.

Briefly, it is now accepted that neurosecretory material is synthesized in the large cell somata of the supraoptic and paraventricular neurons in relation to the endoplasmic reticulum, further elaborated in the Golgi complex, and then transported along the axons and their branches, to be released at the axon terminals, and then to be taken up by the blood which is percolating through adjacent capillaries. Further, there is some evidence that, whilst both the supraoptic and paraventricular nuclei are associated with the production of the hormones vasopressin and oxytocin, vasopressin is predominantly a product of the supraoptic nucleus and oxytocin of the paraventricular nucleus. However, many questions remain unanswered.[605] For example, the precise chemical constitution of the neurosecretory material remains to be determined, and it appears that the chemically related hormones oxytocin and vasopressin are transported in a relatively non-active form, probably conjugated with a polypeptide carrier which is termed *neurophysin*. Secondly, the rate and mechanism of transport, presumably involving some form of axoplasmic flow, remains to be defined accurately. Finally, the manner in which the hormones are released at the axonal terminals is not understood, although suggestions have been made that both calcium ions and the local release of acetylcholine by the synaptic terminals may be involved. The special vascular relationships of the supraoptic and paraventricular nuclei are discussed in some further detail below.

In addition to the production of posterior lobe hormones oxytocin and vasopressin, neurosecretory pathways are also considered to play an important role in the control of secretory activity by the anterior lobe of the hypophysis. Much evidence supports the view that groups of hypothalamic cells produce a variety of *releasing hormones* which are transported along their axons and then discharged into the upper radicles of the portal system of blood vessels, by which means they are carried to the vascular bed which permeates the anterior lobe, where they reach and influence the appropriate glandular cells. The term releasing hormone is not, however, entirely appropriate; some inhibit the release of hormone by anterior lobe cells, whilst others stimulate synthesis of the hormone, as well as promoting its release. They include *releasing hormones* for corticotrophin, luteinizing hormone, follicle stimulating hormone, thyrotrophin and somatotrophin, and *release inhibiting hormones* for prolactin and the melanocyte stimulating hormone. The parvocellular neurosecretory pathway provided by the *tuberoinfundibular tract* has been proposed as the main route for the synthesis and transmission of these releasing hormones to the portal blood flow. However, some fibres in the tract also have particularly high concentrations of acetylcholine, whilst others are rich in catecholamines, and this is paralleled by the ultrastructural appearances of their end bulbs (p. 1370). Some contain small clear synaptic vesicles, whilst others contain larger dense-cored vesicles, and yet others contain a mixed population. There are no morphological evidences of the typical large, electron-dense, membrane-bound granular masses which characterize the magnocellular pathway. Accordingly, it has been proposed that the fibres of the tuberoinfundibular tract carry releasing hormone in a dispersed, active, form, and may also carry catecholamines or acetylcholine.

Finally, it must be emphasized that many of the axonal terminals of the magnocellular pathway also end in the upper infundibulum and may also be involved in control of the anterior lobe of the hypophysis. For these reasons, the magnocellular and parvocellular pathways may not be as functionally independent as has been envisaged by some investigators.

## FUNCTIONS OF THE HYPOTHALAMUS

Clinically it had long been recognized that lesions in the hypothalamus often lead to widespread and bizarre combinations of symptoms and signs, which stem from endocrine, metabolic, visceral and behavioural disturbances. However, it has been widely assumed that such combinations result from the interruption of control pathways for these various 'functions' which, although largely independent, are closely related topographically either in or near the hypothalamus. In particular, although the general significance of the hypophysis cerebri as an endocrine gland was gradually emerging in the closing decades of the last century and the opening ones of the twentieth,[606] it is only in the last forty years that the interrelation of the hypophysis and nervous system has been firmly established.[602] Thus, the science of *neuroendocrinology* has emerged[605] and has made increasingly rapid progress, complementing the widely accepted role of the hypothalamus as the 'head ganglion' of the autonomic nervous system (Sherrington[607]). More recently, intensive investigation has not only confirmed in greater detail the controls exerted by the hypothalamus on the *endocrine system* and the *lower autonomic centres*, but has also emphasized that hypothalamic action depends upon afferent information channels, both nervous and vascular, and that it is interlocked, both structurally and functionally, with higher regions of the nervous system. The latter include the complex of structures which many authors group as the *limbic lobe* or *system* (p. 930), and the prefrontal regions of the cerebral cortex.

Reference has been made elsewhere (p. 746) to one possible approach to the study of nervous systems in general, namely, that they operate in more complex animals as controllers of the *homeostatic cycles* which tend to preserve the individual and the species within a fluctuating environment. In mammalia, the frontal cortex, limbic system, hypothalamus, and lower regions of the brainstem and spinal cord are conveniently regarded as forming a hierarchy of controls particularly directed towards those homeostatic cycles, which are mediated by the autonomic nervous system, the endocrine system, and the locomotor patterns associated with them. The concept of such a hierarchy is important because of the widespread use of the terms lower, intermediate and higher 'centres' for a variety of visceral (and locomotor) controls. The term centre is largely a product of the available methods of analysing central nervous activities—usually by the focal stimulation or ablation of more or less discrete patches of nervous tissue, usually by electrical or chemical means. Such experimental manœuvres are then combined with other forms of observation—biochemical or cytological analysis, changes in general metabolic status, growth or behaviour patterns, electrophysiological recording and so forth. Whilst it is undoubtedly true that focal stimulation or ablation may cause dramatic changes in a particular group of responses, and that some regions exhibit apparently spontaneous and sometimes rhythmic electrical changes when isolated, great caution must be used before regarding such regions as independent, autonomous, controlling centres of particular activities. The bulk of the available evidence indicates that such 'centres' are best regarded as *nodal regions* of nervous tissue which, by virtue of their chemical constitution,

[605] B. T. Donovan, *Mammalian Neuroendocrinology*, McGraw-Hill, London. 1970.
[606] H. Cushing, *The Pituitary Body and its Disorders*, Lippincott, Philadelphia. 1912.
[607] C. S. Sherrington, *The Integrative Action of the Nervous System*, 2nd ed., Yale University Press, New Haven. 1947.

intrinsic geometry and connexions, and extrinsic connexions, nervous or vascular, are essential for the normal range of certain responses which follow particular patterns of inflowing information. It must be appreciated that the various other regions of the nervous system from which afferent information channels converge upon the 'centre', whilst often less dramatic in their effect upon the responses in question when individually modified, are nevertheless collectively as important as the so-called centre itself. Further, particularly within a confined region such as the hypothalamus, to and from which numerous pathways converge and diverge, and which is composed of many rather ill-defined neuron groups, some of which have diffuse patterns of connexions, it is found that many of the functional 'centres' of different investigators overlap or virtually coincide. For these reasons, many investigators prefer to discuss the effects of stimulation or ablation of general zones of the hypothalamus, e.g. lateral, posterior, preoptic, mamillary, etc., rather than attempting to ascribe particular functional roles to individual hypothalamic nuclei. Partial exceptions to this are the well-recognized neurosecretory nuclei with specific cell products which pass into the bloodstream in the infundibulum or posterior lobe of the hypophysis, but even in these cases their afferent neural and vascular connexions are incompletely understood.

In general terms, experiments in animals involving transection of the nervous system at various levels demonstrate that as progressively higher levels are included below the plane of section, more complex and effective homeostatic readjustments can be carried out.[608] Decerebrate preparations with transection at upper midbrain levels can perform individual minor reflex readjustments of the cardiovascular, respiratory and alimentary systems, but these are not integrated and normal body temperature is not maintained. When transection is performed cranial to the hypothalamus, separating it from the limbic system, but retaining the connexions between the hypothalamus, hypophysis, brainstem and spinal cord, a completely different picture emerges. Quite effective homeostasis is maintained over a moderate range of environmental conditions. The various visceral and endocrine control systems are integrated into more ordered patterns of responses; furthermore, 'innate drives' and 'motivated behaviour patterns' make their appearance, including forms of feeding, drinking, apparent satiation, copulatory responses, and so forth. However, the homeostatic mechanisms break down if the environmental stresses involved exceed a certain range, e.g. persistent fairly high or low environmental temperatures. In addition, the motivated behaviour patterns become abnormal under stress, the animal may attack, attempt to eat, drink, or copulate with a bizarre range of objects. If, however, the connexions between the limbic system (p. 930) and hypothalamus are also preserved, and only neocortical regions are ablated, highly effective homeostatic responses occur under a wide range of adverse environmental conditions.

An enormous research literature has accumulated concerning the functional roles of the hypothalamus and the subject of neuroendocrinology, which cannot be reviewed in this volume; and the footnote references should be consulted for details and an introduction to extensive bibliographies. In summary, therefore, animal experimentation, usually involving focal stimulation or ablation of the hypothalamus, has emphasized its intimate relationship to the following activities.

(1) **Endocrine control** by the formation of releasing factors or release-inhibiting factors which influence the production of thyrotrophin, corticotrophin, somatotrophin, prolactin, luteinizing hormone, follicle stimulating

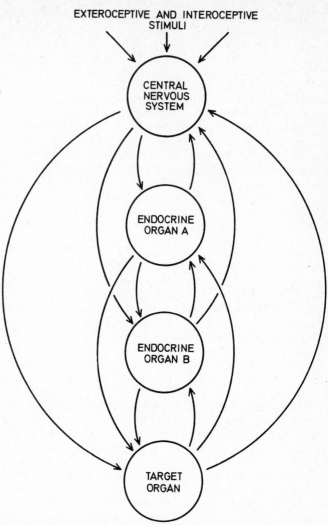

EXTEROCEPTIVE AND INTEROCEPTIVE STIMULI

7.106 A flow diagram showing a stimulus pattern impinging on the central nervous system, and the possible interactions of the latter with endocrine organs A and B and a target tissue. Note the different orders of feed-forward and feed-back pathways envisaged. From *Neuroendocrinology* by E. Scharrer and B. Scharrer, Columbia University Press, 1963 By courtesy of the authors and publishers.

hormone, and melanocyte stimulating hormone, by the cells of the *anterior pituitary*. Some of these affect target cells in the general body tissues directly, whilst others do so through the intermediary of a second endocrine organ, e.g. the thyroid gland, adrenal cortex, or the gonads. In the latter instances the sequence of control mechanisms is illustrated diagrammatically in 7.106. Neural pathways converge upon, and are integrated within, the hypothalamus, and modify its production of releasing or inhibiting factors (p. 909). In turn, these modify the activities of endocrine glands A and B, and ultimately the target tissues. Each of the intermediate levels in the chain are also modified by the operation of negative or positive feed-back loops which depend upon the blood concentration of the secretory products of subsequent stages in the chain. (For further details consult footnote references [604, 605, 609].)

(2) **Neurosecretion**[610, 611] of oxytocin and vasopressin (antidiuretic hormone, ADH) directly into the bloodstream of the infundibulum and posterior lobe of the hypophysis. Despite its name, whether vasopressin exerts

[608] B. K. Anand, in: *Control Processes in Multicellular Organisms*, eds. G. E. W. Wolstenholme and J. Knight, Churchill, London. 1970.

[609] E. Scharrer and B. Scharrer, *Neuroendocrinology*, Columbia University Press, N.Y. 1963.

[610] H. Heller and R. B. Clark, *Neurosecretion*, Mem. Soc. Endocr., Academic Press, London, N.Y. 1962.

[611] M. Gabe, *Neurosecretion*, Pergamon Press, London, Paris, N.Y. 1966.

any significant effect on vascular non-striated muscle under physiological conditions remains uncertain. However, it has a powerful effect on the reabsorption of water by the kidney, whilst oxytocin causes contraction of uterine and mammary smooth muscle which may be of importance during suckling, coitus and parturition.[605] Stimulation of neural pathways from the nipples and genitalia causes an increase in the rate of oxytocin release. The rate of release of vasopressin is determined, in part, by the tonicity and osmotic pressure of the blood perfusing *osmoreceptor sites* both within the hypothalamus[612] and in the peripheral circulation—probably in the hepatic portal vein.[613] From the latter, lengthy nervous pathways are involved before the impulse pattern generated reaches the hypothalamus. Similarly, a reduced blood volume is considered to stimulate *volume receptors* in the great veins and the walls of the atria of the heart, thus causing an increased release of vasopressin.[614] Finally, pain, and a variety of emotional states and conditions of stress, greatly modify the rate of release of the hormone.

(3) **General autonomic effects.** It has long been held that cranial zones of the hypothalamus mediate general parasympathetic activity, whilst caudal zones mediate sympathetic activity. Whilst there is undoubtedly a preponderance of one or other effect in these zones, there is much interaction and overlap between the effects in different regions, and a rigid distinction between parasympathetic and sympathetic 'centres' cannot be maintained. However, focal stimulation or ablation of the hypothalamus shows that it is intimately concerned with *cardiovascular*, *respiratory* and *alimentary* control. A detailed analysis cannot be given here, but such experiments are often accompanied by profound changes in heart rate, cardiac output, vasomotor tone and peripheral resistance, blood pressure, differential blood flow through different organs, and also in the frequency and depth of ventilatory excursions of the thorax, and in the motility and secretory activity of the stomach and intestines.

(4) **Temperature regulation.** In all warm blooded animals a critical balance is achieved between the overall heat production and loss of the body, and the hypothalamus provides a central regulating mechanism for this. A raised body temperature is depressed by vasodilatation, with an increased cutaneous blood flow, sweating, panting, and reduced heat production, whilst with a lowered body temperature the converse conditions apply, with shivering and, if prolonged, an increase in the activity of the thyroid gland. Information concerning body temperature reaches the hypothalamus via neural pathways from peripheral *thermodetectors* for cold and heat, and from thermodetector neurons within the hypothalamus itself. The latter monitor the prevailing temperature of the blood perfusing the hypothalamus, whilst other hypothalamic neurons are chemoreceptors which react specifically to the presence of blood-borne viruses, toxins, pyrogenic drugs etc. These converging flows of information are passed to regions of the hypothalamus which then set in train the appropriate autonomic, endocrine and muscular responses. It has been proposed that an *antirise* region exists in the cranial hypothalamus which controls vasodilatation, sweating, panting and possibly reduction of heat production, whilst the caudal hypothalamus houses an *antidrop* region controlling vasoconstriction, shivering and other means of raising heat production. The topographical limits and degree of separation of this *dual hypothalamic thermostat* cannot yet be regarded as finally settled. Some investigators[615] consider that a *dual chemical thermostat* is interposed between the inflow of information and the antirise and antidrop regions of the hypothalamus, consisting of groups of neurons containing 5-hydroxytryptamine, or norepine-

phrine (and possibly dopamine). Warmer blood, impulses from heat receptors, antipyretic substances or anaesthetics, are thought to cause the release of norepinephrine (or dopamine) which in turn stimulates the antirise mechanisms. Cooler blood, impulses from cold receptors, or pyrogenic substances, stimulate a release of 5-hydroxytryptamine which causes activation of the antidrop mechanisms.

(5) **Regulation of food and water intake.** Many investigations[616, 617] have demonstrated that there exist regions with opposing actions in the medial and lateral zones of the hypothalamus. Ablation of the medial zone leads to over-eating or *hyperphagia*, eventually leading to gross obesity, whilst ablation of the lateral zone leads to *hypophagia* or even complete *aphagia* with death from starvation. Conversely, stimulation of the medial zone causes the animal to eat less, whilst lateral stimulation initiates eating or increases and prolongs the food intake. Thus, a laterally placed *hunger* or *feeding* 'centre' balanced against a medially placed *satiety* 'centre' have been proposed. Neurons which are specifically sensitive to the concentration of glucose in the circulating blood have been demonstrated in the medial zone of the hypothalamus and are probably important in the operation of the satiety centre.

Water balance and the osmolality of the blood are in part controlled by the osmoreceptor/volume receptor—vasopressin—renal system described previously, which determines the rate of water loss in the urine. Coupled with this is a *thirst* or *drinking centre* in the lateral zone of the hypothalamus which regulates water intake. Experimental stimulation of this region causes immediate and copious drinking, and, if the stimulation persists, gross over-hydration results.

(6) **Sexual behaviour and reproduction.** Through its control of gonadotrophin production by the anterior pituitary, the hypothalamus controls many aspects of reproductive physiology, including gametogenesis, cyclic variations in the reproductive tracts, and the maturation and maintenance of secondary sexual characteristics. Furthermore, hypothalamic stimulation may induce receptivity of the male in the female, and simple copulatory movements in the male, and it has also been shown that some hypothalamic neurons are sensititive to the circulating level of oestrogen or testosterone.

It should be noted at this point that whilst the elementary *drives* associated with hunger, thirst and sex may be considered to stem in part from an intact hypothalamus, for their full integration into complex behaviour patterns, a two-way commerce between the hypothalamus and limbic system is necessary (p. 938). Such patterns include searching for and procuring a mate, food and drink, home-building, rearing of young, etc.

(7) **Biological clocks**. Many tissues, organs and systems in the body show a cyclic variation in some of their functional activities, the cycle having a periodicity of approximately twenty-four hours. Well-known examples of such *circadian rhythms* include regular fluctuations in the body temperature, the concentration levels of a number of plasma constituents, the eosinophil count, adrenocortical secretory activity, and renal secretory mechanisms. In some cases the rhythm is partly an intrinsic property of the organ or tissue itself, but in many cases an overall control is exerted by an intact hypothalamus.

[612] E. B. Verney, *Proc. R. Soc. B.*, **135**, 1947.
[613] F. J. Haberich, *Fedn Proc. Fedn Am. Socs. exp. Biol.*, **27**, 1968.
[614] O. H. Gauer, *Fedn Proc. Fedn Am. Socs. exp. Biol.*, **27**, 1968.
[615] R. D. Myers, in: *The Hypothalamus*, eds. W. Haymaker, E. Anderson and W. J. H. Nauta, Thomas, Springfield, Illinois. 1969.
[616] B. K. Anand and J. R. Brobeck, *Yale J. Biol. Med.*, **24**, 1951.
[617] B. K. Anand, *Physiol. Rev.*, **41**, 1961.

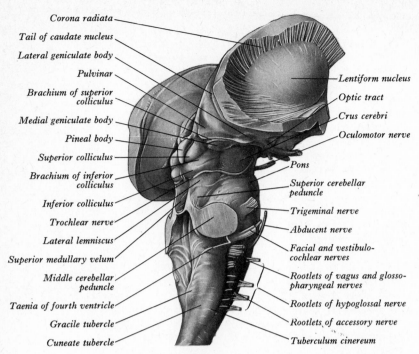

Corona radiata
Tail of caudate nucleus
Lateral geniculate body
Pulvinar
Brachium of superior colliculus
Medial geniculate body
Pineal body
Superior colliculus
Brachium of inferior colliculus
Inferior colliculus
Trochlear nerve
Lateral lemniscus
Superior medullary velum
Middle cerebellar peduncle
Taenia of fourth ventricle
Gracile tubercle
Cuneate tubercle

Lentiform nucleus
Optic tract
Crus cerebri
Oculomotor nerve
Pons
Superior cerebellar peduncle
Trigeminal nerve
Abducent nerve
Facial and vestibulo-cochlear nerves
Rootlets of vagus and glosso-pharyngeal nerves
Rootlets of hypoglossal nerve
Rootlets of accessory nerve
Tuberculum cinereum

7.107A   Posterolateral aspect of the hindbrain and midbrain, exposed by removal of the cerebellum and most of the cerebrum.

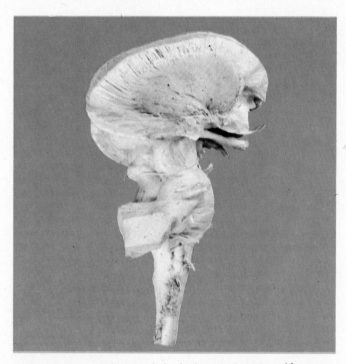

7.107B   Right lateral view of the brainstem; compare with 7.107A. (Dissection by Dr. E. L. Rees.)

Widespread lesions in other parts of the nervous system leave the biological timing mechanism unaffected, but hypothalamic lesions alone cause serious disturbances of rhythm.

The periodic conditions of sleeping and wakefulness are an outstanding example of a circadian rhythm. In recent years a large volume of investigation has been directed towards an understanding of the mechanisms of sleep (see footnote references[618-620] for an introduction to the literature). Briefly, sleep is no longer regarded as a passive 'switching off' process whereby there is simply a reduction in the activity of a cerebral activating system. Two principal states of sleep are now recognized. During the waking state, the electroencephalogram is charac-terized by a low-amplitude wave pattern with a frequency of about 10 cycles per second, upon which background there are bursts of irregular 'random' activity. With the onset of sleep, the waveform changes to one which is *synchronized*, of a large amplitude and a slow frequency. This state of *slow* or *light sleep* is one from which the subject is aroused relatively easily; it is a dreamless condition. After some time the condition of slow sleep is interspersed with bouts of *fast*, *deep*, or *paradoxical sleep*. The electroencephalogram shows fast, low-amplitude, *desynchronized* waves. Muscle tone is in general reduced, particularly in the neck musculature, but there occur characteristic rapid eye movements (so-called REM sleep), during which the subject is difficult to rouse, and experiences dreams. Three or four sessions of REM sleep occur each full night. It is generally thought that the level and type of sleep depends upon the balance between two opposing systems, which are disposed throughout much of the brainstem and include parts of the thalamus, hypothalamus and limbic system. On the one hand there is the *reticular activating* or *arousal system*, with its cranial extensions to the cerebral cortex, stimulation of which leads to wakefulness and desynchronization of cerebral activity. On the other hand, there has been demonstrated a series of *hypnogenic zones* in the medulla, pons, midbrain, thalamus, hypothalamus and basal limbic structures, the stimulation of which leads to synchronization of cerebral cortical activity, and a variety of induced sleep-like states, which differ in their detailed characteristics. The precise manner in which these opposing, hierarchical systems of sleep-controlling regions interact awaits further investigation, but in general the thalamohypothalamic centres seem dominant whilst those in the medulla, pons and midbrain are subordinate. It is of interest that intact centres in the neighbourhood of the locus coeruleus, rich in catecholamines, seem to be important in the generation of paradoxical sleep. Furthermore, the overall circadian rhythm of sleeping and waking is seriously disturbed with lesions in the cranial hypothalamus, and the rhythm is paralleled by corresponding fluctuations of serotonin (5-hydroxytryptamine) concentration in the hypnogenic zones of the brainstem and diencephalon. Whether the serotonin functions as a humoral sleep-inducing and maintaining factor, or as a neural transmitter in the hypnogenic system, remains to be determined.

(8) **Emotion, fear, rage, aversion, pleasure and reward.** The emotional content of an individual consists of two main elements: the *subjective feeling state* or *affective tone*, and the *objective physical accompaniments* which constitute *emotional expression*. For the full integration of both these aspects of emotion, with changes in the internal and external environment, and with other cerebral activities, the essential neurological structures are an intact hypothalamus, limbic system, and prefrontal cortex. With such a complex and interlocked system it is impossible to ascribe specific functional roles to individual subregions. Nevertheless, some elementary responses can be elicited by focal stimulation or ablation of the hypothalamus both in the intact animal (or human being during neurosurgery), or after the experimental removal of higher centres. The early classical experiments were carried out on decorticate dogs[621] and subsequently analysed in greater detail on decorticate cats.[622] In the

[618] M. Jouvet, *Archs ital. Biol.*, **100**, 1962; *Acta neurochir.* **12**, 1964; *Prog. Brain Res.*, **18**, 1965.
[619] G. F. Rossi, *Acta neurochir.*, **12**, 1964.
[620] W. P. Koella, in: *The Hypothalamus*, eds. W. Haymaker, E. Anderson and W. J. H. Nauta, Thomas, Illinois. 1969.
[621] F. Goltz, *Pflügers Arch. ges. Physiol.*, **51**, 1892.
[622] W. B. Cannon and S. W. Britton, *Am. J. Physiol.*, **72**, 1925.

latter mild peripheral stimulation evoked a condition of *sham rage*, with hissing, growling, baring of claws and fangs, piloerection, arching of the back, dilatation of the pupils, striking at objects and lashing of the tail. The term 'sham' was used because it was assumed that feeling states and directed behaviour could not occur in the decorticate animal. Later it was shown that the sham rage was abolished by obliteration of the caudal hypothalamus, but could be elicited by stimulation of the latter in intact animals.

Many subsequent studies have demonstrated that stimulation or ablation of different hypothalamic regions cause changes in the emotional accompaniment of the basic drives of sex, hunger and thirst, whilst other regions are related to the behavioural and (in man) the subjective aspects of rage, fear and pleasure. Particular emphasis has recently been placed upon the existence of centres which are broadly opposed in their actions—*positive* and *negative reward centres*. Stimulation of the former leads to 'pleasurable sensations' or the gratification of an intense drive—with an appropriate experimental situation, an animal will repeatedly self-stimulate its hypothalamus until exhausted, even ignoring food and drink after prolonged periods of deprivation. Stimulation in man often causes a general sensation of well-being, and on some occasions it has a strong erotic content. Such *positive reinforcement* may be used to expedite the responses of experimental animals in situations which demand learning. Conversely, stimulation of the negative reward centres presumably causes pain or 'displeasure' and the experimental animal will go to considerable effort and complex patterns of behaviour to avoid repetitive stimulation.

## The Metathalamus and Visual Pathway

**The optic chiasma** (**7**.108A) is a flattened, somewhat quadrilateral bundle of nerve fibres situated at the junction of the anterior wall of the third ventricle with its floor. Its anterolateral angles are continuous with the optic nerves, the posterolateral angles with the optic tracts. The lamina terminalis (p. 919) is continuous with its upper surface and is crossed, just above the chiasma, by the anterior communicating artery. Inferiorly the chiasma usually rests on the diaphragma sellae a short distance posterosuperior to the optic groove of the sphenoid bone. In about 10 per cent of subjects it is either more anterior and in the groove or altogether more dorsal in position. It is always in close relation to the hypophysis (**8**.196). Posteriorly it is related to the tuber cinereum and the infundibulum below, and to the third ventricle above. Laterally it is related to the termination of the internal carotid artery and the anterior perforated substance. A small recess of the third ventricle, the *optic recess*, passes ventrocaudally over its superior surface as far as the lamina terminalis (**8**.196).

Most of the fibres of the optic chiasma start in the retina and reach the chiasma through the optic nerves. In the chiasma the fibres from the nasal half of each retina, including the nasal half of the macula, cross the median plane and enter the optic tract of the opposite side, while the fibres from the temporal half pass backwards in the optic tract of the same side. The crossed fibres loop for a short distance into the ipsilateral optic tract before crossing in the chiasma or into the contralateral optic nerve after crossing. The macular fibres, and those from the central area in the immediate vicinity of the macula, form a flattened band which occupies almost two-thirds of the central region of the chiasma. This bundle is superior to all peripheral decussating fibres. Inferior to this are the

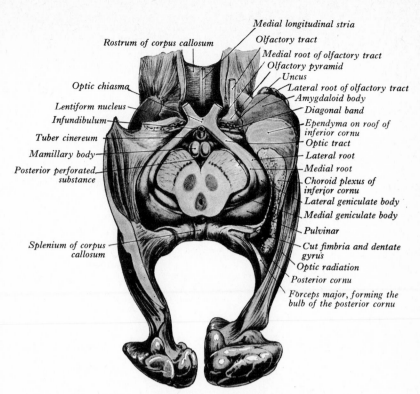

*Rostrum of corpus callosum* — *Medial longitudinal stria* — *Olfactory tract* — *Medial root of olfactory tract* — *Olfactory pyramid* — *Uncus* — *Lateral root of olfactory tract* — *Amygdaloid body* — *Diagonal band* — *Ependyma on roof of inferior cornu* — *Optic tract* — *Lateral root* — *Medial root* — *Choroid plexus of inferior cornu* — *Lateral geniculate body* — *Medial geniculate body* — *Pulvinar* — *Cut fimbria and dentate gyrus* — *Optic radiation* — *Posterior cornu* — *Forceps major, forming the bulb of the posterior cornu*

*Optic chiasma* — *Lentiform nucleus* — *Infundibulum* — *Tuber cinereum* — *Mamillary body* — *Posterior perforated substance* — *Splenium of corpus callosum*

**7**.108A A ventral dissection of the brain showing the metathalamus and the optic tracts. On the right side of the figure the inferior horn of the ventricle is exposed. The floor has been removed but the choroid plexus is *in situ* and obscures most of the roof.

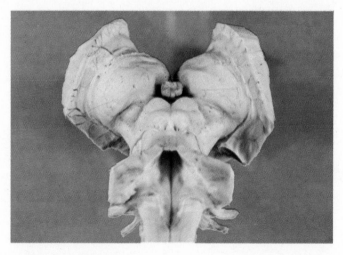

**7**.108B An oblique view of the dorsal aspect of the brainstem looking cranially. In the foreground is the floor of the rhomboid fossa, bounded laterally by the sectioned white matter of the cerebellum containing the dentate nuclei; the cranial recess of the fourth ventricle passes inferior to the superior medullary velum to continue into the aqueduct of the midbrain. More cranially, the emerging trochlear nerves, the colliculi, superior and inferior brachia, the medial and lateral geniculate bodies, and the pineal body may be identified. Lateral to the pineal body on each side is the rounded pulvinar of the dorsal thalamus, skirted laterally by the curving body and tail of the caudate nucleus, whilst most laterally is the cut surface of the corona radiata. (Dissection by Dr. E. L. Rees.)

fibres from the extramacular parts of the nasal half of the retinae. Most inferior are the nasal fibres concerned with the monocular fringes of the binocular visual field. Dorsal to and within the optic chiasma are bundles of fibres which are not derived from the optic nerve and form no part of the visual pathway. Although these are termed, collectively, the supraoptic commissures, they are not really commissures but decussations. One of these is the *supraoptic commissure* (of Gudden), which was formerly, but incorrectly, believed to connect the medial geniculate

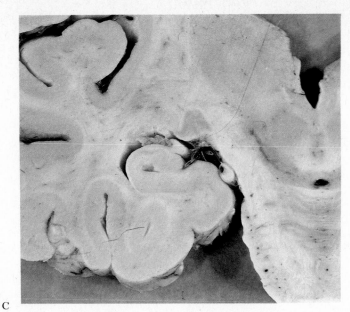

C

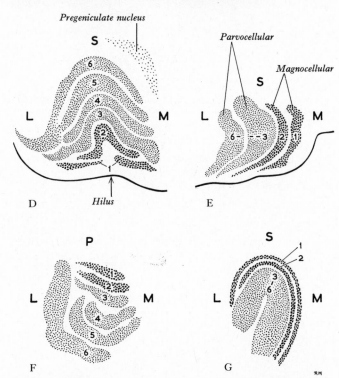

*Pregeniculate nucleus*

S

6
5
4
3
2
1

L        M

D        *Hilus*

*Parvocellular*

*Magnocellular*

S

L        M

6  3  2  1

E

P

L        M

1
2
3
4
5
6

F

S

1
2
3
6

L        M

G        RM

7.108 C–G  (C) The lateral geniculate body, shown in coronal section in the human brain to display its general position and orientation—it is the cap-shaped mass of grey and white matter near the centre of the field. Note its relationship to the inferior horn of the lateral ventricle, the structures visible on the sectioned surface of the midbrain tegmentum, and the dorsal thalamus. Even at this low magnification the lamination of the lateral geniculate body is visible. The four diagrams show the right lateral geniculate nucleus in section: (D) a mature human nucleus in coronal section near its central region and (E) near its posterior pole. Note the reduction in the number of discernible laminae in the latter. The lamination is also visible (F) in an approximately horizontal section at the time of birth. In some primates, for example *Tarsius* (G), the magno-cellular layers (1 and 2) are curved externally around the parvocellular layers (3–6); the higher primate arrangement is almost the reverse of this when examined in the coronal plane. See text for further details, and consult footnote references [630, 632, 634].

bodies of the two sides. Its connexions are not fully known, but evidence, from work on animals, suggests that its fibres arise in the brainstem and spinal cord; its existence, in man, is denied by some authorities. The so-called supraoptic commissure is only one of at least three dorsal connecting pathways described in the optic chiasma. They are reputed to terminate in such cell

groups as hypothalamic nuclei and the subthalamus in some animals, such as the cat, but it appears improbable that they are in any way associated with visual functions. Similarly, detached bands of nerve fibres have been noted as leaving the optic tract to pass dorsally across the cerebral peduncle inferior to the main tract. Such bundles as the *transverse peduncular tract* and various other *accessory optic tracts*, though present in some lower mammals and infra-mammalian forms, are stated to be absent in primates by some authorities (but see p. 882). According to this view all the myelinated fibres of the optic tracts in man pass either to the lateral geniculate body or to the superior colliculus and pretectal nucleus.[623]

The optic chiasma is supplied from the network of arteries in the investing pia mater. This network receives branches from the superior hypophysial, internal carotid, posterior communicating, anterior cerebral and anterior communicating arteries. The veins drain into the basal veins and the anterior cerebral vein above.

**The optic tracts** (7.108, 109) are continued dorso-laterally from the posterolateral angles of the chiasma. Each passes between the anterior perforated substance and the tuber cinereum, as the anterolateral boundary of the interpeduncular fossa. The tract becomes flattened and winds round the upper part of the cerebral peduncle, to which it adheres. In this part of its course it is hidden from view on the basal surface of the cerebrum by the uncus and parahippocampal gyrus. Reaching the lateral geniculate body the optic tract divides into medial and lateral "roots". The medial of these is believed to contain supraoptic commissural fibres; the lateral root or ramus consists of afferent fibres which arise in the retina and undergo partial decussation in the optic chiasma, as already described, but it also contains a few fine efferent fibres which are passing forwards to terminate in the retina. Most of the fibres of the lateral ramus are found to end in the lateral geniculate body (p. 917); some sweep medially below the pulvinar and gain the superior colliculus and the pretectal nucleus (pp. 888, 999). The detailed arrangement of retinal fibres in the optic chiasma and tract has been worked out in the monkey,[623] and clinical observations suggest a very similar form of organization in the human structures.[624] Illustration 7.109 shows these details. A notable feature is that nerve fibres derived from the macula, which occupy a central position in the optic nerve and chiasma, assume an eccentric and dorsolateral location in the optic tract, where fibres from both retinae mingle. As will be detailed later, this re-arrangement is a prelude to the mode of spatial representation in the lateral geniculate body (p. 918), the superior colliculus and visual cortex (p. 961).

Further fibres arise from nerve cells in the lateral geniculate body, and pass through the posterior limb of the internal capsule. Emerging from the capsule as a broad bundle termed the *optic radiation*, the fibres of the second visual neurons curve backwards and medially to reach the cortex of the occipital lobe of the cerebrum, where the cortical visual apparatus is situated (p. 960). On their way they are separated from the posterior horn of the lateral ventricle only by the tapetum of the corpus callosum.

Some of the fibres in the optic radiation take an oppo-site course, arising from the cells of the occipital cortex and passing to the superior colliculus, which therefore receives cortical in addition to retinal fibres. From the superior colliculus further fibres travel by the tecto-bulbar tracts to reach the nuclei of the third, fourth, sixth

[623] S. Polyak, *The Vertebrate Visual System*, University of Chicago Press, Chicago. 1957.
[624] H. M. Traquair, *An Introduction to Clinical Perimetry*, 5th ed., Kimpton, London. 1948.

and eleventh cranial nerves, and the anterior grey column of the spinal cord. Recent studies suggest that such 'oculomotor' connexions are doubtful in primates, including man (p. 887).

## The Metathalamus—the Geniculate Bodies

The metathalamus (7.108, 109) consists of the *medial* and *lateral geniculate bodies*, bilateral eminences on the inferior aspect of the thalamus lateral to each side of the midbrain. As this collective term suggests, they are relatively late specializations of the vertebrate thalamus in both phylogenetic and ontogenetic senses. Their basic roles as relay nuclei on the acoustic (medial geniculate) and visual (lateral geniculate) pathways have long been recognized; but more recent evidence shows that their connexions, and hence their functions, are much more complex than this. In particular, there exists in both pathways—as in most, if not all sensory projections—a corticofugal or efferent component, modulating the patterns of centripetal inputs, which can hence no longer be regarded as arrays of simple responses to stimulation of peripheral receptors, proceeding independently along completely separated parallel channels. For example, neuronal mechanisms exist, as elsewhere, for collateral inhibition and probably for interaction between different modalities of sensibility.

### THE MEDIAL GENICULATE BODY

The medial geniculate body (7.108, 120) projects from the inferior surface of the pulvinar of the thalamus (7.108), lateral to the superior colliculus. Its contour is ovoid, with the long axis directed anterolaterally. The inferior brachium (p. 881) ascends with a ventrolateral inclination to reach the lateral geniculate body, passing between it and the pulvinar; it contains nerve fibres from the ipsilateral lateral lemniscus (derived in part from the opposite superior olive) and from both inferior colliculi.

In its **internal structure** the medial geniculate nucleus exhibits no clear-cut division into sub-nuclei; the entire mass presents a knee-shaped profile in section and hence its name. On the basis of size its cells are largely segregated into a dorsal, *parvocellular part*, or principal division, and a smaller ventromedial division, the *pars magnocellularis*, which in fact contains an admixture of the smaller cell type. Wedged between the pulvinar and the pretectal region, dorsomedial to the medial geniculate body, is a small mass of nerve cells, the *suprageniculate nucleus* of some forms; its connexions are uncertain, but it probably receives fibres from reticular elements in the lateral tegmental region of the midbrain and pons concerned in other modalities of sensation, including pain (p. 888). Closer study of the constituent nerve cells of the medial geniculate nucleus, particularly of their dendritic organization and their connexions in the cat, has prompted a more complex partition into regions and component nuclei.[625] In this animal the medial geniculate nucleus has been allotted dorsal, ventral and medial divisions, with further subdivisions, one of which—the 'ventral nucleus' of the ventral division—has a laminar structure. This is a detail of special interest, because this part of the geniculate body receives most of the inferior collicular projection in the cat;[626] and, as will be described below, the lateral geniculate body is also laminated, this pattern being clearly associated with a spatial organization of sensory terminals. In the same feline schema, the medial division is regarded as the terminus of direct lateral lemniscal fibres, and evidence is growing that these are, in the cat

and monkey, spinal afferents concerned in modalities of sensibility other than acoustic, ending in the magnocellular (ventromedial or medial) part of the medial geniculate body. It has hence been suggested that this, and perhaps the suprageniculate nucleus, may be involved in integrations between visual, auditory, general somatic and even visceral inputs.

The role of the medial geniculate body in the acoustic pathway is still in many details obscure, apart from its function as a relay nucleus. This is in large part due to its relative inaccessibility to the recording electrode or destructive probe, neither of which can be accurately placed without marked difficulties of approach. By analogy the laminar appearance of the ventral division, and the existence of a tonotopical organization at cortical level, both suggest similar arrangements in the medial geniculate body; and evidence both in favour of this and against it has been adduced in experimental animals. It is clearly not yet justifiable to suggest tonotopical representation in man. The efferent auditory projection is considered to be derived directly from the small-celled regions of the medial geniculate nucleus, terminating in the temporal lobe, in an area in monkeys corresponding to area 41 in man (p. 963)—part of the superior temporal gyrus. Other acoustic areas have been delineated by animal experimentation, and they may also exist in man (p. 963). A primary acoustic area (designated AI in the cat) is directly connected to the medial geniculate body; secondary acoustic areas (AII and others) may also receive projections from the same parvocellular parts of the geniculate complex, or from its magnocellular part. All these areas may be concerned in various aspects of acoustic function (p. 963), and there is abundant evidence of tonotopical representation of the spiral organ of the cochlea in area AI. The role of the medial geniculate body, however, in determination of frequencies of sounds remains *sub judice*, the evidence being largely negative.[627] Lesions of the medial geniculate body do not lead to pronounced deafness unless they are bilateral, since both cochlear organs are represented in each lateral lemniscus (p. 853).

### THE LATERAL GENICULATE BODY

The lateral geniculate body is a small nuclear complex distinguishable on the surface as a small ovoid projection from the inferior aspect of the posterior region of the thalamus (7.108, 120). Its long axis is approximately sagittal, and its anterior pole blends with the larger, lateral moiety of the optic tract, the medial 'root' or ramus of which separates the geniculate elevation from the lateral aspect of the crus cerebri. The medial geniculate body is, of course, medial to it, but in a more dorsal position. The inferior or superficial aspects of both geniculate bodies are obscured from view by the medial region of the temporal lobe, the parahippocampal gyrus being the immediate relation (p. 929). Proceeding dorsally from the posteromedial region of the lateral geniculate body, to reach the pretectal area and lateral side of the superior colliculus, is a narrow linear elevation, the *superior brachium* (7.107). This contains uninterrupted retinal nerve fibres which mediate optic reflexes through the pretectal and thence via the oculomotor nuclei and tectospinal tracts (p. 887). The superior brachium is between the medial geniculate body and the pulvinar in much of its extent. From comparison of the lateral ramus of the optic tract and superior brachium, whose relative

---

[625] D. K. Morest, *J. Anat.*, **98** and **99**, 1964 and 1965.

[626] R. Y. Moore and J. M. Goldberg, *J. comp. Neurol.*, **121**, 1963.

[627] I. C. Whitfield, *The Auditory Pathway*, Arnold, London. 1967.

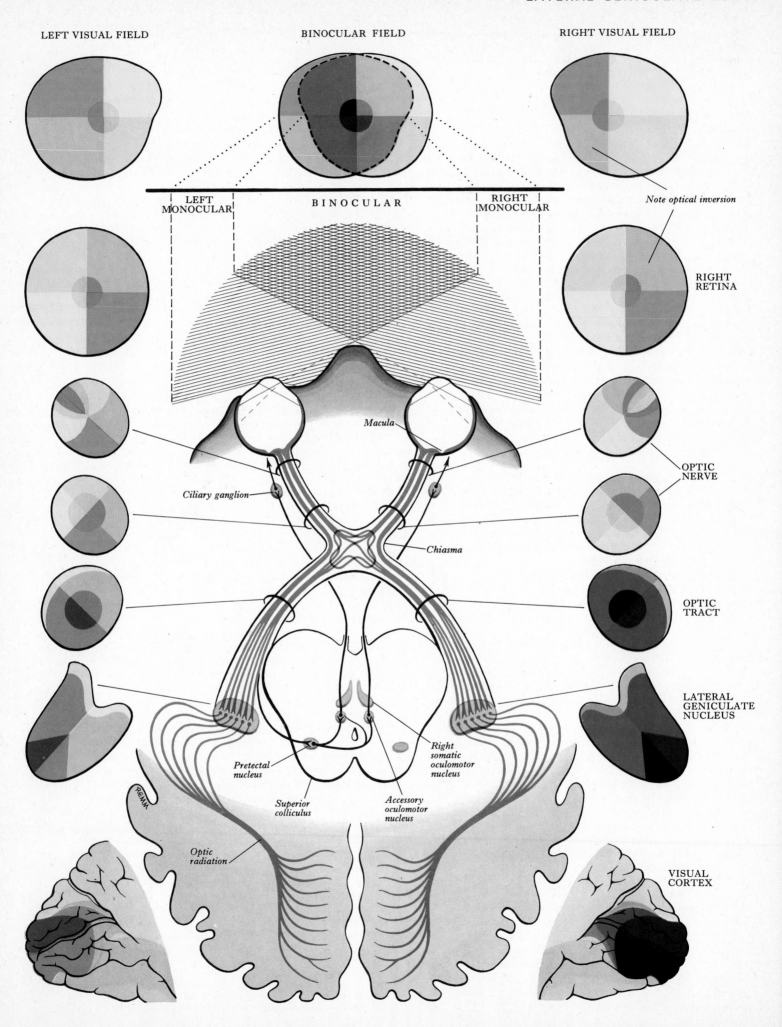

LEFT VISUAL FIELD

BINOCULAR FIELD

RIGHT VISUAL FIELD

LEFT
MONOCULAR

BINOCULAR

RIGHT
MONOCULAR

*Note optical inversion*

RIGHT
RETINA

*Macula*

*Ciliary ganglion*

OPTIC
NERVE

*Chiasma*

OPTIC
TRACT

*Right
somatic
oculomotor
nucleus*

LATERAL
GENICULATE
NUCLEUS

*Pretectal
nucleus*

*Superior
colliculus*

*Accessory
oculomotor
nucleus*

*Optic
radiation*

VISUAL
CORTEX

sizes represent the balance between the forebrain and midbrain destinations, it is obvious that the phylogenetically older, mesencephalic termination is greatly reduced in man, as in other primates, but to a lesser degree in mammals in general. The emergence of the lateral geniculate body was during sub-mammalian evolution, at a stage where the optic tract contains only contralateral nerve fibres from the eye. This decussation is basic in vertebrates, and while it is possible to formulate various explanatory hypotheses to account for it—like other central nervous decussations—these must remain speculative.[628, 629] The advent of an element of uncrossed retinal connexions in mammals—especially developed in the primates and others with forward looking eyes and overlap of visual fields—can be associated with an increasing specialization of the *dorsal part* of the *primitive lateral geniculate body*, which forms by volume the main part of the structure in higher mammals, including man. It is in this region of the whole nuclear mass that a laminar organization appears, perhaps in direct association with the terminals of ipsilateral and contralateral retinal projections (*vide infra*). The *ventral part* of the mammalian lateral geniculate body is also known in many forms as the *pregeniculate nucleus*, which is in man represented by a small, but not exiguous group of nerve cells,[630] medial to the main laminar nucleus in its ventral third or so. Medially, the cells of the pregeniculate nucleus extend in a scattered array towards the subthalamic region, marking the evolutionary and embryonic origin of this part of the lateral geniculate complex. It receives a bilateral retinal projection (possibly as collaterals from fibres passing to the tectum and to the main nucleus); this projection is said to be limited to the central region of the retina and to form part of the light reflex pathways through a *pregeniculo-mesencephalic connexion*.[628] Such an arrangement has a particular clinical interest to explanations of the Argyll-Robertson phenomenon (p. 1129). A cortical connexion with the pregeniculate nucleus has not been established, and it is to be emphasized that some workers deny that optic nerve fibres terminate in this nucleus in primates, in which it is nevertheless a well-developed entity.

**The dorsal or main lateral geniculate nucleus** exhibits a well-known laminar structure, there being six (and perhaps seven) layers of nerve cells discernible in some part of the nucleus in higher primates, such as the rhesus macaque (the subject of much experimental study) and mankind. It should be noted at once, however—particularly in respect of proposals to equate this pattern with functional ideas, such as trichromatic theories of colour vision[631]—that the number and arrangement of laminae varies in different mammals, being three in the cat (another much used experimental animal). The laminar pattern also displays regional degrees of elaboration in the geniculate nucleus in most species, including man. Phylogenetically, an original division into two laminae has been suggested, concerned with separate terminations of ipsi- and contra-lateral retinal fibres.[628] Nevertheless, all six layers appear together in human

embryonic development.[632] With the development of two major classes of neurons, large and small, a splitting of these primary layers may have occurred. In this connexion it is pertinent to note that interlaminar strata of larger cells occur between the three recognized laminae in the feline lateral geniculate nucleus.[633]

In describing the human lateral geniculate body, particularly as regards its intrinsic and external interconnexions and their functional interpretation, it is necessary to remember that such details are almost entirely extrapolated from experimental results observed chiefly in cats and monkeys, together with a considerable volume of comparative structural study in mammals, including many primates.[630] Nevertheless, the commonly used experimental animals, especially monkeys, display such a similarity of structural organization in the lateral geniculate body that it is unlikely that data established thus cannot be extended, in most instances, to mankind.

The appearance and orientation of the laminae of the human lateral body are shown in illustration 7.108C–G. This orientation is often confusingly presented in textbooks and other accounts (consult references [632, 634]), its relation to other structures being obscured by omission of reference data. Often depicted in coronal sections (7.108C), it is also sometimes shown in sagittal section, and in both views the lamination is apparent, since the laminae are somewhat like a series of caps set one upon another. The lamination is best displayed in coronal sections from the central region of the nuclear mass and in a direction towards its posterior (caudal) pole. Anteriorly or cranially, i.e. near the entry of the optic tract, the layers are blended together into a common mass, and at the posterior extremity the number is reduced to four—in a region of the nucleus which is considered to be monopolized by terminating macular fibres. As illustration 7.108C shows, the laminae are curved, with a ventral concavity forming a kind of 'hilus', at which some of the retinal efferents enter from the adjacent optic tract. This hilus is much more prominent in the monkey than in man. Dorsally, the nucleus is dome-shaped and projects towards the thalamus; from this aspect the majority of the fibres of the optic radiation, or *geniculostriate projection*, emerge from the nucleus. Both medially and laterally the laminae blend, as if at the edge of the cap-shaped mass; and the lateral border is sharp; the blending layers reverse their curvature here, becoming ventrally convex, or upturned like the peak of a cap. It is also noteworthy that concave contours of the laminae are also reversed in the posterior (macular) part of the geniculate nucleus. As a result, the profiles of the laminae, in the coronal plane, are slightly sinuous on the lateral side. (Some of the confusion concerning the lamination of the lateral geniculate body is due to the fact that the order of the layers is reversed in some lower primates, the large celled laminae 1 and 2 being *external* and *dorsal* to the others—on the outer aspect of the curvature of the entire laminar structure. In *Tarsius* the situation is extreme, the layers being an inverted replica of the human situation—or vice versa. In the lemuroids transitional states occur. Much controversy has been entailed by the use of the terms inversion and eversion, which need not detain us here.)

---

7.109 A diagram of the visual pathway to show the spatial arrangement of nerve cells and their fibres in relation to the quadrants of the retinae and visual fields. The proportions at various levels are not exactly to scale, and in particular the macula has been exaggerated in size in the visual fields and retinae. In each quadrant of the visual field, and the parts of the visual pathway subserving it, two shades of the respective colour are used—the paler for the peripheral fields and a darker shade for the macular part of the quadrant. From the optic tract onwards these two shades are both made more saturated to denote intermixture of neurons from both retinae, the palest shade being reserved for parts of the visual pathway concerned with monocular vision. The path of the light reflex has also been indicated.

[628] S. Polyak, *The Vertebrate Visual System*, University of Chicago Press, Chicago. 1957.
[629] W. S. Duke-Elder, *Textbook of Ophthalmology*, Vol. I, Kimpton, London. 1932.
[630] W. E. Le G. Clark, *Br. J. Opthalmol.*, **16**, 1932.
[631] W. E. Le G. Clark, *Nature, Lond.*, *146*, 1940; and *Documenta ophth.*, **3**, 1949.
[632] E. R. A. Cooper, *Brain*, **68**, 1945.
[633] B. D. Thuma, *J. comp. Neurol.*, **46**, 1928.
[634] L. W. Chacko, *J. Anat. Soc. Ind.*, **4**, 1955.

The most careful estimates suggest that there are about 1 million nerve cells in the human lateral geniculate body, corresponding closely to the count of fibres in the optic nerve and tract.[635] (Estimates in the macaque monkey are as much as 1·8 million,[636] but only 1·2 million in the optic nerve.[637] *See*, however, reference[638].) This 1:1 ratio in man does not, however, imply that each optic nerve fibre connects with only one geniculate cell. This relationship may be the case in respect of the macula, but such details are still uncertain. It has long been established[636, 639, 640] that each fibre, derived from the retinal ganglion cells, ends by dividing into no more than five or six terminals connecting with a corresponding number of geniculate nerve cells in *one* lamina. (The geniculate cells may connect with terminals from more than one retinal fibre.) The laminae are usually numbered 1 to 6, starting from the concave, ventral, or hilar aspect of the nucleus. Fibres from the *contralateral* optic nerve end in layers 1, 4 and 6, *ipsilateral* fibres in layers 2, 3 and 5. Early recognition that transneuronal degeneration (p. 762) occurs in the lateral geniculate body,[640] coupled with an adequate terminal degeneration technique,[641] has lead to the detailed elucidation of this bilateral representation of the retinae in each lateral geniculate body. Even with the Marchi degeneration technique alone it had been possible to show in monkeys[642]—by studying the results of small retinal lesions—that fibres from different quadrants of the retinae are located correspondingly in the optic nerve (p. 997 and **7.**109), macular fibres occupying a central position. Similarly, an orderly but somewhat different arrangement was demonstrated in the optic chiasma and tract (**7.**109), with the difference that in the tract, fibres from corresponding quadrants in both retinae occupy the same location. This pattern is carried into the lateral geniculate body, where the macular fibres terminate in the central and posterior part of the nucleus, the peripheral fibres in its anterior part, the upper retinal quadrants ending medially, the lower ones laterally (**7.**109). Transneuronal techniques enabled much more precise plotting of the retinogeniculate connexions,[643] and since the cortical projection fibres of the affected geniculate nerve cells also degenerate, it was demonstrable that the same kind of a precise point-to-point connexion continues through the optic radiation to the striate cortex (p. 762). The precision of this topical organization in the visual pathway has been repeatedly confirmed in cats and monkeys.[628, 644] As will be detailed elsewhere (p. 962), ablation of small parts of the striate cortex in the occipital lobe leads to highly localized patches of degenerating geniculate cells in *six layers* on the same side. These effects appear in a columnar representation of corresponding points of the two retinae, each in *three* of the six geniculate laminae.

So far this account has considered the visual pathway as a series of parallel conducting pathways, with no mention of possible interaction between them—whether from the same retina or from both. In fact, it has for long been assumed that, apart from inevitable convergence of activities in the far more numerous rods and cones of the retina upon the more limited population of optic nerve neurons (retinal ganglion cells—p. 1117), the remainder of the visual pathway consists of functionally isolated conductors, with a simple relay in the lateral geniculate body. This simple view has been customary textbook teaching, with the modification that the bringing together of fibres from both retinae in the geniculate body constitutes subcortical 'fusion'. The latter would be a naïve assumption in the absence of data beyond those recounted above. The neuronal organization of the retina itself is, of course, complex; there is clear evidence, both anatomical and physiological (p. 1111), of interaction between its neurons.

Hence the pattern of impulses in the optic nerve is not the simple result of a mosaic of receptor responses, like the signals in a cable between a television camera and its monitor—even if the effects of corticofugal connexions are ignored (p. 1118). Integrative activities in the cat's lateral geniculate body have also been demonstrated[645] between corticofugal fibres and the incoming sensory projection, as in other sensory pathways. While unit recording has also shown the existence of lateral inhibition and of units responsive to specific modes of stimulation, there is apparently no clear evidence to indicate that individual geniculate cells receive impulses from both retinae.[646]

An increasing elaboration of cytological detail, particularly in respect to dendritic fields and synaptic characteristics, has been recorded in the cat[647] and monkey. It is not yet possible to correlate these findings either functionally or structurally into a fully connected model of geniculate activity, but it is obvious that the view of this as a comparatively simple relay mechanism is completely demolished. Three major elements are involved: (*a*) *afferents* from the retinae—to which may be added corticofugal fibres and perhaps fibres from the ubiquitous reticular system; (*b*) the *efferent geniculostriate projection*; and (*c*) the *intrinsic neuronal population*, consisting largely of Golgi type II nerve cells, not all the axons of which are confined to a single lamina, and hence might mediate connexions between bilateral retinal afferents. Most accounts say little of the precise arrangement of the cells (Golgi type I) whose axons stream dorsally through intervening laminae to form the geniculostriate pathway; attention has been predominantly concentrated—both in light and electron microscope studies—upon dendritic morphology and the distribution and functional attributes of synapses. The profusion of the resultant neuropil is in itself suggestive evidence of highly complex interneuronal mediation between the afferents and efferents of the lateral geniculate body. One particularly interesting feature is the occurrence of *glomeruli*—conglomerations of synapses between dendritic and axonal terminals, the latter in part derived from optic nerve fibres.[647, 648] These are similar in some respects to the synaptic glomeruli described in the cerebellum (p. 869), and in other thalamic 'relay' nuclei (p. 895), and are likely to subserve the same kind of integrative function. The glomeruli are highly complex structures consisting of a main and peripheral axons, a main and peripheral dendrites, and various other neuronal and glial elements (see also p. 776). Some axons may be involved in the formation of several glomeruli; others, morphologically distinguishable, occur in the periphery of the glomerulus, making synaptic contacts not only with the dendrites in it but also with the central axon within its core. The latter type of synapse, like other *axoaxonal* connexions, is probably inhibitory.[649] Dendrodendritic synapses have also been identified (for further details see p. 773). Such observations probably provide the anatomical substrate for the

[635] C. Kupfer, L. Chumbley and J. de C. Downer, *J. Anat.*, **101**, 1967.
[636] W. E. Le G. Clark, *J. Anat.*, **75**, 1941.
[637] S. R. Bruesch and L. B. Arey, *J. comp. Neurol.*, **77**, 1942.
[638] K. L. Chow, J. S. Blum and R. A. Blum, *J. comp. Neurol.*, **92**, 1950.
[639] P. Glees, *J. Anat.*, **75**, 1941.
[640] M. Minkowski, *Arb. hirnanat. Inst., Zürich*, **7**, 1913.
[641] P. Glees, *Nature, Lond.*, **146**, 1946.
[642] B. Brouwer and W. P. C. Zeeman, *Brain*, **49**, 1926.
[643] W. E. Le G. Clark and G. G. Penman, *Proc. R. Soc. B.*, **114**, 1934.
[644] T. H. Meikle and J. M. Sprague, *Int. Rev. Neurobiol.*, **6**, 1964.
[645] D. H. Hubel and T. N. Wiesel, *J. Physiol., Lond.*, **155**, 1961.
[646] P. Glees, in: *The Visual System*, eds. R. Jung and H. Körnmuller, Springer, Berlin. 1961.
[647] A. Peters and S. L. Palay, *J. Anat.*, **100**, 1966.
[648] J. A. Campos-Ortega, P. Glees and V. Neuhoff, *Z. Zellforsch. mikrosk. Anat.*, **87**, 1968.
[649] J. C. Eccles, *The Physiology of Synapses*, Springer, Berlin. 1964.

occurrence of inhibitory as well as excitatory receptive field effects identified by unit recording in the lateral geniculate nucleus.[645] Glomerular structures of a similar nature have been identified in the monkey.[650] Such *synaptic* glomeruli are not to be confused with clusters of nerve cells, also called glomeruli, described at a much earlier date;[651] these exist in all the laminae of the monkey's geniculate nucleus, the number in the clusters increasing from 12–15 in layer 1 to 60–100 in layer 6. It has recently been suggested[647] that the somata of the neurons whose neurites are involved in a *synaptic glomerulus* may be clustered together as a *cellular glomerulus*, a view which tentatively equates the latter with the nerve cell groups described above. Electron microscope evidence suggests that the synaptic glomeruli may become more complex in the outer layers of the lateral geniculate nucleus. However this may be, the intricate synaptic relationships thus established provide an illuminating prelude to full structural delineation of the integrative mechanisms in the lateral geniculate nucleus.

The findings so far noted on the whole indicate only *intra*laminar integration; the question of *inter*laminar interaction is of special interest with regard to integration of information from both eyes. Since each retinal ganglion cell fibre terminates, as far as is known, merely in one lamina, any interaction between fibres derived, as is presumed, from the same locus in one retina but ending separately in three geniculate laminae, would require some form of interlaminar connexion. Even were such connexions unsupported by anatomical evidence, the results of unit recording at the geniculate level would strongly indicate their existence. The same reasoning appertains to interaction between impulses derived from corresponding loci in *both* retinae. Again, as far as is known, each lamina projects separately to the striate cortex—and not, as some diagrams loosely depict, by a fictitious form of neuron with a soma in each lamina and a single conjoined axon projecting to the cortex! Physiological evidence has tended to corroborate the view that impulses from the two retinae are integrated only at the level of the striate cortex.[652] However, it has been claimed recently that unit recording demonstrates binocular interaction at the geniculate level; and electron microscope observations suggest that in the fibre zones between laminae are synapses between neurons intrinsic to the lateral geniculate nucleus.[653] Neurons in the laminae—probably second order interneurons—have also been shown to mediate interlaminar connexions;[654, 655] these *could* be concerned in channelling effects from both retinae into single geniculostriate fibres. Certainly, the neuronal independence of the geniculate laminae seems to have been finally dismissed.

## The Third Ventricle

The third ventricle (**7**.97, 110), which is the derivative of the primitive forebrain vesicle, is a median cleft between the two thalami. It communicates posteriorly with the fourth ventricle through the cerebral aqueduct, and anteriorly with the lateral ventricles through the interventricular foramina. It has a roof, a floor, anterior and posterior boundaries, and two lateral walls.

The *roof* is formed by a layer of ependyma which stretches between the upper edges of the lateral walls of the cavity and is continuous with the rest of the ependymal lining of the ventricle. It is covered by, and adherent to, a fold of pia mater, named the *tela choroidea* of the third ventricle, from the inferior surface of which a pair of vascular fringed processes, the *choroid plexuses of the third ventricle*, project downwards, one on each side of the median plane, and invaginate the ependymal roof into the ventricular cavity (**7**.157).

The *floor* (**7**.110) descends ventrally and is formed mainly by structures which belong to the hypothalamus; ventrodorsally these are: the optic chiasma, the infundibulum and tuber cinereum, and the mamillary bodies. Posterior to the last-named, the floor is formed by the posterior perforated substance and by the tegmentum of the cerebral peduncles. The ventricle is prolonged downwards into the infundibulum as a funnel-shaped *infundibular recess*. The hypophysis is attached to the apex of the infundibulum.

The *anterior boundary* (**7**.110) is inferiorly the *lamina terminalis*, which represents the cranial terminal of the primitive neural tube. It forms a thin layer of grey matter stretching from the superior surface of the optic chiasma to the rostrum of the corpus callosum. In its superior part the anterior boundary is formed by the columns of the fornix, which diverge as they descend into the lateral walls of the ventricle, and by the anterior commissure (p. 937), which crosses the median plane anterior to them. At the junction of the floor and anterior wall, immediately above the optic chiasma, the ventricle presents a small angular diverticulum, the *optic recess*. At the junction of the roof with the anterior and lateral limits of the ventricle is the *interventricular foramen*, through which the third and the lateral ventricles communicate with one another. It represents the site of the original diverticular outgrowth from the telencephalon which forms the cerebral hemisphere, and is relatively large and circular in a 10 mm human embryo. In the adult, however, it is reduced to a somewhat crescentic slit, bounded anteriorly by the curving column of the fornix and posteriorly by the convex anterior tubercle of the thalamus.

The *posterior boundary* (**7**.110) consists of the pineal body, the posterior commissure and the cerebral aqueduct. A *pineal recess* projects into the stalk of the pineal body, whilst anterosuperior to the latter is a second, *suprapineal recess*, consisting of a diverticulum of the epithelial ventricular roof.

Each *lateral wall* consists of an upper part formed by the medial surface of the anterior two-thirds of the thalamus, and a lower formed by the hypothalamus and continuous with the grey matter of the ventricular floor. These two regions of the lateral wall are separated by the *hypothalamic sulcus*, which extends from the interventricular foramen to the cerebral aqueduct, but is not always an obvious feature. As noted previously (p. 891), the hypothalamic sulcus can be regarded as dividing the diencephalon into two. Above (dorsal to) the sulcus is the *pars dorsalis diencephali* consisting of the dorsal thalamus and the epithalamus, below (ventral) is the *pars ventralis diencephali* which constitutes the hypothalamus and subthalamus. Each lateral wall of the third ventricle is limited superiorly by the ridge covering the stria medullaris thalami (p. 892). The columns of the fornix curve ventrally cranial to the interventricular foramina, and then run in the lateral walls of the ventricle, where, at first, they form distinct prominences, but subsequently sink into them. The lateral walls are joined to each other across the cavity of the ventricle by a band of grey matter, the *interthalamic adhesion* (p. 892). The hypothalamus has been described on p. 904.

[650] M. Colonnier and R. W. Guillery, *Z. Zellforsch. mikrosk. Anat.*, **62**, 1964.

[651] R. P. Taboada, *Trab. Lab. Invest. biol. Univ. Madr.*, **25**, 1927.

[652] D. H. Hubel and T. N. Wiesel, *Nature, Lond.*, **221**, 1969.

[653] R. W. Guillery and M. Colonnier, *Z. Zellforsch. mikrosk. Anat.*, **103**, 1970.

[654] R. W. Guillery, *J. comp. Neurol.*, **128**, 1966.

[655] R. W. Guillery, *Brain Res.*, **28**, 1971.

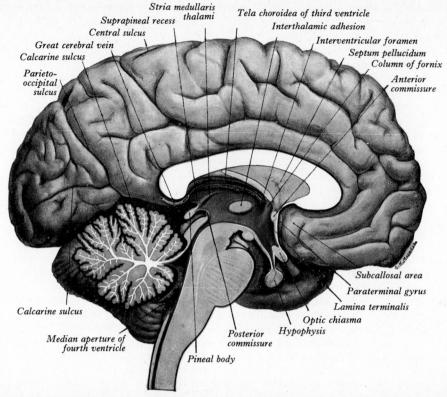

Stria medullaris thalami
Suprapineal recess
Central sulcus
Great cerebral vein
Calcarine sulcus
Parieto-occipital sulcus
Tela choroidea of third ventricle
Interthalamic adhesion
Interventricular foramen
Septum pellucidum
Column of fornix
Anterior commissure
Calcarine sulcus
Median aperture of fourth ventricle
Posterior commissure
Pineal body
Hypophysis
Optic chiasma
Lamina terminalis
Paraterminal gyrus
Subcallosal area

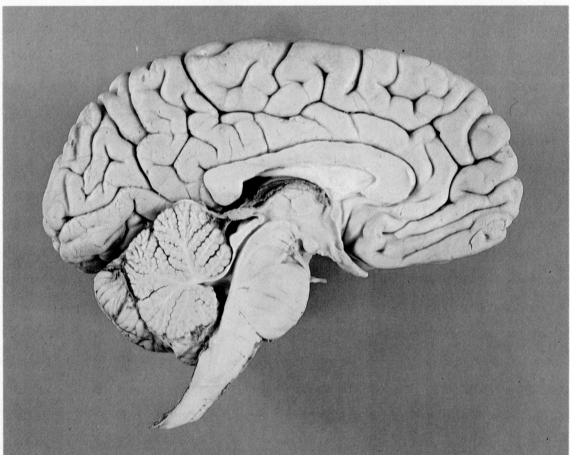

7.110A *above*   Median sagittal section of the brain to show the third and fourth ventricles. The pia mater is indicated in red, the ependyma is shown in blue.

7.110B *below*   A median sagittal section through the brain. For detailed labelling of the structures visible on this specimen compare with 7.110A, 7.114 and 8.195. (Dissection by Dr. E. L. Rees.)

**The interpeduncular fossa** (7.55, 104, 111) is a trapezoid area of the cerebral base, limited anteriorly by the optic chiasma, posteriorly by the anterosuperior surface of the pons, anterolaterally by the converging optic tracts, and posterolaterally by the diverging cerebral peduncles. The structures contained in it have been described elsewhere; dorsoventrally they are the posterior perforated substance (p. 904), mamillary bodies (p. 905), tuber cinereum (p. 904), infundibulum and hypophysis cerebri (p. 1367).

920

# THE TELENCEPHALON OR 'ENDBRAIN'

The expansion of the telencephalon and the development of the two cerebral hemispheres have already been described (p. 138). In primitive vertebrates each cerebral hemisphere is predominantly concerned with olfactory impulses, which enter it rostrally at the *olfactory lobe*. This lobe may be drawn away to form an *olfactory bulb* which remains connected to the rest of the hemisphere by a stalk, the *olfactory tract*. In the basal parts of each hemisphere masses of grey matter, the *basal nuclei*, are present and form an early motor centre. The wall of the hemisphere constitutes the *pallium*, wherein olfactory and other flows of information are presumed to be integrated. In the course of evolution visual, auditory and other conduction paths have been transferred, through the thalamus, to the pallium of the cerebral hemispheres, an instance of encephalization. Consequently, each cerebral hemisphere enlarges as a result of the formation of an additional region, the *neopallium*, the predominantly olfactory pallium being confined to a *piriform lobe* inferolateral in site. The medial wall of the hemisphere becomes specialized to form the *hippocampal formation*. This was for long also regarded as primarily part of the olfactory mechanism, but in recent years this view has become untenable (see p. 931). In higher mammals the neopallium is greatly enlarged; the piriform lobe, in contrast, is relatively reduced. With the growth of the neopallium motor pathways are developed from this, but the basal nuclei remain as essential parts of the motor control apparatus. The greatly increased growth of the neopallium in mammals is due to the formation of *association areas* concerned with the interaction of its multiplicity of afferent and efferent connexions. (It should be noted that the hippocampal formation is often termed the *archipallium*, or *primal* cortex, and the piriform lobe the *paleopallium*, or *ancient* cortex. Some authorities, however, group both these regions under the term *archipallium*.)

The telencephalon includes: (1) the cerebral hemispheres, the commissures which connect them, and the cavities which they contain; and (2) the anterior parts of the third ventricle, including the preoptic regions in the telencephalon impar, already described (p. 905). Each cerebral hemisphere consists of an outer layer of grey matter, termed the *cortex*, an inner mass of white fibres (*centrum semiovale*), the deeply situated *basal nuclei* and a cavity, the *lateral ventricle*.

# THE CEREBRAL HEMISPHERES

The cerebral hemispheres form the largest part of the brain, and, when viewed together from above, assume the outline of an ovoid mass broader behind than in front, the greatest transverse diameter corresponding with a line connecting the two parietal tuberosities. The hemispheres are incompletely separated by a deep median cleft, named the *longitudinal cerebral fissure*, and each possesses a central cavity, the *lateral ventricle*.

**The longitudinal fissure of the cerebrum** contains a sickle-shaped process of dura mater, the *falx cerebri*, and the anterior cerebral vessels. Anteriorly and posteriorly, the fissure completely separates the cerebral hemispheres from each other; centrally, however, it only extends down to a great central white commissure, named the *corpus callosum*, which connects the hemispheres across the median plane.

## The Surfaces of the Cerebrum

Each cerebral hemisphere presents three surfaces: superolateral, medial and inferior.

The *superolateral surface* is convex in adaptation to the concavity of the corresponding half of the vault of the cranium. The *medial surface* is flat and vertical and is separated from that of the opposite hemisphere by the longitudinal fissure and the falx cerebri. The *inferior surface* is of an irregular form, and may be divided into two parts: orbital and tentorial. The orbital part, being the orbital surface of the frontal lobes, is concave, and rests on the orbital roofs and the nose; the tentorial part is concavoconvex, and is the inferior surface of the temporal and occipital lobes; anteriorly it is adapted to the corresponding half of the middle cranial fossa; posteriorly it rests upon the tentorium cerebelli, which intervenes between it and the superior surface of the cerebellum.

The three surfaces are separated by the following borders: (*a*) *superomedial*, between the superolateral and medial surfaces; (*b*) *inferolateral*, between the superolateral and basal surfaces; the anterior part of this border separates the superolateral from the orbital surface of the frontal lobe, and is known as the *superciliary* border; (*c*) *medial occipital*, between the tentorial part of the inferior and the medial surface; and (*d*) *medial orbital*, separating the orbital part of the inferior from the medial surface. The anterior end of the hemisphere is named the *frontal pole*, the posterior, the *occipital pole*; and the anterior end of the temporal lobe, the *temporal pole*. About 5 cm anterior to the occipital pole on the inferolateral border there is an indentation, the *pre-occipital incisure* or notch.

A paramedian line drawn from a point a little superolateral to the inion, forwards to a point just superolateral to the nasion, corresponds to the superomedial margin. The superciliary border follows the curve of the eyebrows at a slightly higher level as far as the zygomatic process of the frontal bone and then ascends to the pterion. The temporal pole can be indicated on the surface of the head by a line drawn, with a forward convexity, from the pterion to the middle of the upper border of the zygomatic arch, and this line, continued backwards just above the zygomatic arch and crossing the auricle a little above the external acoustic meatus, corresponds to the inferolateral margin of the hemisphere, which then curves downwards to reach the posterior end of the superomedial border (**6.**119).

The surfaces of the hemispheres are moulded into a number of irregular eminences, named *gyri* or *convolutions*, and separated by furrows termed *sulci* or *fissures*.

The irregular character of the surfaces of the cerebral hemispheres is a very prominent feature, but up to the end of the third fetal month these surfaces are smooth and unbroken, like the surfaces of the brains of reptiles and birds. Thereafter localized depressions become apparent, and they deepen and extend over the surfaces to form the sulci (*see* p. 140 and **2.**89A–G). Each sulcus corresponds to an infolding of the cortex; thereby the total amount of grey matter is about three times as much as might be inferred from the surface area of the hemisphere. In certain situations the sulci develop along lines separating areas which differ from one another in the details of their microscopic structure and in the functions which they predominantly subserve.[656] Such sulci may therefore be termed *limiting sulci,* since they establish the limits of certain functional areas. The central sulcus is an example of a limiting sulcus, for it is set between two areas of cortex which differ in thickness so notably that this can be appreciated with the naked eye (**7.**115A). In other situations sulci develop in the long axis of a rapidly growing homogeneous area and are termed *axial sulci.* The posterior part of the calcarine sulcus is in the centre of the striate area and is merely a fold in the visual cortex. In other situations, again, a sulcus may be situated between two surface areas of cortex which are structurally different, but its lip and not its floor may form the dividing line between the two areas. In these cases a third area may be present in the walls of the sulcus without appearing on the surface at all. Such a sulcus is termed an *operculated sulcus,* and this type is represented in the human brain by the lunate sulcus, which separates the striate from the peristriate areas on the surface, and contains in its wall the submerged parastriate area, which really intervenes between them. These three varieties include all the sulci which develop on the surface of the brain, with the exception of the lateral sulcus and the parieto-occipital sulcus. The former is the result of the slower expansion of the cortex of the insula and its consequent submersion by the adjoining cortical areas, which eventually come into contact with one another so as to delimit the lateral sulcus. The latter is brought about subsequent to the development of the corpus callosum. The posterior end of this great commissure has to convey not only the fibres from the occipital lobes of the brain but also a large number of fibres from its temporal lobes. As a result, a number of smaller axial and limiting sulci become crowded together and some of them become buried within the walls of the parieto-occipital sulcus. These two are really secondary sulci, since their occurrence depends on factors other than exuberant growth in closely adjoining areas.

Some of the sulci which indent the cerebral surface are deep enough to produce corresponding elevations in the walls of the lateral ventricles. The anterior part of the calcarine sulcus, which produces the calcar avis of the posterior horn, and the collateral, which produces the collateral eminence in the inferior horn, are therefore termed *complete fissures or sulci.* There is, however, no special morphological or functional significance to be attached to the fact that while some sulci are complete others are incomplete. (All the features mentioned in the above account can easily be identified in the illustrations in this section.)

The gyri and their intervening sulci are fairly constant in arrangement; at the same time they vary within certain limits, not only in different individuals, but in the two hemispheres of the same brain.

The convolutional pattern of the cerebral cortex is an inevitable concomitant of the much greater increase in volume of the pallium or mantle of nerve cells in the cortex as compared with the lesser increase in volume of the subjacent white matter. The actual area of the human cortex is about 2,200 cm², and only a third of this is visible on the surface, the rest being obscured from view in the sulci and fissures. By this form of evolution a large increase in cortical area is possible without great change in cranial capacity, but it would be misleading to explain the arrangement in this teleological manner, as is sometimes done. Similarly, any presumed association of high intelligence with great complexity of convolutional pattern is also fallacious. The most intricate arrays of sulci and gyri occur in the cerebra of the elephant and the whale, both of

which have in addition much larger brains than man, though not so in relation to their total size. No close relationship between convolutional complexity and brain size with cerebral abilities has been established in man himself; abundant examples of highly able individuals with relatively small brains and the reverse of this have been attested. Attempts to draw deductions from the endocranial casts of fossil forms of man—as an indication of the development of certain gyri and hence abilities (such as the capacity for speech)—have likewise proved misleading and have been largely abandoned.

It is convenient for description and reference to separate the surfaces of the cerebral hemisphere into a number of lobes, but it must be remembered that this division is purely one of convenience; moreover the lobes do not precisely correspond in surface extent to the cranial bones from which their names are derived.

## THE SUPEROLATERAL SURFACE OF THE CEREBRAL HEMISPHERE

Two sulci, viz. the *lateral sulcus* and the *central sulcus,* take a large part in forming the boundaries of the lobes into which this surface is divided (**7.**111A, B).

**The lateral sulcus** (**7.**111, 115) is a deep cleft situated on the inferior and lateral surfaces of the cerebral hemisphere. It consists of a short stem which ends by dividing into three rami. The *stem* commences on the inferior surface at the anterior perforated substance and extends laterally between the orbital surface of the frontal lobe and the anterior part of the temporal lobe. It is occupied by the posterior border of the lesser wing of the sphenoid bone and the sphenoparietal venous sinus. On reaching the lateral surface it divides into anterior horizontal, anterior ascending and posterior rami. The *anterior ramus* runs forward for 2·5 cm or less into the inferior frontal gyrus, while the *ascending ramus* runs upwards for about an equal distance into the same gyrus. The *posterior ramus* is the longest division. It courses posteriorly and slightly upwards across the lateral surface for about 7 cm before turning upwards to end in the parietal lobe. The floor of this sulcus is formed by the limen insulae and the insula, and it conducts the middle cerebral vessels from the inferior to the superolateral aspect of the hemisphere. It can be represented on the side of the head by a line drawn backwards and slightly upwards for 7 cm from the pterion and then curving upwards to end under the parietal eminence.

**The central sulcus** (**7.**111) commences in or near the superomedial border of the hemisphere a little posterior to the mid-point between the frontal and occipital poles. It runs sinuously downwards and forwards for about 8 to 10 cm and ends a little superior to the posterior ramus of the lateral sulcus, from which it is always separated by an arched gyrus. The general direction of the sulcus makes an angle of rather less than 70° with the median plane (**7.**111). It lies at the junction of the motor and sensory areas of the cortex (pp. 954 and 958).

When the central sulcus is opened up, the opposed walls are found to be marked by a number of small gyri which interlock with one another after the manner of gears in mesh, and are therefore termed *interlocking gyri.* This arrangement provides additional cortex without any corresponding increase in the surface area of the hemisphere. Another feature is brought to light by opening up the sulcus. The floor is not the same depth throughout, for a little inferior to the middle of the sulcus its walls are usually connected to each other by a buried, transverse

[656] W. E. Le G. Clark in: *Essays on Growth and Form,* eds. W. E. Le G. Clark and P. B. Medawar, Clarendon Press, Oxford. 1945.

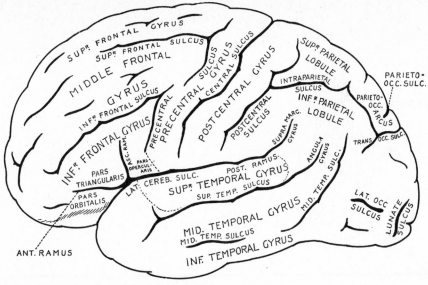

**7.111A** Lateral aspect of the superolateral surface of the left cerebral hemisphere.

gyrus. The explanation of this condition is found in the mode of development of the central sulcus. When it makes its appearance in the sixth month, it does so in two distinct parts, superior and inferior, which are at first separated by a transverse gyrus connecting the precentral convolution to the postcentral. The two parts occasionally remain separate, but as a rule they run into each other, and the transverse gyrus becomes buried as a *deep transitional gyrus*.

**The frontal lobe** is the anterior part of the hemisphere. On the superolateral surface it is bounded behind by the central sulcus, above by the superomedial border and

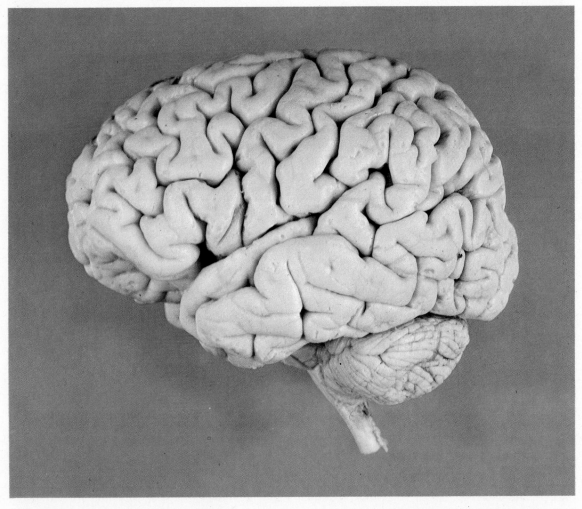

**7.111B** A left lateral view of the brain to show the pattern of gyri and sulci on the superolateral aspect of the cerebral hemisphere. Compare with **7.111A**, which was drawn from a different specimen, for labelling of the many structures visible. Note also the contrasting cortical patterns of the cerebrum and cerebellum. (Dissection by Dr. E. L. Rees.)

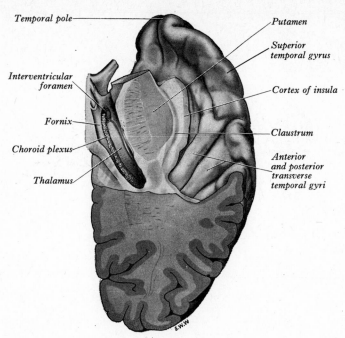

Temporal pole

Interventricular foramen

Fornix

Choroid plexus

Thalamus

Putamen

Superior temporal gyrus

Cortex of insula

Claustrum

Anterior and posterior transverse temporal gyri

7.112 Horizontal section showing the superior surface of the right temporal lobe.

cortex of this gyrus gives origin to some of the fibres of the important corticonuclear and corticospinal (pyramidal) motor tracts (p. 820).

The *superior frontal gyrus* is above the superior frontal sulcus, and is continuous over the superomedial margin of the hemisphere with the medial frontal gyrus on the medial surface. It may be divided by an incomplete sulcus (7.111).

The *middle frontal gyrus* lies between the superior and the inferior frontal sulci.

The *inferior frontal gyrus* is inferior to the inferior frontal sulcus and is invaded by the anterior and ascending rami of the lateral sulcus. The areas grouped around these two rami constitute the *speech area of Broca* (areas 44 and 45) and are associated with the motor element of speech (p. 956). The region lying below the anterior ramus is termed the *pars orbitalis*, and it curves round the superciliary margin to the orbital surface of the frontal lobe. The area between the ascending and the anterior rami is termed the *pars triangularis*, while the area posterior to the ascending ramus forms the *pars opercularis (posterior)* and is continuous posteriorly with the inferior limit of the precentral gyrus.

**The temporal lobe** is inferior to the lateral sulcus. Posteriorly, it is limited by an arbitrary line from the preoccipital notch (p. 921) to the parieto-occipital sulcus, where it cuts the superomedial margin about 5 cm anterior to the occipital pole. The lateral surface of the temporal lobe is divided into three parallel gyri by two sulci.

The *superior temporal sulcus* begins near to the temporal pole and runs posteriorly and slightly upwards parallel to the posterior ramus of the lateral sulcus. Its posterior end curves up into the parietal lobe. The *inferior temporal sulcus* is subjacent and parallel to the superior sulcus. It is broken up into two or three short sulci, but its posterior end ascends into the parietal lobe, posterior and parallel to the upturned end of the superior sulcus.

In this way the lateral surface of the temporal lobe is

below by the superciliary border and the stem of the lateral sulcus.

The superolateral surface of the frontal lobe is traversed by three sulci which divide it into four gyri. The *precentral sulcus* runs parallel to the central sulcus, and is separated from it by the precentral gyrus. It is usually divided into upper and lower parts, but the two may be confluent. The *superior frontal sulcus* curves forwards from about the middle of the upper part of the precentral sulcus, while the *inferior frontal sulcus* is parallel to it at a lower level. The area of the frontal lobe which lies anterior to the

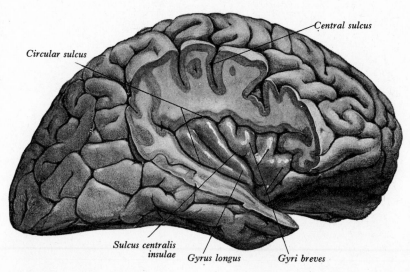

Circular sulcus

Central sulcus

Sulcus centralis insulae

Gyrus longus

Gyri breves

7.113A The right insula, exposed by the removal of its opercula.

precentral sulcus is thus divided into the superior, middle and inferior frontal gyri. An incomplete sulcus often divides the middle frontal gyrus (7.111).

The *precentral gyrus*, bounded posteriorly by the central sulcus and anteriorly by the precentral sulcus, extends from the superomedial border of the hemisphere, where it is continuous with the paracentral lobule on the medial surface, to the posterior ramus of the lateral sulcus. The

divided into three parallel gyri, the *superior*, *middle* and *inferior temporal gyri*. Along its superior margin the superior temporal gyrus is continuous with the gyri in the floor of the posterior ramus of the lateral sulcus. These are three or four in number, and they extend obliquely forwards and laterally from the *circular sulcus* which surrounds the insula. They are termed the *transverse temporal gyri* (7.112). The anterior transverse temporal gyrus and

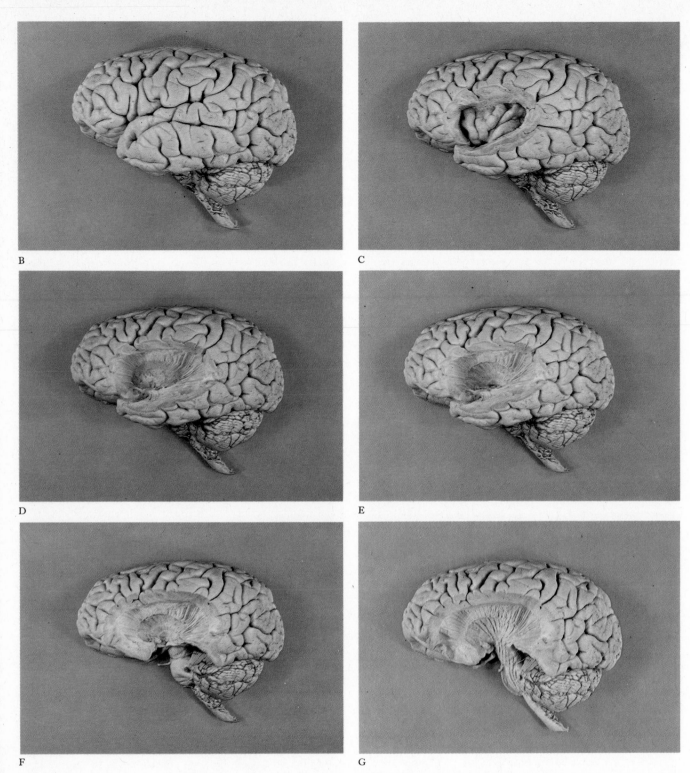

B

C

D

E

F

G

7.113 B–G  A series of dissections of the left cerebral hemisphere at progressively deeper levels to demonstrate the insula and subjacent structures. B  the intact brain; note the position of the posterior ramus of the lateral cerebral sulcus on which the dissections are centred; C  the cortical gyri of the insula exposed by removal of the frontal, temporal and parietal opercula; D  the removal of the insular cortex, extreme capsule, claustrum and external capsule has exposed the lateral aspect of the lentiform nucleus (the putamen); E  removal of the lentiform nucleus displays fibres of the internal capsule coursing across its medial aspect; F  removal of part of the temporal lobe shows the internal capsular fibres converging on the crus cerebri of the midbrain; G  removal of the optic tract, and superficial dissection of the pons and upper medulla, emphasizing the continuity of the corona radiata, internal capsule, crus cerebri, longitudinal pontine fibres, and the medullary pyramid. (Dissection by Dr. E. L. Rees.)

the part of the superior temporal gyrus with which it is in continuity are auditory in function (p. 963).

**The parietal lobe** is bounded anteriorly by the central sulcus and posteriorly by the line joining the pre-occipital incisure to the superomedial margin at the point where it is cut by the parieto-occipital sulcus. Its inferior limit is the posterior ramus of the lateral sulcus and a line drawn to the posterior boundary from the point where the ramus

ascends. Thus, both the posterior boundary and the posterior part of the inferior boundary of the parietal lobe on this surface of the hemisphere are arbitrary.

The lateral aspect of the parietal lobe is subdivided into three areas by the *postcentral* and *intraparietal sulci*.

The *postcentral sulcus* (7.111 A, B), which may be divided into upper and lower parts, is posterior and parallel to the central sulcus. Inferiorly it ends above the posterior ramus of the lateral sulcus and in front of its upturned end. It divides the parietal lobe into an anterior part, the postcentral gyrus, and a large posterior part which is further subdivided by the intraparietal sulcus. The *intraparietal sulcus* usually commences in the postcentral sulcus about its middle or at the superior end of its lower subdivision. It extends postero-inferiorly across the posterior part of the parietal lobe, dividing it into superior and inferior parietal lobules. Posteriorly, as the occipital ramus, it extends into the occipital lobe, where it joins the transverse occipital sulcus at right angles.

The *postcentral gyrus* lies between the central and postcentral sulci. Its cortex receives somatic sensory impulses (p. 958).

The *superior parietal lobule* is between the superomedial margin of the hemisphere and the intraparietal sulcus. Anteriorly, it is continuous with the postcentral gyrus round the upper end of the postcentral sulcus, while posteriorly it frequently runs into the arcus parietooccipitalis, which surrounds the lateral part of the parietooccipital sulcus (7.111 A, B).

The *inferior parietal lobule* is inferior to the intraparietal sulcus and posterior to the lower part of the postcentral sulcus. It is divided into three parts. The *anterior part* is the *supramarginal gyrus* and arches over the upturned end of the lateral sulcus; it is continuous anteriorly with the lower part of the postcentral gyrus and below and behind with the superior temporal gyrus. Occasionally it is limited posteriorly by a small *sulcus intermedius primus*, which descends from the intraparietal sulcus. The *middle part* or *angular gyrus*, the cortex of which is believed to be concerned with the visual element in stereognosis (p. 960), arches over the upturned end of the superior temporal sulcus and is continuous behind and below with the middle temporal gyrus; sometimes a small *sulcus intermedius secundus* forms its posterior boundary. The anterior and middle parts of the inferior parietal lobule are subjacent to the parietal tuberosity (p. 261). The *posterior part* arches over the upturned end of the inferior temporal sulcus and extends on to the occipital lobe.

**The occipital lobe** lies behind the line joining the preoccipital incisure to the parieto-occipital sulcus. The *transverse occipital sulcus* descends from the superomedial margin posterior to the parieto-occipital sulcus and is joined about its middle by the intraparietal sulcus. Its superior part is the posterior boundary of the *arcus parieto-occipitalis*, an arched gyrus which surrounds the end of the parieto-occipital sulcus. The *lateral occipital sulcus* is a short horizontal sulcus on the lateral aspect of the occipital lobe dividing it into *superior* and *inferior occipital gyri* (7.111 A, B). The *lunate sulcus*, when present, is just in front of the occipital pole. It is placed vertically and sometimes joins the calcarine sulcus, although the two are more often separated from each other. The lips of the lunate sulcus, which is operculated in type, separate the striate from the peristriate area of the cortex, but the parastriate area is buried within the walls of the sulcus and intervenes between them. The lunate sulcus is the posterior boundary of the *gyrus descendens*, which lies behind the superior and inferior occipital gyri. Two curved sulci, named the superior and inferior polar sulci, are often present near the extremities of the lunate sulcus. The *superior polar sulcus* arches upwards on to the medial aspect of the occipital lobe from the neighbourhood of the upper limit of the lunate sulcus; the *inferior polar sulcus* arches downwards and forwards on to the inferior aspect from the lower limit of the same sulcus. These two polar sulci enclose semilunar extensions of the striate area (p. 960) and indicate the expansion of the visual cortex associated with the formation of its large macular area[657] (p. 961).

**The insula** (7.113 A–D) is deep in the floor of the lateral sulcus and is almost surrounded by a *circular sulcus*. It has been overlapped by the overgrowth of the cortical areas which adjoin it, and can only be seen when the lips of the lateral sulcus are widely separated. These areas of the cortex are therefore termed the *opercula of the insula*, and they are separated from each other by the ascending and posterior rami of the lateral sulcus. The *frontal operculum* or lid lies between the anterior and ascending rami, and is formed by the pars triangularis of the inferior frontal gyrus. It may be of small size in cases where the two rami between which it lies arise by a common stem. The *frontoparietal operculum* is between the ascending and the upturned end of the posterior ramus of the lateral sulcus. It is formed by the pars posterior of the inferior frontal gyrus, by the lower ends of the precentral and postcentral gyri, and by the lower end of the anterior part of the inferior parietal lobule. The *temporal operculum* is below the posterior ramus and is formed by the superior temporal gyrus and the transverse temporal gyri. Anteriorly the inferior part of the insula adjoins the pars orbitalis of the inferior frontal gyrus.

When the opercula are removed, the insula is seen as a pyramidal eminence, the apex of which is directed inferiorly towards the anterior perforated substance (7.113). Here the circular sulcus is deficient and the medial part of the apex is termed the *limen insulae* (*gyrus ambiens*). The surface of the insula is divided into a larger anterior and a smaller posterior part by the *sulcus centralis insulae*, which runs up and back from the apex of the insula. The anterior part is divided by shallow sulci into three or four *short gyri*, while the posterior part is formed by one *long gyrus*, which is often divided at its upper end. The cortical grey matter of the insula is continuous with that of the various opercula round the bottom of the circular sulcus. The insula overlies, and is more or less co-extensive with the claustrum and the putamen of the lentiform nucleus (7.113 B, C, D).

## THE MEDIAL SURFACE OF THE CEREBRAL HEMISPHERE

The medial surface (7.114 A, B) cannot be examined until the two cerebral hemispheres have been separated from each other by the division of (1) the commissures which connect them and (2) the roof, floor, anterior and posterior walls of the third ventricle (7.114 A, B). The most conspicuous feature on this surface is the great commissure which is termed the *corpus callosum*. It forms a broad arched band which lies in the floor of the central part of the longitudinal fissure (7.110). The recurved, anterior end of the corpus callosum is termed the *genu*. Below, it is continuous with the *rostrum*, which narrows rapidly as it passes backwards to become connected to the upper end of the lamina terminalis; above, it is continuous with the *trunk* or main 'body' of the commissure, which arches upwards and backwards to end in a thick, rounded posterior extremity, the *splenium*. To the concave surfaces of the trunk, genu and rostrum are attached the laminae of the septum pellucidum, which occupy the interval between them and the fornix—a curved, flattened band of white fibres inferior to it. Immediately in front of the lamina terminalis and almost co-extensive with it, there is a narrow, triangular field of grey matter, the *paraterminal gyrus* (p. 937). Anteriorly it is separated from the rest of the cortex by a shallow *posterior parolfactory sulcus*. A little anterior to this a second, short, vertical sulcus may be present and is termed the *anterior parolfactory sulcus*. The portion of cortex which lies between these two sulci is

[657] G. E. Smith, *J. Anat.*, **64**, 1930.

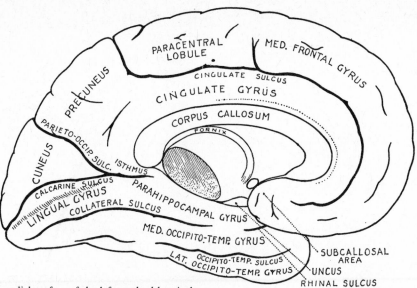

**7.114A** Diagram of the medial surface of the left cerebral hemisphere, after sagittal section of the brain, and removal of the brainstem.

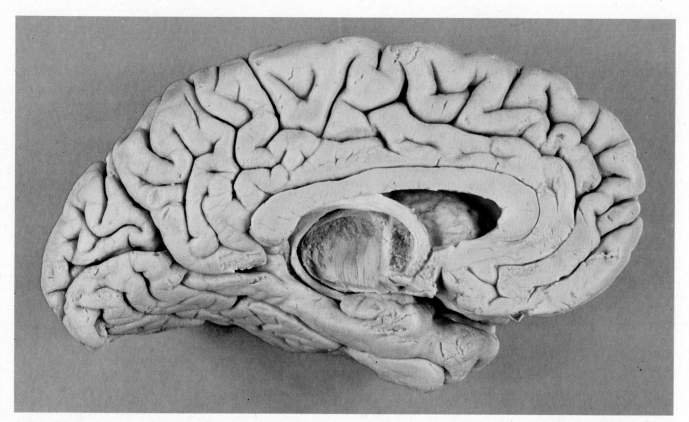

**7.114B** The medial surface of the left cerebral hemisphere after sagittal section of the brain, followed by removal of the brainstem and septum pellucidum. (For identification of the principal gyri and sulci of the cerebral cortex, compare with **7.114A**.) The dissection has been deepened in the region of the dorsal thalamus and hypothalamus to demonstrate the column, body, crus and fimbria of the fornix, and the mamillothalamic fasciculus (compare with **7.117A** and B). The head of the caudate nucleus is visible bulging into the floor of the anterior horn of the lateral ventricle. (Dissection by Dr. E. L. Rees.)

the *subcallosal area* (*parolfactory gyrus*) (**7.110, 119**). The anterior sloping edge of the paraterminal gyrus is sometimes called the *prehippocampal rudiment* (p. 937).

The anterior part of the medial surface of the hemisphere is divided into an outer and an inner zone by the curved *cingulate sulcus*. This commences below the rostrum of the corpus callosum and passes first forwards, then upwards and finally backwards, conforming with the curvature of the corpus callosum. Its posterior end turns up to reach the superomedial margin of the hemisphere, about 4 cm behind the mid-point between the frontal and occipital poles, and is posterior to the upper extremity of

the central sulcus (**7.110, 114**). The outer zone demarcated by the cingulate sulcus forms, with the exception of its extreme posterior end, a part of the frontal lobe. It is subdivided into larger anterior and smaller posterior parts by a short sulcus ascending from the cingulate sulcus above the middle of the trunk of the corpus callosum. The larger anterior region is the *medial frontal gyrus*, while the smaller posterior area is termed the *paracentral lobule*. The superior end of the central sulcus usually cuts into the posterior part of the paracentral lobule and the precentral gyrus is directly continuous with the cortex of the lobule. This area mediates control of movements of

927

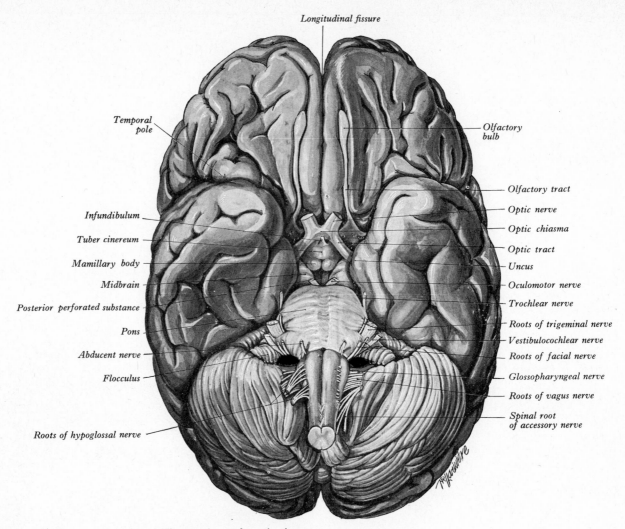

Longitudinal fissure

Temporal pole

Infundibulum

Tuber cinereum

Mamillary body

Midbrain

Posterior perforated substance

Pons

Abducent nerve

Flocculus

Roots of hypoglossal nerve

Olfactory bulb

Olfactory tract

Optic nerve

Optic chiasma

Optic tract

Uncus

Oculomotor nerve

Trochlear nerve

Roots of trigeminal nerve

Vestibulocochlear nerve

Roots of facial nerve

Glossopharyngeal nerve

Roots of vagus nerve

Spinal root of accessory nerve

7.115A Basal aspect of the brain. The anterior perforated substance (unlabelled) is between the diverging lateral and medial roots of the olfactory tract and anterolateral to the optic tract.

the lower limb and perineal region of the opposite side, and clinical evidence suggests that it exercises voluntary control over the defaecation and micturition reflexes (p. 1335).

The zone within the curve of the cingulate sulcus is the *cingulate gyrus*. Commencing below the rostrum this gyrus follows the curve of the corpus callosum, from which it is separated by the *callosal sulcus*, and it continues round the splenium on to the inferior surface of the hemisphere to become continuous with the parahippocampal gyrus through the narrow *isthmus* (7.117A). It is connected with the anterior nuclear group of the thalamus by both afferent and efferent pathways.

The line of the cingulate sulcus is interrupted posterior to the paracentral lobule, but is partially continued by a short variable *subparietal* (*suprasplenial*) *sulcus*.

The posterior part of the medial surface of the hemisphere is traversed by two deep sulci which converge anteriorly and meet a short distance posterior to the splenium of the corpus callosum. These are the parieto-occipital and the calcarine sulci. The *parieto-occipital sulcus* commences on the superomedial margin of the hemisphere about 5 cm anterior to the occipital pole and is directed downwards and slightly forwards to meet the calcarine sulcus. When the lips of the sulcus are separated it will be found that, although on the surface of the hemisphere the parieto-occipital and the calcarine sulci are apparently continuous, they are in reality separated from each other by the deeply situated *cuneate gyrus*. In

addition, the walls of the sulcus show the presence of two or more vertically disposed sulci. These were originally exposed on the medial surface of the hemisphere, but they were included in the parieto-occipital sulcus owing to the growth of the splenium (p. 140). The walls of the parieto-occipital sulcus thus resemble those of the lateral sulcus, although the contained sulci and gyri are fewer in number and smaller in extent.

The *calcarine sulcus* commences near the occipital pole. Although it is usually restricted to the medial surface of the hemisphere its posterior end may extend on to the lateral surface. It runs anteriorly a little above the inferomedial margin of the hemisphere, taking a slightly curved course with an upward convexity, and joins the parieto-occipital sulcus at an acute angle a little posterior to the splenium of the corpus callosum. Continuing forwards the calcarine sulcus crosses the inferomedial margin and gains the inferior aspect of the hemisphere, where it forms the inferolateral boundary of the *isthmus*, which connects the cingulate with the parahippocampal gyrus. At its junction with the parieto-occipital sulcus the floor of the calcarine sulcus is crossed by the buried anterior cuneolingual gyrus. The posterior part of the calcarine sulcus, behind its junction with the parieto-occipital, is an axial sulcus, set in the long axis of the visual cortex (p. 960), but the anterior part is a limiting sulcus and separates the striate, visual cortex from that of the isthmus. The anterior part conforms to the definition of a complete sulcus, since it produces an elevation in the medial wall of the posterior cornu or horn of the lateral ventricle (the calcar avis).

The quadrilateral area, bounded anteriorly by the upturned end of the sulcus cinguli, posteriorly by the parieto-occipital sulcus, superiorly by the superomedial margin and inferiorly by the suprasplenial sulcus, is termed the *precuneus* and, together with the part of the paracentral lobule posterior to the central sulcus, constitutes the medial surface of the parietal lobe.

The wedge-shaped area bounded in front by the parieto-occipital sulcus, below by the calcarine sulcus and above by the superomedial margin, is termed the *cuneus*. Its surface is usually indented by one or two small irregular sulci, and forms the medial surface of the occipital lobe.

## THE INFERIOR SURFACE OF THE CEREBRAL HEMISPHERE

This surface is divided into a smaller part, anterior to the stem of the lateral fissure, and a larger part posterior to it (**7.**115 A, B; 116). The anterior region forms the orbital part of the inferior surface of the cerebral hemisphere. It is concave from side to side and rests on the cribriform plate of the ethmoid bone, the orbital plate of the frontal and the lesser wing of the sphenoid bone. An antero-posterior sulcus traverses this surface near its medial margin and, since it is overlapped by the olfactory bulb and tract, it is termed the *olfactory sulcus*. The medial strip of cortex which it marks off is the *gyrus rectus*. The rest of this surface is marked by irregular sulci, the *orbital sulci*, generally H-shaped, dividing it into a number of *orbital gyri*. Four can usually be recognized, named, according to their position, anterior, medial, posterior and lateral orbital gyri (**7.**116).

The larger, posterior region of the inferior cerebral surface is its tentorial part since it is immediately superior in part to the tentorium but also to the middle cranial fossa. It is traversed by two anteroposterior sulci, the collateral and occipitotemporal. The *collateral sulcus* commences near the occipital pole and extends anteriorly, roughly parallel to the calcarine sulcus, from which it is separated by the *lingual gyrus*. Anteriorly the collateral sulcus may be continued into the *rhinal sulcus*, but the two are usually separated. The *rhinal sulcus* runs forwards in the line of the collateral sulcus and separates the temporal pole from a somewhat hook-shaped projection posteromedial to it and termed the *uncus*. This fissure marks the lateral limit of the piriform lobe of the cortex (**7.**119).

The *occipitotemporal sulcus* is parallel to the collateral sulcus and lateral to it. As a rule it does not extend as far as the occipital pole, and it is frequently divided into two or more parts.

The *lingual gyrus* lies between the calcarine and collateral sulci. Anteriorly it passes without interruption into the *parahippocampal gyrus*, which commences at the *isthmus*, where it is directly continuous with the cingulate gyrus, and then passes forwards medial to the collateral and rhinal sulci. Anteriorly the parahippocampal gyrus becomes continuous with the uncus, its medial edge being lateral to the midbrain. The *uncus* is the hook-like, anterior end of the parahippocampal gyrus and forms the posterolateral boundary of the anterior perforated substance. The medial part of the uncus extends laterally above its lateral part and will be described later (**7.**119); its inferior surface cannot be exposed completely until its lateral and more superficial part has been removed (**7.**120). The uncus forms part of the *piriform lobe*, which is part of the olfactory system (*vide infra*) and is phylogenetically one of the oldest parts of the pallium. (For further details of the uncal region, and the complex terminology applied to this and surrounding areas,

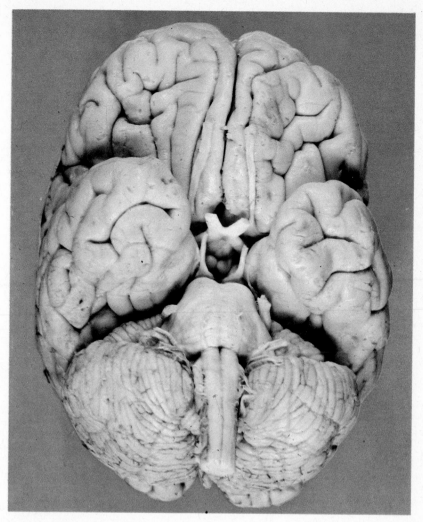

**7.**115 B   The base of the brain. For labelling compare with **7.**56, 115 A. (Dissection by Dr. E. L. Rees.)

consult illustrations **7.**117 A and **7.**119.)

The *medial occipitotemporal gyrus* extends from near the occipital to the temporal pole. It is limited medially by the collateral and rhinal sulci and laterally by the occipito-temporal sulcus. The lateral part of this area forms the *lateral occipitotemporal gyrus*, which is continuous round the inferolateral margin of the hemisphere with the inferior temporal gyrus.

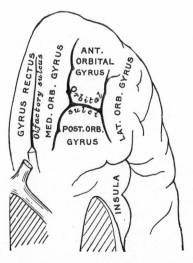

**7.**116   The orbital surface of the left frontal lobe.

# THE LIMBIC LOBE AND OLFACTORY PATHWAYS

During development the superolateral surfaces of the diencephalon gradually merge with the central areas of the inferomedial surfaces of the two cerebral hemispheres (p. 140). Completely bordering the area of fusion on each side, a series of structures develop in the wall of the hemisphere and constitute the **limbic lobe**—a term introduced in 1878 by Broca[658] on comparative anatomical grounds. Many of the structures constituting the limbic lobe (literally the *bordering* lobe) are phylogenetically old, and have a highly arched form; topographically they are interposed between the diencephalon and the massive neopallial areas of the cerebral hemisphere (7.117). Interest in the limbic lobe was heightened when Papez in 1937 suggested its role in emotional behaviour.[659, 660] Since that time an ever-increasing volume of research has emphasized that the lobe has profuse interconnexions

balance between aggressive and social behaviour in community living.[661, 662]

The terminology applied to these regions is complex; alternative schemes are in use, and common agreement in terms of a rational basis for scientific definition has proved impossible to achieve (see discussions in footnote references [61, 660, 663]). Broadly, however, the increasingly widespread use of the terms limbic lobe and limbic system indicate that, at the present state of our knowledge, many investigators believe that such collective names serve a useful purpose, despite differences in detailed application of the terms by some workers, and the strong opposition to their use at all by a minority.[61] Most authorities include a series of subcortical nuclei and their connexions, the phylogenetically older areas of cortex, the archipallium and paleopallium, and the immediately adjacent border of

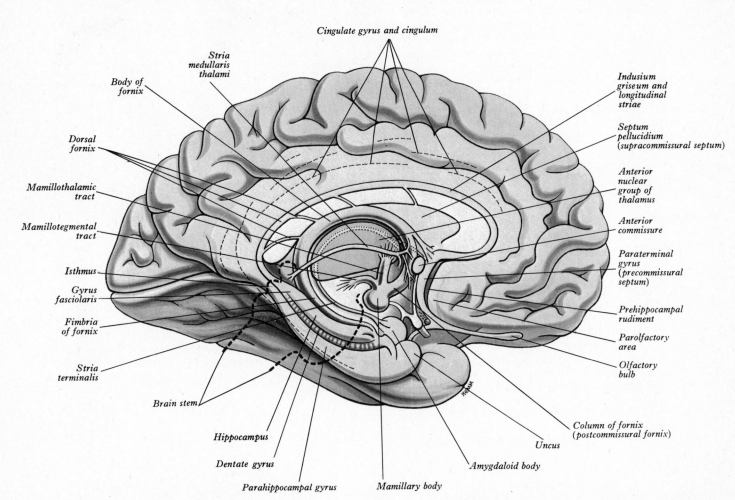

**7.117A** A diagram of a dissection of the medial aspect of a cerebral hemisphere to demonstrate the majority of the structures included under the term limbic system in the present account; these are coloured yellow. The anterior nuclear group of the dorsal thalamus is coloured orange and included with the limbic system; the remainder of the dorsal thalamus is magenta. The approximate position of the brainstem which was removed in the course of dissection is outlined in a heavy interrupted line. This diagram should be compared with the colour photograph of a dissection prepared from the *lateral* aspect of a hemisphere (7.117B).

with the olfactory system, the hypothalamus, thalamus, epithalamus and, to a lesser extent, areas of the neocortex. It is intimately associated with the higher integration of visceral, olfactory and somatic information, and the patterning of complex long and short term homeostatic responses. The latter include seeking and capturing prey, courtship, mating, rearing of young, the subjective and expressive elements in emotional responses, and the

[658] P. Broca, *Revue Anthrop.*, **1**, 1878.
[659] J. W. Papez, *Archs Neurol. Psychiat., Chicago.*, **38**, 1937.
[660] L. E. White, Jr., *Int. Rev. Neurobiol.*, **8**, 1965.
[661] P. D. Maclean, *J. nerv. ment. Dis.*, **127**, 1958; and in: *The Hypothalamus*, eds. W. Haymaker, E. Anderson and W. J. H. Nauta, Thomas, Illinois. 1969.
[662] R. B. Livingston, in: *Control Processes in Multicellular Organisms*, eds. G. E. W. Wolstenholme and J. Knight, Churchill, London. 1970.
[663] W. Bargmann and J. P. Schadé, *Prog. Brain Res.*, **3**, 1963.

the neopallium—the cingulate and parahippocampal gyri, and their associated fibre tracts. Difficulties arise when attempts are made to place precise boundaries between these regions and adjacent ones, with which some of them are functionally interconnected. For example, opinions differ concerning what areas of frontal cortex should be included, and whether or not the intimately related hypothalamus should be embraced by the term. Of greater practical importance is the need for an agreed international nomenclature for as many orders of subdivision of the brain as possible, based upon the most widely acceptable criteria currently available, with a continuous process of revision as further knowledge accumulates. In the present account the terms limbic lobe and system are included, and the structures described under these headings will be listed below.

Even greater terminologic difficulty attaches to the widely used name **rhinencephalon**.[663] Traditionally, the name was used to indicate all those brain structures associated with olfaction, and for many years it was assumed that most of the structures of the limbic lobe were primarily olfactory pathways and centres of integration. However, with advancing researches in comparative and developmental neurology, olfactory physiology, more detailed neuroanatomical studies, together with behavioural and other functional studies on the limbic system and hypothalamus, there has been a considerable change of emphasis. Since the term rhinencephalon has many shades of meaning in the hands of different workers using different approaches, and when investigating different species, it will not be included in this account.

The structures mentioned or described here or elsewhere in this volume, which are included in the limbic system are:

(1) The olfactory nerves, bulb and tract (together with the nervus terminalis, and the transient accessory olfactory bulb and vomeronasal nerve).

(2) The anterior olfactory nucleus.

(3) The medial, intermediate and lateral olfactory striae and the medial and lateral olfactory gyri.

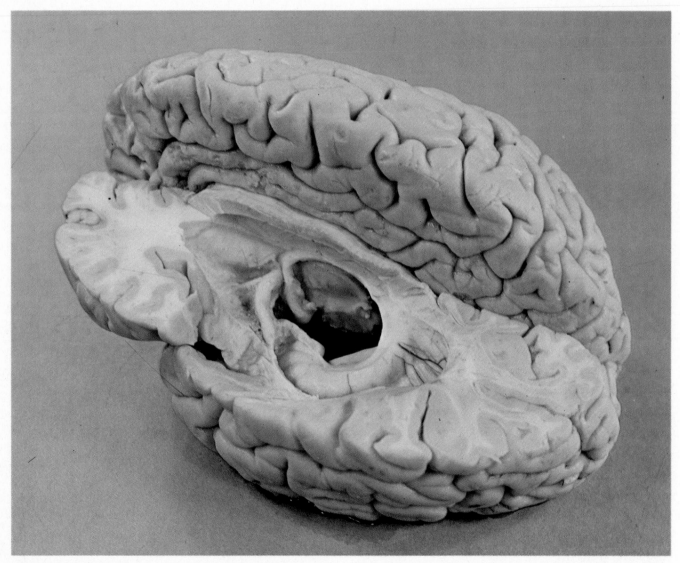

**7.117B** A dissection of the left cerebral hemisphere from the supero-lateral aspect to demonstrate various structural features of the limbic system. The corpus callosum is divided sagittally in the region of its body only; the frontal, temporal and occipital lobes have been sectioned horizontally and their superior parts removed. The left lentiform nucleus, much of the caudate nucleus and dorsal thalamus have been removed, and the floor of the inferior horn of the lateral ventricle laid open. Note: (1) the horizontally sectioned head of the caudate nucleus; (2) the spiral disposition of the fornix as it curves from the mamillary body through its left column, body, crus and fimbria; (3) the curved elevation of the hippocampus projecting into the floor of the inferior horn of the ventricle, and ending anteriorly as the grooved pes hippocampi; (4) the anterior commissure entering the left hemisphere immediately anterior to the column of the fornix, and passing laterally, to diverge into small anterior and large posterior components; between the latter the deep aspect of the anterior perforated substance is visible; (5) within the curve of the fornix the medial aspect of the *right* thalamus crossed superiorly by the stria medullaris thalami; (6) coursing above the corpus callosum a longitudinal white stria is visible, and above this arches the right gyrus cinguli. Compare with **7.117A**. (Dissection by Dr. A. M. Seal, Department of Anatomy, Guy's Hospital Medical School.)

(4) The olfactory trigone, the anterior perforated substance with the olfactory tubercle, and the diagonal band of Broca.

(5) The piriform lobe which includes: (*a*) the lateral olfactory gyrus continuing into the gyrus ambiens—together forming the prepiriform cortex; (*b*) the lateral olfactory stria continuing into the gyrus semilunaris (periamygdaloid area); (*c*) the uncus hippocampi including the uncinate gyrus, the tail of the dentate gyrus (band of Giacomini), and the intralimbic gyrus; (*d*) the entorhinal area (area 28)—the cranial part of the parahippocampal gyrus.

(6) The amygdaloid complex of nuclei.

(7) The septal areas, including the septum pellucidum, and the septum verum—a nuclear complex much of which is deeply placed but in part corresponds to the paraterminal gyrus.

(8) The hippocampal formation which includes: (*a*) the prehippocampal rudiment, the indusium griseum and longitudinal striae; (*b*) the gyrus fasciolaris, Ammon's horn, the dentate gyrus, the subiculum, and related regions.

(9) The fornix and its various ramifications and divisions.

(10) The stria terminalis.

(11) The stria habenularis.

(12) The cingulate and parahippocampal gyri.

The hypothalamus, medial part of the thalamus, prefrontal cortex, and the anterior commissure, all of which are intimately related to the foregoing structures, are described elsewhere in the present section.

## THE OLFACTORY BULB

The olfactory bulb (7.115 A) is a flattened, oval, reddishgrey mass which lies superior to the medial edge of the orbital plate of the frontal bone near the lateral margin of the cribriform plate of the ethmoid. It is inferior to the anterior end of the olfactory sulcus, on the orbital surface of the frontal lobe of the brain; the gyrus rectus is directly superior to the cribriform plate.

The olfactory nerve fibres which are the central processes of the olfactory cells of the nasal mucosa (p. 1089) converge upon the inferior surface of the cribriform plate and collect into about twenty bundles which pass through the foramina in the plate, and then continue to enter the inferior surface of the bulb.

As described previously (p. 139) the olfactory bulb and tract develop as a hollow diverticulum from the anteromedial part of the floor of the primitive cerebral hemisphere. With growth, the basal part of the diverticulum elongates to form the olfactory tract and, in the human embryo, the cavity of the terminal olfactory bulb (the 'olfactory ventricle') and that of the elongating tract are gradually obliterated by approximation and subsequent fusion of their walls. However, the site of the original cavity is sometimes marked by deeply-placed vestigial aggregations of modified ependymal cells. Thus, the olfactory bulb has a radial organization consisting of a number of superimposed layers with increasing depth from the surface. This laminar pattern is particularly well defined in many mammals other than man, and also in the human fetus, but often becomes less distinct as the brain matures. The detailed histology of the olfactory bulb, as revealed by the light microscope after staining with the Nissl and Golgi methods, has been known since the turn of the century,[664–667] and this has been supplemented by experimental studies using degeneration techniques, e.g. [668–670], physiological studies, e.g. [671, 672], and more recently, by detailed ultrastructural analyses.[673]

From the surface, and progressing towards the central

core, the olfactory bulb consists of: (1) the olfactory nerve fibre layer; (2) the layer of synaptic glomeruli and interglomerular spaces; (3) the molecular and external granular layer; (4) the mitral cell layer; (5) the internal granular layer; and (6) the fibres of the olfactory tract.

**The neurons** of the olfactory bulb comprise: (1) the large characteristically shaped *mitral cells* which form a layer only one or two cells thick; (2) internal, middle and external *tufted cells*, analogous to, but smaller than, the mitral cells, and progressively reducing in size throughout the thickness of the molecular layer from the superficial aspect of the mitral layer to the deep aspect of the glomeruli; (3) numerous small round or stellate *internal granule cells*; (4) various types of small *periglomerular cell* distributed around, within, and deep to the synaptic glomeruli. The periglomerular cells and the small external tufted cells constitute the *external granular layer* of the earlier histologists.

It is now clear that previous accounts of the mechanism of the olfactory bulb as a simple relay between incoming olfactory nerve fibres and the dendrites of mitral cells, the axons of which proceed into the olfactory tract, were a gross over-simplification. The bulb is a region of great structural complexity to which only brief reference can be made here (see the footnote references quoted for details). In particular the following features are to be noted: (1) there is a great *convergence* of olfactory nerve fibres on to the dendrites of the mitral and tufted cells which occupy much of the synaptic glomeruli (*vide infra*); (2) a number of cell types, mitral, tufted and others, contribute axons to the olfactory tract which proceed to other brain centres; (3) a number of different types of interneuron provide pathways for complex patterns of interaction between the main conduction channels, and also complicated feedback paths; and (4) transmission in the bulb is modulated by centrifugal axons which converge on it from the contralateral olfactory bulb, anterior olfactory nucleus and other centres (*vide infra*). Some of these features are summarized in illustration 7.118.

It is convenient to consider first the main conduction path through the bulb, followed by the complications introduced by local interneurons and centrifugal pathways.

In addition to *basal* dendrites which establish synaptic connexions with granule cell processes, both the large mitral cells (the shape of their somata resembling a bishop's mitre) and the more prominent external tufted cells possess large *apical* dendrites which pass superficially towards the glomerular layer where they branch and form rich arborizations in a number of synaptic glomeruli. The incoming olfactory nerve fibres converge upon the glomeruli, and form numerous axodendritic synapses with the apical dendrites of the mitral and tufted cells, whilst the axons of the latter pass through the inner granular layer, giving off a number of collateral branches,

[664] S. Ramon y Cajal, *Gazz. sanit.*, Barcelona, 1890; *Histologie du système nerveux de l'homme et des vertebrés*, Maloine, Paris. 1911; *Studies on the Cerebral Cortex (Limbic Structures)*, trs. L. M. Kraft, Lloyd-Luke, London. 1955.

[666] T. Blanes, *Revta trimest. microgr.*, **3**, 1898.

[666] W. E. Le Gros Clark, *J. Neurol. Neurosurg. Psychiat.*, **14**, 1951; *Yale J. Biol. Med.*, **29**, 1956; *Proc. R. Soc. B.*, **146**, 1957.

[667] F. Valverde, *Studies on the Piriform Lobe*, Harvard University Press, Mass. 1965.

[668] T. P. S. Powell and W. M. Cowan, *Nature, Lond.*, **199**, 1963.

[669] J. L. Price, *Brain Res.*, **7**, 1968.

[670] L. Heimer, *J. Anat.*, **103**, 1968.

[671] W. Sem-Jacobsen, M. C. Petersen, H. W. Dodge, Q. D. Jacks, J. A. Lazarte and C. B. Holman, *Am. J. med. Sci.*, **232**, 1956.

[672] K. B. Døving, in: *Chemistry and Physiology of Flavors*, eds. H. W. Schultz, E. A. Day and L. M. Libbey, Avi, Connecticut. 1967.

[673] A. J. Pinching and T. P. S. Powell, *J. Cell Sci.*, **9**a, b, c, 1971.

before continuing into the deep zone of nerve fibres to form the main constituents of the olfactory tract.

**The synaptic glomeruli** of the olfactory bulb are large, roughly spherical territories, often exceeding 100 μm in diameter, containing many thousands of nerve cell processes from various sources, with a wide variety of types of synaptic interconnexion between them. In addition to the large dendrites of the mitral and internal tufted cells just described, the glomerulus also receives dendrites from various types of *periglomerular cell* (including the external granule cells, the external tufted cells, and

dritic synapse from an olfactory nerve axon terminal. Finally, the dendrites of the periglomerular cells receive a number of axodendritic synapses from the axons of other periglomerular cells.

**The interglomerular spaces** are occupied, in part, by the cell somata of the different categories of periglomerular cell and their processes. Some of these cells have dendrites which ramify both in the spaces and also in the glomeruli as described above. Other interneurons which have been designated short-axon cells have dendritic trees which are wholly extraglomerular. The

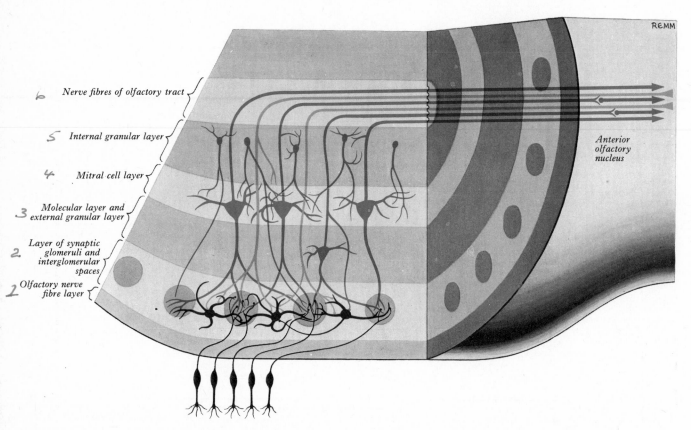

Nerve fibres of olfactory tract

5   Internal granular layer

4   Mitral cell layer

3   Molecular layer and external granular layer

2   Layer of synaptic glomeruli and interglomerular spaces

1   Olfactory nerve fibre layer

Anterior olfactory nucleus

REMM

**7.118** A scheme of the olfactory bulb based upon neurocytological and experimental studies in a number of mammalian types. The radial organization of the bulb into 'layers', with their principal neuron types, and an approximate indication of their main connectivity patterns, is shown. They 'layers' of the bulb which receive the names indicated are, of course, merely a convenient descriptive frame of reference; they should not obscure the functionally essential interconnexions which cross the boundaries between these zones. The colours used indicate—*red:* mitral and tufted neurons and their processes; *blue:* internal granule neurons; *purple:* periglomerular neurons; *black:* olfactory receptor neurons and their processes. Note that the olfactory tract consists of (1) centripetal axons of mitral and tufted cells, some of which synapse with neurons in the anterior olfactory nucleus, and (2) centrifugal axons (yellow) which terminate in the different zones indicated. Refer to text for a more detailed description of both the organization of the bulb, and the destinations of olfactory tract fibres.

the superficial short-axon cells of different authors[673]). In all, about 100 individual neurons contribute dendrites to each glomerulus, and (in the rabbit) each receives the terminals of some 25,000 olfactory nerve axons. Further, the axonal terminals of a number of periglomerular cells also penetrate the glomerulus. Detailed analyses of the synaptic contacts between these different elements, and their possible modes of operation, are still in progress;[673, 674] in outline, the following synaptic contacts have been described.

The terminal parts of the olfactory nerve axons do not receive axoaxonic (presynaptic) contacts from other sources, but they establish the axodendritic contacts with mitral and tufted cell dendrites mentioned above, and also with the dendrites of periglomerular cells. The periglomerular cell dendrites also form complex reciprocal dendrodendritic contacts with mitral and tufted cell dendrites; often one or both of the elements in such a double dendrodendritic contact also receive an axoden-

interglomerular spaces are also penetrated by mitral cell dendrites, many of the axonal ramifications and terminals of the periglomerular cells themselves, and the termination of centrifugal axons from the olfactory tract. Again, reciprocal dendrodendritic contacts between periglomerular cell dendrites and those of mitral and tufted cells are found, together with axodendritic contacts between either extrinsic or intrinsic axons and the periglomerular cells. The details of these contacts and the other varieties described, will not be pursued further here (for these see footnote reference [673]).

**The internal granular layer** which lies deep to the mitral cell layer consists of large numbers of microneurons or *amacrine granule cells*,[674] which possess no true axon. Their dendrites branch repeatedly, some spreading locally, whilst others pass deeply into the molecular layer where, once again, reciprocal dendrodendritic synapses

[674] J. L. Price and T. P. S. Powell, *J. Cell Sci.,* **7**a and b, 1970.

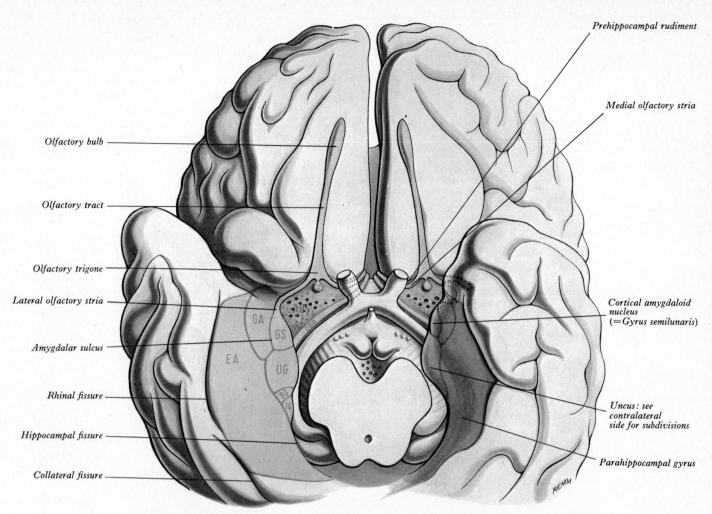

*Prehippocampal rudiment*

*Medial olfactory stria*

Olfactory bulb

Olfactory tract

Olfactory trigone

Lateral olfactory stria

Amygdalar sulcus

Rhinal fissure

Hippocampal fissure

Collateral fissure

*Cortical amygdaloid nucleus (=Gyrus semilunaris)*

*Uncus: see contralateral side for subdivisions*

*Parahippocampal gyrus*

7.119   A diagram of structures on the inferior aspect of the human brain in the area immediately surrounding the optic nerves, chiasma, optic tracts and interpeduncular fossa. Many of these structures are intimately related to the olfactory and limbic systems; they are coloured blue. The right temporal pole has been displaced laterally to expose underlying structures. In addition to the features which have been labelled fully, the abbreviations used have the following significance: OT —olfactory tubercle; APS—anterior perforated substance; DBB—diagonal band of Broca. The uncus hippocampi is divided into three areas; IG—the intra-limbic gyrus; BG—the band of Giacomini; and UG—the uncinate gyrus. The lateral olfactory stria continues into the gyrus semilunaris (GS); this is bordered laterally by the gyrus ambiens (GA); whilst further laterally is the entorhinal area (EA) which is the cranial extension of the parahippocampal gyrus. Note the curved extensions of the prehippo-campal rudiments, medial olfactory striae, and diagonal bands of Broca on to the medial aspect of the hemisphere. The triangular midline zone between the converging diagonal bands, and superior to the optic chiasma, is the lamina terminalis. The occasional intermediate olfactory stria which merges with the olfactory tubercle, is illustrated but unlabelled. (After Kuhlenbeck: redrawn and modified form: *The Hypothalamus*, with the permission of the authors W. J. H. Nauta and W. Haymaker, and the publishers Charles C. Thomas, Springfield, Illinois.)

are established with the dendrites of mitral and tufted cells. The granule cell dendrites also receive axodendritic synapses from recurrent collateral branches of mitral and tufted cell axons, and also from many of the terminals of centrifugal axons in the olfactory tract.

In short, the neurons of the olfactory bulb and their processes present some of the most complex sets of synaptic patterns yet described in the nervous system. The granule and periglomerular cells are considered to be inhibitory interneurons, and by their geometric organization and array of contacts, they provide the substrate for interaction between the principal conduction channels through the bulb. Thus, they mediate feed-forward, lateral and feed-back inhibitory processes, and also inhibitory effects by the centrifugal axons which pass into the bulb from the opposite olfactory tract. Much remains to be determined concerning the detailed operation of these various elements.

In many non-primate mammals, and submammalian forms, a diverticulum lined by specialized epithelium called the *vomeronasal organ* (of Jacobson) lies on each side of the nasal septum. The nerve bundles from this epithelium run with the ventral groups of olfactory nerve fibres and then converge to form the *vomeronasal nerve*,

which ends in an *accessory olfactory bulb*, situated on the dorsomedial aspect of the main bulb. Although an accessory bulb and vomeronasal nerve are present on one or both sides in a proportion of human embryos, both structures degenerate with increasing maturity of the nervous system.[675–677]

## THE OLFACTORY TRACT

The olfactory tract (7.115, 119) is a narrow white band which issues from the posterior aspect of the olfactory bulb and continues posteriorly on the inferior (orbital) surface of the frontal lobe, where it covers the line of the olfactory sulcus. The tract is triangular in outline in transverse section, its narrow apex being recessed into the olfactory sulcus. It consists of the centrally directed axons of the mitral and tufted cells of the bulb, and also some centrifugal axons which have crossed from the opposite bulb and anterior olfactory nucleus in the anterior commissure, and other centrifugal axons arising from neurons

[675] D. C. Hume, *J. comp. Neurol.*, **73**, 1940.
[676] R. E. McCotter, *Anat. Rec.*, **6**, 1912; **9**, 1915.
[677] E. C. Crosby and T. Humphrey, *J. comp. Neurol.*, **74**, 1941.

in or near the anterior perforated substance (*vide infra*). The precise contribution of these and other possible sources to the centrifugal outflow is still under active investigation.[678 – 682]

### The Anterior Olfactory Nucleus

At the posterior end of the olfactory bulb its various characteristic cell layers disappear, but the deeply placed granule cell layer is replaced throughout the length of the olfactory tract by scattered groups of medium-sized multipolar neurons which constitute the *anterior olfactory nucleus*. Posteriorly, these groups of neurons continue into the olfactory striae and trigone (*vide infra*) to abut on or become continuous with the grey matter of the prepiriform cortex, the anterior perforated substance and the precommissural septal areas. Many of the centripetal axons from mitral and tufted cells which constitute the olfactory tract relay in, or give collaterals to, the anterior olfactory nucleus, and then the axons of the latter continue with the direct fibres from the bulb to form the olfactory striae.

## THE OLFACTORY STRIAE AND TRIGONE

Posteriorly, as the olfactory tract approaches the anterior perforated substance, it flattens and becomes splayed out into a smooth *olfactory trigone* (olfactory pyramid) from the caudal angles of which the fibres of the tract continue as separate diverging bundles, the *medial* and *lateral olfactory striae* which border the anterior perforated substance (7.119). In some brains a small *intermediate stria* can be distinguished passing from the centre of the trigone to sink into the anterior perforated substance.

**The lateral olfactory stria** courses along the anterolateral margin of the anterior perforated substance as a whitish bundle distinguishable by the naked eye. It continues into the limen insulae (p. 926), at which point it makes an abrupt bend posteromedially to merge with an elevated region of grey matter called the gyrus semilunaris which bounds the cranial margin of the uncus hippocampi (7.119). The gyrus semilunaris incorporates part of the *corticomedial* subdivision of the *amygdaloid complex* of nuclei (*vide infra*). A tenuous layer of grey matter which clothes the lateral olfactory stria is called the *lateral olfactory gyrus* and this merges laterally with grey matter of the *gyrus ambiens* which in part forms the limen insulae. The lateral olfactory gyrus and gyrus ambiens, together, constitute the *prepiriform region* of the cortex which passes caudally into the *entorhinal area* of the parahippocampal gyrus.

The prepiriform region, the periamygdaloid region and the entorhinal area (area 28) together comprise the **piriform lobe** of the cerebrum; it is bounded laterally by the *rhinal sulcus* and is relatively more prominent in macrosmatic mammals, and during the early fetal stages of human brain development. The relative positions of these structures and their surroundings are more easily appreciated by reference to illustration 7.119.

**The medial olfactory stria**, covered by a thin veil of grey matter—the *medial olfactory gyrus*—passes medially along the cranial boundary of the anterior perforated substance and converges towards the medial continuation of the diagonal band of Broca (*vide infra*). Together they curve superiorly on the medial aspect of the hemisphere, anterior to the line of the lamina terminalis (7.119). The diagonal band continues into the paraterminal gyrus, whilst the medial stria becomes indistinct from surface view as it approaches the boundary zone which includes the paraterminal gyrus, parolfactory gyrus, and between them, the narrow prehippocampal rudiment. (See illustration 7.117 A.)

## THE ANTERIOR PERFORATED SUBSTANCE

This is an important topographic landmark on the base of the brain. It lies caudal to the olfactory trigone and the diverging medial and lateral olfactory stria, in the angle between the optic chiasma and tract medially, and the uncus caudally (7.119). Medially, it is continuous above the optic tract with the grey matter of the tuber cinereum, and more anteriorly, with the paraterminal gyrus. Laterally, it reaches the limen insulae, where it is continuous with the prepiriform cortex, and more caudally it merges with the periamygdaloid area (gyrus semilunaris). Superiorly, it is continuous with the grey matter of the corpus striatum and claustrum through the aggregations of grey and white matter which form the *substantia innominata*. Part of the latter, together with fascicles of the ansa lenticularis and anterior commissure separate the anterior perforated substance from the globus pallidus.

The inferior aspect of the anterior perforated substance is related to the termination of the internal carotid artery and the origins of the anterior and middle cerebral arteries; from the latter a number of central arteries pierce the surface of the brain and supply deeper structures (p. 984), and when removed during dissection their paths form the perforations from which the region derives its name.

Immediately caudal to the olfactory trigone the anterior perforated substance presents a small *olfactory tubercle* which varies in its prominence, and into the base of which the occasional intermediate olfactory stria sinks. The tubercle is a large structure in macrosmatic animals but is greatly reduced and sometimes indistinguishable in man. Similarly, the intermediate stria, although sometimes absent, is occasionally represented by two or three fine intermediate striae which radiate into the perforated substance. The caudal zone of the anterior perforated substance where it abuts on the optic tract, is formed by the smooth surface of the *diagonal band of Broca*. Caudolaterally, the band is continuous with the periamygdaloid area, whilst craniomedially it continues above the optic chiasma to merge with the paraterminal gyrus (precommissural septum).

The variations in cytoarchitectonic patterns, and the numerous and sometimes divergent views concerning the connexions of these various regions cannot be reviewed in detail here; for this the reader should consult original papers and large works devoted exclusively to neuroanatomy. In summary, the following points may be noted.

The six laminae, which, although varying in their prominence in different regions, are widely held to characterize the neocortex (p. 950), are not found in the same form in the archipallial and paleopallial regions of the limbic system. In some areas of the latter a laminar pattern is either absent or scarcely distinguishable, whilst in other areas an obvious but distinctive lamination exists, varying from a primitive three-layered to a transitional six-layered variety, where limbic cortex adjoins and merges with neopallial regions. Thus, the medial and lateral olfactory gyri, prepiriform cortex and indusium griseum consist of isolated patches or a thin veil of grey matter and associated fibre bundles, with no laminar pattern. Similarly, the cranial and caudal zones of the anterior perforated substance, the diagonal band of Broca, paraterminal gyrus and the periamygdaloid cortex are poorly differentiated without an obvious laminar pattern, but specific cell aggregations occur in some of

[678] B. G. Cragg, *Expl Neurol.*, **5**, 1962.
[679] T. P. S. Powell and W. M. Cowan, *Nature, Lond.*, **199**, 1963.
[680] T. P. S. Powell, W. M. Cowan and G. Raisman, *J. Anat.*, **99**, 1965.
[681] J. L. Price, *Brain Res.*, **7**, 1968.
[682] L. Heimer, *J. Anat.*, **103**, 1968.

them. These include the *nucleus of the lateral olfactory tract* in the periamgdaloid region, and the *nucleus of the diagonal band of Broca*. The central zone of the anterior perforated substance is better differentiated and presents three layers—an outer plexiform, an intermediate pyramidal and a deep polymorphic layer. This region also has a number of characteristic cup-shaped aggregations of granule cells in the pyramidal layer and sometimes extending into the plexiform layer. These are the *islands of Calleja*, which vary considerably in size, the medial being the largest—it is closely related to another prominent group of larger pleomorphic cells, the *nucleus accumbens septi*. The structure of the hippocampal formation is further discussed below, but it may be noted at this point that the dentate gyrus and Ammon's horn both consist of a primitive trilaminar type of cortex which shows a gradual transition through the subicular region until a modified six-layered variety is found in the entorhinal area of the parahippocampal gyrus.

## THE TERMINATION OF THE OLFACTORY TRACT

The areas of termination of olfactory tract fibres have been widely studied experimentally in mammals including monkeys, and despite minor differences in some accounts, substantial agreement has been reached. What obtains in the human brain is, of course, less certain.

As we have seen, the olfactory tract fibres are the axons of mitral and tufted cells in the olfactory bulb, some of which synapse with cells in the anterior olfactory nucleus, the axons of the latter then continuing with the direct fibres of the tract. Through the medium of the lateral olfactory stria, tract fibres reach and synapse with neurons in the lateral part of the anterior perforated substance, the lateral olfactory gyrus, the prepiriform cortex and in the corticomedial group of amygdaloid nuclei (*vide infra*). These regions are often grouped as the **primary olfactory cortex**, and it should be noted that in contrast to all other sensory pathways, fibres reach these cortical areas directly without a synapse in one of the thalamic nuclei. The entorhinal area (area 28) of the parahippocampal gyrus, which occupies the caudal part of the piriform lobe, receives few or no tract fibres directly, but receives profuse connexions from the primary cortex; accordingly, it is sometimes called the **secondary olfactory cortex**. It is thought that the primary and secondary olfactory cortices are the principal areas responsible for the subjective appreciation of olfactory stimuli.

The variable intermediate olfactory stria ends in the anterior perforated substance, but the destination of fibres in the medial stria is much less certain. Some of the latter also end in the anterior perforated substance, whilst others have been described as reaching the paraterminal gyrus and adjacent regions, but such claims cannot be regarded as established in the human brain. A number of fibres in the medial olfactory stria cross the midline in the anterior commissure for distribution to the contralateral anterior olfactory nucleus and olfactory bulb.

In addition to the entorhinal area, the primary olfactory cortex also projects to the basolateral part of the amygdaloid complex, the septal areas, the nucleus medialis dorsalis of the thalamus, and to many of the hypothalamic nuclei.

## THE AMYGDALA

The amygdala (amygdaloid body, amygdaloid nuclear complex), so named because its general shape resembles that of an almond, consists of a series of neuronal masses and associated nerve fibres in the dorsomedial part of the temporal pole of the cerebrum. It forms the ventral,

superior and medial walls of the ventral tip of the inferior horn of the lateral ventricle. Its topographical relationships are complicated. Superiorly, it is partly continuous with the inferomedial margin of the claustrum, and fibres of the external capsule and substriatal grey matter incompletely separate it from the putamen and globus pallidus; it is closely applied to the optic tract. The amygdala is partly deep to the gyrus semilunaris, the gyrus ambiens and the uncinate gyrus (7.119A); transitional zones connect it with the anterior perforated substance, prepiriform cortex and parahippocampal gyrus. Caudally, it is closely related to the ventral part of the hippocampus; it fuses with the tip of the tail of the caudate nucleus, which has coursed ventrally in the roof of the inferior horn of the lateral ventricle; the stria terminalis issues from its caudal aspect.

### Divisions of the Amygdala

The amygdaloid complex is divided into two main groups of nuclei, *corticomedial* and *basilateral*, together with junctional zones where these adjoin or partly fuse with adjacent areas. A detailed account of the subdivisions, connexions and homologies of these groups will not be attempted here (see footnote references [29, 683]) and only some of the main points will be outlined.

**The corticomedial amygdaloid complex** consists of the *central, medial* and *cortical amygdaloid nuclei*, the *nucleus of the lateral olfactory stria*, and a transitional poorly differentiated *anterior amygdaloid area*. The cortical nucleus, as its name suggests, may be regarded as a rudimentary cortex, with irregular groups of pyramidal and granule cells; it occupies the surface elevation of the gyrus semilunaris.

The corticomedial complex is continuous through transitional zones with the anterior perforated substance, the diagonal band of Broca, the substantia innominata, and with the putamen, caudate nucleus, and surrounding cortical areas of the uncus and parahippocampal gyrus. It is relatively small in the human brain.

**The basolateral amygdaloid complex**, large and well differentiated in the human brain, consists of *lateral, basal* and *accessory basal amygdaloid nuclei*. It is partly continuous with the claustrum, and, through a cortico-amygdaloid transitional zone, with the cortex of the parahippocampal gyrus.

### The Connexions of the Amygdaloid Complex

These are incompletely established for the human brain, most of the available information stemming from degeneration and electrophysiological studies in a variety of mammals, including monkeys (see, for example [684–688]).

Briefly, **afferent connexions** reach the corticomedial complex via the lateral olfactory stria from the olfactory bulb and anterior olfactory nucleus, whilst the basilateral complex receives many afferents from the cortex of the piriform lobe (p. 932). Other afferents converge on the amygdala from the hypothalamic nuclei, both specific and non-specific thalamic nuclei, the brainstem reticular formation, and probably a number of areas of neocortex (*vide infra*).

The best understood *outflow* from the amygdaloid nuclei occurs via the stria terminalis to the septal areas,

[683] E. C. Crosby and T. Humphrey, *J. comp. Neurol.*, **74**, 1941.
[684] W. E. Le G. Clark and M. Meyer, *Brain*, **70**, 1947.
[685] A. C. Allison, *J. Anat.*, **88**, 1954.
[686] T. P. S. Powell, W. M. Cowan and G. Raisman, *J. Anat.*, **99**, 1965.
[687] P. Gloor, in: *Handbook of Physiology*, Vol. II, Section I, *Neurophysiology*, eds. E. J. Field, H. W. Magoun and V. E. Hall, Am. Physiol. Soc., Washington. 1960.
[688] R. Wendt and D. Albe-Fessard, in: *Physiologie de l'hippocampe*, Centre National de la Recherche Scientifique, Paris. 1962.

the preoptic and adjacent regions of the hypothalamus, whilst some continue into the stria medullaris to reach the habenular nucleus. Other *amygdalofugal fibres* do not run with the stria terminalis, but follow more ventrally placed direct routes (p. 907) to reach many of the hypothalamic nuclei, the cortex of the piriform lobe, the nucleus medialis dorsalis of the thalamus, and the reticular formation of the midbrain tegmentum. Reciprocal connexions probably exist between the amygdaloid complex and the orbitofrontal, cingulate and temporal regions of the neocortex, whilst *interamygdaloid fibres* run with the other components of the anterior commissure (*vide infra*). Some functional associations of the amygdala are mentioned with those of the limbic system as a whole (p. 943).

## THE STRIA TERMINALIS

This is a small, discrete bundle of fine myelinated nerve fibres, which is visible to the unaided eye throughout much of its course. Fibres pass in both directions within the bundle to a number of different destinations. Topographically, the stria issues from the posterior aspect of the amygdaloid complex and runs caudally in the roof of the inferior horn of the lateral ventricle, on the medial side of the tail of the caudate nucleus. It follows the curve of the nucleus and then passes ventrally in the floor of the body of the ventricle, occupying the groove which separates the caudate nucleus from the thalamus, where it is closely related to the thalamostriate vein. It passes inferior to the interventricular foramen to approach the region of the anterior commissure, where it diverges into a series of components which are supracommissural, commissural, and subcommissural in position. As the stria nears the anterior pole of the thalamus, within its various subdivisions scattered groups of small neurons are found; these constitute the *bed nucleus of the stria terminalis*, within which a number of its fibres relay. Many of the fibres in the supra- and sub-commissural components are amygdalofugal, and are passing to the septal areas (*vide infra*), the preoptic and anterior hypothalamic nuclei, whilst others descend to the anterior perforated substance and adjacent regions of the piriform lobe. Some of the subcommissural fibres recurve to join the column of the fornix, and yet others pass caudally with the stria medullaris to the habenular nucleus. It is probable that reciprocal connexions are established between some of these regions and the amygdaloid nuclei, by fibres which pass in the reverse direction through the stria. It will be appreciated that interamygdaloid fibres pursue a most intricate topographical course. Leaving one amygdaloid complex they pass through almost the whole length of the highly curved stria terminalis to reach the anterior commissure, where they cross the midline and then curve in the reverse direction through the contralateral stria to reach the opposite amygdaloid complex.

## THE ANTERIOR COMMISSURE

The anterior commissure is a compact bundle of myelinated nerve fibres which crosses the midline anterior to the columns of the fornix, embedded in the lamina terminalis, where it forms part of the anterior wall of the third ventricle some 1·5–2·0 cm superior to the optic chiasma (7.110, 114, 141). When seen in sagittal section it is oval in shape with its long diameter (about 2·5 mm) placed vertically. Traced laterally, its fibres are twisted and entwined like the strands of a rope; further laterally, it separates into two principal bundles. The smaller *anterior bundle* curves forwards on each side towards the anterior perforated substance and olfactory tract. The large *posterior bundle* curves backward and laterally on each side

and for some distance is lodged in a deep groove on the antero-inferior aspect of the lentiform nucleus. Beyond the latter, the posterior bundle forms a fan-shaped radiation into the anterior part of the temporal lobe including the parahippocampal gyrus. Commissural fibres have been described in various mammals, including primates, as interconnecting the following structures with their fellows—(1) the olfactory bulb and anterior olfactory nucleus; (2) the anterior perforated substance, olfactory tubercle and diagonal band of Broca; (3) the prepiriform cortex; (4) the entorhinal area and adjacent parts of the parahippocampal gyrus; (5) part of the amygdaloid complex—in particular, the nucleus of the lateral olfactory stria; (6) the bed nucleus of the stria terminalis, and the nucleus accumbens septi; (7) the middle and inferior gyri of the temporal lobe in their anterior regions; and (8) possibly other neocortical areas, including small regions of the frontal lobe.

The intertemporal neocortical connexions form the largest component of the anterior commissure in primates, including the human brain. However, in the latter many of the detailed connexions of the fibres in the commissure remain to be elucidated. Further, a proportion of its fibres may not be truly commissural, but decussating pathways between dissimilar centres on the two sides.

## THE SEPTAL AREAS

In subprimate mammals, the *septal areas* consist of the thick medial walls of the cerebral hemispheres situated immediately anterior and superior to the lamina terminalis and anterior commissure. They consist of nuclear masses of grey matter together with relatively coarse bundles of white fibres, and according to their relationship to the anterior commissure may be divided into *pre-* and *supra-commissural* parts.

In higher primates and particularly in the human brain, the septal areas are considerably modified in association with the great expansion of the neocortex and corpus callosum in these forms. The supracommissural septum now corresponds in large measure to the bilateral thin laminae of white fibres, sparse grey matter and neuroglia, which form the right and left halves of the septum pellucidum. The precommissural septum (*septum verum* of some authors) in contrast, consists of relatively well-defined dorsal, ventral, medial and caudal *groups of nuclei* —each of these may be subdivided into a series of individual nuclei, but these will not be detailed here. However, the precise topographical limits of the human septum verum, and the terminology applied to the surface topography and nuclear groups of this region, have been the source of some confusion and disagreement. (For detailed reviews consult footnote references [689–691].)

Most authorities agree that the precommissural septum corresponds in part to the paraterminal gyrus. The latter has been mentioned elsewhere (p. 926) as a narrow vertical strip which lies between the anterior surface of the lamina terminalis and the posterior parolfactory sulcus. The anterior slope of the gyrus which passes into the sulcus is sometimes called the *prehippocampal rudiment*. Inferiorly, the gyrus and rudiment are continuous with the diagonal band of Broca and with the medial olfactory stria (7.119B). Superiorly, they narrow, and spread around the rostrum and genu of the corpus callosum to become continuous with the indusium griseum (p. 938). However, some investigators hold that only the prehippocampal rudiment is continuous with the indusium

[689] H. Stephan and O. J. Andy, *J. Hirnforsch.*, **5**, 1962.
[690] O. J. Andy and H. Stephan, *J. comp. Neurol.*, **133**, 1968.
[691] W. J. H. Nauta and W. Haymaker, in: *The Hypothalamus*, eds. W. Haymaker, E. Anderson and W. J. H. Nauta, Thomas, Illinois. 1969.

griseum, whilst the detailed connexions of the medial olfactory stria are uncertain in the human brain.

Whilst some of the septal nuclei are located within the paraterminal gyrus, others are more deeply placed[689–691] and are interspersed with fibres of the precommissural fornix (p. 942). Scattered cell groups interconnect the precommissural septum with the septum pellucidum, the substantia innominata and the anterior perforated substance.

**The main afferent connexions** to the septal nuclei are from: (1) the amygdaloid complex via the diagonal band and stria terminalis; (2) the anterior perforated substance by fibres which probably run with the medial olfactory stria; (3) the hippocampus via the fornix; (4) the midbrain reticular formation and hypothalamic nuclei through ascending fibres in the medial forebrain bundle.

**The main outflows** from the septal nuclei are—(1) fibres which return to the hippocampal formation in the fornix; (2) descending fibres in the medial forebrain bundle which are distributed to many of the hypothalamic nuclei and to the midbrain reticular formation; (3) fibres which pass in the stria medullaris thalami to the habenular nuclei.

Finally, interconnexions are probably established between the septal areas and the vestigial indusium griseum and also with the cingulate gyrus, but details of these remain uncertain.

Thus, the septal areas are important focal zones through which many of the principal limbic and hypothalamic structures are interconnected. For long thought to be reduced, atrophic, and perhaps functionless in primates, recent studies have demonstrated that in fact the septal nuclei have increased in prominence throughout the primates and reach their highest degree of primate development in the human brain.[690]

## The Hippocampal Formation

The hippocampal formation develops in the medial pallial fringe of the cerebral hemisphere, immediately adjacent to the outer convex border of the choroidal fissure (p. 980), where, with progressive development, it assumes a highly arched form extending from the interventricular foramen to the ventral extremity of the inferior horn of the lateral ventricle. The modifications in the superior part of the formation, which accompany the expansion of the neopallium and the corpus callosum, have also been discussed previously (p. 140). Essentially, the hippocampal formation consists of a curved band of phylogenetically ancient cortex (the *archipallium*), limited on its concave aspect by the choroidal fissure, and merging on its convex aspect with surrounding areas of *neopallium*. Traced in a radial direction from the choroidal fissure towards the neopallium, three main zones may be distinguished within the archipallium, namely, the *dentate gyrus*, the *cornu ammonis* and the *subiculum*. The dentate gyrus and cornu ammonis show some contrasting structural features, but are generally regarded as the most primitive *trilaminar* types of cortex, whilst the subiculum shows a graded variation in structure from a four, through a five, to a modified six-layered type of cortex where it merges with the surrounding neocortex. With further development profound growth changes cause an infolding of these archipallial zones towards the neighbouring cavity of the lateral ventricle. To assist understanding, these zones and their changes in relative position, are shown in a highly simplified manner in illustration **7**.121. The general form of infolding is similar throughout Mammalia. However, its degree, and the areas of hemisphere wall in which a well-differentiated hippocampal formation persists, varies greatly in different groups. These variations will not be detailed here, but they reflect the differences in relative expansion of the neopallium, corpus callosum and temporal lobe in the different groups. In the human brain, that part of the hippocampal arch related to the medial wall and roof of the body of the lateral ventricle becomes greatly reduced in association with the relatively enormous size of the corpus callosum, a well-developed hippocampal formation being confined to the floor and medial wall of the inferior horn of the ventricle.

Anteroinferiorly, the extremities of the archipallial arch are continuous with the septal area including the paraterminal gyrus, the anterior perforated substance and parts of the piriform lobe (p. 932). Further, the topographical limits of the structures to be included in the hippocampal formation vary somewhat in the accounts of different authorities. Here it is considered to include— (1) the indusium griseum, and the longitudinal striae and their extensions; (2) the gyrus fasciolaris; (3) the dentate gyrus, cornu ammonis and subiculum; (4) parts of the uncus. The term *hippocampus* is often used to denote the macroscopic swelling in the floor of the inferior horn of the lateral ventricle consisting of the interlocked dentate gyrus, cornu ammonis and related structures.

What follows is a brief topographical account of these regions, some further structural details of the hippocampus, and a description of the functionally related fornix.

### THE INDUSIUM GRISEUM

The indusium griseum or *supracallosal gyrus*, is a thin, poorly differentiated veil of grey matter which covers the superior surface of the corpus callosum. Laterally, on each side, it passes into the callosal sulcus to become continuous with the cortex of the cingulate gyrus. Anteriorly, it sweeps around the genu and rostrum of the corpus callosum to merge, on each side, with the superior end of the paraterminal gyrus. It will be recalled that the latter is continuous inferiorly with the diagonal band of Broca and, through this, with the anterior perforated substance and periamygdaloid area. Posteriorly, the indusium griseum passes on to the splenium of the corpus callosum where it diverges to become continuous with the right and left *gyrus fasciolaris* (*splenial gyrus*). The latter is a delicate strip of grey matter which curves downwards, forwards and laterally, to blend with the posterior extremity of the *dentate gyrus*. Embedded in the indusium, and causing a ridging of its free surface, are two narrow bundles of white fibres on each side, the *medial* and *lateral longitudinal striae* (of Lancisi) (**7**.139). The medial striae course near the midline whilst the lateral striae are in the depths of the callosal sulci. The striae are regarded as the reduced white matter of the vestigial indusium. Anteriorly, they pass towards the paraterminal gyri, whilst posteriorly they continue through the gyrus fasciolaris to reach the fimbriae of the fornix (*vide infra*). The detailed connexions of the striae are uncertain, but in the supracallosal part of their course they probably contribute fibres which pierce the corpus callosum and form part of the *dorsal fornix* (p. 942).

### THE HIPPOCAMPUS

As noted above, the hippocampus consists of the complex interfolded layers of the dentate gyrus and cornu ammonis, the latter being continuous through the subicular region with the cortex of the parahippocampal gyrus. The name hippocampus stems from the supposed resemblance of these cell laminae, when viewed in coronal section, to the outline of a sea-horse. Grossly, the hippocampus is superior to the subiculum and medial part of the parahippocampal gyrus, where it forms a curved elevation about 5 cm long extending throughout the entire length of the floor of the inferior horn of the lateral ventricle. Its anterior extremity is expanded, and at this point its margin sometimes presents two or three shallow grooves with intervening elevations giving a paw-like appearance—the so-called *pes hippocampi*. The ventricular surface is convex in coronal section and, of course, covered by ependyma, beneath which pass tangential white fibres of the *alveus* converging medially upon a longitudinal projecting bundle of white fibres, the *fimbria of the fornix*. The general relationships of these various cell layers and fibre bundles as seen in coronal section are best appreciated by preliminary references to a simplified diagram (**7.**121). It will be noted that passing *medially* from the line of the collateral sulcus, the neocortex of the *parahippocampal gyrus* merges with the transitional cortex of the *subiculum*. The latter curves superomedially to reach the inferior surface of the *dentate gyrus*, and then continuing to curve laterally becomes continuous with the cell laminae of the *cornu ammonis*. The latter continues to curve, first superiorly and then laterally above the dentate gyrus, and finally ends pointing towards the centre of the superior surface of the dentate gyrus. However, it should be appreciated that the degree of curvature of these regions varies somewhat along the length of the hippocampus and also in different specimens.

Topographically, the *dentate gyrus* (**7.**120) is a crenated strip of cortex which is related inferiorly to the subiculum, laterally to the cornu ammonis, and superiorly to the recurved part of the cornu ammonis, the alveus and, more medially, to the fimbria of the fornix (**7.**121). However, the distribution and form of the fimbria is quite variable (*vide infra*), but medially it is separated from the notched medial margin of the dentate gyrus by the *fimbriodentate sulcus*. The *hippocampal sulcus*, of variable depth, intervenes between the dentate gyrus and the subicular extension of the parahippocampal gyrus. Posteriorly, as noted above, the dentate gyrus is continuous with the gyrus fasciolaris, and through this, with the indusium griseum. Anteriorly, the dentate gyrus is continued into the notch of the uncus, where it makes a sharp bend medially across the central part of its inferior surface. This transverse part is smooth and featureless, being termed the *tail of the dentate gyrus* (band of Giacomini), and it becomes indistinguishable on the medial aspect of the uncus. The tail separates the rest of the inferior surface of the uncus into an anterior *uncinate gyrus* and a posterior *intralimbic gyrus* (**7.**119, 120).

## THE STRUCTURE OF THE HIPPOCAMPUS

Since the extensive pioneering researches of Cajal[664] and Lorente de Nó[692] a vast literature has accumulated concerning the structure and connexions of the hippocampus. Only a few salient points can be mentioned here, and for details texts devoted wholly to neuroanatomy (e.g. [28, 29, 61]) and original papers should be consulted. Detailed reviews of the complex terminologies proposed for the various laminae and their subdivisions are to be found in the writings of Lorente de Nó,[692] Rose,[693] and Gastaut and Lammers.[694] Examples of the many investigations into the connectivity patterns of the hippocampus using degeneration techniques may be found in footnote references [695–697], using ultrastructural techniques [698–701], and neurophysiological recording methods.[702, 703]

Some aspects of the terminology used and some of the main structural features are shown in outline in illustration **7.**122.

It should be noted that because of the form of cortical folding which occurs during development, the original *external* surfaces of the dentate gyrus and subiculum (the *strata moleculare*) are closely applied to each other in the depths of the sulcus hippocampi (or along the obliterated line of the sulcus). Throughout much of its extent, the subicular region merges laterally with the modified six-layered cortex of the *entorhinal area* of the parahippocampal gyrus. (Some authorities prefer to include the subiculum with the parahippocampal gyrus, rather than with the hippocampal formation.) As noted above, during its curved course from the entorhinal area to the beginning of Ammon's horn, the subiculum exhibits a gradual change in its structure from a modified six-layered to a four-layered type of cortex, with accompanying differences in its patterns of connectivity. Accordingly, the subiculum is often divided into four zones, the *parasubiculum, presubiculum, subiculum* and the *prosubiculum*.

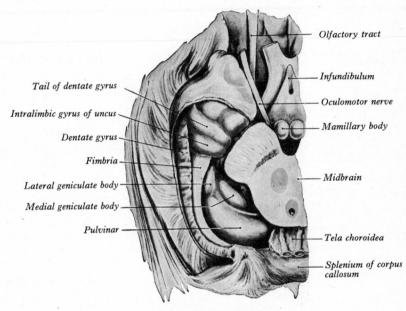

Tail of dentate gyrus

Intralimbic gyrus of uncus

Dentate gyrus

Fimbria

Lateral geniculate body

Medial geniculate body

Pulvinar

Olfactory tract

Infundibulum

Oculomotor nerve

Mamillary body

Midbrain

Tela choroidea

Splenium of corpus callosum

**7.**120  Basal aspect of part of the brain dissected to display the uncus, dentate gyrus, fimbria, etc.

Their structural differences will not be detailed here, but it should be appreciated that the prosubiculum merges into the cornu ammonis which, using the same criteria, may be regarded as a primitive trilaminar cortex possessing *molecular, pyramidal* and *polymorphic* layers from its original external surface towards its ventricular surface. However, using other methods and criteria, many more sub-layers are often described in Ammon's horn (*vide infra*). Further, although the general cytoarchitectonic pattern is roughly similar throughout Ammon's horn,

[692] R. L. de Nó, *J. Psychol. Neurol., Lpz.*, **46**, 1934.

[693] M. Rose, *J. Psychol. Neurol. Lpz.*, **34**, 1926; **35**, 1927.

[694] H. Gastaut and H. J. Lammers, *Anatomie du rhinencéphale. Les grandes activités du rhinencéphale*, Masson, Paris. 1960.

[695] T. W. Blackstad, *J. comp. Neurol.*, **105**, 1956; *Acta anat.*, **35**, 1958.

[696] G. Raisman, W. M. Cowan and T. P. S. Powell, *Brain*, **88**, 1965; **89**, 1966.

[697] L. E. White, *J. comp. Neurol.*, **113**, 1959; and *Int. Rev. Neurobiol.*, **8**, 1965.

[698] T. W. Blackstad, in: *The Neuron*, ed. H. Hydén, Elsevier, Amsterdam. 1967.

[699] T. W. Blackstad and A. Kjaerheim, *J. comp. Neurol.*, **117**, 1967.

[700] T. W. Blackstad and P. R. Flood, *Nature, Lond.*, **198**, 1963.

[701] L. H. Hamlyn, *J. Anat.*, **96**, 1962.

[702] P. Andersen, T. W. Blackstad and T. Lømo, *Expl Brain Res.*, **1**, 1966.

[703] P. Andersen, J. C. Eccles and Y. Løyning, *J. Neurophysiol.*, **27**, 1964a and b.

there are regional differences in its detailed structure and connexions. For these reasons, different investigators have proposed various methods and criteria for subdividing this region into a series of radially disposed fields (7.122). These include the **cornu ammonis fields CA1 to CA4** of Lorente de Nó,[692] and the **hippocampal fields H1 to H5** of Rose.[693] Unfortunately, these do not correspond; the former, as the name implies, are limited to Ammon's horn, whilst the H1 field of Rose includes part of the subiculum, the prosubiculum, and part of Ammon's horn.

**The cornu ammonis**, following the intensive studies of Cajal,[664] is usually considered to consist of the following sub-layers starting on its ventricular aspect—(1) the *ependyma*; (2) the *alveus*; (3) the *stratum oriens*; (4) the *stratum pyramidalis*; (5) the *stratum radiatum*; (6) the *stratum lacunosum*; and (7) the *stratum moleculare*. Many authors group the last two sub-layers as a single stratum lacunosum-moleculare.

**The alveus** is a subependymal layer of white fibres both entering and leaving the hippocampus. The efferent fibres are predominantly the axons of the large neurons of the stratum pyramidalis, together with a smaller number from some cells of the stratum oriens and dentate gyrus. These axons converge to form the large efferent component of the *fimbria of the fornix* (*vide infra*), but before joining it they give rise to fine collateral branches which re-enter the hippocampus. Afferent fibres from other regions of the nervous system, including commissural fibres from the opposite hippocampal formation, also

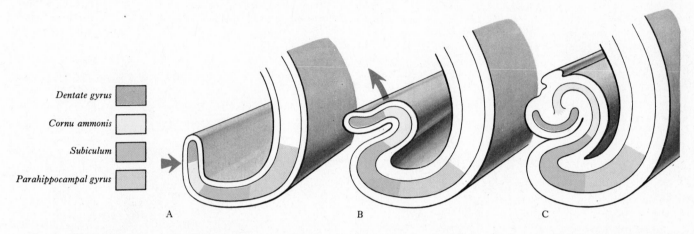

Dentate gyrus

Cornu ammonis

Subiculum

Parahippocampal gyrus

A    B    C

**7.121 A–C** The hippocampus and related structures seen in coronal section. A, B and C are a series of diagrams to assist understanding of the assumption of the definitive positions of the dentate gyrus, cornu ammonis, subiculum and parahippocampal gyrus, in the floor of the inferior horn of the lateral ventricle in the human brain. Note that these are not tracings from a series of embryonic sections, and that they have

been somewhat simplified in the interests of clarity. Note also that the amount of curvature and infolding which occurs varies along the length of the hippocampus, and in different specimens. It is important to appreciate that following folding, the original *external* surfaces of the dentate gyrus and part of the subiculum are in contact, and that the degree of tissue fusion which occurs along the line of the hippocampal sulcus is quite variable.

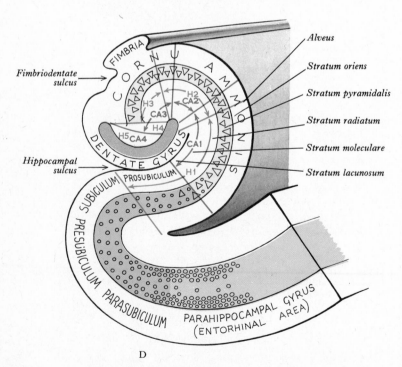

Fimbriodentate sulcus

Hippocampal sulcus

FIMBRIA

CORNU    AMMONIS

H2 CA2
H3
CA3
H4
H5 CA4
CA1
H1

DENTATE GYRUS

SUBICULUM    PROSUBICULUM

PRESUBICULUM    PARASUBICULUM    PARAHIPPOCAMPAL GYRUS (ENTORHINAL AREA)

Alveus

Stratum oriens

Stratum pyramidalis

Stratum radiatum

Stratum moleculare

Stratum lacunosum

D

**7.121 D** An analysis of the major topographical zones and the complex terminology applied to the hippocampus and related structures seen in a coronal section of the floor of the inferior horn of the lateral ventricle in a mature human brain. Colour code for tissue zones as in A–C. The approximate limits of the various subdivisions of the subiculum are labelled. CA 1–4 are the cornu ammonis fields of Lorente de Nó[692], and H 1–5 are the hippocampal fields of Rose.[693]

approach the cell layers of the hippocampus through the alveus.

*The stratum oriens* is interlaced with the axons and collateral branches of fibres entering and leaving the hippocampus; it is penetrated by some of the basal dendrites of the large pyramidal cells of the adjacent layer, and it contains the cell somata and dendrites of relatively small, irregularly shaped neurons, some of which are termed *basket cells*. These small cells have been shown to be inhibitory interneurons. They receive axosomatic and axodendritic synapses from some of the afferent fibre collaterals to the hippocampus, and also collaterals from efferent fibres. Some of the axons of these interneurons penetrate the radiate and molecular layers establishing axodendritic contacts with pyramidal cells, but the most distinctive terminals are those of the basket cells, which form numerous, crowded, axosomatic synapses on the cell bodies of the pyramidal neurons.

*The stratum pyramidalis* is a particularly well-defined double layer of both large and small pyramidal cells. Their bases face the stratum oriens and alveus, whilst their apices point towards the stratum radiatum. The axon of a pyramidal cell issues from its base or from a basal dendrite, and passes into the alveus, where it gives collateral branches and then continues into the fimbria of the fornix. Some of these collateral branches end on cells in the stratum oriens, but many (the *Schaffer collaterals*) pursue a recurrent course to the stratum moleculare where they terminate on the apical dendrites of adjacent pyramidal cells. The dendritic tree of a pyramidal cell has two main components, basal and apical. The *basal dendrites* radiate into the neighbouring pyramidal layer, but the majority pass into the stratum oriens and overlying alveus; they are beset with dendritic spines. The *apical dendrites* pass deeply, and together with associated axons and a few pyramidal cells, make up the bulk of the *stratum radiatum*. On reaching the *stratum lacunosum-moleculare*, the apical dendrites branch profusely, and these terminal branchlets, together with their stem dendrite, are also covered with dendrite spines. Thus, these deepest layers consist of the terminal dendrites of the pyramidal cells, axonal terminals of various afferents to the hippocampus, the recurrent (Schaffer) collaterals mentioned above, and the cell bodies, dendrites and axonal arborizations of the scattered, deeply placed interneurons, from which the stratum lacunosum receives its name. Whilst the con-

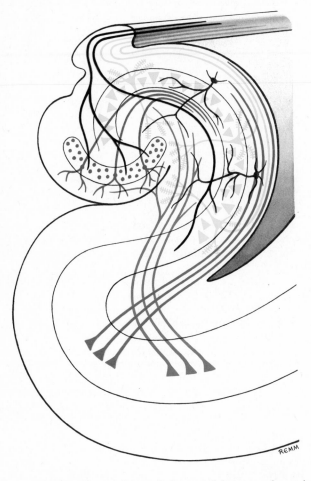

7.122  A diagram of some of the main features of the neuronal organization and connectivity patterns of the dentate gyrus, cornu ammonis, subiculum and parahippocampal gyrus. The cell somata, dendrites and axons of the pyramidal neurons of the cornu ammonis are yellow; their axons form the efferent hippocampal fibres of the alveus and fimbria. Afferent fibres to the cornu ammonis from the fimbria are purple, those following the alvear path are green, whilst those following the perforant path are blue. Basket neurons are in black. The neurons of the dentate gyrus, and their axons which form the mossy fibres of the hippocampus, are in magenta. See text for further details.

nexions of the hippocampus are treated in a subsequent paragraph, it may be noted here that the various zones of the dendritic tree of the pyramidal cell receive distinctive types of axonal terminal. Thus, commissural fibres from corresponding regions of the opposite hippocampus end upon basal dendrites, whilst those from non-corresponding regions end on the apical dendrites in the strata lacunosum and moleculare. Afferents from the entorhinal cortex form synapses with the most terminal branches of the apical dendrites in the molecular layer, whilst the

synaptic endings of the Schaffer collaterals are found in the stratum lacunosum. The mossy fibres derived from dentate gyrus cells form large synaptic terminals which enclose the prominent dendritic spines of the apical dendrites in the stratum radiatum, but as noted above, basket cell terminals form a dense population of axosomatic synapses. Attempts have been made to correlate these interesting zonal variations in axonal terminals with differences in the character of the electrical recordings made with microelectrodes inserted to varying depths in Ammon's horn.[702, 703] Thus, many of the afferent systems, and the pyramidal cells themselves, are now known to be excitatory, and some of the interneurons, particularly the basket cells, are known to be inhibitory in their action.

**The dentate gyrus** is less well understood, but is considered to be a trilaminar cortical structure. Extending deeply from the line of the hippocampal sulcus it consists of: (1) a superficial *molecular layer*; (2) an intermediate *granular layer*; and (3) a deep *polymorphic cell layer*. These will not be considered in detail here. Briefly, the various cell types in the three laminae have spine-studded dendritic trees which either radiate locally or pass in the superficial layer. They receive synaptic terminals from some of the afferent fibres to the hippocampus from extrinsic sources, and also from the axons of neighbouring neurons. Some of the cells are Golgi type II neurons with axons which terminate locally; others have much longer axons which, after collateral branching, run to join the efferent fibres in the fimbria of the fornix. The most distinctive axons, however, are called *mossy fibres*. They arise from many of the cells in the granular layer and then pass through the polymorphic layer giving collateral branches to its neurons. The mossy fibres then proceed along a curved course in the superficial part of the stratum radiatum of the cornu ammonis, where they make a series of very large synaptic contacts with the spines on the initial segments of the apical dendrites of the pyramidal cells.

## THE CONNEXIONS OF THE HIPPOCAMPUS

**Afferent pathways** to the hippocampus arise in: (1) parts of the cingulate gyrus; (2) the septal nuclei; (3) the entorhinal cortex; (4) the indusium griseum; (5) commissural fibres from the opposite hippocampal formation, and (6) possibly some fibres from the prepiriform cortex.

The fibres from the cingulate gyrus reach the hippocampus via the cingulum (p. 971) and are distributed both directly to the cornu ammonis, and indirectly after relays in the subicular region. The afferents from the septal nuclei retrace the curved path of the fornix back to the hippocampus. The commissural fibres from one hippocampal formation pass through the fimbria and crus of the fornix on the same side to reach, and cross the midline in, the commissure of the fornix (*vide infra*). Thereafter, they recurve back through the opposite crus and fimbria to reach the contralateral hippocampus. Some fibres derived from cells in the indusium griseum run posteriorly in the longitudinal striae, with which they pass through the gyrus fasciolaris to reach the fimbria, which conducts them to the hippocampus.

The most profuse afferent connexions of the dentate gyrus and the cornu ammonis, however, are derived from the entorhinal cortex and subicular regions, and they pass by two distinct routes. Fibres from the medial part of the entorhinal area and parasubiculum follow an *alvear path* through the prosubiculum to reach the alveus and stratum oriens of the cornu ammonis. In contrast, the afferents derived from the lateral part of the entorhinal area follow a *perforant path* through the subiculum, which crosses the alvear path, and continues into the stratum lacunosum-moleculare of the cornu ammonis and adjacent parts of the dentate gyrus. These routes, and those entering from the fimbria are shown in illustration **7.122**.

## THE FORNIX

In addition to the afferent hippocampal fibres and commissural fibres described above, the fornix constitutes the sole **efferent system** from the hippocampus. These efferent fibres are mainly the continuations of the axons of the pyramidal cells of Ammons's horn, but a small

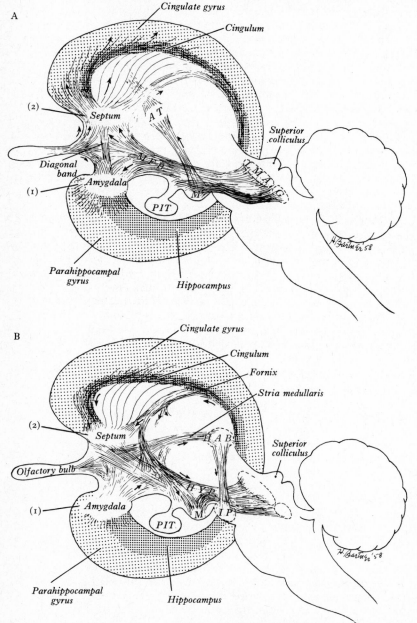

**7.123**A and B  Schematic drawings of one concept of the 'limbic lobe' (after MacLean) in which emphasis is placed upon the medial forebrain bundle (MFB) as a major line of communication between the limbic cortex, the hypothalamus and the midbrain. Note the relationship between the fornix and the cingulum. The limbic cortex, which is considered as a hierarchical system of concentric strips, is indicated by heavy and light stipple. The neocortex is not included. A   The ascending pathways to the limbic structures, with emphasis on the divergence of fibres from the medial forebrain bundle to the amygdala (1) and to the septal area (2). Note also the input from the olfactory bulb and tract. B   Descending pathways from the limbic system. AT: anterior group of thalamic nuclei; CG: central grey matter of the midbrain; DB: diagonal band of Broca; G: tegmental reticular nuclei; HAB: habenular nucleus; HYP: hypothalamus; IP: interpeduncular nucleus; LMA: limbic midbrain area (of Nauta); M: mamillary body; PIT: hypophysis cerebri; SC: superior colliculus. (From P. D. MacLean in: *The American Journal of Medicine*, **25**, 1958; by courtesy of the author and publishers.)

proportion are derived from neurons in the stratum oriens and the dentate gyrus. These various axons pass through the alveus and converge upon the medial border of the ventricular surface of the hippocampus to form the *fimbria*. The latter is a flattened band of white fibres which lies superior to the dentate gyrus and forms the inferior boundary of the choroidal fissure. The disposition of the fimbria is variable. It may project above the dentate gyrus with a free medial edge, the *taenia fornicis*, and a lateral border which merges into the alveus; alternatively, its free border may be twisted over towards the lateral side, uncovering the dentate gyrus (**7.140**). Anteriorly, the fimbria continues into the hook of the uncus (**7.120**). Traced posteriorly on the floor of the inferior horn of the ventricle, it ascends towards the splenium and the majority of its fibres now pass anteriorly below the splenium, and then curve forward above the thalamus, forming the *crus of the fornix*. The two crura are closely applied to the inferior surface of the corpus callosum and are connected to each other by transverse fibres which pass between the hippocampal formations of the two sides and form the *commissure of the fornix* (hippocampal commissure). The commissure is a thin triangular sheet which, together with the converging crura, is sometimes termed the *lyra* or *psalterium* (an instrument resembling a harp). Between the commissure and the corpus callosum, a horizontal cleft (the so-called *ventricle of the fornix*) is sometimes found. Anteriorly, the two crura come together in the median plane to form the *body of the fornix* which is really a symmetrically disposed bilateral structure. The body of the fornix lies above the tela choroidea and the ependymal roof of the third ventricle (**7.157**) and is attached to the inferior surface of the corpus callosum and, more anteriorly, to the inferior borders of the laminae of the septum pellucidum. Laterally, the body of the fornix overlies the medial part of the upper surface of the thalamus, and the choroidal fissure is placed below its free lateral edge. Through this fissure the choroid plexus in the lateral margin of the tela choroidea passes into the body of the lateral ventricle (**7.157**). Anteriorly, above the interventricular foramina, the body of the fornix diverges into right and left bundles which curve inferiorly towards the anterior commissure forming the anterior boundary of the foramina. As each bundle approaches the commissure it divides around it into two components—a *precommissural fornix*, and a *postcommissural fornix* (column of the fornix). Each column continues to curve infero-posteriorly and gradually sinks into the corresponding part of the lateral wall of the third ventricle to reach the superior aspect of the mamillary body.

In addition to the foregoing bundles, some fibres leave the fimbria near the splenium to run anteriorly with the supracallosal medial and lateral longitudinal striae, where they are joined by others arising from the indusium griseum. Some fibres of the striae then pass inferiorly between the fibre bundles of the corpus callosum, where they are joined by other fascicles which pass straight into the corpus callosum from the fimbria. These various fascicles, which intersect the callosal bundles, constitute the *dorsal fornix*. Some fibres of the dorsal fornix relay in the scattered patches of grey matter in the septum pellucidum, whilst others course directly on through the septum; both direct and indirect fibres largely rejoin the main body of the fornix.

Thus, following these different bundles of the fornix, *hippocampal efferents* pass to: (1) the gyrus fasciolaris, indusium griseum, cingulate gyrus, and the septum pellucidum via the *dorsal fornix*; (2) to the precommissural septum, the preoptic and anterior hypothalamic nuclei via the *precommissural fornix*; (3) during its descent the *postcommissural column of the fornix* gives direct fibres to the anterior nuclei of the thalamus and to many of the hypothalamic nuclei (p. 907), before proceeding to its main termination in the medial mamillary nucleus; (4) other fibres curve caudally from the column of the fornix to join the stria medullaris thalami to reach the habenular nuclei, whilst yet others continue into the reticular formation of the midbrain tegmentum.

In summary, illustrations **7**.123 A and B show the main inflow and outflow pathways associated with the limbic system (based upon footnote reference [661]).

## THE ROLE OF THE LIMBIC SYSTEM

An immense volume of research has been directed towards a better understanding of the biological roles of the various complex and interconnected structures which are often grouped together under the term limbic system, described in the previous pages. Despite this, their significances can, at present, only be described in the most general terms. Even a brief review of the experimental results is beyond the scope of the present volume but, in summary, the following points may be noted.

(1) Many of the structures such as the amygdaloid and septal complexes and the hippocampal formation were for long regarded as primarily olfactory integration centres. However, it is now widely accepted that only those regions included under the terms *primary* and *secondary olfactory cortices* (p. 936) are intimately concerned with olfaction. After olfactory bulb stimulation, only weak electrical discharges, occurring after a long latency, can be recorded from the hippocampus, cingulate gyrus, etc. Thus, perhaps higher order olfactory information does reach these areas to be integrated with information from many other sources which is also projected to them.

(2) An intact limbic system, hypothalamus and brainstem are necessary for fully integrated and *effective homeostatic responses* to occur under a wide range of environmental conditions (see also p. 909).

(3) Stimulation or ablation of different regions in experimental animals such as the amygdala, septal areas or hippocampus, lead to a variety of *complex changes in behaviour* involving locomotor, autonomic and endocrine effects.

Thus, for example, stimulation of the amygdaloid region[704, 705] often leads initially to what has been termed the *arrest reaction* and the *attention responses*. Movement patterns already in progress are inhibited. Changes have been demonstrated in reflex or cortically induced movements, in cardiovascular, respiratory, gastro-intestinal, genital and urinary activities. Searching movements, with turning of the head and eyes to the opposite side, and movements of chewing, licking and swallowing often occur. More prolonged stimulation may lead to a *fear* or *flight response* with increased searching movements and finally withdrawal with attempts to hide, or to a *rage* or *defence reaction* with hissing, crouching, clawing and piloerection. Conversely, ablation of the amygdaloid regions on both sides leads, in general, to placid, 'sociable' forms of behaviour, and a loss of aggression in previously savage animals. Accompanying this, bizarre forms of hypersexual behaviour occur, together with persistent oral examination of the environment, non-discriminative swallowing of liquids and solids, and an indifference to normally pain-producing stimuli.

Reference has already been made to the presence within the hypothalamus of so-called positive and negative reward centres (p. 912). Similarly, following stimulation in the septal areas, certain hippocampal areas and related structures, there occur a variety of locomotor and general visceral effects, together with an apparent *pleasure reaction* with docility, repetitive grooming and often penile erection—obvious preludes to copulatory behaviour. Ablation of the hippocampal structures on both sides in experimental animals, and occasionally as a result of disease or surgical intervention in man, sometimes results in disturbances of *recent memory*. To what degree the hippocampus itself, or in association with related structures, is normally involved in the establishment of short- or long-term memory traces remains conjectural, and the detailed mechanisms which operate are, of course, unknown.

(4) In short, therefore, the limbic structures are widely regarded as involved in both *brief* and *prolonged homeostatic responses*.[661, 662] The long-term responses have been grouped into those mainly directed at *preservation of the individual* and those concerned more with *preservation of the species*. The former include searching for and securing food and drink, and aggressive, defensive or flight responses. The latter include mating, rearing of young, 'home' building and other forms of social behaviour. The limbic structures are also intimately involved in *emotional behaviour*, both in terms of subjective feeling states such as fear, rage, pleasure and so forth, and also in the physical expression of these states. Finally, they may be involved in the establishment of *memory patterns*.

---

[704] G. V. Goddard, *Psychol. Bull.*, **62**, 1964.

[705] B. Kaada, in: *Aggression and Defence. Neural Mechanisms and Social Patterns*, eds. C. D. Clemente and D. B. Lindsley, University of California Press, Berkeley. 1967.

# THE CEREBRAL CORTEX

## Introduction

The cerebral cortex has been studied over several centuries, with increasing momentum. It was examined by the first microscopists, and as early as 1776 the stria in the occipital cortex named after him was noted by Gennari, this being the first recorded structural detail. Only with the advent of improved microscopes in the 1830's and later did effective investigation of cortical organization begin; it has continued uninterruptedly since then, producing an increasing number of papers which has become an almost unmanageable deluge in this century. Consequently, no more than the most outstanding contributions can be mentioned here, and emphasis must be chiefly upon reports of work done in recent decades. However, it is important to note the basic discoveries from which the intricate knowledge of today has expanded, if only to maintain a wider perspective amid the flood of detailed description and speculation which renders current activity so interesting and yet confusing in its constant sallies and revisions. The accent of endeavour has naturally varied with the availability of techniques; but the major aims have been and remain the elucidation of the *modus operandi* in the cerebral cortex and the localization of different forms of activity in it.

Earlier investigations, inevitably microscopic, were stimulated by the techniques of Nissl, Golgi, Cajal, and Weigert (**7**.124), amongst others. Even prior to this, with

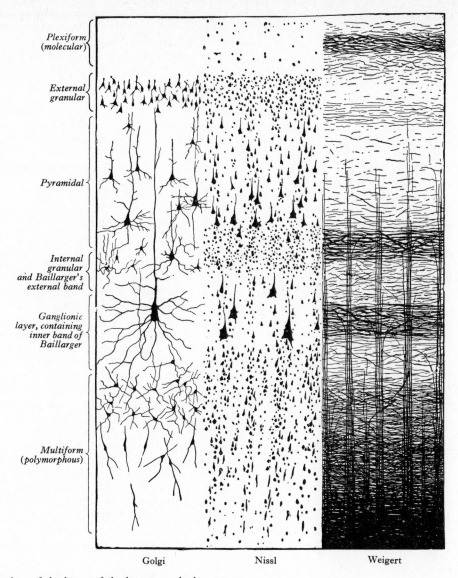

Plexiform (molecular)

External granular

Pyramidal

Internal granular and Baillarger's external band

Ganglionic layer, containing inner band of Baillarger

Multiform (polymorphous)

Golgi          Nissl          Weigert

**7.124** Representations of the layers of the human cerebral cortex, as stained by the techniques of Golgi, Nissl and Weigert.

less satisfactory methods, Baillarger[706] and Meynert,[707] had ascribed a laminar pattern to the cortex, with particular emphasis upon fibre structure—*myeloarchitecture*. Subsequent workers using newer techniques[708–714] confirmed this, but with notable variations and disagreements now largely overlooked. A six-layered schema prevailed (Brodmann), although this was based upon Nissl-stained material alone, in which all the highly significant details of dendrites studied by other workers were invisible; moreover, the data were accumulated from a comparative series which, although including simian brains, did not include the human cortex. These studies, in which a six-layered pattern became almost a dogma, led to the recognition of great variations in this theme in different cortical regions or 'areas', no less than fifty-two being distinguished. These results, embodied in the familiar 'Brodmann maps'—still widely current—were transferred somewhat arbitrarily to man by others, and they gained much credence amongst physiologists, perhaps because they provided a useful numerical reference guide to the cortex (**7.125** A, B) as they still do today.

Techniques such as Nissl's merely reveal the morphological variations and distribution of nerve cell bodies, and this *cytoarchitectural* mode of study requires *myeloarchitectural* methods to display myelinated nerve cell processes. Only with both methods of examination,

coupled with axonal staining by such techniques as the Golgi method—to which must be added the more recent availability of electron microscopy and refined experimental degeneration techniques—only with all these can the finer details of cortical organization be defined. Unfortunately, the Nissl-based cytoarchitectonic mapping of the cerebral cortex initially attracted more attention than other available techniques, and its continued use, together with myelin staining, has led to an almost excessive parcellation of the cortex into different areas, few of which can be accorded clear physiological significance. One useful outcome of these somewhat unfruitful studies was the diversion of interest among younger workers to

[706] J. G. F. Baillarger, *Mém. Acad. roy. Méd., Paris*, **8**, 1840.

[707] T. Meynert, *Vjschr. Psychiat., Vienna*, **1** and **2**, 1867–8.

[708] W. B. Lewis, *Brain*, **1**, 1878.

[709] A. W. Campbell, *Histological Studies on the Localisation of Cerebral Function*, University Press, Cambridge. 1905.

[710] S. R. y Cajal, *Histologie du système nerveux, de l'homme et des vertébrés*, Maloine, Paris. 1909–11.

[711] K. Brodmann, *Vergleichende Lokalisationslehre der Grosshirnrinde*, Barth, Leipzig. 1909.

[712] C. Vogt and O. Vogt, *Naturwissenschaften*, **14**, 1926.

[713] C. von Economo and G. N. Koskinas, *The Cytoarchitectonics of the Human Cerebral Cortex*, University Press, Oxford. 1929.

[714] R. Lorente de Nó, in: *Physiology of the Nervous System*, ed. J. F. Fulton, Oxford University Press, New York. 1949.

physiological studies. The rapid advance in this field of cortical investigation gradually lead to much discordance between the results of stimulation studies and architectonic mapping (except in broad details), and this has prompted several notable critical reviews.[715, 716] These have not entirely deterred the 'architectonicians', and it must be stated that in the *broader* aspects of their schemata there is considerable accord between their structurally established areas and the results of physiological experimentation.

The definition of five or six major types of cortical organization (cf. Campbell[709] and von Economo and Koskinas[713], **7**.126 A, B) has proved valid in functional terms, but the excesses of architectonics are reminiscent, except in their admittedly serious structural basis, of the multi-faculty maps of phrenology. The division of the cortex into such a multiplicity of 'organs' seems basically improbable. As the critics of such concepts have stressed, variations in a single area in different individuals of the same species, the effects of cortical development and folding, and other factors, particularly the pattern of subcortical connexions, may all contribute to variable structural appearances in the cortex—and to variations which are not uniform. The need for a more quantitative approach to the problem has also been emphasized by the same critics, but this remains largely an exhortation, though its ultimate necessity is generally recognized.

That a laminar appearance characterizes the cerebral cortex cannot be denied, but dogmatic views on the number of layers in this neuronal continuum, or upon the variations in, and equivalence of, the customarily numbered six layers in different areas, have been shown to be of little or no functional significance, if pushed to excess. Nevertheless, the Brodmann schema of numbered layers is still almost universally employed, perhaps as a mere convenience, and it will perforce be described below. Localization of function to a considerable degree—inasmuch as some areas receive or project large and easily identifiable subcortical connexions—also remains undeniable, and the polemics which this concept occasioned in the late nineteenth century are largely forgotten.[717] But the original extents of such 'motor' and 'sensory' areas, as defined (and perhaps artificially confined) by architectonic studies, have been markedly modified and augmented by physiological investigations, and also by the results of degeneration experiments.

Studies of the cortex by Golgi and silver-staining methods, though originally somewhat obscured by work based on Nissl technique, have received a renewed impetus with the recent development of micro-recording from the larger individual nerve cells of the cortex. Prior to this the elaborate structural studies of the neurites of cortical neurons, which have been available for half a century, could not be equated with the results of physiological experimentation; but, as has been mentioned elsewhere (p. 765), during the last decade or so the intimate arrangement of neurons and their individual activities have shown a growing correlation in elaborating concepts of the mode of action of small volumes of nervous tissue, in a variety of sites in the central nervous system, including cerebral cortex.

While classical cyto*architectonic* teaching has become perhaps little more than a useful mode of geographical definition of cortical areas (and a source of some confusion in the 'translation' of areas from species to species of experimental animals), cyto*architectural* details, as revealed by the methods of Golgi and Cajal, are beginning to fit the observed behaviour of individual 'units' in the living cortex. Classical neurite studies of the cerebral cortex—chiefly in lower mammals, such as rodents (see, for example, reference [718])—have led to recognition of a large

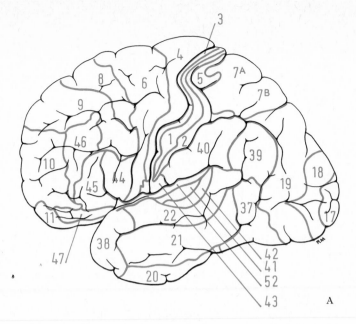

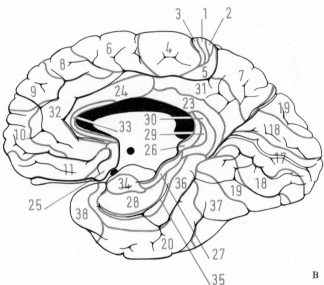

**7**.125 A and B  The superolateral (A) and medial (B) surfaces of the human cerebral hemisphere demonstrating the cytoarchitectonic areas identified and designated numerically by K. Brodmann (1909). See text for further details and references. Compare with **7**.126.

number of nerve cell types. The familiar pyramidal and stellate (granule) cells of Nissl-stained material were chiefly differentiated by relative size into a few unsatisfactory categories, subjectively assessed as large, medium, or small, and so on, with few attempts at measurement. The comparatively unilluminating results of this kind of study are well represented in **7**.126 B. This should be compared with **7**.127 B which illustrates the much more useful information afforded by techniques capable of revealing the interconnexions between cortical neurons. It is upon such criteria that a much larger range of neuronal differentiation can be based; and since it is ultimately interneuronal connexions which must be correlated with their activities in life, this approach to cortical structure is inevitably more appropriate than cytoarchitectonic

[715] K. S. Lashley and G. Clark, *J. comp. Neurol.*, **85**, 1946.

[716] D. A. Sholl, *Organisation of the Cerebral Cortex*, Methuen, London. 1956.

[717] E. Clarke and C. D. O'Malley, *The Human Brain and Spinal Cord*, University of California Press, Los Angeles. 1968.

[718] R. L. de Nó, *J. Psychol. Neurol., Lpz.*, **46**, 1934.

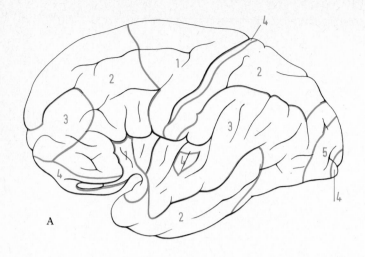

A

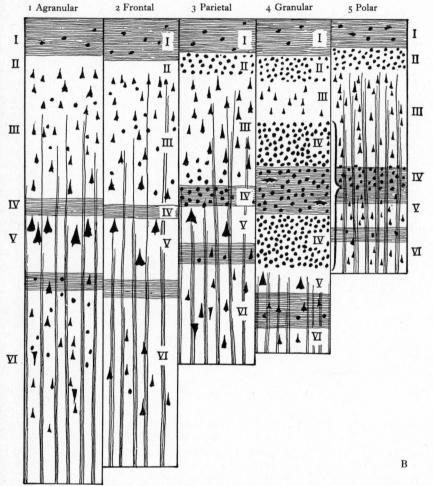

| 1 Agranular | 2 Frontal | 3 Parietal | 4 Granular | 5 Polar |

B

7.126 A and B. The distribution of the five major types of cerebral cortex, as projected on to the superolateral surface of the hemisphere, according to C. von Economo and G. N. Koskinas (1931). The numbering of cortical areas (A) corresponds to the cytoarchitectonic types (B). See text for further details and references. Compare with 7.125.

study of Nissl-stained material. Broadly the results of the two methods do not conflict, but one is overwhelmingly more informative. Even though light microscopy proved unequal to the task of full visualization of synapses in the cerebral cortex, the patterns of interconnexion of cortical neurons were in major details well clarified many years before electron microscopy became available.

The termination of afferent nerve fibres in the superficial layers of the cortex, nearer the surface than the

946

somata of efferent neurons, the existence of recurrent axon collaterals from the latter which turn back superficially to form contacts through interneurons with their own dendrites, and the existence of a marked 'vertical' organization in the cortex—these and other features were all available as the basic cortical 'circuitry' before the refined microelectrode techniques of recent years began to seek a structural background to their recordings. As will be apparent later, the 'chains' of neurons, emphasized by Lorente de Nó, arranged in innumerable cortical units, repeated through the cortex, have fitted particularly well into physiological studies of the postcentral and striate regions (pp. 959, 961).[719, 720]

As elsewhere in the central nervous system, unit recording and more precise physiological study of the transmission processes of excitatory and inhibitory synapses have generated a renewed demand for the finest details of connexions between neurons. Various forms of synapse and their ultrastructural features are given full description elsewhere (p. 773); though identification of these structures in the cerebral cortex was achieved comparatively late,[721] a large literature concerning cortical synaptology has now accumulated. Axodendritic and axosomatic synapses predominate in the cerebral cortex, and may be the only types present; but the profusion of synapses, especially in relation to the dendritic spines of pyramidal cells, obviously provides a structural *mélange* for most complex interactions, however far we may yet be from anything more than the simplest interpretations of the full significance of such arrangements. Nevertheless, structure and function are rapidly progressing together in cortical study; and even if the joint 'models' of cortical activity which are currently evolving evince a somewhat hectic tendency to change, almost from week to week, this is surely a healthier state than the stagnating dogma which has sometimes becalmed neurological research.

In the relatively simple account of the cerebral cortex and its specific areas which follows, space will not permit an adequate reflexion of the intense activity in current research; for this the reader must consult recent original papers and surveys, e.g.[722] It may be noted here that vascular patterns[723] and distribution of enzymes[724] have been used as criteria of differentiation of 'areas' in the cerebral cortex: The 'chemical architecture' of the cerebral cortex has also been discussed.[725]

## QUANTITATIVE ASPECTS OF CORTICAL STRUCTURE

Quantitative studies of the cerebral cortex have been comparatively few; the first serious attempt to ascribe numerical values to its features was made by Economo and Koskinas,[713] who recorded data on variation in cortical depth which remain the most detailed for man. They also computed the total surface areas as 220,000 mm², a more recent figure being 285,000 mm²,[716] with a volume of 300 cm³. Naturally the total number of cortical nerve cells has attracted much interest and computation, and figures of 14,000 million,[713] 6,900 million,[726] 5,000

[719] V. B. Mountcastle, *J. Neurophysiol.*, **20**, 1957.
[720] D. M. Hubel and T. N. Wiesel, *J. Physiol., Lond.*, **160**, 1962.
[721] E. G. Gray, *J. Anat.*, **93**, 1959.
[722] M. L. Colonnier, in: *Brain and Conscious Experience*, ed. J. C. Eccles, Springer, Berlin. 1966.
[723] R. A. Pfeifer, *Die angioarchitektonische Areale Gliederung der Grosshirnrinde*, Thieme, Leipzig. 1940.
[724] A. Pope, *Archs Neurol. Psychiat., Chicago*, **16**, 1967.
[725] D. B. Tower, in: *Handbook of Physiology*, Sect. I, Vol. III, ed. J. Field, Am. Physiol. Soc., Washington. 1960.
[726] G. A. Shariff, *J. comp. Neurol.*, **98**, 1953.

million,[716] and 2,600 million[727] are representative, and illustrate a downward trend which may be due to improving technique. Such numbers are beyond real comprehension, and it is easier to grasp the magnitude of such a cell population by its proportions in a smaller sample. For example, a column of cells 1 mm square and 2·5 mm deep may contain as many as 60,000 neurons; and in one study of the motor cortex (precentral gyrus) each neuron was considered to take part in about as many synapses and to connect with some 600 other nerve cells.[728] Such a small volume of cortex, in itself containing perhaps $3 \times 10^9$ synapses, might be multiplied a quarter of a million times to represent the whole cortex. The wealth of interconnexions of such huge numbers of cells is clearly very great. In the striate area,[729] where about one-tenth of the cortical neurons are said to be concentrated, the dendrites of a single neuron may connect with 2–4,000 other cells, and an incoming afferent projection fibre may ramify through a volume of cortex containing 5,000 cells. Even the figures

that the ratio shows a phylogenetic increase up to man, due to an increase in the amount of neuroglia.

Various other quantified data regarding the mammalian cortex are scattered through the literature, which should be consulted for further details. In general—apart from an impression of the enormous potentialities for interconnexion and interaction—such figures have no immediate usefulness. The knowledge that each afferent or efferent projection fibre may have upwards of 1,000 neurons associated with it, more or less remotely, merely emphasizes the general truism of an extremely intricate field of interaction between them. The time may be far off when happenings in such large numbers of neurons can be defined in precise spatial and temporal terms, if indeed this can ever be expected in other than generalized statistical approximations. For the present, the limited events in minuscule volumes of cortex offer a more promising and primarily essential field of investigation. Examples of such studies will be mentioned in connexion with the

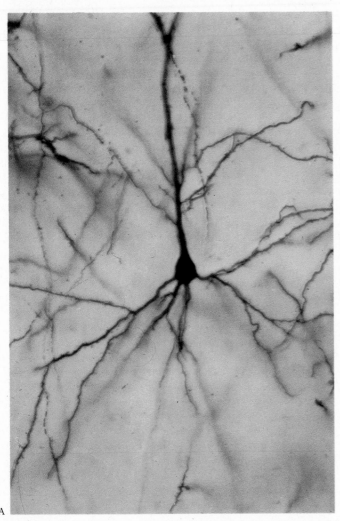

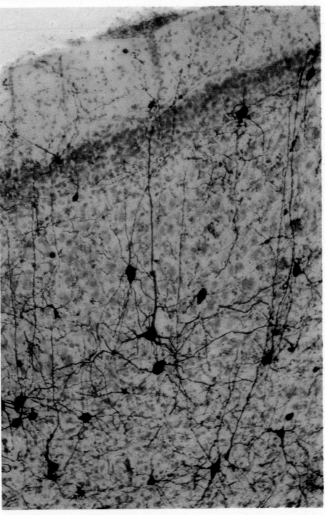

A

B

7.127A and B Preparations contrasting the Golgi and Nissl methods of staining nerve cells in the cerebral cortex. In A a single pyramidal cell stands out amongst many unstained elements. In B isolated Golgi-stained neurons are prominent amongst the remaining Nissl-stained cortical elements. (Preparations provided by Dr. A. R. Lieberman, University College, London.)

given above are, however, dwarfed by the cerebellar neuronal population—see p. 869.

The density of packing of nerve cells in different areas and their laminae shows much variation, being most dense in the striate area and perhaps least so in the precentral gyrus. The ratio by volume of the somata of neurons to all other constituents in the cortex (the grey/cell coefficient) has been estimated, and average ratios of 27:1[730] and 70:1[731] for man have been cited. It is claimed

particular cortical areas in which they have been most successful. Arising from such research, a profusion of concepts of neuronal 'circuitry', diagrams to illustrate

[727] M. Pakkenberg, *J. comp. Neurol.*, **128**, 1966.
[728] B. G. Cragg, *J. Anat.*, **101**, 1967.
[729] D. A. Sholl, *J. Anat.*, **89**, 1955.
[730] C. von Economo and G. N. Koskinas, *Die Cytoarchitektonik der Hirnrinde*, Springer, Berlin. 1925.
[731] H. Haug, *J. comp. Neurol.*, **104**, 1956.

947

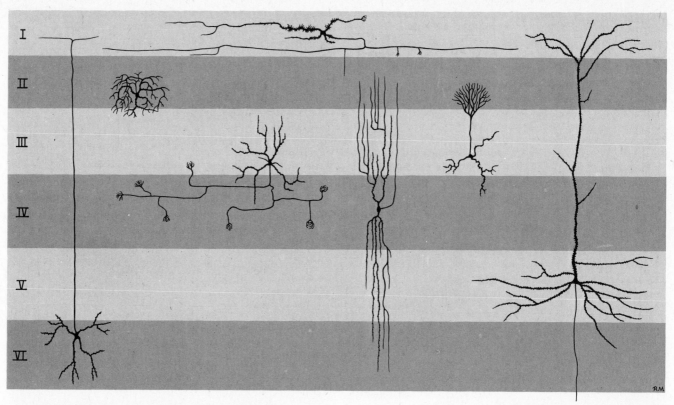

**7.128A** Typical outlines of characteristic neocortical neurons as seen in sections prepared by the metallic impregnation techniques introduced by Golgi and Cajal. From left to right are shown Martinotti, neurogliaform,

basket, horizontal, fusiform, stellate, and pyramidal types of neuron. Many other forms and variants have been described. See text for literature.

these, and even models employing artificial 'neurons' have appeared in recent literature, e.g.[732–738] Naturally, these speculations undergo rapid change and modification as knowledge in the very active fields of synaptology and unit recording advances; and hence, despite their great interest, it is as yet premature to include such details here.

## The Structure of the Cerebral Cortex

To the unaided eye the cerebral cortex forms a complete mantle or *pallium* covering the hemisphere and obviously variable in thickness (1·5 to 4·5 mm) when seen in section. It is thicker on the exposed convexities of gyri than in the depths of sulci, in which the larger part of the cortex is hidden from surface view. Such variations in thickness might well correspond to structural variations in the pallium; and it has in fact been suggested that the positioning of gyri and sulci is conditioned by such structural differences,[739] but this cannot be claimed with respect to the *functionally* differentiated areas, which in many instances depart in their outlines from the sulcal pattern. In freshly cut cerebral cortex laminar details can often be appreciated even without a simple magnifying lens (e.g. the visual stria of Gennari); and by such means horizontally disposed layers of nerve fibres, the inner and outer bands of Baillarger (p. 950), can usually be discerned. It has even been claimed that using such simple methods more than a score of structurally distinct areas of cortex can be identified.[740]

In its **microscopic structure** the cortex of the cerebrum, like 'grey matter' elsewhere, consists of an intricate blending of nerve cells and fibres, neuroglia and blood vessels. Neuroglial cells and the vascular arrangements have been dealt with in other sections (pp. 778 and 781). The features of the neurons and their interconnexions and distributions must now be considered. It should, how-

ever, be noted here that variation in the distribution of the blood vessels has been utilized as a criterion in differentiating cortical areas.[741]

The neurons of the pallium have been described and categorized in great detail, but they can be assigned to a relatively small number of classes, the great majority in fact falling into two such groups, the *pyramidal* cells and the *stellate* (granule) cells. Both types may be assorted into a variable number of subdivisions on the basis of size and the appearances of their neurites (7.128). Both types are found at most levels in the cortex and in almost all areas, though their numbers and distribution vary greatly from place to place. (These variations, together with alterations in size, provide the criteria for distinguishing different cortical areas in Nissl-stained material, of course.) Other types of cells commonly distinguished are *fusiform*, *horizontal*, and *neurogliaform cells*, and the *cells of Martinotti*.

**Pyramidal nerve cells**, so named from the shape of their somata (7.15), vary from small elements measuring about 10 $\mu$m across to the giant pyramidal cells (of Betz) which reach 70 $\mu$m and more. Their apices are usually orientated towards the surface of the cortex, and from this region of the cell a thick *apical dendrite* ascends a variable distance, giving off collateral branches and often ending

---

[732] W. G. Walter, *The Living Brain*, Duckworth, London. 1953.

[733] N. Wiener and J. P. Schadé (eds.), *Nerve, Brain and Memory Models*, Elsevier, London. 1963.

[734] N. K. Taylor, *Proc. R. Soc. B.*, **159**, 1964.

[735] J. Z. Young, *A Model of the Brain*, Clarendon Press, Oxford. 1964.

[736] M. Arbib, *Brains, Machines and Mathematics*, McGraw-Hill, N.Y. 1964.

[737] W. R. Ashby, *Design for a Brain*, Wiley, N.Y. 1960.

[738] M. Minsky, *Matter, Mind and Models*, Spartan books, Washington. 1965.

[739] W. E. Le G. Clark, in: *Essays on Growth and Form*, eds. W. E. Le G. Clark and P. B. Medawar, University Press, Oxford. 1945.

[740] G. E. Smith, *J. Anat.*, **41**, 1907.

[741] R. A. Pfeifer, *Die angioarchitektonische Areale Gliederung der Grosshirnrinde*, Thieme, Leipzig. 1940.

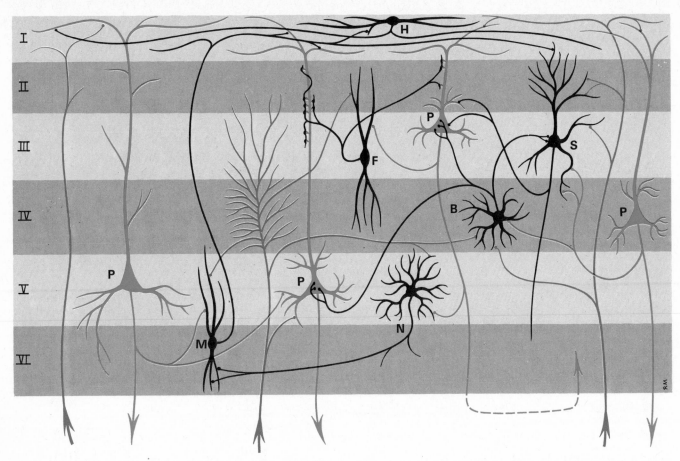

7.128 B  A diagrammatic representation of the most frequent types of neocortical neuron, showing typical connexions with each other and with afferent fibres (*blue*). Neurons limited to the cortex in their distribution are indicated in *black*. Efferent neurons are in *magenta*. The right and left afferent fibres are association or cortico-cortical connexions, the central afferent is a specific sensory fibre. Neurons are shown in their characteristic lamina, but many types have somata in more than one layer. They are indicated thus: P=pyramidal, M=Martinotti, F=fusiform, H= horizontal, N=neurogliaform, B=basket, S=stellate. See text for details and compare with the stereodiagram in 7.132.

in a complex spray of terminal dendritic twigs. From the other, basal angles of the cell body *basal dendrites* sprout, spreading laterally into the surrounding neuropil to form dendritic fields of varying shapes and extents.[742] A statistical analysis of the branching of such dendrites and those of the stellate cells in the visual cortex has been attempted,[743] but this quantitative kind of dendrological study is still a neglected and indeed difficult field. On the whole, the vertical extent of the dendritic extensions of pyramidal cells is markedly greater than it is in the horizontal or tangential direction. The dendrites are beset, especially in their smaller branches, with very large numbers of *dendritic spines* (p. 773), which are now known to be the sites of axodendritic synapses.[744] Since the number of these synapses, even by the crudest estimates, is very large, it is at once evident that there is a physical basis for the most elaborate interneuronal reactions in the cortex. The axons of pyramidal cells, which are invariably much smaller in calibre than the trunks of their main dendrites, behave in a variety of manners. From larger elements, chiefly in lamina V (*vide infra*), *projection axons* extend centripetally out of the cortex to reach more or less distant subcortical structures, such as the basal ganglia, brainstem nuclei, and the grey matter of the spinal cord. Some may pass back into more or less distant parts of the cortex as *long* or *short association fibres*. The axons of smaller pyramidal cells usually ramify entirely within the cortex, and even those which leave it commonly divide by giving off a small number of collaterals which remain as intrinsic or *intracortical axons*. These latter may extend horizontally, but they more often pursue an obliquely recurrent course towards the more superficial laminae of the cortex. Even from this brief description it is clear that the larger pyramidal cells, whose somata appear in Nissl-stained sections to be sited in a single lamina, in fact extend through most and often all levels of the cortex, since their apical dendrites frequently reach the superficial, *plexiform lamina* (*vide infra*). Thus, each pyramidal neuron forms a species of columnar unit extending through the cortex together with its numerous connexions, including other pyramidal elements, many forms of interneuron, and afferent projection fibres. Lateral interconnexions are mediated by various forms of intracortical horizontal neurons and by association neurons.

**Stellate nerve cells**, often called *granule cells* because of their small size and appearance in Nissl-stained material, appear in variable density of distribution in all the cortical laminae except the most superficial (lamina I); but they are usually concentrated in greater abundance in laminae II and IV (*vide infra*). Like pyramidal cells, stellate neurons would probably have been designated as multipolar if they had not first been described in Nissl-stained sections. They are small, of the order of 6 to 10 $\mu$m in diameter, with a rounded soma drawn out at numerous angles by their richly branching dendrites and a single, relatively short axon. They are hence members of the Golgi type II series of neurons. Their dendrites carry numbers of spines, indicating abundant synapses with other neurons. A wide variety of stellate cells have been distinguished, principally upon the behaviour of their

[742] M. L. Colonnier, *J. Anat.*, **98**, 1964.
[743] D. Sholl, *J. Anat.*, **87**, 1953.
[744] E. G. Gray, *J. Anat.*, **93**, 1959.

axons. These, though confined to the cortex, may travel considerable distances in it, chiefly in a vertical direction but also horizontally in some instances. The vertical axons may be centripetal or centrifugal in direction, the latter reaching as far as lamina I. One particular type of stellate cell, the *basket cell*, which is horizontally extended, has a short vertical axon which almost immediately divides into a horizontal family of collaterals. These end in pronounced terminal tufts or arborizations, forming synapses with the somata cells and proximal parts of the dendrites of pyramidal cells. Such cells have a particular interest, in their horizontal extension, because of the perhaps excessive attention at present concentrated on vertical organization in the cerebral cortex (p. 959). Another type of stellate cell is in fact *fusiform* in appearance, due to the emergence of two large dendrites which sprout from opposite poles of the soma, dividing at once into elaborate bouquets of branches which extend vertically in the cortex. The 'dendrite' which extends centrifugally towards lamina I is in fact the axon. The entire neuron may stretch through the whole thickness of the cortex, probably establishing synaptic contacts with a number of pyramidal cells. The *neurogliaform stellate cells* are small, with a dense and localized dendritic arborization, within which the short axon also usually ramifies.

**The horizontal cells** (of Cajal) are confined to the plexiform lamina I; they are small and fusiform and their dendrites spread short distances in two opposite directions in the plexiform layer. Their axons, often derived from one of the dendrites, divide into two branches which depart from each other to travel to much greater distances in the same layer. **The cells of Martinotti** occur at most levels in the cortex. They are small and multipolar, with a localized dendritic field and a long axon which runs centrifugally to the plexiform lamina, producing a few short horizontal collaterals *en route*. The so-called **pleomorphic cells** are considered to be modified pyramidal cells with axons entering the white matter. Their somata are variously shaped, perhaps in accord with differences in their dendritic sproutings; the dendrites spread widely into the cortex.

Many other forms of nerve cell have been detailed in the cerebral cortex, but since even the array of types mentioned above cannot yet be linked into a fully co-ordinated scheme of interaction, it is merely confusing to multiply the details. It should never be overlooked that the most intensive studies of cortical neurons have been carried out on subprimate mammals; and although appearances in the primate cortex, as chiefly pursued in material from macaque monkeys, are similar, investigations of even 'cold' structural arrangements in the human cortex have been remarkably few.[713, 745]

## Laminar Pattern of the Cerebral Cortex

The cortex or pallium of the cerebrum may be conveniently divided into an older and original part, the *allocortex*, consisting of the archicortex and paleocortex (also known as the archipallium and paleopallium), which are considered elsewhere (p. 921), and a newer development, the *neocortex* (isocortex or neopallium). The latter may be equated with those systems of sensory and motor activity which originally had little or no connexions with the fore-brain, but have acquired these over evolutionary time by the process of prosencephalization. The remarks which follow apply only to the neocortex.

As already stated in the Introduction to this section (p. 944), the customary description of a six-layered cortical structure successfully promulgated by Brodmann and his followers has, by its general acceptance, obscured earlier disagreements and widespread dissatisfaction with its arbitrary nature. The same strictures must be applied to excessively detailed architectonic mapping of the cortex which has stemmed from the same somewhat dogmatic views. However, Brodmann's numbered layers and areas provide a reference grid of considerable practical value and are widely used; and therefore, until some more intellectually satisfying system emerges, the details— insofar as they are useful—must be repeated here. The six laminae (7.124, 126) may be described as follows:

I. **The plexiform lamina** (molecular or zonal layer) contains the sparsely scattered horizontal cells (of Cajal), and consists apart from this of a dense mat of tangentially orientated fibres, derived from pyramidal cells (apical dendrites), stellate cells (vertical axons), cells of Martinotti (centrifugal axons), and other elements, including cortical afferent fibres, both projection and associational.

II. **The external granular lamina** contains the somata of stellate and small pyramidal cells, usually packed densely, though this varies, like other laminar details, in different areas of the cortex. Passing through the lamina are vertically arranged dendrites and axons from subjacent layers, intermingling with the dense neuropil of local dendrites and axons. Ascending afferent fibres make extensive multiple synaptic contacts with the apical dendrites of large pyramidal cells (with somata in lamina V) in this and the subjacent layer.

III. **The pyramidal lamina** contains the cell bodies of medium-sized pyramidal cells, the smaller of which are situated nearer to lamina II. Some stellate cells also occur in this layer, including horizontally disposed basket cells and vertically orientated fusiform cells, their dendrites and axons extending far beyond the layer itself.

IV. **The internal granular lamina** is usually narrower than other layers, except lamina I, and is chiefly characterized by the somata of stellate cells, with occasional small pyramidal cells. The cells are densely aggregated and the lamina is traversed by a concentration of horizontally arranged fibres, long known collectively as the *external band of Baillarger*. As in the case of other laminae, the layer also contains large numbers of vertically orientated neurites derived from nerve cells in others parts of the cortex, in subcortical regions, and in adjoining layers.

V. **The ganglionic lamina** contains the largest pyramidal cell somata, but smaller elements of the same type also occur, the actual dimensions of these cells varying in different cortical areas. In any particular area, however, the largest pyramidal cells are in lamina V. Small numbers of stellate cells may also occur. The layer is, of course, permeated by a dense neuropil of dendrites and axons derived both from its intrinsic elements and cells in other laminae. It is also traversed by ascending and descending projection fibres and by association fibres. A considerable complement of horizontally deployed fibres is apparent in lamina V, corresponding, in sections stained to display myeloarchitectural details, to the *internal band of Baillarger*.

VI. **The multiform lamina** contains a considerable range of cell types, as judged by their somata and processes, the variable shape of the former reflecting to some extent the variations in their dendritic arrays. Most of the cells are small and are considered to be modified pyramidal elements, despite the fusiform, triangular, ovoid and other profiles of their somata. The small, multipolar Martinotti cells are often prominent in this lamina. Lamina VI is not always well demarcated from the subjacent cortical zone of fibres approaching or departing from the cortex itself.

[745] P. Bailey and G. von Bonin, *The Isocortex of Man*, University of Illinois Press, Urbana. 1951.

The numbering and nomenclature of cortical laminae set out briefly above is in the style of Brodmann. Many synonyms for their names are in circulation, derived from the work of such investigators as Campbell and Cajal; the Vogts also introduced another, somewhat more awkward nomenclature, based on myeloarchitectonic studies, in which the fibre structure is emphasized. Views as to the number of layers have varied widely, and much subdivision has been suggested. For example, lamina VI has been divided into VIa and VIb on the distribution of triangular and fusiform cells, and into no less than four sublaminae (VIa$^1$, VIa$^2$, VIb$^1$ and VIb$^2$) in material stained to show fibre structure. All layers except lamina II have been further analysed in this manner, as many as sixteen laminae in total being recognized by the Vogts. The usefulness of such minute dissection has been severely criticized, and these details are only mentioned here as examples. Similar remarks are applicable to much of the work in the field of cortical architectonics. Here again the Brodmann maps have achieved most attention. Their early transference, in a form elaborated further by the Vogts but still not worked out in man, to the human cortex by Foerster has overshadowed the contribution of Economo and Koskinas. In one respect this is fortunate, because the latter chose to designate areas by letters, as has Conel,[746] and these, and other nomenclatures, would have proved much less manageable than Brodmann's simple numbers. However, in recent years, new views on the extent of the major sensory and motor areas of the cortex have generated the need for a more appropriate terminology than Brodmann's.[747] The new series of symbols suggested will be referred to in connexion with cortical areas involved; many of them are already in wide use in experimental studies, but since a lack of uniformity persists in this, and since such terms are only beginning to penetrate into clinical neurology, the customary numerical designation of cortical areas must be retained for the present.

## REPRESENTATIVE VARIANTS OF CORTICAL STRUCTURE

While it is obviously impossible, and probably unprofitable, to detail and discuss here the almost endless nuances of cortical structure in full-blown architectonics, it is necessary to allude to a smaller number of basic variant types of cortex. These were recognized in the classical pioneer studies of Campbell[709] and consolidated by Economo and Koskinas.[713] Five fundamental types are described (7.126) in the neocortex, and while all are considered to develop from the same six-layered or *sesquilaminar pattern*, two of them are regarded as lacking certain laminae when fully differentiated, and are hence described as *heterotypical*; these are the *granular* and *agranular* types. The *homotypical* variants, in which all six laminae are discernible, are called *frontal* (premotor), *parietal* (postcentral), and *polar* (visuopsychic)—names which link them with specific regions in a somewhat misleading manner, as illustration 7.126 shows. For example, the frontal type occurs in the parietal and temporal lobes.

**The agranular type** of cortex is considered to be lacking in the granular laminae (II and IV), but it does usually display scattered stellate nerve cells. The predominant neuronal type is, however, pyramidal, and it is in this form of cortex that the greatest densities and largest sizes of pyramidal cells occur. Originally identified in the precentral gyrus (area 4), it also occupies areas 6, 8 and 44 (7.125) and occurs in other regions, including parts of the limbic system (p. 930). It is characterized by the projection of large concentrations of efferent fibres from the pyramidal cells, and agranular cortex can thus be equated with the 'motor' areas—with the proviso that

such areas are now known to receive afferent projections in addition, as will be detailed in connection with the individual areas.

**The granular type** of cortex (koniocortex) may be regarded as at the opposite extreme of the main categories of cortical structure. The granular layers are maximally developed in such areas and contain densely packed stellate cells, amongst which are nevertheless a variable but small number of pyramidal cells. Laminae III and IV are poorly developed or unidentifiable. This type of cortex is associated with afferent projections but, here again, there is evidence of a lesser number of efferent fibres, derived from the few pyramidal cells usually to be found in this otherwise 'granular' cortex. Despite the relative lack of different laminae, the granular and agranular types of cortex exhibit little qualitative distinction, being rather at the opposite extremes of a gradation, in which the pyramidal and stellate series of cell types are reciprocally developed. Typical granular cortex is formed in the postcentral gyrus, striate area, and in the superior temporal gyrus (acoustic area); it also occurs in small parts of the hippocampal gyrus (p. 939). Despite the very large number of stellate cells packed into this form of cortex, especially in the striate area, it is the thinnest of the five main recognized types. In the striate cortex the external band of Baillarger (lamina IV) is particularly well defined, as the *stria of Gennari* (or Vicq d'Azyr).

The remaining three types of cortex may be regarded as intermediate forms. In the **frontal type** large numbers of small and medium-sized pyramidal cells occur in laminae III and V, the granular layers (II and IV) being less prominent. The relative numbers of these two major forms of nerve cell vary reciprocally in the different areas in which this form of cortex exists. It is not confined to the frontal region of the cerebrum (7.126). The **parietal type** of cortex contains less pyramidal cells, which are mostly smaller in size than in the frontal type; the granular laminae are, on the contrary, wider and contain more abundant stellate cells. This kind of cortex occupies large areas in the parietal and temporal lobes (7.126). The **polar type** is classically identified with small areas near the frontal and occipital poles of the hemisphere, and hence its name. Apart from granular cortex, it is the thinnest form of the five types. All six laminae are represented in it, but the pyramidal layer (III) is reduced in width, but is not so extensively invaded by stellate cells as in the granular type of cortex. As in the latter, the multiform layer (VI) is more highly organized than in other forms of cortical structure.

While further subdivision of the above five basic types of cortical 'organization' may be useful for specific experimental purposes, it must be emphasized again that in the microscopic sections in which they are customarily distinguished—whether stained to show cell somata or their processes—the finer and more significant details of true organization are not apparent in studies of the whole thickness of the cortex. The functional organization is naturally linked to the spatial distribution of the cells, but it is in their actual patterns of connexion that any real enlightenment as to cortical mechanisms must be sought. Golgi preparations in particular have yielded an immense amount of information indicating the probable designs of neuronal interaction. Functional hypotheses deduced from such merely structural data, however intricate, require confirmation in terms of the precise nature of synapses both in their distribution and mode of

[746] J. Le R. Conel, *The Postnatal Development of the Human Cerebral Cortex*, Vol. I, Harvard University Press, Cambridge, Mass. 1939.

[747] C. N. Woolsey, in: *Cerebral Localization and Organization*, eds. G. Schaltenbrand and C. N. Woolsey, University of Wisconsin Press, Madison. 1964.

action. Details of this kind depend upon electron microscopy and unit recording. Unfortunately, such techniques deal only with much smaller volumes of cortical tissue, but most exciting results are apparent in the research in this field in the last decade or so, as will be seen in various sections of this account of the central nervous system. The cytoarchitectural approach to the problems of cortical activity was a necessary prelude, and the resultant definition of various forms of organization in structural terms remains as a necessary schema of orientation to which the finer ultrastructural details must be constantly referred.

# THE MAIN CORTICAL AREAS

Before describing the major areas customarily distinguished, on functional and structural data, in the human cerebral cortex—such as the somatomotor, somatosensory, visual and auditory areas—some preliminary general remarks are necessary. As has already been emphasized, the somewhat extreme parcellation of the cortex deriving from the studies of Brodmann has a limited usefulness and is frankly misleading if regarded as more than a reference grid in defining parts of the cortex. Even the simpler differentiation of the cortex into *sensory* areas receiving afferent projection fibres and *motor* areas projecting efferents—the remainder being regarded as 'silent' or *associational*—can no longer be considered appropriate, being itself an inaccurate over-simplification.

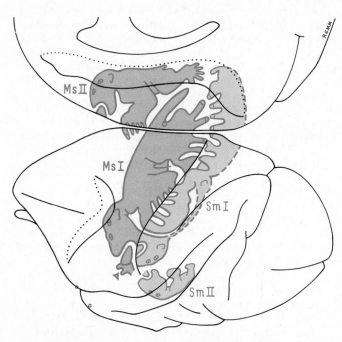

7.129 The main sensorimotor areas projected diagrammatically upon the superolateral surface of the simian cerebral hemisphere. Note the somatotopic arrangement in all four areas. (Adapted from C. N. Woolsey, 1964—see text for details and references.)

Evidence has accumulated during the last three decades to show that the areas receiving or originating projection fibres are much more extensive than the initial classical studies indicated. Furthermore, the division into 'receiving' and 'originating' projection areas is by no means so distinct as at first appeared. Thus, the postcentral gyrus is not the only area to which a somatosensory thalamic projection is directed; at least two other areas of cortex are similarly involved, as will be detailed later in this section. In the same way, the precentral gyrus is supplemented by a second 'motor' area. It is necessary to qualify the term 'motor' because the distinction of motor and sensory areas still customary in simpler accounts of the cerebral cortex is erroneous, and has indeed been known to be so

for many years. As long ago as 1933 motor responses to stimulation of the 'sensory' areas were demonstrated,[748] and projection of efferent ('pyramidal') fibres from the same postcentral area was established shortly afterwards.[749] Since these pioneer studies a mass of confirmatory evidence in various experimental animals has extended these findings to other areas. Moreover, clinical and experimental observations in mankind suggest that similar arrangements obtain. It is hence more appropriate to speak of the pre- and post-central areas as being *sensorimotor*; and since a mixture of afferent and efferent connexions has been shown to exist also in respect to the projection fibres of the acoustic and visual 'sensory' areas, they also are more accurately described as sensorimotor in character.

The recognition that the corticospinal or 'pyramidal' pathway is derived from nerve cells in a much larger area than the precentral gyrus is paralleled by similar findings in regard to the various thalamic and geniculate projections upon the cortex; these terminate in considerably wider regions of the cortex than originally described. For example, the classical somatosensory area in the postcentral gyrus is supplemented by a second area, inferior to it, and by a third, on the medial aspect of the hemisphere, which is also a motor area (*vide infra*). Similarly, the lateral and medial geniculate bodies are now known to project to other regions of the cortex beyond the visual and auditory areas of conventional description. Not only the striate cortex (area 17, visuosensory area), but also the para- and peri-striate areas around it (areas 18 and 19—the 'visuopsychic' cortex) receive projection fibres; and in cats the acoustic radiation has been shown to terminate not only in the *first acoustic area* (41), but also in several other regions in the temporal cortex.

These modifications of the originally simple motor and sensory areas require a revision of terminology. The most widely used[750] (7.129), though not entirely satisfactory or as yet accurately adapted to the human cortex, divides the main sensorimotor area into a part in the precentral gyrus termed MsI, because it is the main or *first* predominantly *M*otor area but to a lesser extent also *sensory*. Conversely, in the postcentral gyrus, SmI is the primary *S*ensory area, though also partly *motor*. On the medial surface of the cerebrum is a further sensorimotor area, which, being largely motor, is called the *supplementary motor area*, MsII. Despite this, Ms*II* is sometimes known as the *third* somatomotor area, because there is a second sensorimotor area, SmII (7.129), inferior to SmI. It would, of course, have been easier to regard MsII as the second somatomotor area and SmII the third, as some authorities do, but this merely shifts the numerical confusion. Some authors surmount the difficulty by disregarding the useful abbreviations and speaking of first, second and third

[748] J. G. Dusser de Barenne, *Archs Neurol. Psychiat., Chicago,* **30,** 1933.
[749] P. M. Levin and F. K. Bradford, *J. comp. Neurol.,* **68,** 1938.
[750] C. N. Woolsey, in: *Cerebral Localization and Organisation,* eds. G. Schaltenbrand and C. N. Woolsey, University of Wisconsin Press, Madison. 1964.

motor or sensory areas; but this obscures the fact that strictly there are *four* sensorimotor areas covered by this terminology, MsI, MsII, SmI and SmII, each of which is to some extent motor and sensory in activity. This terminology is admittedly a little perplexing, but its shortcomings are merely incidental to the important fact that the frontoparietal sensorimotor region is a complex of areas, each with its own degree of somatotopic organization.

In the occipital lobe the striate, parastriate and peristriate regions of the cortex (areas 17, 18 and 19) are likewise termed the *first*, *second* and *third visual areas*, or visual areas I, II and III. A more complex array of terms[751] applied in particular to the feline cerebrum is current to

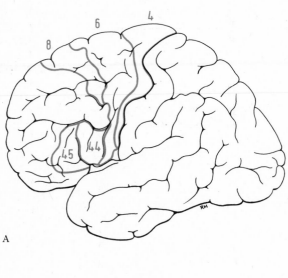

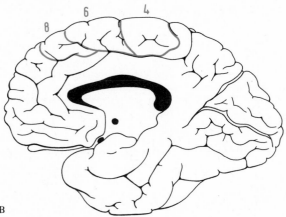

7.130A and B   Superolateral (A) and medial (B) surfaces of the cerebral hemispheres, showing approximate correspondence of the Brodmann areas to the main motor area (4) or MsI, the premotor area (6, 8) and motor speech area of Broca (44, 45). See text for details and compare with 7.125, 134, 135A and B.

describe the four temporal areas considered to receive auditory projection fibres in cats. These are the *first acoustic area* (AI)—the auditory area of usual description—the *second acoustic area* (AII), and the *anterior* and *posterior ectosylvian areas* (Ea and Ep). The accessory acoustic areas can only be indicated in a tentative manner in the human cortex (7.138), partly because the acoustic parts of the temporal lobe are entirely superficial in the cat, whereas they are partly folded into the inferior lip of the lateral sulcus in mankind. All the sensory areas named above not only receive projection fibres from particular nuclei of the thalamic complex (though this is not completely established with respect to the ectosylvian

acoustic areas), they also project back to the same regions, and perhaps in some instances to other nuclei at lower levels in the central nervous system—connexions which in each modality are probably concerned with inhibitory and sometimes facilitatory effects in their own sensory pathway. It is this afferent-efferent character of most, and probably all, the sensorimotor areas which makes the concept of distinguishable motor and sensory parts of the cortex anatomically invalid and functionally misleading.

It is clear from the above remarks that much less of the cerebral cortex remains to be dubbed as 'associational', in the vague but well-established meaning of the term. Nevertheless, large regions in all the lobes of the cerebrum are not accounted for by the sensorimotor areas. In regard to the human brain, much clinical evidence strongly suggests that such so-called 'silent' areas are indeed concerned in the further elaboration and interpretation of sensory information, and in the combination of its different modalities. Much less is known of the connexions of these parts of the cortex, whether by association or commissural fibres. For these reasons, less can be said of these areas than the sensorimotor domains of the cortex. Nevertheless, ablation experiments coupled with tracing of degenerating axons and with observation of disturbed behaviour, and similar deductions in human patients affected by damage, disease or surgical intervention, are beginning to provide more coherent concepts of the activities of the association areas, as will become apparent below.

Though it might be regarded as functionally appropriate to consider first the predominantly sensory areas of the cortex and then those which are mainly motor, the widespread involvement of many parts of the cortex in even the simplest of activities and the sensorimotor nature of the areas concerned render any such considerations of priority almost meaningless. The main areas will therefore be described on the basis of the lobes in which they are located, and in the arbitrary order—frontal, parietal, occipital and temporal.

## THE FRONTAL LOBE

The cortex of the frontal lobe may be divided for convenience into two main regions, *precentral* and the unfortunately named *prefrontal*. The former is largely sensorimotor, the latter 'association' cortex.

**The precentral area** includes the whole of the precentral gyrus and the posterior (caudal) parts of the superior, middle and inferior frontal gyri (Brodmann areas 4 and 6). The whole of this region (7.130) is characterized by the almost complete absence of the granular layers. Intracortical fibres are very numerous and the plexiform layer is particularly densely packed. The precentral area has been divided into posterior and anterior parts, *motor* (area 4) and *premotor* (area 6), but the distinction between these layers differs, according to whether cytoarchitectural or physiological data are applied. As comparison of illustrations 7.125 and 7.130A shows, the boundary between areas 4 and 6 descends through the precentral gyrus, whereas the entire gyrus is regarded as the *motor area*. Hence it is less confusing to disregard the Brodmann numeration of areas, or to use it as a merely approximate indication of the situation of areas. Thus, the premotor area occupies parts of the three frontal gyri, corresponding largely to area 6, but including parts of areas 8, 44 and 45 (7.130A). For the present, it is simpler and more direct to designate the whole precentral area

[751] J. E. Rose and C. N. Woolsey, *Cortical Connexions and Functional Organization of the Thalamic Auditory System of the Cat*, University of Wisconsin Press, Madison. 1958.

as the *first* or leading **somatomotor area** (MsI), remembering that functional variations occur within it and that these may to some extent coincide with cytoarchitectonic differences.

A feature of the whole precentral area (MsI) is the prominence of pyramidal nerve cells of all sizes. The largest of these, the *giant pyramidal cells of Betz*, vary in height from 30 to 120 μm and in breadth from 15 to 60 μm, being most numerous in the medial part of the first somatomotor area, where it extends over the superomedial border of the hemisphere into the paracentral lobule (7.130 B). They become progressively less frequent as the precentral gyrus is followed downwards towards the lateral fissure.

area involved is intimately involved in the mediation of voluntary movements. The order of loci, starting from the paracentral lobule, is associated with the lower limb, the trunk (in the upper part of the precentral gyrus), the upper limb, neck, and head (7.131 A). Much greater detail of this bodily 'representation' has accumulated, of course, and it has been established that the amount of cortex mediating movement in any particular region of the body is proportional not to the bulk of muscle involved but to the skill with which it is customarily used. All these details can be better appreciated by consulting 7.131 A. It is perhaps more important to emphasize that even in the earliest studies of the excitability of the 'motor cortex', it was recognized that

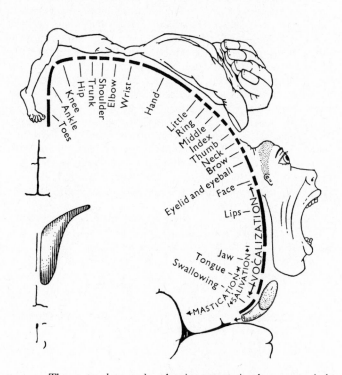

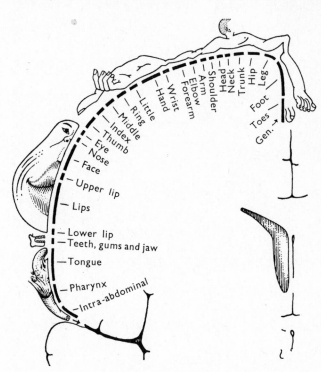

**7.131 A** The *motor homunculus* showing proportional somatotopical representation in the main motor area. (After W. Penfield and T. Rasmussen, *The Cerebral Cortex of Man*, Macmillan, 1950.)

**7.131 B** The *sensory homunculus* showing proportional somatotopical representation in the somesthetic cortex. (After W. Penfield and T. Rasmussen, *The Cerebral Cortex of Man*, Macmillan, 1950.)

They also extend less and less forwards in the gyrus in the same direction, following the boundary of area 4, to which they are largely limited, being absent from the premotor or anterior part of the first somatomotor area. In view of the mode of somatotopical arrangement now to be described in this region, it is tempting to suppose that the size of the larger pyramidal cells is associated with the length of their axons. The number of giant pyramidal cells in the human motor cortex has been estimated as between 25,000 and 30,000,[752, 753] a figure which conflicts with the million or so fibres in the medullary pyramid.[754, 755] It is clear that the huge majority of corticospinal and probably corticobulbar fibres are derived from smaller pyramidal cells. As is now known, many such fibres do not originate in area 4 at all, and it is interesting to note here that ablation of this area in monkeys reduces the fibres in the pyramid by a mere 25 per cent.[755] Obviously the majority of 'pyramidal' fibres have other origins, as will be detailed below.

The recognition that *contralateral movements*, simple in type, can be elicited in different parts of the body by electrical stimulation of separate loci in the region of the central sulcus dates from the pioneer study of Fritsch and Hitzig in dogs.[756] This discovery has been confirmed in innumerable subsequent studies in primates,[757] including man,[758, 759] and it has become a tenet of neurology that the

movements could be elicited from the postcentral gyrus, as well as from the precentral, and that the same movement could be excited in the same experimental animal's brain from different loci at different times. More careful control of the parameters of stimulation in later investigations has confirmed this apparent 'plasticity',[760] which is, of course, difficult to represent in textbook illustrations. This and other factors have obscured to some extent these early findings, and the polemics associated with the great volume of reports on cerebral motor function, especially regarding discrepancies between clinical observations and experimental findings, were only useful insofar as they refocused attention on facts rather than theories.[761]

[752] A. W. Campbell, *Histological Studies on the Localisation of Cerebral Function*, Cambridge University Press, Cambridge. 1905.
[753] A. M. Lassek, *Archs Neurol. Psychiat., Chicago*, **44**, 1940.
[754] A. M. Lassek and G. L. Rasmussen, *Archs Neurol. Psychiat., Chicago*, **42**, 1939.
[755] A. M. Lassek, *J. nerv. ment. Dis.*, **95**, 1942.
[756] G. Fritsch and E. Hitzig, *Arch. Anat. Physiol.*, **37**, 1870.
[757] A. S. Leyton and C. S. Sherrington, *Q. Jl exp. Physiol.*, **11**, 1917.
[758] D. Ferrier, *Proc. R. Soc. B.*, **22**, 1874.
[759] W. Penfield and T. Rasmussen, *The Cerebral Cortex of Man*, Macmillan, New York. 1950.
[760] E. G. T. Liddell and C. G. Phillips, *Brain*, **73**, 1950.
[761] P. C. Bucy (ed.), *The Precentral Motor Cortex*, University of Illinois Press, Urbana. 1944.

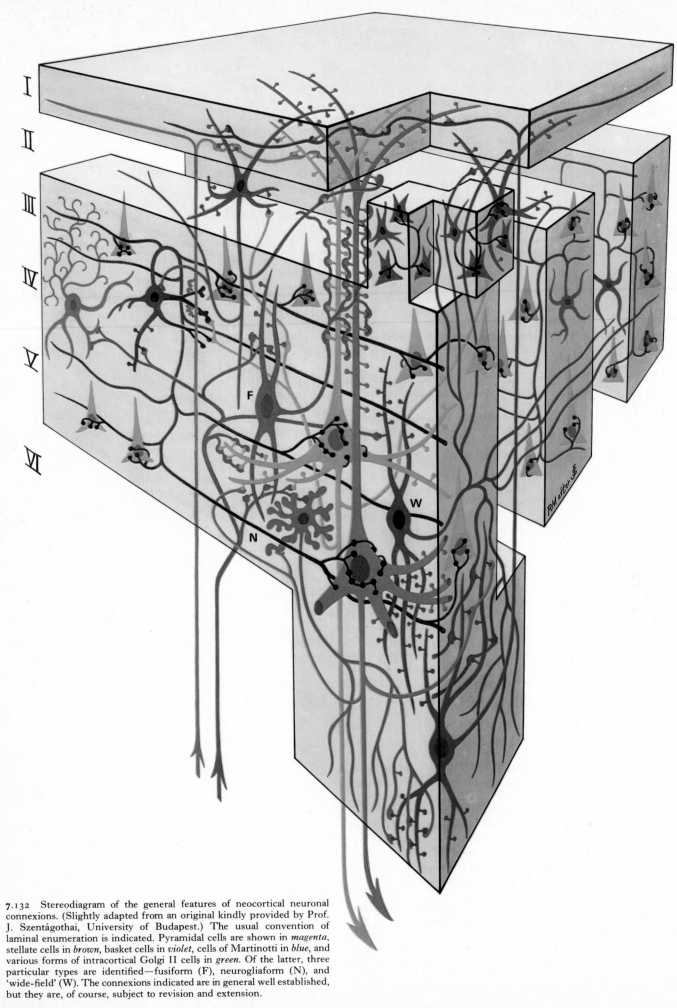

**7.132** Stereodiagram of the general features of neocortical neuronal connexions. (Slightly adapted from an original kindly provided by Prof. J. Szentágothai, University of Budapest.) The usual convention of laminal enumeration is indicated. Pyramidal cells are shown in *magenta*, stellate cells in *brown*, basket cells in *violet*, cells of Martinotti in *blue*, and various forms of intracortical Golgi II cells in *green*. Of the latter, three particular types are identified—fusiform (F), neurogliaform (N), and 'wide-field' (W). The connexions indicated are in general well established, but they are, of course, subject to revision and extension.

As a result of much painstaking work it is well established that while the whole first somatomotor cortex (MsI = areas 4 *and* 6) is a source of corticospinal fibres, it is not the only one. Both in monkeys[762] and man[763] the first somatosensory area (SmI = areas 3, 1 and 2) in the parietal lobe is also a source of corticospinal fibres, and there is some evidence that the second somatosensory area (SmII, approximately equal to areas 40 and 43—*see* p. 960), below the first area and just above the lateral fissure (posterior limb), also contributes 'pyramidal' fibres. Smaller contributions from the occipital and temporal lobes have also been described, in the cat.[764] Physiological evidence is largely in accord with these anatomical findings. The fibres descending from this extensive origin vary much in calibre. In the human pyramid 90 per cent were estimated to be 1–4 $\mu$m in diameter, while only about 2 per cent were 11–22 $\mu$m, a fraction corresponding closely with the number of giant pyramidal cells.[765] Up to 94 per cent of the fibres are myelinated in man.[766]

**The primary, first somatomotor area** or MsI receives fibres from the cerebellum, which relay in the nucleus ventralis lateralis of the thalamus (p. 898), and these are distributed particularly to its anterior region (area 6), and to the prefrontal area (area 8). It also receives afferents concerned in other *sensory* modalities, probably via the thalamus also, but in addition from the hypothalamus and from other parts of the cortex. Physiological studies suggest that the corticospinal neurons are influenced not only by somatosensory impulses but also by visual, acoustic and 'nonspecific' thalamic afferents (p. 898). The interactions of all these influences on the pyramidal neurons inevitably demands a most intricate deployment of axons, dendrites and their synapses in the cortex. Illustration **7**.132 is a tentative epitomization of the kind of structure involved. It is basically columnar in arrangement as in other parts of the cerebral cortex, the pyramidal neurons being extended vertically through the cortex and making abundant vertical associations with afferents and also horizontal connexions with intracortical interneurons. This concept tallies to some extent with recent studies of individual motor neurons by microelectrode techniques in the monkey[767] and cat.[768] These indicate that some motor neurons at least, though excitable from a considerable area, can be most easily stimulated within a cylindrical section of cortex about 1 mm in diameter.

However the so-called *plasticity* of the 'motor' cortex may be explained, the anatomical evidence favours a fixed and specific relation between the pyramidal cells and the effectors which they influence. At all levels of the corticospinal pathway a highly specific somatotopical arrangement has been demonstrated. In this connexion it should be emphasized that stimulation of cortical areas is an artificial method, which does not distinguish between direct excitation of pyramidal cells, or even their axons, and of the innumerable intracortical elements which interconnect with them. It is all the more interesting to note that studies employing microelectrode techniques are nevertheless beginning to point in the same direction.

Before dealing with certain specific regions of the somatomotor cortex, it is necessary to point out that stimulation of the cortex in experiment never produces elaborate coordinated movements, but only simple combined activities between synergists and antagonists. The movements elicited bear no relation to the particular skills or motor experience of the individual. This is to be expected, because such stimulation leaves out of account not only other efferent pathways but also the wide range of afferents from the cerebellum, thalamus and other cortical areas mentioned above.

Extending forwards into the middle frontal gyrus from the part of the precentral gyrus concerned with facial movements is the **frontal eye field**; it occupies a considerable part of the Brodmann area 8, invading area 6 behind and probably area 9 in front (**7**.133). Stimulation, which is most effective in area 8, elicits conjugate or binocular movements of the eyes, especially towards the contralateral side, but perhaps also in other directions. Movements of the head and pupillary dilatation may also be elicited from the frontal eye field. For a review of work on these responses see reference[769]. Little is known with certainty concerning the efferent projection from this area; degenerating fibres have been traced from it in monkeys as far as the midbrain, but their ultimate destination is not established. None have been traced with certainty to the nuclei of the motor nerves of the extrinsic

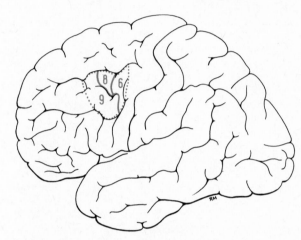

**7**.133 Superolateral surface of left cerebral hemisphere showing the frontal motor eye field, corresponding to parts of Brodmann areas 6, 8 and 9 (compare with **7**.125). The perimeter of this area is delineated by an interrupted line to indicate uncertainty as to its precise extent.

ocular muscles, and it has been hypothecated that they influence these through intermediary cell masses or 'centres' in the brainstem. There is, however, no doubt that voluntary and reflex eye movements are mediated by the frontal eye field and its projection. Like the rest of the first somatomotor area, this region of it also receives association fibres, probably from the occipital cortex, and in addition thalamic afferents from the juxtalamellar part of the dorsomedial nucleus,[771] to which the central zone of the frontal eye field (area 8) reciprocally projects.[772] A **second frontal eye field**, roughly anterior to the above has been demonstrated in monkeys, and hypothecated in man.[770]

**The motor speech area** of Broca is an extension of the primary somatomotor cortex into the inferior frontal gyrus, coinciding approximately with area 44 and part of 45 (**7**.134). Little reliable knowledge is available concerning its anatomical connexions, although subjacent to it are large concentrations of association fibres effecting interconnexions between many other parts of the cortex.

[762] P. M. Levin and F. K. Bradford, *J. comp. Neurol.*, **68**, 1938.
[763] H. G. J. M. Kuypers, *Brain*, **81**, 1958.
[764] F. Walberg and A. Brodal, *Brain*, **76**, 1953.
[765] A. M. Lassek, *J. comp. Neurol.*, **76**, 1942.
[766] W. DeMeyer, *Neurology, Minneap.*, **9**, 1959.
[767] S. Landgren, C. G. Phillips and R. Porter, *J. Physiol, Lond.*, **161**, 1962.
[768] H. Asanuma and H. Sakata, *J. Neurophysiol.*, **30**, 1967.
[769] E. C. Crosby, *J. comp. Neurol.*, **99**, 1953.
[770] E. C. Crosby, R. E. Yoss and J. W. Henderson, *J. comp. Neurol.*, **97**, 1952.
[771] G. Scollo-Lavizzari and K. Akert, *J. comp. Neurol.*, **121**, 1963.
[772] E. Rinvik, *Expl Brain Res.*, **5**, 1968.

Most information as to its functional significance is derived from the results of ablation or stimulation in experimental animals and man.[773] Ablation may abolish vocalization and usually produces a motor or expressive *aphasia*, or paralysis *of speech* in man, if carried out in the left or *dominant* hemisphere. In some individuals the leading speech area is, however, on the right, and it is considered that in some there is no such dominance.

It is to be emphasized that damage to the motor speech area does not entail *paralysis* of the *musculature* involved, all of which is in any case also amenable to stimulation of appropriate parts of the primary motor area in the precentral gyrus. Stimulation of the area may lead to a variety of effects, according to the parameters employed; speech in conscious patients may be actually inhibited, or simple acts of vocalization, such as the utterance of a vowel sound, may ensue. The response in experimental animals consists of simple movements of the face, lips and larynx and perhaps vocalization. In man also it is to be emphasized that the responses are, as in the case of the somatomotor cortex, always simple. In stimulation studies of the human cortex very similar effects can be elicited from two other areas, one in the frontal lobe, the supplementary motor area (MsII), and another curving round the posterior extremity of the lateral sulcus and occupying a large region in the parietal and, more extensively, temporal lobes. This latter area is sometimes known as the **second motor speech area of Wernicke**. All three regions, which may be named the *anterior, posterior* and *superior motor speech areas*, develop in the dominant hemisphere in each individual; and while the corresponding parts of the cortex in the opposite hemisphere have in some human patients apparently taken over the functions of a damaged area in the dominant hemisphere, they are perhaps in ordinary circumstances uncommitted in the activities of speech.

Illustration 7.134 shows the positions of these areas, but it must be said at once that other and often far more complex 'maps' of the cortical areas reputed to be concerned in speech have been propounded. Language, in all its permutations of speaking, listening, reading and writing, is obviously a most intricate activity, and it would be surprising if this, the major form of human communication and perhaps the main distinction of mankind, did not in fact involve widespread and voluminous parts of the brain and central nervous system. In view of the lack of information concerning the connexions of the various cortical areas believed to mediate these activities, it is hardly to be expected that other, subcortical mechanisms will have yet been implicated, despite the intensely active speculation prompted by study of the various forms of aphasia; but the pulvinar of the thalamus has recently been associated with the speech 'centres'.[774] However, the inconclusive nature of the evidence in this highly interesting field must limit further pursuit of the subject here, and the reader should consult the excellent reviews available.[775-777]

**The supplementary motor area** (MsII) must now be briefly considered, before passing on to the remainder, the 'prefrontal' region of the frontal lobe. This is, like other projection areas, sensorimotor in nature, but being predominantly motor and in the frontal lobe it is most conveniently described here; its sensory activities, about which less is known, will be merely alluded to in connection with the somatosensory cortex. The situation of this supplementary motor area, on the medial surface of the hemisphere has already been stated (p. 960); it is anterior to, and probably confluent with, the medial extension of the first somatomotor area into the paracentral lobule which mediates leg and perineal movement. It is thus in the medial frontal gyrus in man (area 6 and probably in

part area 8). Movements of the contralateral limbs can be elicited from the supplementary motor area in monkeys and in man,[778] but higher thresholds obtain than in the primary somatomotor cortex, as in the case of other accessory areas, and the movements are sometimes ipsilateral or bilateral. A somatotopic pattern has been established in monkeys (7.129),[779] but has not as yet been demonstrated in man. Efferent fibres from this area have been traced into the spinal cord in cats,[780] most of these ending contralaterally. There is also a bilateral projection to the thalamus, and to the gracile, cuneate and pontine nuclei, contrasting with the similar but unilateral projections from the primary somatomotor cortex. In accord with these variations the contributions of these two areas to the integration of movement are probably different, but

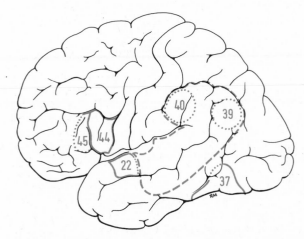

7.134 The superolateral surface of the left cerebral hemisphere showing the motor speech areas of Broca (44, 45) and Wernicke. The latter is variously depicted by different authorities, and is tentatively indicated by the large parieto-temporal area enclosed in an interrupted outline, which itself includes areas 39 and 40. Areas 22 and 37 are considered by some to be respectively auditory and visuo-auditory areas associated with speech and language.

the details are not yet sufficiently well defined to warrant discussion here.[781]

**The second somatosensory area** (SmII), being preponderantly sensory, will be considered in more detail with the primary sensory cortex in the parietal lobe. Since, however, it is also a *somatomotor area*, its less well-established motor characteristics are included here to complete the picture of the 'motor cortex'. Movements of most parts of the body can be elicited from it and the stimulation loci show a somatotopic organization both in subhuman primates and in man.[782] Its projection fibres have been followed as far as cervical spinal segments in monkeys,[783] and to the thalamus and dorsal column and pontine nuclei in cats, in which features it resembles the other somatomotor areas. Little can yet be added with regard to its significance in motor function.

[773] W. Penfield and L. Roberts, *Speech and Brain Mechanisms*, Princeton University Press, Princeton. 1959.

[774] G. A. Ojemann, P. Fedio and J. M. van Buren, *Brain*, **91**, 1968.

[775] R. Brain, *Brain*, **84**, 1961.

[776] W. Penfield, in: *Brain and Conscious Experience*, ed. J. C. Eccles, Springer, Berlin. 1966.

[777] C. H. Millikan and F. L. Darley (eds.), *Brain Mechanisms Underlying Speech and Language*, Grune and Stratton, New York. 1967.

[778] W. Penfield and K. Welch, *Archs Neurol. Psychiat., Chicago*, **66**, 1951.

[779] C. N. Woolsey, P. H. Settlage, D. R. Meyer, W. Spencer, T. P. Hamuy and A. M. Travis, *Res. Publs Ass. Res. nerv. ment. Dis.*, **30**, 1952.

[780] R. Nyberg-Hansen, *Expl. Brain Res.*, **7**, 1969.

[781] A. M. Travis, *Brain*, **78**, 1955.

[782] E. D. Adrian, *J. Physiol., Lond.*, **100**, 1941.

[783] A. Brodal and P. Angaut, *Brain Res.*, **5**, 1967.

**The prefrontal area** corresponds approximately to all parts of the frontal lobe which have not so far been particularized. It hence includes much of the three frontal gyri, the orbital gyri (orbitofrontal area), most of the medial frontal gyrus, and anterior half, approximately, of the cingulate gyrus, etc. It has been said that the great development of the frontal lobe in particular distinguishes the human from other brains. The so-called *silent areas* have long been regarded as a specially notable feature of the human cortex—at least, in their degree of expansion; and the prefrontal area is usually assigned to this category. If, however, silent or association areas are to be regarded as those parts of the cortex whose connexions are predominantly or exclusively mediated by association fibres, the prefrontal region would not qualify. In addition to elaborate afferent and efferent interconnexions with areas of cortex in all lobes of the cerebrum, it also has abundant links with the *thalamus, corpus striatum* and *hypothalamus*, and it projects in addition to the *cerebellum* via the nuclei pontis and perhaps to certain *cranial motor nuclei*.

Through the *superior* and *inferior fronto-occipital fasciculi* the frontal lobe appears to be connected not only with the occipital but also the parietal and temporal lobes. *Commissural* connexions also link corresponding parts of the frontal lobes through the corpus callosum, and there is some evidence that frontal commissural fibres may pass to other lobes. These connexions are said to be largely afferent, but in fact little is known of them in reliable detail, though it is suggested that efferent commissural fibres may also link the frontal lobe to many other parts of the cortex.

Massive *superior* and *inferior thalamic radiations*, principally derived from the nucleus medialis dorsalis (MD) of the medial nuclear group of the thalamus (p. 896) pass to the lateral (areas 9 and 10) and orbital regions of the frontal lobe, both of which in turn project back to the same parts of the thalamus. The anterior thalamic nucleus receives many afferents from the mamillary body and thus from the hippocampus (p. 942), which also connects directly with the anterior thalamus. Connexions of the anterior and medial thalamus with the hypothalamus (p. 907) therefore bring this, in addition, into afferent relation with the prefrontal cortex, from which corticohypothalamic projections have also been described. The *prefrontal corticopontine projection*, though less massive than that from the motor areas of the frontal lobe (4 and 6), is equally well established; both relay with considerable specificity in the paramedian components of the nuclei pontis.[784] The orbitofrontal region in particular projects to the paramedian nucleus of the hypothalamus.

Even this brief survey of the connexions of the prefrontal region suggests highly complex interactions in both *somatic* and *visceral activities*. The orbital surface, or orbitofrontal area, has attracted particular attention among experimenters. Stimulation in monkeys[785] depresses the respiratory rate, blood pressure and gastric motility; inhibition of induced cortical and reflex movements and emotional reactions has also been noted. Ablation of orbitofrontal cortex in primates leads to motor hyperactivity, restlessness, loss of attentiveness; and somewhat similar results follow ablation of the anterior cingulate region. The posterior orbitofrontal cortex and anterior cingulate gyrus are often regarded as parts of the limbic system (p. 932). Behavioural studies of monkeys subjected to *anterior* frontal ablations have adduced similar but often conflicting findings,[786, 787] and the sum total of firmly established fact remains slender.

Some light has been shed on the functional significance of the prefrontal area by the results of lobotomy and leucotomy, performed until recently on human patients in efforts to ameliorate certain mental disorders now treated pharmacologically. The effects of these operations, which were usually bilateral, resembled those caused by extensive disease of the frontal lobes. Abolition of the distressing aspect of illusions and of severe somatic pain were prominent effects, a result which accords with the concept that this part of the cortex is concerned with the 'affective tone' of sensations rather than with any discriminative or localizing aspects of them. Some observers have reported a diminution in intellectual capacity, but limitation of the operation to the orbitofrontal area or the cingulate gyrus is claimed to affect only the emotional balance of personality, suggesting that the superolateral part of the prefrontal area is more concerned with intellectual processes.[788] Patients with extensive frontal lobe damage, from whatever cause, almost always exhibit permanent and on the whole undesirable changes. Though perhaps more tractable and docile, they also show less initiative, untidiness, disregard for others and for general tenets of behaviour, and a marked lack of concentration, all of which can for the moment be summed up as a retrogression from the human condition—a somewhat vague statement but excusable and perhaps appropriate in our present dearth of precise information.

## THE PARIETAL LOBE

Immediately posterior to the central sulcus, occupying most of the postcentral gyrus and also extending over on to the medial surface of the parietal cortex in the paracentral lobule, is the primary or *first somatosensory area* (SmI, areas 3, 1 and 2). Posterior to it is the large 'silent' area of the parietal lobe, taken up in part below by the second speech area (*vide infra*). Inferiorly, in the lowest part of the postcentral gyrus (and extending forwards a little into the precentral gyrus) is the *second somatosensory area* (SmII).

Anterior to its medial extension is the *third somatosensory area*, the supplementary 'motor' area (MsII). It is appropriate here to note that the region of cortex, centrally situated in the cerebral hemisphere, which forms the great arrival station for somatic afferents and similarly for the departure of somatic efferents, consists of four separate, though juxtaposed, sensorimotor areas. Of these, two, the primary and supplementary motor areas are chiefly efferent projection cortex, MsI and II, while two are preponderantly recipients of afferent projection fibres—the primary and secondary somatosensory areas, SmI and II. As 7.129, 135A, B show, all these four areas evince a somatotopic pattern in cats and monkeys, and evidence that this is largely so in man has already been quoted (p. 956). The motor aspects of all four areas have been dealt with above, and it remains to consider their involvement in sensory functions.

**The first somatosensory area** shows interesting cytoarchitectonic variations. Its anterior part (area 3), bordering the central sulcus and extending into its depths to meet the agranular cortex of area 4, is of the granular type but also contains numbers of scattered medium and small pyramidal cells; it is in many respects similar to the striate cortex, the outer band of Baillarger, for example,

[784] O. Nyby and J. Jansen, *Skr. Norske Vidensk.—Akad.*, **1**, 1951.

[785] B. Kaada, in: *Handbook of Physiology*, Sect. 1, Vol. II, eds. J. Field, H. Magoun and V. E. Hall, American Physiological Society, Washington, D.C. 1960.

[786] J. M. Warren and K. Akert (eds.), *The Frontal Granular Cortex and Behaviour*, McGraw-Hill, New York. 1964.

[787] F. Sanides, *J. Hirnforsch.*, **6**, 1964.

[788] W. Lewin, *J. Neurol. Neurosurg. Psychiat.*, **24**, 1961.

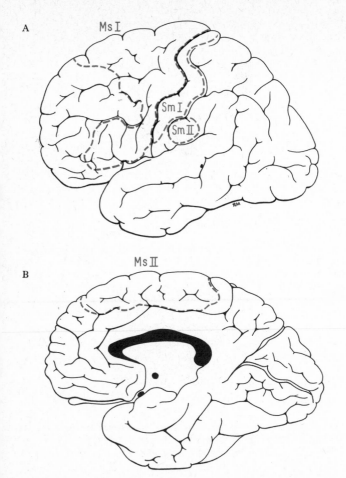

A

B

**7.135A and B** Superolateral (A) and medial (B) surfaces of the cerebral hemispheres showing the sensorimotor areas. See text for details and compare with **7.125, 130**. These areas can only be applied tentatively to the human cortex, and they are hence delineated with interrupted outlines.

being broad but not so prominent as the visual stria. The posterior part of the postcentral gyrus (areas 1 and 2) differs particularly in its smaller content of less densely packed granular or stellate cells (for further details see p. 951). The precise boundary, if such exists, between the pre- and post-central areas in the central sulcus has been a matter of dispute, and may be of some importance in the interpretation of experimental results.[789]

The projection from the *nuclei ventralis posterior lateralis* and *medialis of the thalamus* (VPL and VPM), to the primary somatosensory area is well attested, and it is through this radiation that a wide range of exteroceptive and proprioceptive modalities of sensation are mediated. Unit recording techniques and retrograde degeneration experiments have established that there is a highly specific pattern of localization between the cortex and the thalamus; and this is associated with a somatotopic form of organization in the postcentral gyrus like that in the adjoining first somatomotor area, including an apportioning of cortex in proportion to skill rather than size in the representation of bodily segments. This pattern has been studied in the human cortex by noting the type of sensation and the region to which it is referred when individual loci are stimulated in the exposed cortex at operations.[790] With carefully moderated stimulation very sharp localization can be established. By such means the localization of vesical, rectal and genital sensations to the lowest part of the medial region of the postcentral area has been established in man. The sensations aroused are for the majority of the body contralateral, but may sometimes be referred to the same side (oral region) or they may be bilateral (larynx, pharynx and perineum).

Experimental studies in animals have largely confirmed the localization demonstrated in the human somatosensory cortex. Responses to natural or artificial stimulation of peripheral receptors have also been shown to evoke potentials in the precentral area;[791] and by ablation of the somatosensory cortex it is established that there is a *direct* thalamic radiation to the 'motor' area (p. 898), an elegant demonstration of the latter's sensorimotor nature. Degeneration studies (see, for example, reference [792]) have provided more refined data as to the specificity of the thalamocortical projection; the nucleus ventralis posterior lateralis exhibits a fairly discrete localizational pattern of connexion with areas 3, 1 and 2, suggesting a functional significance in the structural differences between them, as mentioned earlier in this section (p. 898). Unit recording observations have confirmed this, revealing that area 3 is activated only by cutaneous stimuli, whereas area 2 is concerned with impulses from proprioceptors.[791] This implies a transverse deployment of modalities across the long axis of the precentral gyrus.[793] To this is to be added a segmental or dermatomic projection to such transverse strips of cortex, as a further refinement of the somatotopic localization in this area.[794] Moreover, each modality-specific locus appears to be associated with a column of cells vertically arranged through the thickness of the cortex, like the columns described in the visual area (p. 962).

The specificity of the somatosensory neurons concerned with joint receptors appears to be particularly marked, as in the thalamus. Some cortical units respond only to displacement in one direction, and these may continue to discharge even during a statically maintained position of the joint. Such arrangements, if applicable to man, would provide the neuronal basis for the 'joint sense' hypothecated in much earlier studies.[795] Fast adapting units activated by the bending of hairs and others adapting slowly to cutaneous deformation have also been identified. Similar studies suggest that afferents from receptors in striated muscle terminate in units sited in the somato*motor* cortex, and that impulses may reach them by pathways independent of the cerebellum, constituting the mediating basis, in part, for consciousness of stretch in muscles. These experimental findings imply a considerable difference in the sensory properties of the pre- and post-central parts of the main sensorimotor area. The two gyri are, however, linked by numerous short association fibres, conducting in both directions.[796] As is so in most, if not all, the sensorimotor areas, primary or accessory, the first somatosensory area has abundant reciprocal connexions with the thalamus (p. 898), the corticothalamic projection comparing in its specificity of point-to-point linkage with the thalamocortical radiation.[797] In connexion with this specific and apparently unvarying nature, in the spatial sense, of the cerebral level of some modalities in their pathways, a recent study of the cortex in mice is particularly interesting.[798] Barrel-shaped architectonic groupings of nerve cells were detected in the somatosensory area (SmI) and in the part of this related to the head and muzzle. There is some evidence that these

[789] E. Rinvik, *Brain Res.*, **10**, 1968.
[790] W. Penfield and H. Jasper, *Epilepsy and the Functional Anatomy of the Human Brain*, Little, Brown, Boston. 1954.
[791] D. Albe-Fessard and J. Liebeskind, *Expl Brain Res.*, **1**, 1966.
[792] W. E. Le G. Clark and T. P. S. Powell, *Proc. R. Soc. B.*, **141**, 1953.
[793] V. Mountcastle and T. P. S. Powell, *Bull. Johns Hopkins Hosp.*, **105**, 1959.
[794] T. P. S. Powell and V. Mountcastle, *Bull. Johns Hopkins Hosp.*, **105**, 1959.
[795] J. S. B. Stopford, *J. Anat.*, **56**, 1922.
[796] D. N. Pandya and H. G. J. M. Kupyers, *Brain Res.*, **13**, 1969.
[797] E. Rinvik, *Brain Res.*, **10**, 1968.
[798] T. A. Woolsey and H. van der Loos, *Brain Res.*, **17**, 1970.

'barrels' may be units equated with the individual vibrissae of the animal's muzzle. Both this and a study of the spatial distribution of synapses in the same cortical area in neonatal dogs,[799] though of course not immediately applicable to the human cortex, illustrate the intricate and quantitative kind of analysis of the cortex being made in current investigations.

Much less is known of the **second** and **third somatosensory areas** (SmII and MsII). The former is in the superior lip of the posterior limb of the lateral fissure, adjoining the insula in monkeys (**7.**129), and it occupies a similar position in man. Evoked potentials indicate a somatotopic organization in SmII, with the face area most anterior and the leg at the posterior or caudal end of the area. Single units associated with tactile and vibration senses have been identified in the area, and stimulation of Pacinian corpuscles evokes higher potentials than in the primary somatosensory area.[800] The second somatosensory area projects to the thalamus, but its connexions and their reciprocal nature have not yet been studied in detail. It also projects to the dorsal column nuclei, like the other somatosensory areas.

**The third somatosensory area**, which is the equivalent of the supplementary motor area, is in its sensory functions as yet little understood. It is known to receive thalamocortical fibres and projection fibres leave it, some of which are not motor, but details of these connexions are yet to be worked out. Stimulation in conscious human patients is said to evoke generalized sensations referred to the head and abdominal region, but no exact somatotopic pattern can be ascribed to it, as regards its sensory activities.

**The second speech area** of Wernicke (**7.**134), because it is partly in the parietal lobe, must be mentioned here. It occupies a small parietal area, extending more extensively into the temporal lobe (p. 964). The rest of the parietal lobe, between the main somatosensory and visual areas, is 'silent' cortex. This region corresponds more or less to the inferior parietal gyrus, 'areas' 39 and 40.[801] The connexions of this region, as far as they are known, are indeed in part association and commissural, but little clear detail of them has been established; but there is also a reciprocal interconnexion with all the parts of the lateral nuclear group of the thalamus (p. 898). Corticospinal and corticotegmental projections have also been suggested, the latter influencing motor nuclei in the brainstem, and more particularly those of the nerves to the eye muscles, either directly or through intermediary nerve cells. These latter connexions are specially interesting in conjunction with description of a supplementary motor area in areas 5 and 7 in the macaque monkey.[802] The strategic position of the parietal association area close to all the cortical regions concerned with general and special modalities of sensation, coupled with its multifarious connexions, is in itself highly suggestive of complex and integrated activities. Most of the evidence in this regard is derived in man from clinical observations of behavioural defects and distortions consequent upon pathological lesions or surgical ablations, and upon extrapolation of similar results in primates submitted to deliberate experimental damage. The reports available and their results are confusingly numerous and varied. Muscular debility, slowing of reflex activity, disorders of speech (aphasias), loss of awareness of bodily parts and of spatial relation to the environment, and other forms of *agnosia* (a state of absent or defective recognition of the significance of objects and situations), have all been observed. A particular form of agnosia, which has long been associated with parietal lobe damage, is *astereognosis*, a failure to interpret the three-dimensional nature of objects when examined by the hand without the help of vision. *Interpretation* has, indeed, been strongly advocated as the prime parietal activity in man;[803] in connexion particularly with language on the dominant (left) side of the cerebrum and in a more generalized sense on the other side. The parietal lobe is thus perhaps to be regarded as a region of high activity in learning processes, and of uniquely high development in this respect in mankind. In view of the general nature of the evolutionary process it is perhaps unwise and unnecessary to attribute a qualitatively unique nature to the operations of the human parietal area, but its great importance in our behaviour, especially in discrimination and interpretation, is amply attested by clinical evidence and animal experimentation.

## THE OCCIPITAL LOBE

Almost the whole of the occipital lobe is occupied by the Brodmann areas 17, 18 and 19 (**7.**136A, B). Although only area 17, the **striate or visuosensory cortex**, was originally regarded as containing the terminations of the optic radiation, there is now firm evidence that the lateral geniculate body (p. 918) radiates also to areas 18 and 19 in the cat[804] and monkey,[805] and that in these, as in area 17, the spatial arrangement of optic radiation terminals is related to the retinae in an orderly manner.[806] Moreover, all three areas project to the thalamus (lateral geniculate body or pulvinar) and brainstem motor nuclei, or both. Short and long association and commissural fibres link the *three visual areas* together, and to their contralateral equivalents and other parts of the cortex in both hemispheres. (For an exhaustive critique of this and other aspects of visual neuroanatomy consult reference [807].) Occipitopontine fibres have been described, but their status in man is uncertain.

**The striate cortex** (area 17), or **first visual area**, occupies the upper and lower lips and the depths of the posterior part of the calcarine sulcus (**7.**136), extending into much of the cuneus and lingual gyrus. As a cytoarchitectonic area it can easily be defined, both macro- and micro-scopically, by the visual stria and by the thinness of the cortex. Posteriorly the area is limited by the lunate sulcus (and by the polar sulci above and below this), and it thus does not extend beyond the occipital pole in man, though it reaches the lateral aspect of the lobe in other primates. Anteriorly the striate area is bounded by the medial parieto-occipital sulcus, but its lower part, below the calcarine sulcus, may extend somewhat further. The stria becomes less obvious as it is followed posteriorly towards the occipital pole, and this change can be correlated with the retinotopical organization of the area (*vide infra*), its prominence being inversely related to proximity to the central retinal area.

Histologically the area is of the *granular* type, or *koniocortex* (p. 951), in which densely packed stellate cells greatly outnumber the few pyramidal cells present.

[799] M. E. Molliver and H. van der Loos, *Ergeb. d. Anat. u. Entwick.*, **42**, 1970.
[800] A. K. McIntyre, M. E. Holman and J. L. Veale, *Expl Brain Res.*, **4**, 1967.
[801] M. Critchley, *The Parietal Lobes*, Arnold, London. 1953.
[802] E. C. Crosby, T. Humphrey and M. J. Showers, in: *Einige Anordnungen und Funktionen der supplementären motorischen Rinden*, ed. K. F. Bauer, Thieme, Stuttgart. 1959.
[803] W. Penfield, in: *Brain and Conscious Experience*, ed. J. C. Eccles, Springer, Berlin. 1966.
[804] M. R. Glickstein, A. King, J. Miller and M. Berkley, *J. comp. Neurol.*, **130**, 1967.
[805] M. E. Wilson and B. G. Cragg, *J. Anat.*, **101**, 1967.
[806] L. J. Garey and T. P. S. Powell, *Proc. R. Soc. B.*, **169**, 1967; and *J. Anat.*, **102**, 1968.
[807] S. Polyak, *The Vertebrate Visual System*, University of Chicago Press, Chicago. 1957.

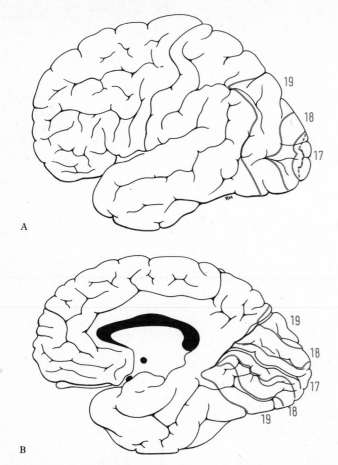

7.136A and B   Superolateral (A) and medial (B) surfaces of the cerebral hemispheres showing the visual areas in the occipital lobe. The striate (17), parastriate (18) and peristriate (19) areas correspond approximately to the Brodmann areas as indicated, and also to visual areas I, II and III. See text for details.

For full details the reader should consult references [807–809]; only salient features will be mentioned here. (a) The deeper stratum of the pyramidal layer (III) contains *large stellate cells*, which almost replace the large pyramidal cells present here in other types, of cortex. (b) The outer band of Baillarger in lamina IV is accentuated as the *visual stria*, consisting of large numbers of terminations of optic radiation and probably association fibres. (c) The ganglionic layer (V), which commonly consists largely of pyramidal cells, including the largest, here contains a few large, scattered *solitary cells (of Meynèrt)*; these are of a modified pyramidal shape, about 30 μm in diameter, and distributed in a single row. Their dendrites extend widely through the cortex and their axons form the projection element of the visual cortex, passing through the optic radiation to reach the superior colliculus and possibly the motor nuclei of the extraocular muscles. (d) The external and internal granular layers (II and IV)—especially the latter—contain larger numbers and more densely packed small stellate cells than any other part of the cerebral cortex.

Although the striate cortex contains only about 3 per cent of the cerebral surface area, approximately one-tenth of all the cortical neurons are said to be concentrated in it. In their cytoarchitectural details, areas 18 and 19 approximate respectively to the polar and parietal types of cortex (p. 951), in which stellate cells are less prominent and pyramidal cells more so. Myelin and axonal stains have been used to investigate the fibre structure of the visual area, especially the striate cortex.[810, 811] In general this resembles arrangements in other cortical areas (p. 949), but dendritic fields in their quantitative aspects

have been studied more intensively in this part of the cortex than perhaps any other excepting the postcentral gyrus. The stimulus to this has been in part the physiological demonstration of a species of columnar organization in the somatosensory area and thereafter in the striate cortex (*vide infra*). So far the physiological techniques in use are providing more illuminating evidence.

The status of area 17 as the primary visual cortical area has long been established, both by electrical stimulation in man and by its connexions with the lateral geniculate body, and through this with the retinae (p. 917). The *retinotopical organization* which exists in the lower parts of the visual pathway have also been shown to be carried through to the cortical level. Each striate area receives impulses from the two ipsilateral half retinae, representing the *contralateral* half of the binocular visual field. As has already been described (p. 918), the patterns of impulses from the retinae do not undergo a simple relay in the geniculate body, where some degree of processing, including probably preliminary integration or at least interaction between impulses from both retinae, has been shown to occur. These activities have been studied even more intensively in the striate cortex, especially by single unit recording technique. The *geniculate radiation* spreads out as it swerves through the white substance of the occipital lobe, its fibres terminating in a strict point-to-point deployment in the striate area, such that the peripheral parts of the retinae activate the most anterior parts of the area, the macular regions activating a relatively large part of the striate cortex adjoining its posterior extremity. Moreover, the superior and inferior retinal quadrants are thus connected with corresponding divisions of the striate area. In the classical studies of the effects of injuries of the occipital lobe in warfare, similar retinotopic results were obtained.[814, 815]

These experimental findings, established in a wide range of mammals and especially primates (see p. 918 for references), have been corroborated by stimulation of the human cortex.[812, 813] The visual impressions thus elicited are simple, such as flashes of light, but they are referred to a specific part of the visual field according to the location of the cortical stimulus. Eye movements are also produced by such stimulation. When similar stimuli are applied to areas 18 and 19 more complex images are reported by the patient, indicating that these regions are concerned in further elaboration of the visual information reaching area 17.

In recent years most interesting results have been obtained by recording the response of single nerve cells to various forms of retinal stimulus; and while these studies have been chiefly pursued in cats,[816] there is little reason to doubt that in principle they are applicable to the human striate cortex, especially since the cytoarchitectonic areas involved in the cat can be equated with those in primates.[817] Briefly, each unit from which recordings are made corresponds to a definite receptive field in the retina, and can presumably be excited only from that area. Units responding to a range of modes of stimulation have been identified; some react to white light, especially in the form

[808] E. C. Crosby, in: *Les grandes activites du lobe occipital*, ed. T. Alajouanine, Masson, Paris. 1960.
[809] M. Colonnier, *J. Anat.*, **98**, 1967.
[810] D. A. Sholl, *J. Anat.*, **89**, 1955.
[811] M. Colonnier, *J. Anat.*, **98**, 1964.
[812] O. Foerster, *J. Psychol. Neurol., Lpz*, **39**, 1929.
[813] W. Penfield and H. Jasper, *Epilepsy and the Functional Anatomy of the Human Brain*, Little, Brown and Co., Boston. 1954.
[814] G. Holmes and W. T. Lister, *Brain*, **39**, 1916.
[815] H. L. Teubér, W. S. Battersby and M. B. Bender, *Visual Field Defects*, Harvard University Press, Cambridge. 1960.
[816] D. H. Hubel and T. N. Wiesel, *J. Physiol. Lond.*, **160**, 1962.
[817] R. Otsuka and R. Hassler, *Arch. Psychiat. Nerven Krankh.*, **203**, 1962.

of stripes or edges between light and dark. This contrasts with the more or less circular receptive fields of excitation demonstrated in the lateral geniculate body. Excitatory units surrounded by inhibitory zones have also been described, but these also evince a strip-like character rather than the circular pattern of the geniculate body. Many units are sensitive to the orientation of the stimulus, responding only to vertical, horizontal or intermediate forms of linear stimulation of the retina. More complex units occur, for example, some responding to the particular direction of a moving stimulus. It is possible that these represent the integration of information from the simpler units mentioned above.

Further work in this field has led to the identification of columnar unitary loci in the striate cortex which respond to stimulation from one retina, although most appear to be excited simultaneously from both; a columnar organization of cells coded according to colour responses has also been advanced.[818, 819] Some of these later results have been obtained in monkeys, with an increased likelihood that they correspond to human visual activities.

These studies, carried out with meticulous reference to the laminar pattern of the striate cortex, suggest a *columnar* form of anatomical arrangement corresponding to the vertical physiological organization in 'units' for which there is such undoubted evidence.[820] The concept of 'chains' of neurons linked by synapses through the vertical dimensions of the cortex is comparatively old (p. 946), and much more recent work, with the advantages of improved staining techniques and electron microscopy, has confirmed and elaborated this view, not only with regard to the striate cortex[821] but also in the case of other areas. Synaptological studies and the results of degeneration experiments indicate clearly that the afferents of such an area as the striate cortex feed their impulses into a limited columnar group of neurons of internuncial type, the resultant of their interactions, excitatory and inhibitory, reaching a pyramidal cell and being thus translated to subcortical neurons or to some other part of the cortex. Such *columnar units* are not, of course, completely independent, being linked to others by recurrent axons, by the tangential fibres in the superficial lamina of the cortex (I), and by actual spatial overlap.[822]

The effects of lesions of the lateral geniculate body in cats provide particularly detailed patterns of the termination of geniculocortical fibres in all three visual areas.[823] In area 17 degenerating terminals are mainly in lamina IV, but a few fine vertical axons reach lamina I to spread tangentially in it. In area 18 the main termination is in lamina IV, while in area 19 the afferent terminations are much less numerous but are spread through layers IV, V and VI. These results not only confirm earlier findings on the wide region of afferent projection in the occipital lobe, but also accord with the divergence of activity in the three parts of the visual cortex. The above experiments entail the infliction of very large, almost total lesions of the lateral geniculate body. Restricted lesions are naturally required to demonstrate the specific point-to-point relationship between the geniculate projection fibres and the visual areas. This specificity can also be shown by making cortical lesions and observing the resultant retrograde degeneration in the geniculate body, where a columnar series of groups of cells in all six layers are affected (p. 918). It is of special interest here that this effect is only achieved when the cortical lesions involve the whole thickness of the cortex.[824] By a similar combined 'attack' the functional details of visual *areas* II and III are being gradually clarified. In both areas evidence of columnar units is accruing, with the difference that the units respond to more complex stimulation and are almost all bi-retinal in respect to their receptive fields.

Parts, at least, of the occipital visual area must be considered as sensorimotor, inasmuch as eye movements can be elicited from them. In monkeys this (third) *occipital eye field* (7.136) is confined to visual areas I and II (17 and 18), stimulation of which produces conjugate deviations in various directions, especially to the opposite side. Head turning, facial movements, and sometimes responses in the upper limbs may occur.[825, 826] This occipital motor eye field (III) is connected reciprocally with the *frontal eye fields* I and II. Such connexions are considered to be involved in the mediation of vision in the voluntary ocular movements which are held to characterize the frontal eye fields. The motor responses from area 18, which include accommodation, are on the contrary thought to be, in natural activities, reflex in nature and involved in following and fixation movements. This area may project to the pulvinar, in which connexion a controversial linkage between the lateral geniculate body and the same part of the thalamus should be noted; projection from the pulvinar to areas 18 and 19 is established in principle, but there is disagreement over details.[827] Efferent projection fibres descend from the occipital motor eye field, particularly from area 19, to the superior colliculus and to the nuclei of the motor nerves of the ocular muscles; but the latter connexion is probably through intermediary nerve cells, such as the para-abducens nucleus (p. 1010) interstitial nucleus of Cajal, nucleus of Darkschewitsch, and the posterior commissural nuclear complex[828]. These descending fibres are to be distinguished from the corticogeniculate projection (pp. 918 and 1118), the evidence for which is chiefly physiological.[829] Such a projection, if substantiated, could account for the cortical modulating effect on geniculate neurons which has been demonstrated by unit recording technique.

The three visual areas are intimately linked by short association pathways, which are probably especially specific in the spatial sense between areas 17 and 18. Association and commissural fibres connect all three areas, but more particularly 18 and 19, to many parts of the ipsi- and contra-lateral hemispheres. Vision and ocular movements may therefore be affected by lesions remote from the visual cortex, or from the recognized motor fields. For example, the course of the optic radiation as it swerves through the temporal lobe (Meyer's 'loop') entails that temporal lesions, such as tumours, may lead to homonymous field defects.[830]

## THE TEMPORAL LOBE

The temporal lobe has lateral and inferomedial surfaces, the former presenting superior, middle and inferior temporal gyri, the latter including the medial and lateral occipitotemporal gyri (sometimes regarded collectively as the fusiform gyrus), which are separated from the parahippocampal gyrus by the collateral fissure (7.114 and

[818] D. H. Hubel and T. N. Wiesel, *J. Physiol., Lond.*, **195**, 1968.

[819] D. H. Hubel and T. N. Wiesel, *Nature Lond.*, **221**, 1969.

[820] D. H. Hubel and T. N. Wiesel, *Nature Lond.*, **221**, 1969.

[821] M. Colonnier, *Archs Neurol. Psychiat., Chicago*, **16**, 1967.

[822] M. Colonnier, in: *Basic Mechanisms of the Epilepsies*, Little, Brown and Co., Boston. 1969.

[823] S. Rossignol and M. Colonnier, *Vision Res., Suppl.* **3**, 1971.

[824] J. E. Rose and L. I. Malis, *J. comp. Neurol.*, **125**, 1965.

[825] N. W. Rieck, *J. comp. Neurol.*, **112**, 1959.

[826] M. B. Bender (ed.), *The Oculomotor System*, Harper and Row, New York. 1964.

[827] S. Locke, *J. comp. Neurol.*, **116**, 1961.

[828] M. B. Carpenter and P. Peter, *J. Hirnforsch.*, **12**, 1971.

[829] L. Widén and C. A. Marsan, in: *Neurophysiologie und Psychophysik des visuellen Systems*, eds. R. Jung and H. Kornhuber, Springer, Berlin. 1961.

[830] M. A. Falconer and J. L. Wilson, *Brain*, **81**, 1958.

119). The temporal lobe is regarded as highly evolved in man and of relatively recent phylogenetic development. In a general way it may be regarded as particularly involved in hearing, language and perception.

Part of the superior temporal gyrus is rolled into the posterior limb of the lateral fissure during human fetal development, and this buries two short gyri which ascend obliquely backwards posterior to the limiting sulcus of the insula. These are the anterior and posterior *transverse temporal gyri* (of Heschl), which correspond to areas 52, 41 and 42 approximately (7.112). A large number of other cytoarchitectonic localities have been described in the temporal lobe; but only those areas just mentioned, together with 22, which adjoins them on the lateral aspect of the superior temporal gyrus, can be reliably equated in man. In the original description of Campbell in 1905 the *acoustic area* of the cortex covered rather more than area 41, to which subsequent observers narrowed it down, thus defining what might be called the classical acoustic area, a leading feature of the temporal gyrus (7.126 A). As will become apparent, Campbell's view has been revived by more recent experimental work.

Area 41 is histologically a variant of the granular type of cortex, but it is thicker than the cortex in the visual and somatosensory areas.[831] Its immediate surroundings, such as area 22 (7.125), are of the parietal type, and beyond this much of the temporal lobe is frontal in type, like the main areas of the parietal and frontal lobes. Both the latter types of cortex show a considerable admixture of pyramidal cells and a diminution in granular elements (stellate cells). For further details consult the authorities referred to on p. 949.

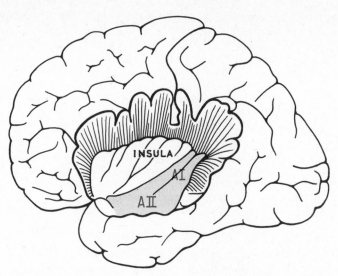

7.138 Superolateral surface of left cerebral hemisphere from which the opercula have been cut away to expose the insula and the adjoining anterior and posterior transverse temporal gyri and their continuity with the superior temporal gyrus. The area shown in blue contains the classical acoustic area, A I (equal to Brodmann area 41 and parts of areas 42 and 52), and the secondary acoustic area, A II (extending into area 22).

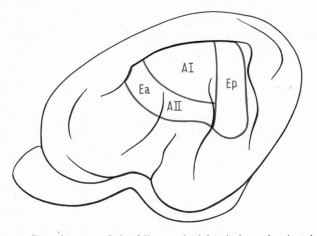

7.137 Lateral aspect of the feline cerebral hemisphere showing the main auditory areas, AI and AII, and accessory areas Ea and Ep. These areas cannot yet be extrapolated with confidence to the human cortex. See text for details. (Adapted from *The Auditory Pathway*, by I. C. Whitfield—see Bibliography.)

**The acoustic area**, as classically defined, is approximately equivalent to area 41; for reasons shortly to be related it is now more properly called the **first acoustic area** (AI). It extends a little into the superior temporal gyrus, but is largely obscured in the lateral fissure, forming the anterior transverse temporal gyrus. The earlier evidence on which the acoustic nature of this area was based may be sought in suitable reviews (see reference[832]). Attempts to define more accurately the area in which projection fibres from the medial geniculate body terminate have extended the area,[833] and the results of cortical stimulation (evoking head and ear movements) and cortical recording of potentials excited by localized stimulation of the cochlea and the cochlear nerve[834] have provided similar evidence. Much of this experimental

work has been carried out on cats, and less often on monkeys. Consequently the details of these accessory areas apply primarily to the feline temporal lobe and cannot be confidently translated in their entirety to man. The **second acoustic area** is often abbreviated to AII and lies inferior to AI in the equivalent of the superior temporal gyrus, in the cat the ectosylvian gyrus. Flanking AII are the *anterior* and *posterior ectosylvian areas*, Ea and Ep, and even further areas have been advanced (7.138). There is some evidence that all the areas named, except Ea, receive projection fibres from the medial geniculate body. Ablation of the first acoustic area, AI, leads to degeneration of cells only in the anterior part of the medial geniculate body, which receives fibres from the inferior colliculus (p. 886); but other parts of the complex of nuclei which make up the body project to all the other areas, except perhaps Ea, but including also part of the insula.[835] It has been suggested that some of the fibres in the acoustic radiation divide and terminate in more than one area, and that this may be in part the cause of the equivocal results of some experimenters. Short association fibres have been shown to link AI to AII and Ep, but not Ea.

The geniculocortical projection has been 'mapped' in the first acoustic area in the chimpanzee,[836] and a topical representation in this[834] was considered at an early date to be *tonotopical*, that is, to indicate a localization pattern on the basis of frequency of sound. This has been strongly denied as a feature of the human first acoustic area,[837] and remains a major controversy.[838] Stimulation in the conscious patient merely produced poorly localized patterns of sound or noise of simple nature, such as buzzing, humming, or ringing, but in the neighbouring areas (which may correspond to those identified in the

[831] P. Bailey and G. von Bonin, *The Isocortex of Man*, University of Illinois Press, Urbana. 1951.
[832] I. C. Whitfield, *The Auditory Pathway*, Arnold, London. 1967.
[833] J. E. Rose and C. N. Woolsey, *J. comp. Neurol.*, **91**, 1949.
[834] C. N. Woolsey and E. M. Walzl, *Bull. Johns Hopkins Hosp.*, **71**, 1942.
[835] D. K. Morest, *J. Anat.*, **98**, 1964.
[836] A. E. Walker and J. F. Fulton, *Brain*, **61**, 1938.
[837] W. Penfield and H. Jasper, *Epilepsy and the Functional Anatomy of the Human Brain*, Little, Brown and Co., Boston. 1954.
[838] E. F. Evans, in: *Hearing Mechanisms in Vertebrates*, Churchill, London. 1968.

cat), more complex acoustic phenomena were elicited. Despite numerous studies of unit recording from the primary acoustic area, this problem has not been settled, but it seems highly likely that there are in fact units which respond to specific frequencies, even if they are not arranged in any particular pattern. Other units which can be excited by variation of frequency with time or direction have been described,[839] and in these specific arrays of units the acoustic area resembles the visual cortex.

The existence of *efferent fibres* descending from the acoustic areas to the brainstem has been alluded to elsewhere (p. 886). These may not only modulate activities in the medial geniculate body but may also mediate various reflexes by forming connexions with motor nuclei of cranial nerves. Some of the fibres probably influence contraction of the stapedius and tensor tympani in the middle ear cavity; experiments suggest that this is increased in association with high-frequency sounds.[840] *Association fibres*, in addition to the short ones alluded to above, link the acoustic areas to the other lobes in their own hemisphere, and perhaps particularly to the frontal pole and the cortex deep in the superior temporal sulcus, which recent work suggests may be special loci of convergence of association fibres from all the sensory areas.[841] Little is known of commissural fibres, but it should be remembered that the lateral lemniscus is a bilateral tract. As a result of this, lesions in man of the medial geniculate body or the acoustic cortex do not lead to noticeable deafness unless they are bilateral—an unusual occurrence. Quite extensive temporal tumours are associated with only minimal effects on hearing, though they may interfere with the acoustic aspects of interpretation of language, especially if in the 'dominant' hemisphere. In connexion with this it is apposite to note that the posterior motor speech area mentioned in the section on the parietal lobe (p. 960) extends markedly into the temporal lobe posterior to the acoustic region, practically surrounding the latter according to some authorities (7.134). This proximity doubtless has its implications in the complex cortical organization of speech, hearing and language, but further comment would be at the present juncture mere speculation.

**The vestibular area** is a matter of uncertainty and disagreement as regards its site, but in the monkey it is said to be located close to the part of the somatosensory area (SmI) concerned with the face in the postcentral gyrus (area 2).[842] Area 2 is a cortical region particularly involved in sensations from deep tissues and joints, and the spatial proximity of a vestibular area to this appears interesting. The area is believed to receive a projection from the vestibular nuclei, but this rests more upon the results of natural or electrical stimulation of the vestibular nerve or its receptors than upon any anatomical demonstration. Unlike the acoustic pathway, the vestibular projection appears to be almost entirely crossed. Indications of some degree of somatotopical specificity in the connexions of the vestibular cortex with parts of the vestibular nuclear complex have been reported,[843] but in view of the lack of anatomical evidence and the conflicting nature of the physiological data, little more can be said until better evidence is available. Another view of the position of the vestibular area must be mentioned; this depends on the recording of equilibratory responses in man, and implicates part of the superior temporal gyrus, anterior to the acoustic areas.[844]

Apart from the acoustic areas, a possible vestibular area, and the extension into it of the posterior motor speech area (of Wernicke), the temporal lobe contains no other functionally designated areas, but it is not therefore to be assumed that all the remainder can be regarded as association cortex. The existence of large numbers of association fibres connecting parts of the temporal lobe to each other and to areas in other lobes is well established, although precise definitions are often lacking. Such connexions with the visual areas—between areas 18 and 19 and 37—and with the parietal lobe—between areas 7 and 40 and 22—are likely to be involved in complex integration between the sensorimotor areas in the temporal, occipital and parietal lobes. Thus, the more posterior region of the temporal lobe is perhaps more concerned with somatic activities, and especially with linguistic communication in its auditory and visual forms. The results of stimulation studies in man naturally provide the chief basis for such views.[845] The anterior region of the temporal lobe appears to be more multiform still in its association with somatic and visceral activities. Apart from intrinsic association connexions, it is linked to the limbic system (p. 930) through the connexions of the parahippocampal gyrus with the hippocampus, and the temporal pole, area 38, is also involved in these interrelationships (p. 941). Effects on blood pressure, respiration, and gastric motility—usually depression—have been elicited by stimulation of this part of the anterior temporal lobe; but the major source of evidence in mankind depends on the defects following limited temporal lobe ablations to relieve epileptiform attacks due to lesions in this region.

Stimulation prior to temporal lobectomy, which usually does not involve removal of either acoustic or motor speech cortex, may elicit complex memories of auditory, visual or combined content. After actual lobectomy a somewhat confusing plethora of manifestations have been described in the extensive clinical literature on this topic, for which the appropriate textbooks should be consulted. Effects on speech, auditory memory, and the interpretation of both auditory and visual phenomena have been noted.[846, 847] A form of visual agnosia, sometimes called 'psychic blindness', in which patients or experimental animals are unable to recognize the visual significance of objects, coupled with a change in dietary habits, tendency to examine objects with the oral region, hypersexual behaviour and loss of emotional responses together constitute a syndrome named after Klüver and Bucy.[848, 849] But in these instances the lobectomy involved the amygdaloid body, hippocampus, and part of the parahippocampal gyrus, and subsequent experiments have shown that these phenomena are only in part due to temporal lobectomy involving neocortex alone (cf. p. 943).

In recent years the temporal lobe has been loosely associated with the activities of memory; but except for the possible participation of the parahippocampal gyrus in what has been ascribed to the hippocampus and other associated structures as 'short term' memory (p. 943), there is little firm evidence of any anatomical entities in the temporal lobe or elsewhere which can be regarded as sites of 'long term' memory.

[839] I. C. Whitfield and E. F. Evans, *J. Neurophysiol.*, **28**, 1965.

[840] P. Carmel and A. Starr, *J. Neurophysiol.*, **26**, 1963.

[841] E. G. Jones and T. P. S. Powell, *Brain*, **93**, 1970.

[842] J. M. Fredrickson, U. Figge, P. Scheid and H. H. Kornhuber, *Expl Brain Res.*, **2**, 1966.

[843] L. C. Massopust and H. J. Daigle, *Expl Neurol.*, **2**, 1960.

[844] W. Penfield, *Ann. Otol. Rhinol. Lar.*, **66**, 1957.

[845] J. S. Blum, K. C. Chow and K. H. Pribram, *J. comp. Neurol.*, **93**, 1950.

[846] B. Milner, in: *Brain Mechanisms Underlying Speech and Language*, ed. F. L. Darley, Grune and Stratton, New York. 1967.

[847] M. A. Falconer, in: *Brain Mechanisms Underlying Speech and Language*, ed. F. L. Darley, Grune and Stratton, New York. 1967.

[848] H. Klüver and P. C. Bucy, *Am. J. Physiol.*, **119**, 1937.

[849] H. Terzian and G. D. Ore, *Neurology, Minneap.*, **5**, 1955.

## OTHER CORTICAL AREAS

**The insula** (7.113A–D) has already been described (p. 926). It is a matter of choice to which lobe it is assigned, since it adjoins and is overlapped by all lobes save the occipital. Histologically it exhibits in its posterior part a type of cortex resembling the parietal (p. 951), whereas its anterior region is variously described as agranular or like the piriform cortex.[850] The fibre connexions of the insula are still largely obscure; short association axons between it and all its opercula have been described, and it is said to be connected to the lateral olfactory gyrus and the piriform lobe (p. 932). Thalamic connexions (to the centromedian nucleus) have also been suggested.[851, 852] Contralateral motor responses in the face and limbs have been elicited by insular stimulation in macaques and gibbons, and a somatotopic pattern may exist in this possible supplementary field.[853] Stimulation in man excites visceral motor and sensory effects, such as belching, gastric movements, nausea and abdominal 'sensations'.[854] Increased salivation in man and experimental animals has also been elicited, and vasomotor effects in the latter. The insula has also been regarded as a gustatory area by some experimentalists. (For a review see reference[855].)

**The 'suppressor areas'** reported by earlier experimenters in various parts of the cortex, particularly a vertical strip anterior to area 4, have been the subject of much controversy and adverse criticism.[856] It is now considered that the suppression of motor activities from such areas is due to a generalized phenomenon of 'spreading depression' which is not associated with any particular areas of cortex. This phenomenon, which has not yet been completely explained, is characterized by a relatively long depression of neuronal activity, which may last several minutes, during which all responses may be suspended or distorted. It has no special anatomical correlates.[857]

**The cingulate gyrus** is discussed elsewhere in connection with the limbic system (p. 895), but certain aspects of its anterior part, corresponding roughly to area 24, must be mentioned here. In its microscopic structure this area has features in common with the pre- and post-central areas. It receives a projection from the anterior nuclear complex of the thalamus which is reciprocated, and it may have connexions with the corpus striatum, hypothalamus and midbrain tegmentum. Commissural fibres through the corpus callosum have been described, and association fibres appear to link it with the frontal and parietal cortex anterior and posterior to the main sensorimotor region.[858]

Stimulation in macaques has been held to evoke bodily movements, both contralateral and bilateral, with some form of somatotopic pattern.[859] This supplementary motor area extends into the posterior part of the cingulate gyrus, but the finding requires confirmation. In human patients stimulation of the anterior cingulate area may elicit changes in pulse, respiration and blood pressure, but the most reliable information has come from the results of surgical division or removal of the anterior cingulate gyrus, which is often involved in frontal leucotomy, performed to alleviate certain mental abnormalities. Cingulectomy alone appears to relieve abnormal aggressiveness and obsessional states, resulting in a milder and more placid personality.[860] Similar effects have been recorded in monkeys subjected to ablations of the anterior cingulate gyrus.[861] More recently, cingulate gyrus ablation has been claimed as a useful manœuvre in relieving intractable pain.[862] This mixture of somatic motor and sensory, emotional and visceral activities is at least in accord with the intermediate position of the anterior cingulate gyrus between the limbic system and the neocortex proper.

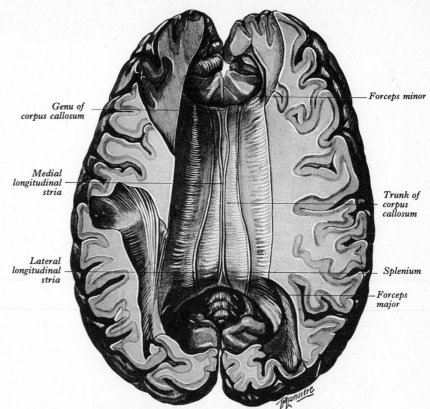

7.139 The corpus callosum, superior aspect, revealed by partial removal and dissection of the cerebral hemispheres.

## The Corpus Callosum

The corpus callosum is the great transverse commissure which connects the cerebral hemispheres and incidentally roofs in the lateral ventricles. Its development in mammals is proportional to the relative volume of the neocortex and is maximal in man.[863] A good conception of its position and size is obtained by examining a median sagittal section of the brain (7.110,114). It forms an arched structure about 10 cm in length, its anterior end being about 4 cm from the frontal poles and its posterior end about 6 cm from the occipital poles of the hemispheres.

The *genu*, which forms the anterior end, inclines postero-inferiorly in front of the septum pellucidum and, diminishing rapidly in thickness, is prolonged posteriorly to the upper end of the lamina terminalis as the *rostrum*. The trunk arches back, convex above, to terminate posteriorly in the *splenium*, which is the thickest part of the corpus callosum.

[850] P. Bailey and G. von Bonin, *The Isocortex of Man*, University of Illinois Press, Urbana. 1951.
[851] W. E. Le G. Clark and W. R. Russell, *J. Anat.*, **73**, 1939.
[852] S. Locke, *J. comp. Neurol.*, **129**, 1967.
[853] M. J. C. Showers and E. W. Lauer, *J. comp. Neurol.*, **117**, 1961.
[854] W. Penfield and T. Rasmussen, *The Cerebral Cortex of Man*, Macmillan, New York. 1950.
[855] B. R. Kaada, in: *Handbook of Physiology*, Sect. 1, Vol. II, eds. J. Field, H. Magoun and V. F. Hall, American Physiological Society, Washington, D.C. 1960.
[856] R. Druckman, *Brain*, **75**, 1952.
[857] A. A. P. Leao, *J. Neurophysiol.*, **7**, 1944.
[858] M. J. C. Showers, *J. comp. Neurol.*, **112**, 1959.
[859] M. J. C. Showers and E. C. Crosby, *Neurology, Minneap.*, **8**, 1958.
[860] P. M. Tow and C. W. M. Whitty, *J. Neurol. Neurosurg. Psychiat.*, **16**, 1953.
[861] P. Glees, J. Cole, C. W. M. Whitty and H. Cairns, *J. Neurol. Neurosurg. Psychiat.*, **13**, 1950.
[862] E. L. Foltz and L. E. White, *J. Neurosurg.*, **19**, 1962.
[863] P. Rakic and P. I. Yakovlev, *J. comp. Neurol.*, **132**, 1968.

The superior surface of the *trunk* of the corpus callosum (7.139) is covered by a thin grey layer, the *indusium griseum* which extends round the genu to the inferior surface of the rostrum to become continuous with the paraterminal gyrus, and in it are embedded two fine longitudinal bundles of fibres on each side, which are termed the medial and lateral longitudinal striae (p. 938); posteriorly the indusium griseum is continuous with the dentate gyrus and the hippocampus through the gyrus fasciolaris (7.140).

In the median plane the trunk of the corpus callosum forms the floor of the longitudinal fissure, and is related to the anterior cerebral vessels and to the lower border of the falx cerebri, which may come into actual contact with it posteriorly (8.31). On each side of the median plane the trunk is overlapped by the gyrus cinguli, from which it is separated by the slit-like callosal sulcus.

The inferior surface of the trunk is concave in its long axis and convex from side to side. In the median plane, the septum pellucidum is attached to it anteriorly,

The *splenium* overhangs the posterior ends of the thalami, the pineal body and the tectum of the midbrain. It is, however, separated from them by a number of structures. On each side of the median plane the crus of the fornix and the gyrus fasciolaris (7.140) curve upwards to reach the splenium. The crus of the fornix continues forwards on the inferior surface of the trunk, but the gyrus fasciolaris passes round the splenium, rapidly tapering off and fading away into the indusium griseum. In the median plane, the tela choroidea of the third ventricle passes forwards below the splenium through the transverse fissure, and the internal cerebral veins emerge from between its two layers and unite to form the great cerebral vein. Above, the splenium is covered with the indusium griseum and is related to the falx cerebri and the inferior sagittal sinus in the median plane, and to the cingulate gyrus on each side. Posteriorly the splenium is related to the free margin of the tentorium cerebelli, the great cerebral vein and the beginning of the straight sinus.

The nerve fibres of the corpus callosum radiate into the

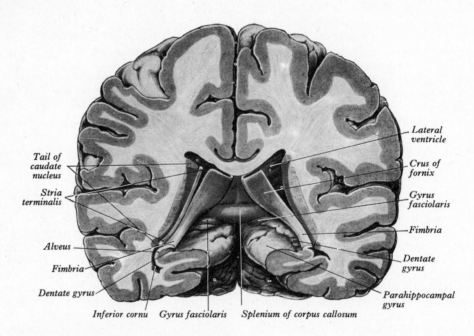

Tail of
caudate
nucleus

Stria
terminalis

Alveus

Fimbria

Dentate gyrus

Inferior cornu    Gyrus fasciolaris

Lateral
ventricle

Crus of
fornix

Gyrus
fasciolaris

Fimbria

Dentate
gyrus

Parahippocampal
gyrus

Splenium of corpus callosum

7.140 Anterior aspect of a coronal section of the cerebrum from which the posterior parts of the thalami have been removed to reveal the splenium and parts of the limbic system. (Note that the dentate gyrus is not equally exposed on the two sides.)

to an extent which depends on the length of the septum (7.110). Posteriorly it is fused with the body of the fornix and the commissure of the fornix. On each side of the median plane, the inferior surface of the trunk forms the roof of the lateral ventricle (7.141) and is covered with the ventricular ependyma.

The *genu* is continuous above with the trunk and below with the rostrum. Its anterior surface, which is related to the anterior cerebral vessels, is covered with the indusium griseum and the longitudinal striae. To its posterior surface is attached the septum pellucidum in the median plane, and on each side it forms the anterior wall of the anterior horn of the lateral ventricle.

The *rostrum* connects the genu to the upper end of the lamina terminalis. In the median plane its superior surface is attached to the septum pellucidum and, on each side, forms the narrow floor of the anterior horn of the lateral ventricle (7.155). On the inferior surface of the rostrum the indusium griseum and the longitudinal striae are carried backwards to the upper end of the paraterminal gyrus.

white core of the hemisphere on each side and disperse to various parts of the cerebral cortex. The rostral fibres extend laterally below the anterior cornua of the lateral ventricles, and connect the orbital surfaces of the two frontal lobes. The fibres of the genu curve forwards and connect the lateral and medial surfaces of the two frontal lobes, as the *forceps minor*. The fibres of the trunk pass laterally and intersect the projection fibres of the corona radiata (7.98). They connect wide cortical areas of the two hemispheres to one another. Those fibres of the trunk and of the splenium which together form the roof and lateral wall of the posterior horn and the lateral wall of the inferior horn of the ventricle constitute the *tapetum* (p. 970). The remaining fibres of the splenium curve backwards and medially into the occipital lobes as the *forceps major*. This large bundle of fibres bulges into the superior part of the medial wall of the posterior horn of the ventricle and forms a curved elevation which is termed the *bulb of the posterior horn*.

Despite the great size of the corpus callosum and the enormous number of commissural fibres that it contains, limited information is available concerning its functional significance, apart from the obvious inference that it links the two hemispheres together and appears to ensure that they act as a single entity. The number of fibres is unknown in man, but in the cat there are 700,000 in each square millimetre.[864] The precise linkages effected by these commissural fibres have not been defined, except in the visual area and the postcentral gyrus.[865] In the somatic sensory areas (SmI and SmII) the connexions are limited to the same area on the opposite side, and the right and left loci concerned with the hand and foot appear to lack such commissural connexion. Where commissural linkages occur they are considered to be highly specific, associating 'corresponding' columnar cortical units in bilateral functions.

'hand area' project commissural fibres, these interhemispheric exchanges of information must first involve transfer from these areas to adjoining parts of the cortex which are so linked. Studies such as these on 'split brain' primates have received interesting corroboration from observation of the effects of callosal division as a means of treatment of some forms of epilepsy in mankind. Contrary to earlier opinions (*vide supra*), profound effects follow extensive interruption of the corpus callosum, though these can only be detected by careful testing. It becomes apparent, for example, that while comprehension of an object can be achieved by both hemispheres, verbal expression of it can only be carried out through the mediation of the *dominant*—usually the left—hemisphere. For further details see footnote references [870, 871].

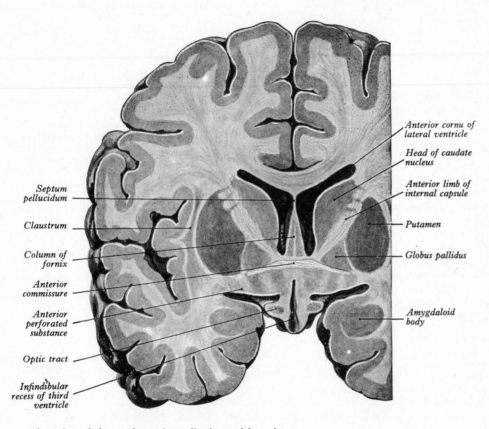

Anterior cornu of lateral ventricle

Head of caudate nucleus

Anterior limb of internal capsule

Putamen

Globus pallidus

Amygdaloid body

Septum pellucidum

Claustrum

Column of fornix

Anterior commissure

Anterior perforated substance

Optic tract

Infindibular recess of third ventricle

**7.141** A coronal section of the cerebrum immediately caudal to the optic chiasma and passing through the anterior commissure.

Cases of complete congenital absence of the corpus callosum are recorded from time to time—the condition is a rare one—but the defect is usually found at autopsy, and the clinical history does not show any characteristic feature which can lead to certain diagnosis during life.[866] In recent years large portions, and in some cases the whole, of the corpus callosum have been divided as a surgical approach with surprisingly little disturbance of function.[867] Subsequently, experimental studies involving the division of the forebrain commissures have demonstrated impairment of the interhemispheric communication concerned in learning processes.[868] Thus, learning reactions in cats (first subjected to midline division of the chiasma) which had been established with one eye, were carried out equally well with the other eye alone, indicating that a transfer of information from one hemisphere to the other had occurred. Transection of the splenial part of the corpus callosum abolished this transfer. Similar observations have been made in chimpanzees,[869] in experiments involving the aquisition of manual skills. Since neither the striate cortex nor the

**The anterior commissure** is described on p. 937, and the *commissure of the fornix* (hippocampal commissure) on p. 942.

## THE SEPTUM PELLUCIDUM

The septum pellucidum is a thin vertical partition (7.110, 114), consisting of two laminae, separated throughout a greater or lesser part of their extent by a narrow interval,

[864] R. E. Myers, *Archs Neurol. Psychiat., Chicago*, **1**, 1959.

[865] E. G. Jones and T. P. S. Powell, *Brain*, **92**, 1969.

[866] F. Unterharnscheidt, D. Jachnik and H. Gött, *Der Balkenmangel. Monographie aus dem Gesamtgebiete der Neurologie und Psychiatrie*, Heft **128**, Springer, Berlin. 1968.

[867] A. J. Akelaitis, *Archs Neurol. Psychiat., Chicago*, **4**, 1942.

[868] C. R. Butler, *Nature, Lond.*, **209**, 1966.

[869] R. E. Myers and C. O. Henson, *Archs Neurol. Psychiat., Chicago*, **3**, 1960.

[870] R. W. Sperry, in: *Brain and Conscious Experience*, ed. J. C. Eccles Springer, Berlin. 1966.

[871] M. S. Gazzaniga and R. W. Sperry, *Brain*, **90**, 1967.

termed the *cavity of the septum pellucidum*, which does not communicate with the ventricles of the brain. The septum is triangular in form, with its base in front and its apex behind. It is attached above to the inferior surface of the trunk of the corpus callosum; below and behind, to the anterior part of the fornix; below and in front to the upper surface of the rostrum of the corpus callosum. The lateral surface of each lamina takes part in the formation of the

medial wall of the anterior horn and central part of the lateral ventricle (7.141), and is therefore covered with ependyma.

The laminae contain both grey and white matter, and for what is known of its connexions see the account of the *septal areas* (p. 937) and the *dorsal fornix* (p. 942). The development of the septum pellucidum is referred to on p. 140.

# INTERNAL STRUCTURE OF THE CEREBRAL HEMISPHERES

In the interior of the hemispheres are the lateral ventricles, the basal nuclei and many fibre tracts, both projection and intrinsic.

## The Lateral Ventricles

The two lateral ventricles (7.142, 143, 144) are irregular cavities situated in the lower and medial parts of the cerebral hemispheres, one on each side of the median plane. They are almost completely separated from each other by the *septum pellucidum*, but each communicates with the third ventricle and indirectly with the other through the *interventricular foramen* (p. 919). They are lined with ependyma and contain cerebrospinal fluid, which, even in health, is secreted in considerable amounts. Each lateral ventricle consists of a *central part* and three *cornua* or *horns*, anterior, posterior and inferior (7.143, 144, 145).

**The central part** (7.144) of the lateral ventricle extends from the interventricular foramen to the splenium of the corpus callosum. It is a curved cavity with a roof, floor and medial wall; on transverse section it is triangular anteriorly and rectangular posteriorly. The *roof* is the inferior surface of the corpus callosum; the *floor*, which is concave superomedially, is formed by the follow-

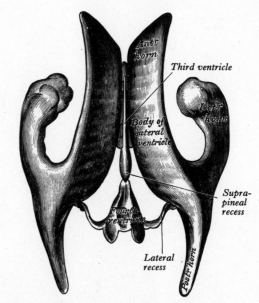

7.143A   A drawing of a cast of the ventricular cavities. Superior aspect. (Retzius.) Note that where the lateral recess joins the fourth ventricle, the lateral dorsal recesses of the roof of the ventricle project dorsally on each side beyond the posterior margin of the median dorsal recess  The superior angle of the fourth ventricle and the aqueduct of the midbrain are hidden by the suprapineal recess.

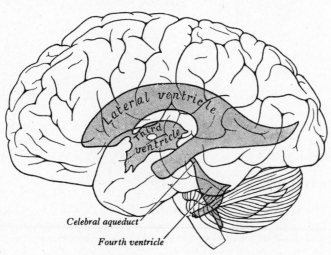

7.142   Projection of the ventricles on to the left surface of the brain.

ing in lateromedial order: the caudate nucleus, the stria terminalis, the thalamostriate vein, and the lateral portion of the upper surface of the thalamus. The caudate nucleus becomes rapidly narrower as it is traced backwards in the floor, and its long axis is directed laterally as well as posteriorly. The stria terminalis, a small bundle of white fibres (p. 937), and the thalamostriate vein occupy a narrow groove which follows the medial border of the

caudate nucleus and separates it from the lateral margin of the superior surface of the thalamus. The latter may be almost entirely hidden by the choroid plexus, which invaginates the ependyma into the cavity through the slit-like interval between the edge of the fornix and the upper surface of the thalamus. This ependymal invagination constitutes the *choroid fissure*. The body of the fornix becomes wider as it is traced backwards, and its thin, lateral margin lies parallel with the groove for the stria terminalis.

The *medial wall* is formed by the posterior part of the septum pellucidum with the body of the fornix in its lower margin. Posteriorly, where the septum pellucidum ends, the roof and the floor meet one another on the medial wall.

**The anterior cornu** (7.141, 142) passes forwards, laterally and slightly downwards, into the frontal lobe. It is continuous behind with the central part at the interventricular foramen. In a coronal section it appears as a triangular slit below the anterior part of the corpus callosum, and it is bounded anteriorly by the posterior surface of the genu and rostrum of the corpus callosum. The *roof* is formed by the anterior part of the trunk of the corpus callosum. The greater part of the *floor* is formed by the rounded head of the caudate nucleus, but, in its medial portion, a small part is formed by the upper surface of the rostrum of the corpus callosum (7.155). The *medial boundary* is formed by the septum pellucidum containing the column of the fornix in its posterior edge.

968

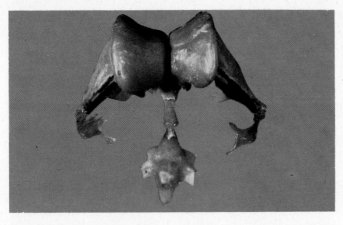

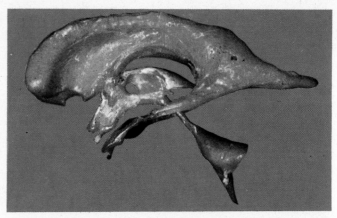

7.143 B and C   Resin casts of the ventricular system of the human brain prepared by Dr. D. H. Tompsett of the Royal College of Surgeons of England. B   Ventral view; C   Left lateral view. Compare with the superior aspect shown in 7.143 A.

**The posterior cornu** curves backwards and medially into the occipital lobe. Its development is very variable and frequently asymmetrical; it may be absent. Its *roof* and *lateral wall* are formed by fibres of the tapetum of the corpus callosum, which separate them from the optic radiation (p. 975). The splenial fibres which constitute the forceps major pass medial to the posterior horn as they sweep backwards into the occipital lobe. In this part of their course they produce a rounded ridge, the *bulb* of the posterior cornu, in the upper part of the *medial wall*. Below

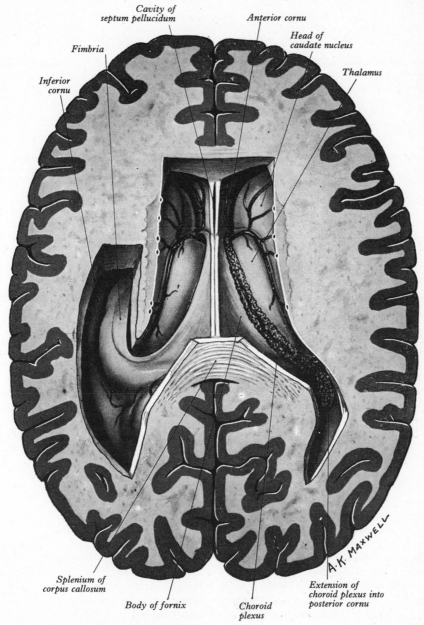

7.144   Horizontal section of the cerebrum dissected to remove the roofs of the lateral ventricles.

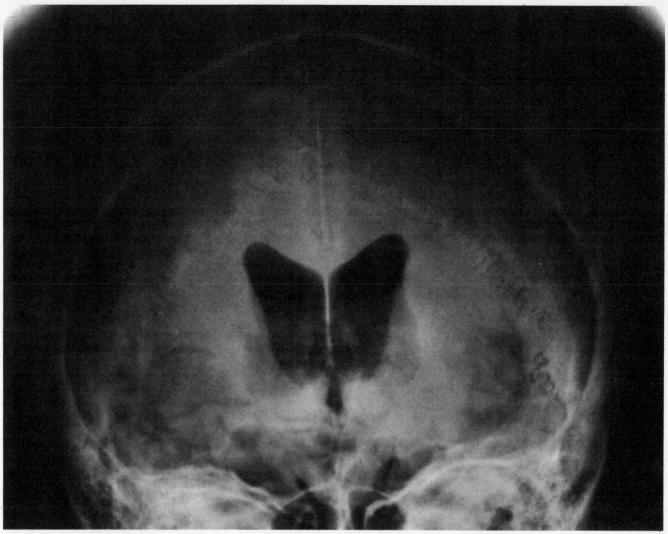

7.145 Anteroposterior radiograph of the head after the introduction of air into the ventricular system of the brain. The outlines of the bodies and anterior horns of both ventricles are separated in the sagittal plane by the shadow of the septum pellucidum; directly inferior to the latter, the outline of the third ventricle can be seen. (Kindly provided by Dr. R. D. Hoare, Dept. of Diagnostic Radiology, Guy's Hospital.)

the bulb, a second elevation may be identified on the medial wall. It is the *calcar avis*, and it corresponds to the infolded cortex of the anterior part of the calcarine sulcus (7.146). Posteriorly the lateral and medial walls meet each other.

**The inferior cornu** (7.144, 147), the largest of the three, traverses the temporal lobe, forming in its course a curve round the posterior end of the thalamus. At first it descends posterolaterally and then curves anteriorly to within 2·5 cm of the temporal pole close to the uncus, its position being fairly well indicated on the surface of the brain by the superior temporal sulcus. A needle introduced at a trephine hole, the centre of which is placed 3 cm behind and 3 cm above the centre of the external acoustic meatus, and passed in the direction of the tip of the opposite auricle, enters the inferior cornu at a depth of 5 cm from the surface.

The *roof* of the inferior cornu is formed chiefly by the inferior surface of the tapetum of the corpus callosum, but the tail of the caudate nucleus and the stria terminalis also extend forwards in the roof, at the extremity of which they are continuous with the amygdaloid body. Its *floor* consists of the collateral eminence laterally and the hippocampus medially; the surface of the latter is covered by the alveus giving rise to the fimbria of the hippocampus, which becomes continuous posteriorly with the crus of the fornix (p. 942). Between the stria terminalis and the fimbria is the inferior, or temporal, part of the choroid

fissure, through which the lower part of the choroid plexus of the lateral ventrical invaginates the ependyma closing the fissure. The choroid plexus covers the upper surface of the hippocampus.

The fimbria and the hippocampus have already been considered (pp. 942 and 938), and a full description of the choroid plexus will be found on p. 980.

The *collateral eminence* (7.147) is an elongated swelling lying lateral to and parallel with the hippocampus. It corresponds with the middle part of the collateral sulcus, and its size depends on the depth and direction of this sulcus. It is continuous behind with a flattened triangular area, named the *collateral trigone*, which forms the floor of the ventricle between the posterior and inferior cornua. The capacity of the lateral ventricles (and the other chambers of the system) can be estimated by anatomical and radiological techniques.[872]

## The Nerve Fibres of the Cerebrum

If the upper parts of the hemisphere be sliced off about 1·25 cm above the corpus callosum, the central white substance of the hemisphere is seen as an oval area surrounded by a narrow convoluted margin of grey matter, and studded with red dots (puncta vasculosa) produced

970

[872] W. Weintraub, *Thèse de l'Université de Genève*, Paris. 1953.

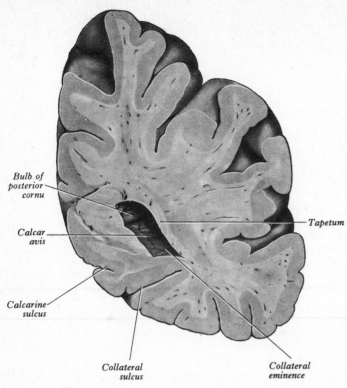

Bulb of
posterior
cornu

Calcar
avis

Tapetum

Calcarine
sulcus

Collateral
sulcus

Collateral
eminence

7.146   Anterior aspect of a coronal section through the posterior cornu of the left lateral ventricle.

by the escape of blood from divided blood vessels. If the hemispheres be sliced off at the level of the corpus callosum, its nerve fibres will be seen in continuity with the white matter of the hemisphere on each side. The white matter contains many myelinated fibres, of varying size, supported by neuroglia. These fibres may be divided, according to their course and connexions, into three systems: (1) The *commissural fibres* connect the two hemispheres to each other, linking corresponding or *homotopic* loci, and also *heterotopic* loci. (2) The *arcuate fibres* connect different cortical areas of the same hemisphere to one another; some of them are collaterals of the projection and commissural fibres, but the majority are independent

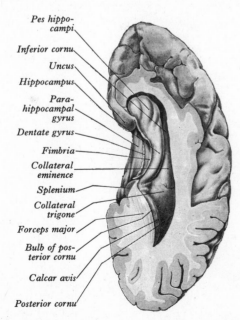

Pes hippo-
campi

Inferior cornu

Uncus

Hippocampus

Para-
hippocampal
gyrus

Dentate gyrus

Fimbria

Collateral
eminence

Splenium

Collateral
trigone

Forceps major

Bulb of pos-
terior cornu

Calcar avis

Posterior cornu

7.147   The posterior and inferior cornua of the right lateral ventricle, exposed from above.

axons. (3) The *projection fibres* connect the cerebral cortex with the grey matter of the brainstem and the spinal cord in both directions.

(1) **The commissural fibres** have already been considered (pp. 901, 937, 942, 965).

(2) **The arcuate (association) fibres** (7.148, 149), which are all ipsilateral, are of two kinds: short arcuate fibres, connecting adjacent gyri to one another; long arcuate fibres, connecting more widely separated gyri to one another. Details of many individual association pathways have already been given in the section on cortical areas.

The *short arcuate fibres* may be intracortical or they may lie immediately beneath the cortex and connect adjacent gyri, some merely passing from one wall of a sulcus to the other.

The *long arcuate fibres* group themselves, somewhat indistinctly, into bundles, which can be dissected in the formalin-hardened brain after the cortex and the subjacent short arcuate fibres have been removed. The fibres in each fasciculus show considerable variation in length, and the longest are always situated in the deepest part of the bundle. Concerning the precise connexions of these fibre bundles very little accurate information is at present available, for histological methods are unable to demonstrate them throughout the whole of their length. The following fasciculi can be distinguished: (*a*) the uncinate fasciculus; (*b*) the cingulum; (*c*) the superior longitudinal fasciculus; (*d*) the inferior longitudinal fasciculus; (*e*) the fronto-occipital fasciculus.

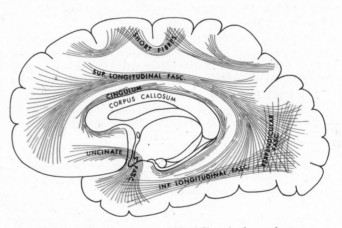

7.148   The principal arcuate (association) fibres in the cerebrum.

(*a*) The *uncinate fasciculus* connects the first motor speech area (p. 956) and the gyri on the orbital surface of the frontal lobe with the cortex of the temporal pole and the area immediately adjoining. The fibres follow a sharply curved course and cross the floor of the stem of the lateral sulcus. They are related to the antero-inferior part of the insular area (7.148, 149).

(*b*) The *cingulum* is a long, curved bundle which commences on the medial surface of the hemisphere below the rostrum of the corpus callosum. It lies within the gyrus cinguli and so follows the curve of that gyrus. Inferiorly it enters the parahippocampal gyrus and spreads out so as to reach the adjoining parts of the temporal lobe. Along its convexity fibres enter and leave it in groups, giving it a spiked irregular appearance.

(*c*) The *superior longitudinal fasciculus* is the largest of all the arcuate fibre bundles. It commences in the anterior part of the frontal region and arches backwards above the insular area and lateral to the lower part of the corona radiata (p. 973). After giving off a number of fibres to the occipital cortex (areas 18 and 19), it curves downwards

971

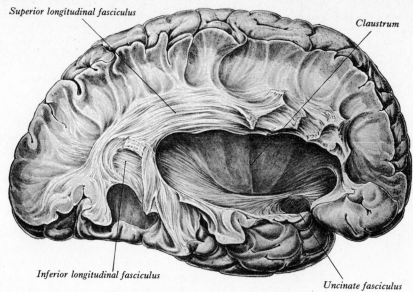

**7.149**  A dissection showing some of the long arcuate fasciculi of the right cerebral hemisphere.

and forwards behind the insular area and spreads out into the temporal lobe. Like the other long arcuate fasciculi, it constantly receives new fibres throughout its whole extent and gives off fibres to the adjoining cortex. Its constituent fibres are so intermingled that it is quite impossible to determine their precise connexions by gross methods (7.149) and for this purpose the dissecting microscope is of no real help.

(d) The *inferior longitudinal fasciculus* commences near the occipital pole and its fibres are derived chiefly from areas 18 and 19. They sweep forwards, separated from the posterior horn of the lateral ventricle by the fibres of the optic radiation and the commissural fibres of the tapetum, and after being crossed by the superior longitudinal fasciculus, they are distributed throughout the temporal lobe.

(e) The *fronto-occipital fasciculus* commences at the frontal pole and passes backwards on a deeper plane than the superior longitudinal fasciculus and separated from it by the lower part of the corona radiata (*vide infra*). It associates itself with the lateral border of the caudate nucleus, and is therefore closely related to the central part of the lateral ventricle. Posteriorly its fibres radiate into the occipital and temporal lobes in a fan-shaped manner, passing lateral to the posterior and inferior horns, and intersecting and mingling with the fibres of the tapetum of the corpus callosum.

The above details are almost entirely based upon the appearances of blunt dissection of the white substance of the cerebrum. Accurate knowledge of the origins and terminations of association fibres can only be established by experimental studies, which have not been carried out

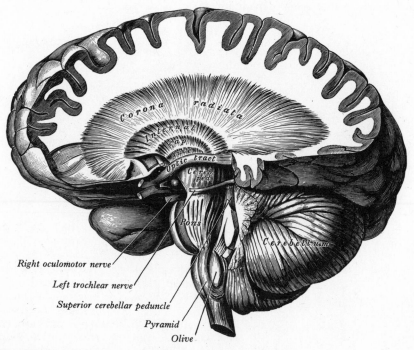

**7.150A**  A dissection showing the convergence of cortical projection fibres through the corona radiata into the cerebral peduncle and pons.

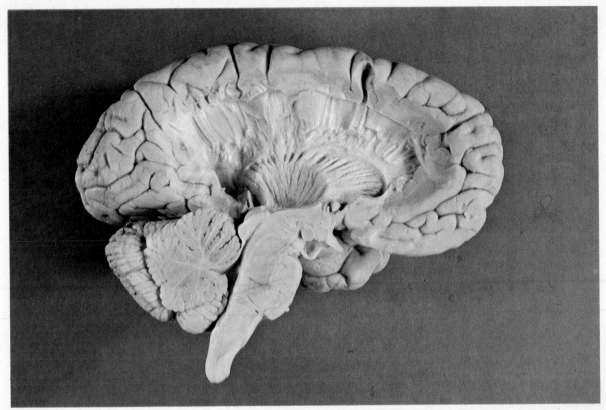

7.150 B After median sagittal section of the brain, the left cerebral hemisphere has been dissected from its *medial* aspect to display the fibre bundles of the corona radiata and internal capsule. This entailed the removal of the cingulate gyrus and subjacent white matter, much of the paramedian corpus callosum and fornix, the dorsal thalamus, and the head and body of the caudate nucleus. The oval depression previously occupied by the dorsal thalamus can clearly be seen within the curved depression left after removal of the caudate nucleus. (Dissection by Dr. Andrew Seal, Dept. of Anatomy, Guy's Hospital Medical School, London.)

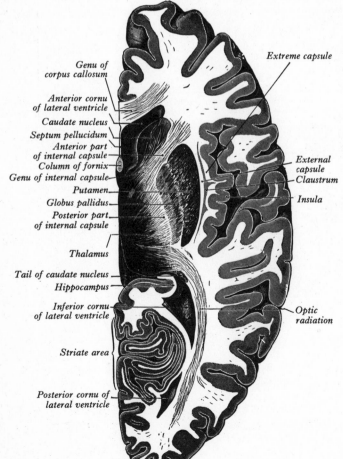

7.151 Superior aspect of a horizontal section through the right cerebral hemisphere.

*Labels (clockwise/top to bottom):*
Genu of corpus callosum
Anterior cornu of lateral ventricle
Caudate nucleus
Septum pellucidum
Anterior part of internal capsule
Column of fornix
Genu of internal capsule
Putamen
Globus pallidus
Posterior part of internal capsule
Thalamus
Tail of caudate nucleus
Hippocampus
Inferior cornu of lateral ventricle
Striate area
Posterior cornu of lateral ventricle
Extreme capsule
External capsule
Claustrum
Insula
Optic radiation

for most regions of the cortex. Studies of the visual areas[873] and the main somatic sensory areas (SmI)[874] suggest a high degree of specificity in such connexions.

(3) **The projection fibres** connect the cerebral cortex with the lower parts of the brain (including the diencephalon) and the spinal cord, and include both *corticofugal* and *corticopetal* fibres.

The projection fibres converge from all directions on the corpus striatum (7.150). For the most part they are internal to arcuate fibres, and they intersect the commissural fibres of the corpus callosum and the anterior commissure. At the periphery of the corpus striatum, they form the *corona radiata*. The medial aspect of the corona radiata is separated from the lateral ventricle by the fronto-occipital fasciculus, and its lateral aspect is covered by the superior longitudinal fasciculus. Below, the corona radiata is directly continuous with the internal capsule, a thick, curved band of white matter which comprises all the projection fibres, and which cuts into the corpus striatum, dividing it almost completely into two parts, the lentiform and the caudate nuclei.

## The Internal Capsule

In horizontal section through the cerebral hemisphere the internal capsule is a broad band of white fibres, bent with a lateral concavity, which accommodates itself to the convex medial surface of the lentiform nucleus (7.151, 152, 153, 154). It can be divided into an *anterior limb*, a *genu*, a *posterior limb*, a *retrolentiform part* and a *sublentiform part*. The anterior limb is interposed between the

[873] W. E. Le G. Clark, *J. Anat.*, **75**, 1941.
[874] E. G. Jones and T. P. S. Powell, *Brain Res.*, **9**, 1968.

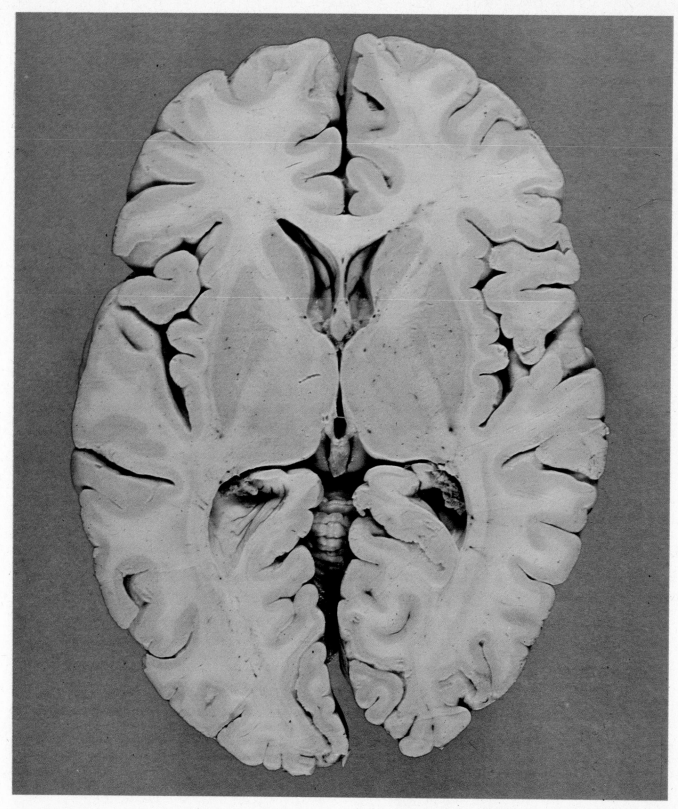

**7.152** A horizontal section through the brain including the frontal and occipital poles of the cerebral hemispheres. Features appearing on this section are discussed at many points throughout the text. For appropriate labelling compare with **7.151**. (Dissection by Dr. E. L. Rees.)

lentiform nucleus on the lateral side and the head of the caudate nucleus on the medial side. The posterior limb has the thalamus on its medial side and the lentiform nucleus on its lateral side. The fibres of the internal capsule continue to converge as they pass downwards, and at the same time the frontal fibres tend to pass backwards and medially, while the temporal and occipital fibres pass forwards and laterally. At the lower limit of the lentiform nucleus, they are crossed by the optic tract and enter the midbrain. The corticofugal fibres enter the crus cerebri,

where the frontal fibres are placed to the medial side and the temporal, parietal and occipital fibres to the lateral side. What follows is a simplified account of the fibre constitution of the internal capsule. A number of other fibre 'systems' are described at points throughout the section on the telencephalon.

The *anterior limb* of the internal capsule contains *frontopontine fibres*, which arise in the cortex of the frontal lobe and synapse about the cells of the nuclei pontis, the axons of which pass to the cerebellar hemisphere of the opposite side. In addition there are the fibres of the anterior thalamic radiation which interconnect the medial and anterior nuclei of the thalamus and the cortex of the frontal lobe.

The *genu* contains the corticonuclear fibres which arise mainly from area 4 of the cerebral cortex and terminate in the motor nuclei of the cranial nerves to the head, mostly of the opposite side. The most anterior fibres of the superior thalamic radiation interconnecting the thalamus and cerebral cortex also extend into the genu.

The *posterior limb* includes the corticospinal tract disposed in scattered bundles, with the fibres concerned with the innervation of the upper limb anteriorly followed by those to the trunk and lower limbs. Other descending fibres here include frontopontine fibres from the frontal lobe, in particular areas 4 and 6, corticorubral fibres from the frontal lobe to the red nucleus and fibres from the globus pallidus contained in the subthalamic fasciculus. The majority of this portion of the internal capsule con-

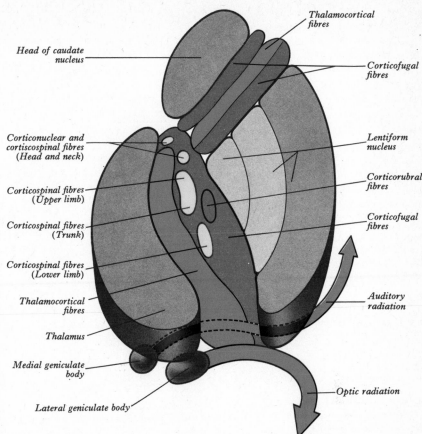

7.154 Diagram of the main components of the internal capsule. Descending motor fibres are shown in yellow, corticofugal fibres to the thalamus and pons, etc. in red, and ascending fibres in blue. (From Strong and Elwyn's *Human Neuroanatomy*—see Bibliography for details.)

tains fibres of the superior thalamic radiation carrying general sensory impulses from the ventral thalamic nuclei to the postcentral gyrus. (For a survey of the posterior limb in the human brain consult reference [875].)

In the *retrolentiform part* are parietopontine and occipitopontine fibres and fibres from the occipital cortex to the superior colliculus and pretectal region. In addition there is the posterior thalamic radiation which includes the optic radiation, and interconnexions between the cortices of the occipital and parietal lobes and the caudal portions of the thalamus, especially the pulvinar.

The fibres of the *optic radiation* arise in the lateral geniculate body and sweep backwards in the angle between the central part and inferior horn of the lateral ventricle. In their course they are intimately related to the superior and lateral surfaces of the inferior horn and lateral surface of the posterior horn of the lateral ventricle, being separated from the latter by the tapetum.

The *sublentiform part* contains the temporopontine and some parietopontine fibres, and the acoustic radiation running from the medial geniculate body to the superior temporal and transverse temporal gyri (areas 41 and 42). There are also a few fibres interconnecting the thalamus with the cortex of the temporal lobe and insula.

The fibres of the *acoustic radiation* sweep forwards and laterally below and behind the lentiform nucleus to reach the cortex.

The connexions between the cortex and the thalamus are discussed on p. 900; corticohypothalamic connexions on p. 907; corticostriate connexions on p. 978.

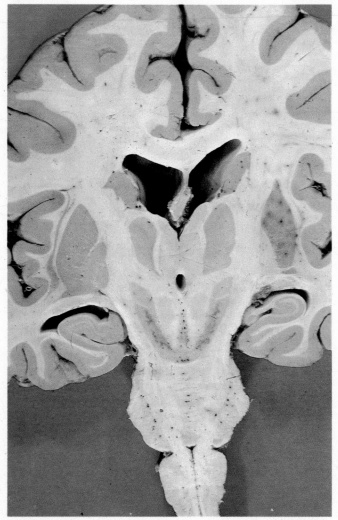

7.153 The central area of the ventral part of the oblique coronal section of the brain shown in 7.95, photographed at higher magnification to show some structural features in greater detail; compare with 7.98 for appropriate labelling. Note in particular: (1) the anterior, medial and lateral parts of the dorsal thalamus, separated by the internal medullary laminae; (2) the relation of the caudate nucleus to the anterior and inferior horns of the lateral ventricle; (3) the lentiform nucleus, divided into an external putamen and an internal globus pallidus; the latter again divided into internal and external parts; (4) the internal capsule, external capsule, claustrum, extreme capsule and insular cortex; (5) the sectioned profiles of the subthalamic and red nuclei, and the substantia nigra; (6) the hippocampus projecting into the floor of the inferior horn of the lateral ventricle. Other structural features on this section are discussed at many points throughout the text. Compare also with 7.152. (Dissection by Dr. E. L. Rees.)

[875] M. C. Smith, in: *Modern Trends in Neurology*, ed. D. Williams, Butterworths, London. 1967.

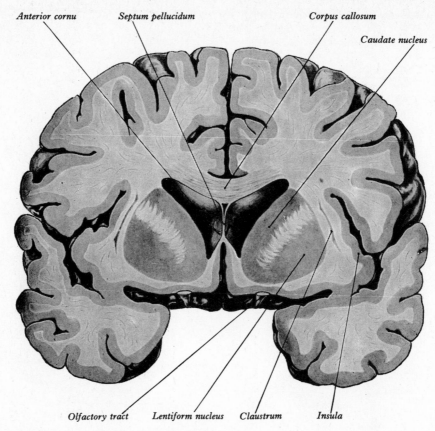

*Anterior cornu*    *Septum pellucidum*    *Corpus callosum*

*Caudate nucleus*

*Olfactory tract*    *Lentiform nucleus*    *Claustrum*    *Insula*

**7.155**   Posterior aspect of a coronal section through the anterior cornua of the lateral ventricles.

## The Basal Nuclei

Situated within each cerebral hemisphere is a series of subcortical nuclear masses of grey matter often loosely grouped under the general term *basal nuclei*. Unfortunately, the structures included vary between workers; but most commonly the term includes the amygdaloid complex, the claustrum, the caudate nucleus and the lentiform nucleus (7.141, 151, 152, 153). These topographical structures are a heterogeneous group with respect to their structural and functional associations and phylogenetic history. Accordingly, a large and often confusing terminology has been generated by different investigators, the various structure being subdivided and regrouped in many different ways. The array of terminologies will not be discussed at length, but some of the more commonly used alternatives are mentioned briefly here. (For a recent critical review of the basal ganglia see footnote reference [876].)

The *amygdaloid body* (amygdaloid nuclear complex, amygdala, or *archistriatum*) is discussed elsewhere in relation to the limbic system (p. 936).

The *claustrum*, a tenuous sheet of grey matter, surrounded by laminae of white matter which separate it from the deep surface of the insula and the external surface of the lentiform nucleus, is further mentioned below.

The *caudate nucleus* and *lentiform nucleus* are commonly grouped together as the *corpus striatum*. The lentiform nucleus is divided into an internal *globus pallidus* and an external *putamen*, which are structurally distinct. The putamen resembles the caudate nucleus in its structure, and together they constitute the *neostriatum*, frequently termed simply the *striatum*. When used in this manner, therefore, striatofugal fibres are those which leave the caudate nucleus or putamen for other destinations, whilst afferents, denoted with the suffix -striate (e.g. thalamo-striate), are those passing to the putamen or caudate nucleus, and not to the *corpus* striatum as a whole. (The terms will be used in the manner just described in this account, but it must be realized that some neuroanatomists refer to the whole corpus striatum when they use these terms, and in other cases, the intended meaning is by no means clear.)

The *globus pallidus* or *paleostriatum* is often referred to simply as the *pallidum*, and hence such terms as pallidal afferents or pallidofugal fibres.

### GENERAL TOPOGRAPHY

**The caudate nucleus** is an arcuate mass of grey matter, which has already been noted in the floor of the anterior cornu and central part of the lateral ventricle and the roof of the inferior cornu (7.141, 144, 151, 152, 153, 156). Its anterosuperior end is massive and termed the *head*. At the interventricular foramen this narrows into the *body* of the nucleus which tapers imperceptibly into the *tail*. The nucleus projects into the floor of the anterior cornu and central part of the lateral ventricle and is continued round into the roof of the inferior cornu of the lateral ventricle, merging at its anterior and lower extremity with the amygdaloid body. In all parts of the ventricle it is covered by ependyma. In the central part and inferior cornu of the lateral ventricle the stria terminalis lies along the medial border of the caudate nucleus. In the central part of the ventricle the stria terminalis lies with the thalamostriate vein in the groove between the caudate nucleus and the thalamus. In the inferior cornu it forms the upper border of the lower part of the choroid fissure.

In the anterior cornu and central part of the lateral

976

[876] F. A. Mettler, in: *Handbook of Clinical Neurology*, eds. P. J. Vinken and G. W. Bruyn, North Holland Publishing Co., Amsterdam. 1968.

ventricle the lateral margin of the caudate nucleus is related to the corpus callosum, being separated from it by the fronto-occipital arcuate bundle (p. 972) and the sub-callosal fasciculus (p. 978). The lateral surface of the nucleus is flat and in contact with the internal capsule. At its anterior end the head of the caudate nucleus is fused below with the putamen of the lentiform nucleus just above the anterior perforated substance. Above this junction strands of grey matter traverse the anterior limb of the internal capsule and connect the putamen of the lentiform nucleus with the head of the caudate nucleus. The striped appearance which this region presents gives origin to the term corpus striatum.

In the inferior cornu of the lateral ventricle the tail curves forwards behind and below the fibres of the internal capsule entering the crus cerebri; these separate it from the thalamus which lies above and medially. Above, the sublentiform part of the internal capsule and fibres from the external capsule separate the tail from the globus pallidus.

**The lentiform nucleus** is shaped like a biconvex lens, but the curvature of its medial surface is sharper than the curvature of its lateral surface (**7**.102, 141, 151, 152, 153, 156). Cut in section, it is seen to consist of two portions, which differ from each other in their colour. The larger lateral portion, which is dark in colour, is termed the *putamen*; the smaller medial portion is of a lighter tint, and is termed the *globus pallidus*.

The lentiform nucleus is completely buried in the substance of the hemisphere. Laterally it is covered by a thin layer of white matter which constitutes the *external capsule*. This sheet is covered on its lateral side by the *claustrum*, which intervenes between it and the subcortical white matter of the insula. Medially the lentiform nucleus is in relation to the internal capsule, which separates it from the thalamus behind, and from the head of the caudate nucleus in front. Round its anterior, superior and posterior margins the nucleus is related to the corona radiata. The inferior part of the lentiform nucleus is deeply grooved by the anterior commissure as it passes backwards and laterally into the temporal lobe (**7**.141), and anteriorly it is continuous with the head of the caudate nucleus. A little in front of the groove, the grey matter of the corpus striatum is continuous with that of the anterior perforated substance, and the lateral striate arteries, which enter the brain at this site, run laterally and then turn upwards in close contact with the lateral surface of the lentiform nucleus, before they pierce its substance. The lentiform nucleus lies above the inferior cornu of the lateral ventricle and is separated from it by the fibres of the external capsule as they pass medially towards the subthalamic region, the sublentiform part of the internal capsule (p. 975), the tail of the caudate nucleus and the stria terminalis. More anteriorly, it is separated from the amygdaloid body by the ansa peduncularis.

## STRUCTURE OF THE CORPUS STRIATUM

The caudate nucleus and putamen are similar in structure, being highly cellular, well-vascularized zones, permeated by delicate bundles of either finely myelinated or non-myelinated, small-diameter fibres. Hence the pinkish-grey colour of these regions when freshly sectioned, in contrast to the pale colour of the globus pallidus which is encapsulated and traversed by numerous, coarse, heavily myelinated fibres.

The neurons of the caudate nucleus and putamen are mainly small multipolar cells, with round, triangular, or spindle-shaped somata, admixed with a small proportion of large multipolar cells, the ratio of the two being roughly

20:1. The small neurons are considered to be receptive and associative interneurons, which receive the synaptic terminals of many of the striatal afferents. The large neurons possess large and roughly spherical or ovoid dendritic trees, and their principal axons are one source of striatal efferents (*vide infra*), but some of the smaller neurons probably also contribute to the striatal outflow. Although the general pattern of connexions of the striatum with extrinsic regions of the nervous region is becoming clearer (*vide infra*) we have, as yet, little knowledge of the detailed morphology of its neurons, intrinsic connexions, and synaptology. Some progress has, however, been made with both the Golgi technique and electron microscopy in various experimental animals,[877, 878] but only some general features have emerged. The dendrites of striatal cells bear dendritic spines, and axodendritic synapses both related to spines and smooth interspine dendritic surfaces, and axosomatic synapses have also been identified.

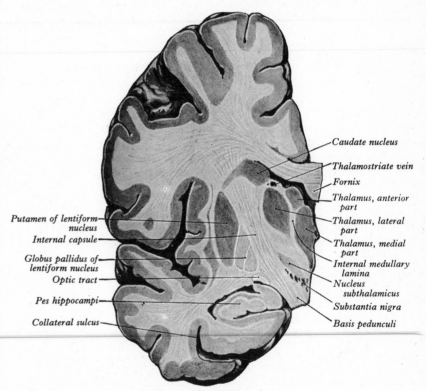

Caudate nucleus
Thalamostriate vein
Fornix
Thalamus, anterior part
Thalamus, lateral part
Thalamus, medial part
Internal medullary lamina
Nucleus subthalamicus
Substantia nigra
Basis pedunculi

Putamen of lentiform nucleus
Internal capsule
Globus pallidus of lentiform nucleus
Optic tract
Pes hippocampi
Collateral sulcus

**7**.156 Anterior aspect of a coronal section through the right cerebral hemisphere.

Further, both asymmetrical (Type I) and symmetrical (Type II) synapses are present. Lesions placed in the cerebral cortex, thalamus, or midbrain, result in degeneration of asymmetrical synapses, which are presumably excitatory, in relation to both dendrites and (after cortical lesions) to the cell somata as well. In contrast, lesions within the caudate nucleus itself cause degeneration in both type I and type II synapses. The latter, which are possibly inhibitory, are distributed on dendrites, somata and the initial segments of axons. In addition, it was shown that the axons of all striatal neurons studied possessed collateral branches and it was thought that the type II synaptic terminals might be derived not only from intrinsic interneurons, but also from the collaterals of neurons projecting to other regions. It is of considerable

[877] J. M. Kemp, *Brain Res.*, **11**, 1968a and b; **17**, 1970.
[878] C. A. Fox, D. E. Hillman, K. A. Siegesmund and L. A. Sether, in: *Evolution of the Forebrain*, eds. R. Hassler and H. Stephan, Thieme, Stuttgart. 1966.

interest that histopharmacological studies[879] have demonstrated that in the caudate nucleus of the rat, many of the synaptic terminals contain dense-cord or 'granulated' vesicles which characterize aminergic neurons (7.19), and are thought, in this site, to represent stores of *dopamine*. The remaining synapses contain the clear spherical small presynaptic vesicles found in cholinergic terminals.

The globus pallidus contains a rather scattered population of large multipolar neurons which in their general cytology closely resemble the lower motor neurons in other situations, and also resemble the large cells of the substantia nigra. Their primary dendrites branch infrequently and possess only occasional small dendritic spines. Their synapses are mainly in relation to these dendrites and are of type II, but scattered between these are a small number of type I. The relatively sparse axosomatic synapses are also of both types. After experimental lesions in the caudate nucleus, numerous degenerating symmetrical (type II) terminals were found in relation to both dendrites and somata in the globus pallidus (and also in the substantia nigra). The axons of the large pallidal neurons give origin to the profuse, well-myelinated, pallidofugal system of fibres (*vide infra*). Topographically, the globus pallidus is separated by a layer of white matter, the *external medullary lamina* or *stria* from the medial aspect of the putamen, whilst an *internal medullary lamina* or *stria* divides it into a smaller, medial, and a larger, lateral part (pallidum I and II respectively).

## CONNEXIONS OF THE CORPUS STRIATUM

In outline, the neostriatum (putamen and caudate nucleus) constitutes the main receiving station; this projects to the globus pallidus, which in turn, gives rise to the main outflow pathways. However, in addition some efferent paths leave the striatum directly, whilst the pallidum also receives other afferent connexions.

**Afferent connexions to the striatum** are derived mainly from the cerebral cortex, thalamus and substantia nigra.

Although their existence was for long in doubt, *corticostriate fibres* have now been shown to constitute a widespread system which is *topically organized* and converges from almost *all parts of the cerebral cortex* on to the caudate nucleus and putamen. The experimental animals used in these studies included rats, rabbits, cats and monkeys to which the degeneration techniques of Glees, Nauta and more recently, ultrastructural methods, have been applied.[880–885] Thus, each part of the cerebral cortex projects to a specific part of the caudate-putamen complex, although some overlap occurs. Most of the projections are derived from the ipsilateral cortex only, but some regions receive bilateral projections from restricted regions of the sensorimotor cortices of both hemispheres. The details of corticostriate projection in these different mammals vary somewhat and will not be given here; obviously they should not be extrapolated directly to the human brain, but it is most probable that broadly similar connexions exist. The most profuse projections are from the sensorimotor cortex, whilst the least prominent are from the visual cortex. Corticofugal fibres reach the striatum through both the internal and external capsules, and from the temporal lobe via sublenticular routes, whilst some of the direct and crossed corticocaudate fibres run with the *subcallosal fasciculus* in association with the fronto-occipital arcuate bundle of fibres. It is at present not clear what proportion of corticostriate fibres have their principal terminations in these nuclei, or whether substantial numbers of them are collateral branches of other corticofugal systems, for example, the corticospinal

tract. As mentioned above, the corticostriate fibres form type I synapses upon the dendrites and somata of the striatal neurons and thus, on morphological grounds, are probably excitatory.

*Thalamostriate fibres* form another profuse afferent system to the striatum and are derived from the nucleus centromedianus, various other intralaminar and midline nuclei, and also from the nucleus medialis dorsalis. Some of these fibres pass directly to the caudate nucleus to terminate there; others traverse the caudate, or skirt it, to reach the internal capsule where they pass between its fibres to reach the putamen. The details of many of these connexions have not been satisfactorily resolved. The nucleus centromedianus has been claimed to project to many parts of the corpus striatum. Studies in the monkey,[886] however, suggested that its projection was topically organized and confined to the putamen, whilst other investigators[887] claimed that its projection was to a band which included the whole mediolateral extent of both putamen and caudate nucleus. The intralaminar and dorsomedial thalamic nuclei are thought to project largely to the caudate nucleus.

*Nigrostriate fibres*, for long considered by some authorities to provide an important afferent system to the striatum and globus pallidus, although doubted by others, have now gained considerable prominence in relation to theories of the genesis of Parkinsonian tremor.[888] An increasing body of evidence, derived from electrophysiology,[889–891] neuroanatomy[892, 893] and neuropharmacology,[888] not only supports the existence of such a pathway, but strongly suggests that its neurons, at least in part, utilize *dopamine* as their neurochemical transmitter.

The nigrostriate fibres take origin from cells in both the pars compacta and pars reticularis of the substantia nigra. They ascend through the caudal subthalamus and reach the internal capsule, where separate bundles of nigrostriate fibres interdigitate with the capsular fibres, giving in histological section an appearance like a hair comb, hence the term *comb bundle* for this tract. Some fibres pass to the caudate nucleus, whilst the remainder continue on to reach the putamen and globus pallidus.

Further afferents may reach the striatum from the subthalamic nucleus and other neighbouring cell groups, but these cannot be regarded as established.

**Striatofugal connexions** are mainly to the *globus pallidus*, but *striatonigral* and *striatothalamic* fibres which retrace the pathways just described, to reach the substantia nigra and thalamus, have also been described. Both the caudate nucleus and the putamen project in a topically organized manner on to the cells of the globus pallidus. The lateral part of the putamen projects only to the external segment of the globus pallidus, whilst the more medial parts of the putamen and the caudate

[879] T. Hökfelt, *Z. Zellforsch. mikrosk. Anat.*, **91**, 1968.
[880] P. Glees, *J. Anat.*, **78**, 1944.
[881] D. G. Whitlock and W. J. H. Nauta, *J. comp. Neurol.*, **106**, 1956.
[882] K. E. Webster, *J. Anat.*, **95**, 1961; **99**, 1965.
[883] J. B. Carman, W. M. Cowan and T. P. S. Powell, *Brain*, **86**, 1963.
[884] J. B. Carman, W. M. Cowan, T. P. S. Powell and K. E. Webster, *J. Neurol. Neurosurg. Psychiat.*, **28**, 1965.
[885] J. M. Kemp and T. P. S. Powell, *Brain*, **93**, 1970.
[886] T. P. S. Powell and W. M. Cowan, *Brain*, **79**, 1956.
[887] W. R. Mehler, in: *The Thalmus*, eds. D. P. Purpura and M. D. Yahr, Columbia University Press, N.Y. 1966.
[888] D. B. Calne, *Parkinsonism*, Arnold, London. 1970.
[889] D. P. Purpura, T. L. Frigyesi and A. Malliani, in: *Neurophysiological Basis of Normal and Abnormal Motor Activities*, eds. M. D. Yahr and D. P. Purpura, Raven Press, N.Y. 1967.
[890] P. Feltz and J. S. Mackenzie, *Brain Res.*, **13**, 1969.
[891] J. D. Connor, *Science, N.Y.*, **160**, 1968.
[892] A. M. Adinolfi and G. D. Pappas, *J. comp Neurol.*, **133**, 1968.
[893] W. J. H. Nauta and W. R. Mehler, in: *Psychotropic Drugs and Dysfunctions of the Basal Ganglia*, eds. G. E. Crane and R. Gardner, U.S. Govt. Printing Office, Washington. 1969.

nucleus project to either both segments of the globus pallidus, or to the internal segment alone.

Other striatofugal connexions have been described, but their status is less certain; these include projections to the subthalamic nucleus and to restricted parts of the inferior olivary nucleus.

**Afferent connexions to the globus pallidus** are principally the topically organized *striatopallidal fibres* from both the putamen and caudate nucleus described above.

Other pallidal afferents include fibres from the subthalamic nucleus, substantia nigra, thalamus and cerebral cortex. The subthalamic fibres reach the globus pallidus (mainly pallidum I) as part of the *subthalamic fasciculus* (p. 902). *Nigropallidal fibres* have been described by a number of authors as part of the comb bundle mentioned above. The neurons forming this tract are dopaminergic, but it is uncertain whether nigrostriate, or nigropallidal fibres predominate in the *human* brain. In addition to the extensive, well-organized corticostriate projection mentioned above, some investigators have described fibres which accompany these from many parts of the cerebral cortex, but terminate directly in the globus pallidus. *Thalamopallidal fibres* may also reach the pallidum from the intralaminar, centromedian and dorsomedial nuclei of the thalamus. It must be emphasized, however, that these somewhat variable results have been obtained with different methods in a number of experimental animals, and the existence of some pathways, and the destination to specific parts of the pallidum of others, have not yet been established in the human brain.

**The pallidofugal system** constitutes by far the quantitatively most important outflow from the corpus striatum. The fibres are coarse and well myelinated, and they form a topographically complex series of pathways which diverge to a number of destinations. The main pathways involved include: (1) the *ansa lenticularis*; (2) the *fasciculus lenticularis*; (3) the *fasciculus thalamicus*; (4) the *fasciculus subthalamicus*; and (5) *descending fibres*. The topography of these tracts was described and illustrated (7.102) with the subthalamus (p. 902) and will not be repeated here.

The main destinations of the pallidofugal fibres are to: (1) the *thalamus*, mainly the *nucleus ventralis anterior*, with smaller contributions to the nuclei ventralis intermedius and centromedianus; (2) the *subthalamic nucleus* and other, smaller, subthalamic centres which include the zona incerta, entopeduncular nucleus and the nucleus of the prerubral field; (3) the *substantia nigra*; (4) the *red nucleus*; (5) the *midbrain reticular formation*; and (6) the *inferior olivary nucleus*.

The following points should also be noted. The external segment of the pallidum projects on to the internal segment, from which most of the pallidofugal fibres originate. The fibres to the subthalamic nucleus, however, arise mainly from the external segment. For long, a *pallidohypothalamic tract* appeared in most accounts of the corpus striatum, but more recent studies using the newer degeneration techniques offered no conclusive evidence that fibres project directly from the globus pallidus to hypothalamic nuclei. The tract described pursues an aberrant course which curves around the column of the fornix; thereafter the majority of its fibres rejoin the main pallidal outflow.

## SUMMARY AND FUNCTIONAL STUDIES

Clearly, the corpus striatum and its associated regions of the nervous system constitute an exceedingly complex set of interconnexions, but their details and our understanding of their function role is still in its infancy.

Broadly, information *converges* on the corpus striatum from most of the cerebral cortex, the thalamus, subthalamus and a number of brainstem centres. After integration within the corpus striatum, information *diverges* again to the thalamus, subthalamus and the various brainstem centres listed above.

For long it was held that the main outflow from the corpus striatum, as part of the classical 'extrapyramidal motor system', *descended*, through various indirect polysynaptic pathways to the lower motor centres. Whilst such descending pathways as the reticulospinal and rubrospinal tracts undoubtedly carry information derived in part from the corpus striatum, it is increasingly clear that the most prominent outflow from the corpus striatum is to the *nucleus ventralis anterior* of the thalamus (p. 898), where, after integration with other channels, *ascending* pathways radiate to the *motor and premotor areas* (areas 4 and 6). Equally important reciprocal interconnexions are established with the *subthalamic nucleus* and *substantia nigra*.

An impressive list of organic nervous diseases has long been known to affect, in varying measure, the different parts of the corpus striatum and their associated nuclei and fibre pathways. These cannot be reviewed here, and the reader should consult texts devoted to clinical neurology and neuropathology. Briefly, in different forms and combinations, these various disease states usually present: (1) *disturbances of muscle 'tone'* or resistance to stretch; sometimes this is reduced, but more commonly some form of *rigidity* is present; (2) diminution or *loss of automatic associated movements* such as arm-swinging during walking, facial expression, etc.; (3) the presence of *unwanted movements* which are uncontrollable and purposeless; these may be *choreiform*, *athetoid*, or *ballistic* (p. 902), or they may take the form of a *tremor* resulting from the fairly rapid alternating contraction of opposing muscle groups. The tremor is usually 'static', that is, present when the limb is otherwise at rest, but occasionally an *intention tremor* is present as in some forms of cerebellar dysfunction (p. 877). Attempts to link the various combinations of symptoms and signs with disease in specific locations have met with limited success. Similarly, experiments with animals have often been uninformative.

Ablation of the putamen, the caudate nucleus, or the globus pallidus, often causes little obvious change in motor behaviour, provided the lesions do not affect surrounding structures. Complete ablation of the globus pallidus on both sides in the monkey, however, results in a general poverty of movement and a reduction in manipulative skills.

Rapid stimulation of the caudate nucleus in unanaesthetized animals sometimes elicits movements of the head and limbs, and some evidences of a somatotopic pattern in the nucleus have been adduced. Low frequency stimulation, or chemical stimulation, at different points in the corpus striatum however, usually results in an inhibition of motor responses. It may induce long periods of immobility, an inhibition of cortically induced movements, or 'arrest reactions' in the unanaesthetized animal. Confirmation of this has been obtained by electrophysiological 'unit' recording from the motor cortex and the ventrolateral thalamus—inhibition of unit activity followed stimulation of the caudate nucleus. Other experiments have demonstrated the inhibition of responses which had been established by learning processes, following caudate nucleus stimulation.

Neurosurgical ablation of the globus pallidus or ventrolateral thalamus has been used, often with considerable success, to diminish contralateral rigidity and tremor in human disease. Thalamic ablations seem more effective in the relief of tremor (including cerebellar tremor) whilst pallidal lesions have a greater effect in reducing rigidity. In addition to their therapeutic value, such manœuvres provide a source of material for histopathological and neuropharmacological study and also allow electrophysiological recording to be carried out. Most interesting in this regard has been the identification of neurons in the ventrolateral thalamus in cases of Parkinsonian tremor, which show a repetitive, rhythmical discharge of impulses, the frequency of which corresponds to that of the tremor.[894-897] Similar findings have been induced experimentally by placing brainstem lesions in the monkey. Intensive experimental analysis involving anatomical, physiological, behavioural and pharmacological methods is now in progress attempting to define the causal mechanism of the rhythmic neuronal discharges. Much interest has been aroused by the demonstration of an *inhibitory dopaminergic nigrostriate pathway* which is probably involved in a proportion of cases of Parkinsonian tremor.[898] Of the various possible mechanisms proposed, it is currently considered most likely that normal striatal function depends upon a balance between the inhibitory afferent pathway just mentioned, and excitatory afferent pathways which are cholinergic. Reduced activity in the inhibitory pathway leads to an excessive excitatory output from the pallidum, which in turn leads to oscillating bursts of activity in ventrolateral thalamic neurons. Finally, the latter through their cortical radiations are thought to generate rhythmical activity in the various corticofugal descending pathways to the lower motor centres. On this view, dopamine is a normal neurotransmitter in the striatum; there is a considerable body of evidence to show that dopamine levels in the striatum are reduced in many cases of Parkinsonism, and this is paralleled by the encouraging clinical responses to replacement therapy in a substantial proportion of patients who have been given L-dopa, a precursor of dopamine.

Despite this dramatic progress in the pharmacological and clinical sphere, however, beyond the long-held view that the corpus striatum is intimately involved in motor control, and the displacement of emphasis from descending pathways to a control of the cerebral cortex by this region of the brain, its precise role in normal behaviour remains conjectural.

**The claustrum** is a thin sheet of grey matter co-extensive with the insula and the putamen of the lentiform nucleus, from which it is separated by the fibres of the external capsule. It is thickest below and in front, where it becomes continuous with the anterior perforated substance, the amygdala, and prepiriform cortex. It has been regarded by some authorities as belonging to the corpus striatum and by others as a detached portion of the insular cortex. However, more detailed studies suggest that it probably consists of at least two structurally and functionally distinct zones. These have been termed the '*insular*' claustrum and the '*temporal*' or '*prepiriform*' claustrum respectively. In experimental animals the insular part of the claustrum has been shown to possess reciprocal, topically organized corticoclaustral and claustrocortical connexions with many regions of the neocortex. Its detailed connexions and functional significance are unknown in the human brain.

**The external capsule** is a thin layer of white matter which is interposed between the lateral aspect of the lentiform nucleus and the claustrum. The fibres of the external capsule are derived from the frontoparietal operculum of the insula and, after passing across the lateral surface of the lentiform nucleus, they turn medially below the nucleus and the ansa lenticularis. Their sub-

thalamic connexions are uncertain. Some of the fibres of the anterior commissure are believed to traverse the external capsule.

## The Choroid Plexus of the Lateral Ventricle

Projecting into the lateral ventricle on its medial aspect is a highly vascularized fringe composed of pia mater and of the ependymal lining of the cavity (7.157, 158). This is the choroid plexus of the lateral ventricle, which is itself only part of a larger structure, the *tela choroidea*, to be described below. The pial basis of the choroid plexus is invaginated during development (p. 137), over a linear region of the medial wall of the hemisphere where no nervous tissue develops. The pia therefore comes into direct contact with the epithelial lining of the ventricle, the *ependyma*, and the two tissues are fused in the structure of the choroid plexus, which otherwise consists chiefly of small blood vessels, capillaries and nerve fibres. The plexus extends anteriorly to the interventricular foramen,

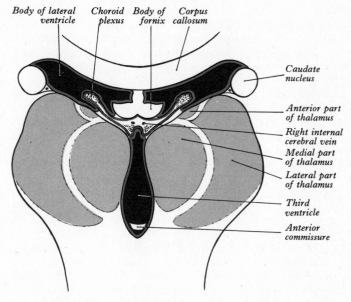

*Body of lateral ventricle*    *Choroid plexus*    *Body of fornix*    *Corpus callosum*

*Caudate nucleus*

*Anterior part of thalamus*

*Right internal cerebral vein*

*Medial part of thalamus*

*Lateral part of thalamus*

*Third ventricle*

*Anterior commissure*

**7.157** Diagram of a coronal section through the lateral and third ventricles. The pia mater of the tela choroidea is shown in red and the ependyma in blue.

where it is continuous across the third ventricle with the choroid plexus of the opposite lateral ventricle. From this point it passes posteriorly above and in contact with the thalamus (7.144) to curve round its posterior end into the inferior cornu of the ventricle, reaching as far as the pes hippocampi (7.147). When the choroid plexus is torn away from the hemisphere, the line of its invagination appears as a narrow cleft, the *choroid fissure*. Through the main part or body of the ventricle the fissure is limited superiorly by the fornix and inferiorly by the thalamus (7.157); in the inferior cornu it is between the stria

[894] G. Guiot, J. Hardy and D. Albe-Fessard, *Neurochirurgia*, **5**, 1962.
[895] G. Guiot, D. Albe-Fessard, G. Arfel and P. Derome, *Neurochirurgia*, **10**, 1964.
[896] H. H. Jasper, *J. Neurosurg.*, **24**, Suppl. II, 1966.
[897] J. A. V. Bates, in: *The Third Symposium on Parkinson's Disease*, eds. F. J. Gillingham, I. M. L. Donaldson, Livingstone, Edinburgh. 1969.
[898] D. B. Calne, *Parkinsonism*, Arnold, London. 1970.

terminalis above and the fimbria (**7**.158). The choroid fissure is the first groove to appear on the surface of the cerebrum (p. 139). In coronal sections of the brain at eight weeks of embryonic development it can already be seen that the choroid fissure is in direct contact with the ependymal roof of the body of the lateral ventricle, and that vascular pia mater is being folded into the fissure. At this stage, before the development of commissures and expansion of the lamina terminalis, only one layer of pia mater extends over the roof of the third ventricle (**2**.86 A). When the corpus callosum expands posteriorly it does so above the level of the choroid fissure, carrying with it a layer of pia on its inferior surface. This overlies the original single pial layer, fusing with it to form the main part of the tela choroidea, lateral extensions of which, also double layered, form the two choroid plexuses in the lateral ventricles. Posteriorly the two layers separate, the inferior (original) layer following the roof of the third ventricle to reach the pineal body and the tectum, the superior cleaving to the corpus callosum and passing round the splenium to the superior surface of the former (**8**.195).

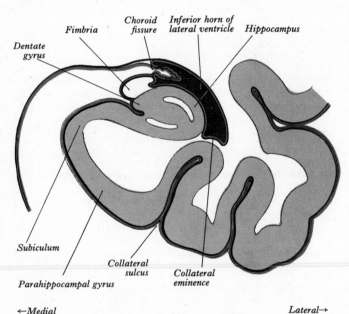

**7**.158 Diagram of a coronal section through the inferior cornu of the lateral ventricle. The pia mater is shown in red and the ependyma in blue.

Where the two layers of pia mater described above are fused they constitute the *tela choroidea of the third ventricle*, as usually defined, although the choroid plexuses of the lateral ventricles are in fact extensions of it. Viewed from above it is a triangular fold, with a rounded apex at the level of the interventricular foramina, often indented by the anterior column of the fornix (**7**.159). Its lateral edges are irregular, due to the contained vascular fringes of the choroid plexuses of the lateral ventricles. At the two posterior or basal angles of the tela choroidea these vascular fringes curve onwards into the inferior cornua of the lateral ventricles, while the wide central part of the base of the tela marks the limit of fusion of the pial layers, which depart from each other here as already detailed. When the tela choroidea has been removed a transverse slit is left between the splenium and the junction of the roof of the third ventricle with the tectum: this is the *transverse fissure*, but it is, of course, not a cerebral fissure in the true sense or usage of the term, for it is not due to a folding of the cerebral cortex. It merely

marks the posterior limit of the extra-cerebral space enclosed by the posterior growth of the corpus callosum above the third ventricle. In the space, enclosed between two layers of pia mater are the choroid plexuses of the third ventricle (p. 919).

**The microscopic structure** of a choroid plexus is essentially as follows. The irregular fringes visible to the naked eye are covered with large numbers of microscopic *villous processes*, each containing afferent and efferent vessels, an intervening capillary plexus, a small amount of supporting connective tissue, and nerve fibres. The villi show varying degrees of complexity (**7**.160), and sections demonstrate the large surface area created in this way. This has been estimated to be at least 200 cm², [899] and this does not allow for the *microvilli* which electron microscopy shows on the ventricular aspect of the ependymal cells. [900] The ependymal microvilli are not as regular in size and distribution as in some other sites, such as the small intestine (p. 1282), being more akin to those seen in the epithelium of the proximal part of the renal tubule. As in the latter, the basal aspect of the ependymal cells present, to a lesser extent, a series of invaginations. [901] These appearances, coupled with absence of secretory granules, unspecialized Golgi apparatus, and other features, suggest a role concerned with water transport rather than secretion. However, physiological studies [902] provide considerable evidence that the cerebrospinal fluid, largely produced by the choroid plexuses, cannot be regarded as a mere filtrate. Ultrastructural studies have also shown that some ependymal cells possess *cilia*, that tight junctions exist between them, and that a distinct *basement membrane* separates them from the adjacent capillaries. [903] The latter are sometimes of the fenestrated type, and recent experiments, [904] in which the protein peroxidase was used as a tracer, showed that, while the capillary endothelium was readily permeable to the tracer, its passage was blocked by the tight junctions between the choroidal ependymal cells. These findings are probably of importance in relation to the concept of a *blood-brain barrier* which is further discussed on p. 36.

The *stroma* of the choroidal villi is derived from the pia mater of the tela choroidea. It consists of pial fibroblasts and few, if any, collagen fibres. The cells are much flattened and do not form complete sheets between the ependyma and the capillary endothelium. Nerve fibres appear to be absent from the actual villi, but in the larger stems from which these branch the amount of connective tissue is greater and myelinated and non-myelinated nerve fibres and small nerve bundles have been identified. [905, 906] The functional significance of these fibres is still uncertain, but the non-myelinated fibres are considered to be vasomotor postganglionic sympathetic elements; others are thought to be derived from the vagus and glossopharyngeal nerves. Comparatively few studies of the nerve supply of the choroid plexuses have been reported and much uncertainty of its distribution and role persists.

The *blood supply* of the choroid plexuses in the tela choroidea is derived from the anterior and posterior choroidal branches (pp. 638, 644), the former being usually a single vessel, the latter three to five in

[899] E. Voetmann, *Acta anat.*, **8**, 1949.
[900] D. S. Maxwell and D. C. Pease, *J. biophys. biochem. Cytol.*, **2**, 1956.
[901] G. D. Pappas and V. M. Tennyson, *J. Cell Biol.*, **15**, 1962.
[902] H. Davson, *Physiology of the Cerebrospinal Fluid*, Churchill, London. 1970.
[903] B. Wislocki and A. J. Ladman, in: *The Cerebrospinal Fluid*, Ciba Foundation Symposium, Churchill, London. 1958.
[904] M. W. Brightman and T. S. Reese, *J. Cell Biol.*, **40**, 1969.
[905] S. L. Clark, *J. comp. Neurol.*, **60**, 1934.
[906] E. R. A. Cooper, in: *The Cerebrospinal Fluid*, Ciba Foundation Symposium, Churchill, London. 1958.

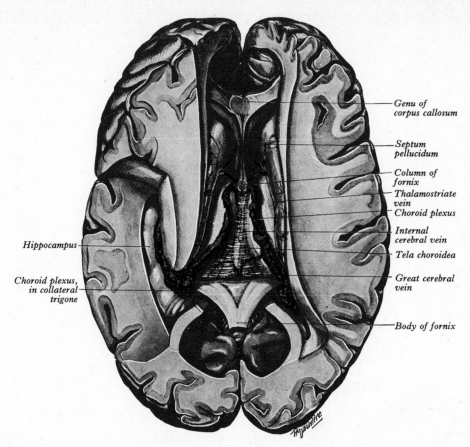

Genu of
corpus callosum

Septum
pellucidum

Column of
fornix

Thalamostriate
vein

Choroid plexus

Internal
cerebral vein

Tela choroidea

Great cerebral
vein

Hippocampus

Choroid plexus,
in collateral
trigone

Body of fornix

7.159 The tela choroidea of the third ventricle and the choroid plexus of the lateral ventricle.

number.[907, 908] The two sets of arteries anastomose to some extent. The capillaries drain into a rich venous plexus, which is served by a single choroidal vein leaving the tela choroidea. This commences in the vicinity of the basal angle of the tela, at the junction of the parts of the choroid plexus in the body and the inferior cornu of the lateral ventricle. This region also corresponds to the frontier between the territories of the anterior and posterior choroidal arteries, and at this point also a solitary glomus (p. 595) is situated. This structure is near the free edge

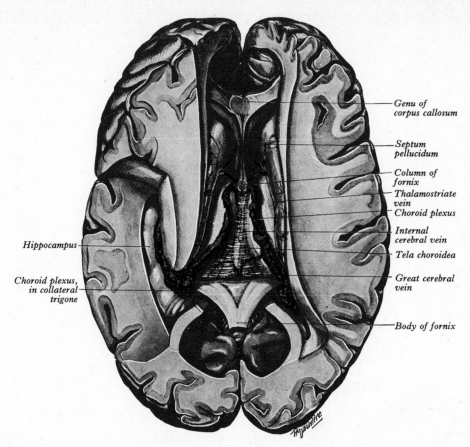

7.160 A section of part of the choroid plexus of the lateral ventricle, stained with haematoxylin and eosin. Note the ependyma lining the ventricular wall above, and covering the loose connective tissue cores of the processes of the plexus, which contain numerous small blood vessels, including many capillaries. A calcareous deposit (dark blue) is present in one process. Owing to the complexity of the ramification of the processes, several appear as disconnected islands of tissue.

of the choroid plexus, and many of the tributaries of the choroidal vein converge towards it. Apart from the occurrence of this body nothing appears to have been established regarding its significance in the plexus.

## Cerebral Dimensions

The human brain has been weighed and measured by many observers; and it has been compared in its volume, weight, relationship to total body weight, and in the proportionate size of its main divisions with the brains of many other vertebrates. Even without actual quantification, such comparisons permit some interesting generalizations regarding the relation between development of brain size and various abilities in mankind and other animals. But even metrical data, where they are available in reliable quantity, are merely estimates of the bulk of nervous tissue, which largely disregard degrees of organization or even the proportions of particular neuronal elements, such as nerve cells, nerve fibres, neuroglia and vascular elements; and such considerations must obviously be taken into account if valid comparisons are to be made. Clearly, therefore, no more than crude deductions are to be expected from data of this kind. Furthermore, available measurements are usually dependent upon small series of observations in any particular species, even sometimes upon a single example. Hence little allowance for individual variation can have been made, whether due to sex, age, or nutritional state, or indeed any other factors which may influence brain size or its relation to body size and weight; and it is particularly

[907] J. W. Millen and D. H. M. Woollam, J. Anat., 87, 1953.
[908] J. W. Millen and D. H. M. Woollam, The Anatomy of the Cerebrospinal Fluid, Oxford University Press, London. 1962.

this ratio which is the focus of most attention. Even in respect to the human, for whom much more adequate series of observations have been recorded, the effects of such factors are often overlooked.

An 'average' human male adult's brain is said to weigh about 1,450 gm and that of his female counterpart about 100 gm less, but such figures are not useful without a corresponding range, which is of the order of 1,240 to 1,680 in males and 1,130 to 1,510 in females. Proportionately males and females differ rather less in brain weight than total body weight. Even the ranges quoted would exclude numbers of famous people whose brain weights lay well outside such extremes, and in both directions. (Consult reference [909] for examples and much other data.) Different ranges for various races have been stated, but the differences between their means are not significant in general, when the much greater variation in body weight is taken into consideration.

Prior to maturity, of course, the human brain varies markedly in weight and in ratio to total body weight,[910] showing throughout its growth, however, the same relatively outstanding development which characterizes the adult. Unlike some other mammals, such as rodents, in which the maximum growth rate may be pre- or post-natal, the cerebral growth spurt in mankind and primates in general is peri-natal—in late fetal development and the first year of extrauterine life. During this first year the brain at least doubles in weight[911] and it reaches about 90 per cent of its final weight by the sixth year. Most of this increase is due to factors such as myelination rather than any augmentation in the number of nerve cells, and for this reason alone any comparison of the growing human brain, on the basis of weight, with the brains of adults or of other species, is pointless where correlation with ability is the criterion.

The human brain is obviously large, both absolutely and relatively; but it is surpassed in both respects by those of certain other mammals. Dolphins, elephants (4,000–5,000 gm) and whales (6,800 gm has been recorded in the blue whale, *Balaenopterus musculus*) have heavier brains than man, although this is offset by brain:body weight ratios of about 1:600 in elephants and of about 1:850 in large whales. However, in dolphins the ratio is approximately 1:40, which is somewhat 'better' than the human average of about 1:50. In some small mammals, such as mice, the ratio may be as low as 1:35, while in smaller primates ratios as low as 1:12 have been estimated (squirrel monkey). Amongst the primates man occupies an almost average position in brain:body weight ratio, the larger apes and monkeys falling much below him in this regard. In absolute size of brain, of course, he much surpasses any other primate; a male gorilla[912] may have a cranial capacity of 412–752 cm³, and while this is only a rough indication of actual brain weight, it is well below the human range (say, 1,200–1,500 cm³). The largest gorilloid brain recorded weighed 750 gm,[913] which is distinctly less than the usual human range. Nevertheless, extremely small brain weights have been recorded in microcephalic idiots; but what is more significant is that brain weights in dwarfs which were *below* the average upper limit for gorillas have nevertheless been recorded in humans possessing at least elementary speech; and the symbolic abstractions of language are widely regarded as correlated with the large absolute size of the human cerebrum. This view has, however, been questioned;[914] and while a certain, as yet indefinable minimal size of brain must be associated with the extraordinary potentialities of mankind in cerebration, it is clear that the kind of data so far mentioned cast little illumination on this problem.

As has already been said above, measurements of brain size and brain:body weight ratio afford no indication of organization within the brain; nor do they take into account the density of packing or total numbers of nerve cells in any particular brain. While it has been said that this density does not vary greatly in mammalian brains when calculated for the whole organ, estimates of this kind are few and subject to much error. Figures for samples taken from the cerebral cortex are perhaps open to the same strictures, but it is of interest to note here that a cubic millimetre of cortex has been estimated to contain as many as 142,000 cells in the mouse, 21,500 in the macaque, and merely 10,500 in man. However, the area of the human cerebral cortex (p. 922) is at least twelve times greater than that of the macaque, which may nevertheless have a brain:body weight ratio similar to man's.

Another mode of approach to the problems of comparison of mammalian and especially primate brains[915] has been to estimate the weights of the main divisions of the brain, such as cerebrum, cerebellum, midbrain, medulla oblongata, olfactory bulb, neocortex, paleocortex, cortex, corpus striatum, and other features, and to express some of these quantities as indices. (As an example of recent studies of this kind consult footnote reference[916].) Large numbers of species of insectivores and primates have been compared in this manner, and although in many instances only one sample from each species has been measured, highly interesting comparisons are possible. While it is, of course, easy to appreciate, without any metrical data, that in the human brain the olfactory structures are small, absolutely and relatively, that the cerebrum-pons-cerebellum complex is markedly developed, or that the cerebral cortex is very extensive in the human brain, quantitative assessment of such statements is much more valuable. In comparing man and the gorilla, for example, the ratio by weight of their medullae oblongatae is approximately 9·6:7, despite the fact that the gorilla weighs at least twice as much as the man. The ratios for the mesencephalon, cerebellum and diencephalon are roughly 2:1, but the human telencephalon is three times as heavy as the gorilloid. The olfactory bulb of the gorilla is almost thrice the size of the human, while the latter's hippocampus is nearly two and a half times as heavy as the gorilla's. Incidentally the ratio of olfactory bulb to hippocampus in the gorilla is hence about 1:15 and in man 1:90, an interesting commentary on the status of the hippocampus in the 'rhinencephalon' (*see* p. 931).

Space does not permit further exploration of such data, and it must be said that though considerations of this kind may have marked significance in evolutionary comparisons between man and other mammals, particularly sub-human primates, they do not provide any clear definition in morphological terms of what it is that is responsible in man's brain for the enormous complexity of his behaviour. Perhaps it is rather in this, and his consequently ever more complex culture, that the essence of humanness can best be defined. It is noteworthy that in assessing the human palæontological record the accent has gradually

[909] S. M. Blinkov and I. I. Glezer, *The Human Brain in Figures and Tables*, Basic Books, New York. 1968.

[910] D. P. Purpura and J. P. Schadé, *Growth and Maturation of the Brain*, Elsevier, Amsterdam. 1964.

[911] M. C. H. Dogson, *The Growing Brain*, Wright, Bristol. 1962.

[912] A. H. Schultze, *The Life of Primates*, Weidenfeld and Nicolson, London. 1969.

[913] R. L. Holloway, *Brain Res.*, 7, 1968.

[914] E. H. Lenneberg, *New Directions in the Study of Languages*, Massachusetts Institute of Technology Press, Cambridge, 1964.

[915] F. Tilney and H. A. Riley, *The Brain from Ape to Man*, Hoeber, New York. 1928.

[916] H. Stephan, R. Bauchot and O. J. Andy, in: *The Primate Brain*, Appleton-Century-Crofts, New York. 1970.

passed from comparison of cranial capacities to that of culture. The *Australopithecinae*, with brains little if at all larger than those of gorillas, may leave us in doubt; but in *Homo habilis*, with—it is true—a considerably larger but still very modest cranial capacity, doubts evaporate as to his humanity; and perhaps most of all because of his ability, as revealed in surviving artefacts. In more recent ancestors also, and again not merely because of increasing *hominoid* brain size (in which *Homo neanderthalensis* even surpassed us, yet is now extinct), but even more because of the increasing evidence of their *human* behaviour are we convinced of their close relationship to ourselves. Their abilities, which from such simple beginnings have led to the great achievement and communication of practical and abstract creation in our own era, are no more likely than our own to be explicable in terms of gross cerebral mensuration. (For important recent discussions of the significance of brain size see footnote references [917], [918].)

## Blood Vessels of the Brain

The arterial supply of the brain (pp. 637, 644) is derived from the **internal carotid** and **vertebral arteries** which lie in the subarachnoid space (p. 990). The vertebral and basilar arteries give branches to the spinal cord, brain-stem and cerebellum, the basilar artery terminating at the upper border of the pons by dividing into two posterior cerebral arteries. The internal carotid artery terminates by dividing into **anterior** and **middle cerebral arteries**. The anterior cerebral arteries are interconnected by the **anterior communicating artery**. Just before terminating, the internal carotid artery communicates through the **posterior communicating artery** with the **posterior cerebral artery**, thus completing a vascular circle, the **circulus arteriosus**, around the interpeduncular fossa (6.61). For details of collateral circulation following blockage of the main feeders of the circle, see footnote reference [919]. From the circulus arteriosus or vessels close to it **central branches** are given off to supply the interior of the cerebral hemisphere and the thalamus. These vessels form six principal groups: (1) an *anteromedial group*, derived from the anterior cerebral and anterior communicating arteries; (2) a *posteromedial group*, from the posterior cerebral and posterior communicating arteries; (3 and 4) right and left *anterolateral groups*, from the middle cerebral arteries; (5 and 6) right and left *posterolateral groups*, from the posterior cerebral arteries after they have wound round the cerebral peduncles. (For details consult footnote reference [920].)

The entire blood supply of the **cerebral cortex** is derived from the **cortical branches** of the anterior, middle and posterior cerebral arteries. They reach the cortex in the pia mater. They divide in its substance, give off branches which penetrate the brain cortex perpendicularly and are divisible into long and short rami. The **long** or **medullary arteries** pass through the grey matter and penetrate the subjacent white matter to a depth of 3 or 4cm[921] without intercommunicating and thus constitute so many independent small systems. **Deep medullary vessels** extending from the central branches towards the cortex have been described, but these are identified as recurrent branches of the long or medullary vessels.[921] The **short arteries** are confined to the cortex, where they form with the long vessels a compact network in the middle zone of the grey matter, the outer and inner zones being sparingly supplied with blood. The vessels of the cortical system are not so strictly 'terminal' as those in the central system[922] but they approach this type closely, for, although neighbouring vessels anastomose with one another on the surface of the brain, they become end

arteries as soon as they pierce its substance. Even the anastomoses on the surface of the brain, however, are in general only between microscopic branches of the cerebral arteries, and there is little clear evidence that they can provide the means of a vicarious circulation in cases of occlusion of larger vessels. Owing to the cellularity of the grey matter, its blood supply is much richer than that of the white. The *lateral surface* of the hemisphere is principally supplied by the *middle cerebral artery*; the area adjacent to the superomedial border as far back as the parieto-occipital sulcus is supplied by the *anterior cerebral artery*, and the occipital lobe and most of the inferior temporal gyrus (excluding the temporal pole) is supplied by the *posterior cerebral artery* (6.59, 60). The *medial* and *inferior surfaces* of the cerebral hemisphere are supplied by the *anterior* and *posterior* cerebral arteries. The area supplied by the anterior cerebral artery extends almost to the parieto-occipital sulcus and includes the medial part of the orbital surface. The remainder of this surface and the temporal pole are supplied by the middle cerebral artery. The rest of the medial and inferior surface is supplied by the posterior cerebral artery (6.59, 60). The junctional zone near the occipital pole between the territories of the middle and posterior cerebral arteries corresponds to the part of the striate cortex concerned with the macula. The phenomenon known clinically as '*sparing of the macula*' is considered to be due to the collateral circulation of blood from branches of the middle cerebral artery into those of the posterior, when the latter vessel is blocked. The middle cerebral artery may in fact itself supply the macular area.[923]

Most of the *corpus striatum* and *internal capsule* is supplied by the medial and lateral striate rami of the central branches of the middle cerebral artery, the remainder being supplied by the central branches of the anterior cerebral artery. One ramus of the middle cerebral is Charcot's artery of cerebral haemorrhage (p. 638).

The *choroid plexuses* of the *third* and *lateral ventricles* are supplied by branches of the internal carotid and posterior cerebral arteries.

The finer details of the vessels of some parts of the diencephalic region have been well explored, particularly in relation to the hypophysis cerebri and its related hypothalamic nuclei (see p. 1371 and footnote reference [924]). Recent studies of the vascularization of the lamina terminalis[925] and of the posterior wall of the third ventricle[926] have been reported. The arterial supply to the lamina is derived from the anterior cerebral arteries and their communicating vessel, and these are described as forming a superficial capillary plexus in the pia mater which drains into a second, more deeply situated plexus of sinusoidal capillaries, characterized by loops or vortices, these draining in their turn into the veins of the hypothalamus. The physiological significance of these arrangements is unknown. The main artery to the posterior parts of the third ventricle is the medial branch of the posterior choroidal artery, and this supplies the posterior commissure, habenular region, the pineal body, and

---

[917] P. V. Tobias, *Am. J. phys. Anthrop.*, **32**, 1970.

[918] H. J. Jerison, in: *The Primate Brain*. See Ref. [916].

[919] W. S. Fields, M. E. Bruetman and J. Weibel, *Collateral Circulation of the Brain*, Williams and Wilkins, Baltimore. 1965.

[920] H. A. Kaplan and D. H. Ford, *The Brain Vascular System*, Elsevier, Amsterdam, London, N.Y. 1966.

[921] O. J. Lewis, *J. Anat.*, **91**, 1957.

[922] S. Sunderland, *J. Anat.*, **73**, 1938.

[923] C. G. Smith and W. F. G. Richardson, *Am. J. Ophthal.*, **61**, 1966.

[924] W. Haymaker, in: *The Hypothalamus*, eds. W. Haymaker, E. Anderson and W. J. H. Nauta, Thomas, Springfield, Illinois. 1969.

[925] H. Duvernoy, J. G. Koritké and G. Monnier, *Z. Zellforsch. mikrosk. Anat.*, **102**, 1969.

[926] C. Plets, *Acta neurochir.*, **21**, 1969.

medial parts of the thalamus, including the pulvinar. The *thalamus* is supplied chiefly by branches of the posterior communicating, posterior cerebral and basilar arteries. The pattern of branches from these main feeders, and the varying details of the angioarchitecture in the different nuclei of the thalamus, have been described *in extenso* in the human brain, together with a full critique of the literature in reference [927].

The *midbrain* is supplied by the posterior cerebral, superior cerebellar and basilar arteries. The crura cerebri are supplied by vessels entering on the medial and lateral sides. The medial vessels pass to the inner side of the crus and also supply the upper and inner part of the tegmentum, including the nucleus of the oculomotor nerve. The lateral vessels supply the lateral part of the crus and the tegmentum. The colliculi are supplied by three vessels on each side from the posterior cerebral and superior cerebellar arteries. There is an additional supply to the crura cerebri and the colliculi and their peduncles from the posterolateral group of central arteries from the posterior cerebral artery.

The *pons* is supplied by the basilar and the anterior, inferior and superior cerebellar arteries. Direct branches from the basilar artery enter along the basilar sulcus. Branches also enter along the trigeminal, abducent, facial and vestibulocochlear nerves and nervus intermedius. There is also a supply from the pial plexus.

The *medulla oblongata* is supplied by the vertebral, anterior and posterior spinal, posterior inferior cerebellar and basilar arteries. Some arteries enter along the anterior median fissure and the posterior median sulcus. Other vessels enter along the rootlets of the last four cranial nerves and intermediately to supply the central substance. In addition there is a supply from the same sources through a pial plexus.

The *cerebellum* is supplied from the cerebellar arteries. The cerebellar arteries, like the cerebral arteries, form superficial anastomoses. Their internal distribution has not been extensively studied, but the possibility of anastomoses of their deeper, medullary branches, as distinct from cortical branches, has been reported.[928]

The *choroid plexus* of the *fourth ventricle* is supplied by the posterior inferior cerebellar arteries.

The blood supplies of the optic chiasma, tract and radiation are of marked clinical interest. The chiasma is supplied in part by the anterior cerebral arteries, but its median zone depends upon rami from the internal carotids which reach it by way of the stalk of the hypophysis cerebri. The anterior choroidal and posterior communicating arteries supply the optic tract, and the radiation receives blood through deep branches of the middle and posterior cerebral vessels. For further details consult footnote references [929, 930].

**The venous drainage of the brain** (pp. 691–698) can be divided into that serving the cerebral hemispheres and that serving the brainstem and cerebellum. The veins are thin-walled, devoid of valves and the majority cross the subarachnoid space to join the dural venous sinuses.

**The veins of the cerebrum** can be divided into external and internal groups. The external cerebral veins are grouped in three sets, the superior which drain forwards into the superior sagittal sinus, the inferior which drain principally into the transverse and cavernous sinuses and the middle which are further subdivided into superficial and deep. The *superficial middle cerebral vein* drains the majority of the lateral surface of the hemisphere, follows the lateral sulcus and terminates in the cavernous sinus. The *deep middle cerebral vein* drains the region of the insula and unites with the *anterior cerebral* and *striate veins* to form the *basal vein*. The areas drained by the anterior cerebral and striate veins correspond approximately with those supplied by the anterior cerebral artery and the central branches entering the anterior perforated substance. The basal vein passes backwards alongside the interpeduncular fossa and midbrain, receives tributaries from this vicinity and joins the *great cerebral vein*.

The two **internal cerebral veins** are formed near the interventricular foramen by the union of the *thalamostriate* and *choroid veins* draining the choroid plexuses of the third and lateral ventricles. They travel backwards parallel to one another between the layers of the tela choroidea of the third ventricle and unite to form the great cerebral vein which enters the straight sinus.

The veins of the *midbrain* join the basal or great cerebral veins.

The veins of the *pons* drain either into the basal vein, cerebellar veins, the petrosal sinuses, transverse sinus or the venous plexus of the foramen ovale.

The veins of the *medulla oblongata* drain into the veins of the spinal cord, the adjacent dural venous sinuses or along the last four cranial nerves by radicular veins to the inferior petrosal sinus or superior bulb of the jugular vein.

The **veins of the cerebellum** drain mainly into the adjacent sinuses or, from the superior surface, to the great cerebral vein.

Although the *innervation* of the intracranial arteries, including those supplying the brain, remains something of a physiological mystery, there is no doubt that a considerable supply of postganglionic sympathetic fibres is distributed along the arterial trees of the internal carotid and vertebral arteries, and that myelinated fibres accompany these in lesser numbers. A parasympathetic supply is supported by more dubious evidence. For a recent review of the literature of this topic, consult footnote reference [931].

There are no lymphatics in the central nervous system. The subarachnoid space is prolonged along the olfactory nerves, thus providing a route between this space and the tissue spaces in the mucoperiosteum of the nasal cavities. The so-called perivascular spaces around brain vessels have been a subject of much controversy (p. 993). Electron microscope appearances confirm the extension of pial elements into the brain around vessels in various mammals such as the rat,[932] and cat.[933] In the latter study the arachnoid 'space' around the small arterioles entering the cortex of the cerebrum was seen to contain electron-dense material, consisting of collagen bundles, pial cells, and cells resembling macrophages, possibly derived from the leptomeninges. These elements do not, apparently, form a complete sheath to the vessels, large areas being seen in which the basement membranes of the brain and vessel are opposed. The 'space' does not extend around capillaries, where the two basement membranes fuse. These observations also entail that the perivascular spaces are not continuous with those around neurons.

[927] C. Plets, J. De Reuck, H. Vander Eecken and R. Van Den Bergh, *Acta neurol. psychiat. belg.*, **70**, 1970.

[928] F. A. Gomes, *O. Medico*, 1969.

[929] A. A. Abbie, *Med. J. Aust.*, **2**, 1938.

[930] R. Bergland and B. S. Ray, *J. Neurosurg.*, **31**, 1969.

[931] E. Nelson and M. Rennels, *Brain*, **93**, 1970.

[932] D. D. Samarasinghe, *J. Anat.*, **99**, 1965.

[933] E. G. Jones, *J. Anat.*, **106**, 1970.

# THE MENINGES

The brain and the spinal cord are enveloped by three membranes (meninges), named from without inwards: the dura mater, the arachnoid and the pia mater.

## THE DURA MATER

The dura mater is a thick and dense inelastic membrane. The portion of it which encloses the brain (*cerebral dura mater*) differs in several particulars from that which surrounds the spinal cord (*spinal dura mater*), and therefore it is necessary to describe them separately; the two parts, however, form one complete membrane, and are continuous with each other at the foramen magnum.

through the foramina at the base of the skull. Outside the skull these sheaths fuse with the epineurium of the nerves, and the sheath of the optic nerve is continuous with the sclera of the eyeball.

The meningeal layer of the cerebral dura mater sends inwards four processes or septa which divide the cranial cavity into a series of freely communicating spaces for the lodgment of the subdivisions of the brain.

(1) *The falx cerebri* (7.161), so named from its sickle-like form, is a strong, arched process of dura mater which descends vertically in the longitudinal fissure between the cerebral hemispheres. It is narrow in front, where it is fixed to the crista galli of the ethmoid bone, and broad

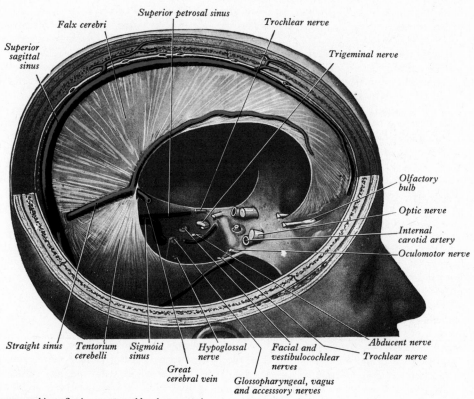

**7.161**   The cerebral dura mater and its reflexions, exposed by the removal of a part of the right half of the skull and brain.

**The cerebral dura mater** lines the interior of the skull, and serves the two-fold purpose of an internal periosteum to the bones, and a supportive membrane for the brain. It is said to be composed of two layers, an inner or meningeal and an outer or endosteal; but these are closely united, except along certain lines where they separate to enclose the venous sinuses which drain the blood from the brain (p. 692). The dura mater adheres to the inner surfaces of the cranial bones, and sends blood vessels and fibrous processes into them, the adhesion being most marked at the sutures, at the base of the skull, and around the foramen magnum. The blood vessels and fibrous processes are torn across when the dura mater is detached from the bones, and consequently the outer surface of the membrane presents a rough and fibrillated appearance; the inner surface is smooth. The endosteal layer of the dura mater is continuous through the sutures and the foramina of the skull with the pericranium, and through the superior orbital fissure with the periosteal lining of the orbital cavity. The meningeal layer provides tubular sheaths for the cranial nerves as the latter pass

behind, where it blends in the median plane with the upper surface of the tentorium cerebelli; the narrow, anterior part is thin, and is frequently perforated by numerous apertures. The upper margin of the falx cerebri is convex, and attached to the inner surface of the skull on each side of the median plane, as far back as the internal occipital protuberance; the superior sagittal sinus (p. 693) runs along this margin. Its lower margin is free and concave, and contains the inferior sagittal sinus. The straight sinus runs along its attachment to the tentorium cerebelli.

(2) *The tentorium cerebelli* (7.161, 162) is a crescentic, arched lamina of dura mater which covers the cerebellum, and supports the occipital lobes of the cerebrum. Its concave, anterior border is free, and between it and the dorsum sellae of the sphenoid bone there is a large oval opening, the *tentorial incisure*, which is occupied by the midbrain and the anterior part of the superior surface of the vermis of the cerebellum. Its convex outer margin is attached (*a*) posteriorly, to the lips of the transverse sulci of the occipital bone and the postero-inferior angles of the parietal bones, where it contains the transverse

sinuses; (b) laterally, to the superior borders of the petrous parts of the temporal bones, where it encloses the superior petrosal sinuses. Near the apex of the petrous part of the temporal bone, the lower layer of the tentorium is pouched forwards and laterally, beneath the superior petrosal sinus, to form a recess between the endosteal and meningeal layers of dura mater of the middle cranial fossa. This recess is called the *trigeminal cave* and envelops the roots of the trigeminal nerve and the posterior part of its sens-

its apex frequently divides into two small folds, which are lost on the sides of the foramen magnum.

(4) *The diaphragma sellae* (7.162) is a small, circular, horizontal fold of dura mater, which forms a roof for the sella turcica and almost completely covers the hypophysis; a small opening in its centre transmits the infundibulum.

The arrangement of the dura mater in the central part of the middle cranial fossa requires further description. As the free rim of the tentorium cerebelli is traced for-

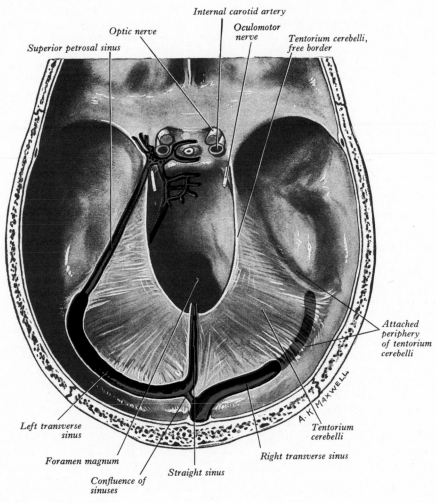

*Internal carotid artery*

*Optic nerve*  *Oculomotor nerve*

*Superior petrosal sinus*  *Tentorium cerebelli, free border*

*Attached periphery of tentorium cerebelli*

*Left transverse sinus*  *Tentorium cerebelli*

*Foramen magnum*  *Right transverse sinus*

*Confluence of sinuses*  *Straight sinus*

**7.162**  The superior aspect of the tentorium cerebelli.

ory ganglion; it is a little more extensive below than above the ganglion. The evaginated meningeal layer terminates by fusing with the anterior part of the ganglion. At the apex of the petrous part of the temporal bone the free border and attached periphery of the tentorium cross each other (7.162); the anterior limits of the free border are fixed to the anterior clinoid processes of the sphenoid bone, whilst those of the attached periphery end on the posterior clinoid processes of that bone. As already described, the straight sinus runs in the line of attachment of the posterior part of the inferior border of the falx cerebri to the tentorium cerebelli.

For details of the comparative anatomy and phylogeny of the tentorium cerebelli see footnote reference [934].

(3) *The falx cerebelli* is a small, sickle-shaped process of dura mater which is situated below the tentorium cerebelli, and projects forwards into the posterior cerebellar notch. Its base, directed upwards, is attached to the posterior part of the inferior surface of the tentorium cerebelli, in the median plane; its posterior margin contains the occipital sinus, and is fixed to the internal occipital crest;

wards, it converges on the attached periphery, and crosses it near the apex of the petrous part of the temporal bone. It is then continued forwards as a clearly visible ridge on the dura mater as far as the anterior clinoid process, to which it is attached. This ridge marks the junction of the roof and lateral wall of the cavernous sinus (7.161).

The attached periphery of the tentorium cerebelli follows the superior border of the petrous part of the temporal bone and, after being crossed by the free border, continues forwards to the posterior clinoid process as a somewhat rounded and indefinite ridge on the dura mater.

An angular interval exists between the anterior parts of the attached periphery and free border (7.162), and in this interval the dura mater forms the roof of the cavernous sinus. In this situation it is pierced in front by the oculomotor and behind by the trochlear nerves. These two nerves remain in close contact with the dura mater after piercing it and are carried forwards and downwards into the lateral wall of the cavernous sinus (6.127).

[934] G. K. Klintworth, *Anat. Rec.*, **160**, 1968.

From the anteromedial portion of the lateral part of the middle cranial fossa the dura mater ascends, forming the lateral wall of the cavernous sinus. When it reaches the ridge produced by the forward continuation of the free border of the tentorium cerebelli, it is carried medially, forming the roof of the cavernous sinus, and is here pierced by the internal carotid artery (7.162).

Medially, the roof of the cavernous sinus is continuous with the upper surface of the diaphragma sellae. At, or just below, the opening in the diaphragma for the infundibulum of the hypophysis, the dura mater, arachnoid and pia mater blend with one another and with the capsule of the hypophysis (p. 1367), so that within the sella turcica it is impossible to differentiate the individual membranes or to recognize the subdural and subarachnoid spaces (6.127).

Apart from its function as the periosteum of the internal surfaces of the cranial bones, the dura mater may act as a steadying influence, through the agency of the tentorium and falx, upon the movement of the brain within the cranial cavity, but this is merely a speculation. A number of venous sinuses are enclosed within its thickness and certain of these are in actual edges of the dural partitions. The junction of the great cerebral vein with the straight sinus in the tentorium cerebelli is a particularly critical point in the venous drainage of the brain. If the relation between these two venous channels is much altered for anything more than short periods of time, as may occur when 'space-occupying' lesions above the tentorium cause a descent of the brainstem relative to the tentorium, obstruction of the great cerebral vein may ensue, with the sequelae of back-pressure, oedema of the choroid plexuses and over-production of cerebrospinal fluid.

**The structure of the dura mater** is basically fibrous, white collagen fibres predominating with an admixture of elastic fibres. The collagen fibres are densely arranged in laminae, in which the fibres are often arranged in a parallel manner, with wide angles between these groupings in adjacent laminae, producing a latticed appearance particularly easy to see in the tentorium cerebelli. The cerebral dura mater is often described as consisting of two layers, an *endosteal* layer acting as the periosteum of the cranial bones to which it is attached, and a *meningeal* or cerebral layer internal to this. This description owes more, perhaps, to the separation where venous sinuses occur and to the splitting of the cerebral dura mater at the foramen magnum and optic canals than to any marked histological differences. The smaller branches of the meningeal vessels are, of course, largely in the endosteal region, since they are, despite their name, primarily periosteal in distribution. Fibroblasts occur throughout the dura mater, but osteoblasts are naturally confined to the endosteal level. The elastic fibres separate the laminae of collagen fibres, which are also and more extensively separated by lacunar spaces considered by some to be continuous with the subdural space (*vide infra*). These spaces are mainly confined to the inner part of the dura mater. In sum, therefore, there are a number of features which distinguish the external from the internal levels of the dura, but there is no discontinuity or any other kind of boundary upon which a clear distinction of a bilaminar nature could be based. At all foramina in the cranium the endosteal element is continuous through them with the external periosteum. At the sutures, before their fusion, the endosteal element is continuous with the sutural membrane, and the dura mater is more strongly attached at these locations. Elsewhere it is more easily detached from the cranial bones. The meningeal element is continuous through the appropriate foramina with the dural sheaths of the spinal cord and the optic nerves. At other foramina it is said to be 'pierced' by the nerve or

vessel passing through them, but it is perhaps more accurately described as becoming continuous with perineurium or adventitial sheaths. Though in close apposition to the arachnoid mater internal to it, the dura mater is very easily separated from the former, as exemplified by the occurrence of subdural haemorrhages between them. Although contrary views have been recorded, there is little doubt that a layer of flattened 'mesothelial' cells is a constant feature of the internal aspect of the dura mater and that small amounts of fluid, though as a mere capillary film, usually exist as a zone of potential separation between arachnoid and dura. (The structure of the subjacent arachnoid is described on p. 993.)

**The arteries of the cerebral dura mater** are very numerous. Those in the anterior fossa of the skull are the anterior meningeal branches of the anterior and posterior ethmoidal and internal carotid arteries, and a branch from the middle meningeal artery. Those in the middle fossa are the middle and accessory meningeal branches of the maxillary artery; a branch from the ascending pharyngeal artery, which enters the skull through the foramen lacerum; branches from the internal carotid artery, and a recurrent branch from the lacrimal artery. Those in the posterior fossa are meningeal branches from the occipital artery, one entering the skull through the jugular foramen, and another through the mastoid foramen; the posterior meningeal branches of the vertebral artery; occasional meningeal branches from the ascending pharyngeal artery, entering the skull through the jugular foramen and hypoglossal canal. The meningeal arteries are chiefly distributed to bone, in contrast to those of the spinal dura mater, and are therefore inappropriately named. Only very fine branches are distributed to the dura itself within the cranium.

The *veins* returning the blood from the cranial dura mater are described on p. 692.

**The nerves of the cerebral dura mater** have been the subject of a number of investigations over a long period.[935-942] The best recognized dural innervation arises from the *trigeminal nerve*, including its ganglion and three principal divisions or their branches, from the upper three *cervical nerves*, and from the *cervical sympathetic* trunk. Other less well-established meningeal branches have been described as arising from the vagus and hypoglossal nerves, and also possibly from the facial and glossopharyngeal nerves (but see below).

In the *anterior cranial fossa* the meningeal nerves are twigs from the anterior and posterior ethmoidal nerves, and anterior filaments from the meningeal branches of the maxillary (*nervus meningeus medius*) and mandibular (*nervus spinosus*) divisions of the trigeminal. The principal area of distribution of the latter two nerves is, however, to the dura of the *middle cranial fossa*, which also receives filaments directly from the trigeminal ganglion. The *tentorium cerebelli* receives on each side the recurrent *tentorial nerve*, a branch of the ophthalmic division of the trigeminal. The dura mater of the *posterior cranial fossa* is innervated by ascending meningeal branches from the upper cervical nerves which enter the cranium through

[935] H. von Luschka, *Die Nerven in der harten Hirnhaut*, Laupp, Tubingen. 1850.
[936] H. von Luschka, *Icones Nervorum Capitis*, Mohr, Heidelberg. 1860.
[937] F. Arnold, *Handbuch der anatomie des Menschen*, Vol. 2, Emmerling und Herder, Freiburg. 1851.
[938] A. Hovelacque, *Anatomie des nerfs craniens et rachidiens et du système grand sympathétique chez l'homme*, Doin, Paris. 1927.
[939] W. Penfield and F. McNaughton, *Archs Neurol. Psychiat.*, Chicago, **44**, 1940.
[940] S. A. Siwe, *Am. J. Anat.*, **48**, 1931.
[941] D. L. Kimmel, *Neurology, Minneap.*, **11**, 1961.
[942] D. L. Kimmel, *Chicago med. Sch. Q.*, **22**, 1961.

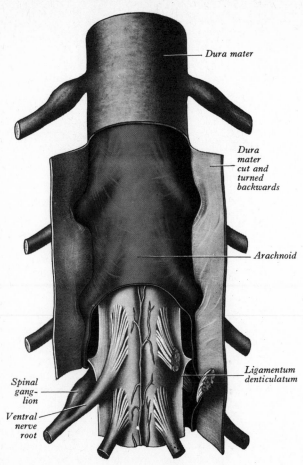

*Dura mater*

*Dura mater cut and turned backwards*

*Arachnoid*

*Ligamentum denticulatum*

*Spinal ganglion*

*Ventral nerve root*

7.163 A part of the spinal cord exposed from the ventral aspect, showing its meningeal coverings.

the anterior part of the foramen magnum (second and third cervical), and through the hypoglossal canal and jugular foramen (first and second cervical nerves). A number of separate filaments enter by each of these routes. Whilst *direct* meningeal branches from the vagus and hypoglossal, and possibly other cranial nerves, cannot be excluded, strong evidence has been accumulated[941, 942] showing that nerves so described are in most cases recurrent filaments from the cervical nerves, which, for a short distance, run within the connective tissue sheath of the cranial nerve concerned.

All the foregoing meningeal nerves contain a post-ganglionic sympathetic component, either derived directly from the superior cervical sympathetic ganglion, or by receiving a communication from one of its perivascular sympathetic nerve extensions into the cranium. These are probably vasomotor fibres, and experiments have been quoted to show that they exert a vasoconstrictor action on pial vessels. Current physiological teaching, however, accords little importance to autonomic control of intra-cranial arteries in general.

Various types of sensory nerve ending, including simple end-bulbs, and Meissner's and Pacinian corpuscles have been described in the dura in various mammals, but little recent information is available concerning man. Thus, the functional role of the sensory and autonomic supply to the dura mater remains uncertain.

**The spinal dura mater** (7.163, 167) forms a loose sheath around the spinal cord, and represents only the inner, or meningeal, layer of the cerebral dura mater; the outer, or endosteal, layer being represented by the periosteum lining the vertebral canal, which is separated from the spinal dura mater by an interval, termed the *extradural space*. The spinal dura mater is attached to the

circumference of the foramen magnum, and to the posterior surfaces of the bodies of the second and third cervical vertebrae; it is also connected by fibrous slips to the posterior longitudinal ligament of the vertebrae, especially near the lower end of the vertebral canal. The subdural cavity ends at the lower border of the second sacral vertebra; below this level the dura mater closely invests the filum terminale of the spinal cord and descends to the back of the coccyx, where it blends with the periosteum. The dura mater gives tubular prolongations to the roots of the spinal nerves and to the spinal nerves themselves as they pass through the intervertebral foramina (7.167). These prolongations are short in the upper part of the vertebral column, but gradually become longer below, owing to the increasing obliquity of the nerve roots (7.37).

**The extradural space** lies between the spinal dura mater and the periosteum and ligaments within the vertebral canal; it contains a quantity of loose fat and areolar tissue and a plexus of veins. The loose fat and areolar tissue of the space, which is known to clinicians as the *epidural space*, extends laterally for a short distance through the intervertebral foramina along the spinal nerves. Dyes or other fluids injected into the sacral hiatus under pressure can spread upwards to the base of the skull in the extradural space, and local anaesthetics injected in the neighbourhood of one spinal nerve immediately outside the intervertebral foramen may spread either upwards or downwards to affect the nerves of adjoining segments, or may spread to the opposite side. In each instance the spread occurs through the extradural space. (For the nerve supply of the spinal dura mater, p. 1032.)

**The subdural space** is a potential space between the dura mater and the arachnoid mater. It contains a film of serous fluid which moistens the surfaces of the opposed membranes. It does not appear to communicate with the subarachnoid space, but is continued for a short distance on the cranial and spinal nerves, and is in free communication with the lymph spaces of the nerves. Around the optic nerve it is continued as far as the back of the eyeball. The significance of the subdural space in terms of function remains a matter of argument rather than demonstration. Possible connexions with venous channels on the one hand and with hypothetical lymph spaces in the substance of the dura mater on the other have been claimed and disclaimed. (See footnote reference [943] for a discussion of these views.) The evidence of electron microscope observations is against the occurrence of any specialized cells of epithelial type in the dura mater, apart from its arachnoid surface, all the dural fibroblasts being of similar appearance. The dural lacunae may in fact be artefacts; certainly the evidence available refutes the passage of significant amounts of a lymphatic fluid from the dura into the subdural or subarachnoid spaces.[944] In the case of the spinal dura mater, however, there is undoubtedly a lymphatic drainage in regard to the extradural adipose tissue, and this may also include the dura itself.[945]

## THE ARACHNOID MATER

The arachnoid is a delicate membrane enveloping the brain and spinal cord and lying between the pia mater internally and the dura mater externally. It is separated from the dura mater by the *subdural space*, but here and there this space is traversed by isolated connective tissue

[943] E. Hoffmann and W. Thiel, *Z. Anat. EntwGesch.*, **119**, 1956.

[944] H. A. Kaplan and D. H. Ford, *The Brain Vascular System*, Elsevier, Amsterdam. 1966.

[945] J. W. Millen and D. H. M. Woollam, *The Anatomy of the Cerebrospinal Fluid*, Oxford University Press, London. 1962.

trabeculae which are most numerous on the posterior surface of the spinal cord. It is separated from the pia mater by the *subarachnoid space*, which is filled with cerebrospinal fluid.

The arachnoid surrounds the cranial and spinal nerves, and encloses them in loose sheaths as far as their points of exit from the skull and vertebral canal.

The *cerebral part of the arachnoid* invests the brain loosely, and does not dip into the sulci between the gyri, nor into the fissures, with the exception of the longitudinal fissure. On the upper surface of the brain it is thin and transparent; at the base it is thicker, and slightly opaque towards the central part, where it extends between the two temporal lobes in front of the pons, so as to leave a considerable interval between it and the pia mater. It cannot be identified in the hypophyseal fossa.

The *spinal part of the arachnoid* (7.163, 167) is a thin, delicate, tubular membrane loosely investing the spinal cord. Above, it is continuous with the cerebral arachnoid; below, it widens out, invests the cauda equina, and ends at the level of the lower border of the second sacral vertebra. (For the structure of the pia-arachnoid see p. 992.)

**The subarachnoid space** is the interval between the arachnoid and pia mater. It contains the cerebrospinal fluid and the larger blood vessels of the brain, and is traversed by a network of delicate connective tissue trabeculae, which connect the arachnoid to the pia mater. The pia mater and the arachnoid are in close contact on the summits of the cerebral gyri; but where the arachnoid bridges the sulci, angular spaces are left, in which the subarachnoid trabecular tissue is found. At certain parts of the base of the brain, the arachnoid is separated from the pia mater by wide intervals, which communicate freely with each other and are named *subarachnoid cisterns*; in these the subarachnoid tissue is scanty and may be absent.

**The Subarachnoid Cisterns** (7.164).

The *cerebello-medullary cistern* (*cisterna magna*) (7.164) is formed by the arachnoid bridging the interval between the medulla oblongata and the under surface of the cerebellum and is triangular on sagittal section; it is continuous below with the subarachnoid space of the spinal cord. The *pontine cistern* (7.164) is an extensive space on the ventral surface of the pons. It contains the basilar artery, and is

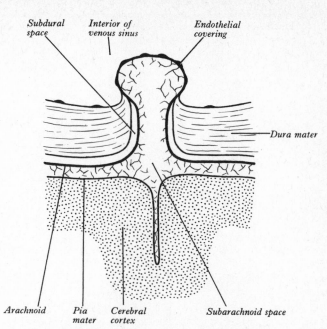

7.165 A diagram to show the structure of a small arachnoid granulation. (After W. E. Le G. Clark.)

continuous below with the subarachnoid space of the spinal cord, behind with the cerebello-medullary cistern, and in front of the pons with the interpeduncular cistern. As the arachnoid extends across between the two temporal lobes, it is separated from the cerebral peduncles and the structures in the interpeduncular fossa by the *interpeduncular cistern*, which contains the circulus arteriosus. Anteriorly the interpeduncular cistern is continued in front of the optic chiasma and is prolonged over the surface of the corpus callosum; here the arachnoid stretches between the cerebral hemispheres immediately below the free border of the falx cerebri, and this leaves a space in which the anterior cerebral arteries are contained. The *cistern of the lateral fossa* contains the middle cerebral artery, and is formed in front of each temporal lobe by the arachnoid bridging the lateral sulcus. The *cistern of the great cerebral vein* (*cisterna ambiens*, or *superior cistern*) occupies the interval between the splenium of the corpus callosum and the superior surface of the cerebellum; it contains the great cerebral vein and the pineal body. It is a widely used neurosurgical landmark.

Other less prominent cisternae have been described; these include the *prechiasmatic* and *postchiasmatic cisterns* related to the optic chiasma, the *cistern of the lamina terminalis*, and the *supracallosal cistern*, all of which, in the above account, were included as extensions of the interpeduncular cistern, and which contain the anterior cerebral arteries.

The subarachnoid space communicates with the general ventricular cavity of the brain by three openings: the *median aperture* (p. 878) is in the median plane in the inferior part of the roof of the fourth ventricle; the two *lateral apertures* are at the extremities of the lateral recesses of that ventricle (p. 878), behind the upper roots of the glossopharyngeal nerves. There is no direct communication between the subdural and subarachnoid spaces. Communications exist between the tissue spaces in the nasal mucous membrane and the subarachnoid space through channels which are present along the course of the olfactory nerves.

The spinal part of the subarachnoid space is a relatively wide interval, and is largest at the lower part of the vertebral canal, where the arachnoid encloses the nerves which form the cauda equina. Above, it is continuous with the

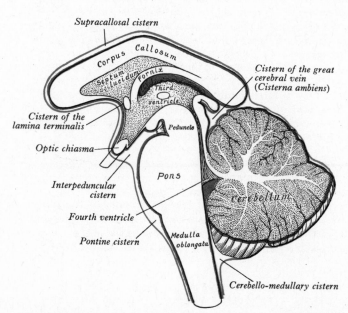

7.164 A diagram showing the positions of the principal subarachnoid cisterns. *Red:* pia mater. *Blue:* arachnoid mater.

cranial subarachnoid space; below, it ends at the level of the lower border of the second sacral vertebra. It is partially divided by two septa, termed, respectively, the subarachnoid septum and the ligamentum denticulatum. Both are described later (p. 992).

**The arachnoid granulations** (7.165, 166) are small fleshy-looking elevations, usually collected in clusters, which are present in the vicinity of the superior sagittal, transverse, and some other sinuses. When the sagittal sinus and the venous lacunae on each side of it are opened, granulations will be found protruding into their interior (7.166). On close inspection they may be seen at the age of eighteen months, and at the age of three they are disseminated over a considerable area; they increase in number and size as age advances. They cause absorption of the bone, and so produce the pits or depressions on the inner aspect of the skull cap. Arachnoid granulations are macroscopic enlargements, or distensions, of minute projections of the arachnoid mater, termed *arachnoid villi*, which are normally present in great numbers in young subjects.

The growth and structure of the arachnoid villi and granulations have been studied in much detail.[946] Histologically each villus appears as a diverticulum of the subarachnoid space, penetrating into the interstices of the dura mater, and covered by a layer of flattened cells containing large oval nuclei and lightly staining protoplasm. In the subarachnoid space there is a reticulum of fine fibrous tissue, the density of which is as a rule greater at the periphery than at the centre of the granulation; in advanced age it frequently contains calcareous nodules.

At the summit of the villus the mesothelial cells proliferate and form a cap which penetrates the surrounding dura mater, and fuses with the endothelial lining of one of the intradural venous sinuses (7.165); in doing so it pulls out a little stalk of arachnoid containing a diverticulum of the subarachnoid space. Except at the point of fusion with the endothelial lining of the sinus, the villus is surrounded by the subdural space and the dura mater; the latter, covered on its cerebral surface by a layer of mesothelium, is invaginated into the venous sinus by the protrusion of the granulation.

Fluid injected into the subarachnoid space passes into these granulations and villi, and it has been found experimentally that fluid passes by osmosis from the arachnoid villi into the venous sinuses of the dura mater.

The *cerebrospinal fluid*[947] is a clear, slightly alkaline fluid, with a specific gravity of about 1007. It contains in solution inorganic salts similar to those in the blood plasma, and also traces of protein and glucose. The cerebrospinal fluid is secreted into the ventricles of the brain by the choroid plexuses and into the subarachnoid space by the plexuses sited in the lateral recesses of the fourth ventricle (p. 879). From the ventricles it passes through the median aperture and the foramina of the lateral recesses of the fourth ventricle and so gains the subarachnoid space in the cerebello-medullary cistern and the pontine cistern. Within the cranium the cerebrospinal fluid flows upwards through the gap in the tentorium cerebelli and then forwards and laterally over the inferior surface of the cerebrum. Finally it ascends over the lateral aspect of each hemisphere to reach the arachnoid villi associated with the superior sagittal sinus, and so is able to pass back again into the bloodstream. It is generally held that within the vertebral canal there is no active flow, but that the process of diffusion and alterations of posture serve to maintain the character of the fluid constant throughout the whole extent of the subarachnoid space. Experimental work[948] suggests that the spinal cerebrospinal fluid may drain back locally into the venous system, through the vertebral venous plexuses, the

intervertebral veins and the posterior intercostal and upper lumbar veins into the azygos and hemiazygos veins. The cerebrospinal fluid supports the brain and spinal cord, and it maintains a uniform pressure upon them. It has been stated that a brain weighing 1500 gm. in air, weighs no more than 50 gm. in cerebrospinal fluid, and through the latter, the total weight of the system is evenly distributed to the meningeal parieties, and their mechanical supports. Our knowledge of the circulation of the cerebrospinal fluid and of the arachnoid villi has, to a large extent, been built up on the work of Weed and his collaborators.[949] Electron microscope studies suggest that there is an open communication between the subarachnoid space and the lumen of the superior sagittal sinus by means of fine tubules, lined by an endothelium, traversing the core of arachnoid granulations in the sheep. A valvular action is hypothecated for these tubules, but this form of drainage, if confirmed, does not exclude filtration.[950]

*Applied Anatomy.* Diseases of the central nervous system and its membranes are often reflected in alterations of the cells which are normally found in the cerebrospinal fluid or in alterations in the concentration of its chemical constituents. Interference with the circulation of the fluid is indicated by variations in the pressure within the meninges. The determination of these alterations and variations is often of service in diagnosis.

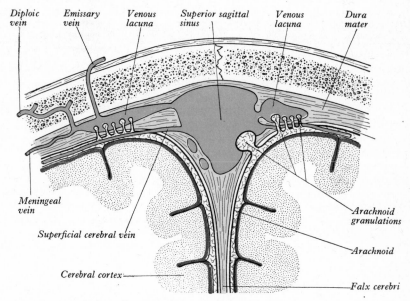

7.166 A coronal section through the vertex of the skull to show the arrangement of the veins and the meninges of the brain and arachnoid granulations.

Specimens of the cerebrospinal fluid may be obtained by the operation of *lumbar puncture*, which is performed through the interval between the laminae or spines of the third and fourth (or fourth and fifth) lumbar vertebrae. A fine trocar and cannula is inserted at the point of intersection of the intertubercular plane with the posterior median line and is passed obliquely upwards and forwards above the upper border of the spine of the fourth lumbar vertebra. It is carried through, or parallel to, the supraspinous and interspinous ligaments into the

[946] W. E. Le G. Clark, *J. Anat.*, **55**, 1920.
[947] H. Davson, *Physiology of the Cerebrospinal Fluid*, Churchill, London. 1970.
[948] F. Howarth and E. R. A. Cooper, *Lancet*, **2**, 1949.
[949] L. H. Weed, *Contr. Embryol.*, **9**, 1920; and *J. Anat.*, **72**, 1938.
[950] A. D. P. Jayatilaka, *J. Anat.*, **99**, 1965.

vertebral canal. The dura mater and the arachnoid are punctured and the instrument is introduced into the subarachnoid space below the lower end of the spinal cord (7.34). When the trocar is withdrawn, the cerebrospinal fluid escapes through the cannula at the rate of one drop per second, under normal conditions, but when the fluid is under increased pressure it escapes in an almost continuous stream. It should also be noted that the introduction of a large needle, such as a trocar, between the vertebral laminae is rather difficult except at lumbar levels. Moreover, the introduction of its point, accurately enough to withdraw fluid, into the narrow subarachnoid space surrounding the spinal cord would be extremely difficult, apart from the danger to the cord itself.

## THE PIA MATER

The pia mater closely invests the brain and spinal cord; it is a vascular membrane, consisting of a plexus of minute blood vessels held together by an extremely fine areolar tissue. The *cerebral pia mater* invests the entire surface of the brain, dips between the cerebral gyri and between the cerebellar laminae, and is invaginated to form the tela choroidea of the third ventricle, and the choroid plexuses

The *ligamentum denticulatum* is situated on each side and the *subarachnoid septum* is present posteriorly (7.167). Below the conus medullaris the pia mater is continued as a longer slender filament, named the *filum terminale* (p. 806).

The pia mater forms sheaths for the cranial and spinal nerves; these sheaths are closely connected with the nerves, and blend with their common membranous investments.

The *ligamentum denticulatum* (7.163, 167) is a narrow, fibrous sheet situated on each side of the spinal cord, between the ventral and the dorsal nerve roots. Its medial border is continuous with the pia mater at the side of the spinal cord. Its lateral border presents a series of triangular tooth-like processes, the points of which are fixed at intervals to the dura mater. These processes are twenty-one in number, on each side. The first process crosses behind the vertebral artery at the point where that vessel pierces the dura mater, and is separated by the artery from the ventral root of the first cervical nerve; it is attached to the dura mater immediately above the margin of the foramen magnum, a short distance behind the hypoglossal nerve, and the spinal part of the accessory nerve ascends on its posterior aspect (7.59). The last process is between the exits of the twelfth thoracic and

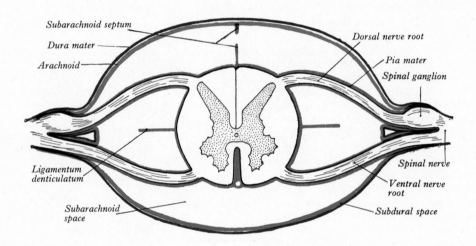

**7.167**　A transverse section through the spinal cord and its membranes. *Black:* dura mater. *Blue:* arachnoid mater. *Red:* pia mater.

of the lateral and third ventricles (pp. 980 and 919); as it passes over the roof of the fourth ventricle, it forms the tela choroidea and the choroid plexuses of this ventricle (p. 879). Upon the surfaces of the hemispheres it gives off from its deep surface a multitude of sheaths around the minute vessels that run perpendicularly for some distance into the cerebral substance. On the cerebellum the membrane is more delicate; the vessels from its deep surface are shorter, and its relations to the cortex are not so intimate. Like the arachnoid, the pia mater cannot be identified in the hypophyseal fossa.

The *spinal pia mater* (7.163, 167) is thicker, firmer, and less vascular than the cerebral pia mater, but like the latter it consists of an outer 'epi-pia' containing the larger vessels, and internal to this a so-called 'pia-glia' or 'pia-intima' in direct contact with the nervous tissue (*vide infra*). Between the layers are cleft-like spaces which communicate with the subarachnoid space, and a number of blood vessels. The spinal pia mater covers the spinal cord, and is intimately adherent to it; in front it dips into the anterior median fissure and lines its walls, the two layers involved being connected by a loose open meshwork of fine fibrous strands (7.167). A longitudinal fibrous band, called the *linea splendens*, extends along the median plane anteriorly.

first lumbar nerves, and consists of a narrow oblique band running downwards and laterally from the conus medullaris (7.163). Changes in the form and position of the denticulate ligament during spinal movements have been demonstrated by cineradiographic techniques.[951]

The *subarachnoid septum* is an interrupted sheet of fibrous tissue, situated in the median plane. It connects the arachnoid to the pia mater opposite the posterior median sulcus (7.167). Incomplete and cribriform in the cervical region, it forms a more complete partition in the thoracic region.

### The Microscopic Structure of the Leptomeninges

The finer structure of the arachnoid and pial meninges is more appropriately described in conjunction.[952] They have a common phylogenetic history, develop embryologically in continuity, and preserve this intimate relationship in their final differentiation to such an extent that they are frequently regarded as a *pia-arachnoid* rather than two separable entities. They will, however, be

[951] B. S. Epstein, *Am. J. Roentg.*, **98**, 1966.
[952] G. Winckler, *Archs Anat. Histol. Embryol.*, **43**, 1960.

described here successively, largely because it is still widely customary to employ separate names for them.

**The structure of the arachnoid mater**, like that of the pia, is essentially that of a loose connective tissue. Both the leptomeninges, like the dura mater, or pachymeninx, are regarded as being of mesodermal origin, though there is some doubt with respect to the innermost region of the pia mater, which may be of ectodermal derivation.[953] In the most primitive vertebrates all three meninges are represented by an undifferentiated *meninx primitiva*; but in tetrapods a distinction into the thick external dura mater and a more delicate internal leptomeninx is established, and in mammals and birds this reaches its most differentiated form. All three meninges develop in the mesenchyme surrounding the central nervous system, with the possible proviso mentioned above.

The *arachnoid mater* consists of collagen, elastin, and reticulin fibres, together with flattened cells usually regarded as mesothelial in type, although there is some disagreement as to this latter point. Both on its dural aspect and on its internal surface, where it forms the external boundary of the subarachnoid space, cells with long cytoplasmic processes and a paler cytoplasm than the fibrocytes of the dura mater are arranged in several layers, with an underlying basement membrane. Tight junctions between some of these cells are demonstrable by electron microscopy,[954] but collagen fibres are interspersed among them and elastic fibres may also appear between the layers of cells. The fibre elements of the arachnoid are of more gracile proportions than those of the dura mater. Fine strands or *trabeculae* of arachnoid tissue extend inwards across the *subarachnoid space*, and these also are usually considered to show a covering of 'mesothelial' cells, within which are collagen fibres and then reticulin fibres surrounding the numerous small vessels which pass through the trabeculae to reach the pia mater and central nervous system. The trabeculae vary much in size and distribution; most are fine strands and they are most numerous in the intracranial part of the subarachnoid space, but are largely absent where this is dilated to form cisternae (p. 990) and are little evident in the spinal region of the space in man. Descriptions of the trabeculae are frequently illustrated from other mammals and this may convey a false or exaggerated impression of their development in mankind. The spaces between the trabeculae are usually extensive and are described as running together to form a single intercommunicating subarachnoid space; but in the human arrangement large stretches of the space are completely free from trabeculae.

Crossing the subarachnoid space the arachnoid trabeculae fuse with the pia mater, which is itself sometimes regarded as divisible into two layers (*vide infra*), the external being a vascularized connective tissue stratum, covered by a mesothelium bounding the subarachnoid space on its internal or cerebral aspect. Some observers regard this stratum of the pia mater as being arachnoid tissue, considering only the avascular layer of collagen and other fibres and their accompanying cells which are immediately adjacent to nervous tissue to represent the true pia. In this case the subarachnoid space is described as being *in* the arachnoid mater. Others prefer to think of the two leptomeninges as a conjoined pia-arachnoid membrane, as stated earlier.

The arachnoid mater is not itself much vascularized, and is often described as avascular; but it does act as a connective tissue support for large numbers of small vessels and their accompanying nerve supplies, traversing the trabeculae to reach the pia mater. Its mesothelial elements and basement membrane, and particularly the tight junctions between the cells, are a barrier to free diffusion of colloidal substances between the subarach-noid space, subdural space, the central nervous system and its non-capillary vessels in both their extra- and intra-cerebral sites. The return of the cerebrospinal fluid is thus largely, if not entirely limited to the arachnoid villi (p. 991), where this permeability barrier is modified and also circumvented by a system of minute valvular canals. The barrier is also absent where the craniospinal nerves pass through fused sleeves of pia and arachnoid as they blend with the perineurium. At these locations cerebro-spinal fluid can diffuse through the arachnoid tissue into neighbouring lymphatics.

**The structure of the pia mater** is also that of a loose connective tissue, containing collagen, elastin and reticulin fibres with flattened 'mesothelial' cells like those of the arachnoid. These cells are considered to be fibrocytic elements by some authorities, especially where they form several layers, associated with reticulin fibres, next to the central nervous system. Here the most internal cells are directly apposed to a convoluted basement membrane, intervening between them and the subjacent end-feet of astrocytes. This relationship is so intimate that the most internal stratum of the pia, together with the basement membrane and the glial processes, is sometimes described as the '*pia-glia*'. It is also sometimes distinguished as the '*pia-intima*', and thus differentiated from the rest of the membrane, the '*epi-pia*', which is the pial element regarded as arachnoid by some, as mentioned above. Sleeves of both pia and arachnoid, with an intervening extension of the subarachnoid space, are carried into the central nervous system around the blood vessels entering or leaving it, forming the perivascular cuffs which have been the subject of so much past disagreement.

The pia mater contains large numbers of blood vessels and their accompanying nerve supplies. On the surface of the spinal cord the more external connective tissue layer of the pia, the epi-pia, is more developed than it is on the cerebral surface, where it is not easily identified. In this stratum the vessels are suspended by trabeculae of pial tissue which meet and blend with arachnoid trabeculae where these are present. Thus many pial vessels project from the surface as they ramify in their pia-arachnoid suspension, and are at least partially surrounded by extensions of the subarachnoid space. Where they turn into the central nervous system prolongations of the space and the two leptomeninges accompany each vessel as far as the commencement of its capillaries. Hence the latter are not separated from nervous tissue by the connective tissue or mesothelial elements which accompany the precapillary vessels; the 'pia-glial' barrier is absent. Current physiological views reject the concept of any significant interchange of fluid between the perivascular extensions of the subarachnoid space and nervous tissue or blood, nor is drainage circulation through them considered likely. It is suggested that these minute fluid-filled spaces merely act as a displaceable medium to accommodate the pulsatile variation in the calibre of the vessels which they surround.

The coverings of the central nervous capillaries are like those in the choroid plexuses (p. 981) in the complete absence of ordinary connective elements from their surroundings. The neuronal level is separated from the blood only by the vascular endothelium, the end-feet of astrocytes, and the basement membrane which they share. While the individual contribution of these structures to the human *blood-brain barrier* cannot yet be stated with certainty, abundant experimental evidence indicates that this is the major and probably the exclusive site of entry of fluid and solutes into the central nervous

[953] J. W. Millen and D. H. M. Woollam, *Brain*, **84**, 1961.
[954] E. Nelson, K. Blinzinger and H. Hager, *Neurology, Minneap.*, **11**, 1961.

tissue, the arachnoid villi providing the main exit for cerebrospinal fluid, and the drainage of fluid from the nervous tissue being partly back into the prevenous ends of the capillaries and perhaps through ependyma into the ventricular system. Experiments in the mouse, using horseradish peroxidase as an electron-dense tracer have, however, shed some light on the problem of the blood-brain barrier.[955] In most of the central nervous situations examined, complete circumferential tight junctions, between adjacent capillary endothelial cells, totally prevent the passage of the tracer. Similar junctions exist between the modified ependymal cells which clothe the choroid plexus. To what extent such findings apply to

other sites, animals and substances, remains speculative.

Apart from their functions in the production, circulation and reabsorption of the cerebrospinal fluid, the meninges also serve as a support to the central nervous system, especially in association with the buoyant effect of the fluid. Like connective tissues elsewhere they also provide routes of access and support for the vessels of the central nervous system, and they constitute at least a mechanical barrier against infection.

[955] M. W. Brightman, I. Klatzo, Y. Olsson and T. S. Reese, *J. Neurol. Sci.*, **10**, 1970.

# THE PERIPHERAL NERVOUS SYSTEM

The peripheral nervous system comprises the afferent, or centripetal, fibres which connect the sensory end organs to the central nervous system, and the efferent, or centrifugal, fibres which connect the central nervous system to the effector apparatus. It includes the twelve pairs of cranial nerves which arise from the brain, and the thirty-one pairs of spinal nerves which arise from the spinal cord. The sympathetic trunks with their various ganglia and branches belong to this system, but they will be dealt with in a separate section (pp. 1065–1083).

7.168 Transverse section of a peripheral nerve (cat). Stained with osmic acid and van Gieson's technique. Note the nerve fasciculi, the epi-, peri- and endo-neurial connective tissue sheaths, and the regional variations in the calibre of the myelinated nerve fibres. Magnification about × 55.

In the most primitive vertebrates the spinal cord gives rise to a series of ventral nerve roots, arising from the anterior grey column and motor in function, and a series of dorsal nerve roots, connected to the posterior grey column and sensory in function. The ventral and dorsal nerve roots do not unite, and they do not correspond in position. The ventral nerve root is segmental and is distri-

buted to the myotome which corresponds to the neuro-mere from which it arises. The dorsal nerve root is inter-segmental in position and runs in the intersegmental connective tissue to reach its cutaneous distribution. In the majority of fishes and in all higher forms the corresponding ventral and dorsal nerve roots which emerge from the spinal cord unite with one another to constitute the individual spinal nerves. The arrangement of the spinal nerves, therefore, follows a very primitive pattern and has not undergone much modification in the process of evolution.

The arrangement of the cranial nerves, on the other hand, has been very profoundly modified. The development and modification of the branchial system and the suppression of segments owing to the elaborate changes which occur in the region of the head have been largely responsible for this modification. In the brain, corresponding ventral and dorsal nerves *never* fuse, although adjoining ventral or dorsal nerves may and actually do unite. Owing to the complete disappearance of certain myotomes the corresponding ventral nerves become completely suppressed. Further, the dorsal nerves, originally sensory nerves supplying chiefly the skin of the head and the mucous membrane of the mouth and pharynx acquire motor fibres which they distribute to the musculature arising in the branchial region (p. 120). With the growth and modification of the brain and the consequent elaboration of the head region, the cutaneous areas of the head are transferred from one nerve to its neighbour, so that the functions of the individual dorsal nerves become altered.

The incorporation of some of the precervical segments in the head leads to the fusion of the corresponding ventral nerves, and the hypoglossal nerve so formed becomes added to the cranial nerves.

**The cerebrospinal nerves**, as we have seen in greater detail elsewhere (p. 783), consist of numerous nerve fibres collected into bundles, which are enclosed in connective tissue sheaths (**7**.168): a small bundle of fibres is called a *fasciculus*. Each fasciculus is surrounded by a connective tissue sheath, named the *perineurium*. Individual nerve fibres are ensheathed, held together and supported within the fasciculus by delicate connective tissue called the *endoneurium*; it is continuous with septa which pass inwards from the perineurium. The collagen fibres of the endoneurium tend to be longitudinally orientated and bundles are sometimes invaginated into the Schwann cells of non-myelinated nerve fibres.[956] If small, the nerve may consist of only a single fasciculus; but if large, it consists of several fasciculi held together and invested by

[956] H. J. Gamble and R. A. J. Eames, *J. Anat.*, **98**, 1964.

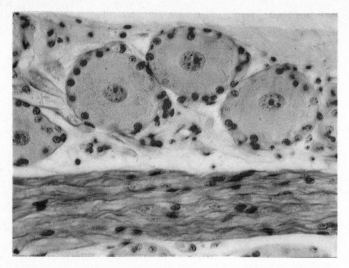

7.169   A typical field in a dorsal spinal nerve root ganglion. Note the characteristic juxtaposition of large ovoid nerve cell somata, and the fascicles of myelinated and non-myelinated nerve fibres. Note also the nuclei of the capsular (satellite) cells which surround each nerve cell. (Grübler's stain—material kindly provided by Mrs. Lyn Gregson.)

connective tissue; this investment is known as the *epineurium*. The cerebrospinal nerves consist both of myelinated and non-myelinated nerve fibres, the proportion of each varying with the functional roles of the nerve concerned.

The blood vessels, supplying a nerve, end in a minute plexus of capillaries which pierce the perineurium, and run, for the most part, parallel with the fibres; they are connected together by short transverse vessels, forming narrow, oblong meshes, similar to the capillary system of muscle. Fine, non-myelinated, vasomotor nerve fibres accompany these vessels, and break up into fine fibrils which form a network around them. Myelinated fibres, termed *nervi nervorum*, run in the epineurium and terminate in oval or bulbous corpuscles (p. 799).

The cerebrospinal nerve fibres pursue an uninterrupted course from the centre to the periphery, but in separating a nerve into its component fasciculi, it is found that bundles of fibres from one fasciculus may join, at a very acute angle, another fasciculus proceeding in the same direction.

In their course, nerves divide into branches, and these frequently communicate with branches of neighbouring nerves; such communications form what is called a *nerve plexus*. Such a plexus is formed by the ventral rami of the trunks of the nerves—as, for example, the cervical, brachial, lumbar and sacral plexuses—or by the terminal funiculi, as in the plexuses formed at the periphery of the body. In the formation of a plexus, the component nerves divide, then join, and again subdivide in such a complex manner that the individual funiculi become intricately interlaced. Hence, each branch leaving a plexus may contain filaments from more than one, and even all of the primary nerves entering the plexus. In the formation also of smaller plexuses at the periphery of the body there is a free interchange of fibres. In each case, however, the individual fibres remain separate and distinct.

Through this interchange of fibres, every nerve leaving a plexus gains a more extensive connexion with the spinal cord than if it had proceeded direct to its distribution without joining other nerves.

**The origin of a nerve** is a phrase usually implying the locus of its emergence from or entry into the central nervous system. This site is sometimes called the *superficial origin*, the *deep origin* being the central group or groups of nerve cells from which the peripheral axons are derived, or to which they are proceeding. The superficial

origin is in some cases single—that is to say, the whole nerve emerges from the central nervous system by a single root; in other instances the nerve arises by two or more roots. The *efferent nerve fibres* are the axons of nerve cells situated in the grey matter of the central nervous system. The *afferent nerve fibres* spring from nerve cells in the organs of special sense (e.g. the retina) or from nerve cells in the ganglia on the cerebrospinal nerves. Having entered the central nervous system they branch and send their ultimate twigs to terminate in synaptic association with nerve cells there.

**The peripheral terminations** of the sensory nerves are dealt with on pp. 794–804, and those of motor nerves on pp. 791, 802.

**Ganglia** are aggregations of nerve cells found on some peripheral nerves. They are present in the dorsal roots of the spinal nerves and the sensory roots of the trigeminal, facial, glossopharyngeal, vagal nerves, and vestibulocochlear nerves. They also occur in association with autonomic nerves (p. 1065). They vary considerably in form and size. Each ganglion is invested by a smooth, firm covering of fibrous connective tissue and associated flattened, fibrocyte-like cells, which is continuous with the perineurium of the nerves, and sends numerous processes into the interior of the ganglion.

Ganglia contain nerve cells and their nerve fibres, and fibres derived from cells elsewhere, which pass right

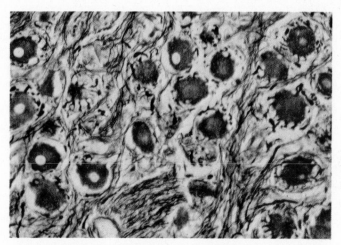

7.170A   Typical field in an autonomic ganglion (human ciliary ganglion), showing nerve cells evenly scattered among fascicles of nerve fibres. (Stained by Bielschowsky's silver and erythrosin technique in material kindly supplied by Dr. N. A. Locket, Institute of Ophthalmology, London.)

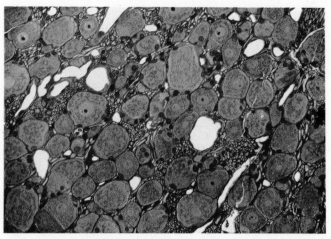

7.170 B   Cells in superior cervical sympathetic ganglion of rabbit. Thin section (*c*. 2μm) of araldite-embedded material stained by toluidine blue. (Material kindly supplied by Dr. J. S. Dixon, Department of Anatomy, University of Manchester.)

through or terminate within the ganglion. Their structure, which is treated briefly here, is considered in greater detail on p. 782. In the spinal ganglia the cells are large, unipolar, and occur in groups round the periphery; in the autonomic ganglia they are multipolar and are scattered more or less uniformly (7.169, 170). Each spinal ganglionic nerve cell has a nucleated capsule (p. 783), which is continuous with the Schwann cells of the nerve fibres connected with the cell. The larger nerve cells in the ganglia of the spinal nerves (7.169) are irregularly spherical in shape, and each gives off a single neurite ('dendro-axonal process') which runs towards the centre of the ganglion, and divides in a T-shaped manner; one limb (axon) of the crossbar enters the spinal cord, the other (dendrite) passes outwards to the periphery. Near its origin the dendro-axonal process is coiled on itself, forming a *glomerulus*. The smaller cells, which are more numerous, and give rise to fine non-myelinated fibres in peripheral nerves and their roots, possess delicate initial

dendro-axonal processes which do not form complicated glomeruli, and pass straight to their T-bifurcation.

Structurally the peripheral division of the process of a unipolar ganglion cell resembles an axon in every respect, but it functions as a greatly elongated dendrite. (It should be noted that the majority of neuroanatomists term all the elongated neurites in a peripheral nerve 'axons' whether they are afferent or efferent.) The somata of afferent neurons in primitive invertebrates, such as *Hydra*, are situated in the ectoderm, with superficial hair-like dendritic processes projecting from them. Such somata are located much deeper in all vertebrates, being close to the central nervous system. Their peripheral processes are presumably the much elongated homologue of the short 'dendrites' of the primitive nerve cells. The primary olfactory neurons retain this primitive position (p. 1089). In the sensory ganglia of the cranial nerves, the nerve cells are also unipolar, though in the ganglia of the vestibulo-cochlear nerve they remain bipolar in type.

## THE CRANIAL NERVES

The craniocaudal sequence of cranial nerves is as follows:

| | | |
|---|---|---|
| 1 Olfactory | 5 Trigeminal | 9 Glossopharyngeal |
| 2 Optic | 6 Abducent | 10 Vagus |
| 3 Oculomotor | 7 Facial | 11 Accessory |
| 4 Trochlear | 8 Vestibulocochlear | 12 Hypoglossal |

These nerves are continuous with the brain and traverse foramina in the base of the cranium. The **motor**, or **efferent**, parts of the cranial nerves arise within the brain from groups of nerve cells which constitute their *nuclei of origin*. They are connected with the cerebral cortex by the corticonuclear fibres; these arise from the cells of the motor areas of the cortex, descend chiefly in the genicular part of the internal capsule to the brainstem, where many, but not all cross the median plane and end by arborizing round the cells of the nuclei of origin of the motor cranial nerves. The **sensory**, or **afferent**, cranial nerves arise from nerve cells outside the brain; these nerve cells may be grouped to form ganglia on the trunks of the nerves, or may be situated in peripheral sensory organs such as the nose, eye and ear. The centrally directed processes of the cells run into the brain and there end by arborizing around nerve cells which are grouped to form their *nuclei of termination*. Fibres arise from the cells of these nuclei and, usually after crossing to the opposite side, run up to connect the nuclei indirectly with the cerebral cortex.

The fibres of most of the cranial nerves begin to acquire their myelin sheaths about the fourteenth week of intra-uterine life. The process is delayed until the twenty-second week in the cases of the sensory part of the trigeminal nerve and the cochlear division of the vestibulo-cochlear. In the case of the optic nerve myelination does not commence until the later stages of gestation.[957]

## The Olfactory Nerves

The olfactory nerves, serving the sense of smell (7.171), commence in the mucous membrane of the olfactory region of the nasal cavity; this region comprises the superior nasal concha and the opposed part of the nasal septum. The nerve fibres originate as the central, or deep, processes of the olfactory cells (7.118) of the nasal mucous membrane, and are collected into bundles which cross one another in various directions, thus giving the appearance

of a plexiform network in the mucous membrane. They are then collected into about twenty branches, which traverse the cribriform plate of the ethmoid bone in lateral and medial groups, and end in the glomeruli of the olfactory bulb (7.118). Each branch has a tubular sheath of dura mater and pia-arachnoid, the former being continued into the periosteum of the nose, the latter into the delicate trabecular connective tissue perineurium (peri-neural sheaths) of the nerve bundles. The tissue spaces in these sheaths are continuous with those of the nasal mucous membrane and with the subarachnoid space above.

The olfactory nerves are not myelinated and consist of bundles of fine axons enfolded within Schwann cells.

The olfactory nerves are unique in that their cells of origin develop in the ectoderm and retain this position throughout life in all vertebrates.

*Applied Anatomy.* In severe head injuries involving the anterior cranial fossa the olfactory bulb may become separated from the olfactory nerves, or the nerves may be torn, thus producing *anosmia*—loss of smell sensibility. Fractures in this situation may also involve the meninges and cerebrospinal fluid may escape into the nose. Such injuries also open up avenues for infection of the meninges from the nasal cavity. The extensions of the subarachnoid space around the bundles of olfactory nerve fibres have been regarded as a potential lymphatic drainage, and on this basis certain meningeal infections are considered to spread along these nerves into the cranial cavity. The evidence for this is still equivocal.

Closely associated with the olfactory nerves is a pair of small nerves named the **nervi terminales**.[958] These nerves were first seen in lower vertebrates, but their presence has been demonstrated in the human embryo and adult. They consist mainly of non-myelinated nerve fibres, and associated with them are small groups of bipolar and multipolar nerve cells. Each nerve runs along the medial side of the corresponding olfactory tract, and its branches traverse the cribriform plate of the ethmoid bone, and are distributed to the nasal mucous membrane. Centrally the nerve is connected to the brain close to the anterior perforated substance and septal areas; in some animals its fibres have been traced to the lamina terminalis, in others

[957] M. F. L. Keene and E. E. Hewer, *J. Anat.*, **66**, 1931.
[958] A. A. Pearson, *J. comp. Neurol.*, **75**, 1941.

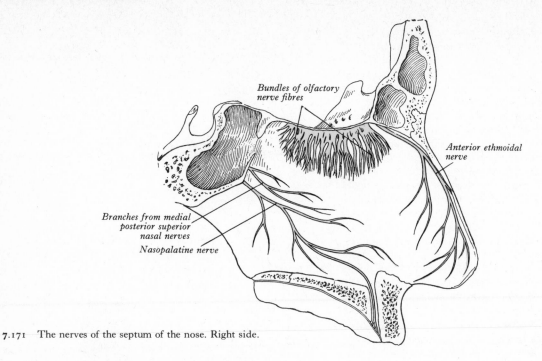

*Bundles of olfactory nerve fibres*

*Anterior ethmoidal nerve*

*Branches from medial posterior superior nasal nerves*

*Nasopalatine nerve*

7.171   The nerves of the septum of the nose. Right side.

to the hypothalamic region. Its function is unknown; some are inclined to view it as a forward extension of the cephalic part of the sympathetic nervous system, which is distributed to the blood vessels and glands of the nasal cavity. The **vomeronasal nerve**, with which the nervus terminalis has been frequently confused, is probably absent in adult man. (See also 934, 1091.)

The detailed architecture and central connexions of the olfactory bulb are described on pp. 932–935, and for the detailed structure of the olfactory mucosa see p. 1089.

## The Optic Nerve

The optic nerve, mediating vision, is distributed to the eyeball. Most of its fibres are afferent and originate in the nerve cells of the ganglionic layer of the retina (p. 1117), but some are efferent, their source of origin being uncertain. Developmentally, the optic nerves and the retinae are parts of the brain (p. 1451), and their fibres are provided with glial and not Schwann cell sheaths.

The fibres of the optic nerve form the innermost layer (*stratum opticum*) of the retina and are the axons of the cells in its ganglionic layer; they converge on the optic disc, and there pierce the outer layers of the retina, the choroid coat, and the lamina cribrosa of the sclera at the posterior part of the eyeball, about 3 or 4 mm to the nasal side of its centre. As the fibres traverse the lamina cribrosa they receive their myelin sheaths, and run in bundles which are collected to form the optic nerve.

The optic nerve, about 4 cm long, is directed backwards and medially through the posterior part of the orbital cavity. It then runs through the optic canal into the cranial cavity and joins the optic chiasma.

The intraorbital part of the nerve is about 25 mm long and has a slightly sinuous course, the length of the nerve being about 6 mm more than the distance between the optic canal and the eyeball. Posteriorly it is closely surrounded by the four recti, but anteriorly is separated from them by a quantity of fat, in which run the ciliary vessels and nerves. The ciliary ganglion lies between the nerve and the lateral rectus. The inferomedial surface of the nerve is pierced, at a distance of about 12 mm behind the eyeball, by the central artery and vein of the retina, which are then directed forwards in the centre of the nerve to the optic disc. In the optic canal, which is about 5 mm

long, the nerve lies above and medial to the ophthalmic artery, and is separated medially from the sphenoidal and posterior ethmoidal sinuses by a thin lamina of bone; in front of the canal the nasociliary nerve and the ophthalmic artery run forwards and medially, crossing above the optic nerve, whilst the branch to the medial rectus from the inferior division of the oculomotor nerve passes below it (7.183).

The intracranial part of the optic nerve, about 10 mm long, runs backwards and medially from the optic canal to the optic chiasma. The posterior parts of the olfactory tract and gyrus rectus, and, near the chiasma, the anterior cerebral artery lie above it. The internal carotid artery is on its lateral side.

The optic nerve is enclosed in three sheaths, which are continuous with the membranes of the brain (7.758), and are prolonged as far as the back of the eyeball. The *outer sheath*, derived from the dura mater, is thick and fibrous, and blends anteriorly with the sclera. The *intermediate sheath*, derived from the arachnoid mater, is thin and delicate. It is separated from the outer sheath by the subdural space, and from the inner sheath by the subarachnoid space. The *inner sheath*, derived from the pia mater, is vascular and closely invests the nerve. From its deep surface septa pass into the nerve and subdivide and reunite to enclose what appear, in transverse sections of the nerve, as polygonal areas, which are occupied by the bundles of nerve fibres. There are about 1,000 such fascicles. From the inner sheath also, an investment is carried on the central vessels of the retina as far as the optic disc.

The ultrastructure of the meninges of the optic nerve resembles that of the meninges elsewhere,[959] but the amount of collagen fibres in the pia and arachnoid is greater than in the general intracranial leptomeninges. Here, as elsewhere, the subarachnoid space is lined completely by epithelial cells of the pia-arachnoid which resemble flattened fibroblasts, forming multilaminar surface membranes of 'mesothelium' or 'meningothelium'.

Close to the eyeball the macular fibres (*papillo-macular bundle*) occupy the lateral part of the nerve, but, as they are traced backwards, they gradually come to lie medially; in front of the chiasma they are close to the medial margin. The fibres from the upper and lower portions of the retina lie above and below respectively; the fibres from the temporal quadrants lie laterally and those from the nasal quadrants medially.

The most recent counts of optic nerve fibres in man[960, 961] give a figure of about 1,200,000 myelinated axons, about 92 per cent of which are small (about 1 $\mu$m in diameter), the rest varying from 2 to 10 $\mu$m. About 53 per cent cross in the chiasma. Most terminate in the lateral geniculate body, but fractions of uncertain size pass to the pretectal nucleus and superior colliculus. A small proportion of the optic nerve fibres are efferent.

The optic nerve is supplied by vessels from the plexus in the investing pia and by direct intraneural branches. The pial plexus receives branches from a superior hypophysial artery and the ophthalmic artery intracranially, from recurrent branches of the ophthalmic artery in the optic canal and from the posterior ciliary arteries and the extraneural part of the central retinal artery in the orbit. The intraneural branches to the nerve arise from the central artery, but their actual contribution to the blood supply of the nerve is probably small[962] (see also footnote reference [963]). The rich blood supply of the optic papilla and the lamina cribrosa has recently been emphasized.[964] The venous drainage is by the central vein of the retina (p. 696).[965]

**The optic chiasma** (p. 913), and the **optic tract** (p. 914), have already been described.

*Applied Anatomy.* The optic nerve is peculiarly liable to neuritis or atrophy in certain affections of the central nervous system, and there are certain points in connexion with the anatomy of this nerve which may throw light upon such associations. (1) From its mode of development, and from its structure, the optic nerve must be regarded as a prolongation of the brain substance, rather than as an ordinary cranial nerve. (2) It receives sheaths from the three cerebral meninges, and these sheaths are separated from each other by spaces which communicate with the subdural and subarachnoid spaces respectively. The innermost sheath sends a process around the arteria centralis retinae into the interior of the nerve, and enters intimately into its structure. Thus inflammatory affections of the meninges or of the brain may readily extend along these spaces, or along the interstitial connective tissue in the nerve.

The *optic neuritis* or *papilloedema* that is often seen in cases of intracranial new growth with increased intracranial tension, is probably caused by increased pressure due to excess of fluid in the general subarachnoid space, since this is in direct communication with a prolongation of the space around the optic nerve as far as the lamina cribrosa (p. 1097).

## The Oculomotor Nerve

The oculomotor nerve (6.123, 124; 7.109, 120, 174, 184) supplies all the extraocular muscles, except the obliquus superior and rectus lateralis; it also supplies, through its connexion with the ciliary ganglion, the sphincter pupillae and the ciliaris, which are, of course, intraocular. It contains about 24,000 fibres.

The fibres of the oculomotor nerve arise from a *complex of nuclei* in the grey matter, ventral to the cranial part of the cerebral aqueduct, which extends cranially for a short distance into the floor of the third ventricle. From this the fibres pass forwards through the tegmentum, the red nucleus and the medial part of the substantia nigra, forming a series of curves with a lateral convexity, and emerge from the sulcus on the medial side of the cerebral peduncle (7.62, 64, 92).

998    **The nuclear complex** from which the fibres of the

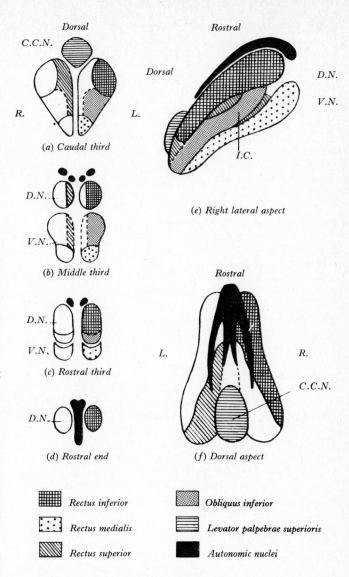

7.172   The constituent parts of the nucleus of the oculomotor nerve in the monkey. (R. Warwick, *J. comp. Neurol.*, **98**, 1953, by courtesy of the publishers.) For significance of abbreviations see footnote reference.[967]

oculomotor nerve are derived consists of a number of paired groups of large multipolar nerve cells, which can be identified in most mammals, together with paired masses of smaller multipolar nerve cells, which are not so easily identified, though well developed in primates and many other mammals, and which are the source of the parasympathetic outflow in the oculomotor nerves. On each side of the midline the large-celled oculomotor mass is topographically divided into **dorsolateral, intermediate** and **ventromedial nuclei** (7.172), which are extended in a columnar form approximately in the long axis of the midbrain.[966, 967] These sub-nuclei become clearly identifiable in early fetal life in man.[968] According to experimental evidence in monkeys they are the motor pools of the *rectus inferior, obliquus inferior* and *rectus medialis*, in that dorsoventral order (7.172). Dorsal to the right and left large-celled masses, and at a level corre-

[960] O. Oppel, *Albrecht v. Graefes Arch. Ophthal.*, **166**, 1963.
[961] C. Kupfer, L. Chumbley and J. de C. Downer, *J. Anat.*, **101**, 1967.
[962] J. François and A. Neetens, *Documenta ophth.*, **26**, 1969.
[963] N. Belmonte, *Archos. Soc. oftal. hisp.-am.*, **28**, 1968.
[964] P. Henkind and M. Levitsky, *Am. J. Ophthal.*, **68**, 1969.
[965] E. J. Steele and M. J. Blunt, *J. Anat.*, **90**, 1956.
[966] E. C. Crosby and J. W. Henderson, *J. comp. Neurol.*, **88**, 1948.
[967] R. Warwick, *Brain*, **73**, 1950.
[968] A. A. Pearson, *J. comp. Neurol.*, **80**, 1944.

sponding to their caudal extremities, is a median nucleus, composed of similar large multipolar nerve cells, the **caudal central nucleus**, which in the same experimental study was observed to be the conjoined motor pool of the two *levators* of the upper eyelids.[967, 969] Dorsal to the right and left main oculomotor nuclei are the two **accessory** or **autonomic nuclei** (of Edinger and Westphal), composed of somewhat smaller multipolar nerve cells, whose axons travel out in the oculomotor to relay in the ciliary ganglion.[970] These accessory nuclei are best developed at cranial oculomotor levels, where they fuse together and arch ventrally over the cranial end of the main oculomotor nuclei (**7.**172); in their more caudal, paired parts these autonomic columns frequently show a tendency to further splitting in man and other primates.

Although a median group of larger motor nerve cells has been a standard feature of oculomotor topography for many decades, this 'central nucleus of Perlia' is a most variable entity in mammals, and indeed in the same species. The function of convergence was loosely ascribed to it at an early date on inadequate and fallacious evidence. Its degree of development in primates is not commensurate with its supposed function, nor is it possible to equate its size with binocular vision.[971] Topographic observers have described it as frequently absent from the human midbrain.[972, 973] There are always a few scattered large motor cells in the midline raphe between the right and left oculomotor masses, but these never constitute a clear nuclear mass, like the caudal central nucleus; in any case, such nerve cells appear to innervate the superior rectus, and not the medial rectus.[974]

Other views of the topographical arrangement of the motor pools of the extraocular muscles have been advanced,[975, 976, 977] all of which suggest a craniocaudal pattern, rather than the dorsoventral scheme described here; but in both forms of organization, which are very different in other ways, there is general agreement that the issuing oculomotor fibres, somatic and autonomic, are almost completely ipsilateral in their midbrain course. At the most some axons from the median raphe and the caudal central nucleus may cross into the opposite oculomotor nerve to innervate the rectus superior and the levator palpebrae superioris; but the extensive crossing of oculomotor axons which is a usual tenet of textbook accounts is not supported by any of the experimental studies quoted here, almost all of which were carried out in primates.

For a discussion of the claims of other nuclei in the vicinity of the oculomotor complex to be included with it, consult footnote reference [978].

**Connexions** of the oculomotor nucleus include fibres from: (1) the corticonuclear tracts of *both* sides; some fibres leave the tracts at the level of the oculomotor nucleus but some (aberrant pyramidal fibres) leave at a higher level and thereafter descend in the medial lemniscus; they end either directly on the cells of the nucleus or are linked to them via interneurons; (2) the medial longitudinal fasciculus by which it is connected to the nuclei of fourth, sixth and eighth cranial nerves (p. 885); (3) the tectobulbar tract, by which it is connected to the visual cortex through the medium of the superior colliculus; and (4) the pretectal nucleus of both sides for the light reflex. For much information on such connexions and their functional significances consult footnote reference [979], and for further comments see p. 1028.

**Course.** On emerging from the brain, the nerve, invested by pia mater, lies in the subarachnoid space. It passes between the superior cerebellar and posterior cerebral arteries (**8.**196), and runs forward in the interpeduncular cistern on the lateral side of the posterior communicating artery. It then perforates the arachnoid

and lies in the triangular interval between the free and attached borders of the tentorium cerebelli. Piercing the inner layer of the dura mater on the lateral side of the posterior clinoid process the nerve traverses the roof, and further forwards descends into the lateral wall of the cavernous sinus, where it lies above the trochlear nerve (**6.**127). In this situation it receives one or two filaments from the internal carotid plexus of the sympathetic, and communicates with the ophthalmic division of the trigeminal. It then divides into a superior and an inferior ramus, which enter the orbit through the superior orbital fissure, within the anulus tendineus communis to which are attached the four recti; here the nasociliary nerve is placed between the two rami (**7.**176, 269).

The *superior ramus*, the smaller, ascends on the lateral side of the optic nerve, and supplies the rectus superior and levator palpebrae superioris. The *inferior ramus* divides into three branches. One passes below the optic nerve to the rectus medialis; another goes to the rectus inferior; the third and longest runs forwards between the rectus inferior and rectus lateralis, to the obliquus inferior. The branches enter the muscles on their ocular surfaces, with the exception of that to the obliquus inferior, which enters the posterior border of the muscle.

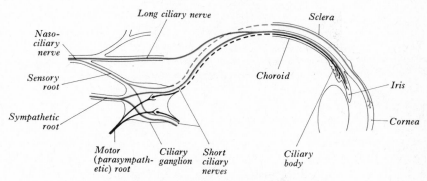

**7.**173 A diagram showing the ciliary ganglion, with its roots and branches of distribution. *Magenta:* sympathetic fibres. *Heavy black:* parasympathetic fibres. *Blue:* sensory (cerebrospinal) fibres. Alternative pathways are given for the sympathetic fibres to the dilatator pupillae. A schematic parasagittal section is shown of the upper lateral quadrant of the eyeball, but the retina has not been included.

From the nerve to the inferior oblique a short thick branch (sometimes represented by two or three separate branches) passes to the lower part of the ciliary ganglion and forms its *motor* or *parasympathetic root*. It consists of finely myelinated fibres, derived from the accessory oculomotor nucleus, which synapse about cells in the ganglion, whence postganglionic fibres pass in the short ciliary nerves to supply the sphincter pupillae and ciliaris (pp. 1103, 1107).

**The ciliary ganglion** (**7.**173, 176) is a small, flattened ganglion of a reddish-grey colour and about the size of a pin's head; it is situated near the apex of the orbit in some loose fat between the optic nerve and the rectus lateralis, lying usually on the lateral side of the ophthalmic artery.

[969] R. Warwick, *J. comp. Neurol*, **98**, 1953.
[970] R. Warwick, *J. Anat.*, **88**, 1954.
[971] W. E. Le G. Clark, *J. Anat.*, **60**, 1926.
[972] V. Tsuchida, *Arb. hirnanat. Inst., Zürich*, **2**, 1906.
[973] E. C. Crosby and R. T. Woodburne, *J. comp. Neurol.*, **78**, 1943.
[974] R. Warwick, *Brain*, **78**, 1955.
[975] B. Brouwer, *Zentbl. ges. Neurol. Psychiat.*, **40**, 1918.
[976] J. Szentágothai, *Arch. Psychiat. NervenKrankh*, **115**, 1942.
[977] M. B. Bender and E. A. Weinstein, *Archs Neurol. Psychiat., Chicago*, **49**, 1943.
[978] R. Warwick, *J. Anat.*, **87**, 1953.
[979] M. B. Bender (ed.), *The Oculomotor System*, Hoeber, New York. 1964.

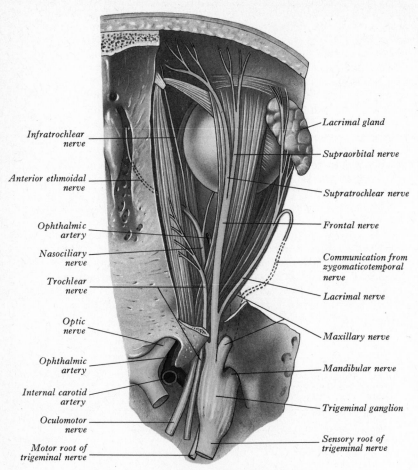

Infratrochlear
nerve

Anterior ethmoidal
nerve

Ophthalmic
artery

Nasociliary
nerve

Trochlear
nerve

Optic
nerve

Ophthalmic
artery

Internal carotid
artery

Oculomotor
nerve

Motor root of
trigeminal nerve

Lacrimal gland

Supraorbital nerve

Supratrochlear nerve

Frontal nerve

Communication from
zygomaticotemporal
nerve

Lacrimal nerve

Maxillary nerve

Mandibular nerve

Trigeminal ganglion

Sensory root of
trigeminal nerve

7.174    The nerves of the right orbit, superior aspect.

It is a peripheral ganglion of the parasympathetic system and its constituent cells are multipolar. These cells are not typical of autonomic ganglia in general, being much larger in dimensions; a very small number of nerve cells of typical autonomic type are also present.[980]

Its *connexions* or *roots* (7.173) enter or leave it posteriorly, but only its parasympathetic function is basic; the sympathetic and sensory fibres merely pass through it, and are absent in some mammals. The *motor* or *parasympathetic root* is derived from the nerve to the inferior oblique and consists of preganglionic fibres which arise from the cells of the accessory (Edinger-Westphal) nucleus (7.109). These fibres are relayed in the ganglion and the postganglionic fibres travel in the short ciliary nerves to supply the sphincter pupillae and ciliaris. More than 95 per cent of these fibres supply the ciliaris, which is much the larger muscle in volume;[980] hence this motor pathway is much more concerned with focusing of the eye than with the light reflex. The *sympathetic root* is a branch from the internal carotid plexus. It may pass direct to the ganglion or it may join the sensory root and reach the ganglion indirectly. It consists of postganglionic fibres from the superior cervical ganglion which traverse the ciliary ganglion without being interrupted, to emerge in the short ciliary nerves. They are distributed to the blood vessels of the eyeball and they may include the fibres which supply the dilatator pupillae when these fibres do not follow their usual course in the ophthalmic, nasociliary and long ciliary nerves. The *sensory root* is formed by a *ramus communicans* to the nasociliary nerve. It contains sensory fibres from the eyeball, which reach the ganglion in the short ciliary nerves and pass through it without being interrupted. It leaves the ganglion posteriorly and runs backwards to join the nasociliary nerve near the point where that nerve enters the orbit.

The *branches* of the ganglion are delicate filaments, eight to ten in number, which emerge from the front of the ganglion in two bundles, of which the lower is the larger. They are termed the *short ciliary nerves*. The postganglionic parasympathetic fibres in them are myelinated. In company with the ciliary arteries they run forwards in a wavy course, one set above the optic nerve, the other below. They subdivide into about fifteen to twenty branches, which pierce the sclera around the entrance of the optic nerve and pass forwards in delicate grooves on the inner surface of the sclera. They contain both motor and sensory fibres; the former are distributed to the sphincter pupillae and ciliaris and to the blood vessels of the eyeball; the latter supply the cornea, iris and choroid. The existence of proprioceptive fibres in the oculomotor nerve can no longer be doubted, in view of the occurrence of stretch endings in the extraocular muscles (p. 1029). How far such fibres travel centripetally in the nerve, and where they terminate centrally are still unsettled problems (but see p. 1002).

*Applied Anatomy.* Division of the oculomotor nerve leads, when complete, to (1) ptosis, or drooping of the upper eyelid, on account of paralysis of the levator palpebrae superioris; (2) lateral strabismus (or squint), on account of the unopposed action of the rectus lateralis and obliquus superior, which are not supplied by the oculomotor nerve and are therefore not paralysed; (3) dilatation of the pupil, because the sphincter pupillae is paralysed; (4) loss of power of accommodation and of contraction on exposure to light, as the sphincter pupillae and the ciliaris are paralysed; (5) slight prominence of the eyeball, owing to most of its muscles being relaxed; and (6) diplopia, or double vision, the false image being higher than the true. Occasionally paralysis may affect only a part of the nerve—for example, there may be a dilated and fixed pupil, with ptosis, but no other signs. Irritation of the nerve causes spasm of one or other of the muscles supplied by it; thus, there may be medial strabismus from spasm of the medial rectus, accommodation for near objects only, from spasm of the ciliaris, or a contracted pupil owing to irritation of the sphincter pupillae.

## The Trochlear Nerve

The trochlear nerve (7.174, 176), the most slender of the cranial nerves, supplies the superior oblique muscle of the eyeball. It contains about 3,400 fibres.

It arises from a nucleus situated in the floor of the cerebral aqueduct, opposite the upper part of the inferior colliculus (7.62, 64, 91). This nucleus lies in line with the ventromedial part of the oculomotor nucleus, and occupies the position of the somatic efferent column. The medial longitudinal fasciculus is ventral to the trochlear nucleus. The oculomotor and trochlear nuclei often overlap a little and can only be distinguished by the slightly smaller size of the trochlear nerve cells.

**Connexions.** The nucleus receives fibres from: (1) the corticonuclear tracts of *both* sides, probably in a manner similar to those of the oculomotor nerve nucleus (p. 999); (2) the medial longitudinal fasciculus, by which it is connected with the nuclei of the third, sixth and eighth cranial nerves (p. 885); (3) from the tectobulbar tract, through which it receives impulses from the visual cortex through the medium of the superior colliculus (p. 887). (See also p. 1028.)

**Course.** After leaving the nucleus the fibres of the trochlear nerve pursue a very unusual course (p. 883). They first run downwards and laterally through the

[980] R. Warwick, *J. Anat.*, **88**, 1954.

tegmentum and then turn backwards round the central grey matter into the upper part of the anterior medullary velum. Here they decussate with the contralateral fibres, and, having crossed the median plane, emerge from the surface of the velum at the side of the frenulum veli, immediately below the inferior colliculus (7.90) It is the only cranial nerve that emerges from the brainstem on its dorsal aspect.

The nerve is directed laterally across the superior cerebellar peduncle, and then winds forwards round the cerebral peduncle immediately above the pons, and between the posterior cerebral and superior cerebellar arteries. It appears between the upper border of the pons and the temporal lobe, and pierces the inner stratum of the dura mater immediately below the free border of the tentorium cerebelli, a little behind the posterior clinoid process. It then passes forwards in the lateral wall of the cavernous sinus, below the oculomotor nerve and above the ophthalmic division of the trigeminal nerve (6.127). In this part of its course it is closely adherent to the tentorial branch of the ophthalmic nerve, which lies below it. Near the front of the sinus it crosses over the oculomotor nerve, and enters the orbit through the superior orbital fissure, above the orbital muscles, and medial to the frontal nerve (7.174). In the orbit it passes medially, above the origin of the levator palpebrae superioris, and finally enters the orbital surface of the obliquus superior (7.176).

In the lateral wall of the cavernous sinus the trochlear nerve communicates with the ophthalmic division of the trigeminal nerve, and with the internal carotid plexus of the sympathetic. In the superior orbital fissure it occasionally gives off a branch to the lacrimal nerve. Although an exchange of fibres through communications in the cavernous sinus has been denied,[981] more recent evidence,[982] based on nerve fibre analysis in human material, suggests that a substantial component of fairly large nerve fibres, possibly proprioceptive in nature, are present in the trochlear nerve distal to the cavernous sinus. This part of the nerve contained 3,500 fibres, whereas proximal to the sinus the count was only about 2,400.

*Applied Anatomy.* When the trochlear nerve is interrupted the superior oblique is paralysed so that the patient is unable to turn his eye downwards and laterally. Should the patient attempt to do this, the eye of the affected side is rotated medially, producing *diplopia* or double vision. Single vision exists in the whole of the field so long as the eyes look above the horizontal plane; diplopia occurs on looking downwards. To counteract this the patient holds his head forwards, and also inclines it to the sound side.

## The Trigeminal Nerve

The trigeminal is the largest cranial nerve. It is the sensory nerve of the face, the greater part of the scalp, the teeth, the mouth and the nasal cavity, and the motor nerve of the muscles of mastication and some other muscles. It also contains proprioceptive fibres from the masticatory and probably from the extraocular muscles. It divides into three branches, ophthalmic, maxillary and mandibular.

It is attached to the ventral surface of the pons, near its upper border, by a large sensory and a small motor root—the latter being placed medial and anterior to the former.

The fibres of the *sensory root* arise from the cells of the **trigeminal (semilunar) ganglion.** This ganglion (7.174, 177) occupies a recess (*trigeminal cave*) in the dura mater covering the trigeminal impression near the apex of the petrous part of the temporal bone (p. 276). It lies at a depth of 4·5–5 cm from the lateral aspect of the head, at

the posterior extremity of the zygomatic arch. The ganglion is crescentic in shape, with its convexity directed anterolaterally; on its surface are visible a number of interlacing nerve fascicles. Medially it is in relation with the internal carotid artery and the posterior part of the cavernous sinus, inferiorly, with the motor root of the nerve, the greater (superficial) petrosal nerve, the apex of the petrous part of the temporal bone, and the foramen lacerum. It receives filaments from the internal carotid plexus of the sympathetic, and gives twigs to the tentorium cerebelli.

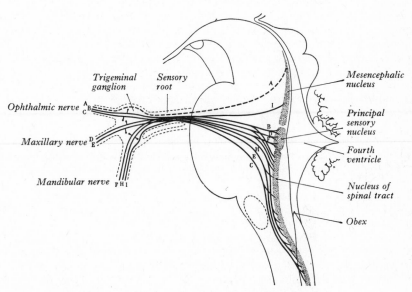

7.175 The nuclei receiving the primary afferent fibres of the trigeminal nerve. A: proprioceptive fibres from ocular muscles. B: tactile and pressure fibres from ophthalmic area. C: pain and temperature fibres from ophthalmic area. D: tactile and pressure fibres from maxillary area. E: pain and temperature fibres from maxillary area. F: tactile and pressure fibres from mandibular area. H: pain and temperature fibres from mandibular area. I: proprioceptive fibres from muscles of mastication. Proprioceptive fibres are believed to occur in all three divisions of the trigeminal nerve.

The branches of the unipolar cells of the trigeminal ganglion divide into peripheral and central branches. The former are grouped to form the *ophthalmic* and *maxillary* nerves, and the sensory part of the *mandibular* nerve. The central branches constitute the fibres of the sensory root of the nerve, which leaves the concave margin of the ganglion, runs backwards and medially below the superior petrosal sinus and the tentorium cerebelli, and enters the pons. Some fibres from proprioceptor endings in the masticatory and extraocular muscles may pass through the semilunar ganglion without connexion with nerve cell somata.

On entering the pons the fibres of the sensory root course dorsomedially towards the **principal sensory nucleus** situated at that level (7.70). On approaching the nucleus about 50 per cent of the fibres divide into ascending and descending branches; the others ascend or descend without division. The descending fibres, which are predominantly finely myelinated or non-myelinated, form the **spinal tract of the trigeminal nerve** which descends into the upper cervical part of the spinal cord. As the tract descends terminals and collaterals are given off to synapse with the cells of the **spinal nucleus of the trigeminal nerve** (7.60–63, 66, 68, 175). The nucleus consists of small- and medium-sized cells and is continuous below with the substantia gelatinosa. The tract embraces the nucleus on its dorsolateral aspect. In the

[981] S. Sunderland and E. S. R. Hughes, *Brain*, **69**, 1946.
[982] W. Zaki, *Archs Anat. Histol. Embryol.*, **43**, 1960.

lower part of the medulla oblongata it is superficial and lies under the tuberculum cinereum. The fibres which synapse in the nucleus are concerned predominantly (but not exclusively) with painful and thermal sensibility. It has been demonstrated experimentally that (1) the fibres of the ophthalmic nerve are placed ventrally in the tract and descend to the lower limit of the first cervical segment of the spinal cord; (2) the fibres of the maxillary nerve lie in the central part of the tract and do not extend below the medulla oblongata; (3) the fibres of the mandibular nerve are placed in the dorsal part of the tract and do not extend much below the middle of the medulla oblongata (7.175). This experimental evidence is confirmed by the clinical results after section of the spinal tract[983-985] in cases of severe trigeminal neuralgia. Section of the tract 4 mm below the level of the obex renders the ophthalmic and maxillary areas analgesic but tactile sensibility, apart from the abolition of 'tickle', is much less affected. When it is desired to include the mandibular area as well, the section must be made at the level of the obex itself. In addition, as a result of this operation, the mucous membrane of the tonsillar sinus, the posterior third of the tongue and the adjoining parts of the pharyngeal wall (glossopharyngeal nerve) and the cutaneous area supplied by the auricular branch of the vagus nerve are also rendered analgesic; it may, therefore, be inferred that the fibres concerned join the spinal tract of the trigeminal nerve and end in its nucleus. During the course of these operations the laminated character of the tract has also been confirmed. A small group of sensory cells, associated with the glossopharyngeal nerve, but related to the spinal trigeminal tract, has been described.[987] As well as the trigeminal, vagal and glossopharyngeal afferents to the spinal nucleus, others reach it from the sensory root of the facial nerve, the dorsal roots of the upper cervical nerves, and descending fibres from the sensorimotor regions of the cerebral cortex (see also p. 1029).

Some of the ascending trigeminal fibres, many of which are heavily myelinated, synapse around the small cells of the principal sensory nucleus which lies lateral to the motor nucleus and intervenes between the latter and the middle cerebellar peduncle: it is continuous below with the nucleus of the spinal tract (7.62, 175). It is considered to be concerned mainly with tactile sensibility.

Other ascending fibres enter the **mesencephalic nucleus**. This nucleus is composed of a column of *unipolar* cells. It is believed that their peripheral branches convey proprioceptive impulses from the muscles of mastication and it is also alleged that proprioceptive impulses travel to the mesencephalic nucleus from the teeth and from the facial and ocular muscles[986, 989] (7.62, 91, 155). The neurons of the mesencephalic nucleus are unique in being the only primary sensory neurons whose cell bodies are within the central nervous system.[988] Small multipolar cells, possibly interneurons, occur near the unipolar neurons.

**Connexions.** The majority of the fibres which arise in the sensory nuclei of the trigeminal nerve cross the median plane and ascend in the trigeminal lemniscus (p. 1029) to the nucleus ventralis posterior medialis of the thalamus (p. 896), from which fibres are relayed to the cortex of the postcentral gyrus (areas 3, 1 and 2, p. 959). Some, however, ascend to the thalamus on the ipsilateral side. It is probable that collateral branches of both primary and secondary afferent trigeminal neurons reach many other central regions such as the cranial nerve nuclei, the reticular formation, cerebellum, tectum, subthalamus, hypothalamus, etc, but their details have not been established in the human brain. (See also p. 1029.)

The nerve fibres which ascend to the nerve cells of the mesencephalic nucleus may afford collaterals to the motor trigeminal nucleus and the cerebellum. They are, of course, morphologically dendrites; the true axons of the mesencephalic neurons possibly descend in part to the principal trigeminal sensory nucleus, but little is known of them.

**The motor nucleus** of the trigeminal nerve gives rise to the fibres of the motor root. It is ovoid in shape with typical large multipolar cells interspersed with smaller multipolar cells. It lies in the upper part of the pons on the medial side of the principal sensory nucleus, which is separated from it by the fibres of the trigeminal nerve. It occupies the position of the branchial (special visceral) efferent column (7.62, 64, 70). Detailed analysis has shown that the motor nucleus of the trigeminal consists of a number of relative discrete sub-nuclei, the axons of which innervate individual muscles.[990]

**Connexions.** The motor nucleus receives fibres from the corticonuclear tracts of *both* sides; these fibres leave the tracts at the level of the nucleus or at a higher level in the pons (aberrant pyramidal fibres) and descend in the medial lemniscus. They may end on the cells of the nucleus or are linked to them by interneurons. The motor nucleus receives fibres from the sensory nuclei of the trigeminal nerve, and, as stated above, possibly some from the mesencephalic nucleus, forming monosynaptic reflex arcs for the proprioceptive control of the muscles of mastication. It also receives fibres from the reticular formation, red nucleus and the tectum, from the medial longitudinal fasciculus and possibly fibres from the locus coeruleus, by which salivary secretion and mastication are correlated.

## THE OPHTHALMIC NERVE

The ophthalmic nerve (7.174, 179, 182) the superior division of the trigeminal nerve, is wholly sensory. It supplies branches to the eyeball, the lacrimal gland and the conjunctiva, to a part of the mucous membrane of the nasal cavity, and to the skin of the nose, eyelids, forehead and scalp. It is the smallest division of the trigeminal nerve, and arises from the anteromedial part of the trigeminal ganglion as a flattened band, about 2·5 cm long, which passes forwards in the cavernous sinus close to its lateral wall and below the oculomotor and trochlear nerves (6.127); just before entering the orbit through the superior orbital fissure, it divides into three branches, viz. *lacrimal*, *frontal* and *nasociliary*.

The ophthalmic nerve is joined by filaments from the internal carotid plexus of the sympathetic, and communicates with the oculomotor, trochlear and abducent nerves, a route by which the proprioceptive fibres of these nerves may pass into the trigeminal. It supplies a recurrent meningeal branch (*tentorial nerve*), which crosses below and adheres to the trochlear nerve, and is distributed to the tentorium cerebelli (p. 988).

**The lacrimal nerve** (7.174) is the smallest of the main branches of the ophthalmic nerve. It sometimes receives a filament from the trochlear nerve, but possibly this filament consists of fibres which have previously passed from the ophthalmic to the trochlear nerve. The lacrimal nerve enters the orbit through the lateral part of the superior orbital fissure (7.177), runs along the upper border of the rectus lateralis with the lacrimal artery, and receives a twig from the zygomaticotemporal branch of

[983] G. E. Smyth, *Brain*, **62**, 1939.
[984] A. Brodal, *Archs Neurol. Psychiat., Chicago*, **57**, 1947.
[985] M. A. Falconer, *J. Neurol. Neurosurg. Psychiat.*, **12**, 1949.
[986] K. B. Corbin and F. Harrison, *J. Neurophysiol.*, **3**, 1940.
[987] J. Bossy, *Acta anat.*, **70**, 1968.
[988] J. B. Johnston, *J. comp. Neurol.*, **19**, 1909.
[989] A. A. Pearson, *J. comp. Neurol.*, **90**, 1949.
[990] J. Szentágothai, *J. comp. Neurol.*, **90**, 1949.

the maxillary nerve, often said to contain secretomotor fibres for the lacrimal gland (see, however, p. 1067). It enters the lacrimal gland and gives off several filaments to the gland and the conjunctiva. Finally it pierces the orbital septum, and ends in the skin of the upper eyelid, joining with filaments of the facial nerve.

The lacrimal nerve is occasionally absent, and its place is then taken by the zygomaticotemporal branch of the maxillary nerve. Sometimes the latter branch is absent and is replaced by a branch of the lacrimal nerve.

**The nasociliary nerve** (7.174, 176) is intermediate in size between the frontal and lacrimal nerves, and is more deeply placed. It enters the orbit through the medial part of the superior orbital fissure within the common tendinous ring, which gives origin to the recti muscles of the eyeball, and here it is situated between the two rami of the oculomotor nerve (7.176). It crosses the optic nerve with the ophthalmic artery, and runs obliquely below the rectus superior and obliquus superior, to the medial wall of the orbital cavity. Here, under the name of the *anterior*

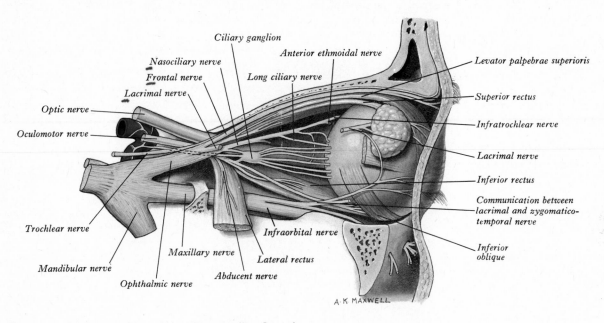

7.176   The nerves of the right orbit, and the ciliary ganglion. Lateral aspect.

**The frontal nerve** (7.174, 176) is the largest branch of the ophthalmic division. It enters the orbit through the superior orbital fissure (7.174) above the muscles, and runs forwards between the levator palpebrae superioris and the periosteum. About midway between the apex and base of the orbit it divides into a small supratrochlear and a large supraorbital branch.

The *supratrochlear nerve* runs medially and forwards, passes above the trochlea of the obliquus superior, and gives off a descending filament to join the infratrochlear branch of the nasociliary nerve. The nerve then emerges from the orbit between the trochlea and the supraorbital foramen, curves upwards on the forehead close to the bone in company with the supratrochlear branch of the ophthalmic artery, and sends filaments to the conjunctiva and skin of the upper eyelid; it then ascends under cover of the corrugator and the frontal belly of the occipitofrontalis and divides into branches which pierce these muscles and supply the skin of the lower part of the forehead close to the median plane.

The *supraorbital nerve* runs forwards between the levator palpebrae superioris and the roof of the orbit, passes through the supraorbital notch or foramen, and gives off palpebral filaments to the upper eyelid and conjunctiva. It then ascends upon the forehead with the supraorbital artery, and divides into a smaller medial and a larger lateral branch, which supply the skin of the scalp, reaching nearly as far back as the lambdoid suture. These two branches are at first situated deep to the frontal belly of the occipitofrontalis; the medial branch perforates this muscle, the lateral branch pierces the epicranial aponeurosis. Both branches supply small twigs to the mucous membrane of the frontal sinus and to the pericranium.

*ethmoidal nerve*, it passes through the anterior ethmoidal foramen and canal and, entering the cavity of the cranium, runs forwards in a shallow groove on the upper surface of the cribriform plate of the ethmoid bone, beneath the dura mater; it then descends through a slit at the side of the crista galli into the nasal cavity, and lies in a groove on the inner surface of the nasal bone. It supplies two *internal nasal branches*—a medial to the mucous membrane of the front part of the nasal septum, and a lateral to the anterior part of the lateral wall of the nasal cavity. Finally it emerges, as the *external nasal branch*, at the lower border of the nasal bone, and, passing down under cover of the transverse part of the nasalis, supplies the skin of the ala, apex and vestibule of the nose.

The nasociliary nerve communicates with the ciliary ganglion, and gives off the long ciliary, the infratrochlear and the posterior ethmoidal nerves.

The *ramus communicans with the ciliary ganglion* (p. 999, 7.173) usually joins the nasociliary nerve as the latter enters the orbital cavity. It lies on the lateral side of the optic nerve, and emerges from the posterosuperior angle of the ciliary ganglion (7.173); it is sometimes joined by a filament from the internal carotid plexus of the sympathetic, or from the superior ramus of the oculomotor nerve.

The *long ciliary nerves*, two or three in number, are given off from the nasociliary nerve, as it crosses the optic nerve. They accompany the short ciliary nerves from the ciliary ganglion, pierce the sclera near the attachment of the optic nerve, and, running forwards between the sclera and the choroid, are distributed to the ciliary body, iris and cornea. They usually contain the sympathetic fibres for the dilatator pupillae (p. 1107);

1003

these are postganglionic fibres and have their cells of origin in the superior cervical ganglion. In view of the susceptibility of the exposed epithelium of the cornea to damage, the corneal distribution of the long ciliary nerves is of pre-eminent importance.

The *infratrochlear nerve* is given off from the naso-ciliary nerve near the anterior ethmoidal foramen. It runs forwards along the medial wall of the orbit above the upper border of the rectus medialis, and is joined, near the pulley of the obliquus superior, by a filament from the supratrochlear nerve. It then escapes from the orbit below the trochlea; it supplies branches to the skin of the eyelids and side of the nose above the medial angle of the eye, the conjunctiva, lacrimal sac and lacrimal caruncle.

The *posterior ethmoidal nerve* leaves the orbital cavity through the posterior ethmoidal foramen and supplies the ethmoidal and sphenoidal sinuses. It is frequently absent.

## THE MAXILLARY NERVE

The maxillary nerve (7.176, 177), the intermediate division of the trigeminal nerve, is wholly sensory. It is intermediate in position and size between the ophthalmic and mandibular nerves. It begins at the middle of the trigeminal ganglion as a flattened plexiform band, and, passing horizontally forwards along the lower part of the lateral wall of the cavernous sinus (6.127), leaves the skull through the foramen rotundum, where it becomes more cylindrical in form and firmer in texture. It then crosses the upper part of the pterygopalatine fossa, inclines laterally on the posterior surface of the orbital process of the palatine bone and on the upper part of the posterior surface of the maxilla, and enters the orbit through the inferior orbital fissure. It is now named the **infraorbital nerve** and, having traversed the infraorbital groove and canal in the floor of the orbit, it appears on the face through the infraorbital foramen. At its termination the nerve lies under cover of the levator labii superioris, and divides into branches which are distributed to the ala of the nose, the lower eyelid, the skin and mucous membrane of the cheek and upper lip, and which communicate with filaments of the facial nerve.

In view of the fact that the mouth is generally regarded as representing a pair of fused visceral clefts, the maxillary nerve can be described as the pretrematic and the mandibular nerve as the post-trematic branch of the trigeminal nerve. In early fetal life the maxillary nerve primarily supplies the constituent structures of the maxillary process, but later it extends its territory of innervation into the adjoining frontonasal process (*see* p. 118 and 7.182).

The *branches* of the maxillary nerve may be divided into four groups, according to their origin in the cranium, in the pterygopalatine fossa, in the infraorbital canal, or on the face.

| In the cranium | Meningeal | 1 |
| In the pterygopalatine fossa | Ganglionic | 2 |
| | Zygomatic | 3 |
| | Posterior superior alveolar | 4 |
| In the infraorbital canal | Middle superior alveolar | 5 |
| | Anterior superior alveolar | 6 |
| On the face | Palpebral | 7 |
| | Nasal | 8 |
| | Superior labial | 9 |

The **meningeal nerve**[941, 942] (sometimes termed the *nervus meningeus medius*) is given off from the maxillary near the foramen rotundum; it receives a communication from the internal carotid sympathetic plexus and then accompanies the frontal branch of the middle meningeal artery and supplies the dura mater of the middle cranial fossa. Its most anterior twigs, however, reach the anterior cranial fossa.

**The ganglionic branches**, two in number, connect the maxillary nerve to the pterygopalatine (spheno-palatine) ganglion, which lies immediately below it in the pterygopalatine fossa (7.177). They contain the secreto-motor fibres for the lacrimal gland (*vide infra*), and sensory fibres from the orbital periosteum and the mucous membranes of the nose, palate and pharynx (p. 1249).

**The zygomatic nerve** (7.177) arises in the pterygo-palatine fossa, enters the orbit by the inferior orbital fissure, courses along the lateral wall of the orbit, and divides into two branches, zygomaticotemporal and zygomaticofacial.

The *zygomaticotemporal branch* skirts the inferolateral wall of the orbit, sends a branch to join the lacrimal nerve (p. 1002), and, passing through a canal in the zygomatic bone, enters the temporal fossa. It ascends between the bone and the temporalis, pierces the temporal fascia about 2 cm above the zygomatic arch, and is distributed to the skin of the temple. It communicates with the facial nerve and with the auriculotemporal branch of the mandibular nerve. As it pierces the temporal fascia, it sends a slender twig between the two layers of the fascia towards the lateral angle of the eye. The communication with the lacrimal nerve conveys parasympathetic postganglionic fibres from the pterygopalatine ganglion to the lacrimal gland.

The *zygomaticofacial branch* passes along the infero-lateral border of the orbit, emerges upon the face through a foramen in the zygomatic bone, and, perforating the orbicularis oculi, supplies the skin on the prominence of the cheek. It forms a fine plexus with the zygomatic branches of the facial nerve and the palpebral branches of the maxillary nerve.

**The superior alveolar (dental) nerves** (7.177) arise from the maxillary nerve before it leaves the pterygo-palatine fossa, or as it lies in the infraorbital groove or canal. They are termed the posterior, the middle and the anterior superior alveolar (dental) nerves.

**The posterior superior alveolar (dental) nerve** arises from the maxillary in the pterygopalatine fossa and runs downwards and forwards to pierce the infratemporal surface of the maxilla (p. 1221) and descend under the mucous lining of the maxillary sinus. After supplying the sinus the nerve divides into small branches which link up to constitute the molar part of the *superior dental plexus* supplying twigs to the molar teeth. In addition, it supplies a branch to the upper gum and the adjoining part of the cheek.

**The middle superior alveolar (dental) nerve** arises from the infraorbital as it passes along the infra-orbital groove, and runs downwards and forwards in the lateral wall of the maxillary sinus. Like the posterior, it terminates in a number of small branches which link up with the superior dental plexus, and these give off twigs to supply the upper premolar teeth. This nerve is variable in its behaviour. It may be duplicated or triplicated or it may be absent.[991, 992]

**The anterior superior alveolar (dental) nerve** (7.177) leaves the lateral side of the infraorbital nerve near the midpoint of the infraorbital canal, and runs in the canalis sinuosus (p. 1221) in the anterior wall of the maxillary sinus. At first it curves beneath the infraorbital foramen and passes medially towards the nose; it then turns downwards and divides into branches which supply

[991] F. Wood Jones, *J. Anat.*, **73**, 1939.
[992] M. J. T. FitzGerald, *J. Anat.*, **90**, 1956.

the incisor and canine teeth. It takes part in the formation of the superior dental plexus, and gives off a *nasal branch*, which passes through a minute canal in the lateral wall of the inferior meatus, and supplies the mucous membrane of the anterior part of the lateral wall (as high as the opening of the maxillary sinus) and the floor of the nasal cavity, communicating with the nasal branches from the pterygopalatine ganglion. Its terminal branch emerges near the root of the anterior nasal spine and supplies the adjoining part of the nasal septum.

(7.177, 179) is the largest of the peripheral ganglia of the parasympathetic system. It is deeply placed in the pterygopalatine fossa, close to the sphenopalatine foramen and in front of the pterygoid canal. It is somewhat flattened, of a reddish-grey colour, and is situated just below the maxillary nerve as it crosses the fossa. Although it is *connected functionally with the facial nerve*, its topographical relations with the maxillary nerve and its branches are so intimate that it may conveniently be described at this stage.

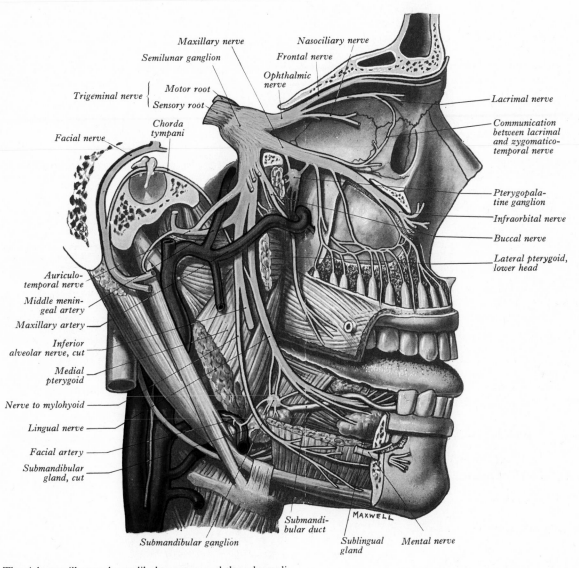

**7.177**   The right maxillary and mandibular nerves, and the submandibular ganglion.

**The palpebral branches** ascend deep to the orbicularis oculi. They soon pierce the muscle to supply the skin of the lower eyelid, and join with the facial and zygomaticofacial nerves near the lateral angle of the eye.

**The nasal branches** supply the skin of the side of the nose and of the movable part of the nasal septum, and join with the external nasal branch of the anterior ethmoidal nerve.

**The superior labial branches** are large and numerous; they descend behind the levator labii superioris, and supply the skin of the anterior part of the cheek, the skin of the upper lip, the mucous membrane of the mouth, and the labial glands. They are joined by branches from the facial nerve, and form with them the *infraorbital plexus*.

**The pterygopalatine (sphenopalatine) ganglion**

The *motor or parasympathetic root* is formed by the *nerve of the pterygoid canal* (p. 1012), which enters the ganglion posteriorly. Its fibres are believed to arise from a special lacrimatory nucleus in the lower part of the pons and they run in the sensory root of the facial nerve (nervus intermedius) and its greater petrosal branch (p. 1012) before the latter unites with the deep petrosal nerve (7.179) to form the nerve of the pterygoid canal. These preganglionic fibres are relayed in the ganglion and the postganglionic fibres follow a complicated course to gain their destination. Leaving the ganglion in one of the ganglionic branches, they join the maxillary nerve and pass into its zygomatic branch. Thence they are usually considered to run in the zygomaticotemporal nerve and later leave it in the communicating branch by which it is

1005

connected to the lacrimal nerve (p. 1067). In this way they may reach the lacrimal gland, supplying it with secreto-motor fibres (see, however, below). In addition, secreto-motor fibres—of uncertain origin—for the palatine, pharyngeal and nasal glands are believed to follow a similar route to the ganglion, where they are relayed. Their postganglionic fibres run in the palatine and nasal branches of the ganglion (7.179).

The *sympathetic root* is also incorporated in the nerve of the pterygoid canal. Its fibres, which are postganglionic, arise in the superior cervical ganglion and travel in the internal carotid plexus and the deep petrosal nerve.

The *branches* which appear to arise from the pterygo-palatine ganglion (7.178) are, for the most part, derived from the maxillary nerve through its ganglionic branches, and, though intimately related to the ganglion, do *not* establish any synaptic connexions with its cells. They include orbital, palatine, nasal and pharyngeal branches.

The *orbital branches* are two or three delicate filaments which enter the orbit by the inferior orbital fissure, and are distributed to the periosteum and the orbitalis muscle; some twigs pass through the posterior ethmoidal foramen to the sphenoidal and ethmoidal sinuses. The fibres which supply the orbitalis are directly continuous with the fibres of the sympathetic root of the ganglion. Experiments in monkeys and dissections of human material suggest that the orbital rami of the pterygopalatine ganglion form a plexus with branches of the internal carotid sympathetic nerve. This 'retro-orbital' plexus supplies parasympathetic and sympathetic branches to various orbital structures, including the lacrimal gland (p. 1067).[993]

The *palatine nerves* (7.178) are distributed to the roof of the mouth, the soft palate, the tonsil and the lining membrane of the nasal cavity.

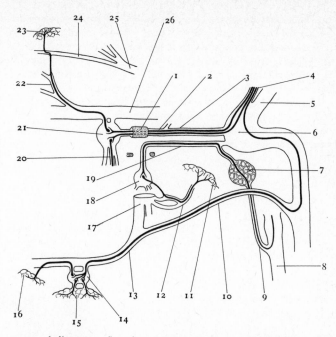

7.179 A diagram to show the parasympathetic connexions of the pterygopalatine, otic and submandibular ganglia. The parasympathetic fibres, both pre- and post-ganglionic, are shown as heavy black lines. The parasympathetic fibres in the palatine nerves (20) are secretomotor to the nasal, palatine pharyngeal glands. Consult text for recent views on the supply to the lacrimal gland.

| | |
|---|---|
| 1. Pterygoid canal. | 14. Submandibular ganglion. |
| 2. Nerve of pterygoid canal. | 15. Submandibular salivary gland. |
| 3. Greater petrosal nerve. | 16. Sublingual salivary gland. |
| 4. Sensory root of facial nerve. | 17. Mandibular nerve. |
| 5. Motor root of facial nerve. | 18. Otic ganglion. |
| 6. Ganglion of facial nerve. | 19. Lesser petrosal nerve. |
| 7. Tympanic plexus. | 20. Palatine nerves. |
| 8. Glossopharyngeal nerve. | 21. Pterygopalatine ganglion. |
| 9. Tympanic nerve. | 22. Zygomaticotemporal nerve. |
| 10. Chorda tympani nerve. | 23. Lacrimal gland. |
| 11. Parotid gland. | 24. Lacrimal nerve. |
| 12. Auriculotemporal nerve. | 25. Ophthalmic nerve. |
| 13. Lingual nerve. | 26. Maxillargy nerve. |

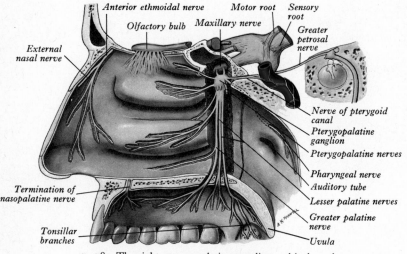

7.178 The right pterygopalatine ganglion and its branches.

The *greater (anterior) palatine nerve* descends through the greater palatine canal, emerges upon the hard palate through the greater palatine foramen, and runs forwards in a groove on the inferior surface of the bony palate, nearly as far as the incisor teeth. It supplies the gums, and the mucous membrane and glands of the hard palate, and communicates in front with terminal filaments of the nasopalatine nerve. While in the greater palatine canal, it gives off *posterior inferior nasal branches*, which emerge through openings in the perpendicular plate of the palatine bone, and ramify over the inferior nasal concha and the walls of the middle and inferior meatuses; at its exit from the canal, palatine branches are distributed to both surfaces of the soft palate.

The *lesser (middle and posterior) palatine nerves* descend through the greater palatine canal, emerge through the lesser palatine foramina and supply branches to the uvula, tonsil and soft palate. The fibres conveying taste impulses from the palate probably pass via the palatine nerves to the pterygopalatine ganglion and thence, without interruption, via the nerve of the pterygoid canal and the greater petrosal nerve to the facial ganglion, where their cells of origin are situated. The central processes of these cells pass through the sensory root of the facial nerve (nervus intermedius) to reach the nucleus of the tractus solitarius (p. 846).

The *nasal branches* enter the nasal cavity through the sphenopalatine foramen. They comprise two sets of nerves. (*a*) The *lateral posterior superior nasal nerves*, about six in number, supply the mucous membrane over the posterior parts of the superior and middle nasal conchae and that lining the posterior ethmoidal sinuses. (*b*) The *medial posterior superior nasal nerves*, two or three in number, cross the roof of the nasal cavity below the opening of the sphenoidal sinus to supply the mucous membrane of the posterior part of the roof of the cavity and of the nasal septum. The largest of these nerves is the *nasopalatine (long sphenopalatine) nerve*, which runs downwards and forwards on the posterior part of the nasal septum, lying in a groove on the vomer. It descends to the roof of the mouth through the incisive fossa in the anterior part of the hard palate. When an anterior and a

[993] G. L. Ruskell, *J. Anat.*, **106**, 1970; **109**, 1971.

posterior incisive foramen (p. 267) are present in this fossa, the left nasopalatine nerve passes through the anterior and the right nerve through the posterior foramen. The nasopalatine nerves furnish a few filaments to the nasal septum and end by supplying the mucous membrane of the anterior part of the hard palate, where they communicate with the anterior palatine nerves.

The *pharyngeal nerve*, a small branch, arises from the posterior part of the ganglion, passes through the palatino-vaginal canal with the pharyngeal branch of the maxillary artery, and is distributed to the mucous membrane of the nasal part of the pharynx, behind the auditory tube.

## THE MANDIBULAR NERVE

The mandibular nerve (7.177, 181, 182) supplies the teeth and gums of the mandible, the skin of the temporal region, part of the auricle, the lower lip, the lower part of the face, and the muscles of mastication; it also supplies the mucous membrane of the anterior, pre-sulcal part of the tongue and the floor of the mouth. The largest division of the trigeminal nerve, it is made up of two roots: a large, sensory root, which proceeds from the lateral part of the semilunar ganglion and emerges almost immediately through the foramen ovale of the sphenoid bone, and a small motor root (the motor part of the trigeminal) which passes below the ganglion, and unites with the sensory root, just outside the foramen ovale, where the nerve lies between the tensor veli palatini medially and the lateral pterygoid laterally. Immediately beyond the junction of the two roots the nerve sends off from its medial side its meningeal branch and the nerve to the medial pterygoid, and then divides into a small anterior and a large posterior trunk. As it descends from the foramen ovale, the mandibular nerve lies at a depth of 4 cm from the surface and a little in front of the neck of the mandible.

**The meningeal branch** (nervus spinosus) enters the skull through the foramen spinosum with the middle meningeal artery. It divides into two branches, anterior and posterior, which accompany the main divisions of the artery and supply the dura mater of the middle cranial fossa, and to a lesser extent that of the anterior fossa and calvarium; the posterior branch also supplies a twig to the mucous lining of the mastoid air cells; the anterior communicates with the meningeal branch of the maxillary nerve. In addition to its sensory fibres the nervus spinosus carries sympathetic postganglionic fibres from the plexus on the middle meningeal artery.

**The nerve to the medial pterygoid** is a slender branch which enters the deep surface of the muscle; it gives one or two filaments which pass through the otic ganglion (p. 1019) without being interrupted and emerge from it to supply the tensor tympani and tensor veli palatini (7.181).

### Anterior Trunk

The small anterior trunk of the mandibular nerve gives off (*a*) a sensory branch named the buccal nerve, and (*b*) motor branches—the masseteric, deep temporal and lateral pterygoid nerves.

**The buccal nerve** (7.180) passes forwards between the two heads of the lateral pterygoid, and then downwards beneath or through the lower part of the temporalis; it emerges from under cover of the ramus of the mandible and the anterior border of the masseter, and unites with the buccal branches of the facial nerve. It furnishes a branch to the lateral pterygoid during its passage through that muscle, and may give off the anterior deep temporal nerve. The buccal nerve supplies the skin over the anterior part of the buccinator, and the mucous mem-

brane lining its inner surface and the posterior part of the buccal surface of the gum.

**The masseteric nerve** (7.180) passes laterally, above the lateral pterygoid, in front of the temporomandibular joint, and behind the tendon of the temporalis; it crosses the posterior part of the mandibular incisure with the masseteric artery, ramifies in the deep surface of the masseter, and gives a filament to the joint.

**The deep temporal nerves** are usually two in number, anterior and posterior. They pass above the upper border of the lateral pterygoid and enter the deep surface of the temporalis. The *posterior branch*, of small size, is placed at the posterior part of the temporal fossa, and sometimes arises in common with the masseteric nerve. The *anterior branch* is frequently given off from the buccal nerve, and then ascends over the upper head of the lateral pterygoid. A third, or middle, branch is often present.

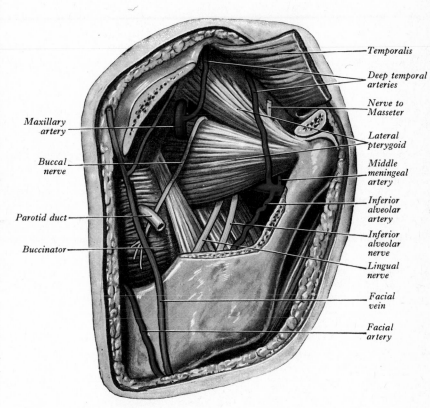

7.180  A dissection of the left pterygoid region, showing some of the branches of the mandibular nerve and the maxillary artery.

**The nerve to the lateral pterygoid** enters the deep surface of the muscle. It may arise separately from the anterior division of the mandibular nerve, or in conjunction with the buccal nerve.

### Posterior Trunk

The posterior trunk of the mandibular nerve is for the most part sensory, but receives a few filaments from the motor root. It divides into auriculotemporal, lingual and inferior alveolar (dental) nerves.

**The auriculotemporal nerve** generally arises by two roots, which encircle the middle meningeal artery (7.177). It runs backwards under cover of the lateral pterygoid on the surface of the tensor veli palatini and passes between the sphenomandibular ligament and the neck of the mandible. It then passes laterally behind the temporomandibular joint in relationship with the upper part of the parotid gland. Finally, emerging from behind the joint, it ascends, posterior to the superficial temporal

1007

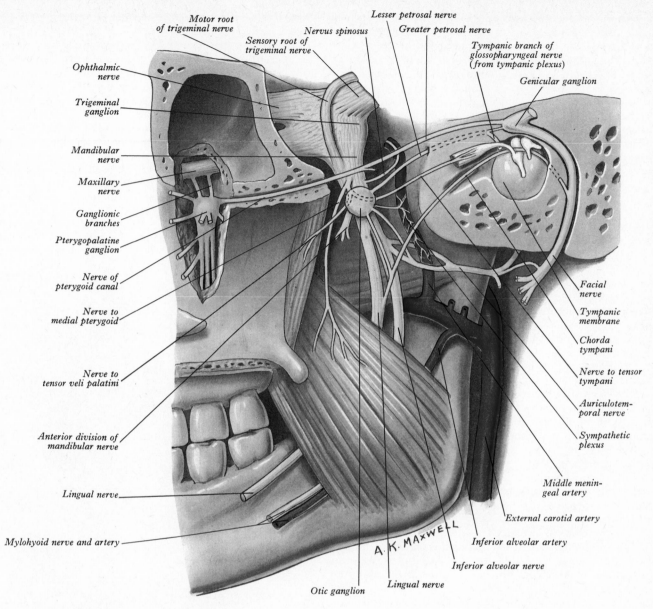

**7.181** The right otic ganglion and its branches displayed from the medial side.

vessels, over the posterior root of the zygoma, and divides into superficial temporal branches.

The auriculotemporal nerve communicates with the facial nerve and the otic ganglion. The branches to the facial nerve, usually two in number, pass forwards and laterally behind the neck of the mandible and join the facial nerve at the posterior border of the masseter. The filaments from the otic ganglion join the roots of the auriculotemporal nerve close to their origin (7.184).

The *branches* of the auriculotemporal nerve are the anterior auricular, branches to the external acoustic meatus, articular, parotid and superficial temporal.

There are usually two *anterior auricular branches*: they supply the skin of the tragus (7.182) and, sometimes, a small part of the adjoining portion of the helix.

The *branches to the external acoustic meatus*, two in number, pass between the bony and cartilaginous parts of the meatus, and supply the skin of the meatus; the upper one sends a twig to the tympanic membrane.

The *articular branches* consist of one or two twigs which enter the posterior part of the temporomandibular joint.

The *parotid branches* convey secretomotor fibres to the parotid gland. The preganglionic fibres are originally derived from the glossopharyngeal nerve through its

tympanic branch and travel by the lesser petrosal nerve to the otic ganglion, whence the postganglionic fibres pass to the auriculotemporal nerve and so reach the gland (7.179). They also convey vasomotor fibres to the blood vessels of the parotid gland. These fibres are directly continuous with the fibres of the sympathetic root of the otic ganglion (p. 1019).

The *superficial temporal branches* accompany the superficial temporal artery and its terminal branches; they supply the skin of the temporal region and communicate with the facial and zygomaticotemporal nerves.

**The lingual nerve** (7.177) is sensory to the mucous membrane of the pre-sulcal part of the tongue, and to the floor of the mouth and the mandibular gums.

It arises from the posterior trunk of the mandibular nerve, and lies at first between the tensor veli palatini and the lateral pterygoid, where it is joined by the chorda tympani branch of the facial nerve, and frequently by a branch of the inferior alveolar nerve. Emerging from under cover of the lateral pterygoid the lingual nerve proceeds downwards and forwards between the ramus of the mandible and the medial pterygoid, lying anterior to, and slightly deeper than the inferior alveolar nerve. It then passes below the mandibular origin of the superior constrictor of the pharynx, and lies against the deep surface of the mandible on the medial side of the roots of the third molar tooth, where it is covered only by the mucous membrane of the gum and can be pressed against the bone by a finger placed inside the mouth. It then leaves the gum and passes on to the side of the tongue, where it crosses the styloglossus, and runs on the lateral surface of the hyoglossus and deep to the mylohyoid; here it is placed above the deep part of the submandibular gland and its duct. It then proceeds forwards on the side of the tongue, lying lateral to the hyoglossus and genioglossus, and divides into its terminal branches, which lie directly under cover of the mucous membrane of the tongue. In the latter part of its course the nerve is in close relation with the submandibular duct; it passes from above downwards and forwards on the lateral side of the duct, and then, winding below it, runs upwards and forwards on its medial side (7.177).

In addition to receiving the chorda tympani and the branch from the inferior alveolar nerve, already referred to, the lingual nerve is connected to the submandibular ganglion (p. 1015) by two or three branches (7.177), and, at the anterior margin of the hyoglossus, forms loops of communication with twigs of the hypoglossal nerve.

The *branches* of the lingual nerve supply the mucous membrane of the floor of the mouth, the lingual surface of the gums, and the mucous membrane of the pre-sulcal part of the tongue, being overlapped to a slight extent by the lingual fibres of the glossopharyngeal nerve (p. 1019); the terminal filaments join, at the tip of the tongue, with those of the hypoglossal nerve. In addition it carries post-ganglionic fibres from the submandibular ganglion (p. 1015) to the sublingual and anterior lingual glands.

**The inferior alveolar (dental) nerve** descends deep to the lateral pterygoid, and then, at the lower border of the muscle, it passes between the sphenomandibular ligament and the ramus of the mandible to the mandibular foramen. Here it enters the mandibular canal, and runs below the teeth as far as the mental foramen, where it divides into an incisive and a mental branch. Below the lateral pterygoid the nerve is accompanied by the inferior alveolar artery. Dissection and radiographic studies show that in a majority of mandibles the inferior dental nerve does not occupy a single canal, but is *plexiform* in arrangement. It is also joined, directly, or through its plexiform branches, by rami entering the bone as parts of neurovascular bundles, derived from attached muscles such as masseter. Such 'accessory' dental nerves ramify particularly in a plane lateral to the molar teeth, and their common occurrence accounts for the incomplete abolition of pain by inferior dental nerve block.[994]

The inferior alveolar nerve gives off the mylohyoid nerve, branches to the molar and premolar teeth of the mandible and the incisive and the mental nerves.

The *mylohyoid nerve* is derived from the inferior alveolar nerve just before the latter enters the mandibular foramen. It pierces the sphenomandibular ligament, descends in a groove on the medial surface of the ramus of the mandible and, passing below the mylohyoid line, it reaches the inferior surface of the mylohyoid, which it supplies together with the anterior belly of the digastric.

The branches to the molar and premolar teeth supply the adjoining gum also. Before they enter the roots of the teeth they communicate with one another and form an inferior dental plexus.

The *incisive nerve* is often described as continuing within the bone to supply the canine and incisor teeth. Alternative views have, however, been expressed: the nerves which supply the incisor teeth form an elaborate plexus on the external aspect of the mandible after emerging from the mental foramen and before they re-enter the bone.[995]

The canine tooth may be supplied either from this incisor plexus or the plexus which innervates the premolars.

The *mental nerve* emerges at the mental foramen, and divides beneath the depressor anguli oris into three branches; one descends to the skin of the chin, and two ascend to the skin and mucous membrane of the lower lip; these branches communicate freely with the facial nerve (mandibular branch).

*Applied Anatomy.* A lesion of the whole trigeminal nerve causes anaesthesia of the corresponding anterior half of the scalp, of the face (excepting a small area near the

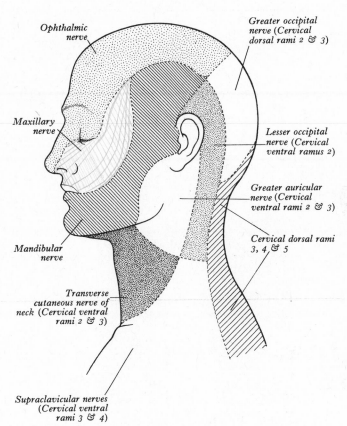

7.182    A diagram showing the cutaneous nerve supply of the face, scalp and neck. Compare with 7.186.

angle of the mandible supplied by the great auricular nerve), of the cornea and conjunctiva, and of the mucous membranes of the nose, mouth and pre-sulcal part of the tongue. Paralysis and atrophy occur in the muscles supplied by the nerve, and when the mouth is opened the mandible is thrust over to the paralysed side. Lesions of the divisions of the nerve give a more limited sensory loss and, if affecting the lingual nerve below the point at which it is joined by the chorda tympani, will be accompanied by loss of taste in the corresponding half of the anterior part of the tongue.

*Pains referred* to various branches of the trigeminal nerve are of very frequent occurrence. As a general rule the diffusion of pain over the various branches of the nerve is at first confined to one only of the main divisions, although in severe cases pain may radiate over the branches of the other main divisions. The commonest example of this condition is the neuralgia which is so often associated with dental caries. Here, although the tooth itself may not appear to be painful, the most distressing referred pains

[994] R. B. Carter and E. N. Keen, *J. Anat.*, **108**, 1971.
[995] C. Starkie and D. Stewart, *J. Anat.*, **65**, 1931.

may be experienced, and these are at once relieved by treatment directed to the affected tooth.

In the area of the ophthalmic nerve, severe supraorbital pain is commonly associated with acute glaucoma or with frontal or ethmoidal sinusitis. Malignant growths or empyema of the maxillary sinus, or unhealthy conditions about the inferior conchae or the septum of the nose, are often found giving rise to 'second division' (maxillary) neuralgia, and should be always looked for in the absence of dental disease in the maxilla. It is in the mandibular nerve, however, that some of the most striking examples are seen. It is quite common to meet with patients who complain of pain in the ear, in whom there is no sign of aural disease, and the cause is usually to be found in a carious tooth in the mandible. Moreover, with an ulcer or cancer of the tongue, often the first pain to be experienced is one which radiates to the ear and temporal fossa, over the distribution of the auriculotemporal nerve.

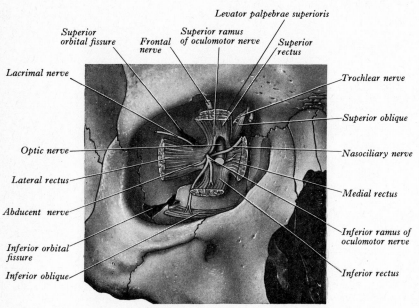

Levator palpebrae superioris
Superior orbital fissure
Frontal nerve
Superior ramus of oculomotor nerve
Superior rectus
Lacrimal nerve
Trochlear nerve
Superior oblique
Optic nerve
Nasociliary nerve
Lateral rectus
Medial rectus
Abducent nerve
Inferior orbital fissure
Inferior ramus of oculomotor nerve
Inferior oblique
Inferior rectus

7.183 A dissection of the right orbit viewed from in front, to show the origins of the orbital muscles and the relative positions of the nerves of the orbit.

The lingual nerve is occasionally divided with a view to relieving the pain in cancer of the tongue. This may be carried out where the nerve lies in direct contact with the mandible below and behind the last molar tooth, covered only by the mucous membrane (p. 282).

In cases of intractable neuralgia of the trigeminal nerve various operative procedures have been introduced from time to time. The trunks of the maxillary and mandibular nerves and the trigeminal ganglion itself have been injected with alcohol with varying degrees of success, and excision of the ganglion, in whole or in part, has frequently been performed successfully, but the last-named operation involves serious risks (laceration of the cavernous sinus, etc.) and is now rarely undertaken. The sensory root of the nerve may be divided behind the ganglion, and this is now the operation of election when the pain is confined to the maxillary and mandibular nerve areas (7.182). Complete division of the sensory root necessarily denervates the cornea completely, and the resulting loss of the corneal reflex leads to neuropathic keratitis. Consequently, in these cases an endeavour is made to preserve the ophthalmic fibres, which lie in the upper and medial part of the root and can be spared if the incision is re-

stricted to the lower and lateral fibres. The motor root of the nerve is left intact.

When the pain is limited to the ophthalmic area or to the ophthalmic and maxillary areas, the operation of election[996] consists in the division of the fibres of the spinal tract of the nerve, where it is most superficial (p. 845) and sometimes forms a recognizable elevation (p. 842) between the lateral margin of the fasciculus cuneatus and the posterior border of the lower part of the olive. Section of the tract 4–5 mm caudal to the obex preserves most, if not all, of the mandibular fibres, because they have entered the cranial part of the nucleus of the tract caudal to this and so escape injury. Following the operation painful and thermal sensibility are lost over the ophthalmic and maxillary areas, but tactile sensibility is retained and the corneal reflex is not abolished.

## The Abducent Nerve

The abducent nerve (7.176) supplies the lateral rectus muscle of the eyeball. Its fibres arise from a small nucleus situated in the cranial part of the floor of the fourth ventricle, close to the median plane and beneath the colliculus facialis (7.62, 64, 68, 69; p. 879). They descend ventrally through the pons, and emerge in the sulcus between the caudal border of the pons and the cranial end of the pyramid of the medulla oblongata (7.55).

The *abducens nucleus* consists of large and small multipolar neurons, the former being sources of the abducent nerve, the latter being known collectively as the *nucleus para-abducens*, which is considered to project to the oculomotor nucleus via the medial longitudinal fasciculus. The total number of cells in the nucleus has been stated to be about 22,000, and only a minority of these can be radicular, since the nerve contains about 6,600 fibres.[997]

*Connexions.* The nucleus of the abducent nerve receives prominent afferent connexions from: (1) the corticonuclear tract principally, but not wholly, of the contralateral side; some of these fibres are aberrant pyramidal fibres which descend from the midbrain to this level in the medial lemniscus (p. 845) and interneurons may link them to the nucleus; (2) the medial longitudinal fasciculus, by which it is connected with the nuclei of the third, fourth and eighth cranial nerves; (3) the tectobulbar tract, by which it is connected with the visual cortex and other centres through the medium of the superior colliculus. (See also p. 887.)

*Course.* After leaving the surface of the brainstem, the abducent nerve runs upwards, forwards and laterally through the cisterna pontis, and usually dorsal to the anterior inferior cerebellar artery. It pierces the dura mater lateral to the dorsum sellae of the sphenoid bone and then bends sharply forwards as it crosses the superior border of the petrous part of the temporal bone close to its apex. In this situation it is inferior to the petrosphenoidal ligament—a fibrous band which connects the lateral margin of the dorsum sellae to the upper border of the petrous part of the temporal bone near its medial end. It next traverses the cavernous sinus, lying at first lateral and then inferolateral to the internal carotid artery (6.127) and enters the orbital cavity through the medial end of the superior orbital fissure. It passes within the common tendinous ring from which the recti of the eyeball arise, lying inferolateral to the oculomotor and nasociliary nerves, and finally sinks into the ocular surface of the lateral rectus (7.183, 269).

996 M. A. Falconer, *J. Neurol. Neurosurg. Psychiat.*, **12**, 1949.
997 B. W. Konigsmark, U. P. Kalyanaraman, P. Corey and E. A. Murphy, *Bull. Johns Hopkins Hosp.*, **125**, 1969.

In the cavernous sinus the abducent nerve is joined by several filaments from the internal carotid plexus, and may communicate with the ophthalmic nerve, though an exchange of fibres has been denied.[998]

*Applied Anatomy.* The abducent nerve is occasionally involved in fractures of the base of the skull. The result of paralysis of this nerve is medial or convergent squint. Diplopia hence follows. The long course forwards of the sixth cranial nerve through the cisterna pontis and its sharp bend over the superior border of the petrous part of the temporal bone make the nerve particularly liable to damage in conditions producing raised intracranial pressure, as a result of which the brainstem is pushed caudally towards the foramen magnum with consequent stretching of the nerve.

## The Facial Nerve

The facial nerve (7.184, 187) possesses a motor and a sensory root, the latter called the *nervus intermedius* (7.55). The two roots appear at the caudal border of the pons just lateral to the recess between the olive and the inferior cerebellar peduncle, the motor part being the more medial; the vestibulocochlear nerve lies immediately to the lateral side of the sensory root. The nervus intermedius usually cleaves to the latter nerve rather than the facial, passing from the eighth to the seventh nerve as they approach the internal acoustic meatus, often as more than one filament. In one-fifth of a series of seventy-three dissections it was not a separate nerve until the meatus was reached, a point of some surgical importance.[999]

The *motor root* supplies the muscles of the face, scalp, auricle, the buccinator, platysma, stapedius, stylohyoid, and posterior belly of the digastric. The *sensory root* conveys from the chorda tympani nerve the fibres of taste for the presulcal area of the tongue, and from the palatine and greater petrosal nerves the fibres of taste from the soft palate; in addition, it transmits the preganglionic parasympathetic (secretomotor) innervation of the submandibular and sublingual salivary glands, the lacrimal gland and the glands of the nasal and palatine mucosae.

**The motor nucleus** from which most of the motor fibres of the facial nerve are derived lies deeply in the reticular formation of the caudal part of the pons (p. 890). It is posterior to the dorsal nucleus of the trapezoid body (7.62, 64, 68) and ventromedial to the nucleus of the spinal tract of the trigeminal nerve. It represents the branchial efferent column, but it lies much more deeply in the pons than might be expected, and its outgoing fibres pursue a most unusual course (7.69). Both these features have been explained by invoking the principle of neurobiotaxis (but see, however, p. 133). The nucleus receives fibres from both corticonuclear tracts in the lower part of the pons or reputedly by aberrant pyramidal fibres which descend in the medial lemniscus. The fibres from the contralateral side contribute to that part of the nucleus which supplies the muscles of the lower part of the face (p. 855). The fibres to that part of the nucleus supplying the muscles around the eyes and forehead are bilateral. In addition, some of the efferent fibres of the facial nerve proceed from the *superior salivatory nucleus (see* p. 855), which is said to be in the reticular formation, dorsolateral to the caudal end of the motor nucleus. The cells of the nucleus have been described as being clustered along the intrapontine part of the facial nerve distal to its loop around the abducens nucleus.[1000] It represents the general visceral efferent column, and it sends its fibres to join the sensory root, by which they are ultimately distributed through the chorda tympani to the submandibular and sublingual salivary glands. From this double origin

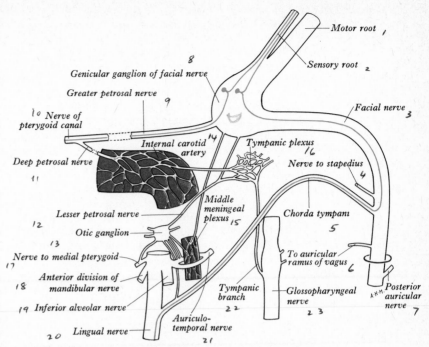

7.184 A plan of the intrapetrous section of the facial nerve, its branches and communications. The course of the taste fibres from the mucous membrane of the palate and from the anterior, oral, or presulcal part of the tongue is represented by the blue lines.

the fibres of the *motor root* pass dorsally and medially, and, reaching the caudal end of the abducent nucleus, they run cranially superficial to this nucleus deep to the colliculus facialis. At the cranial end of the nucleus of the abducent nerve they make a second bend, and run caudoventrally through the pons to the point of emergence between the olive and the inferior cerebellar peduncle (7.55, 69).

Topographically the facial motor nucleus is a complex of smaller nerve cell groups—lateral, intermediate and medial, which have been identified in various mammals including man.[1001, 1002] A further subdivision of the medial nucleus into ventral, dorsal and intermediate sub-nuclei has also been described. (For full details and discussion of the large literature concerning these and other aspects of the facial nucleus, consult footnote reference [1003].) These subsidiary groups of nerve cells extend as craniocaudal columns through the facial nuclear complex, like the columnar groups of the spinal cord or oculomotor nucleus. There is general agreement that the facial subnuclei innervate muscles supplied by individual branches of the facial nerve, or even single muscles, but different observers disagree in details. Retrograde changes due to division of these branches in dogs[1003, 1004] or cats[1002, 1005] have provided most of the evidence, but the effects on motor terminals due to selective lesions of the nucleus have also been studied in cats. General results were that the lateral sub-nucleus innervates the buccal musculature, the intermediate sends axons into the temporal, orbital and zygomatic facial branches, and the medial into the

[998] S. Sunderland and E. S. R. Hughes, *Brain*, **69**, 1946.
[999] A. L. Rhoton, S. Kobayashi and W. A. H. Hollinshead, *J. Neurosurg.*, **29**, 1968.
[1000] E. C. Crosby and B. R. Dejonge, *Ann. Otol. Rhinol. Lar.*, **72**, 1963.
[1001] G. Marinesco, *Presse méd.*, **65**, 1899.
[1002] J. W. Papez, *J. comp. Neurol.*, **43**, 1927.
[1003] G. F. Vraa-Jensen, *The Motor Nucleus of the Facial Nerve*, Munksgaard, Copenhagen. 1942.
[1004] K. Yagita, *Anat. Anz.*, **37**, 1910.
[1005] J. Courville, *Brain Res.*, **1**, 1966.

posterior auricular and cervical rami and probably also into the stapedial nerve. Nuclear lesions produced a roughly similar but more detailed schema.[1006]

**The sensory nucleus** of the facial nerve is the upper part of the *nucleus of the tractus solitarius* of the medulla oblongata (p. 846). It receives afferent fibres from the sensory root and sends efferent fibres to the ventral group of nuclei of the lateral part of the thalamus of the opposite side. As they ascend through the midbrain and subthalamic regions, these fibres are closely related to the median plane.[1007] From the thalamus they are relayed to the inferior part of the postcentral gyrus.

*The sensory root* (*nervus intermedius*) consists of the central processes of the unipolar cells of the genicular ganglion, which leave the trunk of the facial nerve in the internal acoustic meatus and pass centrally as one or more slender bundles between the motor root and the vestibulocochlear nerve or adhering to the latter, to enter the brainstem at the lower border of the pons. The peripheral branches from the processes of the ganglion cells are the taste fibres contained in the chorda tympani and the greater petrosal nerves, and also a few somatic afferent

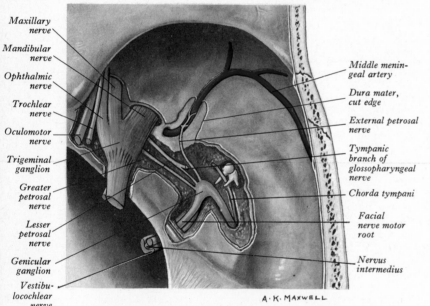

Maxillary nerve
Mandibular nerve
Ophthalmic nerve
Trochlear nerve
Oculomotor nerve
Trigeminal ganglion
Greater petrosal nerve
Lesser petrosal nerve
Genicular ganglion
Vestibulocochlear nerve

Middle meningeal artery
Dura mater, cut edge
External petrosal nerve
Tympanic branch of glossopharyngeal nerve
Chorda tympani
Facial nerve motor root
Nervus intermedius

A·K·MAXWELL

7.185   A dissection of the right middle cranial fossa, showing the course and some of the connexions of the facial nerve within the temporal bone.

fibres from the concha of the auricle (p. 1136). As already stated, the sensory root also contains the efferent preganglionic parasympathetic fibres for the submandibular and sublingual salivary glands, the lacrimal gland, and pharyngeal, nasal and palatine glands.

From their attachments to the brain, the two roots of the facial nerve pass laterally and forwards with the vestibulocochlear nerve to the opening of the internal acoustic meatus. In the meatus the motor root lies in a groove on the upper and anterior surface of the vestibulocochlear nerve, the sensory root being placed between them.

At the bottom of the meatus, the facial nerve enters the facial canal. In this canal the nerve runs at first laterally above the vestibule and, reaching the medial wall of the epitympanic recess, bends sharply backwards above the promontory, and arches downwards in the medial wall of the aditus to the tympanic antrum. Finally it descends to reach the stylomastoid foramen. The point where it bends sharply backwards is named the *geniculum*; it presents a reddish asymmetric swelling named the *genicular ganglion* (7.184). On emerging from the stylomastoid foramen, the facial nerve runs forwards in the substance

of the parotid gland (p. 1210), crosses the styloid process, the retromandibular vein and the external carotid artery, and divides behind the neck of the mandible into branches which pierce the anteromedial surface of the parotid gland and diverge from one another under cover of it. They form a network (*parotid plexus*) and are distributed to the muscles of facial expression. As it emerges from the stylomastoid foramen, the facial nerve lies about 2 cm deep to the middle of the anterior border of the mastoid process. Its course through the parotid gland can be represented by a short horizontal line drawn across the upper part of the lobule of the auricle (6.47).

The facial nerve is supplied by the anterior inferior cerebellar artery in the intracranial part of its course, by the superficial petrosal branch of the middle meningeal artery and the stylomastoid branch of the posterior auricular artery in the intrapetrous part, by branches from the stylomastoid, posterior auricular (or occipital) superficial temporal and transverse facial arteries extracranially. Its venous drainage is into the venae comitantes of the superficial petrosal and stylomastoid arteries.[1008]

**The branches of communication** of the facial nerve may be arranged as follows:

| | |
|---|---|
| In the internal acoustic meatus | With the vestibulocochlear nerve. |
| At the genicular ganglion | With the pterygopalatine ganglion by the greater petrosal nerve. |
| | With the otic ganglion by a branch which joins the lesser petrosal nerve (but see below). |
| | With the sympathetic plexus on the middle meningeal artery. |
| In the facial canal | With the auricular branch of the vagus nerve. |
| At its exit from the stylomastoid foramen | With the glossopharyngeal, vagus, great auricular, and auriculotemporal nerves. |
| Behind the ear | With the lesser occipital nerve. |
| On the face | With the trigeminal nerve. |
| In the neck | With the transverse cutaneous nerve of the neck. |

In the internal acoustic meatus some minute filaments connect the facial nerve with the vestibulocochlear nerve.

**The greater petrosal nerve** arises from the genicular ganglion, and consists chiefly of taste fibres which are distributed to the mucous membrane of the palate; but it also contains preganglionic parasympathetic fibres which are destined for the pterygopalatine ganglion; they are said to be relayed through the zygomatic and lacrimal nerves to the lacrimal gland (but see p. 1004), and through the nasal and palatine nerves to the nasal and palatine mucosal glands (7.179). It receives a twig from the tympanic plexus, passes forwards through the hiatus on the anterior surface of the petrous portion of the temporal bone and runs in a groove on the bone. It passes beneath the trigeminal ganglion and reaches the foramen lacerum. In this foramen it is joined by the **deep petrosal nerve** (7.184) from the sympathetic plexus on the internal carotid artery, and forms the **nerve of the pterygoid canal**, which passes forwards through the pterygoid canal and ends in the pterygopalatine ganglion. The taste fibres pass without interruption through or over the surface of the ganglion into the palatine branches which spring from it.

[1006] J. Szentágothai, *J. comp. Neurol.*, **88**, 1948.
[1007] W. Harris, *Br. med. J.*, **1**, 1952.
[1008] M. J. Blunt, *J. Anat.*, **88**, 1954.

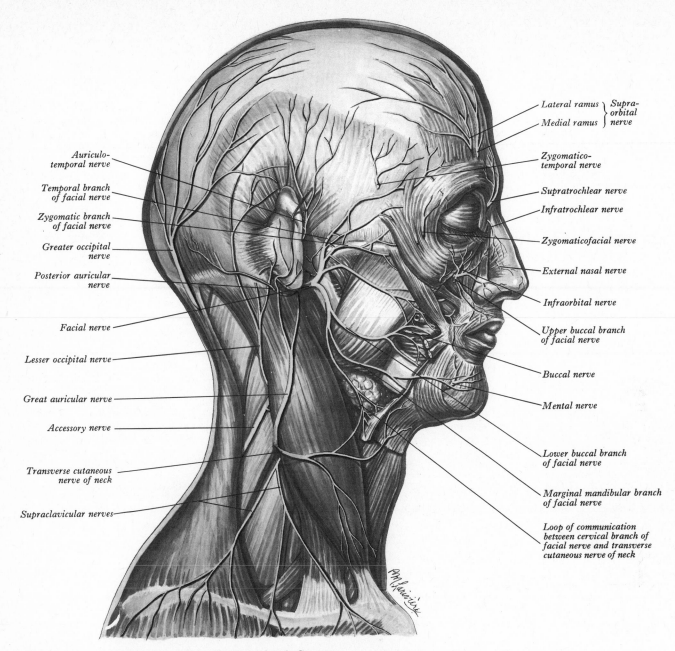

Lateral ramus ⎱ Supra-
Medial ramus ⎰ orbital nerve

Zygomatico-temporal nerve

Supratrochlear nerve

Infratrochlear nerve

Zygomaticofacial nerve

External nasal nerve

Infraorbital nerve

Upper buccal branch of facial nerve

Buccal nerve

Mental nerve

Lower buccal branch of facial nerve

Marginal mandibular branch of facial nerve

Loop of communication between cervical branch of facial nerve and transverse cutaneous nerve of neck

Auriculo-temporal nerve

Temporal branch of facial nerve

Zygomatic branch of facial nerve

Greater occipital nerve

Posterior auricular nerve

Facial nerve

Lesser occipital nerve

Great auricular nerve

Accessory nerve

Transverse cutaneous nerve of neck

Supraclavicular nerves

**7.186** The nerves of the right side of the scalp, face and neck. Compare with **7.182**.

From the trunk of the facial nerve near the genicular ganglion, from the ganglion itself, or from the root of the greater petrosal nerve,[1009] a branch runs to join the lesser petrosal nerve (**7.184**), and is conveyed through this nerve to the otic ganglion. However, the fibres constituting this small communicating nerve do not stem from the facial nerve itself, but from the auricular branch of the vagus. In twenty-four out of twenty-five human dissections the fibres approached the facial nerve through the stapedius muscle, travelling in the muscle's fascial sheath almost as far as the genicular ganglion, before departing to join the lesser superficial petrosal nerve.[1010]

The sympathetic plexus on the middle meningeal artery is joined to the genicular ganglion by an inconstant branch, sometimes named the *external petrosal nerve*.

Before the facial nerve emerges from the stylomastoid foramen, it receives another twig from the auricular branch of the vagus.

After its exit from the stylomastoid foramen, the facial nerve receives a twig from the glossopharyngeal nerve, and communicates with the great auricular and auriculotemporal nerves in the parotid gland, with the lesser

occipital nerve behind the ear, with the terminal branches of the trigeminal nerve on the face, and with the transverse cutaneous cervical nerve in the neck.

**The branches of distribution** (**7.184, 186**) of the facial nerve may be grouped as follows:

| | |
|---|---|
| Within the facial canal | Nerve to the stapedius |
| | Chorda tympani |
| At its exit from the stylo-mastoid foramen | Posterior auricular |
| | Digastric, posterior belly |
| | Stylohyoid |
| On the face | Temporal |
| | Zygomatic |
| | Buccal |
| | Marginal mandibular |
| | Cervical |

**The nerve to the stapedius** arises from the facial nerve opposite the pyramidal eminence on the posterior

---

[1009] B. Vidić and P. A. Young, *Anat. Rec.*, **158**, 1967.
[1010] B. Vidić, *Anat. Rec.*, **162**, 1968.

wall of the tympanic cavity; it passes forwards through a small canal to reach the muscle (p. 1141).

**The chorda tympani nerve** (7.181) arises from the facial nerve about 6 mm above the stylomastoid foramen. It runs upwards and forwards in a canal, and perforates the posterior bony wall of the tympanic cavity through the posterior canaliculus for the chorda tympani nerve, which is situated close to the posterior border of the medial surface of the tympanic membrane and on a level with the upper end of the handle of the malleus. It then passes forwards between the fibrous and mucous layers of the tympanic membrane, crosses the handle of the malleus, and re-enters the bone through the anterior canaliculus for the chorda tympani nerve, which is placed at the medial end of the petrotympanic fissure. The nerve now descends ventrally on the medial surface of the spine of the sphenoid bone (which it sometimes grooves) and passes deep to the lateral pterygoid. In this part of its course the nerve lies

mastoid process; here it is joined by a filament from the auricular branch of the vagus nerve, and communicates with the posterior branch of the great auricular nerve, and with the lesser occipital nerve. As it ascends between the external acoustic meatus and the mastoid process it divides into an auricular and an occipital branch. The *auricular branch* supplies the auricularis posterior and the intrinsic muscles on the cranial surface of the auricle. The *occipital branch*, the larger, passes backwards along the superior nuchal line of the occipital bone, and supplies the occipital belly of the occipitofrontalis.

**The digastric branch** arises close to the stylomastoid foramen, and divides into several filaments which supply the posterior belly of the digastric; one of these filaments joins the glossopharyngeal nerve.

**The stylohyoid branch**, long and slender, frequently arises in conjunction with the digastric branch; it enters the middle part of the stylohyoid.

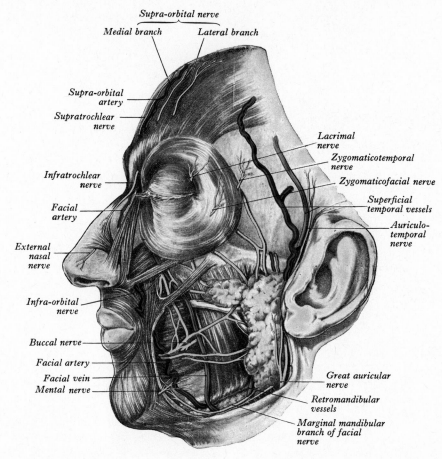

**7.187**   The terminal branches of the left trigeminal and facial nerves in the face.

lateral to the tensor veli palatini and is crossed by the middle meningeal artery, the roots of the auriculotemporal nerve and the inferior alveolar nerve. Finally it joins the posterior border of the lingual nerve at an acute angle. It contains efferent preganglionic parasympathetic (secretomotor) fibres which enter the submandibular ganglion, and are there relayed as postganglionic fibres to the submandibular and sublingual glands; the majority of its fibres are afferent from the mucous membrane covering the anterior, presulcal part of the tongue, save the vallate papillae; they constitute the nerve of taste for this region of the tongue. Before uniting with the lingual nerve the chorda tympani is joined by a small branch from the otic ganglion.

**The posterior auricular nerve** arises close to the stylomastoid foramen and runs upwards in front of the

**The temporal branches** cross the zygomatic arch to the temporal region. They supply the intrinsic muscles on the lateral surface of the auricle, the anterior and superior auricular muscles, and join with the zygomaticotemporal branch of the maxillary nerve, and with the auriculotemporal branch of the mandibular nerve. The more anterior branches supply the frontal belly of the occipitofrontalis, the orbicularis oculi and the corrugator, and join the supraorbital and lacrimal branches of the ophthalmic nerve.

**The zygomatic branches** run across the zygomatic bone to the lateral angle of the eye; they supply the orbicularis oculi, and join with the filaments of the lacrimal nerve and the zygomaticofacial branch of the maxillary nerve.

**The buccal branches** pass horizontally forwards to be distributed below the orbit and around the mouth. The *superficial branches* run between the skin of the face and the superficial muscles, and supply the latter; some are distributed to the procerus, joining with the infratrochlear and external nasal nerves. The upper *deep branches* pass under cover of the zygomaticus major and the levator labii superioris, supplying them and forming an *infra-orbital plexus* with the superior labial branches of the infraorbital nerve; they also supply the levator anguli oris, the zygomaticus minor, the levator labii superioris alaeque nasi and the small muscles of the nose. These branches are sometimes described as lower zygomatic branches. The lower deep branches supply the buccinator and orbicularis oris, and join with filaments of the buccal branch of the mandibular nerve.

**The marginal mandibular branch** runs forwards below the angle of the mandible under cover of the platysma. It lies at first superficial to the upper part of the digastric triangle and then turns upwards and forwards across the body of the mandible to lie under cover of the depressor anguli oris (7.187). It supplies the risorius and the muscles of the lower lip and chin, and joins the mental nerve (p. 1009).

**The cervical branch** issues from the lower part of the parotid gland, runs forwards and downwards under cover of the platysma to the front of the neck. It supplies the platysma and communicates with the transverse cutaneous cervical nerve.

**The submandibular ganglion** is a small, somewhat fusiform ganglion which lies on the upper part of the hyoglossus. There are further ganglion cells in the hilus of the submandibular gland. Like the ciliary, pterygo-palatine and otic ganglia, these are peripheral ganglia of the parasympathetic system. The submandibular ganglion is superior to the deep part of the submandibular gland and below the lingual nerve, from which it is suspended by an anterior and a posterior filament (7.177). Although so intimately related to the lingual nerve, the ganglion is connected functionally with the facial nerve and its chorda tympani branch.

The *motor* or *parasympathetic root* is formed by the posterior filament connecting the ganglion to the lingual nerve. It conveys preganglionic fibres which arise in the superior salivatory nucleus and run in the facial, chorda tympani and lingual nerves to reach the ganglion. There the fibres establish synaptic relations with the cells of the ganglion, and the postganglionic fibres are secretomotor to the submandibular and the sublingual salivary glands. The *sympathetic root* is derived from the plexus on the facial artery. It consists of postganglionic fibres which commence in the superior cervical ganglion and pass through the submandibular ganglion without being interrupted. They are vasomotor to the blood vessels of the submandibular and sublingual glands.

Five or six branches arise from the ganglion and supply the submandibular gland and its duct. Other fibres from the ganglion pass through the anterior filament which connects it to the lingual nerve and are carried to the sublingual and the anterior lingual glands.

**The cutaneous fibres** of distribution of the facial nerve accompany those of the auricular branch of the vagus and probably innervate skin on both aspects of the auricle, in the conchal depression and over its eminence. Details of this innervation are, however, uncertain, as is the question of whether facial fibres reach the external acoustic meatus and tympanic membrane.

*Applied Anatomy.* Facial paralysis is commonly unilateral and may be due to: (1) *supranuclear lesions* of the corticonuclear fibres or of the pathway from the frontal lobe, anterior to the precentral gyrus, to the facial nucleus; (2) *nuclear* or *infranuclear lesions* involving the lower motor neurons.

Facial paralysis due to a supranuclear lesion involving the corticonuclear pathway is usually part of a hemiplegia. The movements of the lower part of the face are usually more severely affected than those of the upper part and voluntary movements are weak or absent whilst emotional and associated movements are little affected. The electrical reactions of the muscles on the affected side are not altered. Occasionally supranuclear lesions result in abolition or weakness of emotional movements with retention of voluntary movements. The dissociation in these forms of paralysis suggests that the supranuclear pathway concerned with emotional movements is distinct from that of the corticonuclear fibres which are concerned with voluntary movements.

The effects of nuclear or infranuclear lesions vary according to the point on its course at which the facial nerve is injured. If the facial nucleus or facial nerve fibres in the pons are involved, neighbouring structures are inevitably involved as well. The facial muscles are represented in cell groups in the nucleus and their degree of involvement will govern the extent of the paralysis which will be ipsilateral: otherwise the symptoms are identical with those seen in more peripheral lesions of the nerve. The associated lesions may thus include paralysis of the lateral rectus muscle of the eyeball due to involvement of the abducent nerve nucleus, around which the facial nerve fibres loop, paralysis of the muscles of mastication due to involvement of the motor nucleus of the trigeminal nerve, sensory loss on the face from implication of the principal sensory nucleus or of the nucleus of the spinal tract of the trigeminal nerve or spinothalamic tract and paralysis of the upper or lower limbs due to lesions of the corticospinal tracts. Due to the proximity of the sensory root of the facial nerve and of the vestibulocochlear nerve, lesions in the posterior cranial fossa or in the internal acoustic meatus may be accompanied by loss of taste in the anterior two-thirds of the tongue and deafness on the same side as the facial paralysis. When the facial nerve is damaged within the temporal bone the chorda tympani nerve is usually involved and in fractures of the petrous temporal bone the vestibulocochlear nerve is also usually implicated. The most common cause of facial palsy is inflammation of the nerve close to the stylomastoid foramen (Bell's paralysis). The cause of this is uncertain, but it results in oedema of the nerve and compression of its fibres in the facial canal or at the stylomastoid foramen. If the lesion is complete the facial muscles are all equally affected, and voluntary, emotional and associated movements of the face suffer equally. There is asymmetry of the face and the affected side is immobile. The eyebrow droops, the lines on the forehead and nasolabial fold are smoothed out and the palpebral fissure is wider than on the normal side due to the unopposed action of the levator palpebrae. Tears fail to enter the lacrimal puncta because they are no longer in contact with the conjunctiva, the conjunctival reflex is absent and efforts to close the eye merely cause the eyeball to roll upwards until the cornea lies under the upper lid. The ala nasi does not move properly on respiration. The lips remain in contact on the paralysed side, but cannot be pursed for whistling; when a smile is attempted the angle of the mouth is drawn up on the unaffected side but on the affected side the lips remain nearly closed, and the mouth assumes a characteristic triangular form. During mastication food accumulates in the cheek, from paralysis of the buccinator, and dribbles or is pushed out from between the paralysed lips. On protrusion the tongue seems to be thrust over towards the paralysed side, but verification of its position by reference to the incisor teeth will·show that this is not really so. The platysma and the muscles of the auricle are paralysed; in severe cases the articulation of labials is impaired. The electrical reactions of the affected muscles are altered (reaction of degeneration), and the degree to which this alteration has taken place after a week or ten days gives a valuable guide to the prognosis. Most cases of Bell's palsy recover completely. For details of variations in the course of the facial nerve in the vicinity of the middle ear, and their surgical importance, consult footnote reference [1011]. Degeneration studies[1012] have shown that the facial nerve contains no fascicular or other pattern corresponding to its peripheral branches, a finding of some significance in suturing the nerve after injury.

## The Vestibulocochlear Nerve

The vestibulocochlear nerve (7.62, 63, 66, 68) appears in the groove between the pons and medulla oblongata, behind the facial nerve and in front of the inferior cerebellar peduncle (7.55). It consists of two sets of fibres, which, although differing in their principal central connexions, are both concerned in the transmission of afferent impulses from the internal ear to the brain. One set of fibres forms the vestibular nerve, or nerve of equilibration, and arises from the cells of the vestibular ganglion situated in the outer part of the internal acoustic meatus; the other set constitutes the cochlear nerve, or nerve of hearing, and takes origin from the cells of the spiral ganglion of the cochlea. Both ganglia consist of bipolar nerve cells; from each cell a central fibre passes to the brain, and a peripheral fibre to the internal ear.

### THE VESTIBULAR NERVE

The fibres of the vestibular nerve enter the brain superomedial to those of the cochlear nerve. They pass backwards through the pons between the inferior cerebellar peduncle and the spinal tract of the trigeminal nerve and divide into ascending and descending branches which mostly end in the vestibular nuclei, although many proceed direct to the cerebellum along the inferior cerebellar peduncle (p. 861).

**The vestibular nuclear complex** comprises the following: (1) The *medial vestibular nucleus* (p. 889), which lies in the vestibular area of the floor of the fourth ventricle, crossed dorsally by the striae medullares. It is the largest subdivision and extends upwards from the medulla oblongata into the pons. (2) The *inferior vestibular nucleus* (p. 890) lies lateral to the medial nucleus and reaches to a lower level in the medulla oblongata. It is placed between the medial nucleus and the inferior cerebellar peduncle, and the descending branches of the incoming vestibular fibres are interspersed among its cells. (3) The *lateral nucleus* (p. 890) lies ventrolateral to the upper part of the medial nucleus, and it is characterized by the large size of its constituent cells. Its upper end becomes continuous with the lower end of (4) the *superior nucleus*, which extends higher into the pons than the other subdivisions and occupies the upper part of the vestibular area. A number of minor subdivisions have been described in the main vestibular nuclei in the cat,[1013] and a somatotopic pattern has been tentatively suggested in the lateral vestibular nucleus.[1014]

*Connexions.* All the vestibular nuclei receive incoming fibres from the vestibular nerve and it is believed that they receive *afferent cerebellovestibular fibres* through the inferior cerebellar peduncle. These fibres are derived, for the most part, from the flocculus and nodule (posterior lobe), but others have been ascribed to the uvula, the lingula and the fastigial nucleus.

From the nuclei *efferent fibres* enter the inferior cerebellar peduncle, most of them being destined for the flocculus and the nodule, though some may pass to the uvula and the lingula, and some have been described as terminating in the fastigial nucleus. As already stated, many of the fibres of the vestibular nerve 'bypass' the nuclei and traverse the inferior cerebellar peduncle to reach the flocculus and the nodule.

As a whole, the vestibular nuclear complex acts as a relay station on an afferent cerebellar pathway, and is in turn a distributing station for efferent cerebellar fibres.

In addition, fibres from the vestibular nuclei enter the medial longitudinal fasciculus (7.94), in which they ascend, or descend, to reach the motor nuclei of the eye muscles and muscles of the neck. Further, from the large cells of the lateral vestibular nucleus, efferent fibres descend to form the vestibulospinal tract (p. 817) and fibres from the other nuclei are believed to join the lateral lemniscus and so may reach the inferior colliculus and the medial geniculate body and, possibly, the cerebral cortex.

Speaking broadly, through its connexions the vestibular system is able to influence the movements of the eyes and head and the muscles of the trunk and limbs, so as to maintain equilibrium when loss of balance is threatened.

### THE COCHLEAR NERVE

As it reaches the brainstem the cochlear nerve (7.62, 63, 66) is placed on the lateral side of the vestibular nerve, but the two nerves soon become separated by the inferior cerebellar peduncle. The cochlear nerve passes round the lateral aspect of the peduncle, while the vestibular nerve penetrates the brainstem on the medial side of that structure.

**The cochlear nuclei** are two in number. The *ventral cochlear nucleus* is placed on the ventrolateral aspect of the inferior cerebellar peduncle, and it receives the larger, ascending branches of the cochlear nerve. The *dorsal cochlear nucleus* lies on the dorsal aspect of the peduncle in the lateral part of the vestibular area of the floor of the fourth ventricle, where it forms the auditory tubercle. It receives the smaller, descending branches of the cochlear nerve. For a detailed experimental analysis of the modes of termination and distribution of the primary cochlear afferent fibres, and a review of the literature, consult footnote reference [1015]. This study demonstrated a consistency between the above details and the tonotopical organization in the cochlear nuclei (p. 853).

Many of the *efferent fibres* from the *ventral cochlear nucleus* (second neuron fibres on the auditory pathway) end in the dorsal nucleus of the trapezoid body, either of the same or of the opposite side. There they are relayed and the tertiary fibres turn upwards, forming an ascending tract, termed the *lateral lemniscus* (7.70, 188). The secondary fibres of the opposite side behave in the same way, and the intersections of the contralateral fibres of the two sides form the *trapezoid body* (7.188). The *efferent fibres* from the *dorsal cochlear nucleus* establish similar connexions (7.188) and the tertiary fibres ascend in the lateral lemniscus of the same and of the opposite side. Many of the cochlear efferents relay in the superior olivary complex (p. 853), the majority from the ipsi-

[1011] D. J. Durcan, J. J. Shea and J. P. Sleeck, *Archs Otolar.*, **86**, 1967.
[1012] W. D. Naoris, *Arch. Otolaryng.*, **88**, 1968.
[1013] A. Brodal and O. Pompeiano, *J. Anat.*, **91**. 1957.
[1014] A. C. Løken and A. Brodal, *Archs Neurol. Psychiat.*, *Chicago*, **23**, 1970.
[1015] K. K. Osen, *Archs ital. Biol.* **108**, 1970.

lateral cochlear nuclei. After relay these pathways join both lateral lemnisci.

Each lateral lemniscus, therefore, consists of tertiary neurons from both sides, and on its upward course to the midbrain some of these have a cell station in a small group of nerve cells, intimately related to the tract and termed the *nucleus of the lateral lemniscus*. On reaching the midbrain, some of the fibres end in the nucleus of the inferior colliculus, but others 'bypass' the nucleus and run in the inferior brachium to reach the medial geniculate body, where they are relayed to the auditory cortex (areas 41, 42 and 22).

Commissural fibres link the two auditory pathways at the level of the inferior colliculi, and auditory reflexes are mediated through the inferior colliculi and the medial longitudinal fasciculi (7.94, 188). An *efferent* component in the acoustic pathway has been noted already (p. 854). Its peripheral fibres are derived from nerve cells in or near the superior olivary complex,[1016, 1017] forming in their central course the *olivocochlear fasciculus*. These fibres terminate in relation to the hair cells of the spiral organ of the cochlea. Functionally, they are probably inhibitory in their actions.[1018] The existence of sympathetic and possibly parasympathetic fibres in the vestibulocochlear nerve has received some support.[1019]

The vestibulocochlear nerve is soft in texture; the axons are ensheathed in glial cells in its proximal part. After leaving the medulla oblongata it passes forwards across the posterior border of the middle cerebellar peduncle, in company with the facial nerve, from which it is partially separated by the labyrinthine artery. It then enters the internal acoustic meatus with the facial nerve. At the outer end of the meatus it receives one or two filaments from the facial nerve, and splits into its *cochlear* and *vestibular* parts, the distribution of which will be described with the anatomy of the internal ear (pp. 1150, 1156, 1157).

*Applied Anatomy.* The vestibulocochlear nerve is frequently injured, together with the facial nerve, in fracture of the middle fossa of the skull implicating the internal acoustic meatus. The nerve may be either torn across, producing permanent deafness, or bruised or pressed upon by extravasated blood or inflammatory exudation, when the deafness will in all probability be temporary. The nerve may also be injured by violent blows on the head without fracture of the skull, and deafness may arise from loud explosions, probably from some lesion of this nerve, which is more liable to be injured than the other cranial nerves on account of its structure. Tumours in the cerebellopontine angle involve the vestibulocochlear and facial nerves, as they lie in relation to the flocculus (7.71) at the lower border of the pons.

## The Glossopharyngeal Nerve

The glossopharyngeal nerve (7.55, 62, 66, 190, 191) contains motor and sensory fibres. It supplies motor fibres to the stylopharyngeus, secretomotor fibres to the parotid gland, and sensory fibres to the pharynx, the tonsil and the posterior part of the tongue; it is also the nerve of taste for this, the postsulcal part of the tongue. It emerges as three or four rootlets from the cranial part of the medulla, in the groove between the olive and inferior cerebellar peduncle above the rootlets of the vagus nerve.

**The sensory nuclei** receive the central processes of the unipolar nerve cells in the superior and inferior ganglia of the nerve; the fibres concerned with taste end in the *nucleus of the tractus solitarius* (p. 846) and those concerned with common sensation probably in the nucleus of the spinal tract of the trigeminal nerve.[1020]

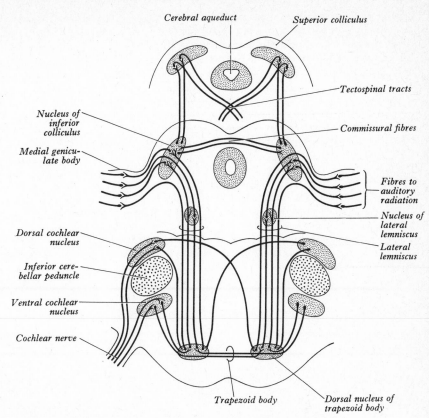

7.188 A simplified diagram to show some of the central connexions of the cochlear nerve and the auditory pathway through the brainstem. Although they are shown in the figure as being of comparable size, the trapezoid body constitutes a much more important and larger commissural bundle than the fibres connecting the nuclei of the two inferior colliculi. Efferent fibres in the cochlear nerve, and *descending* fibres in the auditory pathway have been omitted.

**The motor nucleus** is formed by the rostral part of the *nucleus ambiguus* (p. 848), which lies deeply in the reticular formation of the medulla oblongata. It is connected with the corticonuclear tracts of *both* sides directly and through interneurons. The corticonuclear fibres leave the tract at the level of the nucleus ambiguus or in the pons whence they descend in the medial lemniscus (aberrant pyramidal fibres, p. 1011). The glossopharyngeal part of the nucleus ambiguus sends its efferent fibres to the stylopharyngeus.

In addition, parasympathetic fibres join the motor part of the glossopharyngeal nerve from a representative of the general visceral efferent column which is termed the *inferior salivatory nucleus* (*see* p. 855). This nucleus lies in the reticular formation below the superior salivatory nucleus, and sends its fibres via the tympanic branch of the glossopharyngeal nerve and the tympanic plexus (p. 1018) to the lesser petrosal nerve and the otic ganglion, where they are relayed. The postganglionic fibres pass to the auriculotemporal nerve and so reach the parotid gland (7.179).

From the medulla oblongata the glossopharyngeal nerve passes forwards and laterally towards the triangular depression into which the aqueductus cochleae opens, on the inferior surface of the petrous portion of the temporal bone. It lies at first under cover of the flocculus, and rests on the jugular tubercle of the occipital bone,

[1016] G. L. Rasmussen, *Anat. Rec.*, **82**, 1942.
[1017] G. L. Rasmussen, in: *Neural Mechanisms of the Auditory and Vestibular Systems*, eds. G. L. Rasmussen and W. F. Windle, Thomas, Springfield. 1960.
[1018] I. C. Whitfield, *The Auditory Pathway*, Arnold, London. 1967.
[1019] M. D. Ross, *J. comp. Neurol.*, **135**, 1969.
[1020] A. Brodal, *Archs Neurol. Psychiat., Chicago*, **57**, 1947.

which is sometimes grooved by it. It leaves the skull by bending sharply downwards through the central part of the jugular foramen, anterior to the vagus and accessory nerves, and in a separate sheath of dura mater (7.189). In its transit through the jugular foramen it is lodged in a deep groove leading from the triangular depression for the cochlear aqueduct, and here it is separated by the inferior petrosal sinus from the vagus and accessory nerves. The deep groove is converted into a canal by a bridge which is usually composed of fibrous tissue, but consists of bone in about 25 per cent of skulls. After its exit from the skull it passes forwards between the internal jugular vein and internal carotid artery; it descends in front of the latter vessel, deep to the styloid process and the muscles connected with it, to reach the posterior border of the stylopharyngeus. It then curves forwards, lying upon the stylopharyngeus and either pierces the lower fibres of the superior constrictor of the pharynx or passes between the adjoining borders of the superior and middle constrictors (5.25) to be distributed to the tonsil, the mucous membrane of the pharynx and posterior part of the tongue, and the mucous glands of the mouth.

sympathetic trunk, and with the vagus and facial nerves.

The inferior ganglion is connected by a filament with the superior cervical ganglion of the sympathetic. The branches to the vagus consist of two filaments which arise from the inferior ganglion; one joins the auricular branch, and the other the superior ganglion, of the vagus. The branch to the facial arises from the trunk of the glossopharyngeal nerve below the inferior ganglion; it perforates the posterior belly of the digastric and joins the facial nerve near the stylomastoid foramen.

The *branches of distribution* of the glossopharyngeal nerve are: tympanic, carotid, pharyngeal, muscular, tonsillar and lingual.

**The tympanic nerve** arises from the inferior ganglion of the glossopharyngeal nerve, and ascends to the tympanic cavity through the inferior tympanic canaliculus (p. 294). In the tympanic cavity it divides into branches which form the **tympanic plexus** and are contained in grooves upon the surface of the promontory. This plexus gives off: (1) a branch to join the greater petrosal nerve (p. 1012); (2) branches to supply the mucous membrane lining the tympanic cavity, the auditory tube and the

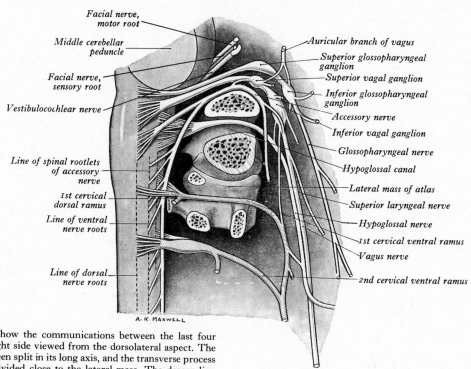

Facial nerve, motor root
Middle cerebellar peduncle
Facial nerve, sensory root
Vestibulocochlear nerve
Line of spinal rootlets of accessory nerve
1st cervical dorsal ramus
Line of ventral nerve roots
Line of dorsal nerve roots

Auricular branch of vagus
Superior glossopharyngeal ganglion
Superior vagal ganglion
Inferior glossopharyngeal ganglion
Accessory nerve
Inferior vagal ganglion
Glossopharyngeal nerve
Hypoglossal canal
Lateral mass of atlas
Superior laryngeal nerve
Hypoglossal nerve
1st cervical ventral ramus
Vagus nerve
2nd cervical ventral ramus

A. K. MAXWELL

7.189 A diagram to show the communications between the last four cranial nerves of the right side viewed from the dorsolateral aspect. The hypoglossal canal has been split in its long axis, and the transverse process of the atlas has been divided close to the lateral mass. The descending branch of the hypoglossal nerve is not shown.

Two ganglia, named the superior and the inferior, are situated on that part of the nerve which traverses the jugular foramen (7.189).

**The superior ganglion** is situated in the upper part of the groove in which the nerve is lodged during its passage through the jugular foramen. It is very small, gives off no branches, and is usually regarded as a detached portion of the inferior ganglion.

**The inferior ganglion** is larger than the superior ganglion and is situated in a notch in the lower border of the petrous portion of the temporal bone (p. 294). Its cells are typical unipolar cells. Their peripheral branches convey taste and general sensibility from the mucous membrane of the posterior third of the tongue, including the sulcus terminalis and the vallate papillae, and general sensibility from the mucous membrane of the pharynx, soft palate and the fauces.

The glossopharyngeal nerve communicates with the

mastoid air cells; and (3) the lesser petrosal nerve. For a recent critique of the final distribution and connexions of this nerve, see footnote reference [1021].

**The lesser petrosal nerve** contains the secretomotor fibres for the parotid gland (*vide infra*). It enters a small canal inferior to that for the tensor tympani, receives a connecting branch from the ganglion of the facial nerve and reaches the anterior surface of the temporal bone through a small opening on the lateral side of the hiatus for the greater petrosal nerve. It then passes through the foramen ovale or the canaliculus innominatus (p. 289) and joins the otic ganglion.

**The carotid branch**, often double, arises just below the skull, and descends on the internal carotid artery to be distributed to the wall of the carotid sinus and to the carotid body. It may communicate with the vagus (inferior

[1021] G. Winckler and B. Cochet, *Bull. Assoc. Anat.*, 1967.

ganglion or one of its branches) and with a branch from the sympathetic (superior cervical ganglion). Another branch, either from the preceding or from the main trunk, joins a fine plexus which also supplies the carotid body. The other branches to this plexus spring from the sympathetic (superior cervical ganglion) and the vagus (p. 1022). For details of the terminal distribution of the carotid sinus nerve consult footnote reference [1022].

**The pharyngeal branches** are three or four filaments which unite, opposite the middle constrictor muscle of the pharynx, with the pharyngeal branch of the vagus nerve and the laryngopharyngeal branches of the sympathetic trunk to form the *pharyngeal plexus*; through this plexus the glossopharyngeal nerve supplies the mucous membrane of the pharynx with sensory branches.

**The muscular branch** supplies the stylopharyngeus.

**The tonsillar branches** supply the tonsil, and form around it a plexus with branches of the middle and posterior palatine nerves; from this plexus filaments are distributed to the soft palate and the region of the fauces.

**The lingual branches** are two in number: one supplies the vallate papillae and the mucous membrane near the sulcus terminalis of the tongue (p. 1237); the other supplies the mucous membrane of the posterior (post-sulcal) part of the tongue, communicating with the lingual nerve. It is the nerve of special sense (taste) and of general sensibility to the posterior region of the tongue.

**The otic ganglion** (7.181, 184) is a small, oval, somewhat flattened ganglion of a reddish-grey colour, situated immediately below the foramen ovale. It is a peripheral ganglion of the parasympathetic system; topographically it is intimately related to the mandibular nerve but, functionally, it is connected with the glossopharyngeal nerve.

It is in relation *laterally* with the trunk of the mandibular nerve at or near the point where it is joined by the motor root of the trigeminal, and it usually surrounds the origin of the nerve to the medial pterygoid; *medially*, with the tensor veli palatini, by which it is separated from the cartilaginous part of the auditory tube; *posteriorly*, with the middle meningeal artery.

The *motor* or *parasympathetic root* of the ganglion is formed by the lesser petrosal nerve, which conveys preganglionic fibres from the glossopharyngeal nerve. These fibres have their origin in the cells of the inferior salivatory nucleus. They are relayed in the otic ganglion and the postganglionic fibres pass by a *communicating branch* to the auriculotemporal nerve. By it they are conveyed to the parotid gland (7.179), to which they supply secretomotor fibres. The *sympathetic root* is derived from the plexus on the middle meningeal artery. It contains postganglionic fibres which arise in the superior cervical ganglion and pass through the otic ganglion without being interrupted. Emerging with the parasympathetic fibres in the communicating branch to the auriculotemporal nerve, they are destined for the supply of the blood vessels of the parotid gland.

*Branches.* A twig connects the ganglion with the chorda tympani nerve and another ascends from it to join the nerve of the pterygoid canal. According to some neurologists these form an additional pathway by which taste fibres from the anterior, pre-sulcal area of the tongue may reach the facial ganglion without passing through the middle ear (p. 1085). The fibres concerned pass through the otic ganglion without being interrupted. Motor branches are supplied to the tensor veli palatini and the tensor tympani, they are derived from the nerve to the medial pterygoid (p. 1007) and have no synaptic relations with the cells of the ganglion.

The glossopharyngeal nerve is the nerve of the third branchial arch, or it would be more nearly correct to describe it as the post-trematic branch of that arch. The pretrematic branch of the second (hyoid) arch is probably the tympanic branch of the glossopharyngeal nerve, but that is uncertain. Like the trigeminal and the facial nerves, the glossopharyngeal corresponds to a dorsal nerve which has acquired special visceral efferent fibres.

## The Vagus Nerve

The vagus nerve (7.55, 62–66, 189–191) is composed of motor and sensory fibres, and has a more extensive course and distribution than any of the other cranial nerves, since it passes through the neck and thorax to the abdomen. It is attached by eight or ten rootlets to the medulla oblongata, below the glossopharyngeal nerve, in the groove between the olive and the inferior cerebellar peduncle.

The fibres of the vagus nerve are connected to four nuclei in the medulla oblongata. (1) **The dorsal nucleus** of the vagus is usually described as a mixed nucleus representing the fused general visceral efferent and general visceral afferent columns. It lies in the central grey matter of the lower, closed, part of the medulla oblongata, and extends upwards into the upper, open, part, where it is placed under the vagal triangle, separated from the hypoglossal nucleus by the nucleus intercalatus (p. 845). The *motor fibres* which arise from it are distributed to the involuntary muscle of the bronchi, heart, oesophagus and stomach, and to the small intestine and part of the large intestine (p. 1067). The particular *sensory fibres* which terminate in the nucleus are uncertain. Although some authorities regard the nucleus of the tractus solitarius (p. 1029) as predominantly a vagal nucleus, there is considerable evidence in favour of the view that afferent fibres from the oesophagus and the abdominal part of the alimentary canal terminate in the dorsal vagal nucleus (see also p. 846). (2) Below the origin of the fibres which join the glossopharyngeal nerve, the neurons of the **nucleus ambiguus** (pp. 848 and 1028) contribute fibres to the vagus nerve which are distributed to striped muscle, viz. the constrictor muscles of the pharynx and the intrinsic muscles of the larynx. It is connected to the corticonuclear tracts of *both* sides and to many other brainstem centres (p. 1028). There have been a number of detailed studies on the architecture and regional localization which occurs in the nucleus ambiguus of man and following experimental analysis in a number of mammals.[1023–1026] As in the case of many of the other cranial nerve motor nuclei, the nucleus ambiguus can be divided into a number of sub-nuclei. The glossopharyngeal fibres arise from a cranial group of cells, whilst the individual laryngeal muscles are innervated by relatively discrete sub-nuclei in more caudal zones; most caudally the cells of the nucleus ambiguus send axons into the cranial part of the accessory nerve (p. 1024). (3) The lower part of the **nucleus of the tractus solitarius** (pp. 846 and 1029) receives those fibres of the vagus which are distributed through the internal laryngeal nerve to the taste buds of the epiglottis and the vallecula. The middle part of the nucleus receives the visceral afferent fibres from the tongue, tonsil, palate and pharynx (glossopharyngeal nerve). The upper part of the nucleus receives the taste fibres from the anterior two-thirds of the tongue and from the soft palate (facial nerve). (4) The vagus contains somatic afferent nerve

[1022] A. G. Willis and J. D. Tange, *Am. J. Anat.*, **104**, 1959.
[1023] J. Szentágothai, *Z. Anat. EntwGesch.*, **112**, 1943.
[1024] B. Getz and T. Sirnes, *J. comp. Neurol.*, **90**, 1949.
[1025] T. Szabo and M. Dussardier, *Z. Zellforsch. microsk. Anat.*, **63**, 1964.
[1026] A. N. Lawn, *J. comp. Neurol.*, **127**, 1966.

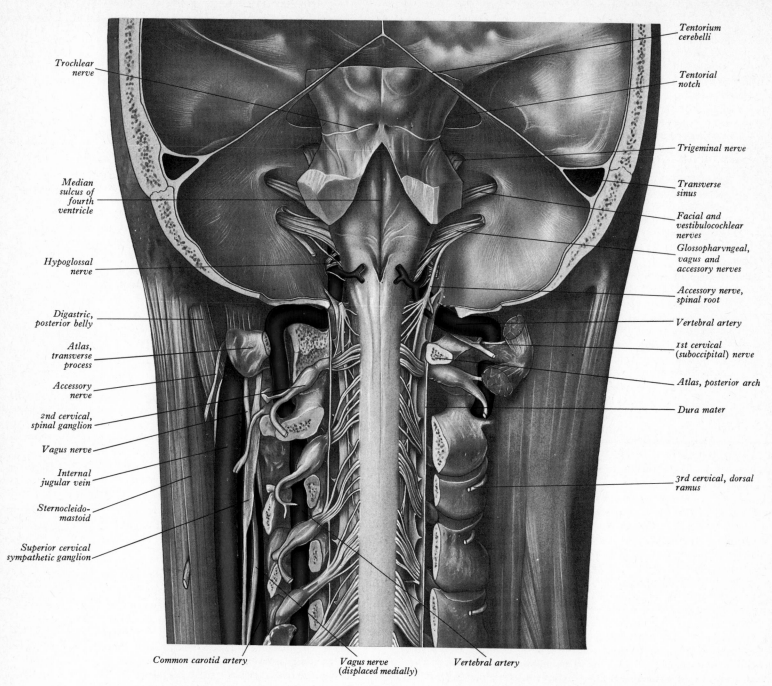

*Trochlear nerve*

*Median sulcus of fourth ventricle*

*Hypoglossal nerve*

*Digastric, posterior belly*

*Atlas, transverse process*

*Accessory nerve*

*2nd cervical, spinal ganglion*

*Vagus nerve*

*Internal jugular vein*

*Sternocleido-mastoid*

*Superior cervical sympathetic ganglion*

*Tentorium cerebelli*

*Tentorial notch*

*Trigeminal nerve*

*Transverse sinus*

*Facial and vestibulocochlear nerves*

*Glossopharyngeal, vagus and accessory nerves*

*Accessory nerve, spinal root*

*Vertebral artery*

*1st cervical (suboccipital) nerve*

*Atlas, posterior arch*

*Dura mater*

*3rd cervical, dorsal ramus*

*Common carotid artery*    *Vagus nerve (displaced medially)*    *Vertebral artery*

7.190 A dissection exposing the brainstem and the upper part of the spinal cord after removal of large portions of the occipital and parietal bones and the cerebellum, together with the roof of the fourth ventricle. On the left side the foramina transversaria of the atlas and the third, fourth and fifth cervical vertebrae have been opened to expose the verte-bral artery. On the right side the posterior arch of the atlas and the laminae of the succeeding cervical vertebrae have been divided and have been removed together with the vertebral spines and the laminae of the opposite side. The tentorium cerebelli and the transverse sinuses have been divided and their posterior portions removed.

fibres, but it is believed that when they enter the medulla oblongata they terminate in the **spinal nucleus of the trigeminal nerve.**

The rootlets of the nerve unite, and form a flat cord which passes below the flocculus of the cerebellum to the jugular foramen, through which it leaves the cranium. In emerging through this opening, the vagus nerve is accompanied by and contained in the same sheath of dura and arachnoid mater as the accessory nerve, a fibrous septum separating them from the glossopharyngeal nerve, which lies in front (7.189). In this situation the vagus nerve presents a well-marked enlargement, named the *superior ganglion.* After its exit from the jugular foramen the vagus nerve enlarges into a second swelling, named the *inferior ganglion.*

**The superior ganglion** is of a greyish colour, spherical in form, about 4 mm in diameter. It is joined by one or two delicate filaments with the cranial root of the accessory nerve; it is connected by a twig with the inferior ganglion of the glossopharyngeal nerve, and with the sympathetic trunk by a filament from the superior cervical ganglion; the auricular branch of the ganglion gives off an ascending twig which joins the facial nerve (p. 1013).

**The inferior ganglion** is cylindrical in form, of a reddish colour, and 2·5 cm long. It is connected with the hypoglossal nerve, the superior cervical ganglion of the sympathetic trunk, and the loop between the first and second cervical nerves. The cranial root of the accessory nerve passes over the ganglion, but is attached to it by fibrous tissue only.

Beyond the inferior ganglion the cranial root of the accessory nerve blends with the vagus nerve; its fibres are distributed principally to the pharyngeal and recurrent laryngeal branches of the vagus nerve.

The cells of both ganglia are unipolar sensory neurons.[1027, 1028] The only evidence to the contrary are some old and unconfirmed electrophysiological experiments and technically unsatisfactory histological observations, both of which have been subsequently refuted. (For details and discussion see footnote references [1029, 1030].) There is no reliable evidence that any significant number of the nerve cells in the ganglion are motor, nor have synapses between pre- and post-ganglionic neurons been demonstrated in it. Indeed, the preganglionic motor fibres, derived from the dorsal nucleus of the vagus, and the special visceral efferents derived from the nucleus ambiguus, which descend to the inferior vagal ganglion, commonly form a band visible to the unaided eye which skirts the ganglion in some mammals[1031, 1032] without passing through it. The disposition of the sensory or motor fibres which do traverse the ganglion is like that of a dorsal root ganglion. It is necessary to emphasize these facts, because there is current in some textbooks an unsupported view that the parasympathetic component of the vagus relays in its inferior ganglion, based with questionable logic upon the presence of large numbers of thinly myelinated and supposedly non-myelinated fibres in the distal parts of the nerve. Even if it were a safe presumption to regard autonomic fibres as postganglionic purely on the basis of their degree of myelination, to do so in this instance would be merely to ignore another tenet of peripheral autonomic morphology, for such a view produces two relays—one in the inferior ganglion, and one in the wall of the target organ. Retrograde degeneration has been demonstrated in the dorsal nucleus of the vagus by division of vagal branches as remote from their origins as the gastric nerves.[1033] Reliable counts and analyses of the nerve fibres in the human vagus are not available, but counts in other mammals do not support the view of the inferior ganglion as a relay station, which seems to be based almost entirely upon a misguided adherence to supposed axioms of autonomic morphology. The extensive factual information quoted above with regard to the structure of the inferior vagal ganglion renders such a view untenable, and it difficult to explain its persistence.

The superior ganglion contains the somata of neurons concerned with general somatic sensation, mediated by the auricular branch of the vagus. The sensory nerve cells in the inferior ganglion are partly concerned with special visceral sensibility (taste) from the epiglottis and vallecula, and partly with general visceral afferent information from the larynx, pharynx, heart, lungs, oesophagus, stomach, small intestine, and part of the colon.

The vagus nerve passes vertically down the neck within the carotid sheath, lying between the internal jugular vein and internal carotid artery as far as the upper border of the thyroid cartilage, and then between the same vein and the common carotid artery until it reaches the root of the neck. The further course of the nerve differs on the two sides of the body.

On the *right side* the vagus nerve continues descending posterior to the internal jugular vein and crosses the first part of the subclavian artery. It enters the thorax and descends through the superior mediastinum, lying at first behind the right brachiocephalic vein, and then to the right of the trachea and posteromedial to the right brachiocephalic vein and the superior vena cava. The right pleura and lung are lateral to the nerve above, but are separated from it below by the azygos vein, which arches forward above the root of the right lung (6.133).

The nerve next passes behind the right principal bronchus to reach the posterior aspect of the root of the

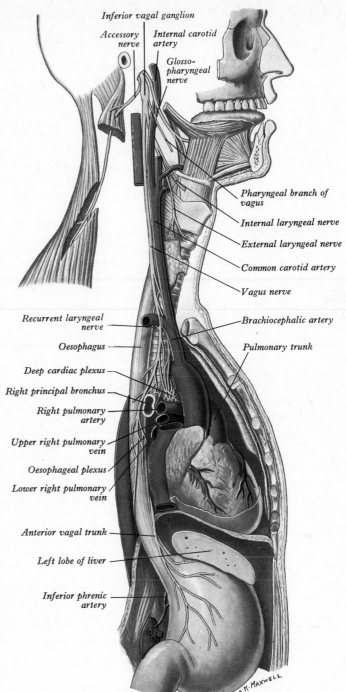

7.191 The course and distribution of the glossopharyngeal, vagus and accessory nerves.

right lung, and there breaks up into posterior bronchial branches, which unite with filaments from the second to fifth or sixth thoracic sympathetic ganglia to form the **right posterior pulmonary plexus**. From the caudal part of this plexus two or three branches descend on the dorsal aspect of the oesophagus, where, with a branch from the left vagus, they form the posterior **oesophageal plexus**; from this a trunk is re-formed which is continued

[1027] A. P. Richardson and J. C. Hinsey, *Proc. Soc. exp. Biol. Med.,* **30**, 1933.

[1028] D. H. L. Evans and J. G. Murray, *J. Anat.,* **88**, 1954.

[1029] G. A. G. Mitchell, *Cardiovascular Innervation,* Livingstone, Edinburgh. 1956.

[1030] A. R. Lieberman, Ph.D. Thesis, *University of London,* 1968.

[1031] H. H. Hoffman and A. Kuntz, *Anat. Rec.,* **127**, 1957.

[1032] N. Mei and M. Dussardier, *J. Physiol. Paris,* **58**, 1966.

[1033] G. A. G. Mitchell and R. Warwick, *Acta anat.,* **25**, 1955.

posterior to the oesophagus to enter the abdomen through the oesophageal opening in the diaphragm. This posterior vagal trunk contains fibres from both vagus nerves (*see* p. 1023).

In the abdomen the **posterior vagal trunk** divides into a small gastric and a large coeliac branch. The gastric branch supplies the postero-inferior surface of the stomach with the exception of the pyloric canal. The coeliac branch ends chiefly in the coeliac plexus, but sends twigs to the splenic, hepatic, renal, suprarenal and superior mesenteric plexuses. (See also p. 1076.)

On the *left side* the vagus enters the thorax between the left common carotid and left subclavian arteries, and behind the left brachiocephalic vein. It descends through the superior mediastinum, crosses the left side of the aortic arch and passes behind the root of the left lung. Just above the aortic arch the nerve is crossed superficially by the left phrenic nerve, and on the arch by the left superior intercostal vein (7.228).

Behind the root of the left lung it divides into posterior bronchial branches, which unite with filaments of the second, third and fourth thoracic sympathetic ganglia and form the **left posterior pulmonary plexus**. From this plexus two branches descend on the front of the oesophagus where, with a twig from the right posterior pulmonary plexus, they form the **anterior oesophageal plexus**; from this plexus a trunk, containing fibres from both vagus nerves, is continued in front of the oesophagus, and enters the abdomen through the oesophageal opening of the diaphragm (see p. 517).

In the abdomen the **anterior vagal trunk** supplies twigs to the cardiac antrum, and then divides into right and left groups of branches. The fibres of the left group follow the lesser curvature of the stomach and supply the anterosuperior surface of this viscus. The right group consists of three main branches. The first, which may be duplicated, proceeds between the layers of the lesser omentum towards the porta hepatis, and divides into (*a*) upper branches which enter the porta hepatis, and (*b*) lower rami which supply chiefly the pyloric canal, the pylorus, the superior and the descending parts of the duodenum, and the head of the pancreas. The second branch is distributed to the anterosuperior surface of the body of the stomach; the third branch follows the lesser curvature of the stomach as far as the angular notch. (See also p. 1275.)

### The Branches of the Vagus Nerve

| | |
|---|---|
| In the jugular fossa | Meningeal |
| | Auricular |
| In the neck | Pharyngeal |
| | Branches to carotid body |
| | Superior laryngeal |
| | Recurrent laryngeal (right) |
| | Cardiac |
| In the thorax | Cardiac |
| | Recurrent laryngeal (left) |
| | Pulmonary |
| | Oesophageal |
| In the abdomen | Gastric |
| | Coeliac |
| | Hepatic |

**The meningeal branch** or branches appear to spring from the superior ganglion of the vagus nerve and are distributed to the dura mater in the posterior fossa of the skull. However, evidence has been presented[941, 942] which suggests that such meningeal branches are in fact recurrent sensory and sympathetic nerves derived from the upper cervical spinal nerves and the superior cervical sympathetic ganglion, which for a short distance run

within the sheath of the upper part of the vagus nerve (pp. 988, 1032).

**The auricular branch** arises from the superior ganglion of the vagus nerve, and is joined soon after its origin by a filament from the inferior ganglion of the glossopharyngeal; it passes behind the internal jugular vein, and enters the mastoid canaliculus on the lateral wall of the jugular fossa. Traversing the substance of the temporal bone, it crosses the canal for the facial nerve about 4 mm above the stylomastoid foramen, and here it gives off an ascending branch which joins the facial nerve. (At this point fibres of the nervus intermedius may pass to the auricular branch of the vagus, providing a possible explanation of the cutaneous vesiculation which sometimes accompanies geniculate herpes.) The auricular branch then passes through the tympanomastoid fissure, and divides into two rami; one is the posterior auricular nerve, the other is distributed to the skin of part of the cranial surface of the auricle and to the posterior wall and floor of the external acoustic meatus and to the adjoining part of the outer surface of the tympanic membrane. The auricular branch of the vagus thus contains *somatic afferent* nerve fibres, but it is believed that when they enter the medulla oblongata they terminate in the spinal nucleus of the trigeminal nerve.

**The pharyngeal branch**, which is the principal motor nerve of the pharynx, emerges superficially from the upper part of the inferior ganglion of the vagus nerve, and consists principally of filaments from the cranial root of the accessory nerve. It passes between the external and internal carotid arteries to the upper border of the middle constrictor muscle of the pharynx, where it divides into numerous filaments which join with branches from the sympathetic trunk, the glossopharyngeal and external laryngeal nerves, to form the *pharyngeal plexus*. Through this plexus vagal fibres are distributed to the muscles of the pharynx, and the muscles of the soft palate, except the tensor veli palatini. A minute filament joins the hypoglossal nerve as the latter winds round the occipital artery, and is often termed the *ramus lingualis vagi*.

**The branches to the carotid body** are minute and variable in number. They may spring from the inferior ganglion or they may travel either in the pharyngeal branch or the superior laryngeal nerve, the latter being most unusual. They form a plexus with rami of the glossopharyngeal nerve and of the cervical part of the sympathetic trunk.[1034] (See also p. 1070.)

**The superior laryngeal nerve**, which is larger than the pharyngeal branch, issues from the middle of the inferior ganglion of the vagus nerve, and in its course receives a branch from the superior cervical ganglion of the sympathetic trunk. It descends, by the side of the pharynx, first posterior, then medial to the internal carotid artery, and divides into the internal and external laryngeal nerves. The human nerve contains about 15,000 fibres.[1035]

The *internal laryngeal nerve* is sensory to the mucous membrane of the larynx as far down as the level of the vocal folds. It also carries afferent fibres from neuro-muscular spindles and other stretch receptors in the larynx.[1036, 1037] It descends to the thyrohyoid membrane, pierces this membrane at a higher level than the superior laryngeal artery, and divides into an upper and a lower branch. The upper branch is directed horizontally, and supplies twigs to the mucous membrane of the pharynx, the epiglottis, the vallecula and the vestibule of the

[1034] D. Sheehan, J. H. Mulholland and B. Shafiroff, *Anat. Rec.*, **80**, 1941.
[1035] J. H. Ogura, J. A. Bello, *Laryngoscope*, St. Louis, **62**, 1952.
[1036] M. F. L. Keene. *J. Anat.*, **95**, 1961.
[1037] J. L. Scheuer, *J. Anat.*, **98**, 1964.

larynx. The lower branch descends in the medial wall of the piriform recess, and gives branches to the aryepiglottic fold, and to the mucous membrane on the back of the arytenoid cartilage. It also supplies one or two branches to the arytenoideus, and these branches unite with twigs from the recurrent laryngeal nerve to the same muscle (*see* p. 1182). The internal laryngeal nerve ends by piercing the inferior constrictor muscle of the pharynx, and unites with an ascending branch from the recurrent laryngeal nerve.

The *external laryngeal nerve*, which is the smaller of the two, descends posterior to the sternothyroid in company with the superior thyroid artery but on a deeper plane; it lies at first on the inferior constrictor of the pharynx, and then, piercing that muscle, winds closely round the inferior thyroid tubercle and reaches the cricothyroid, which it supplies. It gives branches also to the pharyngeal plexus and to the inferior constrictor; behind the common carotid artery it communicates with the superior cardiac nerve, and with the superior cervical sympathetic ganglion.[1038]

**The recurrent laryngeal nerve** differs, as to its origin and course, on the two sides of the body. On the *right* side it arises from the vagus nerve in front of the first part of the subclavian artery; it winds from before backwards, first below and then behind that vessel, and ascends obliquely to the side of the trachea behind the common carotid artery. Near the lower pole of the lobe of the thyroid gland the nerve is always intimately related to the inferior thyroid artery; it may cross either in front of or behind the vessel, or may pass between its branches. On the *left* side, it arises from the vagus nerve on the left of the arch of the aorta, and winds below the arch immediately behind the attachment of the ligamentum arteriosum to the concavity of the arch, and then ascends to the side of the trachea. The nerve on each side ascends in or near the groove between the trachea and oesophagus, and is intimately related to the medial surface of the thyroid gland before it passes under the lower border of the inferior constrictor and enters the larynx behind the articulation of the inferior cornu of the thyroid with the cricoid cartilage. It gives branches to all the muscles of the larynx, excepting the cricothyroid; it communicates with the internal laryngeal nerve, and supplies sensory filaments to the mucous membrane of the larynx below the level of the vocal folds. It also carries afferent fibres from stretch receptors in the larynx.

As the recurrent laryngeal nerve curves round the subclavian artery, or the arch of the aorta, it gives several cardiac filaments to the deep part of the cardiac plexus. As it ascends in the neck it gives branches, more numerous on the left than on the right side, to the mucous membrane and muscular coat of the oesophagus; branches to the mucous membrane and muscular fibres of the trachea and some filaments to the inferior constrictor.

The variations in the relations of the recurrent laryngeal nerves as they approach the larynx are especially important in the surgery of the thyroid gland.[1039, 1040] The nerve does not always lie in a protected position in the tracheo-oesophageal groove, but may lie a little in front of it (slightly more frequently on the right side of the neck) and it may occasionally be some distance lateral to the trachea at the level of the lower part of the lobe of the thyroid gland. On the right side there are almost equal chances of finding the nerve anterior to, or posterior to, or intermingled with the terminal branches of the inferior thyroid artery, while on the left side the nerve is most likely to be posterior to the artery and least likely to be anterior. The nerve may give off extralaryngeal branches which are distributed to the larynx, arising from the nerve before it passes behind the inferior cornu of the thyroid cartilage.

In addition to its true capsule, the thyroid gland is invested with a distinct outer covering formed by the pretracheal fascia (p. 504), which splits into two layers at the posterior border of the lobe of the thyroid gland. One layer clothes the entire medial surface of the lobe and, at and just above the level of the isthmus of the gland, it has a conspicuous thickening, called the lateral ligament of the thyroid gland (p. 1373), which attaches the gland to the trachea and the lower part of the cricoid cartilage. The other layer is more posterior; it passes behind the oesophagus and pharynx and is attached to the prevertebral fascia. By this splitting of the fascia, a fascial compartment is formed on each side of the neck, just lateral to the trachea and oesophagus, and it is in the fat that occupies this space that the recurrent laryngeal nerve and the terminal parts of the inferior thyroid artery lie. The nerve may lie lateral or medial to the lateral ligament of the thyroid gland; sometimes it may be embedded in the ligament.

**The cardiac branches**, two or three in number, arise from the vagus nerve at superior and inferior cervical levels. The small, *superior branches* join with the cardiac branches of the sympathetic trunk. They can be traced to the deep part of the cardiac plexus.

The *inferior branches* arise at the root of the neck. That from the right vagus passes in front or by the side of the brachiocephalic artery, and proceeds to the deep part of the cardiac plexus; that from the left runs down across the arch of the aorta, and joins the superficial part of the cardiac plexus.

Additional cardiac branches arise from the trunk of the right vagus nerve as it lies by the side of the trachea, and from both recurrent laryngeal nerves. They end in the deep part of the cardiac plexus. The cardiac plexus is described on p. 1076.

**The anterior pulmonary branches**, two or three in number and of small size, are distributed on the anterior surface of the root of the lung. They join with filaments from the sympathetic, and form the *anterior pulmonary plexus*.

**The posterior pulmonary branches**, more numerous and larger than the anterior, are distributed on the posterior surface of the root of the lung; they are joined by filaments from the second to fifth or sixth thoracic ganglia of the sympathetic trunk, and form the *posterior pulmonary plexus*. Branches from this plexus accompany the ramifications of the bronchi and supply their constrictor muscles and other pulmonary tissues. (See also pp. 1077, 1190, 1204.)

**The oesophageal branches** are given off both above and below the pulmonary branches; the lower are more numerous and larger than the upper. They form, as already described (p. 1022), the *oesophageal plexus*. From this plexus filaments are distributed to the oesophagus and to the back of the pericardium.

**The gastric branches** are distributed to the stomach, the anterosuperior surface of which is mainly supplied by the left vagus, and the postero-inferior surface mainly by the right. (See pp. 1078, 1275.)

**The coeliac branches** are derived from the posterior vagal trunks: they join the coeliac plexus.

**The hepatic branches** arise from both vagus nerves (p. 1077): they join the hepatic plexus and through it are conveyed to the liver.

**The renal branches** arise from both vagus nerves and join the renal plexus (p. 1078).

[1038] R. Skórnicki, A. Zieniánski and A. Orebowski, *Folia morph.*, **27**, 1968.
[1039] J. L. Doyle, H. O. Watkins and D. S. Halbert, *Tex. Med. J.*, **63**, 1967.
[1040] R. E. M. Bowden, *Br. J. Surg.*, **43**, 1955.

For details of the ultimate distribution of the branches of the vagus nerves in the abdomen, see the section on the Autonomic Nervous System, pp. 1067, 1077, 1079.

*Applied Anatomy.* The trunk of the vagus is not commonly injured, but the functions of the nerve may also be interfered with by damage to its radicular nuclei in the medulla, or during its intracranial course. The symptoms produced by non-functioning of the nerve are palpitation, with increased frequency of the pulse, constant vomiting, slowing of the respiration, and a sensation of suffocation.

'Reflexes' in connexion with the branches of the vagus are not infrequent. The 'ear cough' is perhaps one of the commonest, where a plug of wax in the external acoustic meatus may, by irritating the filaments of the auricular nerve, be responsible for a persistent cough. Syringing the meatus frequently produces cough, and, in children, vomiting is not uncommon. Moreover, syringing of the ear has occasionally been responsible for a sudden fatal reflex cardiac inhibition. Another common example is the persistent cough due to enlarged bronchial lymph nodes in children, which may irritate the recurrent laryngeal nerve.

The anatomy of the laryngeal nerves may also be correlated with some of the morbid conditions of the larynx. When the peripheral terminations of the superior laryngeal nerve are irritated by a foreign body passing over them reflex spasm of the glottis is the result. When the nerve is not functioning there is anaesthesia of the mucous membrane of the upper part of the larynx, so that foreign bodies can readily enter the cavity; since the nerve supplies the cricothyroid, the vocal folds cannot be made tense, and the voice is deep and hoarse. Irritation of the recurrent laryngeal nerves produces spasm of the muscles of the larynx. When both recurrent laryngeal nerves are interrupted, the vocal folds are motionless, in the so-called 'cadaveric position'—in the position in which they also are found in ordinary tranquil respiration—neither closed as in phonation, nor widely open as in deep inspiratory efforts. When one recurrent laryngeal nerve is affected, the vocal fold of the same side is motionless, while the opposite one crosses the median plane to accommodate itself to the affected one; hence phonation is possible, but the voice is altered and weak in timbre. It is generally maintained that in progressive lesions of the recurrent laryngeal nerve the movements of abduction of the vocal cord are abolished before the movements of adduction; conversely, during recovery the movements of adduction are regained before those of abduction (*Semon's law*). There is no direct evidence, however, that the nerve fibres to the abductor muscles have any special grouping in the trunk of the recurrent laryngeal nerve.

## The Accessory Nerve

The accessory nerve (7.62, 64, 189–191) is formed by the union of cranial and spinal roots, but these constituent parts are associated with each other only for a very short part of their course before the cranial part joins the vagus to be distributed through its branches. The cranial moiety should be considered as a part of the vagus nerve; it is a branchial or special visceral efferent nerve in constitution. The spinal 'root' may be either somatic, or special visceral efferent, depending upon the view taken of the evolutionary origin of the sternocleidomastoid and trapezius, which it supplies. This controversy is not likely to be solved, and hence the custom of describing the two parts as a single cranial nerve has been followed here.

**The cranial root** is the smaller; its fibres arise from the cells of the lower end of the **nucleus ambiguus** (p. 848) and possibly from the **dorsal vagal nucleus**. The former

is connected with the corticonuclear tracts of *both* sides. Some of the fibres from this source descend from the midbrain in the medial lemniscus (aberrant pyramidal fibres, p. 845). The fibres of the cranial root emerge as four or five delicate rootlets from the side of the medulla oblongata, below the roots of the vagus. The nerve runs laterally to the jugular foramen, where it is said to interchange fibres with the spinal root, with which it becomes united for a short distance; here it is also connected by one or two filaments with the superior ganglion of the vagus. It passes through the jugular foramen, separates from the spinal portion, and is continued over the inferior ganglion of the vagus, to the surface of which it is adherent. It is distributed principally in the pharyngeal and recurrent laryngeal branches of the vagus. It is probably the source of the motor fibres which run in the former to supply the muscles of the soft palate, with the exception of the tensor veli palatini. Some filaments from it are continued into the trunk of the vagus below the ganglion, to be distributed with the recurrent laryngeal nerve and possibly also with the cardiac nerves.

**The spinal root** is firm in texture, and its fibres arise from an elongated column of motor neurons, *the spinal nucleus*, which is situated in the lateral part of the anterior grey column of the spinal cord, and extends downwards as low as the level of the fifth cervical segment (p. 813). Passing through the lateral white column of the spinal cord, they emerge on its surface midway between the ventral and dorsal nerve roots of the upper cervical nerves (7.189), and unite to form a trunk, which ascends between the ligamentum denticulatum and the dorsal roots of the spinal nerves, and enters the skull through the foramen magnum, behind the vertebral artery (7.190). It is then directed upwards and laterally to the jugular foramen, through which it passes in the same sheath of dura mater as the vagus nerve, but separated from that nerve by a fold of the arachnoid mater. In the jugular foramen, it may receive one or two filaments from the cranial root, or else joins it for a short distance and then parts from it again. At its exit from the jugular foramen, it runs laterally and backwards posterior to the internal jugular vein in about two-thirds of subjects, and anterior to it in about one-third; in rare cases it may pass through the vein. In this situation the accessory nerve crosses the transverse process of the atlas and is itself crossed by the occipital artery. The nerve then descends obliquely, passing medial to the styloid process, the stylohyoid and the posterior belly of the digastric. Together with the superior sternocleidomastoid branch of the occipital artery, it reaches the upper part of the sternocleidomastoid and pierces its deep surface, supplying it and joining with branches from the second cervical nerve. Emerging a little above the middle of the posterior border of the sternocleidomastoid, the nerve crosses the posterior triangle of the neck lying on the levator scapulae (7.186), from which it is separated by the prevertebral layer of the deep cervical fascia and the adipose tissue occupying the triangle. Here it is comparatively superficial, being related to the superficial cervical lymph nodes and receiving communications from the second and third cervical nerves.[1041] Finally, about 5 cm above the clavicle, the accessory nerve disappears under the anterior border of the trapezius and, together with branches from the third and fourth cervical nerves, forms a plexus on the deep surface of the muscle. From this plexus the trapezius receives its innervation. The course of the accessory nerve in the neck can be represented by a line drawn downwards from the lower and anterior part of the tragus to the tip of the transverse process of the atlas, and then downwards and backwards,

[1041] F. Raveau, *Archs Anat. Path.*, **16**, 1968.

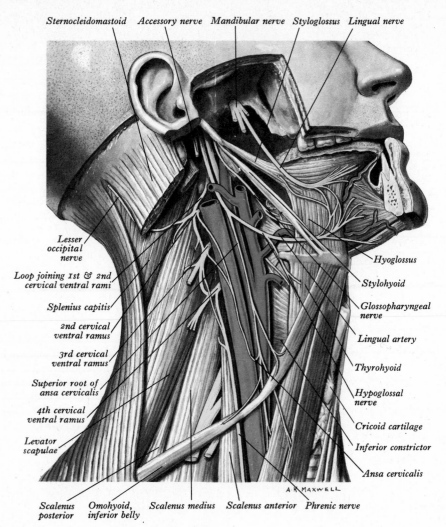

Sternocleidomastoid    Accessory nerve    Mandibular nerve    Styloglossus    Lingual nerve

Lesser occipital nerve

Loop joining 1st & 2nd cervical ventral rami

Splenius capitis

2nd cervical ventral ramus

3rd cervical ventral ramus

Superior root of ansa cervicalis

4th cervical ventral ramus

Levator scapulae

Hyoglossus

Stylohyoid

Glossopharyngeal nerve

Lingual artery

Thyrohyoid

Hypoglossal nerve

Cricoid cartilage

Inferior constrictor

Ansa cervicalis

A K MAXWELL

Scalenus posterior    Omohyoid, inferior belly    Scalenus medius    Scalenus anterior    Phrenic nerve

**7.192** A dissection to show the general distribution of the right hypoglossal and lingual nerves, and the position, constitution and some of the cervical plexus of the right side.

across the elevation produced by the sternocleidomastoid and the depression corresponding to the posterior triangle of the neck, to a point on the anterior border of the trapezius 5 cm above the clavicle. For a discussion of the possible significance of the double nerve supply to trapezius and sternocleidomastoid see footnote reference[1042].

The cranial and spinal roots, after separating from each other, are also known respectively as the *internal* and *external rami* of the accessory nerves. There is general agreement that the spinal root is the sole motor supply to the sternocleidomastoid, the second and third cervical nerves conveying proprioceptive fibres from the muscle. Whether the spinal root is the sole motor supply to the trapezius is uncertain, some maintaining that the third and fourth cervical nerves are purely proprioceptive, while others believe that they supply motor fibres to the lower part of the muscle.

*Applied Anatomy.* The functions of the accessory nerve may be interfered with by central changes; or at its exit from the skull, by fractures running across the jugular foramen; or in the neck, by inflamed lymph nodes, etc. Acute torticollis in children is most commonly due to inflamed lymph nodes. Central irritation causes clonic spasm of the sternocleidomastoid and trapezius, or, as it is termed, spasmodic torticollis. In cases of this affection in which all previous palliative treatment has failed, division or excision of a section of the accessory nerve has been resorted to.

In cases where extensive dissections are undertaken in the posterior triangle of the neck for the excision of pathological nodes, it is essential that this nerve should be sought at the outset and isolated from the mass of diseased nodes so as to preserve its continuity.

## The Hypoglossal Nerve

The hypoglossal nerve (**7.**62, 64, 192, 193) is the motor nerve of the tongue. It is in series with the oculomotor, trochlear and abducent nerves and the ventral nerve roots of the spinal nerves, and represents the fused ventral roots of, probably, four precervical or spino-occipital nerves, the dorsal roots of which have disappeared entirely.

**The hypoglossal nucleus** from which its fibres arise is in line with the modified anterior grey column of the spinal cord. This nucleus is about 2 cm long, and its cranial part corresponds with the hypoglossal triangle of the floor of the fourth ventricle (p. 878). The lower part of the nucleus extends downwards into the closed part of the medulla oblongata, and there lies in the ventral part of the central grey matter, close to the median plane (**7.**61). The fibres from its cells pass ventrally through the medulla oblongata, and emerge as a linear series of 10–15 rootlets through the anterolateral sulcus between the pyramid and the olive (**7.**55).

[1042] J. McKenzie, *J. Anat.*, **89**, 1955.

The hypoglossal nucleus displays a longitudinal division into dorsal and ventral laminae, each of which may be further divided into a mediolateral sequence of relatively discrete sub-nuclei. The latter are considered to correspond to the individual muscles innervated.[1043-1045]

*Connexions.* The nucleus of the hypoglossal nerve receives fibres from the precentral gyrus and adjacent areas of mainly the *opposite* cerebral hemisphere through the corticonuclear tract; some of the latter leave the tract in the pons and travel in the medial lemniscus. They are connected to the nucleus directly or through internuncial neurons. Some evidence has been presented, however, that the most medially situated sub-nuclei receive projection fibres from *both* cerebral hemispheres. The hypoglossal nucleus may connect with the cerebellum via neighbouring perihypoglossal nuclei (p. 845)[1046] and may also be connected with the medullary reticular formation, the sensory nuclei of the trigeminal, and the nucleus solitarius.

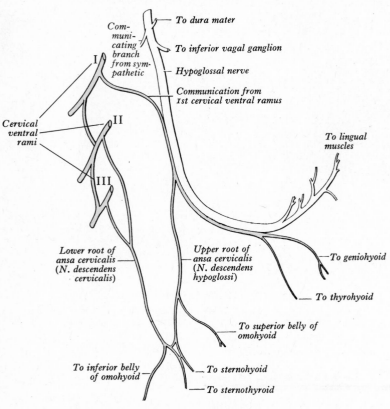

7.193  A plan of the right hypoglossal nerve.

The rootlets of the hypoglossal nerve run laterally behind the vertebral artery, and are collected into two bundles, which perforate the dura mater separately opposite the hypoglossal (anterior condylar) canal in the occipital bone, and unite together after their passage through it; in some cases the canal is divided into two by a small bony spicule. The fact that each fascicle acquires a separate sheath from the dura mater is confirmatory evidence of the composite character of the nerve. On emerging from its canal the nerve lies on a deeper plane than the internal jugular vein, the internal carotid artery, the ninth, tenth and eleventh cranial nerves. It passes laterally, with a downward inclination, behind the internal carotid artery and the glossopharyngeal and vagus nerves to gain the interval between the artery and the internal jugular vein. In this part of its course it makes a half-spiral turn round the inferior ganglion of the vagus, to

which it is united by connective tissue. It then descends almost vertically, lying between the vessels and in front of the vagus nerve, to a point corresponding with the angle of the mandible, and becomes superficial below the posterior belly of the digastric, emerging from between the internal jugular vein and the internal carotid artery. The nerve loops round the inferior sternocleidomastoid branch of the occipital artery (p. 628) and, having crossed the internal and external carotid arteries, it crosses the loop of the lingual artery a little above the tip of the greater cornu of the hyoid bone (7.192), being itself crossed by the facial vein. It inclines upwards as it runs forwards on the hyoglossus, passing deep to the tendon of the digastric, the stylohyoid and the posterior border of the mylohyoid. In the interval between the hyoglossus and mylohyoid the nerve is related above to the deep part of the submandibular gland, the submandibular duct and the lingual nerve. It passes next on to the lateral aspect of the genioglossus and is continued forwards in its substance as far as the tip of the tongue, distributing branches to the muscle.

The hypoglossal nerve communicates with the sympathetic trunk, and with the vagus, first and second cervical, and lingual nerves.

Opposite the atlas the nerve receives branches from the superior cervical ganglion of the sympathetic trunk, and at the same level is joined by a filament from the loop connecting the first and second cervical nerves. This filament soon leaves the hypoglossal and descends as the *upper root* of the *ansa cervicalis* (7.193).

The communications with the vagus nerve take place close to the skull, numerous filaments passing between the hypoglossal nerve and the inferior ganglion of the vagus nerve through the mass of connective tissue which unites them. As the nerve winds round the occipital artery it receives a filament from the pharyngeal plexus, which is termed the *ramus lingualis vagi* (p. 1022).

Near the anterior border of the hyoglossus it is connected with the lingual nerve by numerous filaments which ascend upon the muscle.

The *branches of distribution* of the hypoglossal nerve are:

| | |
|---|---|
| Meningeal | Thyrohyoid |
| Descending | Muscular |

**The meningeal branch** or branches leave the hypoglossal nerve as it passes through the hypoglossal canal; they pursue a recurrent course and then ramify to be distributed to the diploë of the occipital bone, to the dural walls of the occipital sinus, and neighbouring structures including the dura of the inferior petrosal sinus and much of the floor and anterior wall of the posterior cranial fossa. As discussed elsewhere (pp. 988, 1032) these meningeal rami may not be branches of the hypoglossal nerve itself, but ascending, mixed sensory and sympathetic nerves derived from the upper cervical nerves and superior cervical sympathetic ganglion.[941, 942]

**The descending branch** leaves the hypoglossal nerve where the latter turns round the occipital artery, and descends anterior to or in the sheath of the internal and common carotid arteries. It contains no fibres from the hypoglossal nucleus, but only fibres from C1, which constitute the upper root of the ansa cervicalis. After giving a branch to the superior belly of the omohyoid, this nerve is joined by the lower root of the ansa cervicalis from the second and third cervical nerves. The union of the two forms a loop, which is termed the *ansa cervicalis* (ansa hypoglossi). From the convexity of this loop branches pass

[1043] K. Kosaka and K. Yagita, *Jb. Psychiat. Neurol.*, **24**, 1903.
[1044] F. J. Stuurman, *Anat. Anz.*, **48**, 1916.
[1045] J. W. Barnard, *J. comp. Neurol.*, **72**, 1940.
[1046] A. Torvik and A. Brodal, *J. Neuropath. exp. Neurol.*, **13**, 1954.

to supply the sternohyoid, the sternothyroid and the inferior belly of the omohyoid. Another filament has been described which descends in front of the vessels into the thorax, and joins the cardiac and phrenic nerves.

**The nerve to the thyrohyoid** arises from the hypoglossal nerve near the posterior border of the hypoglossus; it runs obliquely across the greater cornu of the hyoid bone, and supplies the thyrohyoid. It is derived from the communication with the first cervical spinal nerve.

**The muscular branches** are distributed to the styloglossus, hyoglossus, geniohyoid and genioglossus. Numerous slender branches pass upwards into the substance of the tongue to supply its intrinsic muscles. Most of these muscular branches are true hypoglossal fibres, but those to geniohyoid stem from the first cervical nerve.

*Applied Anatomy.* When the hypoglossal nerve is injured or diseased, unilateral lingual paralysis follows, together with hemiatrophy of the tongue; the tongue, when protruded, is directed to the paralysed side owing to the unopposed action of the opposite muscles. On retraction, the wasted and paralysed side of the tongue rises up higher than the other. The larynx may deviate towards the sound side on swallowing, due to unilateral paralysis of the depressors of the hyoid bone. If the paralysis is bilateral, the tongue lies motionless in the mouth; taste and tactile sensibility of the organ are perfect, articulation is slow; swallowing is very difficult, and the patient has to throw his head backwards and push the bolus of food back into the pharynx with his finger before he can swallow it.

# MORPHOLOGY OF THE CRANIAL NERVES

It is now possible to group the cranial nerves in a manner which conforms with their phylogenetic history, their individual components and their functions.

*Group I* includes the oculomotor, trochlear, abducent and hypoglossal nerves. These all arise from the cells of the somatic efferent column, and they are distributed to the musculature derived from the *cranial myotomes*. They correspond, therefore, to the *ventral* nerve roots of the spinal nerves, and with the exception of the trochlear, they emerge from the brainstem in line with them. The identification of the individual segments with which each nerve is associated is a matter of considerable difficulty and is not susceptible of proof in the present state of our knowledge, for the precise number of segments represented by the head is still uncertain (p. 87).

*Group II* includes the trigeminal, facial, glossopharyngeal, vagus and accessory nerves. These nerves are concerned with the innervation of the derivatives of the *branchial arches*. They differ from the spinal nerves in possessing motor roots which are distributed to the musculature derived from the *neural crest* (p. 143) and the *lateral plate mesoderm* of the branchial region. Some of these cranial nerves (the trigeminal, vagus and accessory), are compound nerves and have been formed by the fusion of two or more dorsal nerves (p. 994). In the process cutaneous branches, originally connected with the facial, glossopharyngeal and vagus nerves, have been taken over by the trigeminal, so that these nerves in man bear but little resemblance to their homologues in the lower forms of vertebrates and still less to the dorsal nerve roots of the spinal nerves.

On account of the complexity of their components, each nerve may possess more than one nucleus of origin and more than one nucleus of termination. It is noteworthy that the cells of the ganglion of the facial, the inferior ganglion of the glossopharyngeal and the inferior ganglion of the vagus nerve, though derived to a large extent from the neural crest, owe their origin in part to *ectodermal epibranchial placodes* which develop at the dorsal ends of the first three branchial clefts in close relation to the ganglia (p. 143).

Although there are certain difficulties in the way, the homologies of the nerves in Groups I and II are generally accepted, but the allocation of the three remaining cranial nerves is entirely uncertain. On account of its mode of development, the optic nerve is usually regarded as having nothing in common with any of the other cranial nerves except its function as a *special somatic afferent*. The retinal cells, from which its fibres are derived, really constitute an outlying part of the brain, although it may be urged that they are derivatives of the forerunners of the neural crest cells.

The olfactory and the vestibulocochlear nerves may be grouped together or separately, or the vestibulocochlear nerve may be regarded as being homologous with a dorsal nerve. Both nerves arise, in part at least, from ectodermal cells outside the area of the neural tube and crest, but whereas the olfactory cells remain intercalated amongst the epithelial cells of the nasal mucous membrane, the cochlear cells migrate a short distance away from the otic vesicle. It must be explained, however, that many authorities believe that the contribution made by the neural crest is responsible for the formation of the whole of the vestibulocochlear nerve ganglion, and on this account they prefer to regard the vestibulocochlear as a modified dorsal nerve. In comparing the olfactory and vestibulocochlear nerves it must be remembered that the olfactory nerves are restricted in all forms to the region of the head, whereas the vestibulocochlear nerve in man is the sole survivor of a whole series of nerves of the organs of the lateral line, which in lower forms are distributed not only to the head but also to the whole length of the trunk. There is, therefore, considerable justification for the allocation of the olfactory and vestibulocochlear nerves to separate groups.

For a discussion of the phylogeny of the vertebrate cranial nerves consult footnote references[1047-1054].

## General Considerations of the Cranial Nerves

Because of the extremely complex three-dimensional organization of the brainstem, which changes continuously with the level concerned, and the fact that innumerable cell groups and fibre systems exist in relatively small

[1047] D. Black, *J. comp. Neurol.*, **27**, 1917.

[1048] C. J. Herrick, *Introduction to Neurology*, Saunders, Philadelphia. 1922.

[1049] E. S. Goodrich, *Studies on the Structure and Development of Vertebrates*, Macmillan, London. 1958 (Republication of 1930 edition).

[1050] L. Bolk, F. Goppert, E. Kallius and W. Lubosch, *Handbuch der vergleichenden Anatomie der Wirbeltiere*, Vol. 2, Urban und Schwarzenberg, Berlin. 1934.

[1051] C. U. A. Kappers, C. Huber and E. C. Crosby, *Comparative Anatomy of the Nervous System*, Macmillan, New York. 1936.

[1052] C. U. A. Kappers, *Anatomie comparée du système nerveux*, Masson, Paris. 1947.

[1053] P.-P. Grassé (ed.), *Traité de Zoologie*, Vol. XII, Masson, Paris. 1954.

[1054] J. Z. Young, *The Life of Vertebrates*, Clarendon Press, Oxford. 1950.

volumes of nervous tissue, the difficulties of investigation are multiplied, and less detail is known of the intimate arrangement and connexions of many cranial nerve nuclei than is the case with the spinal nerves. Accordingly, the account given of the regional localization and connectivity patterns of many of these cranial nuclei, in general neuroanatomical texts, often conveys a simplicity which is undoubtedly far from reality. It may prove helpful, therefore, at this point to summarize briefly some of the general organizational features which are either emerging, or are suspected by analogy with spinal cord organization, but some of which have not yet been established with certainty in the primate brain. The olfactory, optic and vestibulocochlear nerves, however, are considered in some detail elsewhere in the present volume and will not be pursued further here.

**The motor nuclei of the cranial nerves**, as indicated above, include somatic efferent, special visceral efferent (branchiomotor) and general visceral efferent (autonomic) groups. However, the somatic and special visceral efferent nuclei of the oculomotor, trochlear, trigeminal, abducent, facial, glossopharyngeal, vagus, accessory and hypoglossal nerves may, for present purposes, be grouped, since all innervate *striated muscle*. It will be recalled that the ventral grey matter of the spinal cord consists of a series of longitudinal columns of neurons, as judged by the position of their cell somata; and although their significance is not completely understood (p. 814), they exhibit some degree of somatotopic organization. The cells of the columns include three varieties of motor neuron ($\alpha$, $\beta$ and $\gamma$—p. 829) related to the innervation of extrafusal and intrafusal muscle fibres, and further, the $\alpha$ motor neurons to extrafusal muscle may be divided into 'tonic' and 'phasic' types, whilst 'static' and 'dynamic' types of fusimotor $\gamma$ neurons are also recognized. Between and around these motor neurons are numerous small interneurons, some excitatory, others inhibitory, the latter including the well-known Renshaw cells. Converging on these cell varieties are numerous pathways, completing a wide array of local control loops, both contralateral and ipsilateral, and others descending from supraspinal sources such as the vestibular nuclei, brainstem reticular formation, red nucleus, tectum and tegmentum of the midbrain, and the cerebral cortex. In turn, these parts of the nervous system, which project directly to the lower motor centres, are themselves in receipt of essential control systems from the cerebellum, the corpus striatum, the thalamus and hypothalamus, and many parts of the cerebral neocortex and the limbic system. These have all been considered in detail elsewhere in the present section and no attempt will be made to describe them here. Despite our lack of detailed knowledge of cranial nerve connexions, it seems most probable that comparable control systems operate, and in view of the precision of integrated muscle action involved in phonation, facial expression and ocular movements, the control systems may well be of a *higher* order of complexity than those obtaining at spinal levels.

The trochlear and abducent nerves each innervate a single small muscle, and reflecting this, their motor nuclei are relatively small single groups of neurons. In contrast the oculomotor, trigeminal, facial, glossopharyngeal-vagus-cranial accessory group, and the hypoglossal all innervate complex musculature capable of a highly refined and precise three-dimensional control of their movement patterns. In each case their nuclei can be divided into a series of sub-nuclei which may be related to the major branches of the nerve, or to the innervation of single muscles within the group. In some cases the sub-nuclei show a longitudinal columnar arrangement, the columns varying in their mediolateral and dorsoventral

positioning and in their craniocaudal extent. This somatotopic localization, in terms of the position of cell *somata*, is reminiscent of that existing in the ventral grey column of the spinal cord, and whilst it seems plausible that the delicacy of control may be in some way increased by such grouping, as discussed more fully elsewhere (p. 814), the precise ontogenetic, phylogenetic and functional significance of these groups must await the results of future researches. Also, much less is known in cranial nerve motor nuclei, than in the spinal cord, concerning the quantitative degree of longitudinal and transverse overlap and interlocking of the receptive *dendritic trees* of motor neurons in adjacent nuclei and sub-nuclei. Further, although muscle spindles were for long considered to be absent, or extremely sparse, in facial, masticatory, lingual, laryngeal and extrinsic ocular muscles, their presence has now been amply confirmed in most of these sites (the facial muscles apparently having the least dense population). Nevertheless, the anatomical siting and physiological characteristics of their associated $\gamma$ efferent neurons has not yet been clarified. Similar uncertainty exists concerning the smaller multipolar neurons often found within or in the neighbourhood of cranial nerve motor nuclei, many of which are presumably excitatory or inhibitory interneurons, including Renshaw cells.

The afferent connexions of the motor nuclei of the cranial nerves include components which correspond to all those which converge upon the spinal grey matter, but some are recognized only in outline. The best recognized tract systems associated with these nuclei are: (1) the *medial longitudinal fasciculus*, interlinking the vestibular nuclear complex, a longitudinal series of cranial nerve nuclei and the cervical spinal cord (*see* p. 885); (2) *tectotegmental, tectopontine* and *tectobulbar* projections from the superior and inferior colliculi (p. 886); (3) projections from the *red nucleus* (p. 884); (4) interconnexions with the *brainstem reticular formation* (p. 890); (5) *corticonuclear* projections from the various sensorimotor areas of the cerebral cortex (p. 956); (6) projections from the *sensory nuclei* of other cranial nerves.

It must be emphasized, however, that little is known concerning the detailed mode of termination of these afferent systems, for example, whether they terminate directly on $\alpha$ and/or $\gamma$ motor neurons, or through the intermediary of interneurons, and to what extent they mediate pre- or post-synaptic facilitatory or inhibitory effects. The corticospinal tracts, it will be recalled p. 820), contain fibres predominantly derived from the contralateral cerebral hemisphere, but they also carry a variable proportion of ipsilateral fibres. Similar considerations apply in varying degree to the cranial nerve motor nuclei. Thus, it is widely held that although the corticonuclear fibres to most parts of the hypoglossal nucleus, and that part of the facial nucleus innervating the lower face, are mainly contralateral in origin, whilst those to the trochlear nucleus are predominantly ipsilateral, the remainder, including the most medial parts of the hypoglossal nuclei, receive a *bilateral* corticonuclear projection. The cerebellum, diencephalic centres, and corpus striatum are considered to influence the cranial nerve nuclei through indirect pathways similar to those proposed for the control of spinal motor centres (see the sections devoted to these regions).

**The general visceral efferent nuclei** of the oculomotor, facial, glossopharyngeal and vagus nerves are incompletely understood in terms of their central connexions. (The specific connexions of the accessory oculomotor nucleus related to visual reflexes are discussed elsewhere.) It is presumed that the dorsal nucleus of the vagus and the salivatory nuclei receive the terminals of ascending tracts, and those from other cranial nerve nuclei (particularly the nucleus of the solitary tract), conveying both somatic and visceral information. It is also considered that they establish interconnexions with the brainstem reticular formation, and receive descending pathways, probably polysynaptic, from the hypothalamus, through which, indirectly, the frontal neocortex, the limbic structures, and the thalamus exert their effects. These descending pathways have not been satisfactorily analysed with the neuroanatomical methods currently available. The same uncertainty attaches to the central connexions of the **general visceral afferent pathways** (p. 1081), which physiological studies have shown to influence many brainstem centres, including particularly the brainstem reticular formation, the hypothalamus, the limbic lobe, and the prefrontal neocortex (consult the sections devoted to the connexions of these regions). The proportion of primary general visceral afferent fibres which terminate in either the dorsal nucleus of the vagus, or in the nucleus of the solitary tract, is undetermined, but the latter are accompanied by the **special visceral afferent** (gustatory) fibres of the facial, glossopharyngeal and vagus nerves. These end in a craniocaudal sequence of overlapping zones in the solitary nucleus, where, after synaptic relays, secondary gustatory fibres cross the midline and ascend to terminate in the nucleus ventralis posterior medialis of the thalamus, and also in a number of hypothalamic nuclei. The detailed routes taken by these *solitariothalamic* and *solitariohypothalamic* fibres have not been established in the human brain, but it is thought likely that the former accompany the medial fibres of the *medial lemniscus*, whilst the latter may join the *dorsal longitudinal fasciculus* (p. 886), and the *mamillary peduncle* (p. 907). Collateral branches probably leave these ascending fibres to end in association with the brainstem reticular formation and the nuclei of other cranial nerves. From the caudal regions of the nucleus solitarius fibres descend to the spinal cord as a *solitariospinal tract*. The nucleus solitarius, however, is not to be regarded as a simple relay on the visceral afferent pathways. Other systems converge on the nucleus including ascending fibres from the spinal cord, fibres from the vestibulocerebellum, and descending corticonuclear fibres. Accordingly, interaction between these various information channels probably occurs in the nucleus, and its transmission characteristics are likely to be modulated by activity in the descending fibres from the cerebral cortex.

**The somatic afferent nuclei** of the brainstem constitute the spinal, principal sensory, and mesencephalic nuclei of the trigeminal nerve.

The unique character of the *mesencephalic nucleus* of the trigeminal, which consists of unipolar *primary* sensory neurons, and its probable role as a proprioceptive nucleus have already been described (p. 1002). Electrophysiological investigations support the latter view since rapid responses have been recorded from the nucleus following stretching of the masticatory and extraocular muscles, during passive jaw movement, and following application of pressure to the teeth. Thus, the peripheral processes of the mesencephalic unipolar cells are considered to innervate the muscle spindles of the extraocular and masticatory muscles, the articular tissues of the temporomandibular joint and the periodontal tissues. Possibly they are also the source of the fibres which innervate the muscle spindles of the facial, lingual and laryngeal muscles, but this remains uncertain. Since the cell somata of these primary afferent neurons are deeply embedded in the midbrain, and are arranged as a long, thin, curved lamina of cells on each side, they present particular difficulties to the neuroanatomical investigator, because even the smallest experimental lesions inevitably involve surrounding tissues. Hence, relatively little is known of the central projections of these cells. It has been claimed, however, that some of their central processes descend towards the principal sensory nucleus. Others are thought to project to the motor nucleus of the trigeminal, completing a masticatory reflex loop, whilst collateral branches have been described as entering the cerebellum in a trigeminocerebellar tract (p. 861). Their other connexions remain conjectural.

The manner in which the primary sensory fibres of the three divisions of the trigeminal nerve, which have their cell somata in the trigeminal ganglion, terminate in the *principal sensory* and *spinal nuclei* of the trigeminal nerve have already been described, and only a few further points need be mentioned here. The view, stemming largely from disease of the brainstem or from neurosurgical manœuvres, that the principal sensory nucleus is a simple relay station for tactile information, and the spinal nucleus for thermal and nociceptive information, is certainly an oversimplification. The observation that a large proportion of the sensory radicular fibres *bifurcate* on entering the pons, one branch entering the principal nucleus, and the other the spinal nucleus, has previously been referred to. The *spinal nucleus*, which is continuous caudally with the substantia gelatinosa of the cervical spinal cord, shows a regional variation in its cytoarchitecture (and is sometimes divided for convenience into a craniocaudal sequence of three subnuclei termed *oralis*, *interpolaris* and *caudalis*). Further, the spinal and principal nuclei not only receive the terminals of somatic afferent *trigeminal* fibres, but those of the *facial*, *glossopharyngeal* and *vagus* nerves, in addition to others which ascend from the cervical spinal cord. Both nuclei establish interconnexions with the brainstem reticular formation, and both receive numerous descending corticonuclear fibres from the sensorimotor cortex.

Thus, many information paths converge on both these nuclei, and unit recording with intracellular microelectrodes has confirmed the wide range of different types of cell response in the two nuclei. These vary from rapidly-adapting cells with modality-specific, small receptive fields, to others with multimodal responses and larger receptive fields. Cells responding to light tactile stimuli, and others to nociceptive stimuli were found in *both* nuclei. Some of the units show the phenomenon of inhibitory 'surround' (p. 751), and detailed analyses have shown that both pre- and post-synaptic inhibition and facilitation occur in the nuclei. Their impulse transmission characteristics are modified by stimulation or ablation of the descending corticonuclear tracts, and areas of the brainstem reticular formation. Evidently, the clinical impression of the two nuclei as relatively simple, functionally segregated relay stations, is not supported by experimental evidence, which suggests that they are complex, cooperative, integration centres. In this regard, an interesting analogy has been drawn between the principal sensory nucleus of the trigeminal and the nuclei gracilis and cuneatus, and between the spinal nucleus of the trigeminal and the substantia gelatinosa of the spinal cord, in terms of their structural and functional organization. (See pp. 813, 830, 832–3 for further details of these regions, and a proposed theory of action of the substantia gelatinosa as a 'gate' mechanism controlling sensory input.) Future researches will determine how far such a comparison is justified.

Finally, the statement on p. 1002 that the ascending efferent connexions from the principal and spinal nuclei of the trigeminal consist of crossed fibres which pass to the thalamus as a trigeminal lemniscus may be amplified. Both animal experimentation and observations on human material have shown that multiple trigeminothalamic pathways exist. From the principal sensory nucleus a substantial bundle of fibres cross the midline, whilst a smaller component remains on the ipsilateral side, and they ascend through the upper pons, midbrain and subthalamus, as the *dorsal trigeminothalamic tract* (dorsal division of the trigeminal lemniscus). In the midbrain this tract lies dorsomedial to the red nucleus and medial lemniscus, and it terminates in the nucleus ventralis posterior medialis (VPM) of the thalamus (p. 896). Other fibres from the principal sensory nucleus and from the length of the spinal nucleus mainly cross the midline

and ascend in close company with the fibres of the medial lemniscus; these constitute the *ventral trigeminothalamic tract* (ventral division of the trigeminal lemniscus). Many of these ventral ascending fibres also end in the VPM, but others, mainly from the caudal parts of the spinal nucleus, are described as ending in the medial geniculate body and in the intralaminar nuclei. Collateral branches are considered to leave these ascending pathways to terminate in the brainstem reticular formation, on other cranial nerve nuclei, and some collaterals probably enter into the cerebellum (p. 861).

# THE SPINAL NERVES

The spinal nerves are formed by the union of ventral and dorsal spinal nerve roots which are attached in series to the sides of the spinal cord. There are 31 pairs of these nerves grouped as follows: cervical, 8; thoracic, 12; lumbar, 5; sacral, 5; coccygeal, 1. The abbreviations C, T, L, S and Co., followed by the appropriate numeral are commonly used to identify the individual nerves. They emerge through the intervertebral foramina. The first cervical nerve escapes from the vertebral canal between the occipital bone and the atlas, and is therefore called the *suboccipital nerve*; the eighth issues between the seventh cervical and first thoracic vertebrae.

Each nerve is connected with the spinal cord by ventral and dorsal roots, the latter being characterized by the presence of a *spinal ganglion*.

**The ventral (anterior) roots** contain the axons of cells in the anterior and lateral grey columns of the spinal cord. Each root emerges as a series of rootlets arranged in two or three irregular rows over a distance of about 3 mm across the anterolateral aspect of the spinal cord.

**The dorsal (posterior) roots** contain the processes of cells in the spinal ganglia which are swellings on the roots. Each root consists of two fascicles, medial and lateral, each of which divides into rootlets entering along the posterolateral sulcus. Dissections in a number of different mammals, including man, have shown that the dorsal nerve roots of adjacent segments are often interconnected by fine, oblique bundles of nerve fibres, particularly in the lower cervical and lumbosacral regions of the cord.[1055]

**The spinal ganglia** are collections of nerve cells on the dorsal roots of the spinal nerves. Each ganglion is oval, reddish, and in its size related to that of the nerve root on which it is situated; it is bifid medially where the two bundles of the dorsal nerve root emerge from it to approach and enter the cord. The ganglia are usually in the intervertebral foramina, immediately lateral to the sites where the nerve roots perforate the dura mater (7.37); the ganglia of the first and second cervical nerves, however, lie on the vertebral arches of the atlas and axis, and those of the sacral nerves are inside the vertebral canal, while that of the coccygeal nerve is usually within the dura mater.

The ganglia of the first pair of cervical nerves may be absent, while small *aberrant ganglia* consisting of groups of nerve cells are sometimes found on the dorsal roots of the upper cervical nerves between the spinal ganglia and the spinal cord. (Heterotopic ganglionic neurons are also found in other sites—*see* p. 783.)

Each nerve root receives a covering from the pia mater, and is loosely invested by the arachnoid mater, the latter being prolonged as far as the points where the roots pierce the dura mater. The two roots pierce the dura mater separately, each receiving a sheath from this membrane (7.163, 167); where the roots join to form the spinal nerve

this sheath is continuous with the epineurium of the nerve.

**Size and direction of the spinal nerve roots.** The roots of the upper four *cervical* nerves are small; those of the lower four are large. The dorsal roots of the cervical nerves bear a proportion to the ventral of three to one, which is greater than in the other regions. The dorsal root of the first cervical is an exception to this, being smaller than the ventral root; in about 8 per cent of cases it is absent. The roots of the first and second cervical nerves are short, and run nearly horizontally to their points of exit from the vertebral canal. From the third to the eighth cervical they are directed obliquely downwards, the obliquity and length of the roots successively increasing; the distance, however, between the level of attachment of any of these roots to the spinal cord and the points of exit of the corresponding nerves never exceeds the height of one vertebra.

The roots of the *thoracic* nerves, with the exception of the first, are of small size, and the dorsal roots only slightly exceed the ventral in thickness. They increase successively in length, from above downwards, and, in the lower part of the thoracic region, descend in contact with the spinal cord for a distance equal to the height of at least two vertebrae before they emerge from the vertebral canal.

The roots of the lower *lumbar* and upper *sacral* nerves are the largest, and their individual filaments the most numerous of all the spinal nerves, while the roots of the *coccygeal* nerve are the smallest.

The roots of the lumbar, sacral and coccygeal nerves descend with an increasing degree of obliquity to their respective exits, and since the spinal cord ends near the level of the lower border of the first lumbar vertebra, the lengths of successive roots rapidly increases. As already mentioned (7.35 B), the term *cauda equina* is applied to this collection of *nerve roots*.

From the description given it will be seen that the largest nerve roots, and consequently the largest spinal nerves, are attached to the cervical and lumbar swellings of the spinal cord; these nerves are distributed to the upper and lower limbs.

Immediately beyond the spinal ganglion, the ventral and dorsal nerve roots unite to form the *spinal nerve*, which emerges through the intervertebral foramen, gives off recurrent meningeal branches (*vide infra*), and then divides immediately into a *dorsal* and a *ventral ramus* (7.207). At or immediately distal to its origin the ventral ramus of each spinal nerve is joined by a *grey ramus communicans* from the corresponding ganglion of the sympathetic trunk, while the ventral rami of the thoracic and the first and second lumbar nerves each contribute a *white ramus communicans* joining the corresponding sympathetic ganglion (7.194, 195). The second, third and

---

[1055] W. Pallie and J. K. Manuel, *Acta anat.*, **70**, 1968.

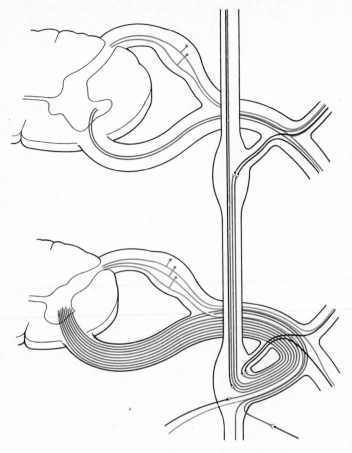

and the first sacral vertebrae, or that between the fourth and fifth lumbar vertebrae. These posterior disc lesions may compress one or more nerve roots as they pass towards their intervertebral foramina, resulting in low back pain ('lumbago'), with or without radiation of the pain to one or both lower limbs ('sciatica'), diminished cutaneous sensibility in the area of supply and weakness of the muscles innervated (e.g. tibialis anterior L. 4; extensor hallucis longus L. 5; flexor hallucis longus S. 1). Less commonly, tumours in the vertebral canal, or spina bifida with meningomyelocoele, may cause lesions of one or more nerve roots of the cauda equina.

### Functional Components and Branches of Spinal Nerves

Each typical spinal nerve contains both somatic and visceral fibres.

**The somatic components** consist of efferent and afferent fibres. The *somatic efferent* fibres for the innervation of skeletal muscles are the axons of $\alpha$, $\beta$ and $\gamma$ neurons in the anterior grey column of the spinal cord. The *somatic afferent* fibres convey impulses towards the central nervous system from a variety of receptors in the skin, subcutaneous tissue, muscles, fasciae, joints, etc (*see* pp. 798–804), and are the peripheral processes of the unipolar cells in the spinal ganglia.

**The visceral components** are also afferent and efferent and belong to the autonomic nervous system (p. 1068). They include sympathetic or parasympathetic fibres at different spinal levels. The preganglionic *visceral*

7.194 A scheme showing the constitution of a typical spinal nerve. In the upper part of the diagram the spinal nerve roots show the somatic components; in the lower part of the diagram the spinal roots show the visceral components. *Red:* somatic efferent and preganglionic sympathetic fibres. *Blue:* somatic afferent and visceral afferent fibres. *Black:* post-ganglionic sympathetic fibres.

fourth sacral nerves also give off visceral branches; these, however, are not connected with the ganglia of the sympathetic trunk, but belong to the parasympathetic part of the autonomic system and run directly into the pelvic plexuses (pp. 1079, 1080).

The cervical spinal nerves increase in size from the first to the sixth. The seventh and eighth cervical and first thoracic nerves are similar in size to that of the sixth cervical. The remaining thoracic nerves are relatively small. The lumbar nerves are large and increase in size from the first to the fifth. The first sacral nerve is the largest of all the spinal nerves, which thereafter decrease in size to the coccygeal, which is the smallest of all the spinal nerves.

In the intervertebral foramen the spinal nerves have important relations. *Anteriorly* are the intervertebral discs and adjacent regions of the bodies of the vertebrae. *Posteriorly* are the joints between which they pass. Each nerve is accompanied by a spinal artery, a plexus of small veins and its own meningeal branch or branches.

*Applied Anatomy.* The nerve roots may be compressed or otherwise irritated in their course from the spinal cord to their exit through the intervertebral foramina. In the cervical region, disease of a vertebral body, degeneration of an intervertebral disc or osteoarthrosis of the intervertebral joints may affect nerve roots as they traverse the intervertebral foramen, causing pain, diminished cutaneous sensibility and some muscular weakness in the field of supply. In the lumbar region, posterior protrusion of an intervertebral disc or rupture of its annular fibres with herniation of the nucleus pulposus is very common, affecting particularly the disc between the fifth lumbar

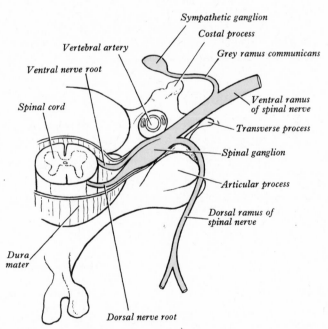

7.195 Scheme showing the relations of a cervical nerve and its ganglion to a cervical vertebra.

*efferent* fibres of the sympathetic component are the axons of cells in the lateral grey column of the thoracic and upper two or three lumbar segments of the spinal cord; they join the sympathetic trunk through the corresponding white ramus communicans and, after establishing synapses, the postganglionic fibres are distributed to non-striated muscle. The preganglionic visceral efferent fibres of the parasympathetic component are the axons of cells in the lateral grey column of the second, third and fourth sacral segments of the spinal cord. They leave the ventral rami of the corresponding sacral nerves to pass to ganglion cells in the pelvis where they synapse. The postganglionic axons of the latter are distributed principally to the smooth muscle in the walls of the pelvic viscera. The *visceral afferent* fibres are also derived from the cells of the spinal ganglia. Their peripheral processes are carried through the white rami communicantes, and after passing without synaptic interruption through one or more sympathetic ganglia end in the tissues of the viscera.

The central processes of the various ganglionic unipolar cells enter the spinal cord through the posterior nerve roots and form synapses around either somatic or sympathetic efferent neurons, thus completing reflex arcs, or they synapse with other neurons in the grey matter of the spinal cord or brainstem which give origin to a variety of ascending pathways. (For further details see the section on the spinal cord, pp. 816–839.)

After emerging from the intervertebral foramen, each spinal nerve supplies small *meningeal* branches and then splits almost immediately into a *dorsal* and a *ventral ramus*, each receiving fibres from both spinal nerve roots.

**The meningeal branches** of the spinal nerves (also known as the *recurrent meningeal nerves* or *sinu-vertebral nerves*) number two to four filaments on each side and are present at all vertebral levels.[1056, 1057] Each receives one or more communications from a neighbouring grey ramus communicans or from a thoracic sympathetic ganglion directly, and the majority then pursue a recurrent (often perivascular) course to re-enter the spinal canal through the intervertebral foramen, passing ventral to the dorsal root ganglion. Here, these mixed sensory and sympathetic nerves divide into transverse, ascending and descending branches where they are distributed to the dura mater, the walls of blood vessels, and to the periosteum, ligaments and intervertebral discs in the ventrolateral region of the spinal canal. Occasionally, fine meningeal branches pass dorsal to the spinal ganglion to be distributed to the dorsally situated dura, periosteum and ligaments, whilst others pass ventrally to reach the posterior longitudinal ligament.

The ascending branches of the upper three cervical meningeal nerves are relatively large and they are distributed to the cerebral dura mater of the posterior cranial fossa (p. 988).

These various meningeal nerves are of importance in relation to the referred pain which characterizes many spinal disorders and also in occipital headache.

---

[1056] D. L. Kimmel, *Neurology, Minneap.*, **11**, 1961.
[1057] D. L. Kimmel, *Chicago med. Sch. Q.*, **22**, 1961.

# DORSAL RAMI OF THE SPINAL NERVES

The dorsal (posterior primary) rami of the spinal nerves are as a rule smaller than the *ventral*. They are directed posteriorly, and, with the exception of those of the first cervical, the fourth and fifth sacral, and the coccygeal, divide into medial and lateral branches for the supply of muscles and skin (7.196) of the posterior regions of the neck and trunk.

## CERVICAL DORSAL RAMI

The dorsal ramus of each cervical spinal nerve, with the exception of the first, divides into a medial and a lateral branch. All these branches innervate muscles but, in general, only the medial branches of the second, third, fourth and, usually, the fifth, supply cutaneous areas. Except for the first and second, each dorsal ramus passes backwards medial to the posterior intertransverse muscle and winds round the articular process into the interval between the semispinalis capitis and the semispinalis cervicis.

**The first cervical dorsal ramus** (the **suboccipital nerve**) (5.40) is larger than the ventral ramus, and emerges superior to the posterior arch of the atlas and inferior to the vertebral artery. It enters the suboccipital triangle and supplies the muscles which bound this region—the rectus capitis posterior major, and the superior and inferior oblique; it gives branches also to the rectus capitis posterior minor and the semispinalis capitis. A filament from the branch to the inferior oblique joins the dorsal ramus of the second cervical nerve (5.40). The nerve occasionally gives off a cutaneous branch which accompanies the occipital artery to the scalp, and communicates with the greater and lesser occipital nerves.

**The second cervical dorsal ramus** is slightly larger than the ventral and all the other cervical dorsal rami. It emerges between the posterior arch of the atlas and the lamina of the axis, below the inferior oblique. It supplies a twig to this muscle, receives a communicating filament from the dorsal ramus of the first cervical, and then divides into a large medial and a small lateral branch. Its ganglion is said to be extradural in position.

The *medial* branch, called from its size and distribution the *greater occipital nerve* (7.196, 198), ascends obliquely between the inferior oblique and the semispinalis capitis, and pierces the latter muscle and the trapezius near their attachments to the occipital bone. It is then joined by a filament from the medial branch of the dorsal ramus of the third cervical, and, ascending in the occipital area with the occipital artery, divides into branches which communicate with the lesser occipital nerve and supply the skin of the scalp as far forward as the vertex of the skull. It gives muscular branches to the semispinalis capitis, and occasionally a twig to the back of the auricle. The *lateral* branch supplies filaments to the splenius, longissimus capitis and semispinalis capitis, and is often joined by the corresponding branch of the third cervical.

**The third cervical dorsal ramus** is intermediate in size between those of the second and fourth. It courses backwards round the articular pillar of the third cervical vertebra, passing medial to the posterior intertransverse muscle, and divides into medial and lateral branches. Its *medial* branch runs between the spinalis capitis and semispinalis cervicis, and, piercing the splenius and trapezius, ends in the skin. While deep to the trapezius it gives a branch, called the *third occipital nerve*, which pierces the trapezius and ends in the skin of the lower part of the occipital region (7.196). It is medial to the greater occipital nerve, and communicates with it. The *lateral* branch often joins that of the second cervical dorsal ramus.

The dorsal ramus of the suboccipital, and the medial branches of the dorsal rami of the second and third cervical nerves are sometimes joined by communicating loops to form the *posterior cervical plexus*.

**The dorsal rami of the lower five cervical nerves** curve backwards round the vertebral articular pillars and divide into medial and lateral branches. The *medial* branches of the fourth and fifth run between the semispinalis cervicis and semispinalis capitis, and, having reached the spines of the vertebrae, pierce the splenius and trapezius to end in the skin (7.196). Sometimes the medial branch of the fifth fails to reach the skin. The medial branches of the lowest three nerves are small, and

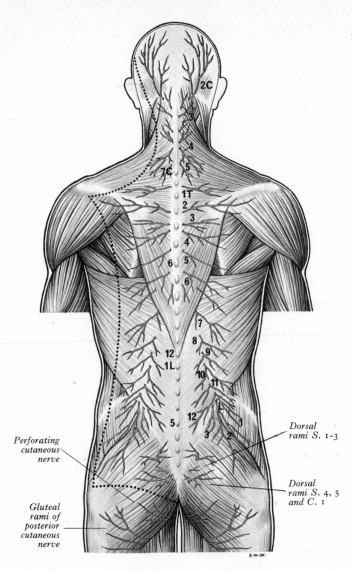

*Perforating cutaneous nerve*

*Gluteal rami of posterior cutaneous nerve*

*Dorsal rami S. 1-3*

*Dorsal rami S. 4, 5 and C. 1*

**7.196** The cutaneous distribution of the dorsal rami of the spinal nerves. The nerves are shown lying on the superficial muscles; on the left side the limit of the skin area supplied by these nerves is indicated by the dotted line. The nerves are numbered on the right side and the spines of the seventh cervical, sixth and twelfth thoracic and first and fifth lumbar vertebrae are labelled on the left side.

end in the semispinalis cervicis, semispinalis capitis, multifidus and interspinales. The *lateral* branches of the lower five nerves supply the iliocostalis cervicis, longissimus cervicis and longissimus capitis.

## THORACIC DORSAL RAMI

The dorsal rami of the thoracic spinal nerves pass backwards close to the joints between the articular processes of the vertebrae and divide into medial and lateral branches. The medial branch emerges between the joint and the medial edge of the superior costotransverse ligament and the intertransverse muscle, but the lateral branch runs laterally in the interval between the ligament and the muscle before inclining posteriorly on the medial side of the levator costae.

The *medial* branches of the *upper six* thoracic dorsal rami run between semispinalis thoracis and multifidus, which they supply; they then pierce the rhomboids and trapezius, and reach the skin by the sides of the vertebral spines (**7.196**). The medial branches of the *lower six* thoracic dorsal rami are distributed chiefly to the multifidus and longissimus thoracis; occasionally they give filaments to the skin near the median plane.

The *lateral* branches increase in size from above downwards. They run through or deep to the longissimus thoracis to the interval between it and the iliocostalis cervicis, and supply these muscles and the levatores costarum; the lower five or six also give off cutaneous branches, which pierce the serratus posterior inferior and latissimus dorsi in a line with the angles of the ribs (**7.196**). The lateral branches of a variable number of the upper thoracic rami also give filaments to the skin. The lateral branch of the twelfth thoracic, after sending a filament medially along the iliac crest, passes downwards to the skin of the anterior part of the gluteal region.

The medial cutaneous branches of the dorsal rami of the thoracic spinal nerves descend for some distance close to the vertebral spines before reaching the skin, while the lateral branches travel downwards for a considerable distance—it may be as much as the breadth of four ribs—before they become superficial; the branch from the twelfth thoracic, for instance, reaches the skin only a little way above the iliac crest.

## LUMBAR DORSAL RAMI

The dorsal rami of the lumbar spinal nerves pass back medial to the medial intertransverse muscles and at once divide into medial and lateral branches.

The *medial* branches run close to the articular processes of the vertebrae and end in the multifidus.

The *lateral* branches supply the erector spinae (sacrospinalis). In addition the upper three give off cutaneous nerves which pierce the aponeurosis of the latissimus dorsi at the lateral border of the erector spinae and cross the posterior part of the iliac crest to reach the skin of the gluteal region (**7.196**), some reaching as far as the level of the greater trochanter.

## SACRAL DORSAL RAMI

The dorsal rami of the sacral spinal nerves are small, and diminish in size from above downwards; with the exception of the fifth, they emerge through the dorsal sacral foramina. The *upper three* are covered at their points of exit by the multifidus, and divide into medial and lateral branches.

The *medial* branches are small, and end in the multifidus.

The *lateral* branches join with one another and with the lateral branches of the dorsal rami of the last lumbar and fourth sacral to form loops on the dorsal surface of the sacrum. From these loops branches run to the dorsal surface of the sacrotuberous ligament and form a second series of loops under the gluteus maximus. From this second series of loops the *gluteal branches*, two or three in number, arise and at once pierce the gluteus maximus along a line drawn from the posterior superior iliac spine to the apex of the coccyx; they supply the skin over the posterior gluteal area (**7.196**).

The dorsal rami of the *lower two* sacral nerves are small and lie below the multifidus. They do not divide into medial and lateral branches, but unite with each other and with the dorsal ramus of the coccygeal nerve to form loops on the back of the sacrum; filaments from these loops supply the skin over the coccyx.

## COCCYGEAL DORSAL RAMUS

The dorsal ramus of the coccygeal spinal nerve does not divide into a medial and a lateral branch, but receives, as already stated, a communicating branch from the last sacral; it is distributed to the skin over the back of the coccyx.

The ventral rami of the spinal nerves supply the limbs and the anterolateral aspects of the trunk; they are for the most part larger than the dorsal rami. In the thoracic region they run independently of one another, retaining, like all the dorsal rami, a more or less segmental distribution. In the cervical, lumbar and sacral regions, however, they unite near their origins to form plexuses. It is to be noted that the dorsal rami of the spinal nerves do not enter into the formation of these plexuses; their distribution has already been described (p. 1032).

## CERVICAL VENTRAL RAMI

The ventral rami of the cervical nerves, with the exception of the first, appear between the corresponding anterior and posterior intertransverse muscles. The ventral rami of the *upper four* nerves unite to form the *cervical plexus*; those of the *lower four*, together with the greater part of the ventral ramus of the first thoracic nerve, join to form the *brachial plexus*.

Each nerve receives at least one grey ramus communicans, the upper four from the superior cervical ganglion, the fifth and sixth from the middle cervical ganglion, and the seventh and eighth from the cervicothoracic ganglion of the sympathetic trunk (*see* p. 1073).

The ventral ramus of the *first cervical (suboccipital) nerve* appears above the posterior arch of the atlas vertebra, and passes forwards lateral to its lateral mass, and medial to the vertebral artery. It supplies a branch to the rectus lateralis, and, emerging on the medial side of that muscle, descends in front of the transverse process of the atlas and behind the internal jugular vein, and joins with the ascending branch of the second nerve.

The ventral ramus of the *second cervical nerve* issues between the vertebral arches of the atlas and axis and runs forwards between the transverse processes of these two vertebrae; passing in front of the first posterior intertransverse muscle and on the lateral side of the vertebral artery it emerges between the longus capitis and levator scapulae, but when the scalenus medius takes origin from the transverse process of the atlas, it intervenes between the nerve and the levator scapulae. It divides into an ascending branch which joins with the first cervical nerve, and a descending branch which unites with the ascending branch of the third cervical nerve.

The ventral ramus of the *third cervical nerve* appears between the longus capitis and scalenus medius. The ventral rami of the remaining cervical nerves emerge between the scalenus anterior and scalenus medius.

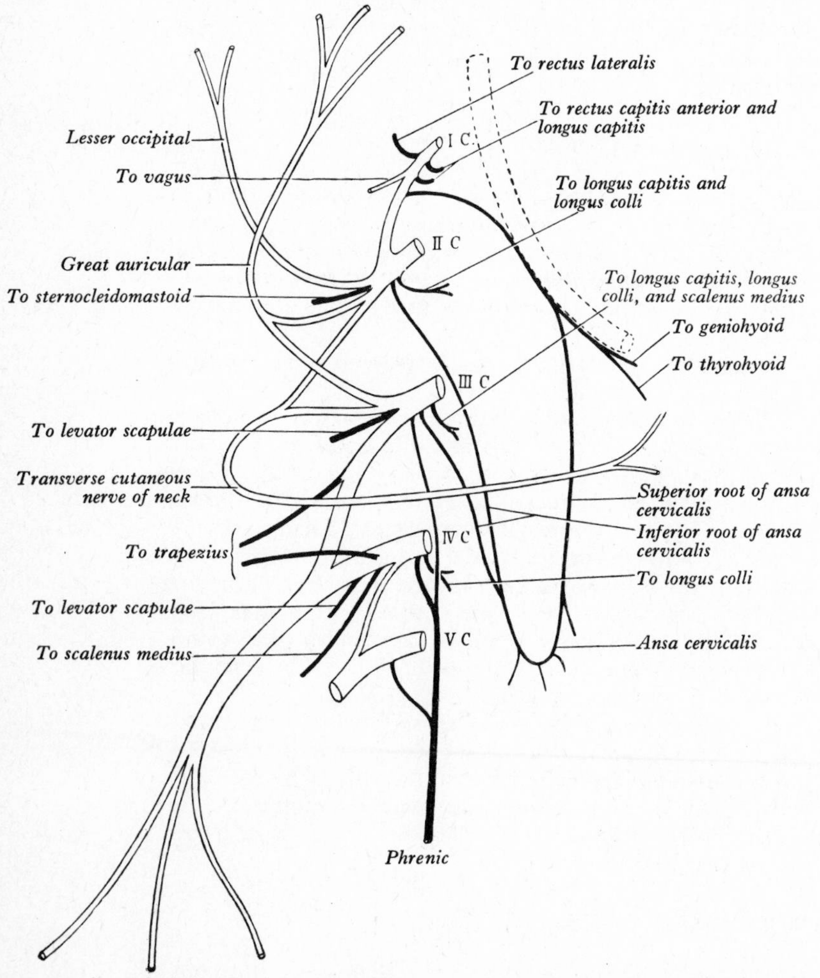

## The Cervical Plexus

The cervical plexus (7.197) is formed by the ventral rami of the upper four cervical nerves; it distributes branches to some of the muscles of the neck and to parts of the integument of the head, neck and chest (7.182). It is placed opposite the first four vertebrae, deep to the internal jugular vein and the sternocleidomastoid, in front of the scalenus medius and levator scapulae. The disposition of the nerves in the plexus is as follows: each nerve, except the first, divides into an ascending and a descending part; these are united in communicating loops with the contiguous nerves. From the union of the second and third nerves, superficial branches are supplied to the head and neck, and from the junction of the third with the fourth arise some of the cutaneous nerves of the shoulder and chest. Muscular and communicating branches spring from the same nerves.

The branches of the plexus may be divided into two sets —a superficial and deep, the superficial consisting of those which perforate the cervical fascia and supply the integument, the deep comprising branches which are distributed for the most part to the muscles. The superficial nerves may be subdivided into ascending and descending, the deep nerves into a medial and a lateral series.

### SUPERFICIAL ASCENDING BRANCHES

The superficial ascending branches of the cervical plexus (7.197–199) include:

| | |
|---|---|
| Lesser occipital | 2 C. |
| Greater auricular | 2, 3 C. |
| Transverse (anterior) cutaneous | 2, 3 C. |

Lesser occipital

To vagus

Great auricular

To sternocleidomastoid

To levator scapulae

Transverse cutaneous nerve of neck

To trapezius

To levator scapulae

To scalenus medius

To rectus lateralis

To rectus capitis anterior and longus capitis

To longus capitis and longus colli

To longus capitis, longus colli, and scalenus medius

To geniohyoid

To thyrohyoid

Superior root of ansa cervicalis

Inferior root of ansa cervicalis

To longus colli

Ansa cervicalis

I C

II C

III C

IV C

V C

Phrenic

Supraclavicular

7.197 A plan of the cervical plexus. The hypoglossal nerve is shown by interrupted lines and the muscular branches by solid black lines. The roman numerals and letters I C to V C indicate the *ventral rami* of these cervical spinal nerves.

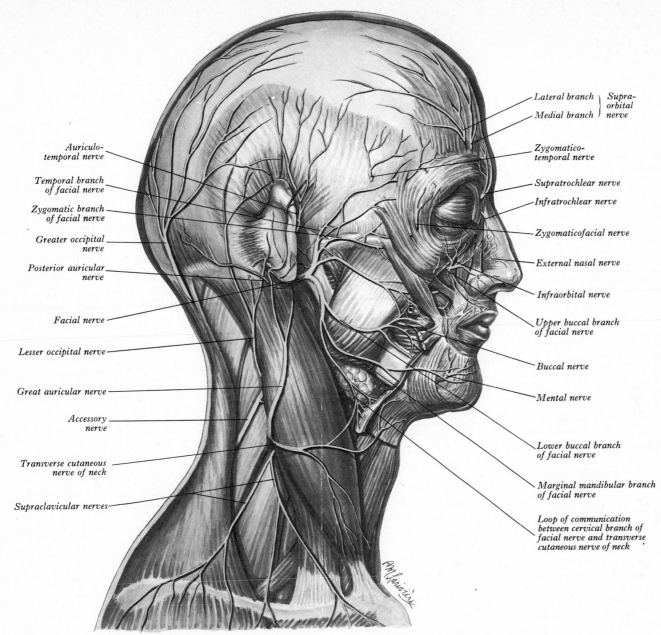

Auriculo-
temporal nerve

Temporal branch
of facial nerve

Zygomatic branch
of facial nerve

Greater occipital
nerve

Posterior auricular
nerve

Facial nerve

Lesser occipital nerve

Great auricular nerve

Accessory
nerve

Transverse cutaneous
nerve of neck

Supraclavicular nerves

Lateral branch } Supra-
Medial branch } orbital
               } nerve

Zygomatico-
temporal nerve

Supratrochlear nerve

Infratrochlear nerve

Zygomaticofacial nerve

External nasal nerve

Infraorbital nerve

Upper buccal branch
of facial nerve

Buccal nerve

Mental nerve

Lower buccal branch
of facial nerve

Marginal mandibular branch
of facial nerve

Loop of communication
between cervical branch of
facial nerve and transverse
cutaneous nerve of neck

**7.198**   The nerves of the right side of the scalp, face and side of neck.

**The lesser occipital nerve** (7.197, 198) arises from the second cervical nerve, sometimes also from the third; it curves around the accessory nerve and ascends along the posterior border of the sternocleidomastoid. Near the cranium it perforates the deep fascia, and is continued upwards on the side of the head behind the auricle, supplying the skin and communicating with the great auricular and greater occipital nerves, and with the posterior auricular branch of the facial nerve. The lesser occipital nerve varies in size, and is sometimes duplicated.

It sends off an *auricular branch* which supplies the skin of the upper third of the cranial surface of the auricle, and communicates with the posterior branch of the great auricular nerve. The auricular branch is occasionally derived from the greater occipital nerve.

**The great auricular nerve** (7.197, 198) is the largest of the ascending branches. It arises from the second and third cervical nerves, encircles the posterior border of the sternocleidomastoid, and, after perforating the deep fascia, ascends upon that muscle beneath the platysma in company with the external jugular vein. It passes on to the parotid gland, where it divides into an anterior and a posterior branch.

The *anterior branch* is distributed to the skin of the face over the parotid gland, and communicates in the substance of the gland with the facial nerve.

The *posterior branch* supplies the skin over the mastoid process and on the back of the auricle, except at its upper part; a filament pierces the auricle to reach its lateral surface, where it is distributed to the lobule and the concha. The posterior branch communicates with the lesser occipital nerve, the auricular branch of the vagus nerve, and the posterior auricular branch of the facial nerve.

**The transverse (anterior) cutaneous nerve of the neck** (7.197, 198) arises from the second and third cervical nerves, turns round the posterior border of the sternocleidomastoid about its middle, and runs obliquely forwards, deep to the external jugular vein, to the anterior border of the muscle. It perforates the deep cervical fascia, and divides beneath the platysma into ascending and descending branches, which are distributed to the anterolateral parts of the neck.

The *ascending branches* pass upwards to the submandibular region, and form a plexus with the cervical branch of the facial nerve, beneath the platysma; others

1035

pierce that muscle, and are distributed to the skin of the upper and front parts of the neck.

The *descending branches* pierce the platysma, and are distributed to the skin of the side and front of the neck, as low as the sternum.

## SUPERFICIAL DESCENDING BRANCHES

These are: Supraclavicular (3, 4 C)—medial, intermediate and lateral.

**The supraclavicular nerves** (7.197, 198) arise by a common trunk derived from the third and fourth cervical nerves. This trunk emerges from beneath the posterior border of the sternocleidomastoid, descends under cover of the platysma and deep cervical fascia, and divides into medial, intermediate and lateral (posterior) branches, which diverge from one another and pierce the deep fascia a little above the level of the clavicle.

The *medial supraclavicular nerves* run obliquely downwards and medially, crossing the external jugular vein and the clavicular and sternal heads of the sternocleidomastoid, to supply the skin as far as the median plane and as low down as the second rib. They furnish one or two filaments to the sternoclavicular joint.

The *intermediate supraclavicular nerves* traverse the clavicle, and supply the skin over the pectoralis major and deltoid as low down as the level of the second rib, immediately adjoining the area supplied by the second thoracic nerve (7.221). The amount of overlapping in this situation is minimal.

The *lateral (posterior) supraclavicular nerves* descend obliquely across the superficial surface of the trapezius and the acromion, and supply the skin of the upper and posterior parts of the shoulder.

## DEEP BRANCHES—MEDIAL SERIES

These include the following communicating and muscular branches:

| | | |
|---|---|---|
| Communicating branches with | Hypoglossal | 1, 2 C. |
| | Vagus | 1, 2 C. |
| | Sympathetic | 1, 2, 3, 4 C. |
| Muscular branches to | Rectus capitis lateralis | 1 C. |
| | Rectus capitis anterior | 1, 2 C. |
| | Longus capitis | 1, 2, 3 C. |
| | Longus colli | 2, 3, 4 C. |
| | Inferior root of ansa cervicalis | 2, 3 C. |
| | Phrenic | 3, 4, 5 C. |

**The communicating branches** consist of several filaments which pass from the loop between the first and second cervical nerves to the vagus, hypoglossal and sympathetic. The branch to the hypoglossal ultimately leaves that nerve as a series of branches, viz. the meningeal, the *superior root of the ansa cervicalis*, the nerve to the thyrohyoid and, probably, the nerve to the geniohyoid (p. 1026). A communicating branch also passes from the fourth to the fifth cervical nerve, while each of the first four cervical nerves receives a grey ramus communicans from the superior cervical ganglion of the sympathetic trunk.

**Muscular branches** supply the rectus capitis lateralis, rectus capitis anterior, longus capitis and longus colli.

**The inferior root of the ansa cervicalis** (nervus descendens cervicalis) (7.197) is formed usually by the union of two branches, one derived from the second cervical nerve and the other from the third. It passes downwards on the lateral side of the internal jugular vein, crosses in front of this vein a little below the middle of the neck, and continues forwards to join the superior root in

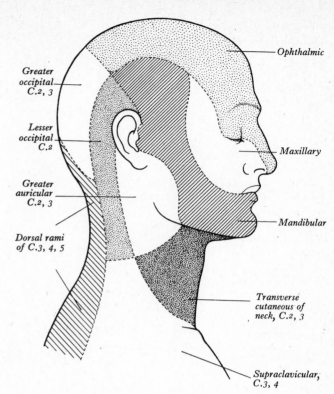

7.199   A diagram showing the cutaneous nerve supply of the face, scalp and neck.

front of the common carotid artery, so forming the *ansa cervicalis (ansa hypoglossi)*. Not infrequently it passes forwards between the internal jugular vein and the common carotid artery to reach the ansa cervicalis (6.46), from which all the infrahyoid muscles, with the exception of the thyrohyoid, are supplied. In a series of 160 dissections of the ansa cervicalis, the inferior root was from the second and third cervical anterior primary rami in 74 per cent, from the second, third and fourth in 14 per cent, from the third alone in 5 per cent, from the second alone in 4 per cent and from the first, second and third in 2 per cent.[1058]

**The phrenic nerve** is the sole motor nerve supply to the diaphragm, but it also contains sensory fibres which have a widespread distribution. It arises chiefly from the fourth cervical nerve but also receives contributions from the third and fifth cervical nerves (7.197). Formed at the upper part of the lateral border of the scalenus anterior, the nerve passes downwards almost vertically across the front of that muscle, *behind the prevertebral fascia* covering the anterior surface of the muscle. The phrenic nerve descends to the root of the neck beneath the sternocleidomastoid, the inferior belly of the omohyoid (near the intermediate tendon of that muscle), the internal jugular vein, the transverse cervical and suprascapular arteries (6.45) and, on the left side, the thoracic duct. It then runs in front of the subclavian artery and behind the subclavian vein, to enter the thorax by crossing from the lateral to the medial side, and in front of the internal thoracic artery (6.67). In the thorax, it descends in front of the root of the lung, between the fibrous pericardium and the mediastinal pleura, to the diaphragm, being accompanied by the pericardiacophrenic vessels. The right and left phrenic nerves differ in their relations.

The *right phrenic nerve*, shorter and more vertical than the left, is separated at the root of the neck from the second part of the right subclavian artery by the scalenus anterior.

---

[1058] N. P. Poriraer and Y. F. Chernikov, *Mat. teoret. Klin. Med.*, **5**, 1965.

It then lies lateral to the right brachiocephalic vein, the superior vena cava, and the fibrous pericardium covering the right surface of the right atrium and of the inferior vena cava.

The *left phrenic nerve*, at the root of the neck, leaves the medial edge of the scalenus anterior and passes in front of the first part of the left subclavian artery and behind the thoracic duct. In the superior mediastinum it lies between the left common carotid and subclavian arteries, and passes medially and forwards superficially to the left vagus nerve just above the aortic arch and behind the left brachiocephalic vein. It then passes superficially to the arch of the aorta and the left superior intercostal vein, in front of the root of the left lung, to lie between the fibrous pericardium covering the left surface of the left ventricle and the mediastinal pleura.

In the neck each nerve receives variable and inconstant communicating filaments from the cervical sympathetic ganglia or their branches. During its course through the thorax, each nerve supplies sensory branches to the mediastinal pleura and to the fibrous pericardium and the parietal layer of the serous pericardium.

*Diaphragmatic relations.*[1059, 1060] The right phrenic nerve passes through the central tendon of the diaphragm, either through the inferior caval orifice or just lateral to it. The left phrenic nerve passes through the muscular part of the diaphragm in front of the central tendon, just lateral to the left surface of the heart and on a more anterior plane than the right phrenic. At the level of the *diaphragm*, or slightly above it, each phrenic nerve gives off a few fine branches which are distributed to the parietal pleura above and the parietal peritoneum below the central part of the diaphragm. The trunk of each phrenic nerve then divides as it passes through the diaphragm into its main branches, which are commonly three in number and arranged in the following way, though variations may occur. (*a*) The anterior (or sternal) branch runs anteromedially towards the sternum and communicates with the corresponding nerve of the opposite side; (*b*) the anterolateral branch runs laterally just in front of the lateral leaflet of the central tendon; (*c*) the posterior branch is short and divides into a posterolateral branch which courses just behind the lateral leaflet of the central tendon, and a posterior (crural) branch that passes to the crural part of the diaphragm. The posterolateral and crural branches may arise separately from the phrenic nerve. These branches are often submerged in the muscular substance of the diaphragm, but may lie to some extent below it, and in addition to supplying motor fibres to the diaphragm they give off sensory fibres to the peritoneum and pleura related to the central part of the diaphragm. The branches also contain proprioceptive sensory fibres from the musculature of the diaphragm. The position of these main branches is of surgical importance in planning incisions through the diaphragm without damage to large branches of the phrenic nerve. The right crus of the diaphragm splits to enclose the oesophagus (p. 517). The right phrenic nerve supplies the part of the right crus that lies to the right of the oesophagus, while the left phrenic nerve supplies the left crus and the part of the right crus that lies to the left of the oesophagus.[1061] (Consult also footnote reference[1062].)

On the inferior surface of the diaphragm, rami of the phrenic nerves communicate with phrenic branches of the coeliac plexus (p. 1077); on the right side, at the junction of the plexuses there is a small *phrenic ganglion*. From these plexuses branches are distributed to the suprarenal glands and, on the right side, to the falciform and coronary ligaments of the liver and the inferior vena cava, and, possibly, through communications with the coeliac and hepatic plexuses, to the gall bladder pp. 1077, 1082).

*Accessory phrenic nerve.* The contribution to the phrenic nerve from the fifth cervical nerve is frequently derived as a branch from the nerve to the subclavius. This is known as the *accessory phrenic nerve*. It lies lateral to the main phrenic nerve and descends behind, or sometimes in front of, the subclavian vein; it usually joins the main nerve about the level of the first rib, though it may not do so until the level of the root of the lung or even lower in the thorax. An accessory phrenic nerve may be derived from the fourth or sixth cervical nerve, or from the ansa cervicalis (p. 1027).

*Applied Anatomy.* The phrenic nerve is the sole motor nerve supply to the diaphragm and section of the nerve in the neck leads to complete paralysis and atrophy of the corresponding half of the diaphragm. If an accessory phrenic nerve is present, section or crushing of the main nerve alone as it lies on the scalenus anterior will not produce complete paralysis of the corresponding half of the diaphragm.

## DEEP BRANCHES—LATERAL SERIES

These include:

| Communicating— | Accessory | 2, 3, 4 C. |
| --- | --- | --- |
| | Sternocleidomastoid | 2, 3, 4 C. |
| Muscular branches | Trapezius | 2 C. |
| | Levator scapulae | 3, 4 C. |
| | Scalenus medius | 3, 4 C. |

**Communicating branches.** The lateral series of deep branches of the cervical plexus communicate with the accessory nerve in the substance of the sternocleidomastoid, in the posterior triangle and under cover of the trapezius.

**Muscular branches** are distributed to the sternocleidomastoid from the second cervical nerve, and to the trapezius, levator scapulae and scalenus medius from the third and fourth cervical nerves. The branches to the trapezius cross the posterior triangle obliquely at a lower level than the accessory nerve.

## The Brachial Plexus

The brachial plexus (7.200) is formed by the union of the ventral rami of the lower four cervical nerves and the greater part of the ventral ramus of the first thoracic nerve (p. 1047); the fourth cervical nerve usually gives a branch to the fifth cervical, and the first thoracic nerve frequently receives one from the second thoracic. The contributions made to the plexus by C. 4 and T. 2 are subject to frequent variation. When the branch from C. 4 is large, the branch from T. 2 is frequently absent and the branch from T. 1 is reduced in size. This constitutes the *prefixed type* of plexus. On the other hand the branch from C. 4 may be very small or entirely absent. In that event the contribution of C. 5 is reduced in size but that of T. 1 is larger and the branch from T. 2 is always present. This arrangement constitutes the *postfixed type* of plexus. These nerves constitute the *roots* of the plexus. The roots are nearly equal in size, but the way in which they form the plexus is subject to some variation. The following is, however, the most constant arrangement. The fifth and sixth cervical nerves unite at the lateral border of the scalenus medius to

[1059] K. A. Merendino, R. J. Johnson, H. H. Skinner and R. X. Maguire, *Surgery Gynec. Obstet.*, **39**, 1956.
[1060] H. Perera and F. R. Edwards, *Lancet*, **2**, 1957.
[1061] J. L. Collis, L. M. Satchwell and L. D. Abrams, *Thorax*, **9**, 1954.
[1062] M. W. Thornton and M. R. Schweisthal, *Anat. Rec.*, **164**, 1969.

form the *upper trunk* of the plexus. The eighth cervical and first thoracic nerves unite behind the scalenus anterior to form the *lower trunk* of the plexus, while the seventh cervical nerve itself constitutes the *middle trunk*. These three trunks run downwards and laterally and just above or behind the clavicle, each splits into an *anterior* and a *posterior division*. The anterior divisions of the upper and middle trunks unite to form a cord, which is situated on the lateral side of the axillary artery, and is called the *lateral cord* of the plexus. The anterior division of the lower trunk passes down at first behind and then on the medial side of the axillary artery, and forms the *medial cord* of the brachial plexus; this cord frequently receives fibres from the seventh cervical nerve. The posterior divisions of all three trunks unite to form the *posterior cord* of the plexus, which is situated at first above and then behind the axillary artery. The posterior division of the lower trunk is very much smaller than the others, and contains few fibres from the first thoracic nerve. It is frequently derived from the eighth cervical nerve before the trunk is formed.

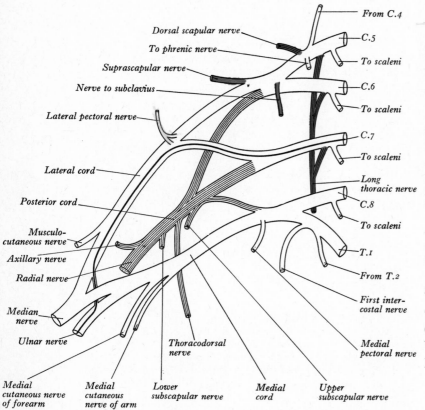

7.200 A plan of the brachial plexus. The posterior divisions of the trunks and their derivatives are shaded and the fibres from C.7 which enter the ulnar nerve are shown as a heavy black line. Letters and numbers C.4–C.8 and T.1–T.2 indicate the *ventral rami* of these cervical and thoracic spinal nerves.

Morphologically the brachial plexus still shows, despite much adaptation to the evolutionary changes in the upper-limb musculature, a clear reflexion of the original flexor-extensor organization of a primitive fin. The posterior cord represents the extensor nerve supply, the medial and lateral cords, the flexor supply. The migration of muscle masses has in some instances modified this basic pattern; for example, the brachialis and the anterior part of deltoid are both supplied (the former only in part) from 'extensor' nerves. For details of the comparative morphology of the plexus consult footnote reference [1063].

## Relations of the Brachial Plexus

*In the neck*, the brachial plexus lies in the posterior triangle in the angle between the clavicle and the lower part of the posterior border of the sternocleidomastoid, being covered by the skin, platysma and deep fascia. When the arm is by the side, it can be felt in this situation as a bunch of tense cords. The plexus is crossed by the supraclavicular nerves, the nerve to the subclavius, the inferior belly of the omohyoid, the external jugular vein and the superficial cervical artery (**6**.64). It emerges between the scalenus anterior and scalenus medius; its proximal part is above the third part of the subclavian artery, while the lower trunk is posterior to the artery; the plexus next passes behind the anterior convexity of the medial two-thirds of the clavicle, the subclavius and the suprascapular vessels, and lies upon the first digitation of the serratus anterior and the subscapularis. *In the axilla* the lateral and posterior cords of the plexus are on the lateral side of the first part of the axillary artery, and the medial cord behind it. The cords surround the second part of the axillary artery on three sides, the medial cord lying on the medial side, the posterior cord behind, and the lateral cord on the lateral side of the artery. In the lower part of the axilla the cords split into the nerves for the upper limb. With the exception of the medial root of the median nerve, the courses of the three cords bear the same relationships to the third part of the axillary artery as the cords from which they spring bear to the second part, i.e. branches from the lateral cord are lateral, branches of the posterior cord are behind, and branches of the medial cord are medial to the artery.

Close to their exit from the intervertebral foramina the fifth and sixth cervical nerves receive grey rami communicantes from the middle cervical ganglion, and the seventh and eighth cervical similar rami from the cervicothoracic ganglion of the sympathetic trunk (p. 1073). The first thoracic nerve also receives a grey ramus from, and contributes a white ramus to, the cervicothoracic ganglion.

**The branches of the brachial plexus** are usually considered, for convenience, as two groups—those arising above the clavicle (*supraclavicular*) and those below it (*infraclavicular*).

## SUPRACLAVICULAR BRANCHES

The supraclavicular branches may be grouped as follows: (*a*) those arising from the roots, and (*b*) those arising from the trunks of the plexus.

| | | |
|---|---|---|
| From the roots of the plexus | 1. To scaleni and longus colli | 5, 6, 7, 8 C. |
| | 2. To join phrenic nerve | 5 C. |
| | 3. Dorsal scapular nerve | 5 C. |
| | 4. Long thoracic nerve | 5, 6, 7 C. |
| From the trunks of the plexus | 1. Nerve to subclavius | 5, 6 C. |
| | 2. Suprascapular nerve | 5, 6 C. |

The branches for the scaleni and longus colli muscles arise from the lower cervical nerves close to their points of exit from the intervertebral foramina.

On the scalenus anterior the phrenic nerve is joined by a branch from the fifth cervical nerve.

**The dorsal scapular nerve** arises from the fifth cervical nerve, pierces the scalenus medius, passes on to the deep surface of the levator scapulae, to which it occasionally gives a twig, and runs in company with the deep course of the dorsal scapular artery on the anterior surfaces of the rhomboids; it ends by supplying these muscles.

[1063] W. Harris, *The Morphology of the Brachial Plexus*, Oxford University Press, London. 1939.

**The long thoracic nerve** (7.204) is usually formed by three roots from the fifth, sixth and seventh cervical nerves, but the root from the seventh nerve may be absent. (A study of seventy dissections of the nerve demonstrated all three roots in only 42 per cent of cases.[1064]) The upper two roots pierce the scalenus medius obliquely, uniting either in the substance of the muscle or on its lateral surface, and the nerve so formed descends dorsal to the brachial plexus and the first part of the axillary artery. Having crossed the upper border of the serratus anterior to gain its outer surface, it is soon joined by the root from C. 7, which emerges from the interval between the scalenus anterior and the scalenus medius at a lower level and descends on the lateral surface of the latter muscle. The nerve is continued downwards to the lower border of the serratus anterior, supplying, in its course, filaments to each of its digitations.

**The nerve to the subclavius** is small and is derived near the point of junction of the fifth and sixth cervical nerves; it descends in front of the plexus and the third part of the subclavian artery, and is usually connected by a filament with the phrenic nerve. It then passes above the subclavian vein and reaches the subclavius, which it supplies.

**The suprascapular nerve** (6.64, 7.205) is a large branch from the superior trunk of the brachial plexus. It runs laterally deep to the trapezius and the omohyoid, and enters the supraspinous fossa through the suprascapular notch, inferior to the superior transverse scapular ligament; it then runs deep to the supraspinatus, and curves round the lateral border of the spine of the scapula in company with the suprascapular artery to gain the infraspinous fossa. In the supraspinous fossa it gives two branches to the supraspinatus and articular filaments to the shoulder joint and acromioclavicular joint; and in the infraspinous fossa it gives two branches to the infraspinatus, besides some filaments to the shoulder joint and scapula.

## INFRACLAVICULAR BRANCHES

The infraclavicular branches are derived from the three cords of the brachial plexus, but their fibres may be traced through the plexus to the spinal nerves from which they originate. They are as follows:

| Lateral cord | Lateral pectoral | 5, 6, 7 C. |
| | Musculocutaneous | 5, 6, 7 C. |
| | Lateral root of median | (5), 6, 7 C. |
| Medial cord | Medial pectoral | 8 C., 1 T. |
| | Medial cutaneous of forearm | 8 C., 1 T. |
| | Medial cutaneous of arm | 8 C., 1 T. |
| | Ulnar | (7), 8 C., 1 T. |
| | Medial root of median | 8 C., 1 T. |
| Posterior cord | Upper subscapular | 5, 6 C. |
| | Thoracodorsal | 6, 7, 8 C. |
| | Lower subscapular | 5, 6 C. |
| | Axillary | 5, 6 C. |
| | Radial | 5, 6, 7, 8 C., 1 T. |

The *pectoral nerves* (7.204) supply the pectoralis major and pectoralis minor.

**The lateral pectoral nerve**, the larger of the two, may arise by two roots from the anterior divisions of the upper and middle trunks, or by a single root from the point where these divisions unite to form the lateral cord of the plexus; it receives its fibres from the fifth, sixth and seventh cervical nerves. It crosses the axillary artery and

vein anteriorly, pierces the clavipectoral fascia, and is distributed to the deep surface of the pectoralis major. It sends a filament to join the medial pectoral nerve and forms with it a loop in front of the first part of the axillary artery (7.204); through this loop the lateral pectoral nerve distributes some fibres to the pectoralis minor.

**The medial pectoral nerve** receives its fibres from the eighth cervical and first thoracic nerves, and arises from the medial cord of the plexus while that cord is still posterior to the axillary artery. It curves forwards between the axillary artery and vein, and unites in front of the artery with a filament from the lateral pectoral nerve. It then enters the deep surface of the pectoralis minor and supplies that muscle. Two or three branches pierce the pectoralis minor, and others may pass round its inferior border, to end in the pectoralis major.

The *subscapular nerves*, two in number, spring from the posterior cord of the plexus, and through it from the fifth and sixth cervical nerves.

**The superior subscapular nerve**, the smaller, enters the subscapularis at a cranial level, and is frequently represented by two branches.

**The inferior subscapular nerve** supplies the caudal part of subscapularis, and ends in teres major; the latter muscle is sometimes supplied by a separate branch.

**The thoracodorsal nerve**, a branch of the posterior cord of the plexus, derives its fibres from the sixth, seventh and eighth cervical nerves; it arises between the upper and lower subscapular nerves and then accompanies the subscapular artery along the posterior wall of the axilla and supplies the latissimus dorsi, in which it may be traced as far as the lower border of the muscle.

**The axillary (circumflex humeral) nerve** (7.205) arises from the posterior cord of the brachial plexus, its fibres being derived from the fifth and sixth cervical nerves. It lies at first on the lateral side of the radial nerve and is placed behind the axillary artery, and in front of the subscapularis. At the lower border of that muscle it winds backwards in close relation to the lowest part of the articular capsule of the shoulder joint, and, in company with the posterior circumflex humeral vessels, passes through a quadrangular space bounded *above* by the subscapularis, in front, and the teres minor, behind, *below* by the teres major, *medially* by the long head of the triceps, and *laterally* by the surgical neck of the humerus. The nerve ends by dividing into an anterior and a posterior branch.

The *anterior branch*, accompanied by the posterior circumflex humeral vessels, winds round the surgical neck of the humerus, deep to the deltoid, as far as the anterior border of the muscle, supplying it, and giving a few small cutaneous branches which pierce the muscle and ramify in the skin covering its lower part.

The *posterior branch* supplies the teres minor and the posterior part of the deltoid; upon the branch to the teres minor an oval enlargement (pseudoganglion) usually exists. The posterior branch pierces the deep fascia at the lower part of the posterior border of the deltoid and is continued as the *upper lateral cutaneous nerve of the arm*, which supplies the skin over the lower part of the deltoid and the skin covering the upper part of the long head of the triceps (7.201).

The trunk of the axillary nerve gives an articular filament which enters the shoulder joint below the subscapularis.

**The musculocutaneous nerve** (7.204) arises from the lateral cord of the brachial plexus, opposite the lower border of the pectoralis minor, its fibres being derived

[1064] J. H. Alexandre, O. Hamonet, P. Lacert and A. M. Moulin, *Archs. Anat. Path.*, **16**, 1968.

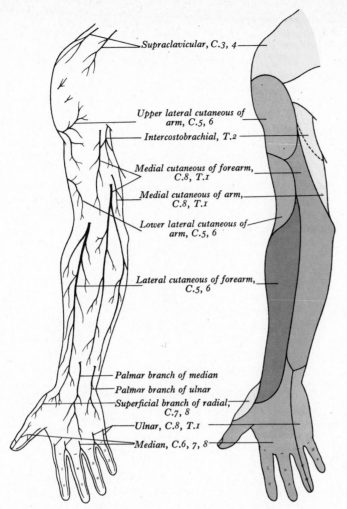

*Supraclavicular, C.3, 4*

*Upper lateral cutaneous of arm, C.5, 6*

*Intercostobrachial, T.2*

*Medial cutaneous of forearm, C.8, T.1*

*Medial cutaneous of arm, C.8, T.1*

*Lower lateral cutaneous of arm, C.5, 6*

*Lateral cutaneous of forearm, C.5, 6*

*Palmar branch of median*

*Palmar branch of ulnar*

*Superficial branch of radial; C.7, 8*

*Ulnar, C.8, T.1*

*Median, C.6, 7, 8*

7.201 The cutaneous nerves of the right upper limb, their areas of distribution and segmental origins, viewed from the anterior aspect.

from the fifth, sixth and seventh cervical nerves. It pierces the coracobrachialis and runs downwards and laterally between the biceps and the brachialis to reach the lateral side of the arm; a little beyond the elbow it pierces the deep fascia on the lateral side of the tendon of the biceps and is continued into the forearm as the *lateral cutaneous nerve of the forearm*. A line drawn distally from the lateral side of the third part of the axillary artery, and laterally across the elevations produced by the coracobrachialis and the biceps, to the lateral side of the biceps tendon of insertion, indicates the position of the musculocutaneous nerve relative to the surface; but variation in the point of entry of the nerve into the coracobrachialis may modify considerably its surface marking.[1065] In its course through the arm it supplies the coracobrachialis, both heads of the biceps and the greater part of the brachialis. The branch to the coracobrachialis leaves the musculocutaneous before that nerve enters the muscle; it receives its fibres from the seventh cervical nerve, and in some instances arises directly from the lateral cord of the brachial plexus. The branches to the biceps and brachialis leave the musculocutaneous nerve after it has pierced the coracobrachialis; that supplying the brachialis gives a filament to the elbow joint. The nerve also sends a small branch to the humerus; this branch enters the bone with the nutrient artery.

**The lateral cutaneous nerve of the forearm** (7.201) passes deep to the cephalic vein, and descends along the radial border of the forearm to the wrist. It supplies the skin over the lateral half of the anterior surface of the forearm and distributes branches which turn round the

radial border of the forearm to communicate with the posterior cutaneous nerve of the forearm and the terminal branch of the radial nerve. At the wrist joint it is placed in front of the radial artery, and some filaments, piercing the deep fascia, accompany that vessel to the dorsal surface of the carpus. The nerve then passes downwards to the base of the thenar eminence, where it ends in cutaneous filaments. It communicates with the terminal branch of the radial nerve, and with the palmar cutaneous branch of the median nerve.

The musculocutaneous nerve presents frequent variations. It may run behind the coracobrachialis or it may adhere for some distance to the median nerve and then pass behind the biceps instead of through the coracobrachialis. Some of the fibres of the median nerve may run for some distance in the musculocutaneous nerve and then leave it to join their proper trunk; less frequently the reverse is the case, and the median nerve sends a branch to join the musculocutaneous nerve. Occasionally it gives a filament to the pronator teres and, sometimes, it may replace the branches of the radial nerve to the dorsal surface of the thumb.

**The medial cutaneous nerve of the forearm** (7.204) arises from the medial cord of the brachial plexus. It is derived from the eighth cervical and first thoracic nerves, and at its commencement is placed between the axillary artery and vein. Near the axilla it supplies a filament which pierces the fascia and is distributed to the skin covering the biceps, almost as far as the elbow. The nerve then runs down the arm on the medial side of the brachial artery, pierces the deep fascia with the basilic vein about the middle of the arm, and divides into an anterior and a posterior branch.

The *anterior branch*, the larger, usually passes in front of, but occasionally behind, the median cubital vein. It then descends on the front of the medial side of the forearm, distributing filaments to the skin as far as the wrist, and communicating with the palmar cutaneous branch of the ulnar nerve (7.201).

The *posterior branch* passes obliquely downwards on the medial side of the basilic vein, in front of the medial epicondyle of the humerus, winds round to the back of the forearm, and descends on its medial side as far as the wrist, distributing filaments to the skin. It communicates with the medial cutaneous nerve of the arm, the posterior cutaneous nerve of the forearm, and the dorsal branch of the ulnar (7.202).

**The medial cutaneous nerve of the arm** is distributed to the skin on the medial side of the arm (7.201). It is the smallest branch of the brachial plexus, and, arising from the medial cord, receives its fibres from the eighth and first thoracic nerves. It passes through the axilla and crosses in front of, or behind, the axillary vein. It then runs on the medial side of this vein, and communicates with the intercostobrachial nerve. It descends along the medial side of the brachial artery and basilic vein (7.204) to the middle of the upper arm, where it pierces the deep fascia, and is distributed to the skin of the medial side of the distal third of the arm, extending on to its anterior and posterior aspects; some filaments reach the skin in front of the medial epicondyle and others over the olecranon. It communicates with the posterior branch of the medial cutaneous nerve of the forearm.

In some subjects the medial cutaneous nerve of the arm and the intercostobrachial nerve are connected by two or three filaments, which form a plexus in the axilla. In others the intercostobrachial nerve is large and may be reinforced by a part of the lateral cutaneous branch of the

---

[1065] M. Latarjet, J. H. Neidhart, A. Morrin and J.-M. Autissier, *C. r. Ass. Anat.*, **138**, 1967.

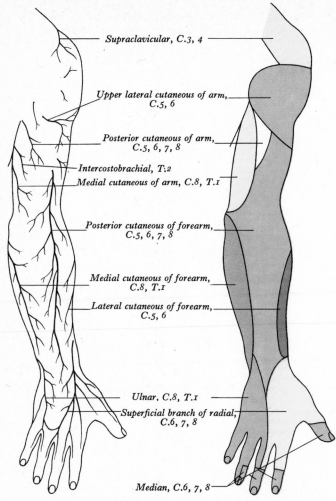

Supraclavicular, C.3, 4

Upper lateral cutaneous of arm, C.5, 6

Posterior cutaneous of arm, C.5, 6, 7, 8

Intercostobrachial, T.2

Medial cutaneous of arm, C.8, T.1

Posterior cutaneous of forearm, C.5, 6, 7, 8

Medial cutaneous of forearm, C.8, T.1

Lateral cutaneous of forearm, C.5, 6

Ulnar, C.8, T.1

Superficial branch of radial, C.6, 7, 8

Median, C.6, 7, 8

7.202  The cutaneous nerves of the right upper limb, their areas of distribution and segmental origins, viewed from the posterior aspect.

third intercostal nerve; it then takes the place of the medial brachial cutaneous nerve, receiving from the brachial plexus a communicating filament which represents the latter nerve; occasionally this filament is absent.

## THE MEDIAN NERVE

The median nerve (7.204) arises by two roots, one from the lateral cord, C. (5), 6, 7, and the other from the medial cord, C. 8, T. 1, of the brachial plexus; the roots embrace the third part of the axillary artery, uniting either in front, or on the lateral side, of the artery. Often some of the fibres derived from C. 7 leave the lateral root in the lower part of the axilla and pass distally and medially behind the medial root and usually in front of the axillary artery to join the ulnar nerve (7.220). These fibres from C. 7 may arise from the lateral cord or even directly from the seventh cervical nerve root of the brachial plexus. On clinical grounds they are believed to be mainly motor fibres to the flexor carpi ulnaris. If the lateral root is small, the musculocutaneous nerve (C. 5, 6, 7) sends a communicating branch to the median nerve in the arm. The median nerve descends into the arm, lying at first lateral to the brachial artery; about the level of insertion of the coracobrachialis it crosses in front of (rarely behind) the artery and descends on its medial side to the cubital fossa, where it lies behind the bicipital aponeurosis and in front of the brachialis, which separates it from the elbow joint. The nerve enters the forearm between the two heads of the pronator teres, crossing from the medial to the lateral side of the ulnar artery, but separated from it by the deep

head of the muscle. (The nerve has been observed to pass instead through the humeral fibres of this muscle.[1066]) It then passes deep to the tendinous bridge that connects the humero-ulnar to the radial head of the flexor digitorum superficialis and descends through the forearm deep to, and adherent to, the flexor digitorum superficialis, lying on the flexor digitorum profundus. About 5 cm above the flexor retinaculum it emerges from behind the lateral edge of the flexor digitorum superficialis and, becoming more superficial just above the wrist, it lies between the tendons of the flexor digitorum superficialis and the flexor carpi radialis, projecting laterally from under cover of the tendon of the palmaris longus (if present). The nerve then passes deep to the flexor retinaculum to gain the palm of the hand. In the forearm it is accompanied by the median branch of the anterior interosseous artery and its course can be represented on the surface by a line running approximately along the midline of the front of the forearm from the medial side of the end of the brachial artery in the cubital fossa (7.203).

### Branches of the Median Nerve in the Arm
These comprise vascular branches to the brachial artery and usually a branch to the pronator teres which is given off at a variable distance proximal to the elbow joint.

### Branches of the Median Nerve in the Forearm
These are muscular, articular, anterior interosseous, palmar cutaneous and communicating. The **muscular branches** are, with one exception, given off in the proximal part of the forearm (near the elbow) to the superficial flexor forearm muscles (except the flexor carpi ulnaris), namely, the pronator teres, flexor carpi radialis, palmaris longus and flexor digitorum superficialis. The branch of the median nerve supplying the part of the flexor digitorum superficialis that passes to the index finger arises near the middle of the forearm and it may be a branch of the anterior interosseous nerve. **Articular branches** arise from the median nerve at, or just distal to, the level of the elbow joint and supply this joint as well as the proximal radio-ulnar joint.

**The anterior interosseous nerve** is given off from the posterior surface of the median nerve as it passes between the two heads of the pronator teres and just distal to the origin of the branches of the median nerve to the superficial flexor forearm muscles described above. Accompanied by the anterior interosseous artery, it passes distally on the front of the interosseous membrane, between and deep to the flexor pollicis longus and the flexor digitorum profundus. It supplies a number of branches to these two muscles; those supplying the flexor digitorum profundus are limited to the lateral part of the muscle which sends tendons to the index and middle fingers. The nerve finally passes beneath the pronator quadratus, supplying a branch that enters its deep surface, and ends by supplying the distal radio-ulnar, radio-carpal and carpal joints.

**The palmar cutaneous branch** of the median nerve commences a short distance above the flexor retinaculum; it pierces the deep fascia or proximal edge of the retinaculum and divides into lateral branches which supply the skin over the thenar eminence and communicate with the lateral cutaneous nerve of the forearm, and medial branches which supply the skin of the central part of the palm and communicate with the palmar cutaneous branch of the ulnar nerve.

**The communicating branch** of the median nerve, which may take the form of a number of slender nerves, is frequently present. It arises from the median nerve (or

[1066] L. J. A. DiDio and J. G. Dangelo, Anat. Anz., 112, 1963.

sometimes its anterior interosseous branch) in the upper part of the forearm and passes distally and medially between the flexor digitorum superficialis and flexor digitorum profundus and behind the ulnar artery to join the ulnar nerve. This communication is of importance in relation to the anomalous nerve supply of certain hand muscles (p. 1044).

### The Median Nerve in the Hand

Just proximal to the flexor retinaculum, the nerve is lateral to the tendons of the flexor digitorum superficialis, but dorsal to the retinaculum it lies immediately deep to the

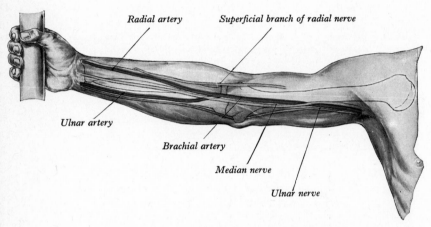

**7.203** The anterior aspect of the right upper limb, showing the position of the principal nerves and vessels projected on to the surface.

retinaculum and on the front of the tendons, in the limited space of the 'carpal tunnel' (*see* p. 1046), i.e. the space bounded in front by the retinaculum and behind by the anterior surfaces of the carpal bones; in certain circumstances the nerve may be compressed in this situation. (*See* carpal tunnel syndrome, p. 1046.) Immediately distal to the flexor retinaculum the nerve becomes enlarged and flattened and usually divides into five or six branches, though the exact mode and level of division of the nerve are variable.

**The muscular branch** is a short stout nerve that arises from the lateral side of the median nerve; it may be the first branch of the median nerve in the palm or it may arise as a terminal branch at the same level as the digital branches. It runs laterally, just distal to the flexor retinaculum, with a slight recurrent curve proximally, lying beneath the lateral portion of the palmar aponeurosis covering the thenar muscles. It winds round the distal border of the flexor retinaculum and comes to lie on the superficial surface of the flexor pollicis brevis, usually giving a branch to this surface of the muscle. It then continues on the superficial surface of the muscle, or it may pass through the muscle itself. It gives a branch to the abductor pollicis brevis, which enters the muscle at its medial edge, then passes deep to this muscle to supply the opponens pollicis, entering the muscle through its medial edge. Rarely, the terminal part of the nerve gives a branch to the first dorsal interosseous, which may be the sole or part nerve supply of this muscle.

The muscular branch may arise in the carpal tunnel and pierce the flexor retinaculum, a point of surgical importance.[1067]

**The palmar digital branches**—most frequently the median nerve divides into four or five digital branches, though it often at first divides into two divisions, a lateral, which provides the digital branches to the thumb and radial side of the index finger, and a medial, which supplies

the digital branches to the adjacent sides of the index, middle and ring fingers. Other variations in the mode of terminal branching of the nerve occur, as well as in the level in the hand at which the branching takes place. The arrangement of the digital nerves is commonly as follows. They pass distally, deep to the superficial palmar arch and its digital branches, lying at first in front of the long flexor tendons. Two proper palmar digital nerves, which may arise by a common stem, pass to the sides of the thumb, the one supplying its lateral side crossing in front of the tendon of the flexor pollicis longus. The proper palmar digital nerve to the lateral side of the index finger supplies a branch to the first lumbrical. Two common palmar digital nerves pass distally between the long flexor tendons, the lateral one dividing in the distal palm into two proper palmar digital nerves traversing the adjacent sides of the index and middle fingers, and the medial one dividing into two proper palmar digital nerves which supply the adjacent sides of the middle and ring fingers. The lateral common digital nerve gives a branch to the second lumbrical, and the medial one receives a communicating twig from the common palmar digital branch of the ulnar nerve and may supply a branch to the third lumbrical. In the distal part of the palm, the digital arteries pass deeply between the divisions of the digital nerves, so that on the sides of the digits the nerves lie immediately in front of the arteries. In most cases the median nerve supplies palmar cutaneous digital branches to the lateral three and one-half digits (thumb, index, middle and lateral side of the ring finger); in some cases the lateral side of the ring finger is supplied by the ulnar nerve. The proper palmar digital nerves that run along the medial side of the index finger, both sides of the middle finger and the lateral side of the ring finger, enter the bases of these digits in the fat between the slips into which the central portion of the palmar aponeurosis divides (p. 553). They pass, with the lumbricals and palmar digital arteries, dorsal to the superficial transverse metacarpal ligament (p. 554) and ventral to the deep transverse metacarpal ligament (p. 440). In the digits, the nerves run distally on the sides of the long flexor tendons, outside their fibrous sheaths, on the plane of the anterior surfaces of the phalanges, and immediately in front of the accompanying digital arteries. Each nerve gives off several branches to the skin on the front and sides of the digit, many of which end in lamellated corpuscles (p. 798), and branches to the metacarpophalangeal and interphalangeal joints. Branches are also supplied to the fibrous sheaths of the long flexor tendons, to the digital arteries (vasomotor), and to the sweat glands (secretomotor). A little beyond the base of the distal phalanx, the digital nerve gives off a branch passing dorsally to supply the nail bed, while the main nerve divides into branches supplying the skin of the terminal part of the digit and the pulp. Just beyond the base of the proximal phalanx, each *palmar* digital nerve gives off a dorsal branch that runs obliquely, distally and dorsally, to supply branches to the skin over the back of the middle and distal phalanges (**7.202**). The proper palmar digital nerves to the thumb and lateral side of the index finger run from beneath the lateral edge of the central part of the palmar aponeurosis, in company with the long flexor tendons to these digits, and in the digits themselves have the same arrangements as described above, but in the case of the thumb small branches from the distal part of the palmar digital nerves are given off to supply the skin on the back of the distal phalanx only.

In addition to the branches of the median nerve described above, variable vasomotor branches pass to supply the radial and ulnar arteries and their branches. Some of the

[1067] B. T. Papathanassion, *J. Bone Jt Surg.*, **50B**, 1968.

intercarpal, carpometacarpal and intermetacarpal joints are said to receive branches from the median nerve or its anterior interosseous branch, though the precise details of the origin and distribution of these branches are uncertain.

## THE ULNAR NERVE

The ulnar nerve (7.204) arises from the medial cord of the brachial plexus, C. 8, T. 1, though, as described above (p. 1041), it often receives fibres from the seventh cervical nerve. It runs distally through the axilla on the medial side of the axillary artery, intervening between it and the axillary vein, and continues distally on the medial side of the brachial artery as far as the middle of the arm. Here it pierces the medial intermuscular septum, and inclines medially, as it descends in front of the medial head of the triceps to the interval between the medial epicondyle and the olecranon, accompanied by the superior ulnar collateral artery. At the elbow it lies in a groove on the dorsum of the medial epicondyle, and as it enters the forearm between the two heads of the flexor carpi ulnaris, it lies on the posterior and oblique parts of the ulnar collateral ligament of the elbow joint. It descends along the medial side of the forearm, lying upon the flexor digitorum profundus; its upper half is covered by the flexor carpi ulnaris; its lower half lies on the lateral side of this muscle, and is covered by the skin and fasciae. In the upper one-third of the forearm, the ulnar nerve is separated from the ulnar artery by a considerable interval, but in the rest of its extent it lies close to the medial side of the vessel (7.204). About 5 cm above the wrist it gives off a dorsal branch, and it is then continued downwards into the hand, passing in front of the flexor retinaculum on the lateral side of the pisiform bone and lying medial to and somewhat behind the ulnar artery. In company with the artery the nerve passes behind the superficial part of the retinaculum and ends by dividing into a superficial and a deep terminal branch. Its relationship to the brachial artery in the arm and to the medial epicondyle at the elbow renders the nerve easy to map out in the upper part of its course; a line drawn from the medial epicondyle to the lateral edge of the pisiform bone represents its course through the forearm (7.203).

The branches of the ulnar nerve are: articular, muscular, palmar cutaneous, dorsal, superficial terminal and deep terminal.

**The articular branches** to the elbow joint are several small filaments which issue from the nerve as it lies between the medial epicondyle and olecranon. Other articular branches are described below.

**The muscular branches**, two in number, begin near the elbow; one supplies the flexor carpi ulnaris (see p. 1041), the other, the medial half of the flexor digitorum profundus.

**The palmar cutaneous branch** arises about the middle of the forearm, and descends on the ulnar artery (7.204), giving some filaments to the vessel. It perforates the deep fascia and ends in the skin of the palm, after communicating with the palmar branch of the median nerve. It sometimes supplies the palmaris brevis.

**The dorsal branch** arises about 5 cm above the wrist; it passes distally and backwards deep to the flexor carpi ulnaris, perforates the deep fascia, and, running along the medial side of the back of the wrist and hand, divides into two, frequently three, dorsal digital nerves: one supplies the medial side of the little finger; the second the adjacent sides of the little and ring fingers. The third, when present, supplies the adjoining sides of the ring and middle fingers, but it may be replaced, wholly or partially, by a branch of the radial nerve, with which it always communicates on the dorsum of the hand (7.202). In the little finger the

dorsal digital nerves extend only as far as the base of the distal phalanx, and in the ring finger as far as the base of the middle phalanx; the more distal parts of these digits are supplied by dorsal branches derived from the proper digital branches of the ulnar and—on the lateral side of the ring finger—median nerves.

**The superficial terminal branch** supplies the palmaris brevis and the skin on the medial side of the hand, and divides into two palmar digital nerves, which can be compressed against the hook of the hamate bone (p. 339). One of these palmar digital nerves supplies the medial side of the little finger; the other (a common palmar digital nerve) sends a twig to join the median

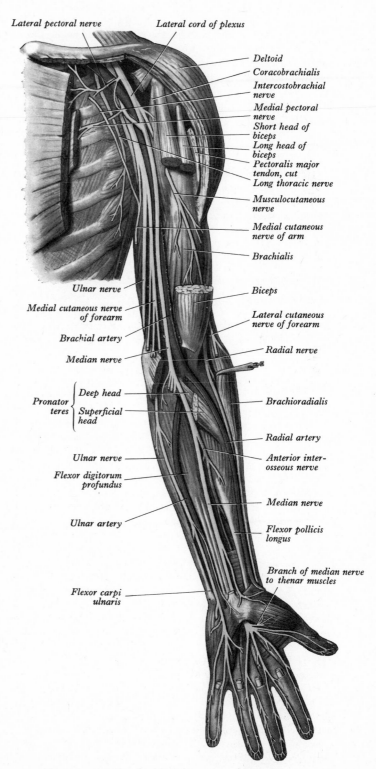

Lateral pectoral nerve    Lateral cord of plexus

Deltoid
Coracobrachialis
Intercostobrachial nerve
Medial pectoral nerve
Short head of biceps
Long head of biceps
Pectoralis major tendon, cut
Long thoracic nerve
Musculocutaneous nerve
Medial cutaneous nerve of arm
Brachialis

Ulnar nerve
Medial cutaneous nerve of forearm
Brachial artery
Median nerve

Biceps
Lateral cutaneous nerve of forearm
Radial nerve

Pronator teres { Deep head / Superficial head
Brachioradialis

Radial artery
Ulnar nerve
Flexor digitorum profundus
Anterior interosseous nerve

Median nerve

Ulnar artery
Flexor pollicis longus

Branch of median nerve to thenar muscles
Flexor carpi ulnaris

**7.204** The nerves of the left upper limb dissected from the anterior aspect.

1043

nerve and then divides into two proper digital nerves for the adjoining sides of the little and ring fingers (7.204). The proper digital branches are distributed to the fingers in the same manner as those of the median nerve.

**The deep terminal branch**, accompanied by the deep branch of the ulnar artery, passes between the abductor digiti minimi and flexor digiti minimi; it then perforates the opponens digiti minimi and follows the course of the deep palmar arch behind the flexor tendons. At its origin it supplies the three short muscles of the little finger. As it crosses the hand, it gives branches to the interossei and to the third and fourth lumbricals; it ends by supplying the adductor pollicis, the first palmar interosseous and, in most cases (p. 556), the flexor pollicis brevis. It also sends articular filaments to the wrist joint.

It has been pointed out that the medial part of the flexor digitorum profundus is supplied by the ulnar nerve; the third and fourth lumbricals which are connected with the tendons of this part of the muscle, are supplied by the same nerve. In like manner the lateral part of the flexor digitorum profundus and the first and second lumbricals are supplied by the median nerve. The third lumbrical frequently receives an additional twig from the median nerve.

The deep terminal branch of the ulnar nerve is said to give branches to some of the intercarpal, carpometacarpal and intermetacarpal joints, though, as in the case of the median nerve, the precise details of the origin and distribution of these branches are uncertain. Vascular (vasomotor) branches are given off from the ulnar nerve in the forearm and hand to supply the ulnar artery and the palmar arteries.

### Anomalous Nerve Supply of Hand Muscles

The nerve supply to the short thenar muscles (flexor pollicis brevis, abductor pollicis brevis and opponens pollicis) is subject to considerable variation. From a study of the results of lesions of the median and ulnar nerves in the forearm,[1068, 1069] the following variations have been deduced, expressed here in percentages of 226 hands examined, relating to the innervation of these thenar muscles by the median nerve, the ulnar nerve or both nerves: flexor pollicis brevis—median 36, ulnar 48, both nerves 17; abductor pollicis brevis—median 95, ulnar 2·5, both nerves 2; opponens pollicis—median 83, ulnar 9, both nerves 7·5. The usual description of the nerve supply to these muscles is that they are all supplied by the median nerve; the results of the investigations cited are probably to be explained by the variable connexions between the median and ulnar nerves in the axilla, arm or forearm, whereby truly median nerve fibres are aberrantly conveyed distally in the ulnar nerve to these muscles.

An arcuate connecting loop has long been known to occur between the median and ulnar nerves in the substance of the flexor pollicis brevis,[1070] either part of which, superficial or deep, may be supplied by fibres from both nerves. In a recent survey[1071] of the considerable literature on this topic, results of dissections of 35 hands showed a loop in 77 per cent of individuals, indicating that it should be a feature of 'normal' description.

Clinically these variations are important in that even with a complete lesion of the median nerve some of these muscles may not be paralysed, and this may lead to the erroneous conclusion that the median nerve has not suffered a complete lesion. Clinical evidence reveals that the short muscles of the thumb, whether apparently supplied by the median or ulnar nerves, receive their segmental supply from the eighth cervical and first thoracic segments of the spinal cord.

## THE RADIAL NERVE

The radial nerve (7.205) arises from the posterior cord of the brachial plexus, C. 5, 6, 7, 8; T. 1. It is the largest branch of the brachial plexus, and it descends behind the third part of the axillary artery and the upper part of the brachial artery, and in front of the subscapularis and the tendons of the latissimus dorsi and teres major. Accompanied by the arteria profunda brachii and, later, its radial collateral branch, it inclines dorsally between the long and medial heads of the triceps. From here it passes obliquely across the back of the humerus, first between the lateral and medial heads of the triceps and then in a shallow groove deep to the lateral head of the triceps muscle. On reaching the lateral side of the humerus it pierces the lateral intermuscular septum and enters the anterior compartment of the arm. It then descends, lying deeply in the intermuscular furrow, which is bounded on the medial side by the brachialis and on the lateral side by the brachioradialis, above, and the extensor carpi radialis longus, below. On reaching the front of the lateral epicondyle, it divides into terminal rami, *superficial* and *deep*.

In the arm the radial nerve is indicated by a line drawn from the commencement of the brachial artery and carried distally and laterally across the elevations produced by the long and the lateral heads of the triceps to the junction of the upper and middle thirds of a line joining the lateral epicondyle to the deltoid tuberosity. The line of the nerve is then continued on the anterior aspect of the arm to the level of the lateral epicondyle, where it lies 1 cm or less to the lateral side of the biceps tendon.

The branches of the radial nerve are: muscular, cutaneous, articular and superficial and deep terminal branches.

**The muscular branches of the radial nerve** supply the triceps, anconeus, brachioradialis, extensor carpi radialis longus and brachialis, and are grouped as *medial*, *posterior* and *lateral*.

The *medial* muscular branches arise from the radial nerve on the medial side of the arm and supply the medial and long heads of the triceps; the branch to the medial head is a long, slender filament, which lies close to the ulnar nerve as far as the distal third of the arm, and is therefore frequently named the *ulnar collateral nerve*.

The *posterior* muscular branch, of large size, arises from the nerve as it lies in the groove. It divides into filaments which supply the medial and lateral heads of the triceps and the anconeus. The branch for the latter muscle is a long nerve which descends in the substance of the medial head of the triceps, and gives numerous branches to it. It is accompanied by the middle collateral branch of the arteria profunda brachii, and passes behind the elbow joint to end in the anconeus.

The *lateral* muscular branches arise from the nerve as it lies in front of the lateral intermuscular septum; they supply the lateral part of the brachialis, the brachioradialis, and the extensor carpi radialis longus.

**The cutaneous branches of the radial nerve** are the posterior cutaneous and the lower lateral cutaneous nerves of the arm and the posterior cutaneous nerve of the forearm.

**The posterior cutaneous nerve of the arm**, of small size, arises in the axilla and passes to the medial side of the arm to supply the skin on its dorsal surface nearly

[1068] T. Rowntree, *J. Bone Jt Surg.*, **31B**, 1949.
[1069] M. H. Day and J. R. Napier, *J. Anat.*, **95**, 1961.
[1070] A. Cannieu, *J. Méd. Bordeaux*, 1886.
[1071] D. Harness and E. Sekeles, *J. Anat.*, **109**, 1971.

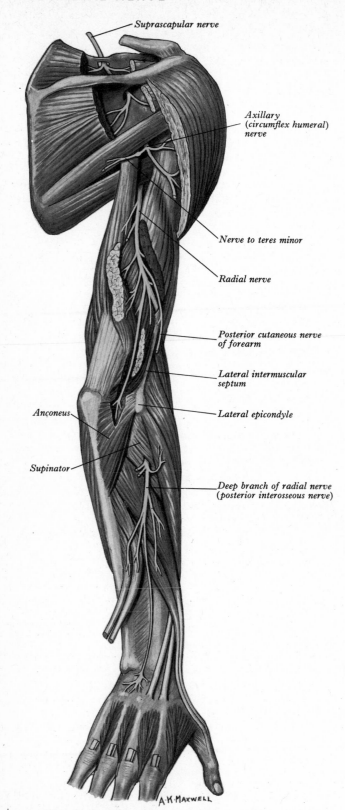

*Suprascapular nerve*

*Axillary (circumflex humeral) nerve*

*Nerve to teres minor*

*Radial nerve*

*Posterior cutaneous nerve of forearm*

*Lateral intermuscular septum*

*Anconeus*

*Lateral epicondyle*

*Supinator*

*Deep branch of radial nerve (posterior interosseous nerve)*

A·K·MAXWELL

**7.205** The suprascapular, axillary and radial nerves of the right upper limb, dissected from the posterior aspect.

as far as the olecranon. It crosses posterior to, and communicates with, the intercostobrachial nerve.

**The lower lateral cutaneous nerve of the arm** perforates the lateral head of the triceps just below the insertion of the deltoid. It then passes to the front of the elbow, lying close to the cephalic vein, and supplies the skin of the lateral part of the lower half of the arm (7.201).

**The posterior cutaneous nerve of the forearm** arises in common with the preceding branch. Perforating the lateral head of the triceps, it descends along the lateral side of the arm, and then along the dorsum of the forearm

to the wrist, supplying the skin in its course, and joining, near its termination, with dorsal branches of the lateral cutaneous nerve of the forearm (7.201).

**The articular branches of the radial nerve** are distributed to the elbow joint.

**The superficial terminal branch** descends from the front of the lateral epicondyle along the front of the lateral side of the upper two-thirds of the forearm, lying at first upon the supinator, lateral to the radial artery and behind the brachioradialis. In the middle third of the forearm it lies behind the brachioradialis, but is now close to the lateral side of the artery. Here it lies first on the pronator teres, next on the radial head of the flexor digitorum superficialis and then on the flexor pollicis longus. It quits the artery about 7 cm above the wrist, passes deep to the tendon of the brachioradialis and, winding round the lateral side of the radius as it descends, pierces the deep fascia and divides into five, sometimes four, dorsal digital nerves.

**The dorsal digital nerves** are small and four or five in number. The first supplies the skin of the radial side of the thumb and the adjoining part of the thenar eminence, communicating with branches of the lateral cutaneous nerve of the forearm; the second supplies the medial side of the thumb; the third, the lateral side of the index finger; the fourth, the adjoining sides of the index and middle fingers; the fifth communicates with a filament from the dorsal branch of the ulnar nerve and supplies the adjoining sides of the middle and ring fingers, but it is frequently replaced by the dorsal branch of the ulnar nerve. On the dorsum of the hand the superficial branch of the radial nerve usually communicates with the posterior and lateral cutaneous nerves of the forearm. The digital nerves to the thumb reach only as far as the root of the nail; those to the index finger as far as the middle of the middle phalanx and those to the middle and ring fingers not farther than the proximal interphalangeal joints. The remaining distal areas of skin on the dorsal surface of these digits are supplied by the palmar digital branches of the median and ulnar nerves (7.202). The superficial radial nerve may supply the whole of the dorsum of the hand; for this and other variations consult footnote reference [1072].

**The deep terminal branch (posterior interosseous nerve)** (7.205) winds to the back of the forearm round the lateral side of the radius between the two planes of fibres of the supinator. It gives a branch to the extensor carpi radialis brevis, and another to the supinator before it enters the latter muscle, and as it traverses its substance it supplies additional branches to it. The branch to the extensor carpi radialis brevis may spring from the commencement of the superficial branch of the radial nerve. As soon as it emerges from the supinator on the back of the forearm the deep branch of the radial nerve gives off three short branches—to the extensor digitorum, extensor digiti minimi and extensor carpi ulnaris—and two long branches—a *medial* to the extensor pollicis longus and the extensor indicis, and a *lateral*, which supplies the abductor pollicis longus and ends in the extensor pollicis brevis. The nerve lies at first between the superficial and the deep muscles of the back of the forearm, but, at the distal border of the extensor pollicis brevis, it passes deep to the extensor pollicis longus and, diminished to a fine thread, runs down on the dorsal aspect of the interosseous membrane of the forearm. Finally it reaches the dorsum of the carpus, where it presents a flattened and somewhat expanded termination ('pseudoganglion') from which filaments are distributed to the ligaments and articulations of the carpus (7.205).

---

[1072] Y. Sayfi, *Archs Anat. Path.*, **15**, 1967.

*Articular branches* from the deep branch of the radial nerve are distributed to the carpal and distal radio-ulnar joints and to some of the intercarpal and intermetacarpal joints, while the digital branches of the radial nerve supply branches to the metacarpophalangeal and proximal interphalangeal joints of the appropriate digits.

*Applied Anatomy.* The brachial plexus may be injured by falls from a height on to the side of the head and shoulder, whereby the nerves of the plexus are violently stretched; the upper trunk of the plexus sustains the greatest injury, and the subsequent paralysis may be confined to the muscles supplied by the fifth nerve—the deltoid, biceps, brachialis and brachioradialis, with sometimes the supraspinatus, infraspinatus and supinator. The position of the limb, under such conditions, is characteristic: the arm hangs by the side and is rotated medially; the forearm is extended and pronated. The arm cannot be raised from the side; all power of flexion of the elbow is lost, as is also supination of the forearm. This is known as *Erb's paralysis*, and a very similar condition is occasionally met with in newborn children, either from injury to the upper trunk from the pressure of the forceps used in effecting delivery, or from traction of the head in breech presentations. A second variety of partial palsy of the brachial plexus is known as *Klumpke's paralysis*. In this it is the eighth cervical and first thoracic nerves that are injured, either before or after they have joined to form the lower trunk. The subsequent paralysis affects, principally, the intrinsic muscles of the hand and the flexors of the wrist and fingers.

The brachial plexus may also be injured by direct violence or gunshot wounds, by violent traction on the arm, or by efforts at reducing a dislocation of the shoulder joint; the amount of paralysis will depend upon the amount of injury to the constituent nerves. When the entire plexus is involved, the whole of the upper extremity will be paralysed and anaesthetic. In some cases the injury appears to be rather a tearing away of the roots of the nerves from the spinal cord than a rupture of the nerves themselves, and where this involves the first thoracic nerve the pupil on the same side may be constricted, on account of damage to the preganglionic fibres emerging in it to supply the dilatator pupillae. The brachial plexus in the axilla is often damaged from the pressure of a crutch, producing the condition known as 'crutch paralysis'. In these cases the radial is the nerve most frequently implicated; the ulnar nerve suffers next in frequency. The median and radial nerves often suffer from 'sleep palsies', paralysis from pressure coming on while the patient is profoundly asleep under the influence of alcohol or some narcotic.

Paralysis of the long thoracic nerve throws the serratus anterior out of action, and may occur in porters who have to carry heavy weights on the shoulder, for the nerve is exposed to injury as it lies in the posterior triangle of the neck. The inferior angle of the scapula is drawn towards the median plane, by the unopposed action of the rhomboids and levator scapulae, and tends to project backwards ('winging' of the scapula) when the arm is held horizontally forwards or when forward pushing movements are attempted against resistance. The arm cannot be raised above the horizontal unless the inferior angle of the scapula is pushed anterolaterally for the patient.

The *axillary* (*circumflex humeral*) nerve, on account of its course round the surgical neck of the humerus, is liable to be injured in fractures of this part of the bone, and in dislocations of the shoulder joint; paralysis of the deltoid, and anaesthesia of the skin over the lower part of that muscle, result. Paralysis of the deltoid renders effective abduction of the arm impossible. The associated paralysis of the teres minor is not easily demonstrated.

The *median nerve* is liable to injury in wounds of the forearm. When it is completely divided proximal to its muscular and anterior interosseous branches, there is loss of flexion of the second phalanges of all the fingers, and of the terminal phalanges of the index and middle fingers. Flexion of the terminal phalanges of the ring and little fingers is effected by the section of the flexor digitorum profundus which is supplied by the ulnar nerve. There is power to flex the proximal phalanges through the interossei. The thumb cannot be opposed or abducted, nor can it be flexed at the interphalangeal joint (*see* p. 1042), and it is maintained in a position of extension and adduction. There is loss in the power of pronating the forearm; the brachioradialis has the power of bringing the forearm into a position of mid-pronation, but beyond this no further pronation can be effected. The wrist can be flexed by the flexor carpi ulnaris, but flexion is combined with adduction of the hand. There is loss or impairment of sensation on the palmar surfaces of the thumb, index, middle, and radial half of the ring fingers, and on the dorsal surfaces of the same fingers over the last two phalanges, except in the thumb, where the loss of sensation is limited to the back of the distal phalanx. Owing to the paralysis of the short muscles of the thumb and the unapposed action of the extensor pollicis longus, an 'ape-like' hand is produced. Injury of the nerve just above the middle of the forearm may result only in weakness of flexion of the index finger ('*pointing*' index finger), since the branch to the part of the flexor digitorum superficialis distributed to that finger arises at about the middle of the forearm (p. 1041). More commonly, however, the nerve is injured proximal to the flexor retinaculum, when the power of flexion of the fingers and pronation of the forearm remains intact, unless the flexor tendons are also divided. The chief effect of lesions here is usually inability to oppose the thumb, though the intact abductor pollicis longus and adductor pollicis may combine to imitate this action. As it lies deep to the flexor retinaculum, the median nerve is situated in the restricted space (carpal tunnel or carpal canal) between the retinaculum and the carpal bones. Any pathological condition which diminishes the size of this tunnel (e.g. carpal dislocation or arthritis, tenosynovitis of the long flexor tendons, etc.) will cause pressure on the nerve with resultant pain and slight sensory impairment in the digits supplied by the nerve and sometimes slight wasting of the thenar muscles, these clinical features constituting the '*carpal tunnel syndrome*'. Most commonly there is no apparent cause for this syndrome and, in any case, complete division of the retinaculum is curative.

The *ulnar nerve* is also liable to be injured in wounds of the forearm. The commonest cause of complete or partial ulnar nerve lesion is injury to the nerve as it lies behind the medial humeral epicondyle. Such injury leads to impaired power of adduction, and, upon an attempt being made to flex the wrist, the hand is drawn to the radial side by the flexor carpi radialis; there is inability to spread out the fingers owing to paralysis of the dorsal interossei, and for the same reason the fingers, especially the ring and little fingers, cannot be flexed at the metacarpophalangeal joints or extended at the interphalangeal joints, and the hand assumes a claw shape from the action of the opposing muscles; there is loss of power of flexion in the fourth and fifth digits; and there is inability to adduct the thumb. The muscles of the hypothenar eminence become wasted. Sensation is lost, or impaired, in the skin supplied by the nerve.

The *radial nerve* also is frequently injured. In consequence of its close relationship to the humerus, it may be injured, but is seldom torn, in fractures of this bone. Callus formation in repair of the fracture seldom interferes with the function of the nerve. In fractures of the middle part of the humerus, the triceps is not paralysed, since its supplying nerves arise from the radial nerve more proximally. It is also liable to be contused against the bone by kicks or blows, or to be divided in wounds of the arm. When paralysed, the hand is flexed at the wrist and lies flaccid. This is known as *wrist drop.* The fingers are also flexed, and when an attempt is made to extend them, the last two phalanges only will be extended, through the action of the lumbrical and interosseous muscles; the first phalanges remain flexed. Extension of the wrist is impossible. Supination is completely lost when the forearm is extended on the arm, but is possible to a certain extent if the forearm be flexed to allow effective action of the biceps. The power of extension of the forearm is lost on account of paralysis of the triceps, if the injury to the nerve has taken place near its origin. As the radial nerve has only a very small area of exclusive supply, the extent of the anaesthesia associated with even severe injuries to it is surprisingly small and is confined to a limited region on the lateral part of the dorsum of the hand.

Dislocations and epiphyseal separations of the elbow and supracondylar fractures of the humerus in children frequently lead to ulnar, median or posterior interosseous injury.

# THORACIC VENTRAL RAMI

The ventral rami of the thoracic nerves (7.206, 207) are twelve in number on each side. The upper eleven lie between the ribs (*intercostal nerves*), while the twelfth lies below the last rib (*subcostal nerve*). Each nerve is connected with the adjoining ganglion of the sympathetic trunk by grey and white rami communicantes: the grey ramus joins the nerve proximal to the point at which the white ramus leaves it. The intercostal nerves are distributed chiefly to the thoracic and abdominal walls. The first two nerves supply fibres to the upper limb in addition to their thoracic branches; the next four are limited in their distribution to the thoracic wall; the lower five supply the thoracic and abdominal walls (p. 1048); the subcostal nerve is distributed to the abdominal wall and the gluteal skin. Communicating branches link the intercostal nerves to one another in the posterior parts of the intercostal spaces and, in addition, the lower five communicate freely as they traverse the abdominal wall.[1073]

### The 1st to 6th Thoracic Nerves

The ventral ramus of the first thoracic nerve divides into a large and a small branch. The large branch ascends in front of the neck of the first rib on the lateral side of the superior intercostal artery, and enters the brachial plexus (p. 1037). The small branch is the *first intercostal nerve*; it runs along the first intercostal space, and ends on the front of the chest as the first anterior cutaneous nerve of the thorax. It furnishes a lateral cutaneous branch which pierces the chest wall in front of the serratus anterior and supplies the skin of the axilla; it may communicate with the intercostobrachial nerve and sometimes join the medial cutaneous nerve of the arm.[1074] The first thoracic nerve frequently receives a connecting ramus from the second; this twig ascends in front of the neck of the second rib.

The ventral rami of the second, third, fourth, fifth and sixth thoracic spinal nerves pass forwards (7.201) in the intercostal spaces below the intercostal vessels. At the back of the chest they lie between the pleura and the posterior intercostal membranes, but in most of their course they run between the internal intercostals and the subcostales and intercostales intimi (7.207). Near the sternum, they cross in front of the internal thoracic artery and transversus thoracis, pierce the internal intercostals, the external intercostal membranes, and the pectoralis major, and their terminal branches form the **anterior cutaneous nerves of the thorax**; they supply the skin of the front of the thorax; the anterior cutaneous branch of the second nerve may be connected to the medial supraclavicular nerves of the cervical plexus. Twigs from the anterior cutaneous branch of the sixth intercostal nerve supply the abdominal skin in the upper part of the infrasternal angle.

*Branches.* Numerous slender muscular filaments supply the intercostals, the serratus posterior superior, and the transversus thoracis. At the front of the thorax some of these branches cross the costal cartilages from one intercostal space to another.

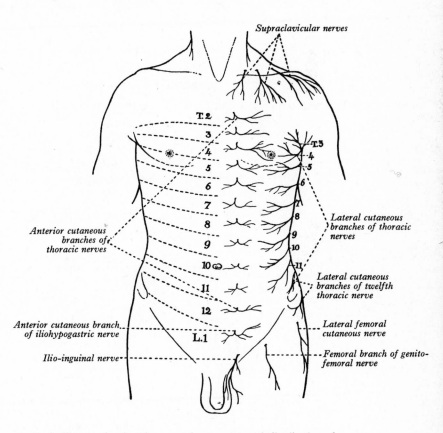

7.206 A diagram showing the approximate segmental distribution of the cutaneous nerves on the front of the trunk. The contribution from the first thoracic spinal nerve is not shown, and the considerable overlap which occurs between adjacent segments is not indicated. For the latter see 7.221.

Each intercostal nerve gives off a collateral and a lateral cutaneous branch before it reaches the angle of adjoining ribs. The *collateral branch* follows the caudal border of the space in the same intermuscular interval as the main trunk, which it may rejoin before it is distributed as an additional anterior cutaneous nerve. The *lateral cutaneous branch* accompanies the main trunk for a time and then pierces the intercostal muscles obliquely. With

[1073] F. Davies, R. J. Gladstone and E. P. Stibbe, *J. Anat.*, **66**, 1932.
[1074] A. J. E. Cave, *J. Anat.*, **63**, 1929.

the exception of the lateral cutaneous branches of the first and second intercostal nerves, each divides into anterior and posterior branches, which subsequently pierce the serratus anterior. The *anterior branches* run forwards over the border of the pectoralis major and supply twigs to the overlying skin; those of the fifth and sixth nerves supply twigs to the upper digitations of the external oblique. The *posterior branches* run backwards, and supply the skin over the scapula and latissimus dorsi.

The lateral cutaneous branch of the second intercostal nerve is named the *intercostobrachial nerve* (7.204). It crosses the axilla to gain the medial side of the arm, and joins with a filament from the medial cutaneous nerve of the arm. It then pierces the deep fascia of the arm, and supplies the skin of the upper half of the medial and posterior parts of the arm, communicating with the posterior brachial cutaneous branch of the radial nerve. The size of the intercostobrachial nerve is in inverse proportion to that of the medial brachial cutaneous nerve. A second intercostobrachial nerve is frequently given off from the anterior part of the lateral cutaneous branch of the third intercostal nerve; it supplies filaments to the axilla and to the medial side of the arm.

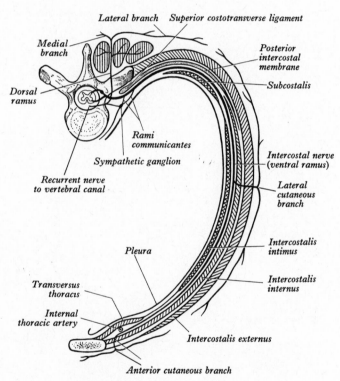

**7.207**  A diagram of the course of a typical intercostal nerve. The muscular and the collateral branches are not shown.

### The 7th to 12th Thoracic Nerves

The ventral rami of the seventh, eighth, ninth, tenth and eleventh thoracic nerves are continued anteriorly from the intercostal spaces into the abdominal wall.

As they approach the anterior ends of the spaces in which they lie, the seventh and eighth nerves curve *upwards* and medially across the deep surface of the costal margin, insinuating themselves between the digitations of the transversus abdominis to gain the deep aspect of the posterior lamella of the aponeurosis of the internal oblique. Having pierced this layer, they lie behind the rectus abdominis and continue upwards and medially (7.208) for a short distance parallel with the costal margin. Both supply the rectus abdominis and, having passed through the muscle near its lateral edge, pierce the anterior wall of

its sheath, to reach and supply the skin. It will be observed that both the seventh and the eighth intercostal nerves cross the costal margin medial to the lateral border of the rectus abdominis and therefore enter its sheath by piercing its posterior wall.

The ninth, tenth and eleventh intercostal nerves pass between the digitations of the diaphragm and transversus abdominis to gain the interval between the latter muscle and the internal oblique. In this intermuscular interval the ninth nerve runs almost *horizontally*, but the tenth and eleventh nerves are inclined caudally and medially. When they reach the lateral edge of the rectus abdominis, they pierce the posterior lamella of the internal oblique aponeurosis and pass behind the muscle. They end like the terminal branches of the seventh and eighth intercostal nerves. The tenth nerve supplies the band of skin which includes the umbilicus (7.206, 221).

The lower intercostal nerves supply the intercostal, the subcostal and the abdominal muscles, and the last three send branches to the serratus posterior inferior. They also supply sensory fibres to the costal part of the diaphragm and the related parietal pleura and peritoneum. Like the upper intercostal nerves the lower intercostal nerves give off *collateral* and *lateral cutaneous branches* before they reach the angles of the ribs. The collateral branch may rejoin the main trunk, but, if it does so, it leaves it again near the lateral border of the rectus abdominis and runs forwards below it (7.208). It pierces the muscle and the anterior wall of its sheath near the linea alba and supplies the skin. The lateral cutaneous branches pierce the intercostals and the external oblique, in the same line as the lateral cutaneous branches of the upper thoracic nerves, and divide into anterior and posterior branches, which are distributed to the skin of the abdomen and back respectively; the anterior branches also supply twigs to the digitations of the external oblique, and extend downwards and forwards nearly as far as the margin of the rectus abdominis; the posterior branches pass backwards to supply the skin over the latissimus dorsi. Each lateral cutaneous branch descends as it pierces the external oblique and the superficial fascia so that it reaches the skin on a level with the corresponding anterior cutaneous branch and the cutaneous branch of the corresponding dorsal ramus (p. 1033 and 7.196).

The ventral ramus of the **twelfth thoracic nerve** (subcostal nerve) is larger than the others, and gives a communicating branch to the first lumbar nerve (sometimes termed the *dorsolumbar nerve*). Like the intercostal nerves it soon gives off a collateral branch. It accompanies the subcostal artery along the lower border of the twelfth rib and passes behind the lateral lumbocostal arch. It then runs behind the kidney (8.148), and in front of the upper part of the quadratus lumborum, perforates the aponeurosis of origin of the transversus and passes forwards between that muscle and the obliquus internus, to be distributed in the same manner as the lower intercostal nerves. It communicates with the iliohypogastric nerve of the lumbar plexus, and gives a branch to the pyramidalis. The *lateral cutaneous branch* of the twelfth thoracic nerve pierces the internal and external oblique muscles, gives a twig to the lowest slip of the latter, descends over the iliac crest about 5 cm behind the anterior superior iliac spine (7.215), and is distributed to the skin of the front part of the gluteal region, some filaments reaching as low as the greater trochanter of the femur.

*Applied Anatomy.* In many diseases affecting the nerve trunks at or near their origins, the pain is referred to their peripheral terminations. Thus, in tuberculosis of thoracic vertebrae, patients often suffer from pain in the abdominal wall. When confined to a single pair of nerves the sensation complained of is often a feeling of constriction, as if a cord were tied round the abdomen, and in these cases the situation of the sense of constriction may serve to localize the disease in the vertebral column. Where the bone disease is more extensive and two or more nerves are involved, a more general, diffused pain in the abdomen is felt.

Again, it must be borne in mind that the nerves which supply the skin of the abdomen supply also the planes of abdominal contents. The importance, therefore, of immediate reflex contraction upon the receipt of an injury cannot be overestimated, and the origin of the cutaneous and motor fibres from the same segments of the spinal cord results in a much more rapid response on the part of the muscles to any peripheral stimulation of the cutaneous filaments than would be the case if the two sets of fibres were derived from independent sources.

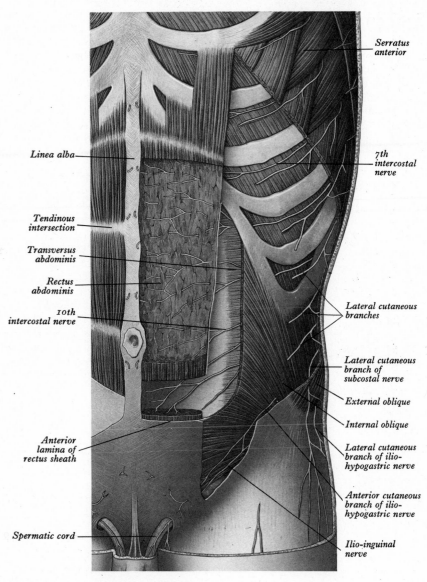

7.208   Diagram to illustrate the course of the lower intercostal and the cutaneous branches of some lumbar nerves. Portions of the muscles of the anterior abdominal wall have been removed, including most of the anterior layer of the rectus sheath and parts of the rectus abdominis.

muscle which constitute the greater part of the abdominal wall, and this is of importance in protecting the abdominal viscera from injury. A blow on the abdomen, even of considerable force, will do no injury to the viscera if the muscles are in a condition of firm contraction; whereas in cases where the muscles have been taken unawares, and the blow has been struck while they were in a state of rest, an injury insufficient to produce any lesion of the abdominal wall has been attended with rupture of some of the

The nerves supplying the abdominal muscles and skin, derived from the lower intercostal nerves, are intimately connected with the sympathetic nerves supplying the abdominal viscera through the lower thoracic ganglia, from which the splanchnic nerves are derived. In consequence of this, in laceration of the abdominal viscera, and in acute peritonitis, the muscles of the belly wall become firmly contracted, and thus as far as possible preserve the abdominal contents in a condition of rest.

The ventral rami of the lumbar nerves increase in size from the first to the last. They are joined, near their origins, by grey rami communicantes from the lumbar ganglia of the sympathetic trunk. These rami consist of long, slender branches which accompany the lumbar arteries round the sides of the vertebral bodies, under cover of the psoas major. Their arrangement is somewhat irregular: one ganglion may give rami to two lumbar nerves, or one lumbar nerve may receive rami from two ganglia: not infrequently the rami leave the sympathetic trunk between two ganglia. The first and second, and sometimes the third, lumbar nerves are each connected with the lumbar part of the sympathetic trunk by a *white ramus communicans*.

The ventral rami of the lumbar nerves pass downwards and laterally into the psoas major. The first three nerves and the greater part of the fourth form the *lumbar plexus*.

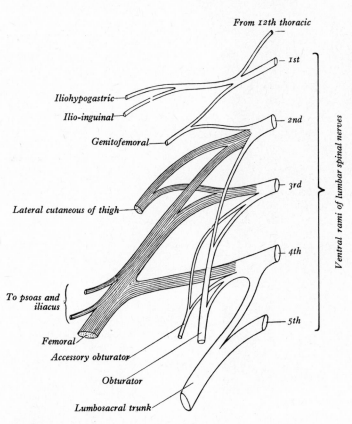

Iliohypogastric
Ilio-inguinal
Genitofemoral
Lateral cutaneous of thigh
To psoas and iliacus
Femoral
Accessory obturator
Obturator
Lumbosacral trunk

*From 12th thoracic*
— 1st
— 2nd
— 3rd
— 4th
— 5th

Ventral rami of lumbar spinal nerves

**7.209** A plan of the lumbar plexus. The *dorsal divisions* of the second, third and fourth lumbar nerves are shaded.

The smaller part of the fourth nerve joins with the fifth to form the *lumbosacral trunk*, which assists in the formation of the *sacral* plexus. The fourth nerve is often termed the *nervus furcalis*, from the fact that it is subdivided between the two plexuses. In most cases the fourth lumbar is the nervus furcalis but this arrangement is frequently departed from. The third is occasionally the lowest nerve which enters the lumbar plexus giving at the same time some fibres to the sacral plexus, and thus forming the nervus furcalis; or both the third and fourth may be furcal nerves. When this occurs, the plexus is termed *high* or *prefixed*. More frequently the fifth nerve is divided between the lumbar and sacral plexuses, and constitutes the nervus furcalis; and when this takes place, the plexus is

distinguished as a *low* or *postfixed* plexus. These variations necessarily produce corresponding modifications in the sacral plexus.

## The Lumbar Plexus

The lumbar plexus (7.209, 210) lies within the posterior part of the psoas major, in front of the transverse processes of the lumbar vertebrae; it is formed by the ventral rami of the first three lumbar nerves and the greater part of the ventral ramus of the fourth; the first lumbar nerve receives a branch from the last thoracic nerve.

Its arrangement varies in different subjects, but the usual condition is the following. The first lumbar nerve, supplemented by a twig from the last thoracic, splits into an upper and a lower branch; the upper, larger branch divides into the iliohypogastric and ilio-inguinal nerves; the lower, smaller branch unites with a branch of the second lumbar to form the genitofemoral nerve. The remainder of the second nerve, the third nerve, and the part of the fourth nerve which joins the plexus, divide into ventral and dorsal branches. The ventral branch of the second unites with the ventral branches of the third and fourth nerves to form the obturator nerve. The dorsal branches of the second and third nerves each divide into a smaller and larger part; the smaller parts unite to form the lateral femoral cutaneous nerve, and the larger parts join with the dorsal branch of the fourth nerve to form the femoral nerve. The accessory obturator, when it exists, arises from the ventral branches of the third and fourth nerves. For details of the blood supply of the lumbar plexus see footnote reference [1075].

The branches of the lumbar plexus may therefore be particularized as follows:

| | |
|---|---|
| Muscular | T. 12, L. 1, 2, 3, 4. |
| Iliohypogastric | L. 1. |
| Ilio-inguinal | L. 1. |
| Genitofemoral | L. 1, 2. |
| **Dorsal divisions** | |
| Lateral cutaneous, of thigh | L. 2, 3. |
| Femoral | L. 2, 3, 4. |
| **Ventral divisions** | |
| Obturator | L. 2, 3, 4. |
| Accessory obturator | L. 3, 4. |

**Muscular branches** are distributed to the quadratus lumborum from the twelfth thoracic and first three or four lumbar nerves; to the psoas minor from the first, to the psoas major from the second, third and, sometimes, from the fourth, and to the iliacus from the second and third lumbar nerves.

**The iliohypogastric nerve** arises from the first lumbar nerve (7.209). It emerges from the upper part of the lateral border of the psoas major, and crosses obliquely behind the lower part of the kidney, and in front of the quadratus lumborum (7.210; 8.148). Just above the iliac crest it perforates the posterior part of the transversus abdominis, and divides between that muscle and the internal oblique into a lateral and an anterior cutaneous branch.

The *lateral cutaneous branch* pierces the internal and external oblique muscles immediately above the iliac crest

[1075] M. H. Day, *J. Anat.*, **98**, 1964.

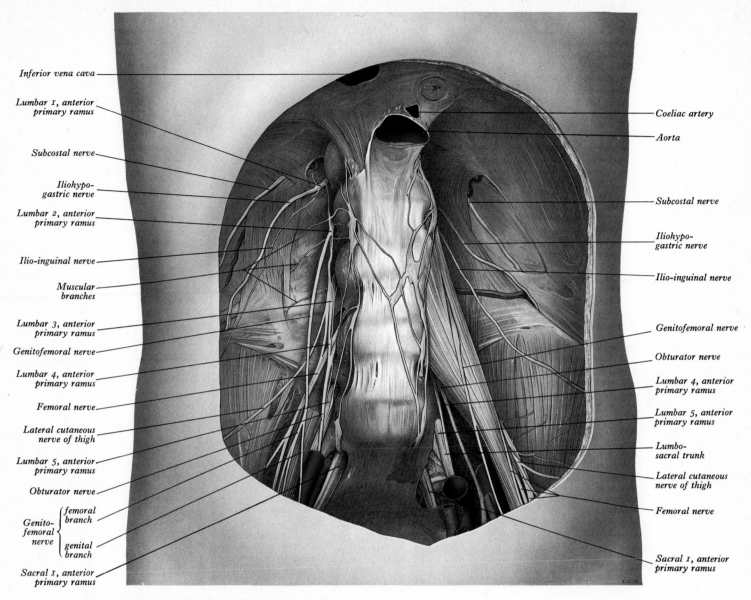

**7.210**  A dissection of the posterior abdominal wall to show the lumbar plexus and sympathetic trunks. The right psoas major has been removed.

at a point a little behind the iliac branch of the twelfth thoracic nerve; it is distributed to the skin of the anterior part of the side of the buttock.

The *anterior cutaneous branch* (**7.206**) runs between the internal oblique and transversus, supplying twigs to both muscles. It then pierces the internal oblique at a point about 2 cm on the medial side of the anterior superior iliac spine, perforates the aponeurosis of the external oblique about 3 cm above the superficial inguinal ring, and is distributed to the skin of the abdomen above the pubis.

The iliohypogastric nerve communicates with the subcostal and ilio-inguinal nerves.

**The ilio-inguinal nerve,** smaller than the iliohypogastric, arises with it from the first lumbar nerve (**7.209**). It emerges from the lateral border of the psoas major, with or just caudal to the iliohypogastric nerve, and, passing obliquely across the quadratus lumborum and the upper part of the iliacus, perforates the transversus abdominis, near the anterior part of the iliac crest, and sometimes communicates with the iliohypogastric nerve. It then pierces the internal oblique, distributing filaments to it, lies below the spermatic cord in the inguinal canal and accompanies it through the superficial inguinal ring. It is distributed to the skin of the superomedial area of the thigh, to the skin over the root of the penis and upper part

of the scrotum in the male (**7.206**), and to the skin covering the mons pubis and adjoining part of the labium majus in the female.

The size of the ilio-inguinal nerve is in inverse proportion to that of the iliohypogastric. Occasionally it is very small, and ends by joining the iliohypogastric nerve; in such cases, a branch from the iliohypogastric takes the place of the ilio-inguinal, or the latter nerve may at times be altogether absent. On the analogy of the intercostal nerves the ilio-inguinal nerve may be regarded as the collateral branch[1076] of the first lumbar nerve, and the iliohypogastric as the main trunk, which gives off the lateral cutaneous branch.

**The genitofemoral nerve** arises from the first and second lumbar nerves (**7.209**). It passes obliquely forwards and downwards through the substance of the psoas major, and emerges on the abdominal surface of the muscle near its medial border, opposite the third or fourth lumbar vertebra; it then descends on the surface of the psoas major, under cover of the peritoneum, and, crossing obliquely behind the ureter, divides at a variable distance above the inguinal ligament into the genital and femoral branches. The genitofemoral nerve frequently divides

[1076] F. Davies, *J. Anat.*, **70**, 1935.

close to its origin, and its two branches then emerge separately through the psoas major.

The *genital branch* crosses the lower end of the external iliac artery, and enters the inguinal canal through the deep inguinal ring; it supplies the cremaster, and gives a few filaments to the skin of the scrotum. In the female, it accompanies the round ligament of the uterus and ends in the skin of the mons pubis and labium majus.

The *femoral branch* descends on the lateral side of the external iliac artery, and sends a few filaments round it; it then crosses the deep circumflex iliac artery, and passing

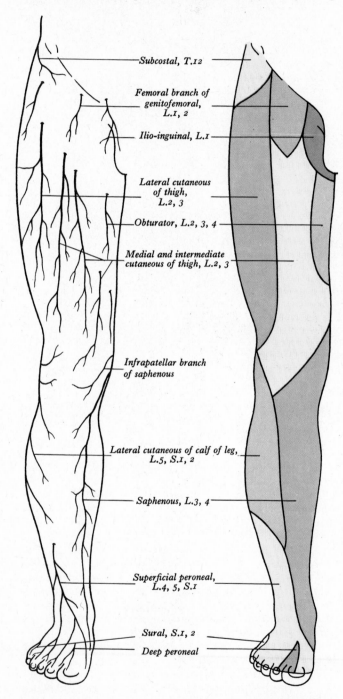

Subcostal, T.12

Femoral branch of genitofemoral, L.1, 2

Ilio-inguinal, L.1

Lateral cutaneous of thigh, L.2, 3

Obturator, L.2, 3, 4

Medial and intermediate cutaneous of thigh, L.2, 3

Infrapatellar branch of saphenous

Lateral cutaneous of calf of leg, L.5, S.1, 2

Saphenous, L.3, 4

Superficial peroneal, L.4, 5, S.1

Sural, S.1, 2

Deep peroneal

7.211 The cutaneous nerves of the right lower limb, their areas of distribution and segmental origins, viewed from the anterior aspect.

behind the inguinal ligament, enters the femoral sheath, lying lateral to the femoral artery. It pierces the anterior layer of the femoral sheath and the fascia lata, and supplies the skin over the upper part of the femoral triangle (7.211). It communicates with the intermediate cutaneous nerve of the thigh, and gives a few twigs to the femoral artery.

**The lateral cutaneous nerve of the thigh** arises from the dorsal branches of the ventral rami of the second and third lumbar nerves (7.209). It emerges from the lateral border of the psoas major, and crosses the iliacus obliquely, running towards the anterior superior iliac spine. It supplies branches to the parietal peritoneum of the iliac fossa. On the right side the nerve passes behind and lateral to the caecum, from which it is separated by the fascia iliaca and the peritoneum; on the left side, it passes behind the lower part of the descending colon. It then passes behind or through the inguinal ligament, at a variable distance medial to the anterior superior iliac spine (commonly about 1 cm), and in front of or through the sartorius into the thigh, where it divides into an anterior and a posterior branch (7.211).

The *anterior branch* becomes superficial about 10 cm below the anterior superior iliac spine, and is distributed to the skin of the anterior and lateral parts of the thigh, as far as the knee. Its terminal filaments communicate with the cutaneous branches of the anterior division of the femoral nerve and with the infrapatellar branch of the saphenous nerve, forming with them the *patellar plexus*.

The *posterior branch* pierces the fascia lata at a higher level than the anterior branch, and subdivides into filaments which pass backwards to supply the skin on the lateral surface of the limb, from the level of the greater trochanter to about the middle of the thigh. It may also supply twigs to the skin of the gluteal region.

## THE OBTURATOR NERVE

The obturator nerve arises from the ventral branches of the ventral rami of the second, third and fourth lumbar nerves (7.209, 210); the branch from the third is the largest, while that from the second is often very small. It descends through the fibres of the psoas major, and emerges from its medial border at the brim of the pelvis, where it passes behind the common iliac vessels, and on the lateral side of the internal iliac vessels. It then runs downwards and forwards along the lateral wall of the lesser pelvis lying on the obturator internus, above and in front of the obturator vessels, to gain the upper part of the obturator foramen, through which it enters the thigh. Near the foramen it divides into an anterior and a posterior branch, which are separated at first by a few fibres of the obturator externus, and lower down by the adductor brevis.

The *anterior branch* (7.212) leaves the pelvis in front of the obturator externus and descends in front of the adductor brevis, and behind the pectineus and adductor longus; at the lower border of the latter muscle it communicates with the medial cutaneous and saphenous branches of the femoral nerve, forming a plexus (termed the *subsartorial plexus*) from which branches are given off to the skin on the medial side of the thigh (7.211). It then descends upon the femoral artery, to which it is finally distributed. Near the obturator foramen this branch gives an articular twig to the hip joint. Behind the pectineus, it distributes branches to the adductor longus, gracilis, usually to the adductor brevis, and often to the pectineus; it receives a filament from the accessory obturator nerve when that nerve is present.

Occasionally the communicating branch to the medial cutaneous and saphenous branches of the femoral nerve is continued down, as a cutaneous branch, to the thigh and leg. When this is so, it emerges from behind the lower border of the adductor longus, descends along the posterior margin of the sartorius to the medial side of the knee, where it pierces the deep fascia, communicates with saphenous nerve, and is distributed to the skin halfway down the medial side of the leg.

The *posterior branch* pierces the anterior part of the obturator externus, and supplies this muscle; it then passes behind the adductor brevis on the front of the adductor magnus, and divides into branches which are distributed to the adductor magnus, and to the adductor brevis when this muscle does not receive a branch from the anterior division of the nerve. It generally gives a slender *articular branch* to the knee joint; this branch perforates the lower part of the adductor magnus or passes through the opening which transmits the femoral artery, and enters the popliteal fossa. Here it descends upon the popliteal artery, to the back of the knee joint, where it pierces the oblique posterior ligament of the knee, and is distributed to the articular capsule. It gives filaments to the popliteal artery.

**The accessory obturator nerve** (7.209) is frequently present. It is of small size, and arises from the ventral branches of the ventral rami of the third and fourth lumbar nerves. It descends along the medial border of the psoas major, crosses the superior ramus of the pubis behind the pectineus, and divides into branches. One branch enters the deep surface of the pectineus; another goes to the hip joint; a third communicates with the anterior branch of the obturator nerve. Occasionally the accessory obturator nerve is very small and supplies only the pectineus.

## THE FEMORAL NERVE

The femoral nerve (7.209, 210), the largest branch of the lumbar plexus, arises from the dorsal branches of the ventral rami of the second, third and fourth lumbar nerves. It descends through the fibres of the psoas major, emerging from the muscle at the lower part of its lateral border, and passes down between it and the iliacus, deep to the iliac fascia; it then passes behind the inguinal ligament to enter the thigh, and splits into an anterior and a posterior division. Behind the inguinal ligament it is separated from the femoral artery by a portion of the psoas major.

Within the abdomen the femoral nerve gives off small branches to the iliacus, the nerve to the pectineus, and a branch which is distributed upon the upper part of the femoral artery; the latter branch may arise in the thigh.

**The nerve to the pectineus** arises from the medial side of the femoral nerve near the inguinal ligament, passes behind the femoral sheath and enters the anterior surface of the muscle.

The anterior division of the femoral nerve gives off the intermediate and medial cutaneous nerves of the thigh (7.211, 212), and muscular branches to the sartorius.

**The intermediate cutaneous nerve of the thigh** pierces the fascia lata about 8 cm below the inguinal ligament, either as two branches, or as a single trunk which quickly divides into two branches; these branches descend vertically on the front of the thigh, and supply the skin as low as the knee. They end in the patellar plexus (p. 1054). The lateral branch of the intermediate cutaneous communicates with the femoral branch of the genitofemoral nerve, and frequently pierces the sartorius, to which it may give a branch of supply.

**The medial cutaneous nerve of the thigh** lies at first on the lateral side of the femoral artery, but at the apex of the femoral triangle it crosses ventral to the artery and divides into an anterior and a posterior branch. Before dividing, the nerve gives off a few filaments which pierce the fascia lata to supply the skin of the medial side of the thigh, in the neighbourhood of the long saphenous vein; one of these filaments emerges through the saphenous opening, and a second becomes subcutaneous about the middle of the thigh. The *anterior branch* runs downwards

on the sartorius, perforates the fascia lata at the junction of the middle with the lower one-third of the thigh, and divides into two branches: one supplies the skin as low as the medial side of the knee; the other crosses to the lateral side of the patella, communicating in its course with the

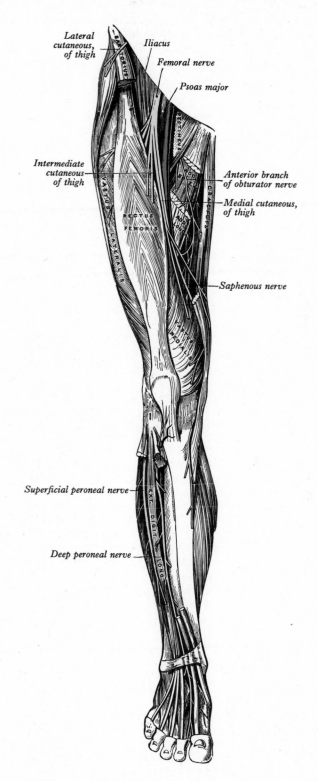

*Lateral cutaneous, of thigh*
*Iliacus*
*Femoral nerve*
*Psoas major*

*Intermediate cutaneous of thigh*
*Anterior branch of obturator nerve*
*Medial cutaneous, of thigh*

*Saphenous nerve*

*Superficial peroneal nerve*

*Deep peroneal nerve*

**7.212**   The nerves of the right lower limb displayed from the anterior aspect.

infrapatellar branch of the saphenous nerve. The *posterior branch* descends along the posterior border of the sartorius to the knee, where it pierces the fascia lata, communicates with the saphenous nerve, and gives off several cutaneous branches. It then descends to supply the skin of the medial side of the leg. Beneath the fascia lata, at the lower border of the adductor longus, it joins to form a plexiform network (*subsartorial plexus*) with branches of the saphenous and obturator nerves. When the communicating branch from the obturator nerve is large and continued to the skin of the leg, the posterior branch of the medial cutaneous is small, and terminates in the plexus, occasionally giving off a few cutaneous filaments.

**The nerve to the sartorius** arises in common with the intermediate cutaneous nerve of the thigh.

The posterior division of the femoral nerve gives off the saphenous nerve, and supplies muscular branches to the quadriceps femoris, and articular branches to the knee joint.

**The saphenous nerve** (7.212) is the largest cutaneous branch of the femoral nerve. It descends on the lateral side of the femoral artery and enters the adductor canal (p. 674) where it crosses in front of the artery obliquely from its lateral to its medial side. At the lower end of the canal it quits the artery, and emerges through the aponeurotic covering of the canal, accompanied by the saphenous branch of the descending genicular artery. It descends vertically along the medial side of the knee behind the sartorius, pierces the fascia lata between the tendons of the sartorius and gracilis, and becomes subcutaneous. It then passes down the medial side of the leg accompanied by the long saphenous vein, descends along the medial border of the tibia, and, at the lower third of the leg, divides into two branches: one continues its course along the medial border of the tibia, and ends at the ankle; the other passes in front of the ankle, and is distributed to the skin on the medial side of the foot, often reaching as far as the metatarsophalangeal joint of the great toe and com-municating with the medial branch of the superficial peroneal nerve.

About the mid level of the thigh, the saphenous nerve gives a branch to join the subsartorial plexus.

After leaving the adductor canal it gives off an *infra-patellar branch* (7.211), which pierces the sartorius and fascia lata, and is distributed to the skin in front of the patella. Proximal to the knee it unites with the medial and intermediate cutaneous nerves of the thigh; below the knee, with other branches of the saphenous nerve; on the lateral side of the joint, with branches of the lateral cutaneous nerve of the thigh, forming a *patellar plexus*.

**The muscular branches** of the posterior division of the femoral nerve supply the quadriceps femoris. The branch to the rectus femoris enters the upper part of the deep surface of the muscle, and supplies a filament to the hip joint. The larger branch to the vastus lateralis forms a prominent neurovascular bundle with the descending branch of the lateral circumflex femoral artery to the lower part of the muscle, and sends an articular filament to the knee joint. The branch to the vastus medialis descends through the upper part of the adductor canal, on the lateral side of the saphenous nerve and the femoral vessels. It enters the muscle about its middle, and gives off a filament which can usually be traced distally on the surface of the muscle to the knee joint. The branches to the vastus intermedius, two or three in number, enter the anterior surface of the muscle about the middle of the thigh; a filament from one of these descends through the muscle to the articularis genus and the knee joint.

**Vascular branches** are given off from the femoral nerve to the femoral artery and its branches (p. 1075).

# SACRAL AND COCCYGEAL VENTRAL RAMI

The ventral rami of the sacral and coccygeal nerves form the sacral and coccygeal plexuses. Those of the upper four sacral nerves enter the pelvis through the pelvic sacral foramina, that of the fifth between the sacrum and coccyx, while that of the coccygeal nerve curves forwards below the rudimentary transverse process of the first piece of the coccyx. The first and second sacral spinal nerves are large; the third, fourth and fifth diminish progressively; the coccygeal nerve is the smallest. Each of these nerves receives a *grey ramus communicans* from the corresponding ganglion of the sympathetic trunk. *Visceral efferent rami* arise from the second, third and fourth sacral nerves; they are named the *pelvic splanchnic nerves* (7.231), and consist of parasympathetic fibres which pass directly to minute ganglia on the walls of the pelvic viscera (p. 1068).

## The Sacral Plexus

The sacral plexus (7.213) is formed by the lumbosacral trunk, the ventral rami of the first, second and third sacral nerves, and part of the ventral ramus of the fourth sacral nerve, the remainder of which joins the coccygeal plexus.

The lumbosacral trunk comprises a part of the ventral ramus of the fourth lumbar nerve, and the whole ventral ramus of the fifth lumbar nerve; it appears at the medial margin of the psoas major and descends over the pelvic brim anterior to the sacro-iliac joint to join the first sacral nerve.

The nerves entering into the sacral plexus converge towards the greater sciatic foramen and unite without much interlacement to form an upper large and a lower small band. The upper band is formed by the union of the lumbosacral trunk with the first, second and the greater part of the third sacral nerves and is continued into the sciatic nerve. The lower band, which has a more plexiform arrangement, results mainly from the junction of the smaller part of the third sacral nerve with the portion of the fourth nerve belonging to the plexus, and is prolonged into the pudendal nerve; it also receives a small contribution from the second sacral nerve. The sciatic nerve is composed of tibial and common peroneal nerves which usually become distinct in the thigh. Above this level, however, these two nerves can be separated to their roots of origin. It is then found that the tibial nerve is formed by the union of ventral divisions of the lumbosacral trunk and first three sacral nerves, while the common peroneal receives the dorsal divisions of the lumbosacral trunk and first two sacral nerves. The component nerves of the sciatic may, however, diverge anywhere along its course from the pelvis. When the division occurs at the plexus the common peroneal usually pierces the piriformis in the greater sciatic foramen. (For details of the blood supply of the sacral plexus see footnote reference [1075].)

## Relations of the Sacral Plexus

The sacral plexus lies on the posterior wall of the pelvic cavity in front of the piriformis (7.214), and behind the internal iliac vessels, the ureter and the sigmoid colon, on the left side, and the terminal coils of the ileum, on the right side. The superior gluteal vessels run between the lumbosacral trunk and the first sacral nerve, or between the first and second sacral nerves, and the inferior gluteal vessels between the ventral rami of the first and second, or second and third, sacral nerves.

## The Branches of the Sacral Plexus

These may be summarized as follows:

|  | Ventral divisions | Dorsal divisions |
|---|---|---|
| To quadratus femoris and gemellus inferior | L. 4, 5, S. 1 | |
| To obturator internus and gemellus superior | L. 5, S. 1, 2 | |
| To piriformis | | S. (1) 2 |
| Superior gluteal | | L. 4, 5, S. 1 |
| Inferior gluteal | | L. 5, S. 1, 2 |
| Posterior femoral cutaneous | S. 2, 3 | S. 1, 2 |
| Sciatic—tibial | L. 4, 5, S. 1, 2, 3 | |
| —common peroneal | | L. 4, 5 |
| | | S. 1, 2 |
| Perforating cutaneous | | S. 2, 3 |
| Pudendal | S. 2, 3, 4 | |
| To levator ani, coccygeus and sphincter ani externus | S. 4 | |
| Pelvic splanchnics | S. 2, 3, (4) | |

**The nerve to the quadratus femoris and gemellus inferior** arises from the ventral branches of the ventral rami of the fourth and fifth lumbar and first sacral nerves (7.213); it leaves the pelvis through the greater sciatic foramen below the piriformis and, descending on the ischium deep to the sciatic nerve, the gemelli and the tendon of the obturator internus, supplies a twig to the gemellus inferior, and enters the anterior surface of the quadratus femoris; it also supplies the hip joint.

**The nerve to the obturator internus and gemellus superior** arises from the ventral branches of the ventral rami of the fifth lumbar and first and second sacral nerves (7.213). It leaves the pelvis through the greater sciatic foramen below the piriformis and gives a branch which enters the upper part of the posterior surface of the gemellus superior. It then crosses the ischial spine lateral to the internal pudendal vessels, re-enters the pelvis through the lesser sciatic foramen, and pierces the pelvic surface of the obturator internus.

**The nerve to the piriformis** arises usually from the dorsal branches of the ventral rami of the first and second sacral nerves, the contribution from the first sacral sometimes being absent; it enters the anterior surface of the muscle.

**The superior gluteal nerve** arises from the dorsal branches of the ventral rami of the fourth and fifth lumbar and first sacral nerves (7.213): it leaves the pelvis through the greater sciatic foramen above the piriformis, accompanied by the superior gluteal vessels, and divides into a superior and an inferior branch. The *superior* branch accompanies the upper branch of the deep division of superior gluteal artery and supplies branches to the gluteus medius and occasionally also to the gluteus minimus. The *inferior* branch runs with the lower branch of the deep division of the superior gluteal artery across the gluteus minimus; it gives twigs to the gluteus medius and gluteus minimus, and ends in the tensor fasciae latae.

**The inferior gluteal nerve** arises from the dorsal branches of the ventral rami of the fifth lumbar and first and second sacral nerves: it leaves the pelvis through the greater sciatic foramen, below the piriformis, and divides into branches which enter the deep surface of the gluteus maximus.

**The posterior femoral cutaneous nerve** arises from the dorsal branches of the ventral rami of the first and

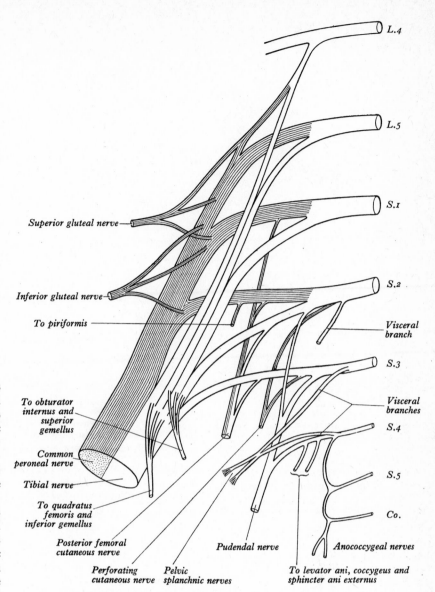

7.213 A plan of the sacral and coccygeal plexuses. L.4–5, S.1–5 and Co., indicate the *ventral rami* of these lumbar, sacral and coccygeal spinal nerves. The *ventral divisions* of these rami are unshaded, the *dorsal divisions* are shaded. The contribution from S.2 to the pelvic splanchnic nerves is shown before joining those from 3 and 4.

second, and from the ventral branches of the ventral rami of the second and third, sacral nerves (7.213), and issues from the pelvis through the greater sciatic foramen distal to piriformis. It then descends under cover of the gluteus maximus with the inferior gluteal artery, lying posterior or medial to the sciatic nerve. It descends the back of the thigh superficial to the long head of the biceps femoris, and deep to the fascia lata: at the back of the knee it pierces the deep fascia and accompanies the short saphenous vein as far as the middle of the calf of the leg, its terminal twigs communicating with the sural nerve.

Its branches are all cutaneous, and are distributed to the gluteal region, the perineum, and the flexor aspect of the thigh and leg.

The *gluteal branches*, three or four in number, turn upwards round the lower border of the gluteus maximus, and supply the skin covering the lower and lateral part of that muscle.

The *perineal branch* distributes twigs to the skin at the upper and medial side of the thigh, and then curves forwards across the origin of the hamstrings, below the ischial tuberosity; it pierces the fascia lata, and runs beneath the superficial fascia of the perineum to the skin

1055

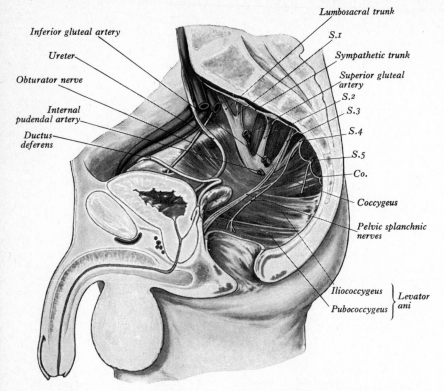

7.214 A dissection of the side wall of the pelvis, showing the sacral and coccygeal plexusis. S.1–5 indicate the anterior rami of the sacral spinal nerves; Co. indicates the ventral ramus of the coccygeal spinal nerve.

of the scrotum in the male, and of the labium majus in the female, joining with the inferior rectal and the posterior scrotal branches of the perineal nerve.

The *branches to the back of the thigh and leg* consist of numerous filaments derived from both sides of the nerve, and distributed to the skin covering the back and medial side of the thigh, the popliteal fossa and the upper part of the back of the leg (7.215).

## The Sciatic Nerve

The sciatic nerve (7.213, 216), the largest in diameter in the body, measures at its commencement 2 cm in breadth. It is the continuation of the upper band of the sacral plexus. It passes out of the pelvis through the greater sciatic foramen, below the piriformis, descends between the greater trochanter of the femur and the tuberosity of the ischium, and along the back of the thigh to about its lower one-third, where it divides into two large branches, named the tibial and common peroneal nerves. The nerve also gives off articular and muscular branches.

In the upper part of its course the nerve is situated deep to the gluteus maximus, and rests first upon the posterior surface of the ischium, the nerve to the quadratus femoris intervening; it then crosses the obturator internus and gemelli, and passes on to the quadratus femoris, by which it is separated from the obturator externus and the hip joint; it is accompanied on its medial side by the posterior cutaneous nerve of the thigh and the inferior gluteal artery. More distally it lies upon the adductor magnus, and is crossed obliquely by the long head of the biceps femoris. It can be represented on the back of the thigh by a broad line drawn distally to the apex of the popliteal fossa from just medial to the midpoint of the line joining the ischial tuberosity to the apex of the greater trochanter.

The *articular branches* of the sciatic nerve arise from the upper part of the nerve, and supply the hip joint by perforating the posterior part of its capsule; they are sometimes derived directly from the sacral plexus.

The *muscular branches* of the sciatic nerve are distributed to the biceps femoris, semitendinosus, semimembranosus and to the ischial head of the adductor magnus (p. 566); the branches to the two latter arise by a common trunk. The nerve to the short head of the biceps femoris comes from the common peroneal division, the other muscular branches from the tibial division of the sciatic nerve.

## THE TIBIAL NERVE

The tibial (medial popliteal) nerve (7.216), the larger, terminal branch of the sciatic nerve, arises from the ventral branches of the ventral rami of the fourth and fifth

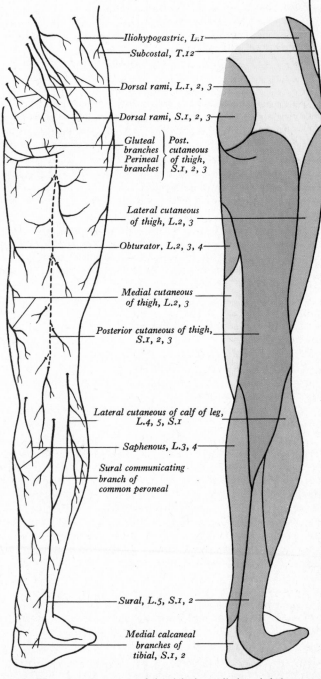

7.215 The cutaneous nerves of the right lower limb and their areas of distribution and segmental origins, viewed from the posterior aspect. The major part of the trunk of the posterior cutaneous nerve of the thigh lies deep to the deep fascia and is therefore shown by an interrupted line.

lumbar and first, second and third sacral nerves. It descends along the back of the thigh and through the middle of the popliteal fossa, to the distal border of the popliteus, where it passes with the popliteal artery deep to the arch of the soleus. Thereafter it is continued into the leg. In the thigh it is overlapped by the hamstring muscles above, but it becomes more superficial in the popliteal fossa, where it lies lateral to, and some distance from, the popliteal vessels; it is superficial to these vessels opposite the knee joint and then crosses to the medial side of the popliteal artery (7.217). In the lower part of the popliteal fossa, the nerve is covered by the contiguous margins of the two heads of the gastrocnemius. It can be represented by a line drawn downwards in the midline of the limb from the apex of the popliteal fossa to the level of the neck of the fibula. Continued downwards to a point midway between the medial malleolus and the tendo calcaneus, the line maps out the whole course of the tibial nerve.

In the leg it descends in company with the posterior tibial vessels to the interval between the heel and the medial malleolus, where it ends under cover of the flexor retinaculum by dividing into the medial and lateral plantar nerves. In proximal section it is covered posteriorly by the soleus and gastrocnemius, but in the distal third of the leg it is covered only by the skin and fasciae, although it is overlapped sometimes by the medial edge of the flexor hallucis longus. Above, it lies on the medial side of the posterior tibial vessels, but it soon crosses behind them and descends to its point of bifurcation along their lateral side. In most of its course it lies on the tibialis posterior, but in the lower part of the leg it comes into relation with the posterior surface of the tibia.

The branches of this nerve are articular, muscular, sural, medial calcanean and medial and lateral plantar.

**Articular branches**, usually three in number, supply the knee joint; one branch accompanies the superior, and another the inferior medial genicular artery; the third branch runs with the middle genicular artery. These branches form a plexus with the articular branch of the obturator nerve, and from the plexus branches are distributed to the oblique posterior ligament of the joint and others accompany the superior and inferior medial genicular arteries and supply the medial parts of the capsular ligament. Another articular branch arises from the nerve just above its terminal bifurcation, and supplies the ankle joint. (For further details of this nerve supply consult footnote reference [1077].)

**The muscular branches** arise from the nerve as it lies between the two heads of the gastrocnemius; they supply that muscle, as well as the plantaris, soleus and popliteus. The nerve to the soleus enters the superficial surface of the muscle. The branch for the popliteus descends, crossing the popliteal vessels obliquely, and turns round the distal border of the muscle to be distributed to its deep surface; it supplies small branches to the tibialis posterior, an articular twig to the upper tibiofibular joint, a medullary branch to the tibia, and an interosseous branch, which descends close to the fibula, and can be traced to the inferior tibiofibular joint.

In the leg, the muscular branches arise either independently or by a common trunk. They supply the soleus, on its deep surface, the tibialis posterior, the flexor digitorum longus and the flexor hallucis longus; the branch to the last muscle accompanies the peroneal vessels.

**The sural nerve** descends between the two heads of the gastrocnemius, and, piercing the deep fascia in the middle or upper part of the back of the leg, is joined by the sural communicating branch of the common peroneal nerve (7.215). It then passes downwards near the lateral margin of the tendo calcaneus, and close to the small saphenous vein, to the interval between the lateral mal-

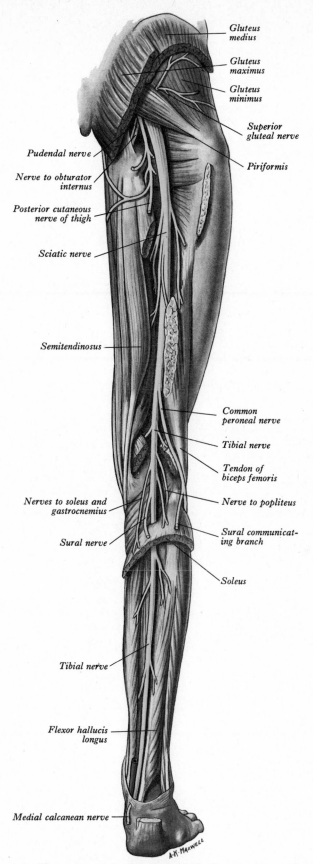

**7.216** The nerves of the right lower limb. Posterior aspect. In this figure the gluteus maximus, the gluteus medius and the superficial muscles of the calf of the leg have been removed and the middle part of the long head of the biceps femoris has been excised.

leolus and the calcaneus; it supplies the skin of the lateral and posterior part of the lower one-third of the leg. It runs forwards below the lateral malleolus, and is continued

[1077] J. Champetier and C. Déscours, *C. r. Ass. Anat.*, **141**, 1968.

along the lateral side of the foot and little toe, communicating on the dorsum of the foot with the superficial peroneal nerve. In the leg, its branches communicate with those of the posterior cutaneous nerve of the thigh. For a recent study of the fibre spectrum and ultrastructure of the fetal sural nerve consult footnote reference [1078].

The *medial calcanean branches* perforate the flexor retinaculum, and supply the skin of the heel and medial side of the sole of the foot.

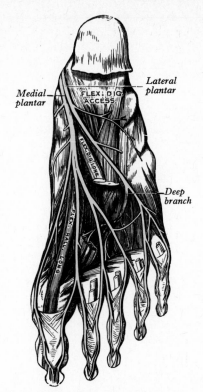

7.218 The plantar nerves of the right foot.

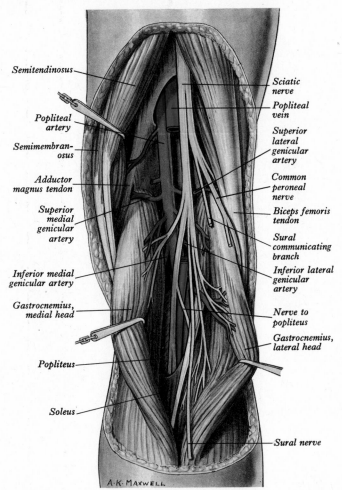

7.217 A dissection of the right popliteal fossa. The two heads of gastrocnemius and the semitendinosus and semimembranosus have been retracted in order to expose the contents of the fossa more fully.

*Vascular branches* are supplied from the tibial nerve and its branches to the arteries which they accompany in the leg and foot (p. 1076).

**The medial plantar nerve** (7.218), the larger of the two terminal divisions of the tibial nerve, accompanies the medial plantar artery and lies on the lateral side of the vessel. From its origin under cover of the flexor retinaculum it passes deep to the abductor hallucis, and, appearing between this muscle and the flexor digitorum brevis, gives off a digital nerve to the medial side of the great toe and finally divides opposite the bases of the metatarsal bones into three plantar digital nerves.

*Branches. Cutaneous branches* pierce the plantar aponeurosis between the abductor hallucis and the flexor digitorum brevis and are distributed to the skin of the sole of the foot.

*Muscular branches* supply the abductor hallucis, the flexor digitorum brevis, the flexor hallucis brevis and the first lumbrical; those for the abductor hallucis and flexor

digitorum brevis arise from the trunk of the nerve near its origin and enter the deep surfaces of the muscles; the branch for the flexor hallucis brevis springs from the digital nerve to the medial side of the great toe, and that for the first lumbrical from the first plantar digital nerve.

*Articular branches* supply the articulations of the tarsus and metatarsus.

The *proper digital nerve of the great toe* supplies the flexor hallucis brevis and the skin on the medial side of the great toe.

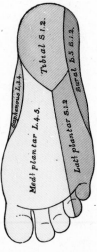

7.219 A diagram showing the distribution of the cutaneous nerves in the sole of the right foot.

The *three common plantar digital nerves* pass between the divisions of the plantar aponeurosis, and each splits into two proper digital branches. Those of the first plantar digital nerve supply the adjacent sides of the great and second toes; those of the second, the adjacent

[1078] J. Ochoa, *J. Anat.*, **108**, 1971.

sides of the second and third toes; and those of the third, the adjacent sides of the third and fourth toes. The third plantar digital nerve receives a communicating branch from the lateral plantar nerve; the first gives a twig to the first lumbrical. Each digital branch gives off cutaneous and articular filaments and opposite the distal phalanx sends upwards a dorsal branch, which supplies the structures around the nail, the continuation of the nerve being distributed to the ball of the toe. It will be observed that

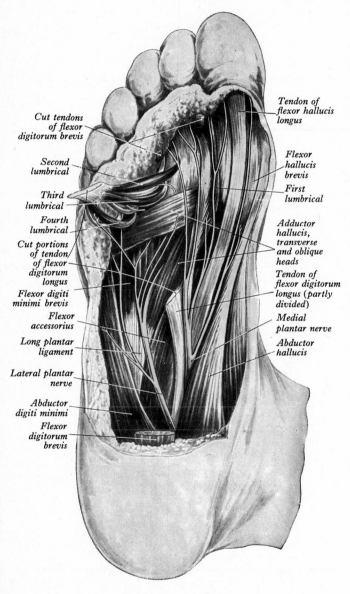

Cut tendons of flexor digitorum brevis

Second lumbrical

Third lumbrical

Fourth lumbrical

Cut portions of tendon of flexor digitorum longus

Flexor digiti minimi brevis

Flexor accessorius

Long plantar ligament

Lateral plantar nerve

Abductor digiti minimi

Flexor digitorum brevis

Tendon of flexor hallucis longus

Flexor hallucis brevis

First lumbrical

Adductor hallucis, transverse and oblique heads

Tendon of flexor digitorum longus (partly divided)

Medial plantar nerve

Abductor hallucis

7.220 A dissection of the lateral and medial plantar nerves of the right foot. Most of the flexor digitorum brevis has been removed. The flexor digitorum longus has been partially divided and its distal end has been displaced together with the second, third and fourth lumbricals.

the digital branches of the medial plantar nerve are similar in their distribution to those of the median nerve in the hand. The muscles supplied by the two nerves also correspond closely. In the hand, the median nerve supplies the abductor and the flexor pollicis brevis, the opponens pollicis and the first and second lumbricals. The opponens is absent in the foot, but the abductor hallucis, flexor hallucis brevis and the first lumbrical are all supplied by the medial plantar nerve. As the flexor digitorum brevis corresponds to the flexor digitorum superficialis (median nerve) of the upper limb, the only difference exists in the innervation of the second lumbrical.

**The lateral plantar nerve** (7.218) supplies the skin of the fifth toe and lateral half of the fourth, as well as most of the deep muscles, *its distribution being similar to that of the ulnar nerve in the hand*. It passes obliquely forwards in company with the lateral plantar artery, which lies on the lateral side of the nerve, and reaches the lateral side of the foot near the tubercle of the fifth metatarsal bone. It passes between the flexor digitorum brevis and the flexor digitorum accessorius, and ends in the interval between the former muscle and the abductor digiti minimi by dividing into a superficial and a deep branch. Before its division, it supplies the flexor digitorum accessorius and abductor digiti minimi and gives off some small cutaneous branches which pierce the plantar fascia and supply the skin of the lateral part of the sole of the foot (7.219).

The *superficial branch* splits into two plantar digital nerves; of these the lateral supplies the lateral side of the fifth toe, the flexor digiti minimi brevis, and the two interosseous muscles of the fourth intermetatarsal space; the medial communicates with the third plantar digital branch of the medial plantar nerve and divides into two branches which supply the adjoining sides of the fourth and fifth toes.

The *deep branch* accompanies the lateral plantar artery on the deep surface of the tendons of the flexor muscles and the adductor hallucis, and supplies the second, third and fourth lumbricals, the adductor hallucis and all the interossei (except those of the fourth intermetatarsal space). The nerves to the second and third lumbricals pass distally deep to the transverse head of the adductor hallucis, and then pass round its distal border to reach the muscles (7.220).

## THE COMMON PERONEAL NERVE

The common peroneal (lateral popliteal) nerve (7.217), about one-half the size of the tibial nerve, is derived from the dorsal branches of the ventral rami of the fourth and fifth lumbar and the first and second sacral nerves. It descends obliquely along the lateral side of the popliteal fossa to the head of the fibula, close to the medial margin of the biceps femoris. It lies between the tendon of the biceps femoris and the lateral head of the gastrocnemius, winds round the lateral surface of the neck of the fibula deep to the peroneus longus, and divides into the superficial and deep peroneal nerves. Its course can be indicated by a line drawn from the apex of the popliteal fossa distally and laterally, along the medial side of the biceps tendon, to the back of the head of the fibula, where the nerve can be rolled against the bone. Previous to its division it gives off articular and cutaneous branches.

The *articular branches* are three in number; of these one accompanies the superior and another the inferior lateral genicular artery. Both may arise by a common trunk. The third, named the recurrent articular nerve, is given off at or near the point of division of the common peroneal nerve; it ascends with the anterior recurrent tibial artery through the tibialis anterior to supply the anterolateral part of the capsular ligament of the knee joint and also supplies branches to the superior tibiofibular joint.

The *cutaneous branches* (7.215), two in number, frequently spring from a common trunk; they are the lateral cutaneous nerve of the calf and the sural communicating branch.

The *lateral cutaneous nerve of the calf* supplies twigs to the skin on the anterior, posterior and lateral surfaces of the proximal part of the leg. The *sural communicating branch* arises near the head of the fibula, runs obliquely across the lateral head of the gastrocnemius to the middle of the leg, and joins with the sural nerve (p. 1057). It may, however, descend as a separate branch as far as the heel.

**The deep peroneal (anterior tibial) nerve** (7.212) begins at the bifurcation of the common peroneal nerve, between the fibula and the proximal part of the peroneus longus, passes obliquely forwards deep to the extensor digitorum longus to the front of the interosseous membrane, where it comes into relation with the anterior tibial artery in the proximal third of the leg; it then descends with the artery to the front of the ankle joint, where it divides into lateral and medial terminal branches. It lies at first on the lateral side of the anterior tibial artery, then in front of it, and again on its lateral side at the ankle joint.

In the leg, the deep peroneal nerve supplies *muscular branches* to the tibialis anterior, extensor hallucis longus, extensor digitorum longus and peroneus tertius, and an *articular branch* to the ankle joint.

The *lateral terminal branch* of the deep peroneal nerve passes across the tarsus, deep to the extensor digitorum brevis and, becoming enlarged by a pseudoganglion like the posterior interosseous nerve at the wrist, supplies the extensor digitorum brevis. From the enlargement three minute *interosseous branches* are given off which supply the tarsal joints, and the metatarsophalangeal joints of the second, third and fourth toes. The first of these sends a filament to the second dorsal interosseous muscle.

The *medial terminal branch* of the deep peroneal nerve runs forwards on the dorsum of the foot, and lies on the lateral side of the dorsalis pedis artery. At the first interosseous space it communicates with the medial branch of the superficial peroneal nerve, and divides into two dorsal digital nerves which supply the adjacent sides of the great and second toes. Before it divides it gives off an *interosseous branch* which supplies the metatarsophalangeal joint of the great toe and sends a filament to the first dorsal interosseous. The deep peroneal nerve may end by dividing into *three* terminal branches.[1079]

**The superficial peroneal (musculocutaneous) nerve** (7.212) begins at the bifurcation of the common peroneal nerve and lies at first deep to the peroneus longus. It then passes forwards and downwards between the peronei and the extensor digitorum longus, pierces the deep fascia in the distal third of the leg, and divides into a medial and a lateral branch. In its course between the muscles, it gives off muscular branches to the peroneus longus and peroneus brevis, and filaments to the skin of the lower part of the leg.

The *medial branch* passes in front of the ankle joint, and divides into two dorsal digital nerves, one of which supplies the medial side of the great toe, the other, the adjacent sides of the second and third toes. It communicates with the saphenous nerve and with the deep peroneal nerve (7.211).

The *lateral branch*, the smaller, passes along the lateral part of the dorsum of the foot, and divides into dorsal digital branches, which supply the contiguous sides of the third and fourth, and of the fourth and fifth toes. It also supplies the skin of the lateral side of the ankle, and communicates with the sural nerve (7.211).

The branches of the superficial peroneal nerve supply the skin of the dorsal surfaces of all the toes excepting the lateral side of the little toe and the adjoining sides of the great and second toes, the former being supplied by the sural nerve, and the latter by the medial terminal branch of the deep peroneal nerve. Frequently some of the lateral branches of the superficial peroneal are absent, and their places are then taken by branches of the sural nerve.

**The perforating cutaneous nerve** usually arises from the posterior aspects of the second and third sacral nerves.

It pierces the lower part of the sacrotuberous ligament, and, winding round the inferior border of the gluteus maximus, supplies the skin covering the medial and lower parts of that muscle.

The perforating cutaneous nerve may arise from the pudendal nerve or it may be absent; in the latter case its place may be taken by a branch from the posterior cutaneous nerve of the thigh or by a branch from the third and fourth, or fourth and fifth, sacral nerves.

**The pudendal nerve** (6.94) derives its fibres from the second, third and fourth sacral spinal nerves (7.213). It leaves the pelvis between piriformis and coccygeus through the lower part of the greater sciatic foramen and enters the gluteal region, crossing the sacrospinous ligament close to its attachment to the ischial spine, being situated on the medial side of the internal pudendal vessels which lie on the ischial spine itself. It accompanies the internal pudendal artery through the lesser sciatic foramen into the pudendal canal (p. 528) on the lateral wall of the ischiorectal fossa; in the posterior part of this canal it gives off the inferior rectal nerve, and then divides into the perineal nerve and the dorsal nerve of the penis (or clitoris).

The *inferior rectal nerve* pierces the medial wall of the pudendal canal, crosses the ischiorectal fossa with the inferior rectal vessels, and is distributed to the sphincter ani externus, to the lining of the lower part of the anal canal and to the skin round the anus. Branches of this nerve communicate with the perineal branch of the posterior cutaneous nerve of the thigh and with the scrotal nerves. The inferior rectal nerve occasionally arises directly from the sacral plexus.

The *perineal nerve*, the inferior and larger terminal branch of the pudendal nerve, runs forwards below the internal pudendal artery. It accompanies the perineal artery and divides into posterior scrotal (or labial) and muscular branches.

The *posterior scrotal branches* number two, medial and lateral. They pierce, or pass superficial to, the inferior fascia of the urogenital diaphragm, and run forwards along the lateral part of the urethral triangle in company with the scrotal branches of the perineal artery; they are distributed to the skin of the scrotum, and communicate with the perineal branch of the posterior cutaneous nerve of the thigh and with the inferior rectal nerve. In the female the corresponding nerves (*posterior labial branches*) supply the labium majus.

The *muscular branches* are distributed to the transversus perinei superficialis, bulbospongiosus, ischiocavernosus, transversus perinei profundus, sphincter urethrae and the anterior parts of the external sphincter and levator ani. A branch, termed the *nerve to the urethral bulb*, is given off from the nerve to the bulbospongiosus; it pierces this muscle, and supplies the corpus spongiosum penis, its terminal fibres ending in the mucous membrane of the urethra.

The *dorsal nerve of the penis* runs forwards above the internal pudendal artery along the ramus of the ischium, and accompanies the artery along the margin of the inferior ramus of the pubis, on the deep surface of the inferior fascia of the urogenital diaphragm. It gives a branch to the corpus cavernosum penis and, at the apex of the membrane, passes through the lateral part of the gap between that structure and the inferior pubic ligament. It then runs forwards, in company with the dorsal artery of the penis, between the layers of the suspensory ligament, to the dorsum of the penis, and ends in the glans penis. In the female the corresponding nerve (*dorsal nerve of the clitoris*) is very small, and supplies the clitoris.

[1079] M. Geller and D. Barbato, *Hospital, Rio de J.*, **77**, 1970.

Clinical evidence indicates that the pudendal nerve supplies sensory branches to the lower inch or so of the vagina, the fibres probably running in the inferior rectal nerve and in the posterior labial branches of the perineal nerve. The pudendal nerves can be infiltrated with a local anaesthetic ('pudendal nerve block') by a needle passed through the vaginal wall and guided by a finger to the ischial spine and sacrospinous ligament, which can be palpated *per vaginam*. For various vaginal operative procedures a general anaesthetic can thus usually be avoided.[1080, 1081]

**The visceral branches** arise from the second, third and fourth sacral spinal nerves, and are distributed to the pelvic viscera. They are termed the *pelvic splanchnic nerves* and are described on p. 1068.

**The muscular branches** are derived from the fourth sacral, and supply the levator ani, coccygeus and sphincter ani externus. The branches to levator ani and coccygeus enter their pelvic surfaces; the ramus to the sphincter ani externus (perineal branch of fourth sacral nerve) reaches the ischiorectal fossa by piercing the coccygeus or by passing between it and the levator ani. Cutaneous filaments from this branch supply the skin between the anus and the coccyx.

**The coccygeal plexus** is formed by a small descending branch from the ventral ramus of the fourth sacral nerve, and the ventral rami of the fifth sacral and coccygeal nerves. The ventral ramus of the fifth sacral nerve emerges from the sacral hiatus and turns forwards round the lateral margin of the sacrum below the cornu. It pierces the coccygeus to gain its pelvic surface and is then joined by a descending filament from the fourth sacral nerve. The small trunk so formed descends on the pelvic surface of the coccygeus and unites with the minute ventral ramus of the coccygeal nerve, which descends from the sacral hiatus, turns round the lateral margin of the coccyx and pierces the coccygeus to gain the pelvis. This small trunk constitutes the *coccygeal plexus*. The *anococcygeal nerves* arises from the plexus, and consist of a few fine filaments which pierce the sacrotuberous ligament and supply the skin in the region of the coccyx.

*Applied Anatomy.* The *iliohypogastric nerve* may be cut, as it lies between the muscles inferiorly in the anterior abdominal wall (p. 1050), by an incision ('McBurney's gridiron') through which the vermiform appendix is approached; the consequent weakness of the muscles in the region of the inguinal canal may predispose to the development of a direct inguinal hernia (p. 1298).

The *lateral cutaneous nerve of the thigh* may be compressed and irritated as it passes through the inguinal ligament (p. 520) or as it pierces the dense fascia lata, and this is said to be one of the causes of a rare condition of pain on the lateral side of the thigh (*meralgia paraesthetica*).

The *femoral nerve* is rarely injured by wounds in the groin or thigh; the result is paralysis of the quadriceps femoris and diminished cutaneous sensibility on the anterior and medial aspects of the thigh.

Surgical division of the *obturator nerve* is sometimes done for relief of spasm of the adductors of the thigh in certain cases of spastic paralysis in children, in paraplegia or in multiple sclerosis. Because of its branches to the hip joint, knee joint and medial side of the thigh, in cases of disease of the hip joint pain may be referred to the medial side of the thigh or to the knee joint.

The *sacral plexus* and *lumbosacral trunk* may be compressed by pelvic tumours, or by the fetal head in pregnancy, and result in pain in the lower limbs which, in the case of malignant growths, may be extremely severe.

The *sciatic nerve* may be injured by posterior dislocations or fracture dislocations of the hip joint; if the lesion of the nerve is complete, which is rare, all muscles below the knee are paralysed and all cutaneous sensibility there is lost, except for the area supplied by the saphenous nerve. In traumatic lesions of the sciatic nerve in middle levels of the thigh, the flexor muscles generally escape because of the high origin of the nerves to these muscles. The surface marking of the sciatic nerve for purposes of injection is given on p. 1056.

The *common peroneal nerve* is the most commonly injured nerve in the lower limb, chiefly because of its exposed position as it winds round the neck of the fibula. Injury here will result in paralysis of all the dorsiflexor and evertor muscles of the foot (tibialis anterior, extensor hallucis longus, extensor digitorum longus, extensor digitorum brevis, peroneus longus and peroneus brevis) producing a '*drop foot*'. There is a variable loss of cutaneous sensibility on the anterolateral aspect of the leg and on the dorsum of the foot.

Owing to its deep and protected position, the tibial nerve is rarely injured. Wounds in the popliteal fossa or posterior dislocation of the knee joint may damage the tibial nerve and produce paralysis of the flexor muscles in the leg and the intrinsic muscles of the sole of the foot, resulting in considerable disability. Furthermore, loss of sensation in the sole of the foot renders its skin liable to 'pressure sores'.

## Morphology of the Spinal Nerves and the Limb Plexuses

The spinal nerves which conform in their behaviour to the more primitive arrangement are the nerves of those segments which have retained to a large extent their *metameric* (segmental) characters, viz. T.2–L.1. These typical spinal nerves are distributed according to a very definite plan. The dorsal ramus passes backwards and downwards lateral to the articular processes and divides into a medial and a lateral branch which penetrate the deep muscles of the back. Both branches innervate the muscles amongst which they lie, and either the one or the other becomes superficial and supplies a band of skin extending from the posterior median line to the scapular line.

The ventral ramus is connected to the corresponding ganglion on the sympathetic trunk by both white and grey rami communicantes. After innervating the subvertebral muscles, it passes round the body wall supplying branches to the lateral muscles of the trunk, and in the neighbourhood of the mid-axillary line gives off a lateral branch which pierces the overlying muscles and divides into an anterior and a posterior division for the supply of the skin. The main trunk is continued forwards in the body wall and, after supplying the ventral muscles, distributes its terminal branches to the skin.

The behaviour of the ventral rami of the spinal nerves of the segments which have lost their obvious metamerism is greatly modified, and the initial modification is seen in the manner in which adjoining nerves unite to form the cervical, brachial, lumbosacral and coccygeal plexuses.

**The cervical plexus.** The cutaneous branches of this plexus are homologous with the anterior terminal and the lateral branches of the ventral rami of the typical spinal nerves. The transverse cutaneous nerve of the neck and the medial supraclavicular nerves represent the anterior terminal branches; the lesser occipital and the lateral supraclavicular represent the lateral branches, while the great auricular and the intermediate supraclavicular probably represent elements of both branches.

[1080] P. J. Huntingford, *J. Obstet. Gynaec. Br. Commonw.*, **66**, 1959.
[1081] T. Nakanishi, *Acta anat. nippon*, **42**, 1967.

**The brachial plexus.** In the formation of the brachial and lumbosacral plexuses the division of the constituent nerves of the plexus into anterior (ventral or flexor) and posterior (dorsal or extensor) branches is characteristic. In the brachial plexus the division affects the three trunks of the plexus (p. 1037) and, to a remarkable extent, it conforms to the differentiation of the primitive musculature of the limb into a flexor (ventral) and extensor (dorsal) group. So far as the cutaneous innervation is concerned, branches of the ventral divisions of the trunks take a large part in the supply of the skin of the dorsal surface of the limb. This problem has been tentatively explained[1082] by assuming that each constituent root of the plexus originally divided into ventral and dorsal branches and that, on the evolution of the human type of plexus, inherently dorsal fibres enter the ventral branches of the trunks. As a result of this rearrangement, fibres of the median and ulnar nerves have a wide area of supply on the dorsal surface of the hand.

The position of the developing limb bud on the ventrolateral aspect of the trunk, and the behaviour of the first and second thoracic nerves, provide support for the view that the constituent nerves of the great limb plexuses represent only the lateral branches of the ventral rami of the typical spinal nerves. The second thoracic nerve sends its lateral cutaneous branch into the upper limb as the intercostobrachial nerve, and the size of this nerve varies inversely with the size of the direct contribution which the second thoracic nerve makes to the brachial plexus. Otherwise the second thoracic behaves like a typical spinal nerve. The first thoracic nerve sends a large contribution to the brachial plexus, and this could be homologous with the lateral branch. The remainder of the nerve, despite its small size, behaves in a typical manner, although its fine anterior cutaneous branch is often absent, and, when present, only supplies a limited area of skin.

**The lumbosacral plexus.** The division of the constituent nerves of the lumbar and sacral plexuses into anterior (ventral or flexor) and posterior (dorsal or extensor) divisions is not so obvious as the corresponding pattern in the brachial plexus, but it can be demonstrated anatomically that the obturator and the tibial nerves arise from ventral and the femoral and peroneal nerves from dorsal divisions. The lateral branches of the twelfth thoracic and first lumbar spinal nerves are drawn over the iliac crest to assist in the innervation of the gluteal skin, but otherwise these nerves behave as typical spinal nerves. The second lumbar nerve behaves in a manner which renders its interpretation difficult, since it not only makes a substantial contribution to the lumbar plexus but also possesses both an anterior terminal branch, the genital branch of the genitofemoral nerve, and a lateral cutaneous branch, represented by the lateral cutaneous nerve of the thigh and the femoral branch of the genitofemoral nerve. The anterior terminal portions of the third, fourth and fifth lumbar and first sacral spinal nerves are suppressed, but the corresponding parts of the second and third sacral nerves supply the skin, etc., of the perineum.

## The Segmental Innervation of Skin

The area of skin supplied by any one spinal nerve, through both its rami, constitutes a **dermatome** and, typically, the dermatomes extend round the body from the posterior to the anterior median line (7.206, 221). The dermatomes of *consecutive spinal nerves* overlap markedly, and this is seen most clearly in those segments of the body which have been least affected by the development of the limbs, i.e. second thoracic to first lumbar (7.221).

In some situations, e.g. the upper part of the anterior

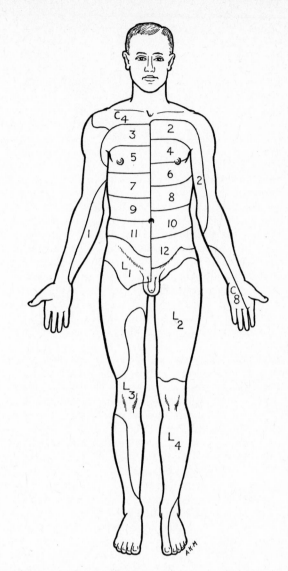

**7.221** The cutaneous areas supplied by the ventral rami of the thoracic and upper four lumbar nerves. (After Foerster.) By comparing both sides the degree of overlapping and the area of exclusive supply of any individual nerve may be estimated. See text for the area supplied by T.1 on the trunk.

thoracic wall, the cutaneous nerves supplying two adjoining areas are not derived from consecutive spinal nerves and the overlap between, above, and below, is minimal. When the second thoracic spinal nerve is severed, the line of anaesthesia is sharply demarcated, although there may be some overlap of the painful and thermal elements. Likewise the results found after section of a peripheral nerve (e.g. the ulnar nerve at the wrist) show that the area of tactile loss is always greater than the area of loss of painful and thermal sensibilities, for the degree of overlap of fibres conveying these types of sensibility is always more extensive than the overlap of fibres conveying tactile sensibility. As a result the area of total anaesthesia and analgesia following section of a peripheral nerve is considerably less than might be anticipated from a knowledge of its anatomical distribution.[1083, 1084]

### Cutaneous Innervation of the Neck and Upper Limb

The first cervical spinal nerve has no cutaneous branches. The second cervical usually supplies the skin of the head,

[1082] W. Harris, *The Morphology of the Brachial Plexus*, Oxford University Press, London. 1939.
[1083] O. Foerster, *Brain*, **56**, 1933.
[1084] H. H. Woollard, G. Weddell and J. A. Harpman, *J. Anat.*, **74**, 1940.

from the vertex backwards to the neighbourhood of the superior nuchal line, the cranial surface and most, if not the whole, of the lateral surface of the auricle, the skin over the angle of the mandible and below the chin (7.182). The third cervical spinal nerve supplies a very oblique band of skin, commencing behind over the back of the scalp and the upper part of the back of the neck and passing forwards and downwards across the side of the neck. The area increases in extent as it is traced forwards, and in the ventral median line extends from the hyoid bone down to the level of the first rib. The fourth cervical spinal nerve supplies the upper half or more of the back of the neck, and the area widens as it is traced downwards and forwards round the side of the neck to the anterior aspect of the trunk. It supplies the skin over the clavicle and first intercostal space, as well as over the acromion and the upper part of the deltoid.

Each of these three areas is overlapped by the succeeding area, but the amount of overlapping is slight and is greater for the dorsal rami than for the ventral rami.

The cutaneous distribution of the spinal nerves which contribute to the brachial plexus becomes intelligible only when reference is made to an early stage in the development of the upper limb. In a human embryo of the fourth week the upper limb is represented by a small, somewhat flattened elevation on the ventrolateral aspect of the trunk opposite to the lower four cervical and the first thoracic segments. The ectoderm covering it is directly continuous with the ectoderm of the trunk and draws its nerve supply from the nerves of the corresponding segments. Similarly, its contained mesoderm is also continuous with the mesoderm of the same segments. The lower limb bud appears at a slightly later stage and always lags behind the upper limb bud in its development.

The limb buds possess ventral and dorsal surfaces and cranial or *preaxial*, and caudal or *postaxial* borders. In the upper limb the *fifth cervical* ventral ramus supplies a strip of skin on both ventral and dorsal surfaces along the preaxial border, and the *first thoracic nerve* has a similar distribution along the postaxial border. The intervening nerves supply approximately parallel strips of skin on both the ventral and dorsal surfaces. As the limb elongates the central nerves of the plexus (C. 6, 7 and 8) become buried proximally and reach the skin only in its more distal part, while the nerves of the adjoining segments (C. 4 and T. 2 and 3) become drawn in to supply the skin at the root of the limb. In the process of growth, the lengthening limb becomes rotated laterally through roughly 90° and adducted to the trunk (p. 123). In the later stages, therefore, the *preaxial border* runs distally along the lateral aspect of the limb to the thumb, which is the *preaxial digit*, while the *postaxial border* runs distally along the medial aspect to the little finger, which is the *postaxial digit*. Accordingly, the cutaneous nerve supply of the lateral aspect of the adult limb is derived from C. 4, which has been drawn in at the root of the limb, C. 5 and C. 6, and its medial aspect from T. 2, T. 1 and C. 8 (7.222). On the *front of the limb* the areas supplied by C. 5 and C. 6 adjoin the areas supplied by T. 2, T. 1 and C. 8 but at the dividing line between them, which is termed the *ventral axial line*, the overlap is minimal, for C. 7 is buried proximally and only reaches the skin a little proximal to the wrist (7.222). On the *back of the limb* the condition is very similar, but C.7 (in the posterior cutaneous nerve of the forearm) reaches the skin at, or a little proximal to the elbow so that the *dorsal axial line* ends at a more proximal level (7.222).

## Cutaneous Innervation of the Trunk

The skin of the trunk is supplied by the spinal nerves T. 1 to L. 1 inclusive (7.206, 221), by the sacral nerves, except the first, and by the coccygeal nerve. These nerves supply

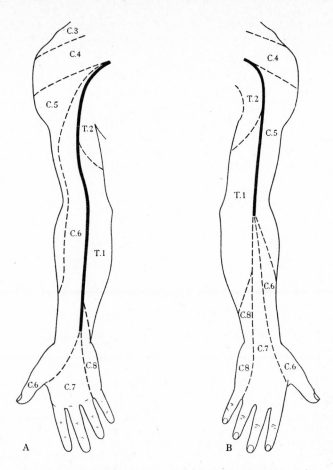

**7.222 A** The arrangement of the dermatomes on the anterior aspect of the upper limb. The *heavy black line* represents the *ventral axial line* and the overlap across it is *minimal*. Across the interrupted lines, the overlap is considerable. B The arrangement of the dermatomes on the posterior aspect of the upper limb. The *heavy black line* represents the *dorsal axial line* and the overlap across it is *minimal*. Across the interrupted lines the overlap may be, and often is considerable.

consecutive curved bands of skin, of which the upper are almost horizontal while the lower are disposed obliquely. The upper half of each band receives additional supply from the nerve above and the lower half from the nerve below, so that no appreciable loss of sensibility follows the section of any individual spinal nerve. It is convenient to remember that the band which includes the subcostal angle is supplied by the seventh thoracic nerve and that the umbilicus lies in the upper part of the band supplied by the tenth thoracic nerve.

The areas supplied by the dorsal rami of these nerves are limited laterally by the dorsolateral line, which commences above on the back of the head and runs downwards and laterally to the medial end of the acromion. It is then continued downwards to the posterior aspect of the greater trochanter of the femur where it curves medially to the coccyx (7.223 B). The cutaneous strips supplied by the dorsal rami do not correspond exactly to the strips supplied by the ventral rami, for they differ both in their breadth and in their position.

On the upper part of the ventral aspect of the thorax the third and fourth cervical areas adjoin the first and second thoracic areas (7.206), owing to the fact that the muscles and skin areas supplied by intervening nerves have grown into the upper limb, and a similar but less extensive gap is found on the posterior aspect of the trunk.

A corresponding arrangement is found in the lower part of the trunk, but it is not so obvious owing to the approximation of the lower limbs to one another, but is still apparent in the gluteal region. The first lumbar area adjoins the second sacral area at the root of the penis and scrotum (*see* p. 1346), for the intervening nerves have been drawn off to supply the lower limb.

### Cutaneous Innervation of the Lower Limb

The skin of the lower limb is innervated by the nerves of the segments from which it is derived, viz. T. 12–S. 3. The arrangement originally is precisely similar to that in the upper limb, but its identification in the adult has been rendered difficult on account of the torsion of the lower limb in the early stages of its development (p. 123).

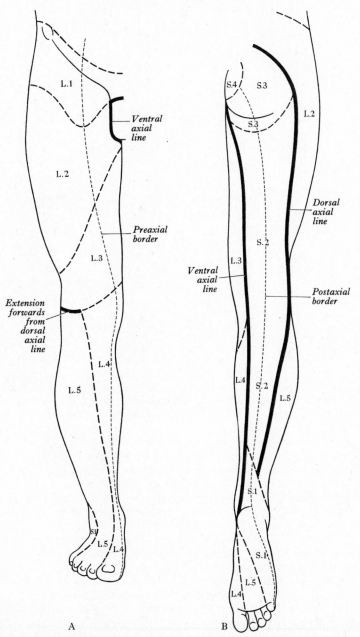

**7.223 A** The segmental distribution of the nerves of the lumbar and sacral plexuses to the skin of the anterior aspect of the lower limb. B The segmental distribution of the nerves of the lumbar and sacral plexuses to the skin of the posterior aspect of the lower limb. For the significance of the markings see **7.222** caption.

Originally the *preaxial border* follows the cephalic border of the limb bud to the hallux, which is the *preaxial digit*, while the *postaxial border* follows its caudal margin to the little toe, which is the *postaxial digit*. As development proceeds, the limb undergoes torsion in a *medial* direction so that the hallux comes to lie on the medial side of the

adult foot and the little toe on its lateral side. The tibia, although homologous with the radius, lies on the medial side of the leg. Since the torsion occurs at the hip joint, the gluteal region retains its dorsal (extensor) situation.

The preaxial border commences above on the middle of the front of the thigh and runs down to the knee. It then curves medially as it descends to the medial malleolus to gain the medial side of the foot and the hallux. The postaxial border commences above in the gluteal region and descends to the popliteal fossa. It then declines laterally as it descends to the lateral malleolus to gain the lateral side of the foot. The *ventral* and *dorsal axial lines* necessarily exhibit a corresponding obliquity. The ventral axial line commences proximally at the medial end of the inguinal ligament and descends the posteromedial side of the thigh and leg to end proximal to the heel. The dorsal axial line commences in the lateral part of the gluteal region and descends on the posterolateral aspect of the thigh to the knee. It then inclines medially and ends before it reaches the ankle (**7.223**).

The segmental cutaneous distribution of the nerves to the lower limb is shown in **7.223**.

Our knowledge of the extent of the individual dermatomes, especially of the limbs, is necessarily based on clinical evidence, and different authorities have mapped out areas which are far from being identical for the same dermatomes. This is due partly to their failure to adopt a common method in the neurological examination of patients and partly to individual differences between patients suffering from similar lesions. There is more disagreement with regard to the dermatomes in the leg, perhaps in part due to the greater frequency of injuries to the brachial plexus, affording more numerous opportunities of correlation between the areas of cutaneous analgesia or anaesthesia and the exact site of damage to the nerve. The figures of the limb dermatomes here inserted are based on those of the Committee appointed by the Medical Research Council, and published in their *Report on Peripheral Nerve Lesions*, 1942.

When studying these figures it must be clearly understood that the *broken lines* indicate that the nerves on each side of them extend considerably beyond them, the amount of such overlapping being often difficult to define. But, along the *ventral* and *dorsal axial lines*, shown in *heavy black*, overlap is minimal, for the nerves on each side of the line are not derived from consecutive spinal nerves, and the intervening nerve or nerves are buried in the substance of the limb in this situation and only reach the skin at a more distal point.

Some observers[1085] maintain that, in the embryonic development of the dermatomes of the limbs, the sensory nerves grow spirally from the dorsal surface of the limb buds around their preaxial and postaxial borders to meet on their ventral surface along the ventral axial line, and they deny the existence of a dorsal axial line. By plotting the areas of hyposensitivity, particularly hypalgesia (diminished sensibility to painful stimuli), following damage to *individual* nerve roots they have constructed charts of the limb dermatomes that differ considerably from those shown in **7.223**.

## The Segmental Innervation of Muscles

Each spinal nerve originally supplies the musculature derived from the myotome of the same segment. In cases where the derivatives of any one myotome persist as separate entities, they retain their original nerve supply, but when derivatives of adjoining myotomes fuse, the

[1085] J. J. Keegan and F. D. Garrett, *Anat. Rec.*, **102**, 1948.

resultant muscle does not necessarily retain its supply from each of the corresponding nerves, although it may and frequently does retain them all. Since the limb muscles develop *in situ* in the mesodermal core of the developing limb, it is impossible to identify the individual segments from which any muscle is derived by the study of its mode of development. The union of the individual spinal nerves and their branches in the brachial and lumbosacral plexuses renders impossible the identification by dissection of the root value of the individual motor nerves.

## Segmental innervation of the Muscles of the Limbs

Most muscles of the limbs are innervated from more than one segment of the spinal cord and the segments involved for individual muscles are indicated in the section on Myology (pp. 532–559). In the list given below, for a given muscle the *predominant segmental origin* of its nerve supply is recorded; damage to these segments or to the motor nerve roots arising therefrom results in maximum paralysis of the appropriate muscles. The information is based chiefly on clinical evidence,[1086–1088] but it must be admitted that there is a difference of opinion in the case of a number of muscles, and not all the muscles of the limbs are included in this list. Moreover, though the evidence for some muscles is incontrovertible, it is scanty and uncertain in many other instances.

### Upper Limb Muscles

C. 3, 4    Trapezius; levator scapulae.

C. 5    Rhomboids; deltoids; supraspinatus; infraspinatus; teres minor; biceps.

C. 6    Serratus anterior; latissimus dorsi; subscapularis; teres major; pectoralis major (clavicular head); biceps; coracobrachialis; brachialis; brachioradialis; supinator; extensor carpi radialis longus.

C. 7    Serratus anterior; latissimus dorsi; pectoralis major (sternal head); pectoralis minor; triceps; pronator teres; flexor carpi radialis; flexor digitorum superficialis; extensor carpi radialis longus; extensor carpi radialis brevis; extensor digitorum; extensor digiti minimi.

C. 8    Pectoralis major (sternal head); pectoralis minor; triceps; flexor digitorum superficialis; flexor digitorum profundus; flexor pollicis longus; pronator quadratus; flexor carpi ulnaris; extensor carpi ulnaris; abductor pollicis longus; extensor pollicis longus; extensor pollicis brevis; extensor indicis; abductor pollicis brevis; flexor pollicis brevis; opponens pollicis.

T. 1    Flexor digitorum profundus; intrinsic muscles of the hand (except abductor pollicis brevis; flexor pollicis brevis; oppenens pollicis).

### Lower Limb Muscles

L. 1    Psoas major; psoas minor.

L. 2    Psoas major; iliacus; sartorius; gracilis; pectineus; adductor longus; adductor brevis.

L. 3    Quadriceps; adductors (magnus, longus, brevis).

L. 4    Quadriceps; tensor fasciae latae; adductor magnus; obturator externus; tibialis anterior; tibialis posterior.

L. 5    Gluteus medius; gluteus minimus; obturator internus; semimembranosus; semitendinosus; extensor hallucis longus; extensor digitorum longus and peroneus tertius; popliteus.

S. 1    Gluteus maximus; obturator internus; piriformis; biceps femoris; semitendinosus; popliteus; gastrocnemius; soleus; peronei (longus and brevis); extensor digitorum brevis.

S. 2    Piriformis; biceps femoris; gastrocnemius; soleus; flexor digitorum longus; flexor hallucis longus; intrinsic foot muscles.

S. 3    Intrinsic foot muscles (except abductor hallucis; flexor hallucis brevis; flexor digitorum brevis; extensor digitorum brevis).

(See also p. 815 for a table of lower limb innervation.)

### Joint Movements

In terms of movements of joints, the segmental innervation of the limb muscles may be expressed in general as follows:

| | | |
|---|---|---|
| Shoulder | Abductors and lateral rotators. | C. 5 |
| | Adductors and medial rotators. | C. 6, 7, 8 |
| Elbow | Flexors. | C. 5, 6 |
| | Extensors. | C. 7, 8 |
| Forearm | Supinators. | C. 6 |
| | Pronators. | C. 7, 8 |
| Wrist | Flexors and extensors. | C. 6, 7 |
| Digits | Long flexors and extensors. | C. 7, 8 |
| Hand | Intrinsic muscles. | C. 8, T. 1 |
| Hip | Flexors, adductors, medial rotators. | L. 1, 2, 3 |
| | Extensors, abductors, lateral rotators. | L. 5, S. 1 |
| Knee | Extensors. | L. 3, 4 |
| | Flexors. | L. 5, S. 1 |
| Ankle | Dorsiflexors. | L. 4, 5 |
| | Plantar flexors. | S. 1, 2 |
| Foot | Invertors. | L. 4, 5 |
| | Evertors. | L. 5, S. 1 |

[1086] O. Bumke and O. Foerster, *Handbuch der Neurologie*, (eds.), Teil 2, Springer-Verlag, Berlin. 1936.

[1087] E. Villiger, *Die Periphere Innervation*, 10th edn, Schwabe, Basel. 1946.

[1088] W. J. W. Sharrard, *J. Bone Jt Surg.*, **37**B, 1955.

# THE AUTONOMIC NERVOUS SYSTEM

The autonomic nervous system includes parts of the central and peripheral nervous systems, the latter being concerned with the innervation of viscera, glands, blood vessels and nonstriated muscle. It is the visceral (splanchnic) component of the nervous system. The term 'autonomic' is convenient rather than appropriate. The *autonomy* of this part of the nervous system is illusory. It is intimately responsive to changes in the somatic activities of the body, and while its connexions with somatic elements are not always clear in anatomical terms, the physiological evidence of visceral reflex activities stimulated by somatic events is abundant. (For general information on the anatomy and physiology of the autonomic nervous system consult footnote references[1089–1094].)

[1089] D. Sheehan, *Archs Neurol. Psychiat., Chicago*, **35**, 1936.

[1090] J. C. White, R. H. Smithwick and F. A. Simeone, *The Autonomic Nervous System*, 3rd edn, Kimpton, London. 1952.

[1091] A. Kuntz, *The Autonomic Nervous System*, 4th edn, Lea and Febiger, Philadelphia. 1953.

[1092] G. A. G. Mitchell, *Anatomy of the Autonomic Nervous System*, Livingstone, Edinburgh. 1953.

[1093] G. A. G. Mitchell, *Cardiovascular Innervation*, Livingstone, Edinburgh. 1956.

[1094] J. Pick, *The Autonomic Nervous System*, Lippincott, Philadelphia. 1970.

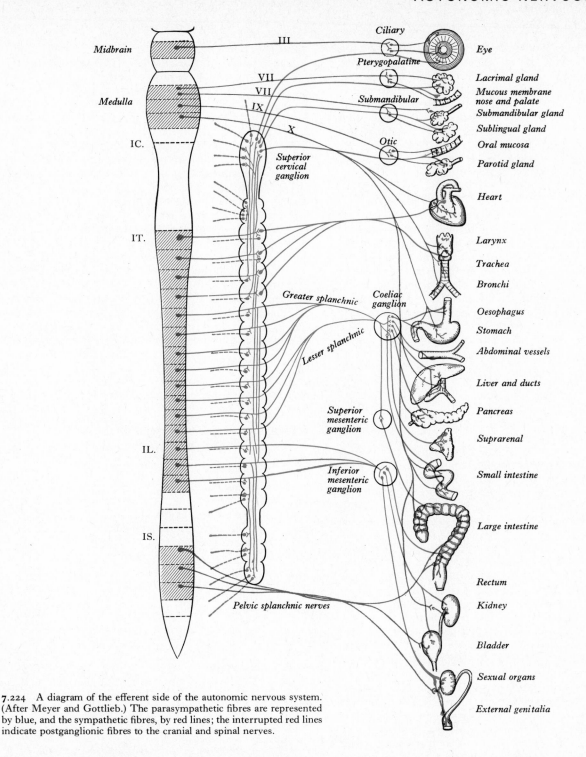

**7.224** A diagram of the efferent side of the autonomic nervous system. (After Meyer and Gottlieb.) The parasympathetic fibres are represented by blue, and the sympathetic fibres, by red lines; the interrupted red lines indicate postganglionic fibres to the cranial and spinal nerves.

Visceral efferent pathways differ from somatic equivalents in being interrupted by peripheral synapses, two neurons being interposed between the central nervous system and the visceral effector organ (7.224). The cells of origin of the primary neurons are sited in the visceral efferent components of cranial nerve nuclei and in the lateral grey columns of the spinal cord. Their axons, which are variably, but usually finely myelinated, traverse the corresponding cranial and spinal nerves to enter ganglia, where they synapse with the somata of the secondary neurons. The axons of the second or excitor neurons are usually nonmyelinated and are distributed to nonstriated muscle or gland cells. There is therefore in the peripheral efferent pathway a *preganglionic neuron* and a *postganglionic neuron*. The latter are more numerous, and one preganglionic neuron may synapse with up to 15 to 20 postganglionic neurons, a circumstance which is associated with the wide diffusion of many autonomic

effects. The disproportion between preganglionic and postganglionic neurons is said to be greater in the sympathetic than in the parasympathetic parts of the autonomic nervous system. (Indeed, in an investigation into the human superior cervical ganglion, a ratio of preganglionic to postganglionic fibres of 1 to 196 was claimed.[1095]) The terminations of the postganglionic neurons are described on p. 791.

The visceral afferent paths resemble somatic ones and the cells of origin of the peripheral fibres are unipolar cells in cranial and spinal nerve ganglia. Their peripheral processes are distributed through the autonomic ganglia or plexuses or possibly through somatic nerves without further synapse. Their central processes (axons) accompany the somatic afferent fibres through dorsal spinal nerve roots to the central nervous system (p. 1081).

1095 S. O. E. Ebbesson, *J. Morph.*, **124**, 1968.

The autonomic nervous system consists of two complementary parts, the *parasympathetic* and the *sympathetic systems* which differ structurally and in their functions. The preganglionic efferent fibres of the parasympathetic nervous system emerge through certain cranial and sacral spinal nerves and constitute the *craniosacral outflow*. On the other hand the preganglionic efferent fibres of the sympathetic nervous system emerge through the thoracic and upper lumbar spinal nerves and constitute the *thoracolumbar outflow*. The cell bodies of the postganglionic neurons in the parasympathetic system are situated peripherally, either as discrete collections forming ganglia nearer to the structures innervated than to the central nervous system, or sometimes dispersed in the walls of the viscera themselves. The cell bodies of the postganglionic neurons in the sympathetic system are generally situated in ganglia on the sympathetic trunk or as ganglia in more peripheral plexuses, almost always nearer to the spinal cord than to the effectors which they innervate.

Physiologically, parasympathetic reactions are generally localized, whereas sympathetic reactions are mass responses. Thus parasympathetic activity results, for example, in slowing of the heart and increase in the glandular and peristaltic activities of the gut; these may be considered as conservation of body energies. Sympathetic activities result, for example, in general constriction of the cutaneous arteries (with consequent increase in the blood supply to the heart, muscles and brain), acceleration of the heart and increase of the blood pressure, contraction of the sphincters and lessening of the peristalsis of the gut, all of which activities mobilize body energies for dealing with any increase in activity.

Whereas the passage of nervous impulses along all preganglionic fibres, parasympathetic postganglionic fibres or along somatic efferent fibres is associated with the liberation of *acetylcholine* in the region of the terminals, in the case of sympathetic postganglionic fibres the substance liberated is *noradrenalin* or *adrenalin*. For this reason the above types of nerves are called *cholinergic* and *adrenergic* respectively. As an exception to this sweat glands are supplied only by postganglionic sympathetic nerves but these are cholinergic.

# THE PARASYMPATHETIC NERVOUS SYSTEM

## Efferent Pathways

The preganglionic parasympathetic fibres are myelinated and occur in (1) the oculomotor; (2) the facial; (3) the glossopharyngeal; (4) the vagus and accessory; and (5) the second, third and fourth sacral spinal nerves. In the cranial part of the parasympathetic system there are four peripheral ganglia which, though small, are readily identified with the naked eye. They are the *ciliary* (p. 999), *pterygopalatine* (p. 1005), *submandibular* (p. 1015) and *otic* (p. 1019) ganglia, all of which have been described in detail with the cranial nerves. These ganglia are concerned solely with efferent parasympathetic pathways, unlike the trigeminal, facial, glossopharyngeal and vagal ganglia, which are all concerned with afferent impulses and contain the cells of origin of sensory fibres only. The cranial parasympathetic ganglia are traversed by afferent fibres, by postganglionic sympathetic fibres and, in the case of the otic ganglion, even by branchial efferent fibres; but in none are the fibres interrupted during their passage through the ganglia. The postganglionic parasympathetic fibres are usually nonmyelinated and shorter than those of the sympathetic system, since the ganglia where their synapses occur are situated in or near the viscera they supply.

(1) The *oculomotor nerve* parasympathetic fibres start in the midbrain, and are derived from the accessory oculomotor (Edinger-Westphal) nucleus (p. 999). The preganglionic fibres travel in the nerve and leave by the branch which it supplies to the inferior oblique to enter the *ciliary ganglion*. There they are relayed, and the postganglionic fibres leave the ganglion in the short ciliary nerves, which pierce the sclera and run forwards in the perichoroidal space, to be distributed to the ciliary muscle (p. 1102) and the sphincter pupillae (p. 1106). These postganglionic fibres are thinly myelinated.

(2) The *facial nerve* contains efferent parasympathetic fibres which are axons of cells in the superior salivatory nucleus (p. 855) and emerge from the brain in the nervus intermedius. They travel in the facial nerve, leaving it a little above the stylomastoid foramen in the *chorda tympani*, which traverses the tympanic cavity and ultimately reaches the *lingual nerve*. In this way they are conveyed to the submandibular region, where they enter the *submandibular ganglion*, in which the postganglionic secretomotor fibres for the submandibular salivary gland arise. Some preganglionic fibres may synapse around cells in the hilus of the gland (see also pp. 1212 and 1213). The secretomotor fibres for the sublingual gland are continued forwards in the lingual nerve after they have arisen in the submandibular ganglion (see also pp. 1212 and 1213). Electrical stimulation of the chorda tympani produces dilatation of the arterioles of both these salivary glands in addition to a secretomotor effect. In addition, the facial nerve has usually been said to contain efferent parasympathetic fibres which are secretomotor to the lacrimal gland, travelling by its greater petrosal ramus and nerve of the pterygoid canal and relaying in the pterygopalatine ganglion. The postganglionic branches are said to travel by the zygomatic nerve to the lacrimal gland (p. 1004) and by branches from the ganglion to glands of the nose and palate. Evidence refuting the former route has recently been reported.[1096] This indicates that direct *lacrimal rami* pass to the gland from a *retro-orbital plexus* composed of direct parasympathetic branches of the pterygopalatine ganglion.

(3) The *glossopharyngeal nerve* contains efferent parasympathetic fibres, which are secretomotor to the parotid gland. They start in the inferior salivatory nucleus (p. 855) and travel in the glossopharyngeal nerve and its tympanic branch. After traversing the tympanic plexus, they enter the lesser petrosal nerve and so reach the otic ganglion. There they are relayed and the postganglionic fibres pass by communicating branches to the auriculotemporal nerve, by which they are conveyed to the parotid gland. Electrical stimulation of the lesser petrosal nerve produces a vasodilator as well as a secretomotor effect.

(4) The *vagus nerve* contains efferent parasympathetic fibres which arise in its dorsal nucleus (p. 846) and travel in the nerve trunk and in its pulmonary, cardiac, oesophageal, gastric, intestinal and other branches. The proportion of efferent parasympathetic fibres in the vagus varies at different levels, but is small in relation to its sensory component. These fibres are relayed in minute ganglia which lie in the walls of the individual viscera.

---

[1096] G. L. Ruskell, *J. Anat.*, **109**, 1971.

The disproportion in the numbers of preganglionic to postganglionic fibres is greater in the vagus than in the efferent parasympathetic components of other cranial nerves and this discrepancy cannot as yet be explained. The cardiac branches are concerned with slowing the rate of the cardiac cycle. They take part in the formation of the cardiac plexuses (p. 1076) and are then relayed in ganglia which are distributed freely over the surfaces of both atria in the subepicardial tissue. The terminal fibres are distributed to the atria and the atrioventricular bundle, and it is only through the latter structure that the vagus can exert any control over the ventricular muscle.[1097] The smaller branches of the coronary arteries are innervated mainly by the vagus, whereas their larger branches, though possessing a double innervation, obtain their chief source of supply from the sympathetic system.[1098] The *pulmonary branches* are motor to the circular non-striated muscle fibres in the bronchi, and are therefore bronchoconstrictor. The synaptic relays are in the ganglia of the pulmonary plexuses. The *gastric branches* are secretomotor to the glands and motor to the muscular coats of the stomach, but they inhibit the action of the pyloric sphincter. The *intestinal branches* have a corresponding action on the small intestine, caecum, vermiform appendix, ascending colon, right colic flexure and most of the transverse colon, being secretomotor to the glands and motor to the muscular coats of the gut, but inhibitory to the ileocaecal sphincter. The synaptic relays, in this case, are situated in the myenteric (Auerbach's) plexus and the plexus of the submucosa (Meissner's plexus), which are described with the structure of the intestines (p. 1284).

(5) The anterior rami of the *second*, *third* and often the *fourth sacral spinal nerves* emit visceral branches passing directly to the pelvic viscera. They constitute the *pelvic splanchnic nerves* (7.231), and they unite with branches of the sympathetic pelvic plexuses. Minute ganglia are situated at the points of union and in the walls of the individual viscera. In these ganglia the sacral preganglionic parasympathetic fibres are relayed.

The pelvic splanchnic nerves supply the rectum with motor fibres, the bladder wall with motor and its sphincter with inhibitory fibres, the erectile tissue of the penis or clitoris with vasodilator fibres, the testes or ovaries probably with vasodilator fibres, and the uterine tubes and uterus with vasodilator and possibly inhibitory fibres. In addition, filaments from the pelvic splanchnic nerves pass upwards through the hypogastric plexus to supply the sigmoid colon, descending colon, left colic flexure and terminal part of the transverse colon with viscero-motor fibres.[1099, 1100] (See also pp. 1078, 1079.)

The nervus terminalis (p. 996) is also considered to contain visceral efferent fibres.

[1097] W. Cullis and E. Tribe, *J. Physiol., Lond.*, **46**, 1913.
[1098] H. H. Woollard, *J. Anat.*, **60**, 1926.
[1099] E. D. Telford and J. S. B. Stopford, *Br. med. J.*, **1**, 1934.
[1100] G. A. G. Mitchell, *Edinb. med. J.*, **42**, 1935.

# THE SYMPATHETIC NERVOUS SYSTEM

The sympathetic nervous system, which is the larger division of the autonomic, includes the two ganglionated sympathetic trunks, their branches, plexuses and subsidiary ganglia. It has a much wider distribution than the parasympathetic system, for it innervates all the sweat glands of the skin, the arrector muscles of the hairs, the muscular walls of many blood vessels, the heart, lungs and other viscera.

### Efferent Sympathetic Pathways

*The preganglionic fibres* are the axons of nerve cells in the lateral column of the grey matter of all the thoracic and upper two or three lumbar segments of the spinal cord where they form the intermediomedial and intermediolateral cell groups (p. 813). These fibres are myelinated and have diameters of 1·5 to 4·0 $\mu$m. They emerge from the spinal cord through the ventral roots of the corresponding spinal nerves and pass into the spinal nerve trunks and the commencement of their ventral rami, which they leave in the *white rami communicantes*, to join either the corresponding ganglia on the sympathetic trunks or their interganglionic parts. Since this outflow is confined to the thoracolumbar region, typical white rami communicantes are also restricted to the fourteen spinal nerves noted above. However, the possibility of a limited outflow of preganglionic fibres in other spinal nerves has been suggested. It is certain that nerve cells of the same type as those in the lateral grey column also exist at other levels, above and below the thoracolumbar outflow,[1101] and that small numbers of their fibres issue in corresponding ventral roots. Dorsal spinal nerve roots may also contain vasodilator fibres. Having reached the sympathetic trunk the preganglionic fibres may behave in a number of different ways (7.225). (*a*) They may end in the corresponding ganglion by arborizing with the dendrites of ganglion cells. (*b*) They may pass through the corresponding ganglion and either ascend to a ganglion at a higher level or descend to one at a lower level before terminating in a similar manner; it is believed that preganglionic fibres do not divide into ascending and descending branches on entering the sympathetic trunk. A single preganglionic fibre may, through its collateral and terminal branches, synapse with nerve cells in several of the ganglia which it traverses; other preganglionic fibres distribute branches to one ganglion only. (*c*) They may pass through the corresponding ganglion and may ascend or descend without being interrupted and then emerge in one of the medially directed branches of the sympathetic trunk to enter the plexus of the autonomic system, where they terminate in relation to the ganglion cells therein. Occasionally the interruption of preganglionic fibres occurs in ganglia situated proximal to the sympathetic trunks; these are known as 'intermediate ganglia' and are most numerous on the grey rami communicantes (*vide infra*) in the cervical and lower lumbar regions.[1102] They may be of microscopic size and are sometimes situated in the ventral roots or trunks of the spinal nerves. Branches from more than one preganglionic fibre may synapse with a single postganglionic neuron.

**The sympathetic ganglia** include collections of cells of the sympathetic trunks, nerve ganglia in the autonomic plexuses and the 'intermediate' ganglia; in addition some ganglion cells are dispersed through the plexuses. Originally the ganglia on the sympathetic trunks correspond numerically to the ganglia on the dorsal roots of the spinal nerves (p. 995); but fusion of adjoining ganglia has occurred and in man there are rarely more than twenty-two or twenty-three and there may be fewer discrete

[1101] G. A. G. Mitchell, *Anatomy of the Autonomic Nervous System*, Livingstone, Edinburgh. 1953.
[1102] J. D. Boyd and P. A. G. Munro, *Lancet*, **2**, 1940.

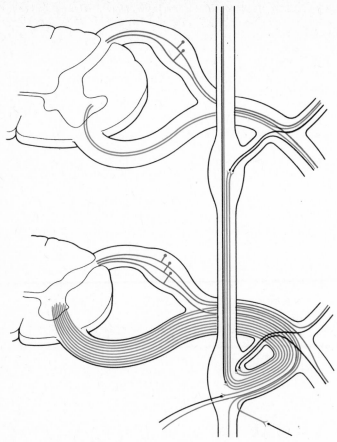

**7.225** A scheme showing the constitution of a typical spinal nerve. In the upper part of the diagram the spinal nerve roots show the somatic components; in the lower part of the diagram the spinal roots show the visceral components. *Red:* motor efferent somatic and preganglionic visceral fibres. *Blue:* afferent somatic and visceral fibres. *Black:* postganglionic visceral fibres.

ganglia. The subsidiary ganglia in the great autonomic nerve plexuses (e.g. coeliac ganglion, superior mesenteric ganglion, etc.) are derivatives of the ganglia of the sympathetic trunks. The nerve cells in the ganglia are multipolar and vary from 15 to 55 $\mu$m in diameter. The cell body is usually surrounded by a capsule of satellite cells but this may be absent. The dendrites are variable in size and distribution. The longer dendrites penetrate the capsule and ramify in the intercellular areas, the shorter dendrites are confined within the capsule. Sometimes the dendrites intertwine to form complex whorls or glomeruli. The terminations of preganglionic fibres are found in proximity to both the intracapsular and extracapsular dendrites. The existence of interneurons in sympathetic ganglion is usually regarded as a matter of doubt.[1103] See, however, footnote reference [1104] for a discussion of the small granule-containing cells described in sympathetic ganglia by a number of workers (e.g. footnote reference [1105]). Similar cells have been noted—in very small numbers—in the ciliary ganglion.[1106] The observation that cells of this kind have short processes, and in particular that afferent and efferent synapses have been identified in relation to them, make it highly probable that they are in fact interneurons. So far, however, they have been studied in a few sites only, and their numbers appear to be small. Further work on this important topic is necessary.

The axons of the ganglion cells are usually fine, non-myelinated fibres and constitute the *postganglionic fibres*. They are distributed to the effector organ in a variety of ways. Postganglionic fibres arising from a ganglion on the sympathetic trunk may (*a*) pass back to the corresponding spinal nerve through a *grey ramus communicans*; this usually joins the spinal nerve trunk just proximal to the white ramus communicans. Its fibres are distributed through the ventral and dorsal rami of the spinal nerves and their branches to the blood vessels, sweat glands and hairs, etc. in their zone of supply. The extent of the segmental area innervated is variable and the territories supplied through adjacent nerves overlap to a considerable degree; the extent of innervation of different effector systems, e.g., sudomotor and vasomotor, by a particular nerve are not necessarily the same. (*b*) They may pass in a medial branch of a ganglion to be distributed to some particular areas or viscera. (*c*) They may pass to blood vessels in the neighbourhood of the sympathetic trunk and supply these or may be carried along the vessels and their branches towards their peripheral distribution. (*d*) They may ascend to a higher level or descend to a lower level before leaving the sympathetic trunk either in one of its medial branches, in a grey ramus communicans or along adjacent blood vessels.

In addition to white and grey rami mixed types are found. Some of these in the thoracic region represent fusion of white and grey rami but some found in the cervical region contain bundles of thick myelinated fibres, which are somatic efferent in character and are utilizing the grey ramus as a convenient route to reach the prevertebral muscle (p. 1070). For a detailed description of rami communicantes and their variations from purely preganglionic to purely postganglionic types consult footnote reference[1107]

After diffusing through the plexuses the postganglionic fibres which arise in or join the plexuses are distributed mainly along blood vessels and some ducts.

**Functional significance.** The efferent postganglionic fibres which pass in the grey rami communicantes to the spinal nerves supply vasoconstrictor fibres to the blood vessels, secretomotor fibres to the sweat glands and motor fibres to the arrectores pilorum muscles in the areas supplied by the corresponding spinal nerve. Those which accompany the motor nerves to voluntary muscles are probably distributed only to the blood vessels supplying the muscles. Thus most, if not all, peripheral branches derived from the spinal nerves contain postganglionic sympathetic fibres. Those which pass to the viscera and other structures are concerned with vasoconstriction, dilatation of the pupils, dilatation of the bronchioles, glandular secretion, movements of the alimentary tract and the urinary bladder (relaxation of the muscle walls and contraction of the sphincters), etc. It is believed that usually, but not invariably, a single preganglionic fibre synapses with the postganglionic neurons innervating one effector system only; therefore a dissociation of sympathetic effects, such as sudomotor and vasomotor activities, can occur. The same is not necessarily true of visceral afferent fibres (p. 834). While in general the sympathetic and parasympathetic systems exert antagonistic influences on the viscera they supply, this is not always so. In the case of the urinary bladder, for instance, the normal emptying and filling of the viscus are controlled only by the parasympathetic system, the sympathetic being concerned with the supply of the blood vessels of the organ.

**Higher autonomic centres.** The peripheral autonomic nervous system is influenced by the activities of higher levels in the brainstem and cerebral hemispheres.

[1103] E. P. Samuel, *J. comp. Neurol.*, **98**, 1953.
[1104] M. R. Matthews and G. Raisman, *J. Anat.*, **105**. 1969.
[1105] T. H. Williams, *Nature, Lond.*, **214**, 1967.
[1106] R. Warwick, *J. Anat.*, **88**, 1954.
[1107] G. Winckler, *Archs Anat. Histol. Embryol.*, **44**, 1961.

The parts of the brain especially concerned have been described in the section on the Central Nervous System and include the brainstem reticular formation, various thalamic and hypothalamic nuclei, the limbic lobe and the prefrontal neocortex, and a variety of ascending and descending pathways which interconnect these regions.

**The sympathetic trunks** are two ganglionated nerve cords which extend from the base of the skull to the coccyx. In the neck the trunk is posterior to the carotid sheath and anterior to the transverse processes of the cervical vertebrae; in the thorax it is anterior to the heads of the ribs; in the abdomen it is anterolateral to the bodies of the lumbar vertebrae, and in the pelvis, anterior to the sacrum, medial to the anterior sacral foramina. Anterior to the coccyx the two trunks meet each other in the unpaired terminal *ganglion impar*.

The cervical ganglia are usually reduced to three by fusion of adjoining units, and from the cranial pole of the superior ganglion the internal carotid nerve commences. This nerve constitutes an ascending continuation of the sympathetic trunk, and it accompanies the internal carotid artery through its canal into the cranial cavity. In the thorax there are usually eleven ganglia, but the number may be ten or twelve. There are usually four ganglia in the lumbar and four or five in the sacral regions.

## CRANIAL PART OF THE SYMPATHETIC SYSTEM

The cranial part of the sympathetic system on each side begins as the **internal carotid nerve**, which is continued up from the superior cervical ganglion of the sympathetic trunk and contains postganglionic fibres derived from its cells. It ascends behind the internal carotid artery, and, entering the carotid canal in the temporal bone, divides into two branches, one of which is lateral and the other medial to the artery.

The *lateral branch*, the larger, gives filaments to the internal carotid artery, and forms the lateral part of the *internal carotid plexus*.

The *medial branch* also supplies filaments to the internal carotid artery, and, continuing onwards, forms the medial part of the internal carotid plexus.

**The internal carotid plexus** surrounds its artery, and occasionally contains a small gangliform swelling on the under side of the vessel, the *carotid ganglion*. In addition to this small ganglion, the rest of the plexus also contains some scattered sympathetic nerve cells. The lateral part of the plexus communicates with the trigeminal and pterygopalatine ganglia, with the abducent nerve and with the tympanic branch of the glossopharyngeal nerve; it distributes filaments to the wall of the internal carotid artery.

The branches communicating with the abducent nerve consist of one or two filaments which join that nerve as it lies upon the lateral side of the internal carotid artery. The communication with the pterygopalatine ganglion is effected by a branch named the *deep petrosal*; this branch perforates the cartilage filling the foramen lacerum, and joins the greater petrosal nerve to form the *nerve of the pterygoid canal*, which passes through the pterygoid canal to the pterygopalatine ganglion. The communication with the tympanic branch of the glossopharyngeal nerve is effected by the *superior* and *inferior caroticotympanic nerves*, which traverse the posterior wall of the carotid canal.

The medial part of the internal carotid plexus is inferomedial to the part of the internal carotid artery which is lateral to the sella turcica, in the cavernous sinus. It gives branches to the internal carotid artery, and communicates with the oculomotor, trochlear, ophthalmic and abducent nerves, and with the ciliary ganglion. It also sends vasomotor twigs along the branches of the internal carotid artery which supply the hypophysis cerebi (p. 1371).

The branch to the oculomotor nerve joins that nerve at its point of division; the branch to the trochlear nerve joins the latter as it lies in the lateral wall of the cavernous sinus; filaments are connected with the medial side of the ophthalmic nerve and one joins the abducent nerve. The filament to the ciliary ganglion arises from the anterior part of the plexus and enters the orbit through the superior orbital fissure; it may join the ganglion directly; it may unite with the communicating branch from the nasociliary nerve to the ganglion (p. 999), or it may travel via the ophthalmic nerve and its nasociliary branch. Its fibres pass through the ciliary ganglion without being interrupted and run in the short ciliary nerves to be distributed to the blood vessels of the eyeball. The fibres which supply the dilatator pupillae usually travel by the ophthalmic, nasociliary and long ciliary nerves. Some fibres may also innervate the ciliaris.[1108, 1109] The preganglionic fibres concerned leave the spinal cord in T. 1, and pass to the cervicothoracic ganglion, through which they pass uninterruptedly. They then ascend in the cervical part of the sympathetic trunk to reach the superior cervical ganglion, where they are relayed. Fibres issuing in the second, third and fourth spinal nerves may also be concerned in the innervation of intra-ocular muscles.

The terminal filaments from the internal carotid plexus are prolonged as plexuses around the anterior and middle cerebral arteries and the ophthalmic artery: along the anterior and middle cerebral arteries they may be traced to the pia mater; along the ophthalmic artery they pass into the orbit where they accompany each of the branches of that vessel. The filaments prolonged on the anterior communicating artery connect the sympathetic nerves of the right and left sides and a small ganglion may be found associated with these filaments. Much of the above detail depends upon comparatively old observations, and it should be noted that more disagreement and discrepancy still obtains in regard to such details than can be considered in a general textbook of anatomy. Consult footnote reference [1101] for an extensive bibliography and discussion.

## CERVICAL PART OF THE SYMPATHETIC SYSTEM

The cervical part of each sympathetic trunk consists of three ganglia distinguished, according to their positions, as the superior, middle and cervicothoracic, connected by intervening cords (7.226). This part sends grey rami communicantes to all the cervical spinal nerves, but receives no white rami communicantes from them; its spinal fibres are derived from the white rami communicantes of the upper thoracic nerves, which enter the corresponding thoracic ganglia of the sympathetic trunk, through which they ascend into the neck. In their course the grey rami communicantes may pierce the longus capitis or the scalenus anterior. (For details of the cervical grey rami see footnote references [1110-1113].)

**The superior cervical ganglion**, the largest of the three, is opposite the second and third cervical vertebrae and is believed to be formed by the coalescence of four ganglia, corresponding with the upper four cervical nerves. It is in relation, in front, with the sheath of the internal carotid artery; behind, with the longus capitis.

[1108] J. M. Génis-Gálvez, *Anat. Rec.*, **127**, 1957.
[1109] G. Törnqvist, *Invest. ophthal.*, **6**, 1967.
[1110] T. K. Potts, *J. Anat.*, **59**, 1925.
[1111] M. Oxford, *J. Anat.*, **62**, 1928.
[1112] J. Pick and D. Sheehan, *J. Anat.*, **80**, 1946.
[1113] S. Sunderland and G. M. Bedbrook, *Brain*, **72**, 1949.

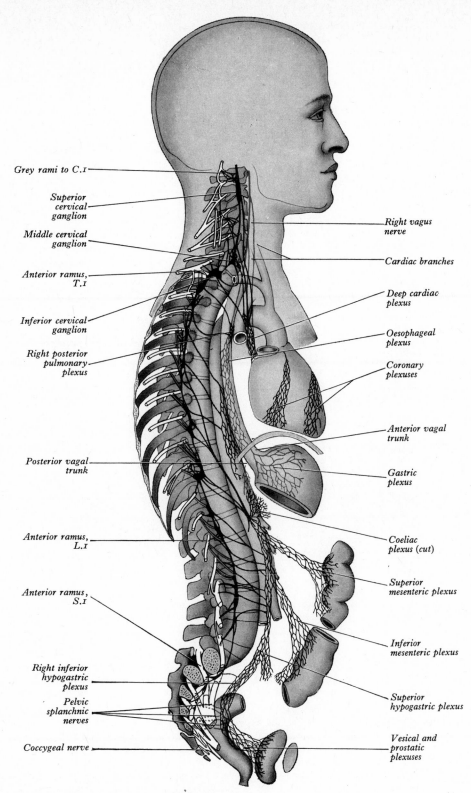

Grey rami to C.1

Superior cervical ganglion

Middle cervical ganglion

Anterior ramus, T.1

Inferior cervical ganglion

Right posterior pulmonary plexus

Posterior vagal trunk

Anterior ramus, L.1

Anterior ramus, S.1

Right inferior hypogastric plexus

Pelvic splanchnic nerves

Coccygeal nerve

Right vagus nerve

Cardiac branches

Deep cardiac plexus

Oesophageal plexus

Coronary plexuses

Anterior vagal trunk

Gastric plexus

Coeliac plexus (cut)

Superior mesenteric plexus

Inferior mesenteric plexus

Superior hypogastric plexus

Vesical and prostatic plexuses

7.226　The right sympathetic trunk and its connexions with the thoracic, abdominal and pelvic plexuses. *Blue:* parasympathetic fibres. *Black:* sympathetic trunk and branches. *Red:* white rami communicantes.

The internal carotid nerve (p. 1070) ascends from the upper end of the ganglion into the cranial cavity; the lower end of the ganglion is united by the connecting trunk with the middle cervical ganglion.

The branches of the ganglion may be divided into lateral, medial and anterior groups.

The *lateral branches* of the superior cervical ganglion consist of grey rami communicantes to the upper four cervical nerves and to certain of the cranial nerves. Delicate filaments run to the inferior ganglion of the vagus, and to the hypoglossal nerve; a branch, named the *jugular*

*nerve*, ascends to the base of the skull and divides into two twigs, one of which joins the inferior ganglion of the glossopharyngeal, and the other the superior ganglion of the vagus; other twigs pass to the superior jugular bulb and to the meninges in the posterior cranial fossa.

The *medial branches* of the superior cervical ganglion are the laryngopharyngeal and cardiac branches.

The *laryngopharyngeal branches* supply the carotid body, and pass to the side of the pharynx, where they join with branches from the glossopharyngeal and vagus nerves to form the *pharyngeal plexus* (p. 1248).

The *cardiac branch* arises by two or more filaments from the lower part of the superior cervical ganglion, and occasionally receives a twig from the trunk connecting the superior with the middle cervical ganglion. It is believed to contain only efferent fibres, the preganglionic outflow being from the upper thoracic segments of the spinal cord, and to be devoid of any visceral pain fibres from the heart (p. 1077). It runs down the neck behind the common carotid artery, and in front of the longus colli; it crosses in front of the inferior thyroid artery and recurrent laryngeal nerve. The course of the nerve of the right side then differs from that of the left. The *right nerve*, at the root of the neck, passes usually behind but sometimes in front of, the subclavian artery, and posterolateral to the brachiocephalic trunk to the back of the arch of the aorta, where it joins the deep (dorsal) part of the cardiac plexus. It is connected with other branches of the sympathetic; about the middle of the neck it receives filaments from the external laryngeal nerve; lower down, one or two vagal cardiac branches join it; and as it enters the thorax it is joined by a filament from the recurrent laryngeal nerve. Filaments from the nerve communicate with the thyroid branches from the middle cervical ganglion. The *left nerve*, in the thorax, runs in front of the left common carotid artery and across the left side of the arch of the aorta, to the superficial (ventral) part of the cardiac plexus. Sometimes it descends on the right side of the aorta and ends in the deep (dorsal) part of the cardiac plexus. It communicates with the cardiac branches of the middle cervical and cervicothoracic sympathetic ganglia, and sometimes with the inferior cervical cardiac branches of the left vagus, and branches from these mixed nerves pass down to form a plexus on the ascending aorta.

The *anterior branches* of the superior cervical ganglion ramify upon the common carotid artery, and upon the external carotid artery and its branches, forming around each a delicate plexus in which small ganglia are occasionally found. The plexus surrounding the facial artery supplies a filament to the submandibular ganglion, and the plexus on the middle meningeal artery sends one ramus to the otic ganglion, and another, termed the *external petrosal nerve*, to the ganglion of the facial nerve. Many of the fibres coursing along the external carotid artery and its branches to supply the sweat glands on the face ultimately leave the blood vessels to be distributed through terminal branches of the trigeminal nerve.

**The middle cervical ganglion** (7.227), the smallest of the three cervical ganglia, is occasionally absent as such, being replaced by minute ganglia in the sympathetic trunk in this region; it may be fused with the superior cervical ganglion. It is usually at the level of the sixth cervical vertebra, anterior or just superior to, the inferior thyroid artery, or it may lie near the cervicothoracic ganglion (p. 1073). It is probably formed by the coalescence of two ganglia corresponding with the fifth and sixth cervical segments, judging by its postganglionic rami, which pass to the fifth and sixth cervical nerves, but also, sometimes to the fourth and seventh. The ganglion also gives off thyroid and cardiac branches. It is connected to the cervicothoracic ganglion by two or more cords, which are very variable in their disposition. The posterior cord usually splits to enclose the vertebral artery. The most anterior cord loops down in front of and then below the first part of the subclavian artery, medial to the origin of its internal thoracic branch, and supplies rami to it. This loop is the *ansa subclavia*. It is intimately related to the cervical pleura, frequently consists of more than one filament, and generally communicates with the phrenic nerve. It is uncertain whether this last connexion indicates a contribution to or from the phrenic nerve. Similarly, a connexion between the ansa subclavia and the vagus nerve, usually described, is of uncertain significance.

The *thyroid branches* run along the inferior thyroid artery to the thyroid gland; they communicate with the superior cardiac, external laryngeal and recurrent laryngeal nerves and send branches to the parathyroid glands. The supplies to the thyroid and parathyroid glands are in part vasomotor, but some fibres reach the secretory cells.[1114]

The *cardiac branch*, the largest of the sympathetic cardiac branches, arises from the middle cervical ganglion, or from the trunk connecting the middle with the cervicothoracic ganglion. On the *right side* it descends behind the

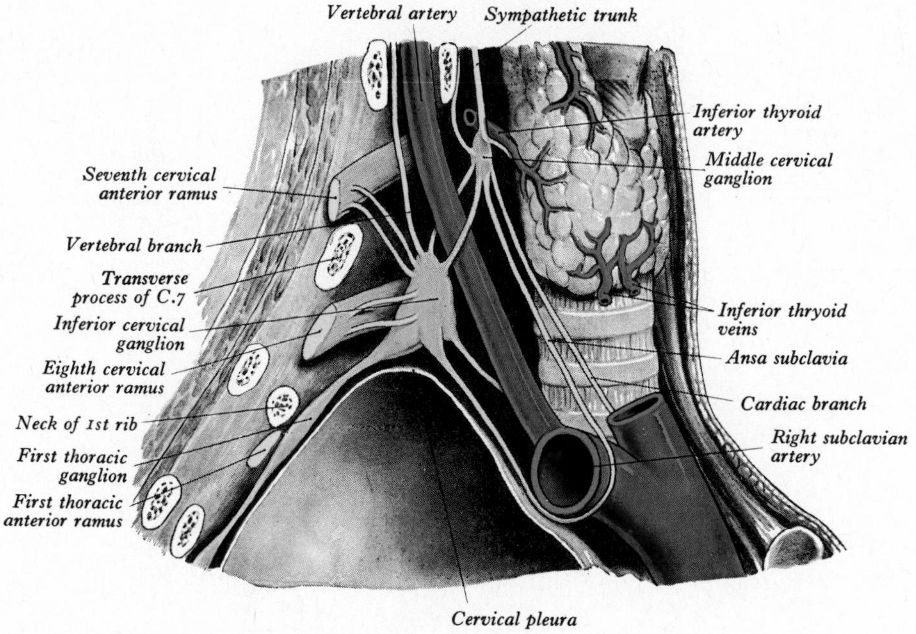
Vertebral artery
Sympathetic trunk
Inferior thyroid artery
Middle cervical ganglion
Seventh cervical anterior ramus
Vertebral branch
Transverse process of C.7
Inferior cervical ganglion
Eighth cervical anterior ramus
Neck of 1st rib
First thoracic ganglion
First thoracic anterior ramus
Inferior thryoid veins
Ansa subclavia
Cardiac branch
Right subclavian artery
Cervical pleura

7.227A The middle and inferior cervical ganglia of the right side. Viewed from the right.

[1114] H. E. Raybuck, *Anat. Rec.*, **112**, 1952.

common carotid artery, and at the root of the neck runs either in front of or behind the subclavian artery; it then descends on the trachea, receives a few filaments from the recurrent laryngeal nerve, and joins the right half of the deep (dorsal) part of the cardiac plexus. In the neck, it communicates with the superior cardiac and recurrent laryngeal nerves. On the *left side*, the nerve enters the thorax between the left common carotid and subclavian arteries, and joins the left half of the deep (dorsal) part of the cardiac plexus.

Fine branches from the middle cervical ganglion also pass to the trachea and oesophagus.

**The cervicothoracic (stellate) ganglion** is irregularly shaped, and much larger than the middle cervical ganglion, being probably formed by the coalescence of the lower two cervical segmental ganglia with the first thoracic. Sometimes the second (and even the third and fourth) thoracic ganglion is fused with the mass; in other instances the first thoracic ganglion is separate and the upper mass then constitutes an *inferior cervical ganglion* (7.226, 227). Owing to the marked change in direction of the sympathetic trunk at the junction of the neck and thorax, the long axis of the cervicothoracic ganglion is almost antero-posterior. The ganglion lies on or just lateral to the lateral border of the longus colli and between the base of the transverse process of the seventh cervical vertebra and the neck of the first rib, which are posterior to it, and the vertebral artery and its associated veins which are anterior. Below it is separated from the posterior aspect of the cervical pleura by the suprapleural membrane; the costo-cervical trunk branches near its lower pole. On its lateral side is the superior intercostal artery.

A small ganglion, the *vertebral ganglion*, may be found on the sympathetic trunk anterior or anteromedial to the commencement of the vertebral artery and directly above the subclavian artery. When present it may give rise to the ansa subclavia and is joined also to the cervicothoracic ganglion by fibres which pass both in front of and behind the vertebral artery. The vertebral ganglion is usually regarded as a detached portion of the middle cervical or cervicothoracic ganglion. Like the middle cervical ganglion it may supply grey rami communicantes to the fourth and fifth cervical spinal nerves.

The cervicothoracic ganglion sends grey rami communicantes to the seventh and eighth cervical and first thoracic nerves, gives off a cardiac branch, supplies branches to neighbouring vessels, and not infrequently sends a branch to join the vagus nerve.

The *grey rami communicantes* to the seventh cervical spinal nerve vary from one to five in number. Two, which is the usual number, are shown in **7.227**. Another often ascends medial to the vertebral artery and in front of the transverse process of the seventh cervical vertebra and, after communicating here with the seventh cervical nerve, sends a small branch upwards through the foramen transversarium of the sixth cervical vertebra in company with the vertebral vessels to join the sixth cervical nerve as it emerges from the intervertebral foramen. Another inconstant branch may pass through the foramen transversarium of the seventh vertebra. The grey rami to the eighth cervical spinal nerve are also multiple and vary from three to six in number.

The *cardiac branch* arises from the cervicothoracic ganglion. It descends behind the subclavian artery and along the front of the trachea, to join the deep part of the cardiac plexus. Behind the subclavian artery it communicates with the recurrent laryngeal nerve and the cardiac branch of the middle cervical ganglion. It is often replaced by a variable number of fine branches derived from the cervicothoracic ganglion and the ansa subclavia.

The *branches to blood vessels* form plexuses on the sub-

clavian artery and its branches. The plexus around the subclavian artery is derived from the cervicothoracic ganglion and the ansa subclavia; it extends to the first part of the axillary artery, but fibres may extend further, though not in large numbers. The plexus on the vertebral artery is derived mainly from a thick branch of the cervico-

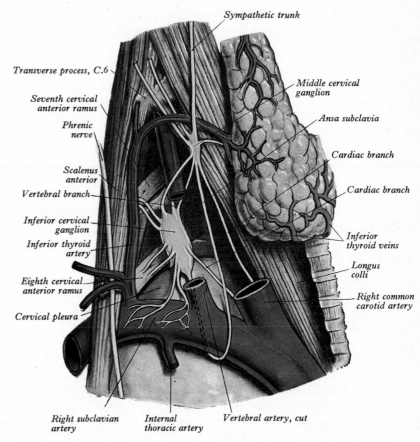

*Sympathetic trunk*

*Transverse process, C.6*

*Seventh cervical anterior ramus*

*Phrenic nerve*

*Scalenus anterior*

*Vertebral branch*

*Inferior cervical ganglion*

*Inferior thyroid artery*

*Eighth cervical anterior ramus*

*Cervical pleura*

*Middle cervical ganglion*

*Ansa subclavia*

*Cardiac branch*

*Cardiac branch*

*Inferior thyroid veins*

*Longus colli*

*Right common carotid artery*

*Right subclavian artery*    *Internal thoracic artery*    *Vertebral artery, cut*

**7.227 B**  Anterior view of the same structures as in **7.227 A**.  Part of the vertebral artery has been excised to show the inferior cervical ganglion. Note the proximity of the inferior cervical and first thoracic ganglia. These are usually fused to form the cervicothoracic ganglion.

thoracic ganglion which ascends behind the vertebral artery to the foramen transversarium of the sixth cervical vertebra, reinforced by branches from the vertebral ganglion or the cervical sympathetic trunk which pass cranially on the ventral aspect of the artery. From the plexus, branches (*deep rami communicantes*) pass to the anterior rami of the upper five or six cervical spinal nerves. The plexus contains a number of nerve cells. The plexus is continued into the skull along the vertebral and basilar arteries and their branches as far as the posterior cerebral artery, where it meets the plexus derived from that on the internal carotid artery. Some authorities consider that the vertebral plexus represents the main intracranial extension of the sympathetic system.[1115, 1116] The plexus on the inferior thyroid artery accompanies the artery to the thyroid gland, and communicates with the recurrent and external laryngeal nerves, with the cardiac branch of the superior cervical ganglion, and with the plexus on the common carotid artery.

The preganglionic fibres for the head and neck leave the spinal cord through the upper five thoracic nerves (mainly the upper three); they pass up the sympathetic

[1115] G. Lazorthes, *Le Système Neurovasculaire*, Masson, Paris. 1949.
[1116] G. A. G. Mitchell, *Nature, Lond.*, **120**, 1952.

trunk to synapse about cells in the cervical ganglia, whence postganglionic fibres are distributed as indicated above.

The preganglionic fibres concerned with supplying the upper limb are derived from the upper thoracic segments of the spinal cord, probably T. 2–6 (or 7). These fibres ascend the sympathetic trunk to synapse with cells mainly in the cervicothoracic ganglion, whence postganglionic fibres pass to the brachial plexus, mainly the lower trunk. Most of the vasoconstrictor fibres supplying the arteries of the upper limb emerge from the spinal cord in the ventral roots of the second and third thoracic nerves. These arteries can thus be denervated surgically by cutting the sympathetic trunk below the third thoracic ganglion, severing the rami communicantes connected with the second and third thoracic ganglia, or cutting (intradurally) the ventral roots of the second and third thoracic spinal nerves. The white ramus to the cervicothoracic ganglion is not cut, partly because it does not convey many vasomotor or sudomotor fibres to the upper limb, but mainly because it contains most of the preganglionic fibres which pass up the sympathetic trunk to the superior cervical ganglion, from which postganglionic branches pass to supply vasoconstrictor and sudomotor nerves to the face and neck, secretory fibres to the salivary glands, the dilatator pupillae (and probably ciliaris oculi), the non-striated muscle in the upper and lower eyelids and the orbitalis. Destruction of this nerve would result in constriction of the pupil, drooping of the upper eyelid (ptosis), enophthalmos and absence of sweating on the face and neck (*Horner's syndrome*), and possibly some disturbance of accommodation. For a review of such procedures consult footnote reference [1117].

The blood vessels of the upper limb beyond the first part of the axillary artery receive their sympathetic nerve supply by means of branches from the brachial plexus through nerves adjacent to the arteries, e.g. the median nerve supplies branches to the brachial artery and palmar arches, the ulnar nerve supplies the ulnar artery and palmar arches and the radial nerve supplies the radial artery.

The first and second (and occasionally the third) intercostal nerves are sometimes connected together in front of the necks of the ribs by filaments which contain postganglionic fibres derived from the grey rami associated with these nerves; these fibres provide another pathway by which postganglionic nerves from the upper thoracic ganglia may pass to the brachial plexus.

## THORACIC PART OF THE SYMPATHETIC SYSTEM

The thoracic part of each sympathetic trunk (7.226, 228) contains a series of ganglia, which usually correspond approximately in number to that of the thoracic spinal nerves, but their number is variable. The first thoracic ganglion is usually fused with the inferior cervical to form the cervicothoracic ganglion. The succeeding ganglion is called the second thoracic ganglion in order that each thoracic ganglion should correspond numerically with the other segmental structures. With the exception of the last two or three, the thoracic ganglia rest against the heads of the ribs, and are posterior to the costal pleura; the last two or three are placed on the sides of the bodies of the corresponding vertebrae. Inferiorly, the thoracic sympathetic trunk passes dorsal to the medial lumbocostal arch (or it may pierce the crus of the diaphragm) to become continuous with the lumbar sympathetic trunk. The ganglia are small and are connected together by the intervening portions of the trunk.

Two or more rami communicantes, white and grey, connect each ganglion with its corresponding spinal nerve,

the white rami joining the spinal nerve farther distally than the grey. Sometimes a grey and white ramus may be fused to form a single 'mixed' ramus (p. 1069).

The *medial branches from the upper five ganglia* are very small; they supply filaments to the thoracic aorta and its branches. On the aorta they form a delicate plexus (*thoracic aortic plexus*) together with filaments from the greater splanchnic nerve. Twigs from the second to fifth or sixth ganglia enter the posterior pulmonary plexus; others, from the second, third, fourth and fifth ganglia, pass to the deep (dorsal) part of the cardiac plexus. Small branches from these pulmonary and cardiac nerves pass to the oesophagus and trachea.

The *medial branches from the lower seven ganglia* are large; they distribute filaments to the aorta, and unite to from the greater, the lesser and the lowest splanchnic nerves, the last of which is not always identifiable.

The *greater splanchnic nerve* consists mainly of myelinated, preganglionic and visceral afferent fibres; it is formed by branches from the fifth to the ninth or tenth thoracic ganglia, but the fibres in the higher branches may be traced upwards in the sympathetic trunk as far as the first or second thoracic ganglion. It descends obliquely on the bodies of the vertebrae, supplies fine branches to the descending thoracic aorta, perforates the crus of the diaphragm, and ends mainly in the coeliac ganglion, but partly in the aorticorenal ganglion and the suprarenal gland. A *splanchnic ganglion* exists on this nerve opposite the eleventh or twelfth thoracic vertebra.

The *lesser splanchnic nerve* is formed by filaments from the ninth and tenth, sometimes the tenth and eleventh, thoracic ganglia, and from the trunk between the ganglia. It pierces the diaphragm with the preceding nerve, and joins the aorticorenal ganglion.

The *lowest splanchnic nerve* (or renal nerve) arises from the last thoracic ganglion. It gains the abdomen with the sympathetic trunk, and ends in the renal plexus.

## LUMBAR PART OF THE SYMPATHETIC SYSTEM

The lumbar part of each sympathetic trunk (7.228, 229) usually consists of four lumbar ganglia, connected together by the intervening portions of the trunk. It is in the extraperitoneal connective tissue anterior to the vertebral column, along the medial margin of the psoas major. Posterior to the medial lumbocostal arch it is continuous with the thoracic part of the trunk and inferiorly, by passing posterior to the common iliac artery, with the pelvic part. On the right side it is overlapped by the inferior vena cava; on the left by the lateral aortic lymph nodes. It lies in front of the lumbar vessels, but some lumbar veins may pass anterior to it.

The first and second, and sometimes the third, lumbar ventral rami send *white rami communicantes* to the corresponding ganglia.

*Grey rami communicantes* pass from all the ganglia to the lumbar spinal nerves. These rami are of considerable length and accompany the lumbar arteries round the sides of the bodies of the vertebrae, medial to the fibrous arches to which the psoas major is attached.

Generally four *lumbar splanchnic nerves* pass from the ganglia to join the coeliac, intermesenteric (abdominal aortic) and superior hypogastric plexuses. The first lumbar splanchnic nerve arises from the first ganglion and joins the coeliac, renal and intermesenteric plexuses. The second nerve arises from the second (and sometimes also the third) ganglion and joins the lower part of the intermesenteric plexus. The third nerve issues from the third

[1117] H. A. Haxton, *Ann. R. Coll. Surg.*, **14**, 1954.

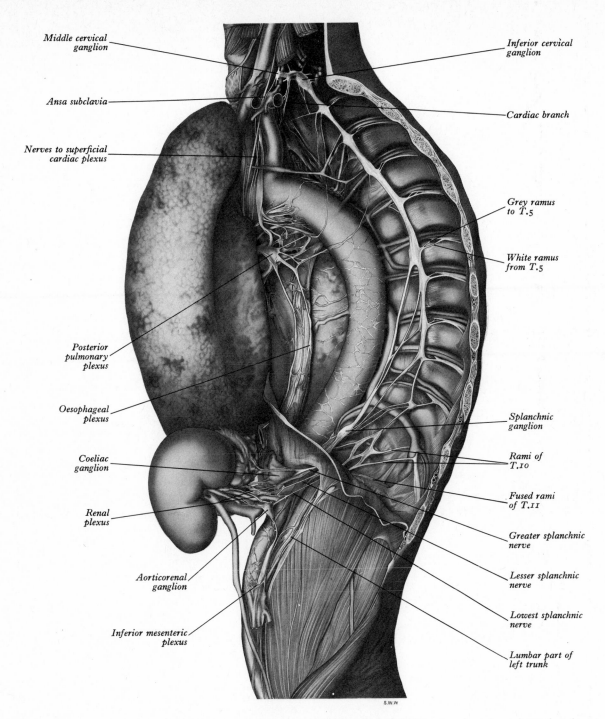

Middle cervical
ganglion

Ansa subclavia

Nerves to superficial
cardiac plexus

Posterior
pulmonary
plexus

Oesophageal
plexus

Coeliac
ganglion

Renal
plexus

Aorticorenal
ganglion

Inferior mesenteric
plexus

Inferior cervical
ganglion

Cardiac branch

Grey ramus
to T.5

White ramus
from T.5

Splanchnic
ganglion

Rami of
T.10

Fused rami
of T.11

Greater splanchnic
nerve

Lesser splanchnic
nerve

Lowest splanchnic
nerve

Lumbar part of
left trunk

S.W.W

7.228   The thoracic part of the sympathetic system of the left side. (Drawn from a dissection by the late Dr. G. D. Channell.) Note that the diaphragm has been divided close to its posterior attachment, and the left lung and the left kidney have been drawn forwards and rotated to the right, so as to expose the posterior surface of the left kidney and suprarenal gland.

or fourth ganglion and passes in front of the common iliac vessels to join the superior hypogastric plexus. The fourth lumbar splanchnic, from the lowest ganglion, goes dorsal to the common iliac vessels to join the lower part of the superior hypogastric plexus or the hypogastric nerve.

*Vascular branches* from all the lumbar ganglia pass to the intermesenteric (aortic) plexus. From the lower lumbar splanchnic nerves, fibres pass to the common iliac arteries, around which they form a plexus continued thence along the internal iliac artery and around the external iliac artery, in the latter case as far as the proximal part of the femoral artery. Many of the postganglionic fibres in the grey rami, connecting the lumbar ganglia to the lumbar spinal nerves, travel in the femoral nerve, and thence in its muscular, cutaneous and saphenous branches, to supply vasoconstrictor nerves to the femoral artery and

its branches in the thigh. Other postganglionic fibres travel in the obturator nerve to the obturator artery. Considerable uncertainties persist with regard to the sympathetic supply to the lower limb (see footnote references [1118, 1119]).

## PELVIC PART OF THE SYMPATHETIC SYSTEM

The pelvic part of each sympathetic trunk (7.229) is situated in the extraperitoneal tissue in front of the sacrum, medial or anterior to the anterior sacral foramina. It comprises four or five sacral ganglia, connected by the intervening sections of the trunk. It is continuous cranially with

[1118] F. R. Wilde, *Br. J. Surg.*, **39**, 1951.
[1119] G. M. Wyburn, *Scot. med. J.*, **1**, 1956.

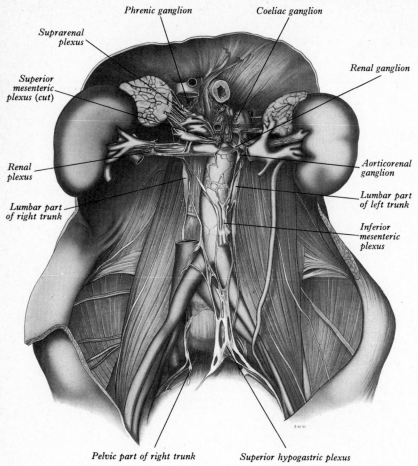

*Phrenic ganglion*  *Coeliac ganglion*

*Suprarenal plexus*

*Superior mesenteric plexus (cut)*

*Renal ganglion*

*Renal plexus*

*Aorticorenal ganglion*

*Lumbar part of left trunk*

*Lumbar part of right trunk*

*Inferior mesenteric plexus*

*Pelvic part of right trunk*  *Superior hypogastric plexus*

**7.229** The abdominal portion of the sympathetic system. (Drawn from a dissection by the late Dr. G. D. Channell.)

the lumbar part, while caudally, the two pelvic sympathetic trunks converge, and unite on the front of the coccyx in the small *ganglion impar*.

*Grey rami communicantes* pass from the ganglia to the sacral and coccygeal spinal nerves. No white rami communicantes pass to this part of the sympathetic trunk.

The *medial branches of distribution* communicate on the front of the sacrum with the corresponding branches from the opposite side; twigs from the first two ganglia join the inferior hypogastric plexus (pelvic plexus) or the hypogastric nerve, and others form a plexus on the median sacral artery. Filaments are distributed to the glomus coccygeum from the loop uniting the two trunks. The 'hypogastric nerve', which is itself usually plexiform, is a somewhat redundant term for the connexions, right and left, which exist between the superior and inferior hypogastric plexuses. (*See* p. 1079.)

*Vascular branches*. Through the grey rami many postganglionic fibres pass to the roots of the sacral plexus, particularly those forming the tibial nerve, to be conveyed to the popliteal artery and its branches in the leg and foot. Others are conveyed by the pudendal and superior and inferior gluteal nerves to the accompanying arteries. Branches to lymph nodes are also described.[1120]

The preganglionic fibres concerned with supplying the lower limb are derived from the lower three thoracic and upper two or three lumbar segments of the spinal cord. They reach the lower thoracic and upper lumbar ganglia through the white rami and some pass down the sympathetic trunk to synapse about cells in the lumbar ganglia, whence postganglionic fibres pass to the femoral nerve to be distributed to the femoral artery and its branches in the thigh; other fibres pass down the sympathetic trunk to synapse with cells in the upper two or three sacral ganglia, whence postganglionic axons pass to the tibial nerve to supply the popliteal artery and its branches in the leg and foot. Sympathetic denervation of the vessels of the lower limb can thus be produced by removing the upper three lumbar ganglia and the intervening parts of the sympathetic trunk, all the preganglionic fibres to the lower limb thus being divided.

[1120] W. Woźniak, *Folia morph.*, **25**, 1966; W. Woźniak and U. Skowrońska, *Anat. Anz.*, **120**, 1967.

# PLEXUSES OF THE AUTONOMIC NERVOUS SYSTEM

The larger plexuses of the autonomic system are aggregations of nerves and ganglia, situated in the thoracic, abdominal and pelvic cavities, and named the cardiac, coeliac and hypogastric plexuses. From the plexuses branches are given to the thoracic, abdominal and pelvic viscera. Extensions from these major perivascular plexuses pass along most of the branches of the large vessels with which they are associated. Such extensions are usually named after the branch artery along which they are distributed. This leads to a plethora of named plexuses, receiving separate description, the details of which may overshadow the essential continuity of the vascular plexuses in the thorax, abdomen and pelvis.

## THE CARDIAC PLEXUSES

The cardiac plexus (**7.226, 228**) is situated at the base of the heart, and is divided into a *superficial* and a *deep* (dorsal) *part*, which are closely connected. Several small ganglia are found in the plexus, the largest and most constant being the *cardiac ganglion* described below.

**The superficial (ventral) part of the cardiac plexus** lies below the arch of the aorta, anterior to the right pulmonary artery. It is formed by the cardiac branch

of the superior cervical ganglion of the left sympathetic trunk, and the lower of the two cervical cardiac branches of the left vagus. A small ganglion, termed the *cardiac ganglion*, is usually present in this plexus, and is situated immediately below the arch of the aorta, on the right of the ligamentum arteriosum. The superficial part of the cardiac plexus gives branches (*a*) to the deep part of the plexus, (*b*) to the right coronary plexus, (*c*) to the left anterior pulmonary plexus.

**The deep (dorsal) part of the cardiac plexus** is situated in front of the bifurcation of the trachea, above the point of division of the pulmonary trunk, and posterior to the aortic arch. It is formed by the cardiac nerves derived from the cervical and upper thoracic ganglia of the sympathetic trunk, and the cardiac branches of the vagus and recurrent laryngeal nerves. The only cardiac nerves which do not join the deep part of the cardiac plexus are those already noted as joining the superficial part of the plexus.

The branches from the *right half* of the deep part of the cardiac plexus pass, some in front of, and others behind, the right pulmonary artery; the former, the more numerous, transmit a few filaments to the right anterior pulmonary plexus, and are then continued onwards to form part of the right coronary plexus; those behind the pulmonary artery distribute a few filaments to the right atrium, and are then continued onwards to form part of the left coronary plexus.

The *left half* of the deep part of the cardiac plexus is connected with the superficial part of the plexus, and gives filaments to the left atrium, and to the left anterior pulmonary plexus, and is then continued to form the greater part of the left coronary plexus.

**The left coronary plexus** is larger than the right, and accompanies the left coronary artery; it is formed chiefly by filaments prolonged from the left half of the deep part of the cardiac plexus, and by a few from the right half. It gives branches to the left atrium and ventricle.

**The right coronary plexus** is formed partly from the superficial and partly from the deep parts of the cardiac plexus. It accompanies the right coronary artery, and gives branches to the right atrium and ventricle.

All the cardiac branches of the vagus and the sympathetic contain both afferent and efferent fibres, except the cardiac branch of the superior cervical sympathetic ganglion which contains efferent (postganglionic) fibres only.

The *efferent* preganglionic sympathetic fibres arise in the upper four or five thoracic segments of the spinal cord; they pass by white rami communicantes to synapse about cells in the upper thoracic ganglia on the sympathetic trunk, though many travel up the trunk to synapse in the cervical ganglia. From the thoracic and cervical ganglia, postganglionic fibres emerge to form the sympathetic cardiac nerves, the functions of which are acceleration of the heart and dilatation of the coronary arteries. Of the sympathetic fibres arising from the first four or five segments of the spinal cord, the upper ones pass to the ascending aorta, pulmonary trunk and ventricles, while the lower ones supply the atria.

The *efferent* parasympathetic fibres are derived from the dorsal nucleus of the vagus and from cells near the nucleus ambiguus, and run in the cardiac branches of the vagus to synapse about cells in the cardiac plexuses and in the walls of the atria. These vagal fibres are concerned with slowing of the heart and with constriction of the coronary arteries (see also p. 1068). In man (and most mammals) the intrinsic cardiac nerve cells are limited to the atria and the interatrial septum;[1121, 1122] they are most numerous in the subepicardial connective tissue and near the sinuatrial and atrioventricular nodes. For an exposition of variations in the human sympathetic cardiac innervation, consult footnote reference [1123].

## THE PULMONARY PLEXUSES

The pulmonary plexuses lie on the anterior and posterior aspects of the bronchial and vascular structures in the roots of the lungs, the anterior pulmonary plexus being much smaller than the posterior. The plexuses are formed by branches from the vagus and the sympathetic. The efferent parasympathetic fibres arise from the dorsal nucleus of the vagus. The efferent sympathetic fibres are postganglionic branches of the second to fifth thoracic ganglia of the sympathetic trunk.

The *anterior pulmonary plexus* is formed by branches from the vagus and from the deep cardiac plexus, the left anterior plexus receiving additional fibres from the superficial cardiac plexus. The *posterior pulmonary plexus* is formed by branches from the vagus, from the deep cardiac plexus and from the second to fifth or sixth thoracic sympathetic ganglia, the left posterior plexus receiving additional branches from the left recurrent laryngeal nerve.

From the plexuses, nerves pass into the lung to form networks around the branches of the bronchi and the pulmonary and bronchial vessels, extending as far as the visceral pleura. On these nerves, near the roots of the lungs, there are minute collections of nerve cells with which the efferent preganglionic vagal fibres synapse. (In a number of organs, notably the small intestine, *interstitial cells* have been described in the terminal autonomic network which is characteristic in many sites. The presence of these in thoracic organs, apart perhaps from the oesophagus, has not been substantiated.[1124]) The efferent vagal fibres are bronchoconstrictor, secretomotor to the mucous bronchial glands and vasodilator in function. The efferent sympathetic fibres are bronchodilator and vasoconstrictor.

## THE COELIAC PLEXUS

The coeliac plexus (**7**.226, 229), the largest of the three great autonomic plexuses, is situated at the level of the last thoracic and the upper part of the first lumbar vertebra, and is a dense network of nerve fibres which unite together two large *coeliac ganglia*. It surrounds the coeliac artery and the root of the superior mesenteric artery. It lies posterior to the stomach and the omental bursa, anterior to the crura of the diaphragm and the commencement of the abdominal aorta, and between the suprarenal glands. The plexus and the ganglia are joined by the greater and lesser splanchnic nerves of both sides and some filaments from the vagus and phrenic nerves and extend as numerous secondary plexuses along the neighbouring arteries.

The *coeliac ganglia* are two irregularly shaped masses placed, one on each side of the median plane, between the suprarenal gland and the origin of the coeliac artery, and in front of the crura of the diaphragm, that on the right side being placed behind the inferior vena cava and that on the left side behind the splenic vessels. The upper part of each ganglion is joined by the greater splanchnic nerve, while the lower part, which is more or less detached and is named the *aorticorenal* ganglion, receives the lesser splanchnic nerve and gives off the greater part of the renal plexus. The position of the ganglion is very variable, being anywhere in the general vicinity of the origin of the renal artery from the aorta. For a recent description and discussion of its connexions, and the distribution of its fibres to tubules and glomeruli, in the kidney, consult footnote reference [1125].

The secondary plexuses springing from or connected with the coeliac plexus are the phrenic, splenic, hepatic, left gastric, intermesenteric, suprarenal, renal, testicular or ovarian, superior mesenteric, and inferior mesenteric.

**The phrenic plexus** accompanies the corresponding inferior phrenic artery to the diaphragm, some filaments passing to the suprarenal gland. It arises from the upper part of the coeliac ganglion, and is larger on the right than on the left side. It receives one or two branches from the phrenic nerve. At the point of junction of the right phrenic plexus with the phrenic nerve there is a small mass, the *phrenic ganglion*. This plexus distributes some branches to the inferior vena cava, and to the suprarenal and hepatic plexuses.

**The hepatic plexus**, the largest derivative of the coeliac plexus, also receives filaments from the left and right vagus and right phrenic nerves. It accompanies the hepatic artery and portal vein and their branches into the liver, and in the liver the nerves are confined to the vicinity

[1121] F. Davies, E. T. B. Francis and T. S. King, *J. Anat.*, **86**, 1952.
[1122] T. S. King and J. B. Coakley, *J. Anat.*, **92**, 1958.
[1123] J. P. Ellison and T. H. Williams, *Am. J. Anat.*, **124**, 1969.
[1124] C. Dijkstra, *Mikroskopie*, **24**, 1969.
[1125] J. E. Norvell, *J. comp. Neurol.*, **33**, 1968.

of the blood vessels. Branches from the plexus accompany all the branches of the hepatic artery. Those passing to the gall bladder form a scanty *cystic plexus*; branches also pass to the bile ducts. The branches accompanying the right gastric artery supply the pylorus. A considerable plexus accompanies the gastroduodenal artery and its branches. From this plexus branches pass to the pylorus and superior part of the duodenum. Many of the nerves pass with the right gastro-epiploic artery to supply the right part of the stomach and the greater curvature. Others pass with the superior pancreaticoduodenal artery and supply the descending part of the duodenum, head of the pancreas and the lower part of the bile duct. The hepatic plexus contains both afferent and efferent sympathetic and parasympathetic fibres, and it is believed that the vagal constituents are motor to the musculature of the gall bladder and bile ducts and inhibitory to the sphincter of the bile duct. A distinct nerve to the sphincter was identified in twenty-three out of twenty-five human dissections.[1126]

**The left gastric plexus** accompanies the left gastric artery along the lesser curvature of the stomach, and joins with the gastric branches of the vagus nerves. The gastric sympathetic nerves are motor to the pyloric sphincter but inhibitory to the muscular coats of the stomach.

**The splenic plexus** is formed by branches from the coeliac plexus, left coeliac ganglion and right vagus nerve. It accompanies the splenic artery to the spleen, giving off, in its course, subsidiary plexuses along the various branches of the artery. The fibres are principally, if not wholly, sympathetic in origin and terminate on the blood vessels and unstriped muscle of the splenic capsule and trabeculae.

**The suprarenal plexus** is formed by branches from the coeliac ganglion, coeliac plexus and the greater splanchnic nerve. Relative to its size, the suprarenal gland has a larger autonomic supply than any other organ. The nerves have hitherto been described as myelinated and preganglionic in nature. In the rat, however, the non-myelinated fibres are ten times as numerous as the myelinated; these non-myelinated fibres are regarded as preganglionic. They terminate in junctions like synapses, often deeply invaginated, in contiguity with chromaffin cells, which are hence homologous with postganglionic sympathetic neurons (p. 1380). A space of 150–200 nm separates the contiguous plasma membranes which often exhibit electron-dense zones. Small vesicles and large vesicles with electron-dense granular contents are present in the endings. Only non-myelinated fibres have been seen innervating chromaffin cells, all of which are related to one or more nerve terminal. Multipolar nerve cell bodies are also found in the adrenal medulla and some of the preganglionic non-myelinated nerve fibres form axodendritic synapses with these cells. The destination of the axons of these nerve cells is not known.[1128] A preponderance of non-myelinated fibres in the suprarenal plexus has also been described in man.[1127-1129]

**The renal plexus** is a rich plexus formed by filaments from the coeliac ganglion, coeliac plexus, aorticorenal ganglion, lowest thoracic splanchnic nerve, first lumbar splanchnic nerve and the aortic plexus. Small collections of nerve cells are found in the plexus, the largest usually lying behind the commencement of the renal artery. The plexus is continued into the kidney around the branches of the renal artery to supply the vessels and the renal glomeruli and tubules, particularly the tubules in the cortex of the kidney. For the main part the renal nerves are vasomotor in function. From the renal plexus branches are given to the ureteric and the testicular (or ovarian) plexuses. The *ureteric plexus* receives fibres from three sources, the upper part by branches from the renal and aortic plexuses, the middle part by branches from the superior hypogastric plexus and the hypogastric nerve, and the lower part by branches from the hypogastric nerve and the inferior hypogastric plexus. The nerves to the ureter are believed to influence its inherent motility.

**The testicular plexus** accompanies the gonadal artery to the testis. Its upper part is formed by branches from the renal and aortic plexuses. Lower down the plexus is reinforced by branches from the superior and inferior hypogastric plexuses. Branches from the plexus pass to the epididymis and the ductus deferens.

**The ovarian plexus** accompanies the ovarian artery and is distributed to the ovary and uterine tube. The upper part of the plexus is formed by branches from the renal and aortic plexuses; lower down it is reinforced from the superior and inferior hypogastric plexuses.

The nerves in the testicular and ovarian plexuses contain efferent and afferent sympathetic fibres; the efferent fibres are vasomotor in nature and are derived from the tenth and eleventh thoracic segments of the spinal cord; the parasympathetic fibres, derived from the inferior hypogastric plexuses, are probably vasodilator in nature.

**The superior mesenteric plexus** is a continuation of the lower part of the coeliac plexus, and receives a branch from the junction of the right vagus nerve with the latter plexus. It surrounds the superior mesenteric artery, accompanies it into the mesentery, and divides into a number of secondary plexuses which are distributed to the parts supplied by the artery—pancreatic branches to the pancreas; jejunal and ileal branches to the small intestine; ileocolic, right colic, and middle colic branches, which supply the corresponding parts of the large intestine. The *superior mesenteric ganglion* is situated in the upper part of the plexus, usually immediately above the origin of the superior mesenteric artery.

The sympathetic nerves to the intestine are motor to the ileocaecal sphincter but inhibitory to the muscle of the gut. In addition, they convey vasoconstrictor fibres.

**The abdominal aortic plexus** (intermesenteric plexus) is formed by branches from the coeliac plexus and ganglia, and receives filaments from the first and second lumbar splanchnic nerves. It is situated upon the sides and front of the aorta, between the origins of the superior and inferior mesenteric arteries. It is not a dense plexus but consists of four to twelve nerves (intermesenteric nerves) connected by obliquely arranged branches. It is continuous above with the coeliac plexus and the coeliac and aorticorenal ganglia, and below with the superior hypogastric plexus. From this plexus parts of the testicular, the inferior mesenteric, the iliac and the superior hypogastric plexuses arise; it also distributes filaments to the inferior vena cava.

**The inferior mesenteric plexus** is derived chiefly from the aortic plexus, but also receives branches from the second and third lumbar splanchnic nerves. It surrounds the inferior mesenteric artery and is distributed along its branches; thus the left colic plexus supplies the left part of the transverse colon, the descending colon and sigmoid colon, and the superior rectal plexus supplies the rectum. Just above, or below, the origin of the inferior mesenteric artery, a ganglion (the *inferior mesenteric ganglion*) may sometimes be found, but more often small discrete ganglia are scattered about the commencement of the artery in the proximal part of the plexus. In one study[1130]

[1126] P. Petkov, *Scripta. med. Varna.*, **7**, 1968.
[1127] R. E. Coupland, *The Natural History of the Chromaffin Cell*, Longmans, London. 1965.
[1128] R. E. Coupland, *J. Anat.*, **99**, 1965.
[1129] K. Grottel, *Pr. Tow. Przyjac. Nauk poznań*, **37**, 1968.
[1130] J. A. Southam, *J. Anat.*, **93**, 1959.

an inferior mesenteric ganglion occurred in every one of twenty-two human stillborn infants examined. The colic sympathetic nerves are inhibitory to the muscular coats of the colon and rectum. Branches from the parasympathetic pelvic splanchnic nerves run up through or near the superior hypogastric and the inferior mesenteric plexuses to supply the large intestine from the left part of the transverse colon down as far as the rectum (p. 1068 and *vide infra*); impulses along these nerves cause contraction of the musculature of the gut.

## THE SUPERIOR HYPOGASTRIC PLEXUS

The superior hypogastric plexus (7.229–231) is situated in front of the bifurcation of the abdominal aorta, the left common iliac vein, the median sacral vessels, the body of the last lumbar vertebra and the promontory of the sacrum, and between the two common iliac arteries. It is often referred to as the presacral nerve, but the plexus is seldom sufficiently condensed to resemble a single nerve and moreover the plexus is prelumbar rather than presacral in position. It lies in the extraperitoneal connective tissue, and the parietal peritoneum can easily be stripped off its anterior surface. The plexus varies in breadth and in the degree of condensation of its constituent nerves, and it often lies a little to one side of the median plane (more often to the left side); the root of the sigmoid mesocolon, containing the superior rectal vessels, lies to the left side of the lower part of the plexus. Scattered nerve cells are found in the plexus.

Above, the plexus is formed by the union of branches from the aortic plexus with the third and fourth lumbar splanchnic nerves. Below, the plexus divides into the right and left hypogastric nerves which descend to the two inferior hypogastric plexuses. The superior hypogastric plexus gives off branches to the ureteric and testicular (or ovarian) plexuses and to that on the common iliac arteries. In addition to the sympathetic fibres which descend to form the superior hypogastric plexus, it may contain parasympathetic fibres (from the pelvic splanchnic nerves) which ascend from the inferior hypogastric plexus, though usually these parasympathetic fibres run up to the left of the superior hypogastric plexus and across the sigmoid vessels and the branches of the left colic vessels. These parasympathetic fibres are distributed partly along the branches of the inferior mesenteric artery, but also as independent retroperitoneal nerves, to supply the left part of the transverse colon, the left colic flexure, the descending colon and the sigmoid colon (*see* p. 1068 and 7.230).

## THE INFERIOR HYPOGASTRIC PLEXUSES

The superior hypogastric plexus divides below into the right and left *hypogastric nerves*, each of which runs down in the extraperitoneal connective tissue into the pelvis, medial to the internal iliac artery and its branches, to become the inferior hypogastric plexus (7.231). Each nerve may be single or may form an elongated narrow plexus consisting of two or three longitudinal nerves connected by anastomosing filaments. (The hypogastric nerves can scarcely be distinguished from their continuations, the inferior hypogastric plexuses. The latter are joined by the pelvic splanchnic nerves, but this distinction is minimized by the fact that both the nerves and the plexuses contain sympathetic and parasympathetic fibres. Some authorities prefer to describe the superior hypogastric plexus as dividing into two inferior hypogastric plexuses.) From each hypogastric nerve branches may pass to the testicular or ovarian plexus, the ureteric plexus, the plexus on the internal iliac artery and to the

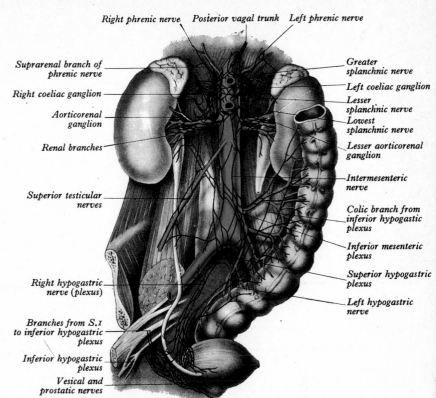

**7.230** Autonomic nerves and plexuses in the abdomen and pelvis. (After G. A. G. Mitchell, *Anatomy of the Autonomic Nervous System*, by courtesy of the author and the publishers.) Note the ascending branches of the inferior hypogastric plexus passing up to supply the descending colon. The sympathetic trunks are not shown on the right side; note the upper, middle and lower ureteric nerves.

*Labels, clockwise from top:*
Right phrenic nerve — Posterior vagal trunk — Left phrenic nerve
Greater splanchnic nerve
Left coeliac ganglion
Lesser splanchnic nerve
Lowest splanchnic nerve
Lesser aorticorenal ganglion
Intermesenteric nerve
Colic branch from inferior hypogastric plexus
Inferior mesenteric plexus
Superior hypogastric plexus
Left hypogastric nerve

*Labels, left side from top:*
Suprarenal branch of phrenic nerve
Right coeliac ganglion
Aorticorenal ganglion
Renal branches
Superior testicular nerves
Right hypogastric nerve (plexus)
Branches from S.1 to inferior hypogastric plexus
Inferior hypogastric plexus
Vesical and prostatic nerves

sigmoid colon, and each nerve may be joined near its commencement by the lowest lumbar splanchnic nerve.

**The inferior hypogastric (or pelvic) plexus** lies in the extraperitoneal connective tissue. In the male it is situated on the side of the rectum, seminal vesicle, prostate and the posterior part of the urinary bladder; in the female, each plexus is placed on the side of the rectum, uterine cervix, vaginal fornix and posterior part of the urinary bladder, and extends into the base of the broad ligament of the uterus. Laterally are the internal iliac vessels and their branches and tributaries, levator ani, coccygeus and obturator internus. Behind are the sacral and coccygeal plexuses and above are the superior vesical and obliterated umbilical arteries. The plexuses contain numerous small ganglia. Each plexus is formed by the hypogastric nerve, which conveys most of the sympathetic fibres to the plexus, and by branches from the ganglia, which convey only a few fibres to the plexus; the parasympathetic fibres in the plexus are derived from the pelvic splanchnic nerves. The preganglionic efferent sympathetic fibres originate in the lower three thoracic and upper two lumbar segments of the spinal cord; some of these relay in the ganglia in the lumbar and sacral parts of the sympathetic trunk, while others synapse about cells in the lower part of the aortic plexus and in the superior and inferior hypogastric plexuses. The preganglionic parasympathetic fibres originate in the second, third and fourth sacral segments of the spinal cord, reach the plexus in the pelvic splanchnic nerves and synapse with cells in the plexus or in the walls of the viscera supplied by the branches of the plexus. From the plexus numerous branches are distributed to the pelvic (and some abdominal) viscera, either directly or by accompanying the branches of the internal iliac artery.

Parasympathetic fibres pass back into the superior hypogastric plexus, or as separate filaments accompanying

1079

it, to reach the inferior mesenteric plexus, through the medium of the aortic plexus. By this route the descending and sigmoid parts of the colon receive a parasympathetic innervation.

**The middle rectal plexus** arises from the upper part of the inferior hypogastric plexus; the fibres pass to the rectum either directly or along the middle rectal artery. The plexus communicates above with branches of the superior rectal plexus and extends inferiorly as far as the internal anal sphincter. The nerve supply of the rectum and anal canal is derived from (*a*) the superior rectal plexus, (*b*) the middle rectal plexus, and (*c*) the inferior rectal (haemorrhoidal) nerves, which are branches of the pudendal nerve. The parasympathetic preganglionic fibres from the superior and middle rectal plexuses synapse with postganglionic neurons in the myenteric plexus, which is well developed in this region. The sympathetic afferents pass through this plexus without interruption. The efferent sympathetic fibres in the rectal plexuses are concerned with inhibition of the expulsive musculature and contraction of the sphincter. Afferent pain impulses pass along both the sympathetic and parasympathetic nerves, but the parasympathetic afferent and efferent fibres are more active in the normal process of defaecation. The inferior rectal nerves supply motor fibres to the external anal sphincter and sensory (somatic) fibres to the lower (ectodermal) part of the anal canal (pp. 175, 1294).

**The vesical plexus** arises from the anterior part of the inferior hypogastric plexus. It is composed of numerous nerves which accompany the vesical arteries to the bladder. Branches from the plexus pass to the seminal vesicles and deferent ducts. Many small collections of nerve cells are present among the nerve fibres in the muscular wall of the bladder. The sympathetic preganglionic efferent fibres in the plexus arise from the lower two thoracic and upper two lumbar segments of the spinal cord; the cells about which they synapse are scattered in the superior and inferior hypogastric plexuses and in the wall of the bladder. The parasympathetic preganglionic efferent fibres arise from the second, third

and fourth sacral segments of the spinal cord and synapse about cells near to or in the walls of the bladder. These neurons convey motor fibres to the muscular coats of the bladder and inhibitory fibres to the sphincter. The efferent sympathetic nerves convey motor fibres to the sphincter and inhibitory fibres to the muscular coats, though some observers maintain that the sympathetic fibres are mainly vasomotor in function and that filling and emptying of the bladder are normally controlled exclusively by the parasympathetic nerves.

**The prostatic plexus** arises from the lower part of the inferior hypogastric plexus and is composed of relatively large nerves which enter the base and sides of the prostate and contain collections of nerve cells. The nerves are distributed to the prostate, seminal vesicles, prostatic urethra, ejaculatory ducts, corpora cavernosa, corpus spongiosum, membranous and penile parts of the urethra and the bulbo-urethral glands. The nerves supplying the corpora cavernosa form two sets, the lesser and the greater cavernous nerves of the penis; these arise from the front part of the prostatic plexus, join with branches from the pudendal nerve and then pass forwards below the pubic arch. The filaments of the *lesser cavernous nerves* pierce the fibrous covering of the penis near its root and supply the erectile tissue of the corpus spongiosum and the penile urethra. The *greater cavernous nerves* run forwards on the dorsum of the penis, communicate with the dorsal nerve of the penis and are distributed to the erectile tissue; some of the filaments pass to the erectile tissue of the corpus spongiosum. The sympathetic nerves supplying the male genital organs produce vasoconstriction, while the parasympathetic produce vasodilatation.

The seminal vesicles are supplied by nerves derived from the vesical plexus, the prostatic plexus and the lower part of the inferior hypogastric nerves. From these nerves, filaments pass to the ejaculatory ducts and to the deferent duct. It is generally believed that constriction of the seminal vesicles and seminal ejaculation are brought about by the sympathetic supply, which also produces inhibition of the bladder musculature and contraction of its sphincter during ejaculation, thus preventing reflex of the seminal fluid into the bladder. It has been, however, suggested that contraction of the seminal vesicles is due to parasympathetic impulses.[1104]

The *uterine nerves* arise from the inferior hypogastric plexus, predominantly from the part of the plexus lying in the base of the broad ligament and known as the **uterovaginal plexus**. From the plexus some nerves pass down with the vaginal arteries, while others pass directly to the cervix uteri, or upwards with or near the uterine arteries in the broad ligament. The nerves passing to the cervix form a plexus in which small paracervical ganglia are found, one ganglion sometimes being large and called the *uterine cervical ganglion*. The uterine nerves passing upwards with the uterine arteries supply branches to the body of the uterus and, in the upper part of the broad ligament, they supply branches to the uterine tube and communicate with the tubal nerves from the inferior hypogastric plexus and with the nerves of the ovarian plexus. The branches of the uterine nerves ramify in the myometrium and endometrium; most of these nerves accompany the vessels. The efferent preganglionic sympathetic fibres supplying the uterus are derived from the last thoracic and first lumbar segments of the spinal cord; the sites of the cells about which they synapse are not known. The preganglionic parasympathetic fibres arise in the second, third and fourth sacral segments of the cord and relay in the paracervical ganglia. While activity of the sympathetic nerves may produce uterine contraction and vasoconstriction, and that of the parasympathetic nerves produce uterine inhibition and vasodilatation, the results

*Left inferior hypogastric plexus*

*Bladder*

*Superior hypogastric plexus*

*Pelvic part of right trunk*

*Pelvic part of left trunk*

*Anterior ramus of S.2*

*Anterior ramus of S.3*

*Pelvic splanchnic nerves*

*Right inferior hypogastric plexus*

*Prostate*

S.W.W

7.231 The pelvic portion of the sympathetic system, viewed from in front and from the right side, a large portion of the right hip bone having been removed. The superior hypogastric plexus is seen to divide below into the right and left hypogastric nerves (which are not labelled), which run down to the inferior hypogastric plexuses. (Drawn from a dissection by the late Dr. G. D. Channell.)

of the activities of these two systems are complicated by the pronounced hormonal control of uterine functions.

The *vaginal nerves* arise from the lower parts of the inferior hypogastric and uterovaginal plexuses, and follow the vaginal arteries and their branches to be distributed to the walls of the vagina, the erectile tissue of the vestibular bulbs and the clitoris (cavernous nerves of the clitoris), the urethra and the greater vestibular glands. The nerves contain numerous parasympathetic fibres which have a vasodilator effect on the erectile tissue.

## Afferent Autonomic Pathways

The efferent autonomic fibres to the viscera and blood vessels are accompanied by others which may be regarded as their sensory counterparts and designated *general visceral afferent* fibres, or perhaps more appropriately as *autonomic afferents*. These nerve fibres are the peripheral processes of unipolar cells in some of the cranial and spinal nerve ganglia. Their central processes (axons) pass in the corresponding nerves to the central nervous system. Their peripheral process (dendrites), which may be myelinated fibres of various sizes or non-myelinated fibres, are distributed with the pre- and post-ganglionic fibres of the parasympathetic and sympathetic subdivisions of the autonomic nervous system, but are not interrupted in autonomic ganglia. Their terminals are variously described as knobs, loops, rings, tendril-like endings and sometimes more elaborate encapsulated endings in the walls of the viscera, including their epithelial lining and serous coverings, and in the walls of blood vessels.

Afferent impulses conducted along these neurons initiate visceral reflexes, but usually these do not reach the level of consciousness. They are also believed to be concerned with organic visceral sensations such as hunger, nausea, sexual sensation, rectal distension, etc. It is also probable that visceral pain fibres follow these peripheral pathways. Although the viscera are insensitive to cutting, crushing or burning, excessive tension and contraction of nonstriated muscle and certain pathological conditions produce visceral pain. It is not always easy to draw a line between what is acceptably pathological and that which is little more than exaggeration of normal activity. 'Abdominal' pain due to excessive intestinal contractions is extremely commonplace. In pathological conditions affecting a viscus vague pain may be felt in the region of the viscus itself (true visceral pain) or in a region of skin or other somatic tissue, the sensory nerve fibres from which enter the same segments of the spinal cord as those which receive pain fibres from the viscus. The latter phenomenon is known as *referred pain*. In addition, if inflammation spreads from a diseased viscus to the parietal serous membrane (e.g. peritoneum) related to it, the somatic pain fibres will be stimulated and cause local somatic pain in this region of the body wall. True visceral pain is poorly localized and dull or heavy. Referred pain is often associated with tenderness of the skin surface at the site of reference.

General visceral afferent fibres occur in the vagus and glossopharyngeal nerves and possibly other cranial nerves, in the second, third and fourth sacral nerves, from which they are distributed with the pelvic splanchnic nerves, and in the thoracic and upper lumbar spinal nerves, where they are distributed through the rami communicantes and along the pathways for efferent sympathetic innervation of the viscera and blood vessels.

The vagus is believed to have a large general visceral afferent component. The fibres have their cells of origin in the superior and inferior ganglia of the nerve, which appear to be predominantly sensory ganglia, despite contrary views in respect of the inferior ganglion (p. 1020). Their central processes terminate in the dorsal nucleus of the vagus in the medulla oblongata, or, according to some authorities, in the nucleus of the tractus solitarius. Their peripheral processes have a wide distribution. Their terminals in the walls of the pharynx and oesophagus, together with the terminals of the general visceral afferent fibres in the glossopharyngeal nerve in the pharynx, are concerned with swallowing reflexes. Afferent fibres are also ascribed to the thyroid and parathyroid glands. In the thorax the general visceral afferent fibres are widely distributed. Some terminate in the heart, walls of the great vessels and aortic bodies; some end in pressor receptors in the walls of the great vessels and are stimulated by distension of the vessel walls resulting from raised intravascular pressure. Fibres from the vagus reach the lungs through the pulmonary plexuses and are distributed to (*a*) the bronchial mucosa; these are probably involved in cough reflexes; (*b*) the bronchial muscle where they encircle the muscle cells and end in tendril-like arrangements which have been regarded as 'muscle spindles' which are believed to be stimulated by alteration in the length of the muscle cells; (*c*) the interalveolar connective tissue where they end in knob-like swellings; these, together with the endings on the smooth muscle cells, may initiate the Herring-Breuer reflex; (*d*) the adventitia of the pulmonary arteries where they may be pressor receptors and the intima of the pulmonary veins where they may function as chemoreceptors. Afferent fibres from the visceral pleura and air passages are also believed to travel with the sympathetic supply to the lungs and to mediate pain sensations.

General visceral afferent fibres in the vagus also terminate in the various coats of the stomach and intestines, the digestive glands and in the kidney. The fibres which terminate in the gut and ducts leading to it are said to be stimulated by distension (stretch) or muscle contraction. Impulses from the stomach may be responsible for the sensations of hunger and nausea.

The general visceral afferent component of the glossopharyngeal nerve includes fibres which innervate the posterior region of the tongue, the tonsil and pharynx; the epithelia of all these parts are derived from endoderm. The innervation of the taste buds in these regions is not included, for these are more properly regarded as *special* visceral afferents, and are treated elsewhere (p. 1084). In addition the glossopharyngeal nerve innervates the carotid sinus and carotid body, the receptors therein being sensitive to tension in the vessel wall and to changes in the chemical composition of the blood respectively. Impulses from these receptors play an essential part in circulatory and respiratory reflexes. The cells of origin of the general visceral afferent fibres lie in the ganglia on the glossopharyngeal nerve, and their terminations in the medulla oblongata are probably similar to those of the general visceral afferent fibres in the vagus nerve.

Sensory fibres coursing in the pelvic splanchnic nerves innervate the pelvic viscera and the distal part of the colon. In the urinary bladder, sensory receptors are described at all levels in its wall. Those in muscle strata are connected with heavily myelinated fibres which reach the spinal cord through the pelvic splanchnic nerves; they are believed to be stretch receptors but may be activated by contraction of the muscle. Pain fibres from the bladder and proximal part of the urethra pass in both the pelvic splanchnic nerves and through the inferior hypogastric plexus, the hypogastric nerves, superior hypogastric plexus and lumbar splanchnic nerves to reach their cells of origin in the ganglia on the dorsal roots of the lower thoracic and upper lumbar nerves. The significance of this double sensory pathway is uncertain; lesions of the cauda equina abolish pain resulting from over-distension of the bladder, but section of the hypogastric nerve is ineffective in relieving pain from the organ.

Though fibres from the pelvic splanchnic nerves, some of which are believed to be afferent, are described in the ovary, no supply from this source to the testis has been demonstrated.

Pain fibres from the body of the uterus pass with sympathetic nerves through the hypogastric plexus and the lumbar splanchnic nerves to cells on the dorsal roots of the lowest thoracic and upper lumbar nerves. Thus, surgical section of the hypogastric nerves has been employed for the relief of dysmenorrhoea. Afferent fibres from the cervix, however, pass in the pelvic splanchnic nerves to their cells of origin in the dorsal roots of the upper sacral nerves. Dilatation (stretch) of the cervix uteri causes pain, but cauterization and removal of small portions of mucosa for biopsy do not.

In general the afferent fibres which accompany the pre- and post-ganglionic fibres of the sympathetic system have a segmental arrangement. They end in the same spinal cord segments as the preganglionic fibres of the efferent pathway to the region or viscus (*vide infra*). The general visceral afferent fibres entering the thoracic and upper lumbar spinal segments are, in the main, concerned with the conduction of pain impulses. Painful sensations from the pharynx, oesophagus, stomach, intestines, kidney, ureter, gall bladder and bile ducts seem to be carried along sympathetic pathways. Such impulses from the heart enter the spinal cord through the first to fifth thoracic spinal nerves. They are carried mainly in the middle and inferior cardiac nerves; a few pass directly into the second to fifth thoracic nerves. There are no general visceral afferent fibres in the superior cardiac nerves. Peripherally the fibres pass through the cardiac plexuses and along the coronary arteries. Anoxia of the heart muscle may give rise to the characteristic symptoms of angina pectoris in which there is presternal pain, referred pain over a large part of the left side of the chest, radiating to the left shoulder and inner side of the left arm, upwards along the left side of the neck to the jaw and occiput and downwards to the epigastrium. Occasionally the pain is felt on both sides or confined to the right side. Afferent fibres from the heart are also carried in the cardiac branches of the vagus nerve. These nerves are concerned with cardiac reflexes depressing the activity of the heart. In some animals (e.g. rabbit) a separate depressor cardiac nerve is present as a branch of the vagus or of the superior laryngeal nerve. In man, the depressor fibres do not form a separate nerve but run in branches of the superior or internal laryngeal nerves which join, in a variable manner, cardiac branches of the vagus or sympathetic.

The pain fibres from the ureter, which also accompany sympathetic fibres, are probably concerned in the painful reflex of renal colic when this duct is obstructed by a calculus.

The afferent (pain) fibres from the testis and ovary run through the corresponding plexuses; their cells of origin are in the ganglia in the dorsal roots of the tenth and eleventh thoracic nerves.

It must be realized that reflex activities in the autonomic nervous system are not initiated solely by impulses conducted through general visceral afferent pathways, nor do impulses travelling in these pathways necessarily activate the general visceral efferent pathways. Indeed, in most situations calling for general sympathetic activity in preparation for effort, the afferent element is almost always somatic, involving either the special senses or skin sensibility. Rises in blood pressure and dilatation of the pupil may result from stimulation of somatic afferent nerves, the receptors of which are located in the skin and other tissues. Conversely, contraction of the rectus abdominis, a somatic structure may result from irritation of abdominal viscera. There is also evidence that reflexes (axon reflexes) may be evoked at the terminals of autonomic postganglionic fibres.

Denervation often has no appreciable effect on the effector organs, nonstriated muscle or glands, innervated by the autonomic system. The contraction of such muscle may be uninfluenced by denervation and no structural changes ensue. This has been variously attributed to the continued activity of ground plexuses or to the intrinsic activity of the visceral muscle cells. In some instances severance of the preganglionic efferent fibres results in hypersensitivity of the postganglionic neurons. In other instances denervation results in cessation of activity, as in the sweat glands, pilomotor muscle, nonstriated muscle of the orbit and in the adrenal medulla.[1131]

## DEGENERATION AND REGENERATION IN THE AUTONOMIC NERVOUS SYSTEM

Though these processes have still to be systematically studied, degeneration in the autonomic nervous system is believed to be similar to that in the cerebrospinal nervous system. There is some evidence that the rate of degeneration differs in different regions or with different types of nerve fibre. Regeneration of preganglionic fibres may be influenced by the site of the lesion and, in the case of postganglionic neurons, regeneration may be followed by reinnervation from neighbouring intact nerve fibres.

As far as available experimental evidence goes, the integrity of Schwann cell sheaths is as important a factor in the regeneration of autonomic nerve fibres, whether myelinated or not, as in the case of somatic fibres.[1132–1135] In some studies observations have suggested that the presence of myelinated fibres in proximity to regenerating non-myelinated fibres is necessary to the latter process.[1132, 1134] To these as yet incomplete studies, it is pertinent to mention earlier experiments in which relatively large defects in the sympathetic trunk, in monkeys and other mammals, have apparently been made good by growth of fibres (which might be pre- or post-ganglionic) across a complete gap in the trunk.[1136, 1137] Conflicting evidence has been derived from human sympathectomies. The functional recoveries sometimes observed may be explained in other ways, such as incomplete interruption of a sympathetic supply, alternative routes of fibres being overlooked. On the whole the experience of surgeons corroborates the experimental findings stated above.[1131]

## SEGMENTAL SYMPATHETIC SUPPLIES

| | |
|---|---|
| Head and neck | T. 1–5 |
| Upper limb | T. 2–5 |
| Lower limb | T. 10–L. 2 |
| Heart | T. 1–5 |
| Bronchi and lung | T. 2–4 |
| Oesophagus (caudal part) | T. 5–6 |
| Stomach | T. 6–10 |
| Small intestine | T. 9–10 |
| Large intestine as far as splenic flexure | T. 11–L. 1 |

[1131] J. Pick, *The Autonomic Nervous System*, Lippincott, Phil. 1970
[1132] D. H. L. Evans and J. G. Murray, *J. Anat.*, **88**, 1954.
[1133] K. Kapeller and D. Mayor, *J. Anat.*, **101**, 1967.
[1134] T. H. Williams, *J. Anat.*, **110**, 1971.
[1135] R. H. M. King and P. K. Thomas, *J. Anat.*, **108**, 1971.
[1136] S. S. Tower and C. P. Richter, *Archs Neurol. Psychiat.*, *Chicago*, **26**, 1931.
[1137] H. A. Haxton, *Ann. R. Coll. Surg.*, **14**, 1954.

| Splenic flexure to sigmoid colon and rectum | L. 1–2 |
| Liver and gall bladder | T. 7–9 |
| Spleen | T. 6–10 |
| Pancreas | T. 6–10 |
| Kidney | T. 10–L. 1 |
| Ureter | T. 11–L. 2 |
| Suprarenal | T. 8–L. 1 |
| Testis and ovary | T. 10–11 |
| Epididymis, ductus deferens and seminal vesicles | T. 11–12 |
| Urinary bladder | T. 11–L. 2 |
| Prostate and prostatic urethra | T. 11–L. 1 |
| Uterus | T. 12–L. 1 |
| Uterine tube | T. 10–L. 1 |

*Applied Anatomy.* Various parts of the sympathetic nervous system are removed surgically in the treatment of a number of clinical conditions. In operations on the efferent side of the sympathetic, ganglia on the sympathetic trunk are removed, or preganglionic fibres cut, rather than postganglionic fibres severed, since the latter procedure may be followed by regeneration of the nerves. For example, the arteries of the limbs may be denervated in conditions of vascular spasm (Raynaud's disease) or in organic arterial disease where spasm is also present; the parts of the system removed are described above (pp. 1074, 1076). In the treatment of essential hypertension, much more extensive sympathectomy has been performed, involving bilateral removal of the sympathetic trunks (from the eighth thoracic to the first lumbar ganglia) and the greater and lesser thoracic splanchnic nerves.

Sympathectomy is also performed for the relief of pain, for example in cases of severe angina pectoris (*see* p. 1082). Division of the superior hypogastric plexus (presacral neurectomy) does not completely relieve pain associated with disease of the pelvic organs, since, as noted above, many of the pain fibres pass in the pelvic splanchnic nerves. The pain fibres from the body of the uterus, however, pass in the sympathetic nerves via the superior hypogastric plexus, so that this operation is successful in cases of intractable painful menstruation (dysmenorrhoea).

In the male, resection of the superior hypogastric plexus is followed by loss of the power of ejaculation and consequent sterility, owing to the interruption of the sympathetic pathway to the seminal vesicles, deferent ducts and prostate. Knowledge of the pathways pursued by these nerves between the ganglia on the sympathetic trunk and the superior hypogastric plexus is less exact and the pathways may vary in different cases, but in certain individuals the outflow from the first lumbar, and possibly the twelfth thoracic, ganglion is of major importance, while in others the fibres from the third lumbar ganglion are chiefly concerned.[1138] For the most recent text on surgical anatomy of the autonomic nervous system consult footnote reference[1139].

[1138] J. C. White, R. H. Smithwick and F. A. Simeone, *The Autonomic Nervous System*, 3rd edition, Kimpton, London. 1952.
[1139] J. Pick, *The Autonomic Nervous System*, Lippincott, Philadelphia. 1970.

# THE PERIPHERAL APPARATUS OF THE SPECIAL SENSES

In the present section the detailed anatomy of the taste buds, the olfactory epithelium and nasal cavity, the eye and the ear are considered. It should also be noted that the development of these structures is treated in the section devoted to Embryology, and their nervous connexions are further detailed in the parts of this volume concerned with the Central Nervous System and with the Cranial Nerves.

## The Gustatory Apparatus

The peripheral gustatory organs are the *taste buds* (*gustatory caliculi*), which are composed of modified epithelial cells arranged in piriform groups (7.232–235) in the epithelium covering the tongue, the inferior surface of the soft palate, the palatoglossal arches, the posterior surface of the epiglottis and the posterior wall of the oral part of the pharynx. They are most numerous on the sides of the vallate papillae of the tongue (7.233), less so on the walls surrounding these papillae; they are plentiful over the folia linguae and the posterior third of the tongue, but are distributed sparingly on the fungiform papillae of the tongue, the soft palate, epiglottis and pharynx. They are more numerous in the infant than the adult and their atrophy increases with age; those in the extreme posterior part of the tongue and in the epiglottis disappear early in life. There are no taste buds in the mid-dorsal region of the oral part of the tongue.

## MICROSCOPIC STRUCTURE OF TASTE BUDS

Each taste bud (7.234) is separated by a basement membrane from the underlying dermis, and opens on to the surface of the epithelium by an aperture termed the

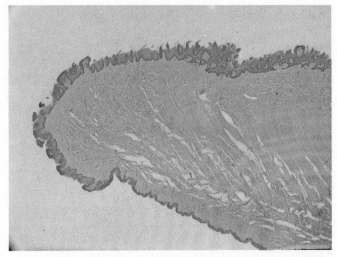

7.232 A low-power light micrograph of a sagittal section through the tip and anterior part of a human tongue, showing: muscle fibres orientated in three different directions; a delicate non-keratinized stratified squamous epithelium on the ventral surface; and a partly keratinized epithelium on the dorsum. The latter is convoluted to produce filiform and fungiform papillae. Dermal papillae project into the deep surface of the epidermal irregularities. Haematoxylin and eosin.

*gustatory pore.* In longitudinal section the cells of the taste bud are crescentic in profile, their pointed apices converging on a small cavity which connects with the gustatory pore (7.234, 235). Some of these cells bear 'gustatory hairs' which, ultrastructurally, are seen to be groups of fine microvilli. The base of each taste bud is penetrated by a group of afferent gustatory nerve fibres which give off branches to ramify and spiral around some of the epithelial cells within the taste bud.

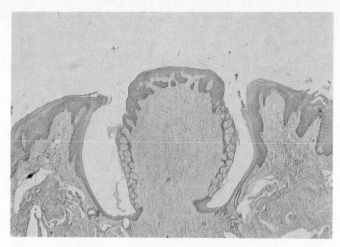

7.233 A medium magnification light micrograph of a human vallate lingual papilla showing numerous taste buds clustered along its lateral surfaces. A connective tissue papilla forms the core of the whole structure, and serous glands, situated between the muscle blocks deep to the corium, open into the lateral recesses of the papilla. Haematoxylin and eosin.

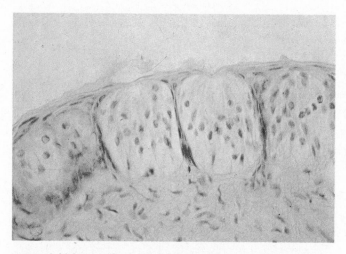

7.234 A high magnification light micrograph of a group of taste buds in a vallate lingual papilla, showing the apical cavity and various fusiform cells within the epithelial capsule. Haematoxylin and eosin.

It has long been known that the gustatory sensory cells are modified epithelial elements which establish contacts like synapses with the terminal branches of the afferent gustatory fibres. The identification of the gustatory cells amongst the other cell types of the taste bud has, however, been the subject of some debate. Recent work involving three-dimensional reconstruction of taste buds from electron micrographs of serial sections[1140] suggests that there are at least five distinct epithelial cell types, two of which appear to be receptor cells and the others supportive, ensheathing or generative in their functions (7.235). The receptor cells are typified by the presence of synaptic contacts with afferent nerve terminals at various points on their surfaces; these show the typical asymmetrical thickening and presynaptic aggregates of small (50 nm) clear synaptic vesicles within the receptor cell, although these appear to be less prominent than in other comparable synapses (p. 774). In addition, one of the epithelial cell types contains dense-cored vesicles about 70 nm in diameter within its cytoplasm, similar to those which have been identified in other sites of the nervous system as catecholamine-containing vesicles (p. 775), whereas in the other cell type these are absent. It is possible that the two cell types represent different stages in the maturation of receptors, which are continually being lost and

replaced (*vide infra*). It is interesting that at the apices of the receptor cells few microvilli are usually present, and the 'gustatory hairs' of light microscopists are mainly to be found on the supporting cells which surround and enwrap the receptors except at their apical surfaces. One of these non-sensory cell types appears to form a peripheral sheath for the whole taste bud, separating it from the surrounding epithelium; another type is basal in position where it probably forms a blastemal cell capable of giving rise to new cells of the other types by mitosis. The third cell type is a true supporting cell which insulates each receptor from its neighbours and also provides sheaths at its basal extremities for the afferent nerve fibres which lose their Schwann sheaths on entering the taste bud. Ultrastructurally the true supporting cell types contain, together with the usual complement of cell organelles, dense bodies of a secretory nature. These are probably the origin of the material rich in polysaccharides which occupies the apical cavity of the taste bud and into which the sensory terminals project. Gustatory molecules must pass through this material before the sensory surface can be reached, and it may play an important, although undetermined, role in the gustatory process.

The nerve fibres which reach the taste bud from the corial plexus are complex in their distribution within the tongue, as deduced by electrophysiological recordings from individual nerve fibres within the more proximal fasciculi of the main gustatory nerves (chorda tympani and glossopharyngeal). Each fibre may possess many terminal branches which spread to innervate widely distant taste buds, and, within these structures, to end in relation to more than one sensory cell. Conversely, each taste bud and each of its contained receptor cells, may be innervated by the terminal branches of several different nerve fibres. This cross innervation of taste buds may be of great physiological importance (*vide infra*).[1141] No evidence has yet emerged concerning the presence of efferent terminals or of inhibitory phenomena in taste buds.

## THE REPLACEMENT OF TASTE BUD CELLS

The cells of the taste bud resemble the cells of the surrounding epithelium in undergoing continual renewal.[1142] Isotopic labelling shows that none of the elements of the taste bud live for more than a few days, except for the basal cells, from which the other cell types are presumably replaced by mitosis. Newly formed sensory cells must therefore make new synaptic contacts with nerve fibre terminals, and experiments indicate that the precise sensitivity characteristics of the sensory cells are determined by the trophic influence of the nerve fibre and not the reverse (*see* p. 794).

The continual degeneration and replacement of taste bud cells means that, within a single bud, cells of different types show a spectrum of morphological appearances which adds to the difficulties of precise identification of cells on structural criteria alone.

## THE PHYSIOLOGY OF GUSTATORY RECEPTORS

In many aquatic vertebrates chemoreceptors with all the characteristics of gustatory endings are widely distributed over the surface of the body; in terrestrial groups this

[1140] R. G. Murray and A. Murray, in: *Taste and Smell in Vertebrates*, Ciba Foundation Symposium, eds. G. E. W. Wolstenholme and J. Knight, Churchill, London. 1970.
[1141] L. M. Beidler, in: *Taste and Smell in Vertebrates*, Ciba Foundation Symposium, eds. G. E. W. Wolstenholme and J. Knight, Churchill, London. 1970.

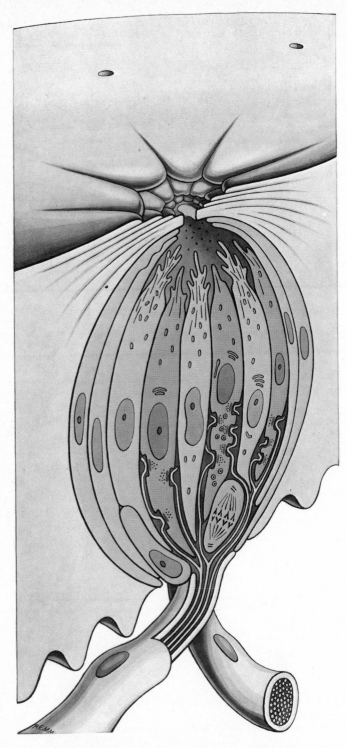

**7.235** A schematic reconstruction of the structure of a taste bud, cut away to expose the various cell types. Presumed sensory cells of two types, one with dense-cored vesicles, the other without, are indicated in purple, and their innervation in yellow. The supporting cells are indicated in magenta, and basal cells in brick red. A dense mucosubstance is present in the apical cavity beneath the apical aperture.

sense is confined to the buccal cavity and adjoining regions of the pharynx. The sense of taste in man, as commonly understood, is largely a result of the activity of lingual receptors, although others which are palatal and laryngopharyngeal in position may also play a significant part. Classically, four groups of subjective taste qualities have been distinguished, each pertaining to zones of special sensitivity on the surface of the tongue, comprising sweet and salt at the tip of the tongue, sour (acid) at the sides, and bitter at the pharyngeal end. Although these qualities

represent subjective sensations, it seemed at one time possible that their special effectiveness in particular areas of the tongue might reflect the presence of receptor cells specific for these general groups. However, the electrophysiological evidence suggests that this is an over-simplified view, since each afferent fibre, subserving widely separated taste buds, responds to a variety of different types of chemical stimuli. Some fibres respond to all four qualities, others to less or only to one. Within a particular class of taste qualities receptors are also differentially sensitive to a wide range of similar chemicals. It would therefore seem likely that the sensation of taste represents the results of the analysis of a complex pattern of differential responses over particular areas of the tongue, so that even if there are only a relatively few specific types of taste receptor cells, much more information may be gained about the precise nature of the taste, and its intensity, than if the innervation were of a simpler kind.[1141 – 1143]

## THE GUSTATORY NERVES

The taste nerve fibres are the peripheral processes of unipolar nerve cells in the geniculate ganglion of the facial nerve, the inferior ganglion of the glossopharyngeal nerve and the inferior ganglion of the vagus. The central processes of these cells form the tractus solitarius (p. 846), and their terminals synapse with the neurons which form the nucleus of that tract. The axons of the latter cross the midline, and many then ascend through the brainstem in the dorsomedial part of the medial lemniscus to approach and synapse with the most medially situated neurons of the *nucleus ventralis posterior medialis* (VPM) of the thalamus (in a region sometimes termed the *accessory arcuate nucleus*). From the VPM axons radiate through the internal capsule to reach the antero-inferior part of the sensorimotor cortex and the region of the limen insulae. Broadly, electrophysiological recording from the VPM and the cerebral cortex confirms these anatomical pathways; some units react to one type of stimulus only, whilst others react to a number of different stimuli. Other ascending pathways have been described as ending in a number of the hypothalamic nuclei, through which gustatory information may reach the limbic system (p. 907), and which allow appropriate readjustments of the autonomic nervous system to be made.

The nerve of taste for the anterior part of the tongue, excluding the vallate papillae, is the chorda tympani (through the lingual nerve); these taste fibres in most individuals pass in the chorda tympani to the ganglion of the facial nerve. In a few individuals, they leave the chorda tympani by anastomotic branches connecting it to the otic ganglion and proceed thence in the greater petrosal nerve to the ganglion of the facial nerve.[1144] This part of the tongue, its *oral* region, is derived from the mandibular branchial arch, and is limited posteriorly by the *sulcus terminalis*. The taste buds in the inferior surface of the soft palate are also supplied mainly by the facial nerve, through the greater petrosal nerve, the nerve of the pterygoid canal and the middle and posterior palatine nerves; the glossopharyngeal also contributes to their supply. The taste buds in the vallate papillae and the pharyngeal part of the tongue, and in the palatoglossal arches and the oral part of the pharynx are innervated by

[1142] L. M. Beidler and R. L. Smallman, *J. Cell Biol.*, **27**, 1965.

[1143] C. Pfaffman, in: *Taste and Smell in Vertebrates*, Ciba Foundation Symposium, eds. G. E. W. Wolstenholme and J. Knight, Churchill, London. 1970.

[1144] H. Schwartz and G. Weddell, *Brain*, **61**, 1938.

the glossopharyngeal, while those in the extreme back part of the tongue and in the epiglottis are supplied by the internal laryngeal part of the superior laryngeal branch of the vagus. These nerve supplies accord with the embryological development of the tongue (p. 169). It is customary to describe the mandibular and glossopharyngeal territories as the 'anterior two-thirds' and 'posterior third' of the tongue. But since there is an easily recognizable boundary between them—the sulcus terminalis—it is uninformative and misleading to divide so variable an organ in this arbitrary and inevitably inexact manner. Pre- and post-sulcal regions are better terms.

# THE OLFACTORY APPARATUS

The peripheral olfactory organs are said to include the *external nose*, and the *nasal cavity*, which latter is divided by a septum into right and left parts. However, the essential olfactory structures are the olfactory epithelium and its nervous connexions.

## THE EXTERNAL NOSE

The external nose is pyramidal, and its upper angle, or *root*, is continuous with the forehead; its free angle or tip is termed the *apex*. Its inferior aspect is occupied by two elliptical apertures, the external *nares* or *nostrils*, which are separated from each other by the septum. The lateral surfaces of the nose form, by their union in the median plane, the *dorsum nasi*, the shape and direction of which varies considerably in different individuals; the upper part of the external nose is kept patent by the nasal bones and the frontal processes of the maxillae. The lateral surfaces end below in the rounded *alae nasi*.

The framework of the external nose (7.236) is composed of bones and hyaline cartilages. The *bony framework*, which supports its upper part, consists of the nasal bones, the frontal processes of the maxillae, and the nasal part of the frontal bone. The *cartilaginous framework* consists of the septal, lateral, and major and minor alar nasal cartilages (7.236, 237). These are connected with one another and with the bones by the continuity of the perichondrium and the periosteum.

The *septal cartilage* (7.236 B, 237), somewhat quadrilateral in form, and thicker at its margins than at its centre, forms almost the whole of the septum between the anterior parts of the nasal cavity. The upper part of its anterosuperior margin is connected to the posterior border of the internasal suture; the middle part is continuous with the lateral nasal cartilages; the lower part is attached to these cartilages by the perichondrium. Its anteroinferior border is connected on each side to the septal process of the major alar cartilage. Its posterosuperior border is joined to the perpendicular plate of the ethmoid bone, and its postero-inferior border is attached to the vomer and to the nasal crest of the maxillae and the anterior nasal spine. The cartilage of the septum may extend backwards (especially in children) as a narrow process, termed the *sphenoidal process*, for some distance between the vomer and the perpendicular plate of the ethmoid bone. The antero-inferior part of the nasal septum between

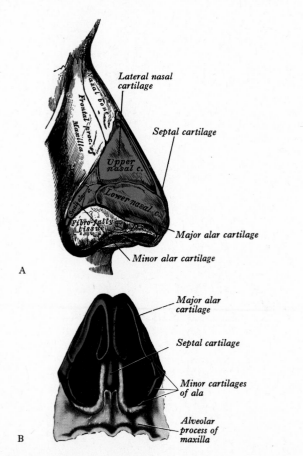

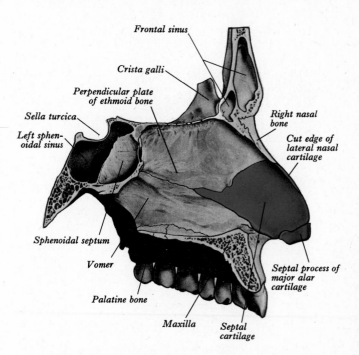

**7.237** The right side of the septum of the nose, showing its constituent bones and cartilages. (Note changes in terminology.)

**7.236 A** The cartilages of the right side of the nose. Lateral aspect. **B** The cartilages of the nose. Inferior aspect. (Note changes in terminology.)

the two nostrils is freely movable, and hence is named the *septum mobile nasi*; it is not formed by the cartilage of the septum, but by the septal processes of the major alar cartilages and by the skin.

The *lateral* (upper) *nasal cartilage* (7.236 A) is triangular in shape. Its anterior margin is thicker than the posterior, and its upper part is continuous with the cartilage of the septum, but its lower part is separated from this cartilage by a narrow fissure; its superior margin is attached to the nasal bone and the frontal process of the maxilla; its inferior margin is connected by fibrous tissue with the major alar cartilage.

The *major alar* (lower) *cartilage* (7.236 A and B) is a thin flexible plate which is situated below the lateral nasal cartilage, and is bent acutely around the anterior part of the naris. The medial part of the plate is narrow, and is termed the *septal process*. The latter is loosely connected by fibrous tissue with that of the opposite cartilage, and to the antero-inferior part of the septal cartilage, thus helping to form the septum mobile nasi. The upper border of the lateral part of the major alar cartilage is attached by fibrous tissue to the lower border of the lateral nasal cartilage. Its posterior, narrow end is connected with the frontal process of the maxilla by a tough fibrous membrane, in which three or four small cartilaginous plates, termed the *minor cartilages of the ala* (7.236 A), are found. Its lower free edge falls short of the lateral margin of the naris, the lower part of the ala nasi being formed by fatty and fibrous tissue covered with skin. In front, the major alar cartilages are separated by a notch which can be felt at the apex of the nose.

The *muscles* acting on the external nose have been described on p. 498.

The *skin* of the dorsum and sides of the nose is thin, and loosely connected with the subjacent parts; but over the apex and alae it is thicker and more firmly adherent, and is furnished with numerous large sebaceous glands, the orifices of which are usually very distinct.

The *arteries* of the external nose are the alar and septal branches of the facial artery, which supply the ala and lower part of the septum, the dorsal nasal branch of the ophthalmic artery, and the infraorbital branch of the maxillary artery, which supply the lateral aspects and the dorsum. The *veins* end in the facial and ophthalmic veins.

The *nerves* for the muscles of the nose are derived from the facial nerve, while the skin receives branches from the ophthalmic nerve, through its infratrochlear branch and the external nasal nerve (p. 1003), and from the infraorbital branch of the maxillary nerve.

## THE NASAL CAVITY

The nasal cavity is divided into right and left halves by the nasal septum (7.238). These two halves open on the face through the nares or nostrils, and communicate behind with the nasal part of the pharynx through the posterior nasal apertures. The *nares* are somewhat piriform apertures, narrower in front than behind. Each measures from 1·5 cm to 2 cm anteroposteriorly, and from 0·5 cm to 1 cm transversely. The *posterior nasal apertures* or *choanae* are two oval openings, each measuring about 2·5 cm in the vertical and 1·25 cm in the transverse direction.

For the description of the bony boundaries of the nasal cavity, *see* p. 278.

Each half of the nasal cavity can be described as having a floor, a roof, a lateral wall and a medial (septal) wall. It consists of three regions—vestibular, olfactory, and respiratory.

The *nasal vestibule* is a slight dilatation just inside the aperture of the nostril (7.239), bounded laterally by the ala and the lateral part of the lower nasal cartilage, and medially by the septal process of the same cartilage; it extends as a small recess towards the apex of the nose. The vestibule is lined with skin, and coarse hairs and sebaceous and sweat glands are found in its lower part; the hairs (vibrissae) curve downwards and forwards to the naris, and tend to arrest the passage of foreign substances

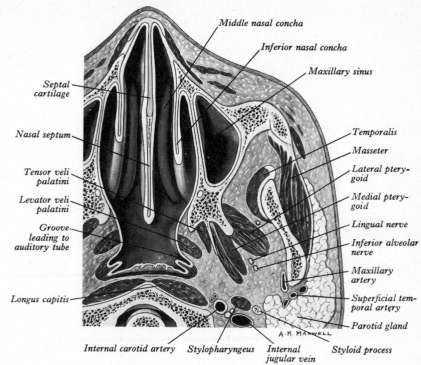

7.238 A transverse section through the anterior part of the head at a level just inferior to the apex of the odontoid process. Superior aspect.

carried with the current of inspired air. In the male, after middle age, they increase considerably in size. The vestibule is limited above and behind by a curved elevation, named the *limen nasi*, which corresponds to the upper margin of the lower nasal cartilage, and along which the skin of the vestibule is continuous with the mucous membrane of the nasal cavity.

The *olfactory region* is limited to the superior nasal concha, the opposed part of the septum and the intervening roof.

The *respiratory region* comprises the rest of the cavity.

**The lateral wall** of the nasal cavity (7.239, 240) is marked by three elevations, the *superior, middle* and *inferior nasal conchae*, and below and lateral to each concha is the corresponding nasal passage or *meatus*. Above the superior concha a triangular fossa, the *spheno-ethmoidal recess*, receives the opening of the sphenoidal sinus. Sometimes a fourth or *highest nasal concha* occurs on the lateral wall of the spheno-ethmoidal recess (7.239); the highest or supreme nasal meatus related to it may contain the opening of a posterior ethmoidal sinus. The *superior meatus* is a short oblique passage extending about half-way along the upper border of the middle concha; the posterior ethmoidal sinuses open, usually by one aperture, into the front part of this meatus. The *middle meatus*, deeper in front than behind, is below and lateral to the middle concha, and is continued anteriorly into a shallow depression situated above the vestibule and named the *atrium* of the middle meatus. Above the atrium an ill-defined curved ridge, termed the *agger nasi* (p. 305), runs forwards and downwards from the upper end of the anterior free border of the middle concha; it is better developed in the newborn child than in the adult. When the middle concha is raised or removed the lateral wall of this meatus is displayed fully. A rounded elevation, termed the bulla ethmoidalis, and, below and extending upwards in front of it, a curved cleft, termed the hiatus semilunaris, form the principal features of this wall. The *bulla ethmoidalis* is caused by the bulging of the middle ethmoidal sinuses, which open on or immediately above it, and the size of the bulla varies with that of its contained

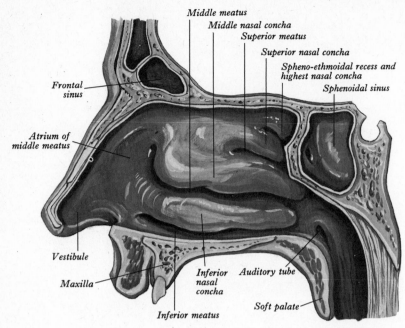

7.239   The lateral wall of the right half of the nasal cavity. Internal aspect.

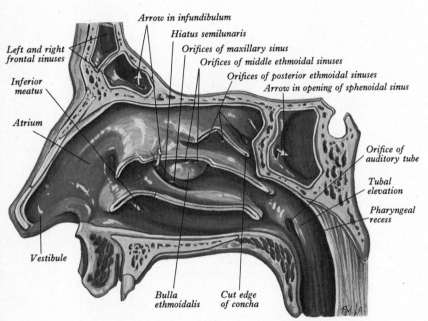

7.240   The lateral wall of the right half of the nasal cavity; the three nasal conchae have been partially removed.

sinuses. The *hiatus semilunaris*, which is bounded inferiorly by a sharp concave ridge produced by the uncinate process of the ethmoid bone, leads forwards and upwards into a curved channel, which is named the *ethmoidal infundibulum*. The anterior ethmoidal sinuses open into the infundibulum, which in rather more than 50 per cent of subjects is continuous with the frontonasal duct or passage leading from the frontal sinus. In other cases the ethmoidal infundibulum ends blindly in front by forming one or more of the anterior ethmoidal sinuses (infundibular sinuses), and the frontonasal duct opens directly into the anterior end of the middle meatus. The opening of the maxillary sinus is situated below the bulla ethmoidalis, and is usually hidden by the flange-like lower edge of the hiatus semilunaris; in a coronal section of the nose this opening is seen to be placed near the roof of the sinus (7.244). An accessory opening of the maxillary sinus is frequently present below and behind the hiatus

semilunaris. The *inferior meatus* is below and lateral to the inferior nasal concha; the nasolacrimal duct opens into this meatus under cover of the anterior part of the inferior concha.

**The medial wall or nasal septum** (7.237) is often deflected from the median plane, thus lessening the size of one half of the nasal cavity and increasing that of the other; ridges or spurs of bone sometimes project from the septum on either side. Immediately superior to the incisive canal at the lower edge of the cartilage of the septum a depression is sometimes seen; it points downwards and forwards, and occupies the position of a canal which connected the nasal with the buccal cavity in early fetal life. On each side of the septum close to this recess a minute orifice may be discerned; it leads backwards into a blind tubular pouch, 2 to 6 mm long, the vestigial *vomeronasal organ*, which is supported by a strip of cartilage named the *vomeronasal cartilage*; it is lined by epithelium consisting mainly of a single layer of tall columnar cells and contains many glands. This organ is well developed in many of the lower animals (e.g. reptiles[1145], [1146]), where it apparently plays a part in the sense of smell, since it is supplied by twigs of the olfactory nerve and is lined with epithelium similar to that in the olfactory region of the nose.

**The roof** of the nasal cavity is narrow from side to side, except at its posterior part, and may be divided, from behind forwards, into sphenoidal, ethmoidal and frontonasal parts, corresponding to the bones which enter into its formation (pp. 115 and 278). The ethmoidal part is almost horizontal, but the frontonasal and sphenoidal parts slope downwards and forwards and downwards and backwards, respectively. The cavity is therefore deepest where its roof is formed by the cribriform plate of the ethmoid bone.

**The floor** is concave from side to side, anteroposteriorly flat and almost horizontal; its anterior three-fourths are formed by the palatine process of the maxilla, its posterior one-fourth by the horizontal part of the palatine bone. About 2 cm behind the anterior end of the floor a slight depression in the mucous membrane overlies the incisive canals (p. 278).

The nasal conchae add greatly to the surface area of the nasal cavity, especially in macrosmatic mammals such as the Carnivora.[1147] This may not only serve to augment the olfactory area but also to increase turbulence and perhaps improve olfaction by somewhat delaying passage of air through the olfactory part of the cavity. Humidification and warming of the inhaled air is also favoured by the increased area of mucous membrane and by turbulence, even in a microsmatic mammal such as man.[1148] Swirling currents also aid in the trapping of particulate material by the mucous secretion.

**The nasal mucous membrane** lines the nasal cavities with the exception of the vestibules, and is intimately adherent to the periosteum or perichondrium. It is continuous with the mucous membrane of the nasal part of the pharynx through the posterior nasal apertures; with the conjunctiva, through the nasolacrimal duct and lacrimal canaliculi; and with the mucous membranes of the sphenoidal, ethmoidal, frontal and maxillary sinuses, through their openings.

The mucous membrane is thickest and most vascular over the nasal conchae, especially at their extremities. It is also thick over the nasal septum, but very thin in the

[1145] A. d'A. Bellairs, *J. Anat.*, **76**, 1942.
[1146] A. d'A. Bellairs and J. D. Boyd, *Proc. zool. Soc. Lond.*, **120**, 1950.
[1147] V. E. Negus, *The Comparative Anatomy and Physiology of the Nose and Paranasal Sinuses*, Livingstone, Edinburgh. 1958.
[1148] P. Cole, *J. Lar. Otol.*, **67**, 1953; **68**, 1954.

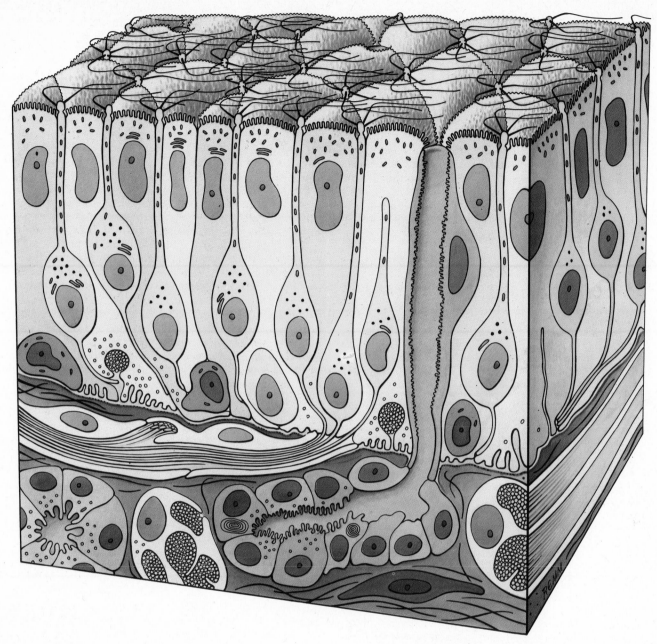

7.241  A schematic reconstruction showing the chief cytological features of the olfactory epithelium. Receptor cells (yellow) are situated among columnar supporting cells. The axons of the receptor cells emerge from the epithelium in groups ensheathed in Schwann cells. Observe the rounded basal epithelial cells and the sub-epithelial glands of Bowman with their intra-epithelial ducts. One of the basal cells is in process of differentiating into a receptor cell. At the surface are cilia of the receptor cells and microvilli of the supporting cells.

meatuses, on the floor of the nasal cavity, and in the various sinuses. The thickness of the membrane reduces materially the size of the bony cavity and the apertures communicating with it. The epithelium of the mucous membrane differs in its characteristics according to the functions of the part of the nose in which it is found. In the *olfactory region*, which extends over the upper 10 mm or so of the septum and over the superior concha and the lateral walls above it, the mucous membrane is yellowish in colour and the epithelium is of a distinctive type.

## STRUCTURE OF THE OLFACTORY EPITHELIUM

The olfactory epithelium is considerably thicker than the surrounding non-sensory epithelium of the nasal cavity, and is composed of three chief cell types, namely the olfactory receptor cells, supporting (sustentacular) cells and basal cells[1149] (7.241, 242).

**The receptor cells** are of particular phylogenetic interest since they are *primary sensory neurons*, the cell bodies of which lie close to the sensory surface, a common feature of invertebrates but unique in the vertebrate classes. These cells are *bipolar* neurons, positioned vertically within the olfactory epithelium, the cell bodies being restricted to the basal two-thirds of the epithelial thickness. Basally, a non-myelinated axon stems from each receptor cell body, to run with other axons in small bundles within the epithelium amongst the processes of supporting and basal cells and, finally, to penetrate the basal lamina, where each bundle becomes ensheathed by Schwann cells.[1150] Such ensheathed bundles (*fila olfactoria*) join with others to form the *fasciculi* of the *olfactory nerve*, and eventually these enter the olfactory bulb, where they synapse with second-order sensory

[1149] D. G. Moulton and L. M. Beidler, *Physiol. Rev.*, **47**, 1967.
[1150] D. Frisch, *Am. J. Anat.*, **121**, 1967.

neurons (mitral cells, basket cells, periglomerular cells, see p. 932). The olfactory axons are amongst the most slender of nerve fibres, being about 0·2 μm in diameter. Within the fila of the olfactory nerve, the axons are typically grouped together in invaginations of the Schwann cell membrane without any intervening Schwann cell processes,[1151] providing possibilities of electrical interaction between adjacent axons.

At the peripheral aspect of the receptor perikaryon (7.243), a single unbranched dendrite extends to the free surface of the epithelium where it expands slightly to form a bulbous olfactory ending (*rod*, *knob*, or *vesicle*), projecting above the general level of the epithelial surface.[1150, 1152–1154] Scattered over the surface of the ending itself are numerous *olfactory cilia* which project into the layer of liquid overlying the epithelium. The cilia possess

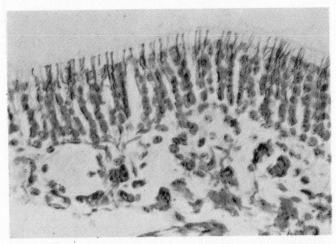

7.242 A vertical section through the olfactory epithelium of the mouse, stained with Holmes' silver method to show the olfactory dendrites and their terminal expansions (above). The nuclei of the receptor neurons are arranged in columns in this preparation; the fila olfactoria can also be seen emerging from the base of the epithelium (below). (Kindly provided by Dr. A. Cuschieri, Depts. of Anatomy, Guy's Hosp. Med. Sch. and Univ. of Malta.)

a '9 plus 2' pattern of microtubules internally, similar to that of motile non-sensory cilia elsewhere (p. 11). Amongst the different groups of vertebrates the length and precise form of the olfactory cilium varies considerably, but in mammals it usually takes the form of a short relatively thick 'shaft' tapering after a few microns to a long, thin, distal tip with reduced numbers of microtubules. Deeper in the dendrite, numerous mitochondria, indicative of high energy consumption, along with other organelles typical of neuronal dendrites—microtubules, smooth and rough coated vesicles, agranular endoplasmic reticulum and ribosomes; centrioles are also often present, especially in young animals. The *perikaryon* is rich in granular and agranular endoplasmic reticulum, Golgi bodies, and lysosomes, all indicating a high level of metabolism. The nucleus is large, rounded and euchromatic.

**The supporting cells** are irregular columnar elements which separate and partially enwrap the receptors. Their elongate heterochromatic nuclei form a distinct layer above the level of the receptor perikarya. The surface of supporting cells is marked by the presence of numerous, long, irregular microvilli which, with the olfactory cilia, form a complex meshwork in the layer of fluid upon the general epithelial surface. Within the cytoplasm are many mitochondria, granular and agranular endoplasmic reticulum and, at the base of the epithelium, lamellated dense bodies which may be similar to the lipofuscin granules of neurons (p. 772), perhaps representing the

remains of autophagic lysosomes. A prominent Golgi apparatus and lysosomes are also found in the apical parts of supporting cells. Near the epithelial surface, fine microfilaments attaching to desmosomes probably give mechanical coherence to the epithelium. Tight junctions are also reported to occur between supporting cells and olfactory receptors at the level of the epithelial surface.[1155]

**The basal cells** are irregular or polygonal in shape, and are confined to the regions abutting the basal lamina of the epithelium. Their nuclei are usually heterochromatic and deeply indented, and their cytoplasm contains numerous microfilaments, often connected to desmosomes, amongst the usual complement of cytoplasmic organelles. Another type of basal cell has also been described, with the appearance of an embryonic blastemal cell, the nucleus being large and euchromatic and the ribosomes unattached to cytoplasmic membranes.

The functions of the supporting and basal cells are not yet fully understood; they undoubtedly have mechanical functions, providing stability to the epithelium, but their role may also be to create the correct metabolic and ionic environment for receptor functioning in a manner analogous to the non-excitable elements of the central nervous system. Mitotic activity occurs at the base of the epithelium well into maturity in many mammals, and is probably associated with the continued histogenesis of supporting and basal cells, although histogenesis of receptors has also been reported for some time after birth. The source of the new cells appears to be pre-existing basal cells, although it is not clear that all basal cells have a capacity for mitosis.[1156]

**The olfactory glands** (of Bowman) (7.241, 242) are branched tubular structures beneath the olfactory epithelium, on to the surface of which they pour their secretions, through narrow, vertical ducts. The secretory acini of these glands are composed of cells with basally placed nuclei and granular cytoplasm. Ultrastructurally, two gland cell types have been reported, both containing dense secretory vesicles, but one showing a denser cytoplasm than the other. Their secretions have been reported in some mammals to contain enzymes (acid phosphatase, esterase) and in mice sulphated acid mucosubstances have been demonstrated as a major component. Since this fluid forms the immediate environment of the receptor endings after it has been secreted, it may play an important part in the diffusion of odours from the air to the olfactory receptors and in regulating the passage of ions to and from the sensory cell during electrical activity. It may also possess bactericidal properties.

In addition to the structures described above, a variable population of lymphocytes is often present, particularly in the basal region of the epithelium, as elsewhere in the upper respiratory tract. During life there is a gradual reduction in the number of olfactory receptors and their axons, up to 1 per cent being lost each year;[1157] the sensory epithelium may be replaced by ciliated columnar epithelium similar to that of the non-sensory respiratory epithelium lining the adjacent regions of the nasal cavity. These changes parallel the gradual loss of the olfactory sense which usually accompanies aging.

[1151] H. S. Gasser, *J. gen. Physiol.*, **39**, 1956.

[1152] T. S. Reese, *J. Cell. Biol.*, **25**, 1965.

[1153] P. C. C. Graziadei, in: *Handbook of Sensory Physiology*, vol. IV: *Chemical Senses*, ed. L. M. Beidler, Springer-Verlag, Berlin. 1971.

[1154] R. Naessen, *Acta Oto-Laryngol.*, **71**, 1971.

[1155] T. S. Reese and M. W. Brightman, in: *Taste and Smell in Vertebrates*, Ciba Foundation Symposium, eds. G. E. W. Wolstenholme and J. Knight, Churchill, London. 1970.

[1156] D. G. Moulton, G. Celebi and R. P. Fink, in: *Taste and Smell in Vertebrates*, Ciba Foundation Symposium, eds. G. E. W. Wolstenholme and J. Knight, Churchill, London. 1970.

[1157] C. G. Smith, *Arch. Otolaryng.*, **34**, 1941.

In the **vomeronasal organ** (of Jacobson), present in most mammals but rudimentary in man (p. 1088), the cellular components are similar to those of the olfactory epithelium except for the reduction or absence of a basal cell layer, the larger size of the receptors, and the presence of microvilli instead of cilia at the sensory endings.[1158] The absence of cilia is particularly interesting since these have been claimed to be the site of chemoreception in the olfactory epithelium; it seems probable that the whole exposed plasma membrane is the chemoreceptive area and that the cilia or microvilli merely serve to increase the surface at which reception of stimuli may take place. Electrical recordings show that vomeronasal receptors respond to odours in much the same way as olfactory receptors, although possibly to a narrower range of chemical types.

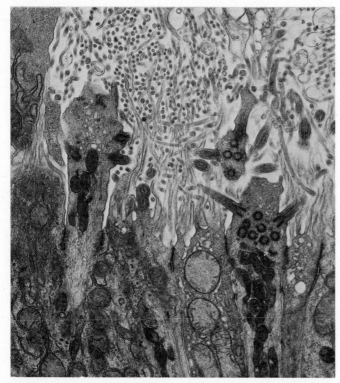

7.243 An electron micrograph showing receptor endings in the olfactory mucosa of a mouse; note the presence of numerous cilia on the sensory terminals, interspersed by numerous microvilli on the surfaces of the supporting cells.

## THE PHYSIOLOGY OF OLFACTORY RECEPTORS

The chemical sense subserved by the olfactory epithelium differs from that of the gustatory and other chemical senses in detecting and discriminating between a wide range of *airborne* molecules at very low concentrations. Although in man the sense of smell is only moderately well developed compared with that of macrosmatic species, in which odours play an important, even dominant role, there is evidence that olfaction may be more significant than previously imagined. In mammals, including primates, the production of specific scents ('pheromones') which affect the social or sexual behaviour of others of the same species is becoming recognized as a common phenomenon, and the close relationship between the olfactory pathways and areas of the brain associated with emotional behaviour in man may be important clues to the significance of odours in general. (See the limbic system, p. 730.)

Turning to more specific aspects of olfaction, the mechanism of odour reception and signalling to the brain have been approached chiefly by the technique of recording electrical changes in or at the surface of the epithelium when it is exposed to odorous stimuli.[1149, 1159] Two types of electrical changes can be recorded, namely a slow negative wave (the *electro-olfactogram*) found at the surface and a short distance below it, representing summated ionic fluxes stemming from many individual receptor dendrites; deeper in the epithelium, and in the olfactory nerve bundles, action potentials representing all-or-none activity in the axons can be detected instead.

Precisely how an array of receptors provides information about the stimulus type and intensity is the subject of much controversy. It might be imagined that individual receptors could be classified into specific types, each responsive to a particular odour. However, it is possible to distinguish between a large variety of different odours, and it would be necessary to postulate a tremendous range of receptor specificity, each group capable of detecting slight differences in molecular properties if there is a one-to-one relationship between receptor type and odour. Electrophysiological recording indicates that single receptors can respond in different ways to a wide variety of odours, and that different receptors exhibit diverse patterns of response to single odours. It seems likely that discrimination in the olfactory system results from the analysis of a pattern of differential activity in a wide range of receptors.

The precise mode of interaction between odours and receptors is also debatable, and many theories have been proposed. The most widely debated theories are those of Amoore[1160] and of Wright.[1161] The stereochemical theory of Amoore suggests that molecular receptor sites on the cell membrane of the receptor interact with specific odorous molecules in the manner of an enzyme with its substrate (a 'key and lock' phenomenon) to cause a change in the permeability properties of the membrane. Alternatively, Wright has argued that receptors may respond to the specific molecular vibrations, at infra-red frequencies, of odorous molecules. Of these two hypotheses the weight of evidence supports some type of action similar to that of the former rather than the latter theory. It can be imagined that receptor sites of various types could be scattered randomly in different combinations over the receptor endings, to give the wide range of differential responses observed in receptor cells electrophysiologically. However, recent analyses suggest that receptor sites may not be placed entirely at random, but that a limited number of combinations may occur to give each receptor sensitivity to a particular group of odours.

## THE RESPIRATORY EPITHELIUM

Those regions of the mucous membrane of the nasal cavity and associated sinuses which are not formed of olfactory epithelium are composed of columnar or pseudostratified ciliated epithelium interspersed with goblet cells collectively termed the *respiratory epithelium*.[1162] In some areas these cells may be low columnar to cuboidal. Beneath the basal lamina are groups of serous and mucous glands which show much variation in cytological detail,

[1158] I. Kolnberger, *Z. Zellforsch. mikrosk. Anat.*, **117**, 1971.
[1159] R. C. Gesteland, J. Y. Lettrin, W. H. Pitts and A. Rojas, in: *Olfaction and Taste* (Proceedings of the first international symposium, Stockholm, 1962), ed. Y. Zotterman, Pergamon, Oxford. 1963.
[1160] J. E. Amoore, in: *Handbook of Sensory Physiology*, vol. IV: *Chemical Senses*, ed. L. M. Beidler, Springer-Verlag, Berlin. 1971.
[1161] R. H. Wright, *Ann. N. Y. Acad. Sci.*, **116**, 1964.
[1162] V. Negus, *The Comparative Anatomy and Physiology of the Nose and Paranasal Sinuses*, Livingstone, Edinburgh. 1958.

opening by branched ducts on to the epithelial surface. The cavernous tissue lying beneath the respiratory mucosa in these areas is extensive (*vide infra*), and vascular disturbances cause alterations in the contours of the epithelial surface visible as swelling or shrinkage of the nasal lining.

The endothelium of these cavernous sinuses is particularly interesting since 'fenestrations' have been demonstrated; it is possible that the muscular coats which are associated with changes in blood pressure in their lumina are under endocrine rather than direct autonomic control.[1163] Immediately basal to the epithelium and its basement membrane there is a fibrous layer infiltrated with lymphocytes, forming in many parts a diffuse lymphoid tissue, and under this is a nearly continuous layer of mucous and serous glands, the ducts of which pass through the lymphoid layer before opening upon the surface. The abundant amount of mucus secreted by the glands and goblet cells makes the surface of the mucosa moist and sticky. Because of this the dust in the inspired air is deposited on the surface and the air is humidified. The rich vascularity of the membrane ensures warming of the inspired air and accounts for its pink colour. The contaminated mucous film covering the membrane is moved by ciliary action downward and backward, away from the olfactory region and into the nasopharynx. Palate movements then transfer it to the oral pharynx and it is swallowed. Some, however, is passed anteriorly into the vestibule of the nasal cavity.

## VASCULATURE AND NERVES OF THE NASAL CAVITY

The *arteries of the nasal cavity* are the anterior and posterior ethmoidal branches of the ophthalmic artery, which supply the ethmoidal and frontal sinuses, and the roof of the nose; the sphenopalatine branch of the maxillary artery, which supplies the mucous membrane covering the conchae, the meatuses, and septum; the terminal part of the greater palatine artery which ascends through the incisive canal (p. 268); the septal ramus of the superior labial branch of the facial artery, which supplies the part of the septum in the region of the vestibule, anastomosing with the sphenopalatine artery, and is a common site of bleeding from the nose (epistaxis); the infraorbital and superior (anterior and posterior) alveolar branches of the maxillary artery which supply the lining membrane of the maxillary sinus; the pharyngeal branch of the same artery, which is distributed to the sphenoidal sinus. The ramifications of these vessels form a close plexiform network, beneath and in the substance of the mucous membrane.

The *veins of the nasal cavity* form a close cavernous plexus beneath the mucous membrane. Arteriovenous communications are present.[1164] The plexus is especially marked over the lower part of the septum and over the middle and inferior conchae. Some of the veins open into the sphenopalatine vein; others join the facial vein; some accompany the ethmoidal arteries, and end in the ophthalmic veins; a few communicate with the veins on the orbital surface of the frontal lobe of the brain, through the foramina in the cribriform plate of the ethmoid bone. When the foramen caecum is patent it transmits a vein from the nasal cavity to the superior sagittal sinus.

The *nerves of the nasal cavity* include branches of the trigeminal and olfactory cranial nerves.

The *lymph vessels* are described on p. 731.

The *nerves of ordinary sensation* (7.171, 178) supplying the nasal cavity are as follows: the anterior ethmoidal branch of the nasociliary nerve, which supplies the anterior and upper part of the septum, the anterior part of the roof

and the anterior parts of the middle and inferior conchae with the lateral wall in front of these; the infraorbital nerve, which supplies the vestibule; the anterior superior alveolar nerve, which supplies the part of the septum and floor near the anterior nasal spine and the anterior part of the lateral wall as high as the opening of the maxillary sinus; the lateral posterior superior nasal and the medial posterior superior nasal nerves (including the nasopalatine nerve), which are branches of the pterygopalatine ganglion, and the posterior inferior nasal branches of the anterior palatine nerve supplying the posterior three-quarters of the lateral wall, roof, floor and septum; branches from the nerve of the pterygoid canal which supply the upper and back part of the roof and septum. It is to be noted that, with the exception of the nasociliary nerve, all the nerves supplying the nasal cavity are derived from the maxillary division of the trigeminal nerve.

Accompanying the sensory fibres in these nerves are postganglionic vasomotor sympathetic fibres to the nasal blood vessels, whilst running with the branches from the pterygopalatine ganglion are postganglionic parasympathetic fibres from the latter which are secretomotor to the nasal glands.

The *olfactory nerves* are, of course, distributed to the olfactory region of the mucosa, and their fibres arise from the bipolar olfactory cells, described above, and are destitute of myelin sheaths. They unite in fasciculi which cross one another in various directions, thus giving rise to the appearance of a plexus in the mucous membrane, and then ascend in grooves or canals in the ethmoid bone; they pass into the skull through the foramina in the cribriform plate of the ethmoid and enter the inferior surface of the olfactory bulbs, in which they ramify and form synapses with the dendrites of the mitral cells, and other varieties of neuron (7.118, see also p. 932). Closely associated with the olfactory nerves are the *nervi terminales* (pp. 934, 996).

## THE PARANASAL SINUSES

The frontal, ethmoidal, sphenoidal and maxillary paranasal sinuses (7.238, 239, 240, 244, 245, 246) vary in size and form in different individuals, and are lined with mucous membrane continuous with that of the nasal cavity, an important fact in connexion with the spread of infections. The mucous membrane resembles that of the respiratory region of the nasal cavity, but is thinner, less vascular and more loosely adherent to the bony walls of the sinuses. The mucus secreted by the glands in the mucous membrane is swept into the nose through the apertures of the sinuses by the movement of the cilia covering the surface. The cilia are not uniformly distributed in the lining mucous membrane but are always present near the opening into the nasal cavity. The function of the sinuses is doubtful. They lighten the skull and add resonance to the voice, but the saving in weight would be trivial, for absence of sinuses does not entail an equivalent volume of *solid* bone, and the weight of trabecular bone which would occupy such a volume is small. It is more probable that some, at least, of the sinuses are manifestations of the exceptional growth pattern of the bones in which they occur. They vary considerably in size in different individuals. Most are rudimentary, or even absent, at birth; they enlarge appreciably during the time of eruption of the permanent teeth and after puberty, and this growth is a factor in the alteration in the size and shape of the face at these times.

[1163] N. Cauna and K. H. Hinderer, *Ann. Otol. Rhinol. Lar.*, **78**, 1969.
[1164] W. F. Harper, *J. Anat.*, **81**, 1947.

**Two frontal sinuses** are posterior to the superciliary arches, between the outer and inner tables of the frontal bone. When of average size, each underlies a triangular area on the surface, the angles of which are formed by the nasion, a point about 3 cm above the nasion and the junction of the medial third with the rest of the supraorbital margin (**3.**116, **7.**245, 246). However, they are rarely symmetrical, because the septum between them frequently deviates from the median plane. Their average measurements are as follows: height, 3·2 cm, breadth, 2·6 cm, depth from before backwards, 1·8 cm. Each extends upwards above the medial part of the eyebrow and backwards into the medial part of the roof of the orbit.

and anterior ethmoidal arteries, and the venous drainage is into the anastomotic vein in the supraorbital notch connecting the supraorbital and superior ophthalmic veins. The lymph drainage is to the submandibular nodes. The nerve supply is derived from the supraorbital nerve.

**The ethmoidal sinuses** (*see* pp. 299–300) consist of thin-walled cavities in the ethmoidal labyrinth, completed by the frontal, maxillary, lacrimal, sphenoidal and palatine bones. They vary in number and size from three large to eighteen small sinuses on each side, and their openings into the nasal cavity are very variable. They lie between the upper part of the nasal cavity and the orbits, and are separated from the latter by the extremely thin orbital

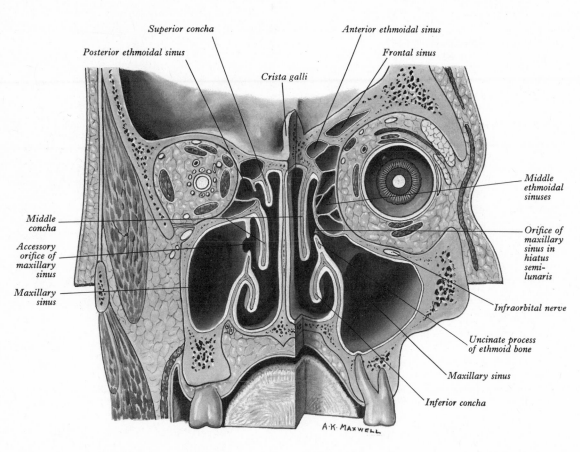

Superior concha

Posterior ethmoidal sinus

Anterior ethmoidal sinus

Frontal sinus

Crista galli

Middle concha

Accessory orifice of maxillary sinus

Maxillary sinus

Middle ethmoidal sinuses

Orifice of maxillary sinus in hiatus semi-lunaris

Infraorbital nerve

Uncinate process of ethmoid bone

Maxillary sinus

Inferior concha

A·K·MAXWELL

**7.**244  A coronal section through the nasal cavity, viewed from the posterior aspect. On the right side the plane of the section is more anterior. The normal orifice of the maxillary sinus is shown on the right side, and the not uncommon accessory orifice on the left side.

The frontal sinus is sometimes divided into a number of intercommunicating recesses by incomplete bony partitions. Rarely, one or both sinuses may be absent, and the degree of prominence of the superciliary arches is no indication of the presence or size of the frontal sinuses. The part of the sinus extending upwards in the frontal bone may be small and the orbital part large, or vice versa. Sometimes one sinus may overlap in front of the other. The sinus may extend posteriorly as far as the sphenoid (lesser wing), but does not invade it. Each opens into the anterior part of the corresponding middle meatus of the nose, either through the *ethmoidal infundibulum* or through the frontonasal duct, which traverses the anterior part of the labyrinth of the ethmoid. Rudimentary or absent at birth, they are generally fairly well developed between the seventh and eighth years, but reach their full size only after puberty (see also p. 307). They are usually more prominently developed in males, giving the profile of the forehead an obliquity which contrasts with the vertical or convex outline usual in children and females. The arterial blood supply of the sinus is from the supraorbital

plates of the ethmoid; infection may spread from the sinuses into the orbit and produce orbital cellulitis. On each side they are arranged in three groups—anterior, middle, and posterior, though some anatomists divide them into two groups, anterior and posterior, the anterior group including those described below as the anterior *and* middle groups. The three groups are not sharply delimited from each other and one group may encroach on the territory generally occupied by another. The groups are really only distinguishable on the basis of their sites of communication with the nasal cavity. In each group the sinuses are partially separated by incomplete bony septa. The *anterior group* vary up to eleven in number and open into the ethmoidal infundibulum or the frontonasal duct by one or more orifices; one sinus frequently lies in the agger nasi and the most anterior sinuses may encroach upon the frontal sinus. The *middle group* (bullar sinuses) generally comprise three cavities which open into the middle meatus by one or more orifices on or above the ethmoidal bulla. The *posterior group* vary from one to seven in number and usually open by one orifice into the superior meatus inferior to the superior concha, though one may open into the highest meatus (when present), and one or more sometimes open into the sphenoidal sinus. The posterior group are very closely related to the optic canal and optic nerve. The ethmoidal sinuses are small, but of clinical importance, at birth; they grow rapidly between the sixth and eighth years and after puberty. They derive their arterial blood supply from the sphenopalatine (p. 631) and the anterior ethmoidal and posterior ethmoidal arteries and are drained by the corresponding veins. The lymphatics of the anterior and middle groups drain into the submandibular nodes and those of the posterior group into the retropharyngeal nodes. The ethmoidal sinuses are supplied by the anterior and posterior ethmoidal nerves and the orbital branches of the pterygopalatine ganglion.

**The two sphenoidal sinuses** (p. 287, **3**.77, 78), are sited posterior to the upper part of the nasal cavity. Contained within the body of the sphenoid bone, they are, therefore, related, above, to the optic chiasma, and the hypophysis cerebri, on each side, to the internal carotid artery and the cavernous sinus. If the sinuses are small, they lie in front of the hypophysis cerebri. They vary in size and shape, and, owing to the lateral displacement of the intervening septum, are rarely symmetrical. Frequently one sinus is much the larger of the two and extends across the median plane behind the sinus of the opposite side; occasionally one sinus may overlap above the other, and rarely there is a communication between the two sinuses. Occasionally one or both sinuses may extend close to and even partially encircle the optic canal on its own side. The following are their average measurements: vertical height, 2 cm; transverse breadth, 1·8 cm; anteroposterior depth, 2·1 cm. When exception-

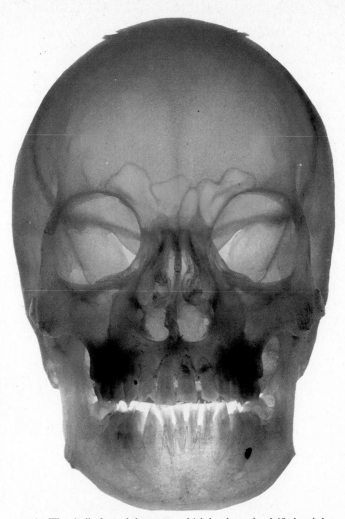

7.246 The skull of an adult woman which has been decalcified and then cleared in methyl salicylate; the specimen was transilluminated and then photographed from the ventral aspect. Note particularly the profiles of the frontal and maxillary paranasal air sinuses, the orbits and superior orbital fissures, and the nasal cavities and conchae. (The specimen was prepared by Dr. D. H. Tompsett of the Royal College of Surgeons of England.)

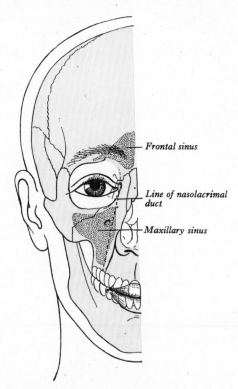

*Frontal sinus*

*Line of nasolacrimal duct*

*Maxillary sinus*

7.245  An outline of the bones of the face, showing the positions of the frontal and maxillary sinuses.

ally large they may extend into the roots of the pterygoid processes or greater wings of the sphenoid, and may invade the basilar part of the occipital bone. Occasionally there are gaps in the bony walls and the mucous membrane may lie directly against the dura mater.

Bony ridges, produced by the internal carotid artery and the pterygoid canal, may project into the sinuses from the lateral wall and floor respectively. A posterior ethmoidal sinus may extend into the body of the sphenoid and largely replace a sphenoidal sinus. Each sinus communicates with the spheno-ethmoidal recess by an aperture in the upper part of its anterior wall. They are present as minute cavities at birth, but their main development takes place after puberty. Their blood supply is by means of the posterior ethmoidal vessels and the lymph drainage is to the retropharyngeal nodes. Their nerve supply is from the posterior ethmoidal nerves and the orbital branches of the pterygopalatine ganglion.

**The two maxillary sinuses**, which are the largest accessory air sinuses of the nose, are pyramidal cavities in the bodies of the maxillae (**3**.117; **7**.244, 245, 246). The base of each is formed by the lateral wall of the nasal cavity; the apex extends into the zygomatic process of the maxilla. The roof, which is the orbital floor, is frequently ridged by the infraorbital canal, while the floor is formed by the alveolar process and is usually about 1·25 cm below the level of the floor of the nose, on a line drawn laterally from the lower border of the ala. Several conical elevations corresponding with the roots of the first and second molar teeth project into the floor, which is sometimes perforated by one or more of these roots. Sometimes the roots of the first and second premolars and the third molar, and occasionally the root of the canine, also project into the sinus (*see* p. 1236). The size of the maxillary sinus varies in different skulls, and even on the two sides of the same skull; when large, its apex may invade the zygomatic bone. The following measurements are those of an average-sized air sinus: vertical height opposite the first molar tooth, 3·5 cm; transverse breadth, 2·5 cm; anteroposterior depth, 3·2 cm. The sinus communicates with the lower part of the hiatus semilunaris through an opening in the anterosuperior part of its base (7.244); a second orifice is frequently seen in, or immediately below, the hiatus. Both are nearer the roof than the floor of the sinus. The maxillary sinus appears as a shallow groove on the medial surface of the bone about the fourth month of intrauterine life, but does not reach its full size until after the eruption of all the permanent teeth. The blood supply of the sinus is by means of the facial, infraorbital and greater palatine vessels; the lymph drainage is to the submandibular nodes. The nerve supply is derived from the infraorbital and the anterior, middle and posterior superior alveolar nerves.

For further details of the human and comparative anatomy of the paranasal sinuses consult footnote reference.[1162]

## RADIOLOGICAL APPEARANCES

Normal sinuses are radiolucent, whereas diseased sinuses show varying degrees of opacity. Radiographs also reveal the extent of development of the sinuses. In anteroposterior view (3.62, 68), the sinuses appear as follows. The frontal sinuses are seen above the nasal cavity and the medial part of the orbits and their asymmetry, vertical extent and the presence of bony septa can be assessed. The ethmoidal sinuses are superimposed on each other as well as on the sphenoidal sinus in the radiograph; they lie between the orbits, below the shadow of the cribriform plate. The sphenoidal sinus is not clear in this view. The maxillary sinus forms a pyramidal-shaped translucent area below the orbit and lateral to the lower part of the nasal cavity; inferiorly it extends into the alveolar process of the maxilla. In lateral view, the extent of the frontal sinus both upwards into the frontal bone and backwards into the orbital roof can be seen. The ethmoidal sinuses are seen extending from the shadow of the frontal process of the maxilla as far back as the sphenoidal sinus,

the latter being clear and distinct below and in front of the fossa for the hypophysis, though of course the areas of the two sphenoidal sinuses are superimposed, and the individual sphenoidal sinuses are best seen in a superior view. The maxillary sinus is well seen in a lateral view; it lies below the orbit and its extent in relation to the roots of the teeth can be clearly seen.

The maxillary and frontal sinuses can also be examined by the method of trans-illumination. In a dark room an electric torch is placed in the mouth, in the case of the maxillary sinus, or against the superomedial angle of the orbital opening, for the frontal sinus. Normally, a red glow is seen in the region of these sinuses, which may be absent where they are diseased. (For a view of the frontal and maxillary sinuses in a cleared preparation see 7.246.)

*Applied Anatomy.* Congenital deformities of the nose occur occasionally, such as complete absence of the external nose, an aperture only being present, or perfect development on one side, and suppression or malformation on the other.

The septum of the nose may be displaced or may deviate from the median plane as a result of an injury or of some congenital defect. Sometimes the deviation may be so great that the septum may come into contact with the lateral wall of the nasal cavity, producing complete unilateral obstruction.

Suppuration in the paranasal sinuses is of frequent occurrence, and it is important to note that the middle meatus is of such a form that pus running down from the frontal sinus or the anterior ethmoidal sinuses is directed by the hiatus semilunaris into the opening of the maxillary sinus, so that the latter sinus may, in some cases, act as a secondary reservoir for pus discharged from these sinuses. All the paranasal sinuses can be infected from the nasal cavity, but it should be noted that in the case of the maxillary sinus, the infection may originate from the vicinity of the teeth (p. 1236). This sinus is the one most frequently the seat of chronic suppuration, which may result in loss of cilia from the surface of the mucosa and hence impairment of mucus flow. The normal opening of the maxillary sinus is high above the floor and is poorly placed for natural drainage. Surgical drainage may be effected by puncturing the lateral wall of the inferior nasal meatus, or the canine fossa on the anterior surface of the maxilla.

# THE VISUAL APPARATUS

## Introduction

Considering the all-pervading medium of sunlight, in which almost all animal and botanical life is immersed, it is inevitable that responses to this form of electromagnetic radiation should occur. The photosynthetic processes widespread in plant forms have a parallel in the photochemical receptors which occur almost universally in the animal kingdom. Although the range of frequencies in solar electromagnetic radiation is much wider, the spectrum of visible light (400–760 nm) is the range within which most animal 'light' receptors or *photoreceptors* function. There is evidence that some animal forms have receptors which react outside this range, either in the ultraviolet or infra-red frequencies; in vertebrates, some vipers and boas[1165] have facial pit organs which respond to infra-red radiation. In general, however, the *visual pigments*, which provide the basis of the photochemical

response, display absorption maxima at various points within the visible spectrum. For example, human *rhodopsin* (visual purple) has a maximum of 497 nm. It is a rod pigment; *iodopsin*, a cone pigment, has been identified in some avian species, and several such pigments are present in human cones, where their differing absorption maxima probably account for colour vision, but full details are not yet available.[1166] The basis of the response is a light-induced 'bleaching' process, during which the pigment changes to another form, with an associated electrical change, which is propagated through the photoreceptors to the first-order neurons. A rapid restoration process is, of course, a *sine qua non*. A multiplicity of visual pigments have been identified and

[1165] G. L. Walls, *The Vertebrate Eye*, Hafner, New York and London. 1963.
[1166] W. A. H. Rushton and G. H. Henry, *Vision Res.*, **8**, 1968.

studied; further details may be obtained in a number of monographs.[1167, 1168]

The next elaboration in visual organs is the introduction of a lens, to concentrate light energy upon the photoreceptor and to impart an element of directional sensibility. Many adaptations of this kind have occurred in invertebrates, mostly in two directions: eyes—as we may now call them—with a large number of separate lens-photoreceptor units, the *compound eyes* familiar in most insects and crustaceans, and the single lens, focusing light on to an array of photoreceptors, as present in snails and squids. It is the latter type of eye which is universal in vertebrates.

True eyes are able not only to respond to variations in *luminance*—a simple function of photoreceptors; by projecting a focused image upon an array of receptors, each with neural pathways of some degree of specificity, a new modality of vision is introduced—sensitivity to *form*. In both cases movement, which is of great biological significance, may be detected, but the vertebrate type of focusing eye has potentialities for much greater precision in this respect.

Primitively, vision appears to be employed as a form of *distance reception* capable of activating warning systems, and of orientating the animal advantageously with regard to light and shade. The paired eyes of most vertebrates are set in a lateral position in the head, permitting an almost panoramic view of the environment. Such *panoramic vision*, coupled with a system of muscles, by which the eye is reflexly rotated towards any object of significance—such as the movement of a predator—is characteristic of most mammals, and clearly provides a valuable 'early-warning' system. In limited groups of mammals, and some raptorial or predatory birds, the position of the orbits has changed, so that the two uniocular fields subtended by each eye overlap to a greater or lesser extent. This entails that the part of the environment in front of the animal is focused by both eyes. By a gradual refinement of the neural control of the ocular muscles, constantly provided with a feedback from the retinae, the eye movements become sufficiently concerted to 'fuse' the two slightly dissimilar images falling on the retinae, leading to the establishment of *binocular vision*. This advance is characteristic of carnivorous mammals, who may track down their prey in part by smell, but must rely upon the much more accurately directional nature of vision to carry out the final attack. Primates also possess forward-looking eyes and hence binocular vision; but in their evolution the effect of an arboreal phase of existence is generally regarded as the operative factor in the elaboration of not merely binocular, but *stereoscopic vision*, which is characterized by a more highly evolved motor 'understanding' of the three-dimensional nature of space. Olfaction is less useful in trees, and the acquisition of great skill in not merely climbing but in swinging or leaping from branch to branch could only occur with the development of stereoscopic vision. The same habitat undoubtedly favoured the retention and elaboration of pentadactyl and grasping extremities; and although man, and perhaps his immediate ancestors, is not an arboreal primate, the terrestrial specialization of his feet has not occurred in his hands. Left free of locomotor influences by the adoption of bipedal gait, the hands have in man formed a highly significant partnership. This, coupled with the development of a particularly large brain, able to process with increasing intricacy the highly detailed information from the eyes, and to control both the eyes and hands in increasingly skilful and subtle tasks, can be regarded as the major factors in the extraordinary evolution of human abilities.

The eye, therefore, is not to be regarded in isolation. Its array of modalities—sensitivity to very small changes in luminosity, particularly in dark-adapted or *scotopic vision*, high discriminativeness as to form and movement and to colour in light-adapted or *photopic vision*—do not merely provide interesting information. The information is vital; it is doubtful whether a blind individual could long survive outside human society. The eyes provide a continuous monitoring of all we do, especially in manual tasks. Visual means of communication have proved more valuable and lasting than auditory means. The gradual evolution of visual signs, reacting with auditory communication, has led to the formation of language in all its permutations. Through language, with all its potentialities for communication of increasingly precise information and conceptual influences, it becomes possible for generation after generation to profit from recorded knowledge and skill. The results of this in human culture have become the mainstream of man's evolution. It is against this background that the structure of the visual apparatus should be studied, as we must now proceed to do.

[1167] W. A. H. Rushton, *Visual Pigments in Man*, University Press, Liverpool. 1962.
[1168] M. A. Pirenne, *Vision and the Eye*, 2nd ed., Chapman and Hall. London. 1967.

# THE PERIPHERAL VISUAL APPARATUS

The eyeball, the peripheral organ of sight, is situated in the cavity of the orbit, the walls of which serve to protect it from injury. The protection is perhaps adventitious, for other considerations, more basic to the function of vision, are more pertinent. It is difficult to imagine how the ocular movements could be controlled in the absence of a socket; nor would the spatial relationship between the two eyes be so precisely preserved in the absence of rigid sockets, a factor of prime importance in animals with binocular vision. Certain accessory structures,—the muscles, fasciae, eyebrows, eyelids, conjunctiva and lacrimal apparatus—are intimately associated with the eyeball and will be described in this section.

**The eyeball** is embedded in the fat of the orbit, but is separated from it by a thin membranous sac, termed the *fascial sheath of the eyeball* (capsule of Tenon) (p. 1128). It is composed of segments of two spheres of different sizes. The anterior segment is one of a small sphere; it is transparent, and it forms about one-sixth of the eyeball. It is more prominent than the posterior segment, which is one of a larger sphere, and is opaque, and it forms about five-sixths of the whole circumference of the eyeball. The term *anterior pole* is applied to the central point of the anterior curvature of the eyeball, and that of *posterior pole* to the central point of its posterior curvature; a line joining the two poles forms the *optic axis*. (By the same convention, the eyeball is considered to have an *equator*, equidistant between the poles; any circumferential line joining the poles is a *meridian*.) The primary axes of the two eyeballs are nearly parallel, and therefore do not correspond with the axes of the orbits, which are directed forwards and laterally. The optic nerves follow the direction of the axes of the orbits, and therefore are not parallel; each nerve enters its eyeball 3 mm to the nasal side of the posterior pole. The vertical diameter (23·5 mm) of the eyeball is rather less than the transverse and anteroposterior diameters (24 mm); the anteroposterior diameter at birth is about 17·5 mm and at puberty from 20 to 21 mm; it may vary considerably from this in *myopia* (29 mm) and *hypermetropia* (20 mm).[1169, 1170] In the female all three diameters are rather less than in the male.

The eyeball comprises three tunics, and the contents enclosed by them. From without inwards the three tunics are: (1) the fibrous tunic, consisting of the *sclera* behind and the *cornea* in front; (2) the vascular, pigmented tunic, comprising, from behind forwards, the *choroid, ciliary body* and *iris*, forming together the *uveal tract*; and (3) the nervous layer, termed the *retina*.

## The Ocular Fibrous Tunic

The fibrous layer of the eyeball (7.247) consists of an opaque, posterior part, the *tunica sclera*, and a transparent, anterior part, the *tunica cornea*.

### THE SCLERA

The sclera, so named from its density and hardness, is a firm membrane which, when distended by the intraocular pressure, serves to maintain the form of the eyeball. It is thickest (about 1 mm) behind, near the entrance of the optic nerve, and thinnest (0·4 mm) at a distance of about 6 mm behind the sclerocorneal junction, in the region of insertion of the recti muscles (p. 1123). Its *external surface* is white, and is in contact with the inner surface of the fascial sheath of the eyeball (p. 1128); it is smooth,

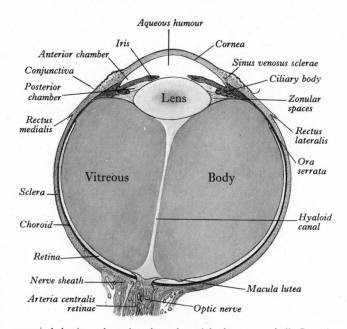

7.247 A horizontal section through a right human eyeball. Superior aspect.

except where the tendons of the orbital muscle are inserted into it; its anterior part is covered by the conjunctival epithelium, reflected on to it from the deep surfaces of the eyelids and continuous anteriorly with that covering the cornea. Its *internal surface* is brown, and is marked by grooves in which the ciliary nerves and vessels ramify; it is separated from the external surface of the choroid by an extensive *perichoroidal space*, which is traversed by an exceedingly delicate cellular tissue, termed the *supra-*

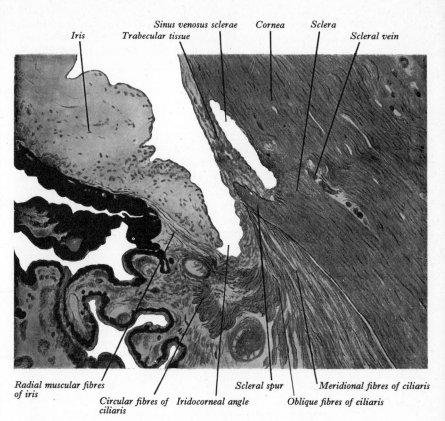

7.248 A general view of a meridional section through the iridocorneal angle.

*choroid lamina* (or *lamina fusca of the sclera*). Posteriorly, the sclera is pierced by the optic nerve, and is continuous through the fibrous sheath of this nerve with the dura mater. Where the optic nerve pierces the sclera, the latter has the appearance of a cribriform plate and is named the *lamina cribrosa sclerae* (7.258); the minute orifices in this lamina transmit the nerve bundles. One opening, larger than the rest, and occupying the centre of the lamina, transmits the central artery and vein of the retina. The lamina cribrosa is the weakest part of the sclera; if the intraocular pressure be raised for some time, as in cases of chronic glaucoma, the lamina cribrosa becomes bulged outwards producing the condition of 'cupped disc'. Around the lamina cribrosa numerous small apertures are present which transmit the ciliary vessels and nerves, and about midway between these and the sclerocorneal junction there are four or five large apertures for the transmission of veins (*venae vorticosae*). In front, the sclera is directly continuous with the cornea, the line of union being termed the *sclerocorneal junction* (or *limbus*). In the substance of the sclera close to this junction is a canal lined with endothelium running circularly, termed the *sinus venosus sclerae*, which in section presents the appearance of an oval cleft. The outer wall of the cleft is formed by a groove in the sclera. Posteriorly the cleft extends as far as a projecting rim of scleral tissue termed the *scleral spur*, which in section is triangular with the apex directed forwards and inwards. The sinus may be double in parts of its course. The inner wall of the scleral sinus, that is, the aspect of the sinus adjoining the aqueous chamber, is formed by a loose trabecular tissue continuous anteriorly with the posterior limiting lamina of the cornea. Between the fibres of this tissue are spaces through which the aqueous humour in the anterior chamber filters into the sinus (7.250), from which it then passes into the

[1169] S. Stenström, *Acta ophthal., Suppl.,* **26**, 1946.
[1170] A. Sorsby and M. Sheridan, *J. Anat.,* **94**, 1960.

bloodstream, since the scleral sinus drains externally into the anterior ciliary veins. Normally the sinus contains no blood; although the communicating channels between the sinus and the anterior ciliary veins contain no valves, these channels are oblique and flattened and may prevent reflux of blood into the sinus. Such a valvular mechanism is dubious, pressure gradients being more likely to prevent reflux of blood, since under conditions of venous congestion blood may pass into·the sinus. The anterior and outer side of the scleral spur gives attachment to most of the fibres of the trabecular tissue mentioned above and the posterior and inner side to the meridional fibres of the ciliaris. The *iridocorneal angle* (**7**.248) of the anterior chamber lies between the trabecular tissue and scleral spur anteriorly and outwards and the periphery of the iris posteriorly and inwards.

Structurally, the sclera is formed of white fibrous tissue intermixed with fine elastic fibres; flattened connective tissue cells, some of which are pigmented, are contained in lacunae between the fibres. The fibres are aggregated into bundles arranged in characteristic patterns in different parts of the sclera. Thus they are circumferential with respect to the optic papilla, but become reticular in arrangement anterior to this, and markedly meridional near the attachments of the four recti.[1171] The individual fibrils vary in diameter from 28 to 280 nm with periodicities of 80 and 21 $\mu$m. Collagen accounts for 75 per cent of the dry weight of the sclera. The sclera acts as a viscoelastic structure—an important factor in relation to intraocular circulation and pressure.[1172, 1173] Its *vessels* are very scanty; its capillaries are small, and unite at wide intervals. Its *nerves* are derived from the ciliary nerves.

## THE CORNEA

The cornea (**7**.247) is the anterior, projecting and transparent part of the external tunic, to which is due the major part of the refraction of the rays of light entering the eye. It is convex anteriorly, and projects as a flattened dome in front of the sclera. Its degree of curvature varies in different individuals, and in the same individual at different periods of life, being more pronounced in youth than in old age. As the curvature of the cornea is greater than that of the rest of the eyeball, a slight furrow, called the *sulcus sclerae*, marks the junction of the cornea and sclera. The cornea is dense and about 1·2 mm thick round its periphery and 0·5–0·6 mm at its centre. Its anterior surface is somewhat elliptical, the transverse diameter being slightly greater than the vertical. Its posterior surface is circular and, because the corneoscleral junction is slightly oblique superiorly and inferiorly, is more extensive than the anterior surface in the vertical axis. The diameter of the cornea is about 11·7 mm on its posterior aspect; anteriorly it is 11·7 mm horizontally but only 10·6 mm in the vertical.

Structurally (**7**.249), the cornea consists from before backwards of five layers—(1) the corneal epithelium, continuous with that of the conjunctiva; (2) the anterior limiting membrane (of Bowman); (3) the substantia propria; (4) the posterior limiting lamina (of Descemet); (5) the endothelium of the anterior chamber.

The *corneal epithelium* covers the front of the cornea and generally consists of five layers of cells. The deepest cells are columnar; their basal surfaces are flat and their outer surfaces rounded, and they contain large round or oval nuclei. The cells of the second layer are polyhedral, with oval nuclei. In the superficial layers the cells become progressively flattened, but, unlike the superficial cells of the epidermis, they contain flattened nuclei and they do not normally become keratinized. Most of the cells

of the corneal epithelium are prickle cells, similar to those of the germinative zone of the epidermis (p. 1162). At the sclerocorneal junction (or limbus), the epithelium becomes thicker (up to ten or more layers of cells) and is continuous with the conjunctiva covering the sclera.

The *substantia propria* is fibrous, tough, unyielding and perfectly transparent. It is composed of about 200–250 flattened, superimposed lamellae which are made up of bundles of modified connective tissue, the fibres of which are continuous with those of the sclera. Each lamella is about 2 $\mu$m thick and of very variable width (10–250 $\mu$m). The fibres of each lamella are mostly parallel, but at obtuse angles to those of adjacent lamellae. Fibres frequently pass from one lamella to the next. The dimensions of the fibres vary in different parts of the cornea, being larger in the vicinity of the posterior limiting membrane. Estimates of diameter vary from 21 to 65 nm with periodicities of 63 and 6 nm.

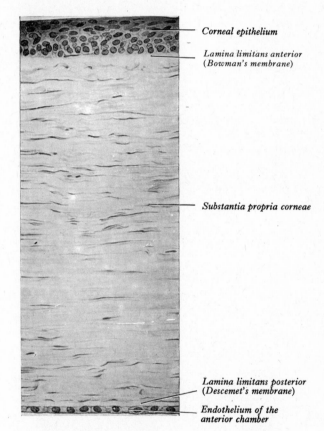

Corneal epithelium

Lamina limitans anterior (*Bowman's membrane*)

Substantia propria corneae

Lamina limitans posterior (*Descemet's membrane*)

Endothelium of the anterior chamber

**7**.249   Radial section through the human cornea. × 128.

Between the lamellae there is a small amount of ground substance, in which fibroblasts occur. These are stellate or dendritic in shape and appear to communicate with one another by numerous offsets. However, electron microscopy shows that there is no syncytial arrangement amongst the corneal cells.

The layer immediately beneath the corneal epithelium is the *anterior limiting lamina*. It consists of fine closely interwoven fibrils structurally similar to those found in the substantia propria, but contains no fibroblasts. It is about 8 $\mu$m in thickness and its collagen fibres are random in arrangement; views on their width vary from 14 to 36 $\mu$m—much less than those of the corneal stroma.

[1171] W. Kokott, *Klin. Mbl. Augenheilk.*, **92**, 1934.
[1172] J. Gloster, E. S. Perkins and M. Pommier, *Br. J. Ophthal.*, **41**, 1957.
[1173] R. St. Helen and W. K. McEwen, *Am. J. Ophthal.*, **52**, 1961.

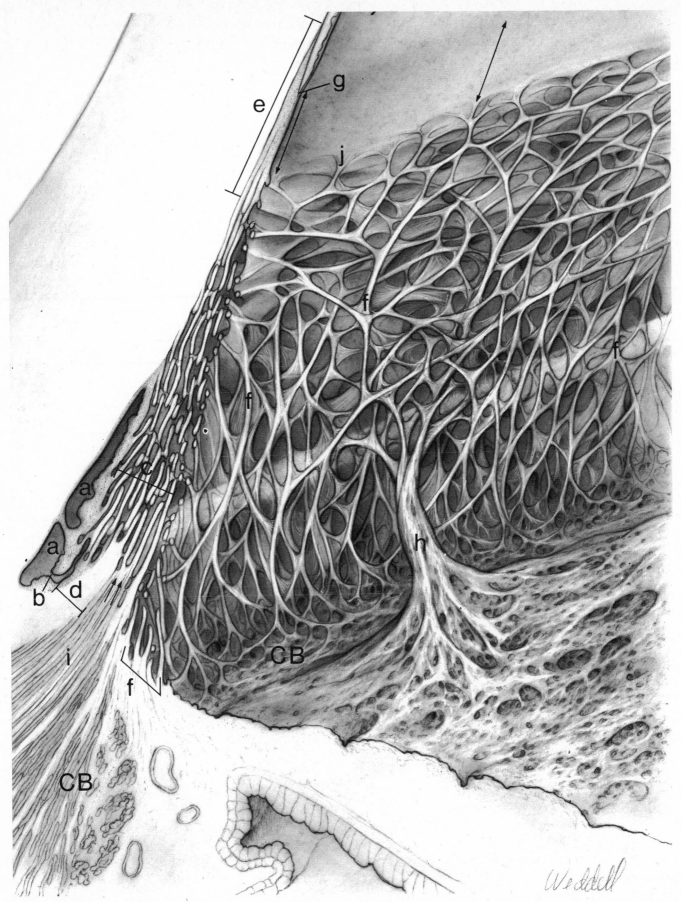

**7.250**  The iridocorneal angle and adjoining structures, showing the proximity of the scleral venous sinus (*aa*) to the pectinate ligament (*ff*). The trabecular meshwork of the latter is partly uveal, being continuous with the iris (*h*) and ciliary body (CB) and muscle (*i*). Anterior to the scleral spur (*d*) scleral trabecular tissue (*c*) is even closer to the scleral venous sinus. Aqueous fluid percolates through this trabecular region, reaching the lumen of the sinus through small apertures (*b*). The pectinate ligament diminishes as it approaches the corneal limbus (*e*), and in this junctional zone the posterior limiting membrane (of Descemet) also terminates (*g*). The endothelium of the anterior chamber (posterior corneal epithelium) is continuous with the endothelium of the trabeculae (*j*) at the limbus. (From *Histology of the Human Eye*, by Drs. Michael J. Hogan and Jorge A. Alvarado, illustrated by Mrs. Joan E. Weddell, published by W. B. Saunders, Philadelphia, 1971—by kind permission of the authors, artist and publishers. **7.**251, 253, 254, 255, 262, and 265 are from the same source.)

The *posterior limiting lamina* covers the posterior surface of the substantia propria, and is a thin, transparent, homogeneous membrane. Ultraviolet and polarization microscopy show that it has a stratified, probably fibrillar arrangement, confirmed by electron microscopy. It is considerably thicker than the endothelium to which it is subjacent and of which it is now regarded to be the basement membrane. It separates easily from both the endothelium and the corneal stroma. At the margin of the cornea it breaks up into fibres which form the trabecular tissue on the inner wall of the sinus venosus sclerae (7.250), the spaces between the trabeculae being termed the *spaces of the iridocorneal angle*; they communicate with the sinus venosus sclerae and with the anterior chamber. Some of the fibres of this trabecular tissue pass on to the internal surface of the scleral spur and are continued into the substance of the iris, forming the *pectinate ligament of the iris*; others are connected with the sloping external surface of the scleral spur and a few reach the anterior part of the choroid. The relationships of the trabecular spaces, anterior chamber, and scleral venous sinus, both in structural and functional terms, are still topics of controversy. See footnote reference[1174] for recent views and discussion.

The *endothelium of the anterior chamber* covers the posterior surface of the posterior elastic lamina, is reflected on to the front of the iris, and also lines the spaces of the iridocorneal angle; it consists of a layer of polygonal, flattened, nucleated cells.

*Vessels and Nerves.* The cornea is a non-vascular structure, the capillary vessels of the conjunctiva and sclera ending in loops at its circumference. Lymph vessels do not occur in the cornea. The *nerves* are numerous and are branches of the ophthalmic nerve, and particularly the long ciliary nerves. Around the periphery of the cornea they form an *annular plexus*, from which fibres enter the substantia propria in a radial pattern. They lose their myelin sheaths and ramify throughout the substantia propria in a delicate network, and their terminal filaments form an intricate plexus beneath the corneal epithelium. This is termed the *subepithelial plexus*, and from it fine, varicose fibrils are given off which pass through the anterior limiting membrane to ramify between the epithelial cells, forming an *intra-epithelial plexus*. Ultrastructural studies[1175] of human corneal nerve fibres show that the perineurium and myelin sheaths are gradually lost as the fibres enter the cornea. There are no specialized end organs, and in their epithelial course the nerve fibres are devoid of Schwann cells; they do not arborize.

The fibrous tunic of the eye is usually dismissed as being merely protective, but its common and continuous functions are to provide a smooth translatable external surface (*vide infra*), a suitable attachment for muscles and a resistance to the intraocular pressure. In this manner the optical shape and dimensions of the eyeball are maintained. For further details of the physiology of the cornea and sclera see footnote references[1176–1178]

## The Vascular Tunic

The vascular tunic or uveal tract of the eye consists of the choroid, the ciliary body and the iris (7.247), forming, of course, a continuous structure.

The choroid covers the inner surface of the sclera, and extends as far forwards as the ora serrata of the retina. The ciliary body continues from the anterior edge of the choroid into the circumference of the iris. The iris is a circular diaphragm behind the cornea, and presents near its centre the rounded aperture of the *pupil*.

## THE CHOROID

The choroid is a thin, highly vascular membrane, of a dark brown or chocolate colour, lining somewhat less than the posterior five-sixths of the eyeball; it is pierced behind by the optic nerve, and in this situation is firmly adherent to the sclera. It is thicker posteriorly. Its external surface is loosely connected with the sclera by the *suprachoroid lamina* (lamina fusca); its internal surface is firmly attached to the pigmented layer of the retina.

Structurally, the choroid consists mainly of a dense capillary plexus, and of small arteries and veins carrying blood to and from it. (In accord with its high vascularity, the blood flow through the choroid is also high, but this is probably to be associated with the effect of the intraocular pressure, some 15–20 mm Hg, which requires a high venous pressure, above 20 mm Hg, if circulation is to be maintained. Metabolic demand is relatively low— the venous blood loses only 3 per cent of its oxygen.[1179] The warming effect of the choroidal circulation may have some importance.) On its external surface is the thin *suprachoroid lamina*, about 30 μm thick, which is composed of delicate non-vascular lamellae, each consisting of a network of fine collagen and elastic fibres, among which are branched cells containing dark-brown pigment granules. Ganglionic neurons and plexuses of nerve fibres are enmeshed in the connective tissue. The mesothelium-lined interstices, sometimes described, are not supported by modern observations; pathological accumulations of fluid may split the lamellae of the suprachoroid. All such potentially weak connective tissue zones are a great attraction to those in search of lymph spaces in the eye.

**The choroid proper** (7.255) is internal to the suprachoroid lamina (which is in part derived from scleral connective tissue. Its layers are variously described, but generally recognized are (*a*) an external *vascular lamina* composed of small arteries and veins and loose supporting connective tissue, in which are scattered pigment cells, (*b*) an intermediate *capillary lamina* (choroidocapillaris), and (*c*) a thin, apparently structureless, *basal lamina* (the membrane of Bruch). The vascular lamina is itself sometimes divided on the basis of the calibre of its vessels, which naturally decreases towards the capillary layer. In general, however, these vessels are relatively small and the capillaries large, and the latter, in any case, dominate the scene. The vascular lamina contains the branches of the short posterior ciliary arteries (p. 636), extending anteriorly in a meridional direction from their entry through the sclera near the optic disc. The veins of the vascular lamina are much larger, and they converge in whorls or vortices upon four or five principal *vorticose veins*, which pass through the sclera to drain into the ophthalmic veins of the orbit. The capillary or choroidocapillary layer, separated from the retina only by the choroidal basal lamina, is almost certainly responsible for the maintenance of the outer layers of the retina, at least in part. It forms a finely meshed network, especially in the posterior region of the eyeball; but the meshes become larger as they approach the ciliary body, where they link up with the capillaries of the ciliary processes. The basal lamina was until recently considered to be a glassy,

[1174] R. C. Tripathi, *Expl Eye Res.*, **10**, 1970.

[1175] H. Matsuda, *Acta Soc. ophthal. jap.*, **12**, 1968.

[1176] H. Davson (ed.), *The Eye*, vol. I., Academic Press, London and New York. 1962.

[1177] M. A. Jakus, *Ocular Fine Structure*, Churchill, London. 1964.

[1178] M. E. Laugham (ed.), *The Cornea*, John Hopkins Press, Baltimore. 1969.

[1179] A. Bill, in: *Adler's Physiology of the Eye*, ed. R. A. Moses, 5th ed., Mosby, St Louis. 1970.

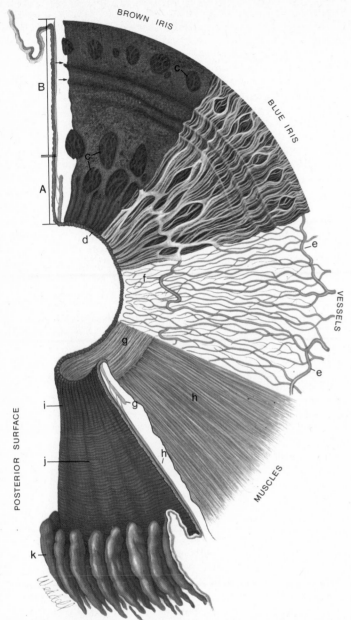

The functions of the pigment cells of the choroid are speculative. Clearly it is plausible to assume that they prevent the passage of light from the exterior of the sclera; but it seems more probable that they absorb light which has passed through the retina, thus preventing reflexion. In many animals, especially in those of nocturnal habit, specialized cells in the choroid form a reflecting structure, the *tapetum*, which is responsible for the greenish glare visible in the eyes of such animals at night.[1182] The significance of this arrangement is uncertain; it may be a mechanism of aggression or it may bring about increased stimulation of the retinal receptors.

## THE CILIARY BODY

The ciliary body is a direct anterior continuation of the choroid, and the iris is a further extension of the ciliary body itself. All three regions of the uveal tract evince certain common features and regional differences dependent on variations in function. The ciliary body is specifically concerned with the suspension of the lens and with the mechanism of accommodation, and this accounts for the accumulation of muscle which causes it to bulge towards the interior of the eyeball (**7.253**). It is also involved in the production of aqueous fluid or humour into the anterior segment of the eye, with which its anterior aspect is related. More posteriorly it is directly contiguous with the vitreous humour, and it is probable that it secretes some of the vitreous mucopolysaccharides. The anterior and the long and short posterior ciliary arteries all meet in the ciliary body (**7.255**), and it is hence a highly vascular region. This rich circulation is concerned not only with the secretory and muscular activities of the body, but also with the supply of the iris and the limbal region. The ciliary body is also traversed by the major nerves supplying all the anterior ocular tissues.

Externally, the ciliary body extends from a point about 1.5 mm posterior to the corneal limbus (which corresponds also to the scleral spur) to a point 7·5 to 8 mm posterior to this on the temporal side of the eyeball and 6·5 to 7 mm on the medial or nasal side. The body is hence a slightly eccentric structure, extending posteriorly from the scleral spur, to which it is attached, with a meridional width varying from about 5·5 to 6·5 mm. As seen from the interior of the eyeball it presents a posterior periphery, where it is continuous with the choroid, which is crenated or scalloped—the *ora serrata*. Its anterior extremity is confluent with the periphery of the iris, and lateral to this it bounds the irido-corneal angle of the anterior chamber. The internal aspect of the ciliary body is grey in colour, due to the pigment in the deeper layer of its epithelium. It is divisible into an anterior ridged or plicated part, the *corona ciliaris* (pars plicata), which surrounds the base of the iris in an annular manner, and posterior to this a relatively smooth annular strip, the *orbiculus ciliaris* (pars plana, ciliary ring). The orbiculus accounts for more than half of the meridional width of the ciliary body, being 3·5 to 4 mm across. The peripheral rim of the orbiculus is the ora serrata, a dentate junction at which the fully developed *optical* or sensory part of the retina is suddenly reduced to two layers of epithelial cells, prolonged over the whole of the ciliary body as the *pars ciliaris retinae* and beyond this on to the posterior surface of the iris. The corona ciliaris, forming a smaller annular region within the orbiculus, is ridged by seventy to eighty *ciliary processes* which radiate in a meridional

**7.251** Composite view of the surfaces and internal strata of the iris. In a clockwise direction from above the pupillary (A) and ciliary (B) zones are shown in successive segments. The first (brown iris) shows the anterior border layer and the openings of crypts (*c*). In the second segment (blue iris), the layer is much less prominent, and the trabeculae of the stroma are more visible. The third segment shows the iridial vessels, including the major arterial circle (*ee*) and the incomplete minor arterial circle (*f*). The fourth segment shows the muscle stratum, including the sphincter (*g*) and dilatator (*h*) of the pupil. The everted 'pupillary ruff' of the epithelium on the posterior aspect of the iris (*d*) appears in all segments. The final segment depicts this aspect of the iris, showing radial folds (*i* and *j*) and the adjoining ciliary processes (*k*). (From *Histology of the Human Eye*—see **7.250**.)

homogeneous layer (lamina vitrea); it is only 2–4 μm in thickness, but electron microscopy has revealed much intimate detail. It consists essentially of a middle stratum of elastic tissue between internal and external collagenous layers, united externally to the basement membrane of the choroidocapillary lamina and internally to the basement membrane of the pigment cells of the retina.[1180, 1181] Its exact functional significance is not certain, but it is obviously related to the passage of fluid and solutes from the choroidal capillaries to the retina, and it is said to provide a smooth surface for the precise orientation of the pigment cells and receptors of the retina, a factor important to precise vision.

[1180] W. Lerche. *Z. Zellforsch. mikrosk. Anat.*, **65**, 1965.
[1181] Y. Nakaizumi, *Archs. Ophthal.*, N.Y., **72**, 1964.
[1182] G. L. Walls, *The Vertebrate Eye*, Hafner, New York. 1963.

direction from the base of the iris towards the orbiculus ciliaris (7.252). Branching from the sides of these processes into the valleys between them are numerous minor ridges, the *ciliary plicae*, forming a complex pattern which, in microscopic preparations, presents highly intricate profiles (7.253). Into the valleys between the ciliary processes groups of fibres of the *zonule* (suspensory ligament) of the lens extend, passing beyond the processes to establish continuity with the basement membrane of the superficial layer of epithelial cells covering the orbiculus ciliaris. The sites of these attachments are marked by striae which pass posteriorly from the valleys of the corona across the orbiculus almost to the apices of the dentate processes of the ora serrata (7.253).

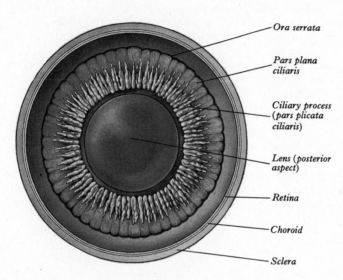

7.252    The interior aspect of the anterior half of the eyeball.

*Ora serrata*

*Pars plana ciliaris*

*Ciliary process (pars plicata ciliaris)*

*Lens (posterior aspect)*

*Retina*

*Choroid*

*Sclera*

For description it is convenient, if arbitrary, to treat of the intimate structure of the ciliary body under three headings: (1) the ciliary epithelium; (2) the ciliary connective tissue and vessels; and (3) the ciliary muscle.

**The ciliary epithelium** is bilaminar, consisting of two layers of simple epithelium superimposed one upon another and representing the two layers of the optic cup. The *superficial lamina* is formed of cells which are columnar over the orbiculus and cuboidal where they cover the ciliary processes, becoming irregular and more flattened in the intervals between the processes. They contain little or no pigment and are the sole anterior continuation of the neural layers of the retina; this excludes the pigment epithelium of the retina, which is itself continuous with the *deeper layer* of the ciliary epithelium. The cells of the latter are also approximately cuboidal and are loaded with pigment granules. The two layers are firmly united, but pathological accumulations of fluid may separate them, just as the retina detaches from its own pigment epithelium. A basement membrane intervenes between the two epithelia, and the basal aspects of the superficial cells are much infolded, as in the case of other secretory epithelia. These superficial cells exhibit junctions of the desmosomal type, and in their cytoplasm mitochondria are numerous and the endoplasmic reticulum is well developed, the latter often forming stacked arrays in the peri-nuclear zone. The Golgi apparatus is not well developed. Lipid and melanin granules are often present but not prominent.

The pigment epithelium is united to the stroma of the ciliary body by its own basement membrane, which is continued posteriorly into the basal lamina of the choroid tunic (p. 1100). The cytoplasm of these cells contains very numerous round or oval granules containing abundant melanin and measuring about 0·6 to 0·8 $\mu$m in diameter. The cells are linked laterally to each other by relatively few desmosomes, these being more numerous between cells in the two strata of the epithelium, despite the intervention of a basement membrane.

**The ciliary stroma** is composed largely of loosely arranged fasciculi of collagen fibres, and these are aggregated into a considerable mass between the ciliary muscle and the overlying ciliary processes, into both of which the connective tissue extends. In this inner stratum of connective tissue are numerous larger branches of the ciliary arteries and veins with a rich interconnecting network of capillaries of comparatively large calibre; the majority of these are adjacent to the epithelium, and are especially concentrated in the ciliary processes. In these sites the capillaries are chiefly of fenestrated type; numerous vessels also enter the ciliary muscle, but the capillaries there evince much less frequent fenestration. Anteriorly, near to the periphery of the iris, is the major arterial circle (7.251, 255), formed chiefly by the long posterior ciliary arteries, branches of the ophthalmic p. 636), which enter the eye well posterior to the equator and pass anteriorly between the choroid and the sclera to reach the ciliary body. The veins of the body, into which those of the iris drain, pass posteriorly to join the vorticose veins of the choroid.

**The ciliary muscle** has been variously described by different authorities, their main divergencies being in the number of divisions or parts recognized in this small annular mass of nonstriated muscle. In most descriptions three parts are usually named—*meridional, radial* or *oblique*, and *circular* or sphincteric—but other views have been stated in recent studies.[1183, 1184] Most and perhaps almost all of the ciliary muscle fibres are attached to the scleral spur (7.254), from which they pass in a variety of directions. It is upon these variations that a somewhat arbitrary division of the whole muscle into parts is dependent. The most external fibres extend in a meridional or longitudinal direction, passing posteriorly into the stroma of the choroid, where many exhibit terminal branchings or *epichoroidal stars*. The most internal fibres swerve acutely as they leave the scleral spur (7.254) and run circumferentially to form a circular or sphincteric element in the muscle, in close proximity to the periphery of the lens. Between these two muscular strata are fibres which cross obliquely from one to the other, often crossing each other in a lattice of interweaving fibres. This part of the muscle is often referred to as radial in disposition. In its ultramicroscopic features the ciliary muscle exhibits some differences from other nonstriated muscle masses. The fibres show distinct cell walls and possess basement membranes, but they contain an unusual abundance of mitochondria and endoplasmic reticulum. A small bundle of fibres is usually surrounded by a common fibroblastic sheath, forming units not encountered in other nonstriated muscles. Junctions between the fibres within a bundle are described, but their precise nature is still uncertain; they are said to resemble intercalated discs. Three types of nerve ending have been observed, the most common being an indirect contact of synaptic membranes with an interposed basement membrane; contact without a basement membrane also occurs, and most rarely larger and more intimate contacts in depressions in the muscle fibre substance.

Both myelinated and nonmyelinated nerve fibres abound in the ciliary muscle and elsewhere in the ciliary body.

[1183] M. Calasans, *An. Fac. Med. Univ. S. Paolo*, **27**, 1953.
[1184] J. Rohen, in: *Handbuch der mikroskopischen Anatomie des Menschen*, Bd III/2, ed. W. W. Möllëndorf, Berlin. 1964.

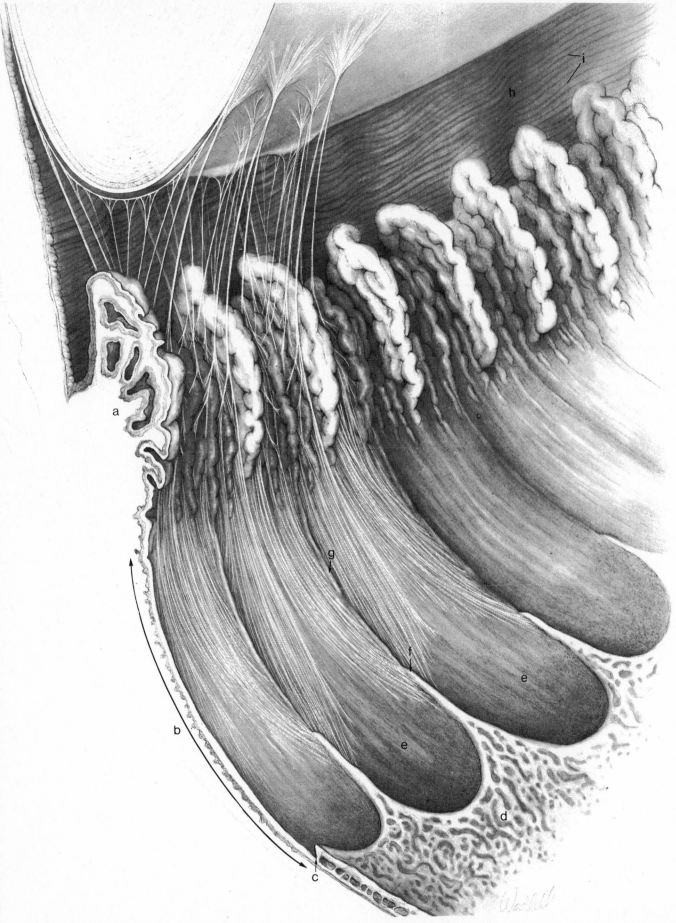

**7.253** A magnified view of the ciliary region seen from the ocular interior. Above is the periphery of the lens, attached by the fibres of the *zonule* (suspensory ligament) to the processes of the *corona ciliaris* (pars plicata) of the ciliary body (a). The *orbiculus ciliaris* or pars plana ciliaris (b) has a scalloped boundary, the *ora serrata* (c), which separates it from the retina (d). Flanking the 'bays' (e) of this are the *dentate* processes (f), with which linear ridges or *striae* (g) are continuous. These striae extend forwards between the main ciliary processes, providing an attachment for the longer zonular fibres. The posterior aspect of the iris shows radial (h) and circumferential (i) sulci. (From *Histology of the Human Eye*—see 7.250.)

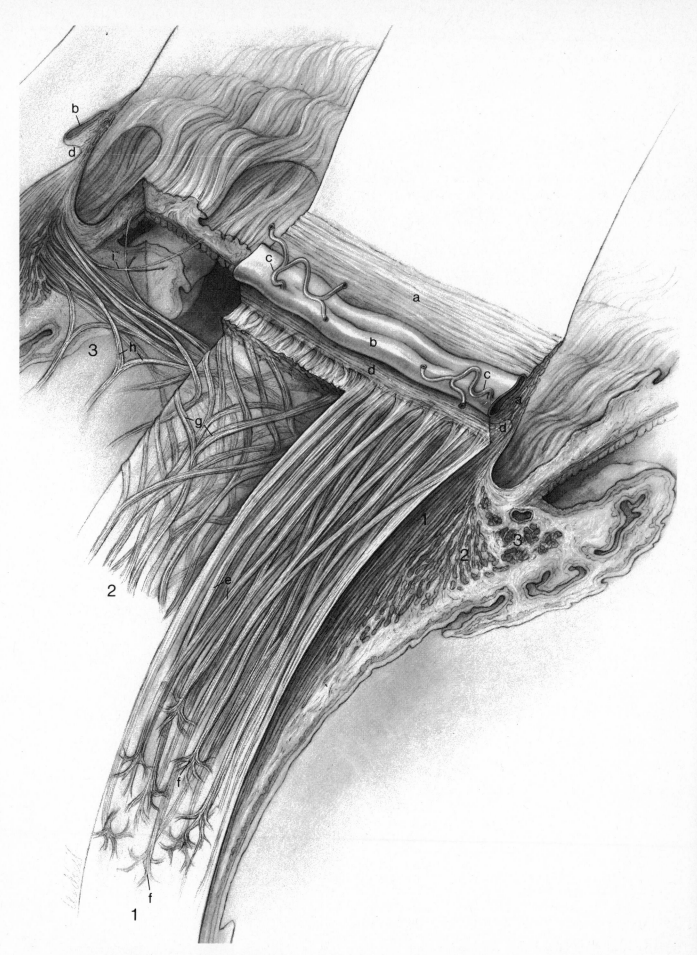

**7.254** The ciliary muscle and its components. The meridional or longitudinal (1), radial or oblique (2), and circular or sphincteric (3) layers of muscle fibres are displayed by successive removal towards the ocular interior. The cornea and sclera have been removed, leaving the pectinate ligament (*a*), the scleral venous sinus (*b*), collecting venules (*c*) and scleral spur (*d*). The meridional fibres often display acutely angled junctions (*e*) and terminate in epichoroidal stars (*f*). The radial fibres meet at obtuse angles (*g*), and similar junctions, at even wider angles (*h*), occur in the circular stratum of the ciliaris. (From *Histology of the Human Eye*—see **7.250**.)

The latter are postganglionic fibres derived from the ciliary ganglion, where they link with the parasympathetic outflow of the oculomotor nerve; but there is considerable evidence that some of these fibres are sympathetic. While it is clear that the former supply stimulates the fibres of the ciliary muscle to contract, the role of the sympathetic supply is still unsettled. Cervical sympathetic stimulation in some experimental animals leads to flattening of the lens, which is tantamount to relaxation of accommodation, but the mechanism of this is uncertain. It may be due to an inhibitory effect on the ciliary muscle; but it has also been suggested that the volume of the ciliary body may be reduced by vasoconstriction, thus resulting in tension on the zonule and through this on the periphery of the lens—the reverse of the slackening effect on the zonule of ciliary contraction.[1185] For a recent critique of this topic consult reference [1186].

## THE IRIS

The iris is the delicate and adjustable diaphragm which surrounds the *pupil*, its central orifice (slightly medial to the true centre), which exerts a considerable control over the amount of light entering the eye. The pupil may vary in diameter over a range of at least 1 to 8 mm, and even more under the influence of drugs. This represents an effective aperture range in excess of $f$ 20 to $f$ 2·5, and a ratio of 32:1 in the amount of light permitted to enter the eye. While this is obviously not enough to save the retina from the effects of very intense illumination, it is a factor in smoothing out the wide range of luminosities encountered in ordinary use and in thus preserving useful vision in highly variable conditions. The pupillary diameters noted above and an average diameter of the iris of about 12 mm are, of course, taken as measured through the cornea, whose dioptric power introduces a magnification factor of about 12 per cent. *Constriction* and *dilatation* of the pupil are self-explanatory terms, for which meiosis and mydriasis are also used clinically, though these are more properly reserved for the extreme limits of contraction and dilatation. For a most erudite discussion of the immense literature on the pupil and its responses and a recent account of iris activity see footnote references [1187, 1188].

Though the iris is named after the rainbow, its range of colour is somewhat less, extending from light blue to a very dark brown. The hue may vary in the two eyes and through the same iris. The colour is due to the combined effects of the iridial connective tissue and pigment cells in absorbing or reflecting different frequencies of light energy in a selective manner. In the absence of significant amounts of pigment, as in the iris of the newborn, the colour is light blue; some degree of pigmentation is necessary to confine light transmission to the pupil and to the centre of the lens, where optical aberrations are least. The concentration of melanocytes is the predominant factor in iris hue, but their distribution is often irregular and may produce in this manner a flecked or maculated appearance.

In shape the iris is not a discoid diaphragm; the anterior convexity of the lens bulges it a little, so that it is more accurately described as a very shallow cone, truncated by the pupillary aperture. It is sited between the cornea and the lens (7.247), immersed in the *aqueous fluid* or humour, and it partially divides the *anterior segment* of the eye into an *anterior chamber*, enclosed by the cornea and iris (which meet at the *iridocorneal angle*) and an unfortunately termed *posterior chamber*, between the iris and the lens. Peripherally, in the latter cavity, the ciliary processes protrude a little between the divisions of the zonular ligament of the lens; and it is here that most of the aqueous fluid is produced, finding its way through the pupil into the anterior chamber and finally to its exit into the scleral venous sinus (p. 1097) at the iridocorneal angle—the 'filtration angle' of clinical parlance.

**The microscopic structure of the iris** displays a number of unusual features (7.251). Its anterior surface, forming the posterior boundary of the anterior chamber, is not covered by a distinct epithelium, despite frequent statements to the contrary; this surface is merely a modified 'anterior border layer' of the general *stroma*, which forms the bulk of the iris. The stroma contains the vessels and nerves of the region and, near the periphery of the pupil, an aggregation of nonstriated muscle fibres forming an annular contractile structure, the *sphincter pupillae*. The posterior aspect of the iris consists of a continuation of the same two layers of epithelium which cover the ciliary body and which represent the internal and external strata of the optic cup. The pupil, through which this epithelium turns round for a short distance on to the *anterior* surface of the iris as the pigment ruff, or 'border', therefore corresponds with the opening of the optic cup. The deeper, and hence in the iris the more anterior of these epithelial layers, is commonly termed, a little confusingly, the *anterior epithelium* of the iris. It should be emphasized to avoid confusion, that this anterior epithelium is immediately *posterior* to the stroma of the iris. Its cells are pigmented, like those of the same layer in the ciliary epithelium; closely associated with them are the radially arranged nonstriated fibres of the dilatator pupillae, which like the sphincter has a most unusual embryological origin in being derived from the neural ectoderm of the optic cup. Superficial and posterior to this layer of cells is a stratum of heavily pigmented cells, forming the so-called *posterior epithelium*. This layer is continuous with the *non-pigmented*, retinal layer of the ciliary epithelium.

The *anterior border layer* or anterior surface of the iris has been much studied at low magnification by slit-lamp microscopy, with which it is seen to display a somewhat fluffy appearance, except in heavily pigmented irides. Depressions or *crypts*, through which vessels may be visible in the stroma, and various radial and circular folds and striae can be observed, but details of this kind should be sought in a suitable authority.[1189] The constituents of the anterior border lamina are chiefly much branched fibroblasts and melanocytes, with no vestige of the endothelium which covers it at birth, and to a rapidly decreasing extent during the first post-natal year.[1190] This is confirmed by electron microscopy.[1191] The fibroblasts form an approximately single continuous layer on the surface, with branching processes which form no actual junctions.[1192] At the peripheral base of the iris they blend with the connective tissue of the trabecular meshwork (pectinate ligament) at the iridocorneal angle. At the pupillary border they come into contact, but again without specialized junctions, with the pigment epithelium of the posterior surface of the iris. The melanocytes also exhibit intricately branched processes, and again

[1185] M. W. Morgan, *Am. J. Optom.*, **21**, 1944.

[1186] M. Alpern, in: *The Eye*, vol. 3, 2nd ed. H. Davson, Academic Press, London. 1969.

[1187] I. E. Loewenfeld, *Documenta ophth.*, **12**, 1958.

[1188] O. Lowenstein and I. E. Loewenfeld, in: *The Eye*, vol. 3, H. Davson, 2nd ed. Academic Press, London. 1969.

[1189] A. Vogt, *Lehrbuch und Atlas der Spaltlampenmikroskopie des lebenden Auges.* Teil 3. *Iris, Glaskörper, Bindehaut*, Ente, Stuttgart. 1942.

[1190] F. Vrabec, *Ophthalmologica*, **123**, 1952.

[1191] A. J. Tousimis and B. S. Fine, *Archs Ophthal., N.Y.*, **62**, 1959.

[1192] G. K. Smelser and T. Ishikawa, *Acta XIX Conc. Ophthal. India*, 1966.

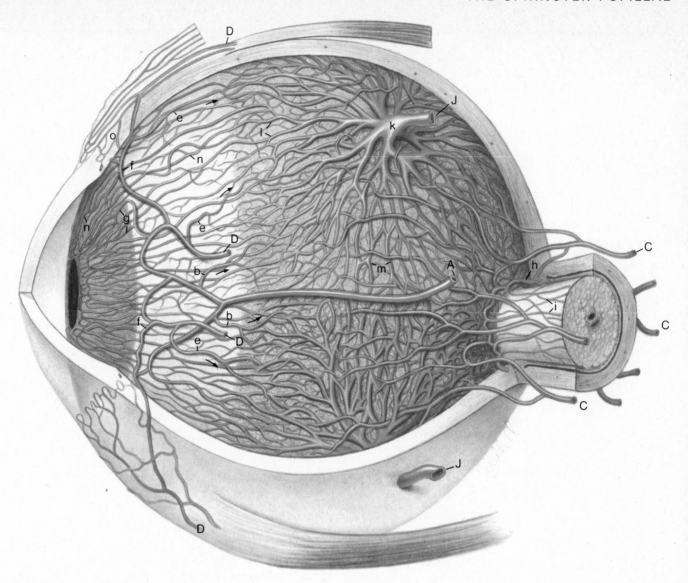

**7.255** The vascular arrangements of the uveal tract. The long posterior ciliary arteries, one of which is visible (A), branch at the ora serrata (bb) and feed the capillaries of the anterior part of the choroid. Short posterior ciliary arteries (CC) divide rapidly to form the posterior part of the choriocapillaris. Anterior ciliary arteries (DD) send recurrent branches to the choriocapillaris (ee) and anterior rami to the major arterial circle (ff). Branches from the circle extend into the iris (g) and to the lim-bus. Branches of the short posterior ciliary arteries (CC) form an anasto-motic circle (h) (of Zinn) round the optic disc, and twigs (i) from this join an arterial network on the optic nerve. The vorticose veins (jj) are formed by the junctions (k) of suprachoroidal tributaries (l). Smaller tributaries are also shown (m, n). The veins draining the scleral venous sinus (o) join anterior ciliary veins and vorticose tributaries. (From *Histology of the Human Eye*—see **7.250**.)

no special junctions have been observed between them. Some capillaries invade the border layer.

Thr *stroma of the iris*, which is derived like the anterior border layer from the mesoderm between the developing lens and optic cup, is also formed by fibroblasts and melanocytes; but in this region there is, in addition, a considerable amount of loose collagenous tissue, whose spaces are filled with fluid and a mucopolysaccharide ground substance. These spaces are apparently in fairly free communication with the fluid in the anterior chamber of the eyeball, and the interchange of fluid between the chamber and the iridial stroma may explain the large changes of volume which appear to accompany con-traction and relaxation of the iris diaphragm. The meso-dermal stroma also contains not only an abundance of blood vessels and nerves, but also the ectodermal sphincter and dilatator muscles. There is no elastic tissue, and any of the elastic recoil which has been attributed to the iris, and sometimes suggested as a dilatation force when the sphincter is relaxed, must reside in other structures, if it in fact exists. The collagen fibrils, which have a diameter of about 60 nm, and a periodicity of 50 to 60 nm, are very loosely arranged, many describing incomplete circum-ferential loops around the pupil as centre. 'Clump' cells, mast cells, macrophages and lymphocytes are said to occur in the stroma, but the reader is referred to larger monographs quoted at the end of this account for fuller details.

**The sphincter pupillae** is an annular flattened band of nonstriated muscle about 0.75 mm in width and 0.15 mm in thickness. Its fusiform cells are closely packed and are often arranged in small groups, as in the ciliary muscle; in accordance with the effect of the muscle on the pupil these fibres are orientated parallel to its margin. Stromal collagen tissue encloses the muscle anteriorly and posteriorly and is particularly dense in the latter situation, where it binds the sphincter pupillae to the pupillary extremity of the dilatator muscle. Ultramicro-scopy shows that the muscle fibre groups noted above are not entered by nerve fibres, only one fibre of the group usually being innervated. It is presumed that the de-polarizing current of contraction spreads to the rest of the fibres through gap junctions. In other details of cytoplasmic organelles, densities resembling Z-bands, and basement membranes, the muscle fibres are like those of nonstriated muscles elsewhere. Small nerves ramify in the connective tissue between the fibre bundles; most of their fibres are nonmyelinated and they are often enclosed as groups of several axons in the same Schwann cell sheath. They do not approach the surfaces of muscle cells more closely than 0·1 μm.

**The dilatator pupillae**, a muscle whose existence has been the subject of a prolonged, vexed and at times almost ridiculous controversy, is now a well-established entity, on microscopic, physiological and pharmacological grounds.[1193, 1194] It is a thin stratum immediately anterior to the deeper, anterior layer of the epithelium of the posterior aspect of the iris. Its fibres are indeed muscular processes of this anterior layer, whose cells are therefore myoepithelial in character. Their apical processes form the epithelium itself (p. 1105). Myofilaments appear in both parts of these cells, but are much more numerous in their basal, muscular processes. The latter are about 4μm thick, 7μm wide, and 60 μm in length. They are fusiform and form a stratum 3 to 5 elements thick through most of the iris, from its periphery to a point near the outer perimeter of the sphincter, which it overlaps a little. Towards this perimeter the dilatator rapidly peters out, sending spurs of muscle processes to blend with it. These processes, unlike the apical parts of the myoepithelial cells of the anterior epithelium, show a clear basement membrane, and they are joined by gap junctions like those in the fibres of the sphincter which probably also serve as points of electrical coupling. Their myofilaments are about 3 nm in diameter and numerous densities resembling Z-discs are evident. Nonmyelinated nerve fibres have been described in relation to the muscular processes or 'fibres', and these terminate very close to the cell membrane, the interval being of the order of 20 nm.

**The arteries of the iris** (7.251, 255, 256) are derived from the long posterior and the anterior ciliary arteries, and from the vessels of the ciliary processes. Each of the two long ciliary arteries, on reaching the attached margin of the iris, divides into an upper and a lower branch; these anastomose with corresponding branches of the artery from the opposite side and with the anterior ciliary arteries, and form a vascular circle (*circulus arteriosus major*). From this circle vessels converge to the free margin of the iris, and there communicate to form a second circle (*circulus arteriosus minor*). This minor circle is incomplete, and some observers regard these vessels as venous. The smaller arteries and veins are very similar in the structure of their walls, and they also share certain peculiarities. Thus, they are often slightly helical—perhaps an adaptation to the great changes in the shape of the iris which occur as the pupil varies in size. Perhaps also to be ascribed to this is the peculiar structure of the vascular wall. All the vessels, including the capillaries, have a non-fenestrated endothelium, with a well-marked and often thick basement membrane. Outside this, in the arteries and veins, there is no elastic lamina, and nonstriated muscle fibres are few, especially in the veins. The connective tissue of the media is loose, and external to this is a remarkably dense collagenous adventitia, which appears to form almost a separate tube outside the endothelium. The loose stratum of the media has been regarded as a lymph space, but this is improbable; it is about 7 μm in width, and contains a matrix probably derived from the basement membrane of the endothelium.[1195]

**The nerves of the iris**, like those of the choroid, are chiefly derived from the branches of the long ciliary rami of the nasociliary nerve and from the short ciliary branches of the ciliary ganglion. The latter contain postganglionic but thinly myelinated fibres which innervate the sphincter pupillae. The dilatator pupillae is

supplied by postganglionic nonmyelinated fibres derived from the superior cervical ganglion of the sympathetic trunk, but the routes by which these reach the muscle are not precisely established, and they may vary in different species of mammals and may be multiple in man. The sympathetic plexus around the internal carotid artery is

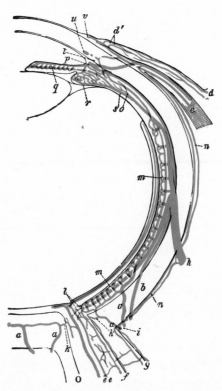

7.256 A diagrammatic representation of the course of the vessels of the eye. Horizontal meridional section. Arteries and capillaries red; veins blue. O. Entrance of optic nerve. *a*. Short posterior ciliary arteries. *b*. Long posterior ciliary arteries. *c*. Anterior ciliary vessels. *d*. Posterior conjunctival vessels. *d'*. Anterior conjunctival vessels. *e*. Central retinal vessels. *f*. Pial vessels. *g*. Dural vessels. *h*. Vorticose veins. *i*. Short posterior ciliary vein. *k*. Branches of the short posterior ciliary arteries to the optic nerve. *l*. Anastomosis of choroidal vessels with those of optic nerve. *m*. choroidocapillary lamina. *n*. Episcleral vessels. *o*. Recurrent artery of the choroid. *p*. Circulus arteriosus major (in section). *q*. Vessels of iris. *r*. Vessels of ciliary process. *s*. Branch from ciliary muscle to vorticose vein. *t*. Branch from ciliary muscle to anterior ciliary vein. *u*. Sinus venosus sclerae. *v*. Capillary loop at margin of cornea.

said to send a branch through the ciliary ganglion, and these postganglionic fibres reach the eyeball through the short ciliary nerves; but some sympathetic fibres may travel to the eye through the long ciliary nerves. (For details of other routes in monkeys, see p. 1006.) The innervation of the muscles of the iris, as that of the ciliaris, is probably more complex, and both the sphincter and dilatator may possess a double autonomic innervation. Histochemical stains for acetylcholine-esterase and fluorescent techniques have demonstrated both cholinergic and adrenergic activity in both iridial muscles.[1196, 1197] Although ganglion cells have occasionally been reported in the iris, it is most likely that all, or almost all the fibres are postganglionic in type, and almost all are also nonmyelinated. They form a plexus at the base of the

[1193] G. W. H. M. Alphen, *Archs Ophthal. Chicago*, **69**, 1963.

[1194] I. E. Lowenfeld, *Documenta ophth.*, **12**, 1958.

[1195] M. J. Hogan, J. A. Alvarado and J. E. Weddell, *Histology of the Human Eye*, Saunders, Philadelphia. 1971.

[1196] B. Ehinger and B. Falck, *Acta physiol. scand.*, **67**, 1966.

[1197] O. Lowenstein and I. E. Loewenfeld, in: *The Eye*, ed. H. Davson, Academic Press, New York. 1969.

iris, and from this small nerves and individual fibres extend not only to the two muscles, but to the vessels and to the anterior border layer and the anterior epithelium (but not the pigment layer) of the posterior surface of the iris. Some fibres may be afferent and some are vasomotor, but little is known of either. (For details of the occurrence and distribution of the nonmyelinated sympathetic and parasympathetic nerve fibres in the choroid consult footnote reference [1198].)

**Pupillary membrane**. In the fetus, the pupil is closed by a delicate, vascular membrane, termed the *pupillary membrane* (p. 146). The vessels of this membrane are partly derived from those of the margin of the iris and partly from those of the capsule of the lens; they end

## The Retina

The retina (7.247) is the neural, sensory stratum of the eyeball. It is very thin, varying from 0·56 mm near the optic disc to 0·1 mm anterior to the equator of the eyeball, continuing at this thickness to the ora serrata. It is, of course, much thinner at the optic disc and the fovea of the macula.[1199] Its external surface is in contact with the choroid, its internal with the hyaloid membrane of the vitreous body. Posteriorly it is continuous with the optic nerve; it gradually diminishes in thickness from the optic disc to the ciliary body; it presents a crenated margin named the *ora serrata* (7.252, 253). Here the nervous tissues

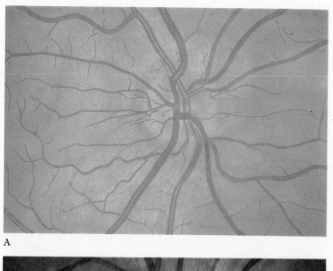

A

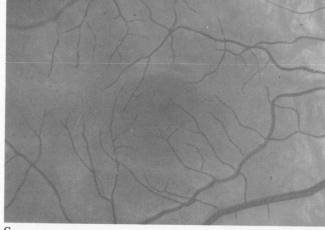

C

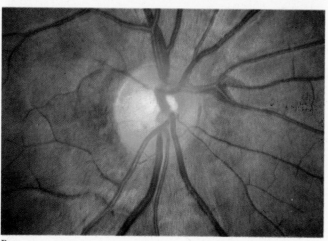

B

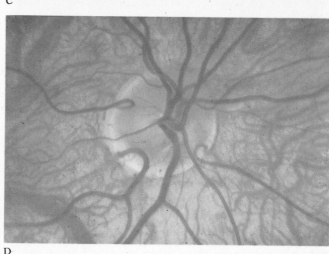

D

**7.257 A–D**  Ophthalmoscopic photographs of the right human retina.

A  Note dichotomous branching of vessels, arteries being brighter red and showing a more pronounced 'reflex' to light, as a pale stria along their length. The veins are also larger in calibre; more of them cross arteries superficially than is usual. The optic disc, around the entry of the vessels, is a light pink, with a surrounding zone of heavier pigmentation. Compare with 7.257 E, from the same Caucasian adult.

B  Appearances in a heavily pigmented individual, with a paler optic disc than in 7.257 A. Note accentuation of the edge of the disc by retinal and choroidal pigmentation. The arteries cross the veins superficially in this retina. Negroid adult.

C  Normal macula of a young Caucasian subject. Note the fovea, showing as a central, paler, circular area. The macular branches of the central retinal artery are approaching from the right. The macula is largely free of vessels of macroscopic size, but the capillaries here form a particularly close network, except at the fovea.

D  The region of the optic disc in an eye with poorly developed pigmentation. Three cilioretinal arteries are curving round the edge of the disc, two on the left, one on the right. Between the two left cilioretinal arteries a single macular artery is apparent. Due to the depressed pigmentation choroidal vessels are also visible, especially veins; and on the left of the photograph two large vorticose venous tributaries can be seen.

in loops a short distance from the centre of the membrane, which is thus left free from blood vessels. About the sixth month of intrauterine life the membrane begins to disappear by absorption from the centre towards the circumference, and at birth only scattered fragments are present; in exceptional cases it persists and may interfere with vision.

of the retina end, but a thin prolongation of the membrane extends forwards over the back of the ciliary processes and iris, forming the *ciliary* and *iridial parts of the retina*.

[1198] G. L. Ruskell, *Expl Eye Res.*, **12**, 1971.
[1199] L. M. Spence, R. Y. Foos and B. R. Straatsma, *Trans. Am. Acad. Ophthal. Oto-Lar.*, **73**, 1969.

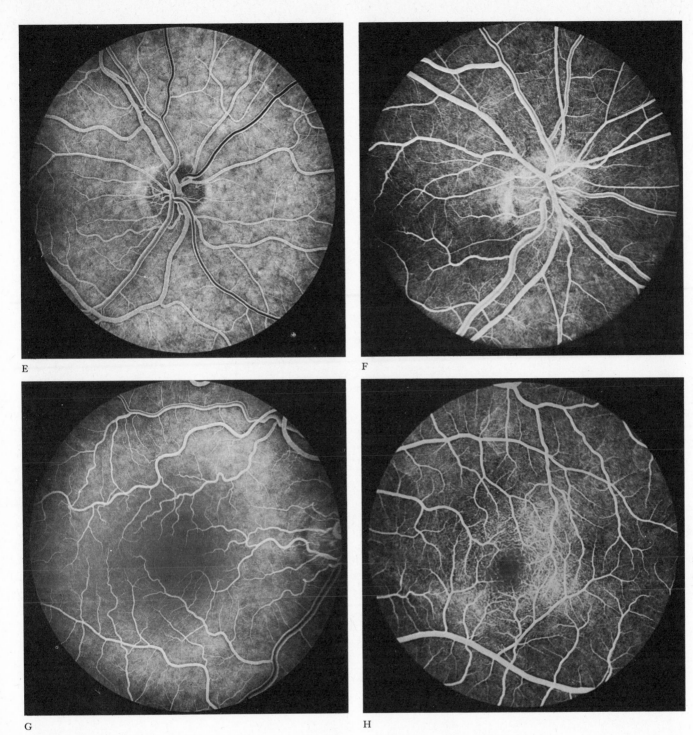

E

F

G

H

**7.257E–H** Fluorescence angiograms of the retina. These are produced by photography with a fundus camera at known periods of time following introduction of fluorescein into the circulation. (For details of the technique consult *Fluorescence Photography of the Eye*, by Emanuel S. Rosen, Butterworths, London, 1969, to whom we are indebted for all the colour photographs and angiograms in this illustration.)

E   Angiogram of the same retina as that appearing in **7.257** A, taken in 'mid-venous' phase. The arteries display an even fluorescence, but the veins appear striped, due to laminar flow. This appearance is the reverse of, and not to be compared with the arterial 'reflex' seen in **7.257** A. The background mottling is due to fluorescence from the choroidal vessels.

F   Angiogram of the left optic disc, showing the major arteries and veins and also their smaller branches. Note particularly the radial pattern in the retinal capillaries. The laminar flow in the veins is less obvious than in **7.257** E.

G   Angiogram showing the macular region of a right eye. The main macular vessels are approaching from the right. The subject was an elderly person with considerable macular pigmentation, which masks fluorescence from the choroidal circulation. Compare with **7.257** H.

H   Angiogram of the macula of a young subject showing the macular capillaries in detail. Note the central avascular fovea. Left eye. Compare with **7.257** G.

This forward prolongation consists of the pigmented layer of the retina together with a deeper stratum of columnar epithelium; in the iridial part of the retina both layers of epithelium are cubical and pigmented. The part of the retina extending from the optic disc to the ora serrata is known as the *optic part of the retina*. The retina is soft, translucent, and of a purple tint in the fresh, unbleached state, owing to the presence of a colouring material, named *rhodopsin*, or *visual purple*; but it soon becomes clouded, opaque, and bleached when exposed to light. (It is, in fact, difficult to prepare an eye in such a way as to demonstrate the purple pigment. In the preserved eyes usually dissected, the *fixed* retina has a cloudy white colour.) Near the centre of the posterior part of

1109

the retina there is an oval, yellowish area, named the *macula lutea* (7.257); it shows a central depression, termed the *fovea centralis*, where visual resolution is highest. At the fovea centralis the retina is exceedingly thin, some of its layers being absent here, and the dark colour of the choroid is distinctly seen through it. About 3 mm to the nasal side of the macula lutea the optic nerve pierces the retina at the *optic disc*, which has a diameter of about 1·5 mm. The circumference of the disc is slightly raised, while the central part presents a slight depression. The centre of the disc is pierced by the central artery and vein of the retina (7.257, 258). The optic disc is insensitive to light, and is termed the 'blind spot'. On ophthalmoscopic examination the normal disc is seen to be pink; it is, however, much paler than the retina and may be grey or almost white. In cases of optic atrophy the capillary vessels disappear and the disc appears white. The name

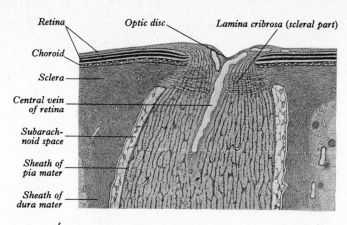

**7.258A** A horizontal section through the optic nerve at its point of exit from the human eyeball.

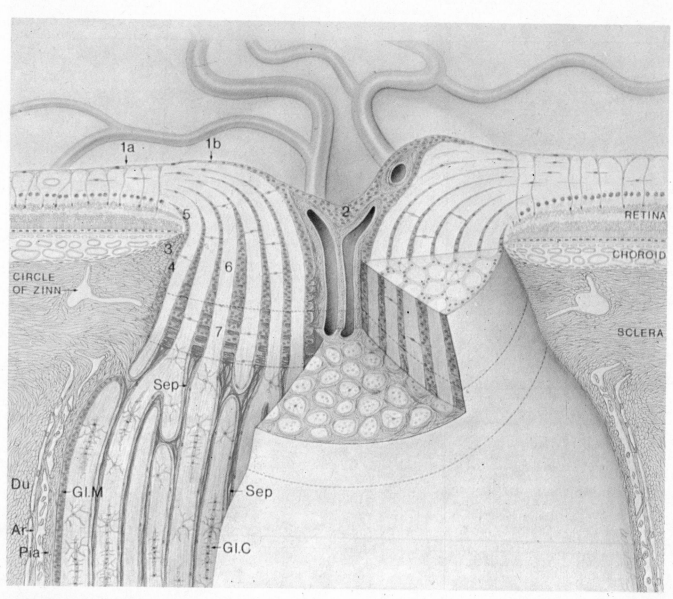

**7.258B** Schematic representation of the exit of the human optic nerve from the eyeball, showing the distribution of collagenous (blue) and neuroglial (magenta) tissues. Sep = septa of collagenous connective tissue carried into the nerve from the pia mater and dividing the nerve fibres into numerous fascicles. Gl.M = astroglial membrane separating nerve fibres from connective tissue. Gl.C = astrocytes and oligodendrocytes among the fibres in their fascicles. 1a is the internal limiting lamina of the retina, which is continuous with an astroglial membrane (of Elschnig) covering the optic disc (1b). An accumulation of astrocytes forms a central meniscus (of Kuhnt) in the centre of the disc (2). The anterior or so-called 'choroidal part' of the lamina cribrosa (6) is separated from the choroid by a spur of collagenous tissue (3). The 'border tissue of Jacoby' (4), which is largely astroglia, frequently extends beyond the choroid (5) to separate much of the retina from the 'retinal part' of the optic nerve head. The posterior part of the lamina cribrosa (7) contains collagenous tissue derived from the optic nerve septa and fenestrated sheets of collagen fibres continuous with those of the sclera. (Reproduced by kind permission of Dr. Douglas K. Anderson and Dr. W. F. Hoyt, *Arch. Ophthal.*, **82** (4), 506–530, 1969. Copyright 1969, American Medical Association.)

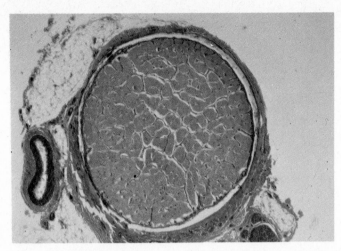

7.258c  A transverse section of the optic nerve and its meningeal coverings posterior or proximal to the entry of the central retinal artery, which is visible at the side of the nerve. The dural and pial sheaths are stained green, the subarachnoid pink. Note the fasciculation of the nerve. (Material stained by Masson's trichrome technique and kindly provided by Dr. N. A. Locket, Institute of Ophthalmology, University of London.)

'optic papilla' applied to the disc is misleading since the normal disc lies in the same plane as the surrounding retina.

## The Structure of the Retina

As has already been stated (pp. 136 and 145), the retina is derived from the two layers of the invaginated optic vesicle, the outer of which becomes the *pigment cell lamina*, the inner developing into the far more complex multilaminar structure containing the *photoreceptors* (rod and cone cells), their *first order neurons* (bipolar cells), the somata and beginnings of the axons of their *second order neurons* (ganglion cells), and *interneurons* arranged across these centripetal pathways (horizontal and amacrine cells). In addition, the retina contains *neuroglial elements* (Müller cells, or sustentacular gliocytes) and a *vascular system* composed chiefly of capillaries. In some descriptions the region of the retina posterior to the ora serrata (*pars optica retinae*)—the region which functions as a sense organ—is separated from its pigment epithelium as 'the retina proper'; but since the epithelium is functionally integrated with the rest of the retina, this arbitrary division into a *stratum pigmentosum* and a *stratum nervosum* will not be followed here. The description will, however, be limited to the sensory region of the retina, whose ciliary and iridial parts have already been considered (pp. 1101, 1102).

It is customary to recognize ten layers in the retina, and this plan will be adhered to in the following pages (7.259–262). It is hardly necessary to add that this is merely a morphological convenience in the primary analysis of the highly integrated nervous elements of the retina.

### 1. THE RETINAL PIGMENT EPITHELIUM

This is a single lamina of cells arranged with marked regularity and extending from the periphery of the optic disc to the ora serrata, anterior to which they continue into the ciliary epithelium (p. 1102). They are approximately flat rectangles in radial sections and hexagonal when seen in tangential aspect. They number about 4 to 6 million in the human eye, becoming more numerous in more aged eyes. Near the macula they measure about

10 and 14 $\mu$m in their radial and tangential dimensions, but become much flattened near the ora serrata.[1200] Their nuclei are in the basal part of the cytoplasm, adjacent to the basal lamina (Bruch's membrane) of the choroid (p. 1100), from which the cells are separated by their own basement membrane. The latter is much infolded into the cytoplasm of the basal aspects of the cells. Their apical regions project between the rod and cone processes as microvilli of 5 to 7 $\mu$m in length. The intermediate cytoplasmic region contains numerous mitochondria and pigment granules. The pigment is melanin, and various other organelles, associated with the formation of this, have been identified in retinal epithelium, including well-developed granular and agranular endoplasmic reticulum in stacked arrays, premelanosomes and melanosomes.[1201, 1202] Lipofuscin also occurs,[1203] probably as a residue representing the end of a phagosomal process. Some recent autoradiographic and ultramicroscopic studies[1204, 1205] suggest that the microvilli of the pigment epithelium cells are concerned in a continuous erosion of the external ends of the rod and cone processes. Lamellar inclusions in the cytoplasm of the microvilli closely resemble the lamellar structures in the outer segments of the photoreceptors; they have been termed phagosomes, and they evince progressive disintegration as they pass deeper into the cytoplasm of the cell.[1206]

A typical cell membrane of 'unit' structure encloses the pigment cells. Basally, as stated earlier, this is much infolded by the basement membrane. The latter has a fibrillar structure, and some of its fibrils join the basal membrane of the choroid, a junction which may explain the adherence of the pigment lamina to the choroid rather than to the rest of the retina. Laterally the membranes of the pigment cells do not interdigitate markedly, and the variable space between them is sealed off from the apical space (between the microvilli and the photoreceptors) by zonulae occludentes. Other forms of junction also occur. A viscous, mucopolysaccharide substance occupies the space, which is embryologically derived from the cerebral ventricles.

Although the *functions of the pigment epithelium* of the retina are still far from elucidated, their ultramicroscopic features strongly suggest a phagocytic activity, possibly a nutritive role, to which may be added a contribution to the spacing and mechanical support of the photoreceptors, and an optical function in absorbing light and preventing back reflexion.

### 2. THE PROCESSES OF THE ROD AND CONE CELLS

The retinal photoreceptor cells (7.259, 260) consist of a cell body containing the nucleus, which will be described in lamina 4 (*vide infra*), an axonal centripetal process which forms synapses with the retinal neurons in lamina 5, and a photosensitive centrifugal or external process which will be the subject of this section. Although intermediate forms exist in various vertebrates, the great majority of these processes, and hence the cells of which they are a part, fall into two categories, *rods* and *cones*, differentiated principally by the cylindrical and conical

[1200] M. O. Ts'o and E. Friedman, *Archs Ophthal., N.Y.*, **78** and **80**, 1967 and 1968.

[1201] A. S. Breathnach and L. M. A. Wylie, *J. Ultrastruct. Res.*, **16**, 1966.

[1202] M. Seiji, in: *Advances in Biology of the Skin*, ed. W. Montagna, Pergamon Press, New York. 1967.

[1203] L. Feeney, J. Grieshaber and M. J. Hogan, in: *The Structure of the Eye*, ed. J. Rohen, Schattauer, Stuttgart. 1965.

[1204] R. W. Young and D. Bok, *J. Cell Biol.*, **42**, 1969.

[1205] M. Spitznas and M. J. Hogan, *Archs Ophthal., N.Y.*, **84**, 1970.

[1206] J. Marshall and P. L. Ansell, *J. Anat.*, **110**, 1971.

form of their processes, but also by the existence of a constricted *outer fibre* connecting the rod process to the soma of its cell (7.260 B), a feature absent from cone cells, though in these a small constriction or waist may be apparent. At the junction of the rod processes with their outer fibres and of the cone processes with their cell bodies is the external limiting membrane, through which the photoreceptor processes appear to be thrust (7.260 B), as if through a sieve; the nature of this structure will be discussed below (see lamina 3).

The rod and cone processes are closely packed in a highly orderly array, but the density of this diminishes throughout the neuroretina to the ora serrata, where they abruptly cease. In the human retina they are most numerous in and near the *macula*, the region at the optical centre of the retina where vision is most discriminative as to form and colour, though least adapted to functioning in low luminosities. They are entirely absent over the whole of the *optic disc*, where the centrifugal fibres of the retina leave the eyeball to form the optic

reference[1207].) The macula and central fovea will be considered further when the general structure of the retina has been described (p. 1118).

The total number of rods in the human retina has been estimated at 110 to 125 million and of the cones at 6·3 to 6·8 million.[1208] Other similar figures have been stated. The distribution of the two types of receptors differs; the cones, which have their densest arrangement at the rod-free foveola (about 147,000 per square millimetre), fall off in numbers very rapidly from this point to a 10-degree circle round the macula to a density of about 5,000 per square millimetre, maintaining this to the ora

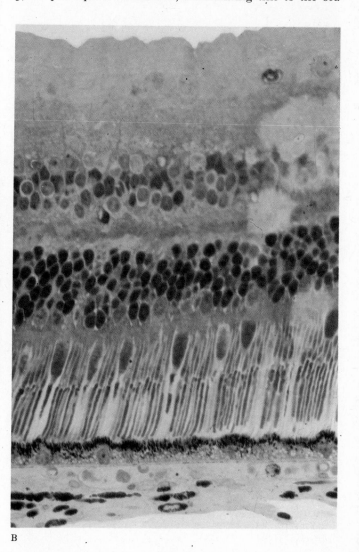

Internal limiting lamina
Lamina of nerve fibres (stratum opticum)
Ganglionic lamina
Internal plexiform lamina
Internal nuclear lamina
External plexiform lamina
External nuclear lamina
External limiting lamina
Lamina of rods and cones
Lamina of pigment cells

A

B

7.259 A–C Sections through the primate retina, from its vitreous aspect (above) to the choroid tunic (below), showing its layered structure some little distance from the macular region. A Diagram to illustrate the customarily recognized strata. B Thin section of simian retina in araldite embedded material, stained by toluidine blue. (Kindly provided by Dr. N. A. Locket, Institute of Ophthalmology, London.) Compare with A. The section in C (kindly provided by Dr. Alan M. Laties, University of Pennsylvania Medical School), shows a region of simian retina freeze-dried and photographed by interference microscopy, primarily to demonstrate the orderly orientation of photoreceptors.

nerve. The *central area* of the retina is a region 5 to 6 mm in diameter, which contains the *macula lutea*, measuring about 2 mm horizontally and 1 mm vertically, its yellow colour being due either to the presence of xanthophyll, a great reduction in the capillary bed, or perhaps to cell inclusions (other than xanthophyll) in the bipolar and ganglion cells. Approximately at the centre of the macula is the *fovea centralis*, a deep conical depression in the retina, where almost all elements except cones are absent, on its floor at least, the diameter of this being said to be no more than 0·4 mm. This *foveola*, as it is sometimes called, is about 4 mm lateral and 1 mm inferior to the centre of the optic disc; the latter corresponds to the 'blind spot' in the uniocular visual field. The extremely small size of the foveola accounts for the accuracy with which the visual axis must be directed to achieve the most discriminative vision. The macula has been further divided into peri- and para-foveal areas, but for such details recent monographs should be consulted. (See also

serrata. The rods, on the other hand, exhibit an almost opposite density, rising from zero at the foveola to an even greater figure than cones at the 10-degree circle (160,000 per square millimetre), and then slowly diminishing in frequency to the periphery of the retina, where there are still estimated to be approximately 30,000 per square millimetre—rods being thus six to thirty times more numerous in the peripheral part of the retina outside the 10-degree circle. This distribution accords well with the phenomena of photopic (cone) and scotopic (rod) vision. Even with light microscopy it is clear that the neurons in the retina are much less numerous than the rod and cone cells; the ganglion cells (*vide infra*, p. 1117), whose axons form the optic nerve, are therefore probably in the region of a million in number in the human retina. It is hence obvious that large numbers of rod and cone cells must

[1207] E. Yamada, *Archs Ophthal., N.Y.*, **82**, 1969.
[1208] G. A. Østerberg, *Acta ophthal., Supp.* **6**, 1935.

activate a single axonal pathway in the optic nerve and beyond.

**The rod and cone processes** exhibit greater differences with light microscopy than with the electron microscope. Even with the former technique both forms of process show an external or peripheral segment, which with ordinary stains is refractile, positively birefringent and PAS-positive, and an internal segment which stains deeply and has a fibrillar structure. The combined segments of the rod process measure about 100 to 120 $\mu$m in the freshly fixed human retina, the cone processes being about 65·to 75 $\mu$m.[1209] These dimensions diminish

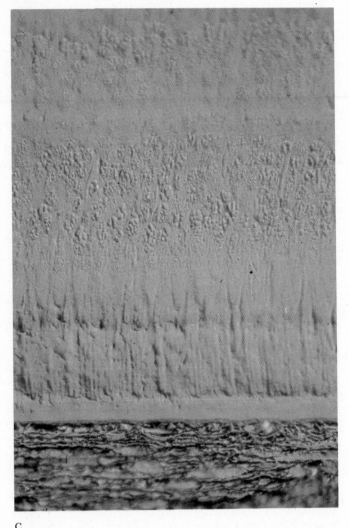

C

towards the ora serrata, especially in the cones, which are in addition much narrower at the fovea, where they closely resemble rods in their dimensions. The outer segment of rods contains the photosensitive pigments named *rhodopsins* (visual purple), and in the cones[1210, 1211] similar pigments have been detected. These substances display different absorption characteristics, and these account for the different behaviour of rods and cones in conditions of high and low luminosity. Different absorption maxima have also been observed amongst cones themselves in the primate retina, and there is at least some degree of accord between these findings and the trichromatic theory of colour vision.

In their *ultrastructural details* the rods and cones are very similar and will be considered together; the rod processes have been more extensively studied.[1212–1217] The rod *outer segment* consists of a remarkably regular series of discoid structures, stacked like thin coins and surrounded by a cell membrane, to the external aspect

of which are applied the microvilli of the pigment epithelial cells (*vide supra*, p. 1110). The electron microscope shows that these *discs*, which number from 600 to 1,000 in various species of vertebrate, are flattened sac-like structures, consisting of two unit membranes continuous at the periphery of the disc and separated by a less electron-dense *intradisc space*, except near the periphery, where the space becomes an annular interval of greater width (7.260 B). In some vertebrates the discs are infoldings of the cell's membrane, but in the human retina this continuity is lost. The dimensions of these discs have been reported in detail in many species, including primates, and details may be sought in the papers quoted. The rod *inner segments* are longer than the outer and somewhat greater in diameter, both differences being even more accentuated in the inner segments of the cones. The inner segment is itself divisible into two regions—an outer *ellipsoid*, which is acidophilic, contains some glycogen, and displays a large number of mitochondria, and an inner *myoid*, adjacent to the soma of the cell, and containing much randomly arranged agranular endoplasmic reticulum and free ribosomes. The myoid is basophilic, and it contains much more glycogen than the ellipsoid. Extending from the inner to the outer segment are bands of the cytoplasm of the ellipsoid, covered with cell membrane, which are closely applied to the outer segment. Another cytoplasmic process connects the ellipsoid to the outer segment, but in this case there is cytoplasmic continuity. This process, the *cilium*, originates in a basal body and has a similar internal structure to a motile cilium.[1218] The cone processes have a very similar structure to that of the rods, the differences being largely dimensional. (For further details see footnote reference[1219].)

Although the structure of the rod and cone processes has now been described in most extensive detail, it is not yet possible to equate their highly remarkable features with functional studies with any degree of confidence. Their stacked discs have been likened to photomultiplier tubes, intensifying the electrical energy derived from photochemical processes, but this is merely an attractive analogy.

## 3. THE EXTERNAL LIMITING LAMINA

At the level of the junctions between rod and cone processes with the outer fibres of the rods and the somata of the cone cells light microscopy shows what appears to be a thin membrane, which is commonly regarded as being fenestrated by the above continuities. It extends throughout the neural retina and has been considered for many decades to consist of the fused terminal expansions of the 'fibres of Müller'. These are elaborate neuroglial elements, with cell bodies in the internal nuclear layer (lamina 6, *vide infra*), and from them long processes stretch radially through almost the whole thickness of the retina, from its vitreal surface almost to the pigment

[1209] D. Eichner, *Z. mikrosk.-anat. Forsch.*, **63**, 1957.
[1210] W. A. H. Rushton, *Visual Pigments in Man*, Liverpool University Press, Liverpool. 1962.
[1211] M. A. Pirenne, *Vision and the Eye*, 2nd edn, Chapman and Hall, London. 1967.
[1212] F. S. Sjöstrand, *J. cell. comp. Physiol.*, **42**, 1953.
[1213] F. S. Sjöstrand, in: *The Structure of the Eye*, ed. G. K. Smelser, Academic Press, New York, 1961.
[1214] G. M. Villegas, *J. Anat.*, **98**, 1964.
[1215] L. Misotten, *Bull. Soc. belge Ophthal.*, **130**, 1962.
[1216] J. E. Dowling, *Science., N.Y.*, **147**, 1965.
[1217] A. I. Cohen, *Anat. Rec.*, **152**, 1965.
[1218] E. DeRobertis, *J. gen. Physiol.*, **43**, 1960.
[1219] C. E. Dieterich and J. W. Rohen, *Albrecht v. Graefes Arch. Ophthal.*, **179** 1970.

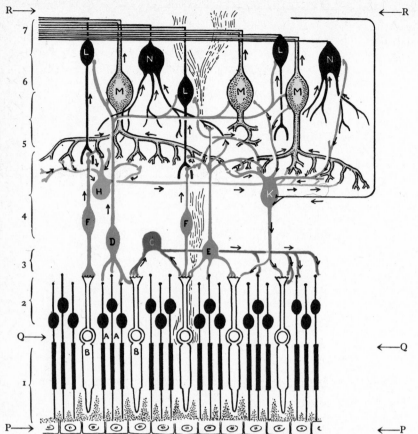

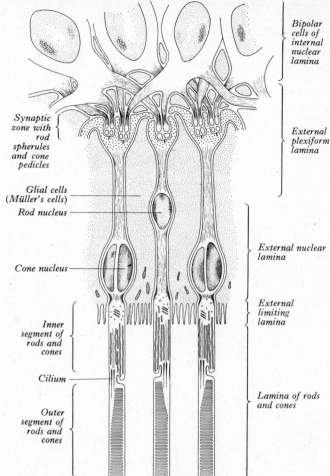

**7.260 A** Scheme of the retinal neurons. (Modified from Polyak.) 1. Rods and cones. 2. External nuclear lamina. 3. External plexiform lamina. 4. Internal nuclear lamina. 5. Internal plexiform lamina. 6. Lamina of ganglia cells. 7. Lamina of nerve fibres, passing to optic disc. P. Pigment cells. Q. Membrana limitans externa. R. Membrana limitans interna. One sustentacular fibre is indicated in the centre of the diagram. AA. Outer rod fibres. BB. Inner cone segments. C. Horizontal cell. D and E. Bipolar cells forming synapses with rods and cones. FF. 'Midget' bipolar cells synapsing only with cones. HK. Amacrine cells. LLL. Midget ganglion cells. MN. Other ganglion cells. Arrows indicate the probable direction of nerve impulses.

**7.260 B** Schematic representation of the ultrastructure of retinal photo-receptors and of their connexions with bipolar nerve cells. Note the stacked discs in the outer segments, and refer to **7.261** and **262** and to the text for further details of the synaptic zone. (Reproduced from F. S. Sjöstrand, in: *The Structure of the Eye*, ed. G. K. Smelser, Academic Press, New York. 1961.)

epithelium. From these vertical fibres large numbers of subsidiary processes spread out horizontally in a dendriform manner into the plexiform layers (laminae 5 and 7) and form meshworks embracing the somata of cells in the nuclear and ganglion cell layers (laminae 4, 6 and 8). Similar 'fibre baskets' also surround the inner segments of the photoreceptors. This structural arrangement has naturally suggested that these *retinal gliocytes* or *Müller cells* supply a physical support to the retina, like neuroglia elsewhere in the central nervous system. Moreover, the processes of these cells form a similar *internal limiting membrane* (lamina 10) on the vitreal aspect of the retina, and hence it is not unreasonable to ascribe a stabilizing role to these glial elements. As long ago as 1932[1220] the external limiting membrane was described as a series of unions between the cell membranes of the rods and cones on the one hand and the 'fibres of Müller' on the other. Ultrastructurally this view has been corroborated (see footnote reference[1221] for a summary of the literature on this topic), but there is much variation in the types of junction described. They occur between the glial processes and the rod and cone inner segments; a recent study of them in the human retina describes them as zonulae adherentes, which also sometimes unite adjoining glial fibres (the classical view) and adjacent photoreceptor processes to each other.[1222]

In the plexiform layers the horizontal branches of Müller's cells are closely related to the dendrites and axons

of the retinal neurons, and may at times form helical lamellae around individual neurites, without, however, the production of myelin. Like other neuroglial cells they also make extensive contacts with blood vessels, especially capillaries; their basement membranes are at these sites fused with those of nonstriated muscle cells in the media of the vessel or with the basement membrane of the endothelium in the case of capillaries. With their very extensive ramifications and widespread contacts with other retinal elements, these gliocytes take up much of the total volume of the retina, also reducing the extracellular space to exiguous proportions. All the glial processes are, of course, cytoplasmic extensions of the cell body, and it is not surprising, therefore, that other than supportive functions have been ascribed to the retinal gliocytes. There is physiological evidence, for example, that they are concerned in the transport of glucose to retinal neurons, and they are able to synthesize and store glycogen.[1223] (For further details see footnote reference[1224].)

[1220] L. B. Arey, in: *Cytology and Cellular Pathology of the Nervous System*, ed. W. Penfield, Hoeber, New York. 1932.
[1221] B. S. Fine and L. E. Zimmermann., *Invest. Ophthal.*, **1**, 1962.
[1222] M. Spitznas, *Albrecht v. Graefes Arch. Ophthal.*, **180**, 1970.
[1223] D. G. Cogan and T. Kuwabara, *Archs. Ophthal.*, N.Y., **79**, 1967.
[1224] M. Radnot and B. Lovas, *Archs. Soc. Am. Ophthal. Optom.*, **6**, 1968.

## 4. THE EXTERNAL NUCLEAR LAMINA

This retinal lamina contains the parts of the rod and cone cells which are not external to the external limiting membrane or in the external plexiform layer, and this implies in particular the somata of these cells. As they traverse the membrane the photoreceptor processes become the narrower 'outer fibres' of the rods and cones, those of the rods being much more slender and elongated (7.260 A). The outer fibres of the cone cells are not much more than a short 'waist' between the process and soma of the cell. The cytoplasm of both types of fibre contains long mitochondria, vesicular agranular endoplasmic reticulum, and many free ribosomes; as it merges into the cell body and spreads round its nucleus, aggregations of microtubules are apparent. The thickness of the external nuclear lamina—and the number of rows of cells in it—varies from 27 $\mu$m in the peripheral retina to 50 $\mu$m in the fovea (p. 1118), representing in the former a single row of cones with four of rod nuclei, and in the latter about ten rows of cone nuclei.

## 5. THE EXTERNAL PLEXIFORM LAMINA

The 'inner fibres' of the rod and cone cells pass centrally (towards the vitreous) and form a most intricate zone of synapses (7.260 B) with the dendrites and axons of the bipolar and horizontal neurons of the internal nuclear layer (lamina 6). The inner fibres of the photoreceptors resemble axons, containing a few mitochondria and vesicles, free ribosomes, microfilaments and microtubules. The rod axons are 15 to 25 nm in diameter and 1 $\mu$m or even more in length, those of the cones being much thicker and containing more microtubules. Rod axons end in an oval, invaginated *rod spherule*, cone axons as conical or pyramidal *cone pedicles*. These terminations form complex multiple junctions with the bipolar and horizontal neurons, the neurites of which approach them from the internal nuclear layer. The external plexiform layer is sometimes regarded as displaying three sublaminae—an outer one of rod and cone inner fibres or axons, an intermediate one of spherules and pedicles, and an internal sub-lamina of bipolar and horizontal cell processes.

**The rod spherule** (7.261)[1225] is part of a synaptic complex consisting of three elements—*presynaptic* (the spherule itself), *synaptic* (contacts of the spherular membrane with those of bipolar dendrites and the neurites of horizontal cells), and *postsynaptic* (bipolar and horizontal cell neurites). The spherule is infolded to form a double-walled structure enclosing in its hollow the terminations of two to seven dendrites or processes. The dendrites are derived from *rod bipolar cells* (*vide infra*) and the processes from horizontal neurons; the latter are probably not polarized, conducting impulses in either direction, and hence their neurites cannot properly be termed axons or dendrites. The cytoplasm of the rod spherule contains many presynaptic vesicles and a peculiar osmiophilic lamellar structure, the *synaptic ribbon* (7.261). The presynaptic (rod) and postsynaptic (bipolar and horizontal cell) membranes are not thickened as in typical synapses, nor does the 15 nm synaptic cleft contain fibrils or other features. Postsynaptic vesicles may also be present.

**The cone pedicle** also displays an invaginated pattern, but of a more complex design (7.261). Its cytoplasmic organelles are like those of the rod spherule. A much larger number of neurites make contacts with it.[1226] These contacts are of three types: (1) deeply infolded synapses, containing three neurite terminals, two more deeply situated than the other, form *triads*, there being about twenty-five such groups to each cone pedicle; (2) slightly depressed contacts, also on the basal aspect of the pedicle, number as many as 500; and (3) inter-receptor contacts connect the periphery of the cone pedicle to adjoining pedicles or rod spherules. The triads contain two 'axon' terminals from horizontal cells and one dendritic terminal from a *midget bipolar neuron* (*vide infra*) or from a horizontal process. (As noted above, some observers consider that the horizontal cell processes cannot be distinguished as axonal or dendritic.) The surface contacts of cone pedicles are synapses with the dendrites of 'flat' bipolar cells (*vide infra*). The inter-receptor contacts are devoid of synaptic vesicles, in contrast with other cone pedicle contacts, but they do contain neurotubules. Each pedicle displays six to twelve such contacts.

From this brief description it is clear that each rod cell has direct connexions with two bipolar and perhaps several cone cells, and also with a horizontal neuron. Cone cells display much more complex and numerous contacts, probably between 575 and 600 in number, and involving midget and flat bipolar cells, horizontal, rod and cone cells. The possible pathways for convergence of activities and interactions between the photoreceptors are obviously numerous.

## 6. THE INTERNAL NUCLEAR LAMINA

This layer is perhaps unfortunately named. In light microscopic preparations the retina contains *three* tiers of 'nuclei' or cell somata; for the ganglion cells provide the most internal, the 'internal' nuclear layer being thus *intermediate* between this and the layer of rod and cone cells. The layer contains the cell bodies of the *retinal gliocytes* (fibres of Müller) and those of the bipolar, horizontal and amacrine neurons. These cellular components of the inner nuclear layer are arranged in orderly strata. Most external are the cell bodies of the *horizontal cells*, whose processes extend into the adjacent external plexiform layer to form synapses with rod spherules and cone pedicles, as already stated above. Internal to this is a stratum of *bipolar neurons*, which are the primary sensory neurons of the retino-geniculate pathway (p. 917); their dendrites connect with the rod and cone cells, and their axons pass centrally into the internal plexiform layer (lamina 7) to form synapses with the ganglion cells (lamina 8). Internal again to the bipolar cells are the somata of the retinal gliocytes, which have been considered earlier (p. 1113). The most internal stratum of the internal nuclear layer consists of the cell bodies of the *amacrine neurons*, with neurites which spread into the adjacent internal plexiform layer to interconnect with the dendrites of ganglion and the axons of bipolar neurons.

Each of the three categories of neurons in the internal nuclear layer—horizontal, bipolar and amacrine—consists of several types, which are distinguished more by the pattern of their connexions than by their cytological differences, which are not easily defined by light or electron microscopy.

**The horizontal neurons** are usually divided into two types[1227]—*rod* and *cone horizontal cells*. They have multipolar somata, from the angles of which extend a single long process and several short ones (seven in cone and ten to twelve in rod horizontals). Their cytoplasm is like that of bipolars (*vide infra*), except that they contain an organelle rich in ribosomes (Kolmer's crystalloid), which

[1225] J. E. Dowling and B. B. Boycott, *Proc. R. Soc. B.*, **166**, 1966.
[1226] L. Missotten and E. Van den Dooren, *Bull. Soc. belge Ophtal.*, **144**, 1966.
[1227] B. B. Boycott and J. E. Dowling, *Phil. Trans. R. Soc. Ser. B.*, **255**, 1969.

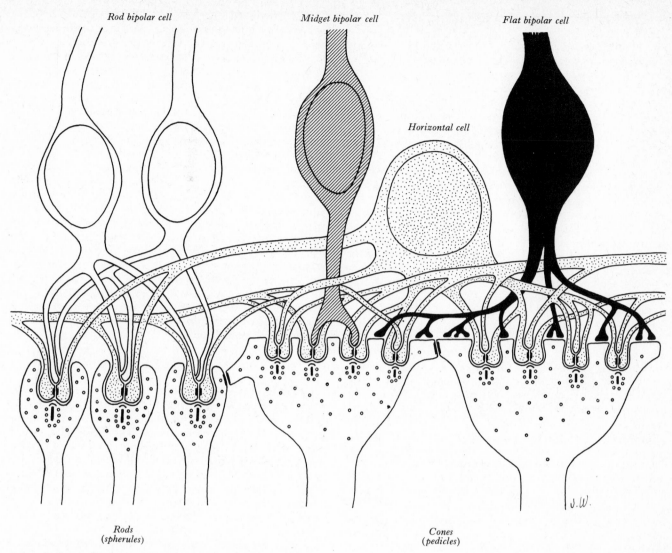

*Rod bipolar cell*   *Midget bipolar cell*   *Flat bipolar cell*

*Horizontal cell*

*Rods (spherules)*   *Cones (pedicles)*

**7.261**  A scheme of the synaptic arrangements involving the rod spherules and cone pedicles of the retina. For details consult text.

is peculiar to them. The long processes may be up to 1 mm in length—a very long neurite by retinal standards —and their branches make contacts with both rod spherules and cone pedicles. The short neurites of the *cone* horizontal neurons form synaptic junctions with seven cone pedicles, taking part in the formation of several of the triads of each (p. 1115). The short processes of the *rod* horizontal cells establish synapses with ten to twelve rod spherules. The long and short neurites of horizontal neurons are not usually classed as either axons or dendrites, and probably transmit impulses in both directions (7.262).

**The bipolar neurons** may be classified as *rod bipolar cells*, forming synapses with a variable number of rod spherules, and *midget* or *cone bipolar cells*, which take part in the triad synapses of cone pedicles (7.261). The axon of each rod bipolar connects with up to four ganglion cells while the midget bipolars connect each with but a single midget ganglion cell (*vide infra*). A third type, the *flat bipolar neuron*, connects by its dendrites with many cone pedicles, and through its axon with all types of ganglion cell. Even with electron microscopy the somata of these three kinds of bipolar neuron are difficult to identify and distinguish. They vary somewhat in size and shape, but all are very similar in their organelles —abundant mitochondria, free ribosomes, agranular endoplasmic reticulum, and microtubules.

**The amacrine neurons** (7.262) are so named because of their lack of a large axonal neurite. All their processes resemble dendrites, but are said to show the cytoplasmic features of both axons and dendrites; the direction of conduction in any process at a particular time will be determined by the polarization of the synapses which are active. Each cell has one or two thick processes from which dendritic trees of variable complexity branch out. It is upon the basis of these patterns that five types of amacrine neuron have been differentiated,[1225] though their somata cannot as yet be distinguished by ultrastructural features. They contain an indented nucleus, many cisternae of granular endoplasmic reticulum, free ribosomes, microtubules and occasionally cytoplasmic crystalline bodies, and surface cilia. Their processes display aggregations of synaptic vesicles at scattered sites, which are presumably points of synaptic contact with bipolar axons and ganglion cell dendrites. *Stratified* and *diffuse* amacrine cell types have been defined on the basis of their dendritic deployment as observed in silver-stained sections; both these types have been further subdivided.

## 7. THE INTERNAL PLEXIFORM LAMINA

Between the internal nuclear layer and the lamina of ganglion cells there is a dense neuropil composed of the interconnecting neurites of bipolar, amacrine and ganglionic neurons; it may also contain occasional displaced

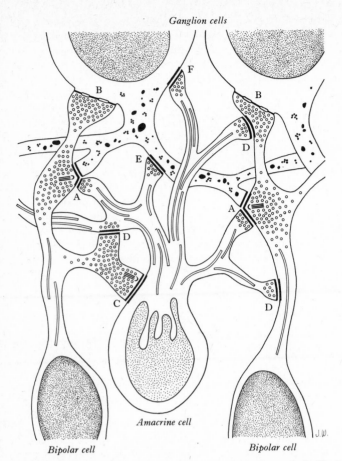

*Ganglion cells*

*Amacrine cell*

*Bipolar cell*          *Bipolar cell*

**7.262** A scheme of the synaptic arrangements in the internal plexiform lamina of the retina. Note that bipolar axonal terminals of three types are shown—*axodendritic* (A) in dyads involving neurites of amacrine and ganglion cells, *axosomatic* involving ganglion cells (B) and amacrine cells (C). Similarly the neurites of amacrine cells also make three types of contact—with the axons of bipolar neurons (D), and with the dendrites (E) and somata (F) of ganglion cells. (Both **7.261** and **7.262** are from *Histology of the Human Eye*—see **7.250**. Modified from J. E. Dowling and B. B. Boycott, *Proc. R. Soc. B.*, **166**, 1966.)

somata of the latter two categories. It is also traversed, like most of the retinal laminae, by the processes of the retinal gliocytes, which fill the spaces between the neurites, coming into close apposition with them. Even in electron microscope studies[1228] the details of the layer are difficult to interpret, but the bipolar axons, amacrine processes, and ganglion cell dendrites can be differentiated, and a wide variety of synaptic contacts can be identified (**7.262**). The bipolar axons form axodendritic and axosomatic synapses with ganglion cells, and axosomatic contacts with amacrine cells. Amacrine cell neurites make synaptic contacts with bipolar cell axons and with the somata of ganglionic cells. These synapses are extremely numerous; in the region of the fovea they are as dense as 2 million per square millimetre.

## 8. THE GANGLIONIC CELL LAMINA

The ganglion cells are the second neurons in the visual pathway. Their dendrites are connected with the processes of bipolar and amacrine cells in the internal plexiform layer, while their axons pass into the layer of nerve fibres (lamina 9), which they form. Here they turn tangentially to approach the optic disc, through which they leave the eyeball as the constituent fibres of the optic nerve. Ganglion cells are arranged in a single stratum through most of the retina, but they are progressively more densely packed from its periphery to the macula. In the vicinity of this they are ranked in about ten rows, diminishing again towards the fovea, in which they are

largely absent. They are multipolar nerve cells and vary from 10 to 30 $\mu$m in diameter; they contain a relatively large nucleus. Ganglion cell dendrites are variable in number and in their patterns of spread and branching; they usually emerge at the opposite pole of the cell with respect to its axon. On the basis of their dendritic patterns ganglion cells have been classified into at least six types (midget, stratified, diffuse, etc.).[1229-1231]

**The midget ganglion cells** are monosynaptic in their connexions, and have relatively simple dendrites. They are the commonest form in the central area of the retina. They make synaptic contact with the axon terminals of the midget bipolar neurons (**7.260, 261**). Since the latter are usually each connected to a single midget ganglion cell centrally, and to a single cone pedicle by their dendrites—especially in the foveal area—these arrangements provide relatively specific pathways for individual cone processes. However, as reference to the connexions of cone cells will show (p. 1115 and **7.261**), this does not entail that a cone cell discharges exclusively through the midget bipolar and midget ganglion cell associated with it. **Polysynaptic ganglion cells** (rod and flat ganglion cells) include all the other types of ganglionic neuron, for details of which the authorities quoted above should be consulted. They have one or two large dendrites which spread much more widely than those of the midget ganglion cells; and they synapse with the axon terminals of many bipolar neurons—probably with hundreds as a rule. Since it is clear, by light microscopy, that the bipolar neurons are more numerous than ganglion cells (though not by two orders of magnitude), it is obvious that many bipolars must transmit to the same ganglion cell; there is also evidence that the reverse relationship obtains. Such intricate interconnexions at least suggest a structural basis for the summation and lateral inhibition long established in general physiological terms, and more recently explored in detail by unit recording techniques.

The cytoplasm of the ganglion cells contains many fibrils and chromatin granules, the latter appearing as aggregations of cisternae of granular endoplasmic reticulum under the electron microscope. Free ribosomes and agranular reticulum are also abundant, as are microtubules. It is not possible, nevertheless, to distinguish the types of ganglion cell by their ultrastructure. Their axons are the main component of the nerve fibre lamina which will now be considered.

## 9. THE NERVE FIBRE LAMINA

The axons of the ganglion cells converge towards the optic disc from all parts of the retina, forming a lamina of nerve fibres (stratum opticum) which is consequently thickest (20–30 $\mu$m) at the periphery of the disc. The axons converge in a simple radial pattern from the medial (nasal) half of the retina, whereas the position of the macular area, inferolateral to the optic disc, somewhat complicates the course of the lateral (temporal) axons. Those from the macula form a *papillomacular fasciculus* which passes directly to the disc, while the more peripheral temporal fibres swerve circumferentially above and below the macula to reach the disc.

The ganglion cell axons are nonmyelinated—an obvious optical advantage, since myelin is highly refractile. The

[1228] R. A. Allen, in: *The Retina*, ed. B. R. Straatsma et al., University of California Press, Los Angeles. 1969.

[1229] S. Cajal, *Histologie du Système Nerveux*, vol. II, Maloine, Paris, 1911.

[1230] S. Polyak, *The Retina*, University of Chicago Press, Chicago. 1941.

[1231] B. B. Boycott and J. E. Dowling, *Phil. Trans. R. Soc. Ser. B.*, **255**, 1969.

myelin sheaths commence as the axons pass into the optic disc to form the optic nerve. Occasionally, small myelinated fibres have been observed in the human retina; myelination is usual in parts of the retina in many other mammals. The axons in the nerve fibre layers are surrounded by processes of retinal gliocytes and of other neuroglial elements, such as astrocytes and microglial cells.[1232] Like the somata of the ganglion cells, their axons vary in size, ranging from 0·6 to 2·0 $\mu$m. (They are, of course, considerably larger when they have acquired their myelin sheaths in the optic nerve.) They have the ultrastructural appearances typical of axons elsewhere (p. 772).

Centrifugal axons have often been described as present in the retina, but this has almost as often been denied. A considerable literature exists on this topic,[1233, 1234] but the existence of such efferent terminals in the human retina is still an open issue. Various sources for efferent retinal fibres have been suggested, including the lateral geniculate nucleus (p. 917), superior colliculus, hypothalamus, and others. They may be vasomotor in nature, but since efferent terminals have been described in relation to amacrine cells by Cajal and others, it is tempting to assume in the visual pathway an efferent analogue to the cortico-olivo-cochlear connexions of the auditory apparatus (pp. 854 and 1156). The majority of studies of this problem have, however, been carried out in birds (Cajal), or mammals remote from man, though this is rarely made plain in textbooks and monographs. There is, nevertheless, good evidence of a corticogeniculate pathway which exerts a modifying influence on the afferent visual pathway (p. 962), and it may be that a so far ill-defined connexion of this kind extends into the retina itself.

## 10. THE INTERNAL LIMITING LAMINA

Classically, the conical branching terminals of the fibres of the retinal gliocytes are said to coalesce at the surface of the vitreous humour to form a continuous membrane, separating the nerve fibre lamina from the vitreous gel, thus 'limiting' the internal aspect of the retina. Some early observers denied this, and considered that the 'membrana hyaloidea'—the limiting surface layer of the vitreous—in reality formed the sole boundary between the retina and vitreous. Electron microscopy of the junction has led to a concept which compounds both the above views. The gliocyte processes have associated with their terminations a basement membrane of about 0·5 $\mu$m, which is sinuously adapted to the glial processes externally but smooth on its internal aspect, where it is adjacent to the vitreous. Collagen fibrils derived from the latter blend with the glial basement membrane, which consequently can be said to have a composite origin. The internal limiting membrane is an obvious factor in the mechanisms of fluid exchange between the vitreous and the retina, and perhaps through the latter, with the choroid.

## PECULIARITIES OF THE MACULAR AREA

The general formation and dimensions of the central, macular and foveal areas have been noted earlier. All the layers of the retina are modified to a greater or lesser degree in this central region of the retina, and to a marked degree in the *fovea*, the central pit of the macula. In the floor of this pit (the *foveola*, p. 1112) there are no rod cells at all, but only about 2,500 closely arrayed and elongated cones, which here greatly resemble rod cells. The somata of even these elements are displaced peripherally to the sloping wall of the fovea, so that only cone *processes* occur in the foveola. Despite the distorting

effect of this arrangement, the foveolar cone processes are nevertheless orientated in a strictly vertical and radial manner, the only other retinal element present (through which light must pass) being the fibrous cytoplasmic processes of the gliocytes, which even here form internal and external limiting membranes. Towards the rim of the conical wall of the foveal pit the other layers begin to appear, and other modifications are also characteristic. Most of the fovea is devoid of rod cells or processes, which only reach its periphery. The rod-free central part of the fovea contains approximately 35,000 cones, and in the whole foveal area (about 1·75 square millimetres) there are in the region of 100,000. Hence, in the fovea, where the cones are most slender and hence most densely aggregated—all other layers being absent—there exist the most favourable conditions for photopic vision. Moreover, the cones in this locality possess the most specific connexions (with individual midget bipolar and ganglion cells), and this accords with the highly discriminative nature of foveal vision.

Because of the general displacement of the outer nuclear lamina towards the periphery of the fovea, the internal fibres or 'axons' of the photoreceptors are stretched out in a tangential direction in the external plexiform layer, and hence no cone pedicles or rod spherules are apparent in the central fovea and foveola. The inner nuclear layer is displaced to the edge of the foveal depression, and the internal plexiform, ganglion cell, and nerve fibre layers are almost absent from the whole fovea. Therefore, even on the wall of the fovea the retina is thinner and more transparent. Capillaries approach as far as the foveal margin, invading only the ganglion cell layer at this circumference. The central fovea is normally devoid of all blood vessels.

The *parafoveal region*, extending for about 0·5 mm around the fovea (diameter = 1·5 mm), is the thickest part of the retina, in part due to heaping up of displaced bipolar and ganglion cells. Around the circumference of the parafoveal area another, *perifoveal region* is described. This is the zone in which the density of cones begins to diminish rapidly, and where the incidence of rods shows an opposite tendency.

## THE OPTIC DISC AND RETINAL BLOOD VESSELS

The retina is interposed between two sets of arteries and veins, the ciliary vessels of the choroid and the branches of the central artery and vein. It is dependent upon both circulations, neither of which is alone sufficient to maintain full visual activity in the retina. The choroidal circulation (p. 1100) and the orbital and intraneural parts of the central retinal vessels have been described elsewhere (pp. 635 and 696).

The **central retinal artery** enters the optic nerve and travels in it to arrive at the 'head' of the nerve, where its constituent fascicles (about 1,000 in man) are passing through the lamina cribrosa—the representative of the sclera in this situation. In fact this region, where the neural tissues of the retina meet the neural elements of the optic nerve (including astrocytes and other glial cells) and also the connective tissues of the sclera and meninges, is highly complex. It is also the entry and exit for the retinal circulation and the only locality in which anastomoses with other arteries (the posterior ciliary arteries, *vide infra*) occur. It can be seen by ophthalmoscopy as the **optic disc** (7.257) or papilla, a region of much clinical interest, since it is here that the central vessels

[1232] J. R. Wolter, *Am. J. Ophthal.*, **48**, 1959.
[1233] P. Bowin, *J. Anat. et Physiol.*, Paris, **31**, 1895.
[1234] N. Mukai, *Can. J. Ophthal.*, **5**, 1970.

enter and leave the eye and can be inspected directly—the only vessels accessible in this way in the whole body. Oedema of the disc (papilloedema) may be the earliest sign of raised intracranial pressure, which is reflected in the subarachnoid space around the optic nerve and may hence compress and obstruct the central retinal vein where it crosses the space. The optic disc is somewhat medial and superior to the posterior pole of the eyeball and hence not on the visual axis. It is round or oval, being usually about 1·6 mm transversely and 1·8 mm in the vertical. Its appearance is very variable and details should be sought in suitable monographs.[1235] In light-skinned races the general retinal hue is a bright terracotta-red, and the pale pink of the optic disc contrasts sharply with this; its central part is usually even paler and may be a light grey colour. These differences are due to the degree of vascularization of the two regions—this being much less at the optic disc—and the total absence of choroidal and retinal pigment cells, these two ocular tunics being represented by little more than the internal limiting membrane of the retina. Even this does not pass far on to the disc, for the retinal gliocytes are here replaced by astrocytes which belong to the optic nerve.[1236] In individuals with considerable skin pigmentation both the retina and the disc display darker hues (7.257). The optic disc does not project at all in many eyes, and rarely enough to justify the term *papilla*. It is usually a little more elevated where the papillomacular fibres turn into the optic nerve on the lateral side; and where the retinal vessels pass through its centre there is usually a slight depression.

The *central retinal vessels* pass through individual apertures in the lamina cribrosa. While still at this level, usually just beyond the reach of the ophthalmoscope, the *central retinal artery* divides into two equal branches, superior and inferior; and these divide dichotomously again, after a course of a few millimetres, into superior and inferior nasal and temporal branches. Each of these four vessels supplies its own 'quadrant' of the retina, their territories being in fact rather more than quadrants, since they ramify beyond the equator as far as the ora serrata. A corresponding system of veins unites to form the central retinal vein, but the venous and arterial vessels do not correspond exactly, and the latter often cross the veins, usually lying superficial to them. At such crossings, in severe hypertension, the arteries may impress the veins and cause visible dilation of them, peripheral to the crossings. Pulsation is usually visible in the arteries. The branching of the central artery is usually dichotomous—two equal rami diverging from each other at an angle of 45–60°, but smaller branches may leave a larger one singly and at right angles to it. The arteries and veins ramify in the nerve fibre layer, close to the internal limiting membrane, which accounts for the clarity with which they can be seen by ophthalmoscopy (7.257). Arteriolar branches pass deeper into the retina and may penetrate as far as the internal nuclear layer, from which venules return to the larger superficial retinal veins. A dense capillary bed extends between such vessels, and this is diffusely arranged and displays no laminar features. In general the structure of the vascular walls is like that of typical vessels of the same calibre, but an internal elastic lamina is lacking in the case of retinal arteries, and muscle cells may appear in their adventitious coat. The capillaries consist of a non-fenestrated endothelium and numerous mural cells or *pericytes*, which extend in the axis of the capillary external to the endothelium, sharing the same basement membrane. The cytoplasm of the two types of cells is similar, but the pericytes do not contain myofilaments; their function remains uncertain. For ultra-structural details of the retinal capillaries see footnote

reference [1237]. Microcirculatory studies of the human retina in flat preparations stained after trypsin digestion have revealed many details of capillary arrangement. This resembles the deployment of capillaries in renal glomeruli, a network of capillaries connecting individual arterioles and venules with little or no interconnexion with neighbouring vessels. The distinction between capillaries is not, however, as exclusive as it is in the vessels which feed them. The whole of the retinal arterial and arteriolar tree is for practical purposes devoid of anastomoses, nor do arteriovenous shunts occur. The territories of the quadrantic arteries, for example, do not overlap, nor do the branches within a given quadrant show any anastomoses. For this reason, any blockage of a retinal artery is followed by loss of vision in the corresponding part of the visual field of that eye. The only exception to the endarterial nature of the retinal arterial system is limited to the vicinity of the optic disc. The posterior ciliary arteries enter the eyeball close to the entry of the optic nerve (7.255), and in addition to branches which supply the adjoining region of the choroid, other rami form an anastomotic circle (of Zinn) in the sclera around the 'head' of the optic nerve. Branches from the circle join the pial arteries supplying the nerve,[1238] and from any of the arteries in this region small rami may pass into the eyeball to anastomose with a retinal artery (7.257). Such a connexion is called a *cilio-retinal artery*; similarly, small retino-ciliary venous anastomotic channels may sometimes be detected. For other details consult footnote reference[1239], in which anastomoses between the central retinal artery and pial branches of the ophthalmic artery within the optic nerve are discussed.

The retinal capillaries, which do not pass beyond the external boundary of the internal nuclear lamina, show regional differences in their density. They are especially numerous in the macula, but absent from the central part of the fovea; they become less numerous in the peripheral retina and are absent from a zone about 1·5 mm wide adjoining the ora serrata.

The central artery is innervated by sympathetic fibres and probably also has a parasympathetic supply.[1240]

## The Ocular Refractive Media

The contents of the eyeball are the aqueous humour, the vitreous body and the lens. All play a part in refracting the rays entering the eye, and the refracting power of the lens can be varied for near or far vision.

### THE AQUEOUS HUMOUR

The aqueous humour fills the anterior and posterior chambers. It is small in quantity and is formed by active transport and diffusion from the capillaries of the ciliary processes, from which it passes into the posterior chamber. Thence it passes into the anterior chamber through the pupillary aperture and escapes from the iridocorneal angle into the anterior ciliary veins, through the spaces of the angle and the sinus venosus sclerae. Interference with the resorption of the aqueous humour into the sinus venosus sclerae results in increase of the intraocular pressure—the condition known as *glaucoma*. The optic disc becomes cupped and resultant degenerative changes

[1235] J. S. Duke-Elder and K. C. Wybar, *A System of Ophthalmology*, vol. II, Kimpton, London. 1961.
[1236] D. R. Anderson and W. Hoyt, *Archs Ophthal., N.Y.*, **82**, 1969.
[1237] Y. L. Tominaga and H. Ikui, *Acta.Soc. Ophthal. jap.*, **68**, 1964.
[1238] S. S. Hayreh, *Br. J. Surg.*, **50**, 1963; *Br. J. Ophthal.*, **53**, 1969.
[1239] S. Singh and R. Dass, *Br. J. Ophthal.*, **44**, 1960.
[1240] G. L. Ruskell, *Expl Eye Res.*, **10**, 1970.

in the nervous and vascular elements of the retina produced by pressure lead to blindness. The operation of iridectomy may re-establish the flow of the aqueous humour from the posterior chamber to the anterior in cases where the disease is due to adhesions between the iris and the lens. The aqueous humour is not only a metabolic avenue for the avascular tissues, the lens and

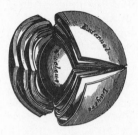

7.263　The human lens, hardened and divided. Enlarged view.

cornea, but is also chiefly responsible for maintenance of the intraocular pressure, and hence the constancy of the optical dimensions of the eyeball. It carries glucose and amino acids and mediates the exchange of respiratory gases. It contains a high concentration of ascorbic acid.

## THE VITREOUS BODY

The vitreous body occupies the vitreous chamber, which constitutes about four-fifths of the eyeball. It fills the concavity of the retina, and is hollowed in front, forming a deep concavity, the *hyaloid (patellar) fossa*, adjacent to the lens. It is a colourless, structureless, transparent gel, consisting of about 99 per cent of water, with some salts and a little mucoprotein (vitrein) and hyaluronic acid. Fibrils of about 16 nm diameter, and a periodicity of 22 nm, and an interfibrillary substance (*vitreous humor*) may be distinguished by electron microscopy.[1241] At its periphery the gel is condensed to form the so-called

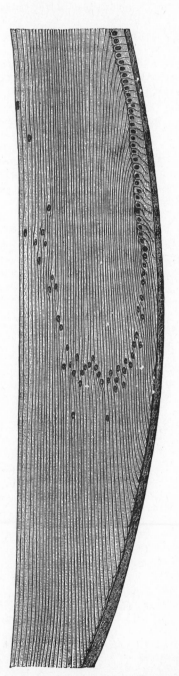

7.264　A section through the margin of the lens, showing the transition of the columnar epithelium into the lens fibres. Note that the lens cells retain their nuclei long after they have assumed the form of a fibre.

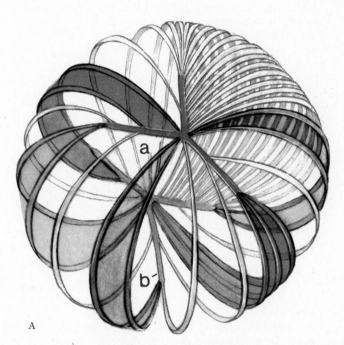

7.265A and B　The structure of the fetal (A) and adult (B) human lens, showing the major details of arrangement of the lens cells or fibres. The anterior (*a*) and posterior (*b*) triradiate sutures are shown in the fetal lens, and it is clear that fibres pass from the apex of an arm of one suture to the angle between two arms at the opposite pole, as shown in the coloured segments. Intermediate fibres show the same reciprocal behaviour, ending nearer to one pole, where they start further from the other, and so on. The suture pattern becomes much more complex as successive strata are added to the exterior of the growing lens, the original arms of each triradiate suture showing secondary and tertiary dichotomous branchings. (From *Histology of the Human Eye*—see 7.250.)

*vitreous (hyaloid) membrane.* A narrow canal, called the *hyaloid canal*, runs from the optic disc to the centre of the posterior surface of the lens. In the fetus the canal is occupied by the hyaloid artery (p. 145), which normally disappears about six weeks before birth. The vitreous membrane is attached to the ciliary epithelium and processes, and to the edge of the optic disc. Anterior to the ora serrata it is thickened by the accession of radial fibres and is termed the *ciliary zonule*. Here the membrane presents a series of radially arranged furrows, in which the ciliary processes are accommodated and to which they

1241 W. Schwarz, in: *The Structure of the Eye*, ed. G. K. Smelser, Academic Press, New York. 1061.

adhere, as is shown by the fact that when they are removed some of their pigment remains attached to the zonule. The ciliary zonule splits into two layers, one of which is thin and lines the hyaloid fossa of the vitreous body; the other, forming a system of *zonular fibres* which collectively comprises the *suspensory ligament of the lens*, is thicker and passes over the ciliary body to be attached to the capsule of the lens a short distance in front of its equator; some of the fibres of the suspensory ligament are attached behind the equator of the lens (**7.253**). Scattered and delicate fibres are also attached to the region of the equator itself. This ligament retains the lens in position, and is relaxed by the contraction of the meridional fibres of the ciliaris, so that the lens is allowed to become more convex (p. 1129). No blood vessels penetrate the vitreous body; so that its nutrition must be carried on by the vessels of the retina and ciliary processes, situated upon its exterior.

The structure of the vitreous body has been studied

The *capsule of the lens* is a transparent, elastic membrane which closely surrounds the lens, and is thicker in front than behind. The lens rests, posteriorly, in the hyaloid fossa of the vitreous body; anteriorly, it is in contact with the free border of the iris, but recedes from it at the circumference, thus forming the posterior chamber of the eye; it is retained in its position chiefly by the suspensory ligament already described.

The *lens* is a transparent, biconvex body, the convexity of its anterior being less than that of its posterior surface. The central points of these surfaces are termed respectively the *anterior* and *posterior poles*; a line connecting the poles constitutes the *axis* of the lens, while the marginal circumference is termed the *equator*. Its dioptric power is much less than that of the cornea. All the optical media of the eye have a refractive index not much removed from that of water ($1 \cdot 33$), but the corneal surface is in contact with air, and the majority of the 58 dioptres of which the eye is capable is effective here. The advantage

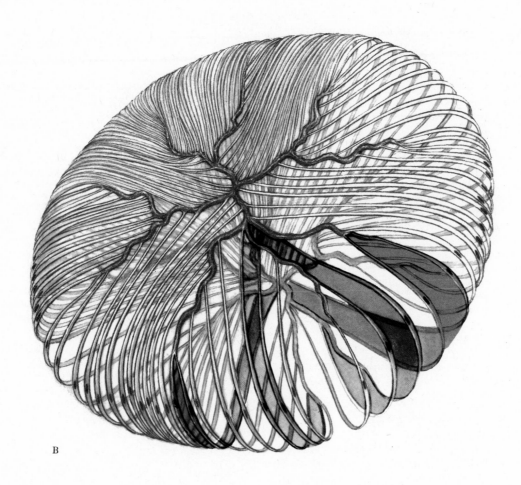

B

in much detail, both by light and electron microscopy, and by X-ray diffraction.[1242-1244] It contains collagen fibrils of 6–15 nm diameter, the arrangement of which shows regional differences, in particular a cortical condensation. Rounded cells can be identified by phase contrast microscopy; for details of such *hyalocytes*, consult footnote reference[1245].

## THE LENS

The lens (**7.263–265**), enclosed in its capsule, is situated immediately behind the iris, in front of the vitreous body, and is encircled by the ciliary processes, which slightly overlap its margin or equator.

of the lens is its potentiality of varying its dioptric power, and this is partly dependent upon a variation in its refractive index from $1 \cdot 386$ in its periphery to $1 \cdot 406$ at its core. The lens contributes about 15 dioptres to the total dioptric power of the eye. The *range* in dioptric power of the lens does not quite reach this, even at birth; most young children show minor refractive errors,[1246] and available

[1242] S. Suguira, *Jap. J. Ophthal.*, **1**, 1957.
[1243] B. S. Fine and A. J. Tousimis, *Archs Ophthal.*, N.Y., **65**, 1961.
[1244] A. Brini, A. Porte and M. E. Stoeckel, *Biology and Surgery of the Vitreous Body*, Masson, Paris. 1968.
[1245] M. J. Hogan, *Invest. Ophthal.*, **2**, 1963.
[1246] A. Sorsby, B. Benjamin, M. Sheridan, J. Stone and G. A. Leary, *M. R. C. Sp. Rep., Lond.*, **301**, 1961.

dioptric range decreases with age, being halved by the age of forty and reduced to 1 or 2 dioptres by sixty. For further information on physiological optics consult footnote references [1247], [1248].

## THE STRUCTURE OF THE LENS

The lens is made up of soft cortical substance and a firm, central part, the so-called nucleus (7.263). Faint sutural lines (radii lentis) radiate from the poles to the equator. In the adult there may be six or more of these lines, but in the fetus there are only three, and these diverge in a Y-shaped manner at angles of 120°; on the anterior surface the Y is upright; on the posterior surface it is inverted.[1249] These lines correspond with the free edges of septa—composed of an amorphous substance, which dip into the substance of the lens. When the lens has been hardened it is seen to consist of a series of concentrically arranged laminae, each of which is interrupted at the septa. Each lamina is built up of a number of ribbon-like lens fibres, the edges of which are more or less serrated—the serrations interdigitating with those of adjacent fibres, which are in part connected by desmosomes,[1250] while the ends of the fibres come into apposition at the sutures. The fibres run in a curved manner from the sutures on the anterior surface to those on the posterior surface (7.265). No fibres pass from pole to pole; they are arranged in such a way that those which begin near the pole on one surface of the lens end near the peripheral extremity on the other, and vice versa. The fibres of the outer layers of the lens are nucleated, and together form a nuclear layer, most distinct towards the equator. The anterior surface of the lens is covered by a layer of transparent, nucleated columnar epithelium. At the equator the cells become elongated, and their gradual transition into lens fibres can be traced (7.264).

*In the fetus*, the lens is nearly spherical and has a slightly reddish tint; it is soft and breaks down readily on the slightest pressure. A small branch (hyaloid artery) from the central artery of the retina runs forwards through the vitreous body to the posterior part of the capsule of the lens, where its branches radiate, forming a plexiform network which covers the posterior surface of the capsule, and is continuous round the margin of the capsule with the vessels of the pupillary membrane and with those of the iris. *In the adult*, the lens is colourless, transparent, firm in texture and devoid of vessels. *In old age*, it is more flattened on both surfaces, slightly opaque, of an amber tint and increased in density. In the condition termed cataract the lens gradually becomes opaque and blindness ensues. In such cases sight may be restored by extraction of the lens and the provision of suitable spectacles.

The dimensions of the lens are of some interest; its diameter at birth is 6·5 mm, increasing to 9·0 mm at fifteen years, after which it continues to grow very slowly throughout life. Its anteroposterior dimension increases from 3·5–4·0 mm at birth to 4·75–5·0 mm at 95(!). Its anterior radius (about 10·0 mm) is greater than the posterior (about 6·0 mm), but both these are reduced during accommodation. The continued growth of the lens is due to the continual slow production of new cells in its epithelium at the lenticular equator. The ultrastructural details of the lens capsule and its epithelium have been studied.[1251], [1252] The capsule consists largely of fine filaments with a periodicity of 60 nm. The lens fibres, which develop from the epithelial cells, are at first nucleated, but their nuclei disappear as the fibre develops and extends. The fibre consists essentially of a fine fibrillary substance. In the adult there are 2,100–2,300 lens fibres; these may be as much as 8–12 mm in length in the cortical zone.

[1247] J. S. Duke-Elder, *The Practice of Refraction*, 8th edn., Churchill, London. 1969.

[1248] A. G. Bennett and J. L. Francis, in: *The Eye*, vol. 4, ed. H. Davson, Academic Press, New York. 1962.

[1249] I. C. Mann, *J. Anat.*, **59**, 1924.

[1250] T. Wanko and M. A. Gavin, *The Structure of the Eye*, ed. G. K. Smelser, New York. 1961.

[1251] T. Wanko and M. A. Gavin, *J. biophys. biochem. Cytol.*, **6**, 1960.

[1252] A. I. Cohen, *Invest. Ophthal.*, **4**, 1965.

# THE ACCESSORY VISUAL APPARATUS

The accessory visual apparatus includes the extraocular muscles, the fasciae, the eyebrows, eyelids, conjunctiva and lacrimal apparatus.

## THE EXTRAOCULAR MUSCLES

The extraocular or extrinsic ocular muscles (7.266, 267) include an elevator of the upper eyelid, the *levator palpebrae superioris*, and six muscles capable of rotating the eyeball in any direction. The latter comprise the four *recti* (*superior, inferior, medialis* and *lateralis*), and the two *obliqui* (*superior* and *inferior*). This is an old pattern of muscles, extending—with slight modifications—through almost the entire vertebrate phylum, apart from the levator palpebrae superioris, which is a later delamination from the rectus superior.

**The levator palpebrae superioris** (7.266, 267) is thin and triangular in shape. It arises from the inferior surface of the lesser wing of the sphenoid bone, above and anterior to the optic canal, from which it is separated by the attachment of the rectus superior. At this posterior attachment it is narrow and tendinous, but soon becomes broad and fleshy, the medial margin of the muscle being almost straight, while the lateral is concave. The muscle ends anteriorly in a wide aponeurosis which splits into two lamellae. Some of the fibres of the superior lamella are attached to the anterior surface of the superior tarsus (p. 1129), while others radiate and pass through the overlying orbicularis oculi to the skin of the upper eyelid. The

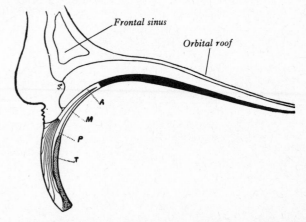

7.266 A diagram of the levator palpebrae superioris, showing its connexions. *A.* Superficial lamella of aponeurosis; *M.* Deep lamella, superior tarsal muscle (of Müller); *P.* Interval between superficial and deep lamellae of aponeurosis; *T.* Tarsus; *S.* Orbital septum.

inferior lamella contains nonstriated muscle fibres form-ing the so-called *superior tarsal muscle*; it is attached directly to the upper margin of the superior tarsus and is covered by conjunctiva on its inferior surface. A less well-marked layer of nonstriated muscle is also present in the lower eyelid; it unites the inferior tarsus to the fascial sheath of the inferior rectus and its expansion to the sheath of the inferior oblique. A further thin layer of non-striated muscle, the *orbitalis*, bridges the inferior orbital fissure; its precise function is uncertain. The *superior* and *inferior tarsal muscles*, just described, presumably assist in elevation of the upper and depression of the lower eyelid. All three nonstriated muscles receive a sympathetic innervation.

The connective tissue on the surfaces of the levator palpebrae superioris and rectus superior fuse. Where the two muscles separate to reach their insertions, the fascia between them forms a thick mass to which is attached the superior conjunctival fornix, and this is described as an additional insertion of the levator palpebrae supe-rioris. When traced laterally the aponeurosis of the levator palpebrae superioris passes between the orbital and palpebral parts of the lacrimal gland and is fixed to a tubercle on the zygomatic bone, just within the orbital margin (p. 310). When traced medially the aponeurosis loses its tendinous nature as it passes over and comes into close contact with the reflected tendon of the obliquus superior, whence it can be followed towards the medial palpebral ligament in the form of loose strands of connec-tive tissue. When the levator palpebrae contracts, the upper eyelid is raised, but the lateral and medial parts of the aponeurosis are stretched and thus limit the action of the muscle; the elevation of the upper eyelid is also considered to be checked by the orbital septum (p. 1130). ('Check' mechanisms abound in the orbit, but there is little or no direct evidence that the connective tissue structures thus implicated do in fact function in this manner. See also p. 1128.)

**The four recti** (7.267, 268) are attached posteriorly to a fibrous ring which surrounds the superior, medial and inferior margins of the optic canal (7.268), and is termed the *common annular tendon*; this fibrous anulus is con-tinued across the lower and medial part of the superior orbital fissure and is attached to a tubercle on the margin of the greater wing of the sphenoid bone. The tendon is closely adherent to the dural sheath of the optic nerve and to the surrounding periosteum; within it are (1) the anterior aperture of the optic canal transmitting the optic nerve and ophthalmic artery, and (2) the medial part of the superior orbital fissure which transmits the two divi-sions of the oculomotor nerve, the nasociliary nerve and the abducent nerve. The superior ophthalmic vein may pass through, or above, the annular tendon, the inferior ophthalmic vein through or below it. Two specialized parts of this fibrous ring may be made out: a lower, which gives origin to the rectus inferior, a part of the rectus medialis and the lower fibres of the rectus lateralis; and an upper, which gives origin to the rectus superior, the other part of the rectus medialis and the upper fibres of the rectus lateralis; a second small tendinous head of origin of the rectus lateralis arises from the orbital surface of the greater wing of the sphenoid bone, lateral to the tendinous ring. Each muscle passes forward in the pos-ition implied by its name, to be attached by a tendinous expansion into the sclera, posterior to the margin of the cornea. The average distances of the insertions of the recti from the margin of the cornea are: medialis, 5·5 mm; inferior, 6·5 mm; lateralis, 6·9 mm; superior, 7·7 mm.

**The obliquus superior** (7.267) is fusiform and occupies a superomedial position in the orbit. It arises

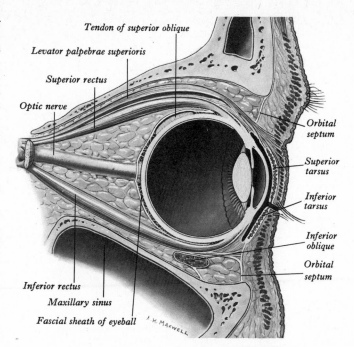

7.267A    A sagittal section through the right orbital cavity.

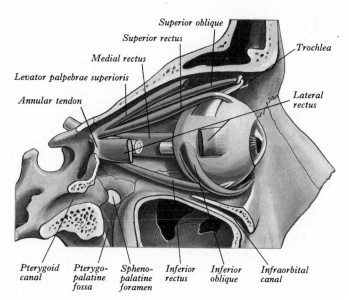

7.267B    The muscles of the right orbit. Lateral aspect.

from the body of the sphenoid superomedial to the optic canal, superior and medial to the origin of the rectus superior, and, passing forwards, ends in a round tendon, which plays in a fibrocartilaginous loop, the *trochlea*, attached to the trochlear fossa of the frontal bone. The contiguous surfaces of the tendon and the trochlea are separated by a delicate synovial sheath. After traversing the trochlea the tendon passes posterolaterally and inferior to the rectus superior to the lateral part of the eyeball, and is inserted into the sclera, behind the equator of the eyeball, in its superolateral posterior quadrant between the rectus superior and rectus lateralis.

**The obliquus inferior** (7.267) is a thin, narrow muscle, near the anterior margin of the floor of the orbit. It arises from the orbital surface of the maxilla lateral to the nasolac-rimal groove. Passing laterally, backwards and upwards, at first between the rectus inferior and the floor of the orbit, and then between the eyeball and the rectus lateralis, it is inserted into the lateral part of the sclera, behind the equator of the eyeball, in its inferolateral posterior quad-rant between the rectus superior and rectus lateralis, near

1123

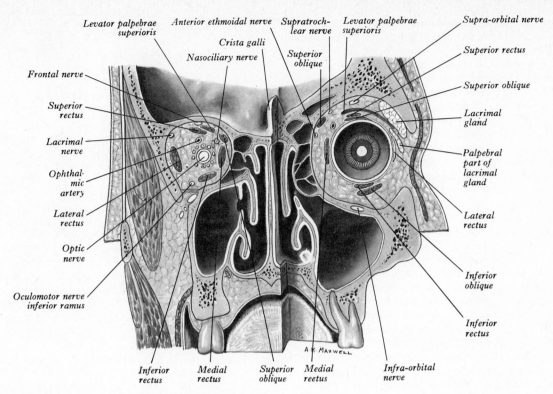

**7.268**   Coronal sections through the two orbits. Posterior aspect. On the left side the plane of the section is more posterior and passes behind the eyeball.

to, but somewhat behind, the insertion of the obliquus superior.

*Nerve supply*. The levator palpebrae superioris, the obliquus inferior, and the recti superior, inferior and medialis are supplied by the oculomotor nerve; the obliquus superior, by the trochlear nerve; the rectus lateralis, by the abducent nerve.

## ACTIONS OF THE EXTRAOCULAR MUSCLES

The *levator palpebrae superioris* elevates the upper eyelid, its antagonist being the orbicularis oculi. The degree of elevation—which, apart from blinking, is maintained for long periods of time during waking hours—is a compromise between adequate exposure of the optical

media and control of light entering the eye. The amount of light, especially in conditions of very bright sunshine, can be reduced by lowering the upper eyelid, thus reducing glare. Although much is known of the physiology of blinking,[1253] and its significance in the distribution of lacrimal secretions, little information is available concerning the continuous activity of the levator to keep the eyelid raised. The respective roles of the main, striated, voluntary part of the muscle and of the small, inferior stratum of nonstriated tissue (the superior palpebral, tarsal, or Müller's muscle) which is innervated by sympathetic neurons, have not been clarified.

The six *extraocular muscles* all *rotate* the eyeball in directions dependent upon the geometrical relationship between their osseous and global attachments (**7.270**), which are, of course, influenced by the ocular movements themselves. Before considering these activities it is important to recognize that the *human* extraocular muscles are not accessible to inspection, and that consequently much opinionation regarding them depends on deductions from disturbances due to lesions of their nerve supplies. A complete assessment of the exact nature of the nerve injury is rarely possible; but this is not to say that, in the vast clinical literature available on this topic, there are not at least some entirely valid observations. It is also essential to note that in any movement of an eyeball, changes in tension may occur in *all six* muscles, although the direct observation of these has rarely been carried out, even in experimental animals.[1254, 1255] It is at least likely that all six muscles are continuously involved, and it is therefore merely a preliminary but necessary exercise to consider each muscle in isolation. Because they form more obvious groupings as antagonists or synergists, it is

**7.269**   Scheme to show the common tendinous ring, the origins of the recti, and the relative positions of the nerves entering the orbital cavity through the superior orbital fissure. (Modified from a figure in Whitnall's *Anatomy of the Human Orbit*, 2nd ed., Oxford, 1932.) Note that the ophthalmic veins frequently pass through the common tendinous ring.

[1253] W. K. McEwen and E. T. Goodner, in: *The Eye*, vol. 3, ed. H. Davson, Academic Press, New York. 1962.
[1254] C. S. Sherrington, *Proc. R. Soc. B.*, **76**, 1905.
[1255] J. Szentágothai, *Sém. Hôp.*, Paris, **26**, 1950.

appropriate to consider the four recti and the two obliques as separate groups, remembering always that they act in concert.

Of the four *recti*, the *medial* and *lateral* muscles exert comparatively straightforward forces on the eyeball. Being approximately horizontal (at least, when the visual axis is in its primary position, directed to the horizon), they rotate the eyeball medially (adduction) or laterally (abduction) about an imaginary vertical axis (7.270). They are antagonists, and by reciprocal adjustment of their lengths the visual axis can be swept through a horizontal arc. When both eyes are involved, as is usual, the four medial and lateral recti can either adjust both visual axes in a *conjugate* movement from point to point at infinity, the axes remaining parallel, or they can *converge* or *diverge* the two axes to and from nearer or more distant objects of interest in the visual field. However, since they do not rotate the eyeball around its transverse axis, the medial and lateral recti cannot make the extremely commonplace action of elevating or depressing the visual axes as the gaze is transferred from nearer to more distant objects or the reverse. This is the contribution of the *superior* and *inferior recti* (aided, as will become apparent, by the two oblique muscles). However, the geometry of these muscles is a little more complex, and the key to the rotational effects which they impart to the eyeball is the obliquity of the orbit (7.270), whose axis does not correspond with the visual axis in its primary position, but is inclined to it by an angle of approximately 23°. The latter value varies somewhat in different individuals, being dependent upon the angle between the two orbital axes (7.270 A). Hence, the simple rotation caused by an isolated *superior rectus*, when analysed with reference to the three hypothetical axes of the eyeball, appears to be complex— being primarily *elevation* (transverse axis), and secondarily a less powerful *medial rotation* (vertical axis), and a slight *intorsion* (anteroposterior axis) in which the upper rim of the cornea (often referred to as 12 o'clock) is rotated medially towards the nose. These actions—which are in fact a simple, single rotation—are easily appreciated as long as it is realized that the direction of traction of the superior rectus runs *posteromedially* from its attachment *anterior* to the equator and *superior* to the cornea, to its osseous attachment near the apex of the orbit (7.270).

The *inferior rectus* pulls in the same direction, but naturally rotates the visual axis downwards about the transverse axis. It is also clear, that if reference is made to the comparable geometry of the situation, that this muscle will also rotate the eye medially about the vertical axis, but that its action around the anteroposterior axis will *extort* the eye, i.e. rotate it so that the 12 o'clock point on the cornea turns laterally. The superior and inferior recti, therefore, both rotate the eyeball medially, and since their turning movements around the transverse and anteroposterior axes are opposed, their combined contraction could rotate the eye medially. In binocular movements they could thus assist the medial recti in converging the visual axes. By reciprocal adjustment the same two muscles can elevate or depress the visual axes. It may be added that, as the eyeball is rotated laterally, the line of traction of the superior and inferior recti more nearly approaches the plane of the anteroposterior axis (7.270), and hence their rotational effects about this and the vertical axis diminish. In abduction to about 20° or so, these two muscles become almost purely an elevator and a depressor of the visual axis.

The *superior oblique muscle* acts on the eyeball from the trochlea, and since the attachment of the *inferior oblique* is for practical purposes vertically inferior to this, both muscles approach the eyeball at the same angle, being attached in approximately similar positions in the *superior*

and *inferior posterolateral* quadrants of the eyeball (7.270). From these attachments it is easy to understand that the superior oblique elevates the *posterior* aspect of the eyeball, the inferior muscle depressing it. Hence, the former rotates the visual axis *downwards*, the latter *upwards*, both movements being around the transverse axis. But the obliquity of both muscles is such that their traction, when the eye is in the primary position, is in a direction posterior to the vertical axis, and thus both rotate the eyeball *laterally* around this axis. In regard to the anteroposterior axis it is not difficult to conclude that in isolation the superior oblique would *intort* the eyeball, the inferior oblique *extorting* it. Like the superior and inferior recti, therefore, the two obliques have a turning movement in common around the vertical axis, but opposed forces in respect of the other two. Acting in concert they could therefore assist the lateral rectus in abduction of the visual axis, as in *divergence* movements of the eyes in transferring attention from near objects to those further away. Just as in the case of the superior and inferior recti, the actions of the oblique muscles also vary with the position of the eyeball; they are more nearly a pure elevator and a depressor as the eye is adducted.

In a short analysis of this kind much must be omitted, and nothing can be said of the defects of ocular movement. For those desiring further information footnote references [1256-1261] will prove useful; for those requiring the barest data, the actions of the extraocular muscles may be summarized as follows:

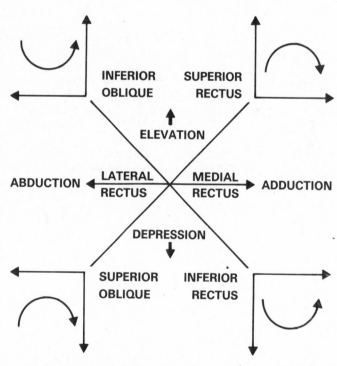

There is a misleading custom of linking extraocular muscles together, usually into pairs—such as the right superior oblique and left inferior rectus—which are supposed thus to deviate both visual axes downwards and to the right, as doubtless they do. Limited views of this

[1256] S. E. Whitnall, *Anatomy of the Human Orbit*, 2nd ed., Oxford University Press, London. 1932.

[1257] S. Cooper, P. D. Daniel and D. Whitteridge, *Brain*, **78**, 1955.

[1258] D. G. Cogan, *Neurology of the Ocular Muscles*, 2nd ed., Thomas, Springfield. 1956.

[1259] A. Schlossman and B. S. Priestley, *Strabismus*, Little, Brown, Boston. 1966.

[1260] M. Alpern, in: *The Eye*, 2nd ed. vol. 3, ed. H. Davson, Academic Press, New York. 1969.

[1261] H. Davson, *Physiology of the Eye*, 3rd ed., Churchill-Livingstone, London. 1972.

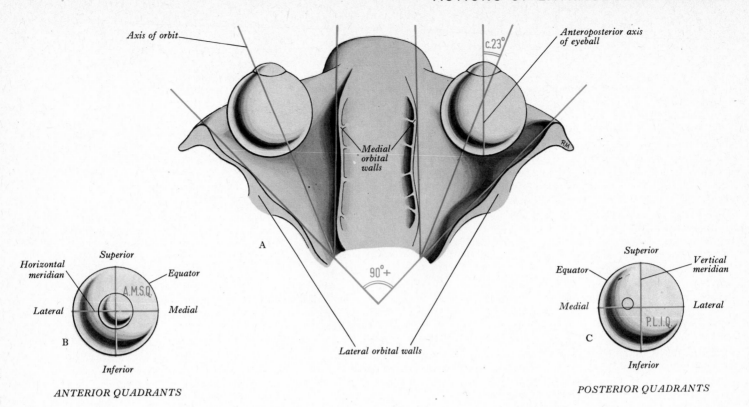

Axis of orbit

Anteroposterior axis of eyeball

c.23°

Medial orbital walls

RM

A

90°+

Lateral orbital walls

Superior

Horizontal meridian

Equator

A.M.S.Q.

Lateral

Medial

B

Inferior

ANTERIOR QUADRANTS

Superior

Equator

Vertical meridian

Medial

Lateral

P.L.I.Q.

C

Inferior

POSTERIOR QUADRANTS

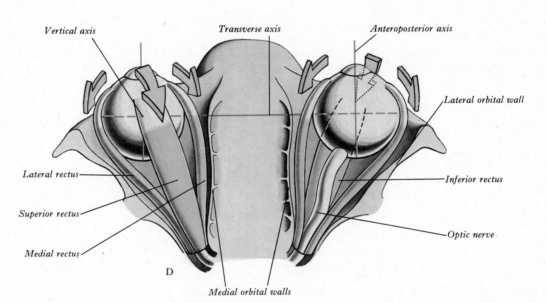

Vertical axis

Transverse axis

Anteroposterior axis

Lateral orbital wall

Lateral rectus

Inferior rectus

Superior rectus

Medial rectus

Optic nerve

D

Medial orbital walls

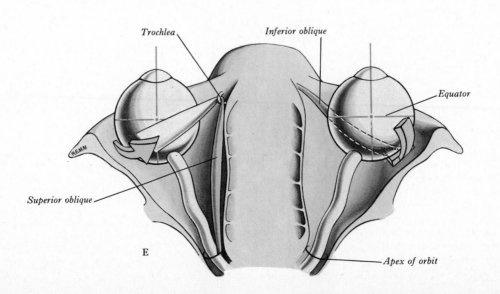

Trochlea

Inferior oblique

Equator

REMM

Superior oblique

E

Apex of orbit

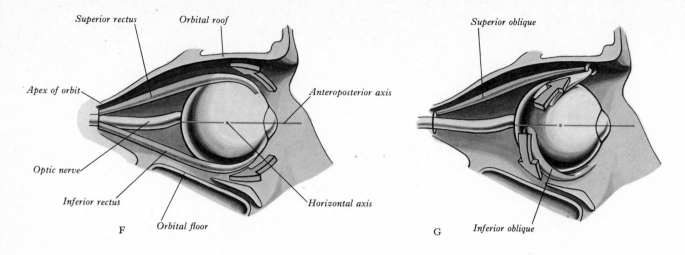

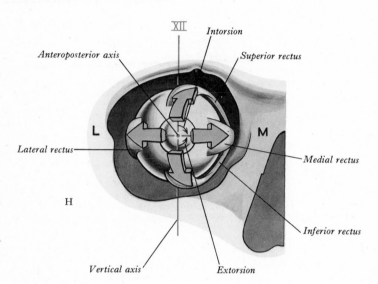

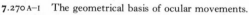

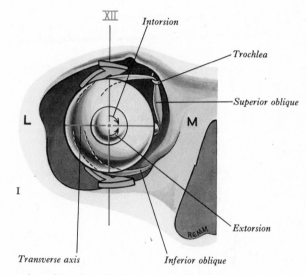

**7.270 A–I**   The geometrical basis of ocular movements.

A   The relationship between the orbital and ocular axes, with the eyes in the primary position of parallel visual axes.

B and C   The ocular globe in anterior and posterior views to show conventional geometry—meridia, equator, etc. AMSQ = anterior medial superior quadrant; PLIQ = posterior lateral inferior quadrant.

D   The orbits from above showing the medial and lateral recti, and the superior rectus (left) and inferior rectus (right), indicating turning moments primarily around the vertical axis.

E   Superior (left) and inferior (right) oblique muscles showing turning moments primarily around the vertical and also anteroposterior axes.

F   Lateral view to show the actions of the superior and inferior recti around the transverse axis.

G   Lateral view to show the action of the superior and inferior oblique muscles around the anteroposterior axis.

H   Anterior view to show the medial rotational moment of the superior and inferior recti around the vertical axis. Conventionally the 12 o'clock position indicated is said to be *intorted* (superior rectus) or *extorted* (inferior rectus) as indicated by the small arrows on the cornea.

I   Anterior view to show the torsional effects of the superior oblique (intorsion) and inferior oblique (extorsion) around the anteroposterior axis, as indicated by the small arrows on the cornea.

kind may have a mnemonic value, but they ignore the inescapable fact that in any ocular rotation *all* six muscles must change in length. Since we do not know enough of the reciprocal innervation circuits of the extraocular muscles, it is impossible to dogmatize as to whether every muscle is contracted precisely in step with the progressive inhibition of an antagonist, although the few experiments previously quoted, in fact, support such a view. However that may be, it would be more useful to link the superior, inferior and medial recti together, as adductors, or *convergence* muscles, and the two obliques with the lateral rectus as abductors, or *divergence* muscles. This is a useful concept in view of the very frequent convergent and divergent movements of the visual axes required in common activities. It is, nevertheless, an over-simplified view; convergence is commonly accompanied by depres-

sion of the visual axes towards objects nearby, and divergence by elevation. In these much more complexly concerted activities, the torsional effects of the muscles become much more important. Analysis shows that in the simple, *cardinal* movements (adduction-abduction, elevation-depression), the torsional effects of the muscles cancel out, and they must also do so in all intermediate positioning of the visual axes to preserve the relationship of corresponding retinal loci and hence binocular (single) vision. So far, no consideration has been given to head movements, but it is common observation that ocular movements are frequently and perhaps usually accompanied by movements of the head, which might be likened to the *coarse* adjustment of an optical instrument such as a microscope, the *finer* adjustments being made by the ocular musculature.

1127

It is interesting to note that while the eye movements are clearly under voluntary control, *torsional* movements cannot be voluntarily incepted. But when the head is tilted relative to the body, reflex torsion movements become apparent, and are in fact necessary to preserve retinal relationships. Any small lapse in the concerted adjustment of the two retinae entails diplopia; it is indeed surprising that such a complex organization of extra-ocular, neck and other muscles is learnt so effectively early in life that diplopia is so rarely experienced by the great majority.

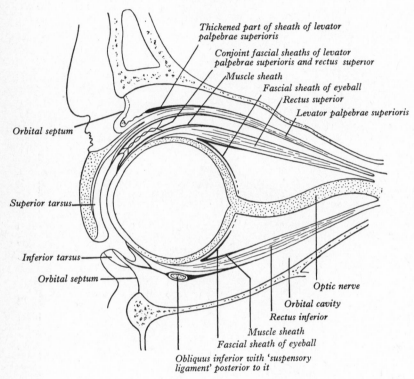

**7.271 A** A scheme of the orbital fascia in sagittal section. (After Whitnall.)

Labels for figure 7.271 A:
Thickened part of sheath of levator palpebrae superioris
Conjoint fascial sheaths of levator palpebrae superioris and rectus superior
Muscle sheath
Fascial sheath of eyeball
Rectus superior
Levator palpebrae superioris
Orbital septum
Superior tarsus
Inferior tarsus
Orbital septum
Optic nerve
Orbital cavity
Rectus inferior
Muscle sheath
Fascial sheath of eyeball
Obliquus inferior with 'suspensory ligament' posterior to it

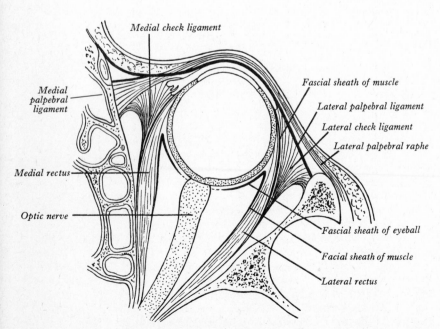

**7.271 B** A scheme of the orbital fascia in horizontal section. (After Whitnall.)

Labels for figure 7.271 B:
Medial check ligament
Medial palpebral ligament
Medial rectus
Optic nerve
Fascial sheath of muscle
Lateral palpebral ligament
Lateral check ligament
Lateral palpebral raphe
Fascial sheath of eyeball
Facial sheath of muscle
Lateral rectus

## THE FASCIAL SHEATH OF THE EYEBALL

A thin fascial membrane envelops the eyeball from the optic nerve to the sclerocorneal junction, separating it from the orbital fat, and forming a socket in which it plays (7.271). Its inner surface is smooth, and is separated from the outer surface of the sclera by the *episcleral space*; this 'space' is traversed by delicate bands of connective tissue which extend between the fascia and the sclera. The fascia is perforated behind by the ciliary vessels and nerves, and fuses with the sheath of the optic nerve and with the sclera around the entrance of the optic nerve. In front it blends with the sclera just behind the sclero-corneal junction. It is perforated by the tendons of the orbital muscles, and is reflected on each as a tubular sheath. The sheath of the obliquus superior is carried as far as the fibrous trochlea of that muscle; that on the obliquus inferior reaches as far as the floor of the orbit, to which it gives off a slip. The sheaths on the recti are gradually lost in the perimysium, but they give off important expansions. The expansion from the rectus superior blends with the tendon of the levator palpebrae superioris; that of the rectus inferior is attached to the inferior tarsus and to the sheath of the obliquus inferior. The expansions from the sheaths of the recti medialis et lateralis are strong and triangular in shape, and are attached to the lacrimal and zygomatic bones respectively; since they may check the actions of these two recti they have been named the *medial* and *lateral check ligaments*. A thickening of the lower part of the fascial sheath of the eyeball, is named the *suspensory ligament of the eye*;[1262] it is slung like a hammock below the eyeball, being expanded in the centre and narrow at its extremities; it is formed by the union of the margins of the sheath of the rectus inferior with the medial and lateral check ligaments. Anomalies of the various parts of the above fascial arrangement may interfere with the normal movements of the eyes and cause various types of squint.[1263] It must be added that, apart from the suspensory ligament, there is little real evidence that any of the so-called check ligaments actually limit eye movements. The connective tissue link between the fasciae covering the superior rectus and levator palpebrae superioris is probably of little functional significance. It certainly does not impede independent movement of the lid and eyeball.

**The orbital fascia** forms the periosteum of the orbit, but is loosely connected to the bones. Behind, it is united with the dura mater and with the sheath of the optic nerve. In front it is connected with the periosteum at the margin of the orbit, and sends off a stratum which assists in forming the orbital septum. From it two processes are given off: one holds the trochlea of the obliquus superior in position, the other, named the *lacrimal fascia*, forms the roof and lateral wall of the sulcus in which the lacrimal sac is lodged (p. 263).

## VISUAL REFLEXES

The impulses concerned with *visual reflexes*, which bring about movements of the eyes, head and neck in response to visual stimuli, follow the pathway provided by the optic nerves and tracts to the superior colliculi. After traversing synapses there, the impulses travel along the tectospinal and tectobulbar tracts to the neurons of the motor columns associated with the spinal and cranial nerves (p. 887).

*Pupil light reflex.* On exposure of the eye to bright light the pupils contract reflexly. The impulses concerned

[1262] C. B. Lockwood, *J. Anat.* **20**, 1886.
[1263] A. B. Nutt, *Ann. R. Coll. Surg.*, **16**, 1955.

travel by the optic nerves and tracts to the pretectal nucleus (p. 888) where secondary neuron fibres arise. These, which are very short and run close to the central grey matter, convey the impulses to the accessory oculomotor (Edinger-Westphal) nucleus (p. 999), whose neurons send preganglionic fibres to the ciliary ganglion through the oculomotor nerve and its branch to the obliquus inferior. The postganglionic fibres from the ganglion traverse the short ciliary nerves to reach the sphincter pupillae. If light be shone into one eye only, both pupils contract (*consensual pupil light reflex*); this is due to the fact that fibres from one optic tract pass to both pretectal nuclei, the crossing fibres passing via the posterior commissure. The dilatator pupillae is supplied by fibres which arise in the superior cervical ganglion of the sympathetic trunk. The preganglionic fibres of this pathway arise from cells of the lateral grey column in the first and second thoracic segments of the spinal cord and pass by the upper thoracic nerves and their white rami communicantes to the sympathetic trunk, in which they ascend to the superior cervical ganglion (p. 1070). As the condition of the pupil at any time is the result of the *balanced action* of these two systems, the pupil becomes dilated when the stimulus of bright light is removed. The pupil will dilate, also, in response to painful stimulation of almost any part of the body. Presumably the fibres of the sensory pathways establish connexions with the efferent preganglionic neurons of the sympathetic described above. Some believe, however, that this reflex dilatation of the pupil is largely due to inhibition of the accessory oculomotor nucleus, though the pathways involved are uncertain. One manifestation of this reflex is the dilatation produced by pinching the skin of the neck; it is termed the *pupillary skin reflex*.

*Accommodation reflexes.* In the process of accommodation for the viewing of near objects the eyes converge and, at the same time, the ciliaris contracts to modify the shape of the lens, and the pupil is constricted to increase the depth of focus. The pathways for the accommodation reflex comprise the optic nerve, optic tract, lateral geniculate body, optic radiation and the visual area of the cerebral cortex. The latter is connected by the superior longitudinal fasciculus to the eye field of the frontal cortex, whence fibres descend through the internal capsule to the nuclei of the oculomotor nerves in the midbrain. From the accessory oculomotor nuclei fibres pass to the ciliaris and sphincter pupillae (relaying in the ciliary ganglion), and from the ventral part of the oculomotor nucleus (*see* p. 998) fibres supply the medial recti for the action of convergence of the eyes (*see* p. 1125). These pathways have not been so definitely established as those for the pupil light reflex, and it has been suggested[1264] that the contraction of the pupil in the accommodation reflex is secondary to the convergence of the eyes and that the afferent impulses arise in the proprioceptor nerve endings in the orbital muscles and travel in the oculomotor nerve direct to the accessory nuclei. In certain diseases of the central nervous system (e.g. tabes dorsalis due to syphilis) the pupil light reflex may be lost while the constriction of the pupil as part of the accommodation reflex is unaffected (Argyll Robertson pupil). The site of the lesion that could produce such an effect is probably located between the accessory oculomotor nucleus and the lateral geniculate body, where the path ways for the two reflexes diverge from each other.

*Conjunctival reflex.* If the conjunctiva be touched lightly, blinking occurs. Afferent impulses travel via the ophthalmic part of the trigeminal nerve and efferent impulses in the branches of the facial nerve to the orbicularis oculi.

## THE EYEBROWS AND EYELIDS

The eyebrows are two arched eminences of skin, which surmount the orbits and support numerous short, thick hairs directed obliquely on the surface. Fibres of the orbicularis oculi, corrugator and frontal belly of the occipitofrontalis are inserted into the skin of the eyebrows.

**The eyelids** or **palpebrae** are two thin, movable folds, placed in front of the eye, and protecting it, by their closure, from injury. The upper eyelid is the larger and more movable, and is furnished with an elevator muscle, the levator palpebrae superioris (p. 1122); the two eyelids are united to each other at their ends, and when the eye is open an elliptical space, termed the *palpebral fissure*, is left between their margins; the extremities of the fissure are called the angles of the eye.

The *lateral angle of the eye* (lateral canthus) is more acute than the medial, and lies in close contact with the eyeball. The *medial angle* (medial canthus) is prolonged for a short distance towards the nose, and is about 6 mm away from the eyeball; the two eyelids are here separated by a triangular space, named the *lacus lacrimalis*, in which a small reddish body, termed the *caruncula lacrimalis*, is situated (7.272). On the margin of each eyelid, at the basal angles of the lacus lacrimalis, there is a small conical elevation, termed the *lacrimal papilla*, the apex of which is pierced by the commencement of the lacrimal canaliculus. This minute orifice (7.272) is known as the *punctum lacrimale*.

The *eyelashes* are attached in the free edges of the eyelids from the lateral angle of the eye to the lacrimal papillae. They are short, thick, curved hairs, arranged in double or triple rows: those of the upper eyelid, more numerous and longer than those of the lower, curve upwards; those of the lower eyelid curve downwards so that the upper and lower eyelashes do not interlace when the lids are closed. A number of enlarged and modified sudoriferous glands, termed *ciliary glands*, are arranged in several rows close to the free margin of each lid and open near the attachments of the eyelashes.

### Structure of the Eyelids.

From without inwards, each eyelid consists of: skin, subcutaneous areolar tissue, fibres of the orbicularis oculi, tarsus and orbital septum, tarsal glands and conjunctiva. The upper eyelid contains, in addition, the aponeurosis of the levator palpebrae superioris (7.273).

The *skin* is extremely thin, and continuous at the margins of the eyelids with the conjunctiva.

The *subcutaneous areolar tissue* is very lax and delicate, and seldom contains any adipose tissue.

The *palpebral fibres of the orbicularis oculi* are thin, pale in colour and parallel with the palpebral fissure. Deep to the muscle there is a layer of loose areolar tissue, which, in the case of the upper eyelid, is continuous with the subaponeurotic layer of the scalp (p. 496), so that effusions of fluid (blood or pus) in this layer of the scalp can pass down into the upper eyelid. It is in this layer of the eyelids that the main nerves lie, so that local anaesthetics have to be injected deep to the orbicularis oculi.

The *tarsi* (7.274) are two thin elongated plates of dense fibrous tissue, about 2·5 cm long; one is placed in each eyelid and contributes to its form and support. The *tarsus of the upper eyelid*, the larger, is of a semi-oval form, about 10 mm in height at the centre, and gradually narrowing towards its extremities. The lowest fibres of the superficial lamella of the aponeurosis of the levator palpebrae superioris are attached to its anterior surface, and the deep lamella of the same aponeurosis is inserted

[1264] H. J. Wilkinson, *Med. J. Aust.*, I, 1927.

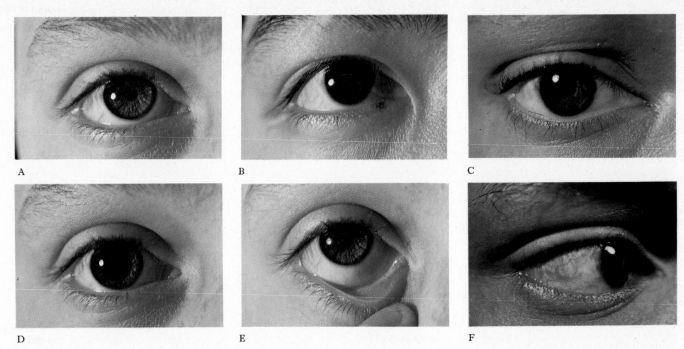

A   B   C

D   E   F

**7.272 A–F** In the top row of photographs the typical appearances of the living eye are compared in a Caucasian female (A), a Mongoloid male (B) and a Negroid male (C). All subjects are about 20 years of age. Note the pale sclera and grey-blue iris in A, the epicanthus overlapping the medial end of the lower eyelid in B, and the dark brown pigmentation of the iris in both B and C, rendering the pupil almost invisible. Compare the size of the pupil in the same eye, photographed under steady bright light in A and by sudden exposure to the same illumination after a period of dark adaptation in D. In E the lower eyelid had been everted somewhat to exhibit the lacrimal punctum and the rich subepithelial network of blood vessels. In F note the circumcorneal pigmentation and the conjunctival blood vessels, deep to which can be seen some details of the episcleral vessels. All photographs are of the right eye.

into its upper margin (7.266). The *tarsus of the lower eyelid*, the smaller, is a narrower plate, the vertical diameter of which is about 5 mm. The free or ciliary margins of the tarsi are thick and straight. The attached or orbital margins are connected to the circumference of the orbit by the orbital septum. The lateral ends of the tarsi are attached by a band, named the *lateral palpebral ligament*, to a tubercle on the zygomatic bone, just within the orbital margin; this ligament is separated from the more superficially placed *lateral palpebral raphe* (p. 497) by a few lobules of the lacrimal gland. The medial ends of the tarsi are attached by a strong tendinous band, named the *medial palpebral ligament*, to the upper part of the lacrimal crest, and to the adjoining part of the frontal process of the maxilla in front of this crest; the lower edge of this ligament is separated from the lacrimal sac by some fibres of the orbicularis oculi, since the latter is attached to the ligament.

The *orbital septum* is a weak membranous sheet, attached to the edge of the orbit, where it is continuous with the periosteum. In the upper eyelid it blends with the superficial lamella of the aponeurosis of the levator palpebrae superioris, and in the lower eyelid with the anterior surface of the tarsus. It is perforated by the vessels and nerves which pass from the orbital cavity to the face and scalp, by the aponeurosis of the levator palpebrae superioris, and by the palpebral part of the lacrimal gland.

The *tarsal glands* (7.275) are embedded in the thickness of the tarsi, and may be visible through the conjunctiva on everting the eyelids; they present an appearance like parallel strings of pearls. They are yellow in colour, arranged in a single row, and number about thirty in the upper eyelid, and somewhat fewer in the lower. They are embedded in grooves on the deep surfaces of the tarsi and correspond in length with the breadth of these plates; they are, consequently, longer in the upper than in the lower eyelid. Their ducts open on the free margins of the lids by minute foramina.

The tarsal glands are modified sebaceous glands, each consisting of a straight tube with numerous small lateral diverticula. The tubes are supported by a basement membrane and are lined at their mouths by stratified epithelium; the deeper parts of the tubes and the lateral offshoots are lined by a layer of polyhedral cells. The secretion of the glands spreads over the margin of the eyelid and tends to prevent the tears from overflowing on to the cheek. It has also been suggested that it spreads over the external surface of the tear film and reduces evaporation.

## THE CONJUNCTIVA

The conjunctiva is the transparent mucous membrane which passes, in a modified form, over the inner surfaces of the eyelids, and is reflected over the front part of the sclera and the cornea.

The *palpebral conjunctiva* is highly vascular, and has numerous subepithelial connective tissue papillae, its deeper part containing a considerable amount of lymphoid tissue, especially near the fornices. It is intimately adherent to the tarsi. At the margins of the lids it is continuous with the skin, with the lining epithelium of the ducts of the tarsal glands, and, through the lacrimal canaliculi, with the lining membrane of the lacrimal sac and naso-lacrimal duct and thence with that lining the nasal cavity. The line of reflexion of the conjunctiva from the eyelids on to the eyeball is named the *conjunctival fornix*, and its different parts are known as the superior and inferior fornices; the ducts of the lacrimal gland open into the lateral part of the superior fornix. Over the sclera the *ocular conjunctiva* is loosely connected to the eyeball; it is thin, transparent, destitute of papillae, and only slightly vascular. Upon reaching the cornea, the ocular conjunctiva continues as the corneal epithelium (p. 1098). The epithelium of the palpebral conjunctiva near the margins of the eyelids is stratified squamous; about 2 mm from the edge of each eyelid there is a groove in which foreign bodies frequently lodge and at which the epithelium comes to consist of two layers, a superficial one of columnar cells and a deeper one of flattened cells. This structure persists throughout most of the palpebral conjunctiva, but as the fornices are approached an intermediate layer of polygonal cells appears and this trilaminar arrangement comprises the structure of the conjunctival epithelium over the sclera. Near the sclerocorneal junction the epithelium changes to the stratified type characteristic of the corneal epithelium (p. 1098). Scattered throughout the conjunctival epithelium there are mucus-secreting goblet cells, but they are few in the palpebral and circumcorneal regions of the epithelium.

The *lacrimal caruncle* (7.272) is a small, reddish, conical body situated in the lacus lacrimalis at the medial angle of the eye; it consists of a small island of skin, and contains sebaceous and sudoriferous glands; a few slender hairs are arrached to its surface. Lateral to, and partly obscured by the caruncle there is a semilunar fold of conjunctiva, the *plica semilunaris*, the concave free lateral edge of which is directed towards the cornea. Its epithelium resembles that of the conjunctiva on the sclera but it contains numerous goblet cells. Beneath the epithelium there is some fat and a little nonstriated muscle. The *nictitating membrane*—present as a conjunctival specialization in some amphibians, reptiles and mammals—may be represented by the semilunar fold; but the homologies of these structures are uncertain.

*Vessels and nerves.* The eyelids receive their blood supply from the medial palpebral branches of the ophthalmic artery and from the lateral palpebral branches of the lacrimal artery (p. 636).

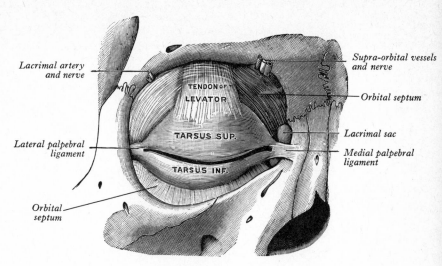

7.274  The tarsi and their ligaments. Anterior aspect.

The ocular conjunctiva is supplied by the ophthalmic division of the trigeminal nerve. The conjunctiva of the upper eyelid is supplied by the ophthalmic nerve, that of the lower eyelid by the maxillary nerve. Many of the nerves to the conjunctiva end in bulbous corpuscles (p. 799).

The lymph vessels of the eyelids and the conjunctiva are described on p. 730.

*Movements of the eyelids.* The position of the lids at any particular time depends on the reciprocal tone of the

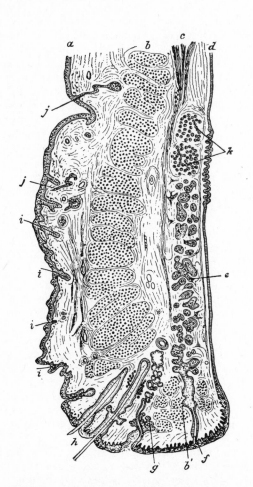

7.273  A sagittal section through the upper eyelid. (After Waldeyer.) *a.* Skin. *b.* Orbicularis oculi. *b′.* Ciliary fasciculi of the orbicularis oculi. *c.* Levator palpebrae superioris. *d.* Conjunctiva. *e.* Tarsal glands embedded in the tarsal plate. *f.* Opening of a tarsal gland. *g.* Sebaceous gland. *h.* Eyelashes. *i.* Small hairs of the skin. *j.* Sweat glands. *k.* Posterior tarsal glands.

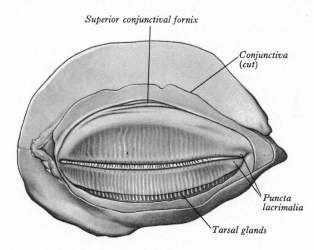

7.275  The posterior surfaces of the upper and lower eyelids of the left side. The orifices of the tarsal glands can be seen on the free margins of the lids.

orbicularis oculi and levator palpebrae superioris and on the degree of protrusion of the eyeball. The usual position when the eyes are open is that the margin of the lower lid crosses the eyeball at the lower edge of the circumference of the iris whilst the upper lid covers about half the width of the uppermost portion of the iris. The eyes are closed by movement of both upper and lower lids produced by contraction of the orbicularis oculi and at the same time the levator palpebrae superioris relaxes. On looking upwards, the levator palpebrae superioris contracts and the upper lid follows the movement of the eyeball. At the same time the eyebrows are raised by the contraction of the frontal bellies of the occipitofrontalis so as to diminish the degree to which the eyebrows jut beyond the eye. The lower lid lags behind the movement of the eye so that much more of the sclera is exposed below the iris and the lid is bulged forwards to some extent by the pressure exerted against its deep surface by the lower part of the eyeball. When the eye is depressed both lids move, the upper retaining its normal relationship to the eyeball and still covering about half the width of the upper portion of the iris. The lower lid is probably dragged downwards by the pull exerted on it by the conjunctiva reflected on to its deep surface from the sclera. In conditions of fear the palpebral fissure is widened by the contraction of the fibres of the nonstriated superior and inferior tarsal muscles, in response to the increased activity of the sympathetic nervous system. For further comments on eyelid movement see p. 1123.

## THE LACRIMAL APPARATUS

The lacrimal apparatus (7.276, 279) consists of (a) the lacrimal gland, which secretes a complex fluid, known as the tears, and its excretory ducts which convey the fluid to the surface of the eye; (b) the lacrimal canaliculi, lacrimal sac, and nasolacrimal duct, by which the fluid is conveyed into the nasal cavity.

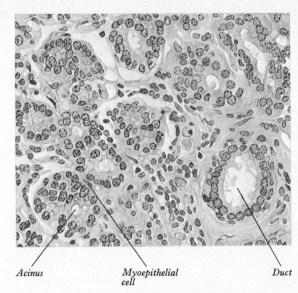

Acinus     Myoepithelial     Duct
                cell

**7.277** A section through a part of the lacrimal gland, showing the acini lined by a layer of columnar cells; a few myoepithelial cells can be seen outside the basement membrane. Magnification about × 320.

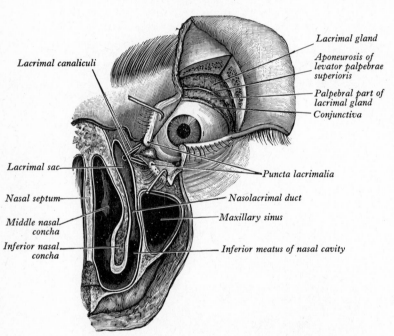

Lacrimal gland

Aponeurosis of levator palpebrae superioris

Palpebral part of lacrimal gland
Conjunctiva

Lacrimal canaliculi

Lacrimal sac

Nasal septum

Middle nasal concha

Inferior nasal concha

Puncta lacrimalia

Nasolacrimal duct

Maxillary sinus

Inferior meatus of nasal cavity

**7.276** The left lacrimal apparatus dissected from the anterior aspect.

**The lacrimal gland** (7.276) is probably homologous with the *Harderian gland* of lower mammals, and is derived from a serous secreting element and a gland secreting an oily material. In primates the lacrimal (serous) element has migrated from its original position in the lower lid to the upper. The human lacrimal gland consists of a larger upper *orbital part* and a lower smaller *palpebral part*, the two parts being continuous with each other posterolaterally around the lateral concave edge of the aponeurosis of the levator palpebrae superioris. The orbital part is about the size and shape of an almond and is lodged in the lacrimal fossa on the medial side of the zygomatic process of the frontal bone, just within the margin of the orbit. It lies above the levator (and, further laterally, above the lateral rectus); its lower surface is connected to the sheath of the levator, its upper surface is connected to the orbital periosteum, its anterior border is in contact with the orbital septum and its posterior border is attached to the orbital fat. The palpebral part, which is about one-third of the size of the orbital part, is subdivided into two

or three lobules and extends below the aponeurosis of the levator into the lateral part of the upper eyelid, where it is attached to the superior fornix of the conjunctiva, through which it can be seen when the eyelid is everted. The ducts of the gland, about twelve in number, open into the superior conjunctival fornix. Those from the orbital part (four or five in number) pass through the palpebral part and are joined by some of the ducts from this latter part, while other ducts of the palpebral part (six to eight in number) open independently. Thus all the ducts pass through the palpebral part, so that excision of this part of the gland is functionally equivalent to removal of the entire gland.

Many small accessory lacrimal glands are present in and near the conjunctival fornices; they are more numerous in the upper lid than in the lower. Their existence may explain why the conjunctiva does not dry up after extirpation of the lacrimal gland proper.

*Structure of the lacrimal gland* (7.277). The gland consists of very small lobules and is a compound tubulo-alveolar gland. The acini are lined by a layer of columnar cells which rest on a basement membrane and contain secretion granules and fat droplets. Outside these there are flattened myoepithelial (contractile) cells. The ducts are lined by a layer of columnar cells, outside which are a few myoepithelial cells. The secretion fluid (tears) contains various salts and an enzyme (lysozyme) which is bacteriocidal. No account of the primate lacrimal gland in terms of its ultrastructure appears to be available. Published accounts are so far chiefly concerned with rodents.[1265, 1266] Mucinogen and zymogen granules have been observed in the secretory cells. The plasma membrane of these cells is extensively infolded on their basal aspects.

The nerve supply of the lacrimal gland is described on p. 1067; it is both sympathetic and parasympathetic. For recent views on the route of the latter supply see footnote reference[1267].

**The lacrimal canaliculi**, one in each eyelid, are about 10 mm long; they commence at the *puncta lacrimalia* (7.272, 276, 278). The *superior canaliculus*, smaller and shorter than the inferior, at first ascends, and then

[1265] B. L. Scott and D. C. Pease, *Am. J. Anat.*, **104**, 1959.
[1266] A. Ichikawa and Y. Nakajima, *Tohoku J. exp. Med.*, **77**, 1962.
[1267] G. L. Ruskell, *J. Anat.*, **109**, 1971.

bends at an acute angle, and passes medially and downwards to the lacrimal sac. The *inferior canaliculus* at first descends, and then runs almost horizontally to the lacrimal sac. At the angles they are dilated into *ampullae*. The mucous lining of the ducts is covered with stratified squamous epithelium, placed on a basement membrane; outside the latter there is a corium rich in elastic fibres (rendering the ducts easily dilatable during the passage of a probe) and a layer of striped muscular fibres which is continuous with the lacrimal part of the orbicularis oculi. At the base of each lacrimal papilla the muscular fibres are circularly arranged and form a kind of sphincter.

**The lacrimal sac** (7.274, 276, 278) is the upper blind end of the nasolacrimal duct, and is lodged in a fossa formed by the lacrimal bone, the frontal process of the maxilla and the lacrimal fascia. It measures about 12 mm in length, its upper, closed end is flattened from side to side, but its lower part is rounded and is continued into the nasolacrimal duct; the openings of the lacrimal canaliculi are situated in its lateral wall slightly below its upper end.

A layer of fascia, continuous with the periosteum of the orbit and named the *lacrimal fascia*, passes from the lacrimal crest of the maxilla to the crest of the lacrimal bone, and forms the roof and lateral wall of the fossa in which the lacrimal sac is sited; between the fascia and the lacrimal sac there is a plexus of minute veins. The lacrimal fascia separates the sac from the medial palpebral ligament in front, and from the lacrimal part of the orbicularis oculi behind. The lower half of the fossa which lodges the lacrimal sac is related medially to the anterior part of the middle meatus of the nasal cavity; the upper half is related to the anterior ethmoidal sinuses. (In an examination of 100 skulls[1268] it was found that in 14 the anterior

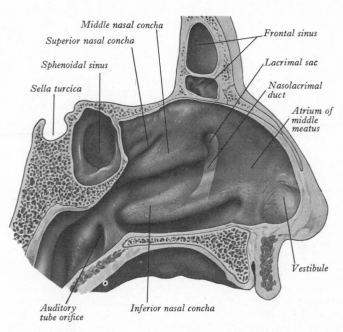

**7.279** The left lateral wall of the nasal cavity viewed from the medial side. The lacrimal sac and the nasolacrimal duct of the left side have been projected on to the lateral wall of the nasal cavity to show their positions relative to the middle nasal concha, the middle meatus and the inferior concha. (After Whitnall.)

through the nasolacrimal duct with the mucous membrane of the nasal cavity.

**The nasolacrimal duct** (7.278, 279) is a membranous canal about 18 mm long, which extends from the lower part of the lacrimal sac to the anterior part of the inferior meatus of the nose, where it ends in a somewhat expanded orifice. A fold of the mucous membrane forms an imperfect valve just above the opening and is known as the *lacrimal fold*. The duct is contained in an osseous canal,

formed by the maxilla, the lacrimal bone and the inferior nasal concha; it is narrower in the middle than at either end, and is directed downwards, backwards and a little laterally. The mucous lining of the lacrimal sac and nasolacrimal duct is covered with two layers of columnar epithelium which in places is ciliated. Around the duct there is a rich plexus of veins, forming an erectile tissue, engorgement of which may obstruct the duct.

Tear fluid secreted by the lacrimal gland enters the conjunctival sac at its superolateral angle and, under the influence of capillarity aided by blinking movements of the eyelids, is carried across the sac to the lacus lacrimalis mainly along the groove between the lower lid margin and the eyeball. From the lacus it passes into the lacrimal canaliculi. Contraction of the orbicularis oculi tends to press the puncta lacrimalia more firmly into the lacus, and capillary attraction serves to suck the lacrimal secretion into the lacrimal sac. The sudden dilatation of the lacrimal sac produced by the lacrimal part of the orbicularis oculi during blinking movements (p. 497) probably assists the process. Under normal conditions the secretion of the tarsal glands prevents the tears from overflowing the lid margins and also covers the capillary film of fluid on the front of the eyeball with a film of oil which delays evaporation.[1269, 1270]

**7.278** Sketch from a coronal section through the right half of the nasal cavity, anterior aspect, to show the relation of the lacrimal passages to the maxillary and ethmoidal sinuses and the inferior nasal concha. The mucous membrane is coloured. (After Whitnall.)

*Lacrimal canaliculi*

*Lacrimal sac*
*Middle meatus*
*Middle concha*
*Nasal septum*
*Nasolacrimal duct*
*Ostium lacrimale*
*Plica lacrimalis*
*Inferior concha*
*Inferior meatus*

ethmoidal sinuses came into relation only in the posterior wall of the fossa; in 32 they reached as far as the suture between the lacrimal bone and the maxilla; while in 54 one large irregular sinus extended as far as the anterior lacrimal crest.)

The lacrimal sac consists of a fibro-elastic coat, lined internally by mucous membrane; the latter is continuous through the lacrimal canaliculi, with the conjunctiva, and

[1268] S. E. Whitnall, *Ophthal. Rev.*, **30**, 1911.
[1269] S. Mishima and D. M. Maurice, *Expl Eye Res.*, **1**, 1961.
[1270] E. Wolff, *Anatomy of the Eye and Orbit*, ed. R. J. Last, Lewis, London. 1968.

# THE AUDITORY AND VESTIBULAR APPARATUS

The peripheral *auditory apparatus* consists of the various parts of the ear, but including in particular, the *cochlear part* of its *membranous labyrinth*. Essentially, each ear is a *distance receptor* concerned with the collection, conduction, modification, amplification and parametric analysis of the complex sound waveforms which impinge on the head. The latter are converted into coded spatio-temporal patterns of nerve impulses in the afferent fibres of the cochlear part of the vestibulocochlear nerve, for onward transmission to the auditory pathways in the central nervous system (pp. 853, 855, 886, 915, 963).

The molecular vibrations of the air which constitute the sound waves approaching the head vary according to: (1) the *direction* and *distance*, or *location* of the source of the waves; (2) the *intensity* or *energy content* of the waves; and (3) the relative purity or admixture of different *frequencies* which make up the wave train. The morphological and functional design of the ears is such that they are, within particular ranges of values, extremely sensitive to differences in frequency and intensity of the sound waves, and together, they are also very effective range and direction finders. Further, they are highly responsive to the *rate of change* of all of these sound wave parameters. The *frequency* of a sound wave is expressed as *cycles per second* or *hertz* (c/s or hz); it is subjectively appreciated as the *pitch* of the sound, and young adult ears are responsive to frequencies of about 20–20,000 hz, although higher or lower values are not uncommon in very young ears. The *intensity* of a sound is expressed as the *quantity of energy* which is transmitted in *unit time* through a *unit area* which is perpendicular to the direction of wave propagation. The subjective appreciation of the intensity of a sound is related to the logarithm of its absolute intensity as defined above, but is also dependent upon the frequency of the sound. The human ear is most sensitive (i.e. has the lowest threshold) for sounds in the 1500–3,000 hz range, and above and below these levels the threshold rises sharply. For example, about 10,000 times more energy is necessary for the equal perception of a sound of 15,000 hz than is for a sound of 2,000 hz. The sensitivity of the ear is indeed astounding; it has been calculated that sounds may be discerned which are due to pressure changes as small as $10^{-10}$ atmospheres—a change equivalent to ascending or descending 1/30,000 of an inch! Because of the great variation in the intensity level of sounds commonly encountered, the concept of the *decibel* has been introduced for convenience. A decibel is defined as 10 times the logarithm of the ratio of the intensity of the sound in question, to the intensity of an accepted reference level. A difference in intensity level of about one decibel is usually just perceptible by the human auditory system.

The *quality* of a sound depends upon the admixture of frequencies it contains. Musical sounds consist of one or more fundamental frequencies each with its mathematically related series of *overtones* or *harmonics*. Mixtures of unrelated or *irregular* frequencies are perceived simply as 'noise'.

The elegant researches into the manner in which the ear operates as a peripheral analyser of frequency and intensity, and how intensity and phase differences impinging on the two ears are related to range and direction finding, can only receive the briefest mention in the present volume. For such details the reader should consult footnote references.[1271-1274]

What follows is a structural account of the human ear, which on phylogenetic, developmental, structural and functional grounds, may be divided into *external*, *middle* and *internal* parts. Intimately associated structurally with the auditory cochlear part of the membranous labyrinth are the sensory receptors in specialized regions of the walls of the utricle and saccule, and in the ampullae of the semicircular ducts. The latter parts of the membranous labyrinth, their contained and surrounding fluids, the bony cavities in which they lie, and the vestibular part of the vestibulocochlear nerve, together constitute the *peripheral vestibular apparatus*. Its essential function is to provide the central nervous system with a constant flow of information concerning the static position of the head in space, or of its state of linear or angular acceleration or deceleration.

## The External Ear

The external ear consists of the *auricle*, or *pinna*, and the *external acoustic meatus*. The former projects from the side of the head and serves to collect the air vibrations which constitute the sound waves; the meatus leads inwards from the bottom of the auricle conducting the vibrations which are thereby transmitted to the tympanic membrane.

### THE AURICLE

The lateral surface of the auricle (7.280) is irregularly concave, looks slightly anteriorly, and presents numerous eminences and depressions. The curved prominent rim of the auricle is called the *helix*; where it turns posteroinferiorly, a small *auricular tubercle* (of Darwin) is frequently seen; this tubercle is very evident about the sixth

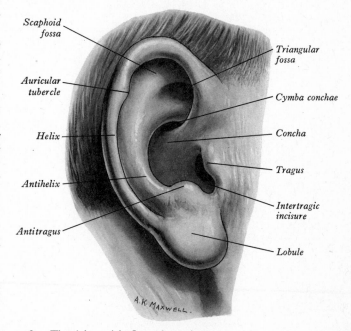

7.280 The right auricle. Lateral aspect.

[1271] G. L. Rasmussen and W. F. Windle (eds.), *Neural Mechanisms of the Auditory and Vestibular Systems*, Thomas, Springfield. 1960.

[1272] I. C. Whitfield, *The Auditory Pathway*, Arnold, London. 1967.

[1273] A. V. S. De Reuck and J. Knight (eds.), *Hearing Mechanisms in Vertebrates*, Ciba Foundation Symposium, Churchill, London. 1968.

[1274] G. E. W. Wolstenholme and J. Knight (eds.), *Sensorineural Hearing Loss*, Ciba Foundation Symposium, Churchill, London. 1970.

month of intrauterine life, when the whole auricle closely resembles that of some adult monkeys. Another curved prominence, parallel with and anterior to the posterior part of the helix, is the *antihelix*; this divides above into two crura, between which is a depressed *triangular fossa*. The narrow curved depression between the helix and the antihelix is the *scaphoid fossa*; the antihelix partly encircles a deep, capacious cavity, the *concha of the auricle*, which is incompletely divided into two by the *crus* or anterior end of the helix. The part of the concha above the crus of the helix is the *cymba conchae*; it overlies, and through it can be felt, the supermeatal triangle of the temporal bone (pp. 265, 292), deep to which lies the mastoid antrum. Below the crus of the helix and in front of the concha, a small, curved flap, the *tragus*, projects posteriorly, partly overlapping the orifice of the meatus. Opposite the tragus, separated from it by the *intertragic incisure*, is a small tubercle, the *antitragus*. The *lobule* lies below the antitragus, and being composed of fibrous and adipose tissues it is soft, unlike the rest of the auricle which is firm and elastic.

The cranial surface of the auricle presents elevations which correspond to the depressions on its lateral surface, and after which they are named, e.g. eminentia conchae, eminentia fossae triangularis, etc.

In addition to acting as a collecting 'trumpet' for sound waves and channelling them into the relatively narrow meatus, the asymmetry of the pinnae and their variations in thickness, probably introduce variable delay paths in sound transmission which may be important in the efficient binaural (and also the cruder monaural) localization of sound sources.

In its **structure** the auricle is composed of a thin plate of elastic fibrocartilage, covered with skin, and connected with the surrounding parts by ligaments and muscles; it is continuous with the cartilaginous portion of the external acoustic meatus, and the latter is joined to the margins of the bony meatus by fibrous tissue.

The *skin of the auricle* is thin, closely adherent to the cartilage, and covered with fine hairs which are furnished with sebaceous glands; these glands are most numerous in the concha and scaphoid fossa. On the tragus and antitragus, and intertragic incisure the hairs are strong and numerous, especially in the male in old age. The skin of the auricle is continuous with that lining the external acoustic meatus.

**The cartilage of the auricle** (7.281) consists of a single piece of elastic fibrocartilage; upon its surface the eminences and depressions described above are found. It is absent from the lobule; it is deficient, also, between the tragus and beginning of the helix, the gap being filled up by dense fibrous tissue. Anteriorly, where the helix bends upwards, there is a small cartilaginous projection, the *spine of the helix*, while at its other extremity the cartilage is prolonged inferiorly as the *tail of the helix*; the latter is separated from the antihelix by the *fissura antitragohelicina*. The cranial surface of the cartilage shows the *eminentia conchae* and the *eminentia triangularis* which correspond to the depressions on the lateral surface. A transverse furrow, the *sulcus antihelicis transversus*, corresponding with the inferior crus of the antihelix on the lateral surface, separates the eminentia conchae from the eminentia triangularis. The eminentia conchae is crossed by an oblique ridge, the *ponticulus*, which gives attachment to the auricularis posterior. There are two fissures in the auricular cartilage, one behind the crus helicis and another in the tragus.

**The ligaments of the auricle** consist of two sets: (1) extrinsic, connecting it to the temporal bone; (2) intrinsic, connecting various parts of its cartilage together.

The *extrinsic ligaments* are two in number, anterior and

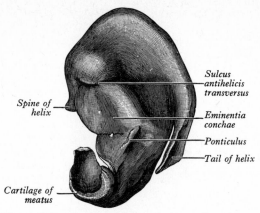

Spine of helix

Cartilage of meatus

Sulcus antihelicis transversus

Eminentia conchae

Ponticulus

Tail of helix

7.281  The medial surface of the right auricular cartilage.

posterior. The *anterior ligament* extends from the tragus and spine of the helix to the root of the zygomatic process of the temporal bone. The *posterior ligament* passes from the posterior surface of the concha to the lateral surface of the mastoid process.

The chief *intrinsic ligaments* are: (*a*) a strong fibrous band, stretching from the tragus to the helix, completing the meatus in front, and forming part of the boundary of the concha; and (*b*) a band between the antihelix and the tail of the helix. Other less prominent bands are found on the cranial surface of the auricle.

## THE AURICULAR MUSCLES

These consist of two sets: extrinsic, which connect it with the skull and scalp and move the auricle as a whole; and intrinsic, which extend from one part of the auricle to another.

**The extrinsic muscles** are the auriculares anterior, superior et posterior.

The *auricularis anterior*, the smallest of the three, is thin, fan-shaped, and its fibres are pale and indistinct. It arises from the lateral edge of the epicranial aponeurosis, and its fibres converge to be inserted into the spine of the helix.

The *auricularis superior*, the largest of the three, is thin and fan-shaped. Its fibres arise from the epicranial aponeurosis, and converge to be inserted by a thin, flattened tendon into the upper part of the cranial surface of the auricle.

The *auricularis posterior* consists of two or three fleshy fasciculi, which arise by short aponeurotic fibres from the mastoid portion of the temporal bone, and are inserted into the ponticulus on the eminentia conchae.

**Nerve supply**. The auriculares anterior et superior are supplied by the temporal branches, and the auricularis posterior by the posterior auricular branch of the facial nerve.

**Actions**. In man, these muscles have very little action; the auricularis anterior draws the auricle forwards and upwards; the auricularis superior raises it slightly; and the auricularis posterior draws it backwards.

**The intrinsic muscles** are helicis major and minor, tragicus, antitragicus, transversus auriculae and the obliquus auriculae. Their effect in modifying the shape of the pinna is minimal or absent in most human ears. Occasional individuals can, however, modify the shape and position of their external ears to a much greater extent.

The *helicis major* is a narrow vertical band situated upon the anterior margin of the helix. It arises from the spine of the helix, and is inserted into the anterior border of the helix, where the latter is about to curve backwards.

1135

The *helicis minor* is an oblique fasciculus, covering the crus helicis.

The *tragicus* is a short, flattened vertical band on the lateral surface of the tragus.

The *antitragicus* arises from the outer part of the antitragus, and is inserted into the tail of the helix and antihelix.

The *transversus auriculae* is placed on the cranial surface of the auricle. It consists of scattered fibres, partly tendinous and partly muscular, extending from the eminentia conchae to the eminentia scaphae.

The *obliquus auriculae*, also on the cranial surface, consists of a few fibres extending from the upper and posterior parts of the eminentia conchae to the eminentia triangularis.

**The nerve supply** to the intrinsic muscles on the lateral surface is provided by the temporal branches of the facial nerve, to the intrinsic muscles on the cranial surface by the posterior auricular branch of the same nerve.

**The arteries of the auricle** are: (*a*) the posterior auricular branch of the external carotid artery, which supplies three or four branches to its cranial surface; twigs from these reach the lateral surface, some by passing through the fissures of the auricular cartilage, and others by turning round the margin of the helix; (*b*) the anterior auricular branches of the superficial temporal artery, which are distributed to the lateral surface; (*c*) a branch from the occipital artery.

**The veins of the auricle** accompany their corresponding arteries. Arteriovenous anastomoses are numerous in the skin of the auricle.

**The lymphatics of the auricle** drain into (*a*) the parotid lymph nodes, especially the node in front of the tragus; (*b*) the upper deep cervical lymph nodes; and (*c*) the mastoid lymph nodes.

**The sensory nerves of the auricle** are: (*a*) the great auricular nerve, which supplies most of the cranial surface and the posterior part of the lateral surface (helix, antihelix, lobule); (*b*) the lesser occipital nerve, which supplies the upper part of the cranial surface; (*c*) the auricular branch of the vagus, which supplies the concavity of the concha and the posterior part of the eminentia; (*d*) the auriculotemporal nerve, which supplies the tragus, the crus of the helix and the adjacent part of the helix; (*e*)

the facial nerve, which in company with the auricular branch of the vagus, probably supplies small areas of skin on both aspects of the auricle—in the conchal depression and over its eminence. The details of this cutaneous innervation by the facial nerve, and whether facial fibres also reach the external acoustic meatus and tympanic membrane, however, remain undetermined.

## THE EXTERNAL ACOUSTIC MEATUS

The external acoustic meatus (7.282, 283) extends from the concha to the tympanic membrane. Its length, measured from the bottom of the concha, is approximately 2·5 cm (measured from the tragus it is about 4 cm long). It consists of two structurally different parts: the lateral third is *cartilaginous*, and the medial two-thirds *osseous*. It forms an **S**-shaped curve, and is directed at first medially, anteriorly and slightly superiorly (*pars externa*); it then passes medially, posteriorly and superiorly (*pars media*), and lastly is carried medially, anteriorly, and slightly inferiorly (*pars interna*). The canal is oval in transverse section, with its greatest diameter obliquely placed with a postero-inferior inclination at the external orifice, but it is nearly horizontal at the medial end. There are two constrictions, one near the medial end of the cartilaginous part, and another, the *isthmus*, in the osseous part, about 2 cm from the bottom of the concha. The tympanic membrane, which closes the medial end of the meatus, is obliquely directed; in consequence the floor and anterior wall of the meatus are longer than its roof and posterior wall.

The lateral *cartilaginous part* of the meatus is about 8 mm long; it is continuous with the auricular cartilage and is fixed by fibrous tissue to the circumference of the medial osseous part of the meatus. The meatal cartilage is deficient posterosuperiorly, the deficiency being occupied by a sheet of collagen; two or three deep fissures are present in the anterior part of the cartilage.

The *osseous part* of the meatus is about 16 mm long, and is narrower than the cartilaginous part. It is directed medially, anteriorly and slightly inferiorly, forming in its course a slight curve the convexity of which is posterosuperior in position. Its medial end is smaller than the lateral end, and it is obliquely placed, with the anterior wall projecting medially about 4 mm beyond the posterior wall; this end is marked, except at its upper part, by a narrow groove, the *tympanic sulcus*, to which the circumference of the tympanic membrane is attached. Its lateral end is dilated, and rough in the greater part of its circumference for the attachment of the cartilaginous meatus. The anterior, inferior and most of the posterior parts of the osseous meatus are formed by the tympanic element of the temporal bone, which, in the fetus, exists only as a *tympanic ring* (p. 295). The posterosuperior region of the osseous part is formed by the squama of the temporal bone.

The skin which envelops the auricle is continued into the external acoustic meatus and covers the outer surface of the tympanic membrane. It is thin, shows no dermal papillae on section, and is closely adherent to the cartilaginous and osseous parts of the tube; hence inflammatory conditions are extremely painful owing to the increased tension in these tissues. In the thick subcutaneous tissue of the cartilaginous part of the meatus there are numerous *ceruminous glands*, which secrete the ear wax or *cerumen*; their coiled tubular structure resembles that of the sweat glands (p. 1169). When active the cells of the secretory part are columnar, but when quiescent they are cuboidal; they are clothed externally by myoepithelial cells. The ducts of the ceruminous glands open either on to the general epithelial surface or into a neighbouring sebaceous gland of a hair follicle. The cerumen prevents maceration

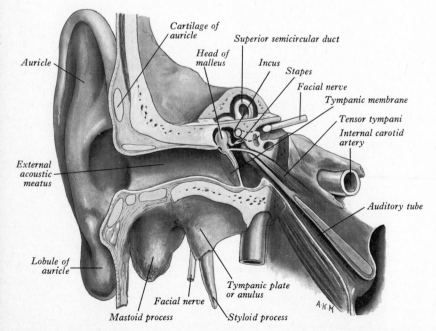

7.282 The external and middle regions of the right ear. Anterior aspect.

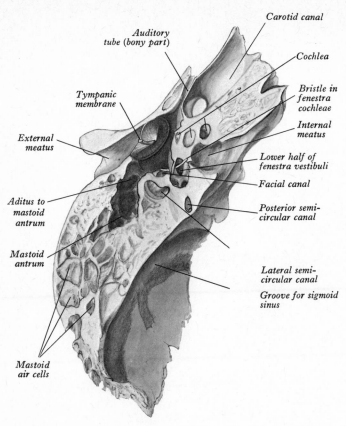

**7.283** An oblique section through the left temporal bone viewed from above. (From a section prepared by Mr. P. F. Milling.) Compare with **7.285** and **7.288**.

of the meatal lining by trapped water, and may discourage epithelial attacks by insects. Over production, or prolonged retention of ear wax may, however, completely block the meatus, or, when in contact with the tympanic membrane, embarass its vibratory responses. The ceruminous glands, as well as hair follicles, are largely limited to the cartilaginous part of the meatus, but a few small glands and fine hairs are found in the roof of the lateral part of the osseous meatus.

In addition to the protective value of the cerumen, and the opposition to the entry of insects and foreign bodies afforded by the meatal hairs, the warm humid environment provided by the relatively enclosed meatal air is essential for the effective mechanical responses of the tympanic membrane.

### Relations of the Meatus

The condyloid process of the mandible is anterior to the meatus, partially separated from its cartilaginous part by a small part of the parotid gland. A blow on the chin may cause the condyle to break into the meatus. The movements of the mandible influence to some extent the lumen of the cartilaginous part. Superior to the osseous part is the middle cranial fossa; behind it are the mastoid air cells, separated from the meatus by a thin layer of bone. The deepest part of the meatus is related superiorly to the epitympanic recess of the tympanic cavity, and posterosuperiorly to the mastoid antrum, the bone separating the antrum being only 1–2 mm thick, so that it can be opened surgically by this 'transmeatal approach'.

The meatal *arteries* are the posterior auricular branch of the external carotid, the deep auricular branch of the maxillary, and auricular branches of the superficial temporal. The *veins* drain into the external jugular and maxillary veins and the pterygoid plexus. The *lymphatics* drain with those of the auricle (p. 729).

The *nerves* supplying the meatus are derived from the auriculotemporal branch of the mandibular nerve, which supplies the anterior and upper walls of the meatus, and the auricular branch of the vagus nerve which supplies the posterior and inferior walls (see also below).

## Clinical Examination of the Meatus

The external acoustic meatus can be examined most satisfactorily by light reflected down a funnel-shaped speculum, when the greater part of the canal and tympanic membrane can be viewed. In using this instrument, the auricle should be drawn upwards, backwards and a little laterally, to render the meatus as straight as possible.

At the point of junction of the osseous and cartilaginous parts of the meatus an obtuse angle projects into the tube antero-inferiorly; this produces a constriction which is important when attempting to remove foreign bodies lodged in the meatus. The shortness of the meatus in children should be remembered when an aural speculum is used, because of the risk of injuring the tympanic membrane; indeed, even in the adult, the speculum should not be introduced beyond the constriction which marks the junction of the osseous and cartilaginous parts. Immediately anterolateral to the membrane there is a marked depression, on the floor of the meatus, bounded laterally by a prominent ridge; here foreign bodies may become impacted. By means of the speculum, combined with traction of the auricle upwards and backwards, the greater part of the tympanic membrane is rendered visible (**7.284**). It is a pearly-grey, slightly glistening membrane, which in the adult is placed obliquely, forming an acute angle of about 55° with the floor of the meatus, while with the roof it forms an obtuse angle. At birth it is more horizontal, situated in almost the same plane as the base of the skull.

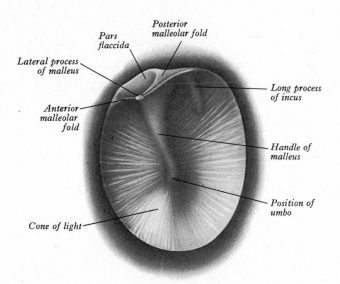

**7.284** The left tympanic membrane, external aspect as seen through a speculum.

A reddish-yellow streak can be seen about midway between the anterior and posterior margins of the membrane which extends from the centre obliquely upwards and forwards; this is due to the handle of the malleus, attached internally to the membrane. At the upper part of this streak, close to the roof of the meatus, a little white, round prominence is clearly seen; this is the lateral or short process of the malleus, projecting against the membrane. The tympanic membrane does not present a plane surface; on the contrary, its centre is drawn inwards, because of its connexion with the handle of the malleus, the centre of the concavity corresponding to the *umbo* (p. 1140) on the deep surface of the membrane. A bright reflected 'cone of light', is seen in the antero-inferior quadrant of the membrane. Anterior and posterior to the short process of the malleus, the variably prominent anterior and posterior malleolar folds are seen, with the flaccid part of the tympanic membrane (p. 1140) between them. Posterior and parallel to the upper part of the handle of the malleus, the long process of the incus is often seen as a whitish streak; sometimes it can be seen to end below near a round spot which is the head of the stapes.

incisions through the membrane should be postero-inferior.

## The Tympanic Cavity

The middle ear or tympanic cavity (**7**.283, 285, 287, 288) is an irregular, laterally compressed space within the temporal bone. It is lined with mucoperiosteum (p. 1145) and filled with air, which is conveyed to it from the nasal part of the pharynx through the auditory tube. It

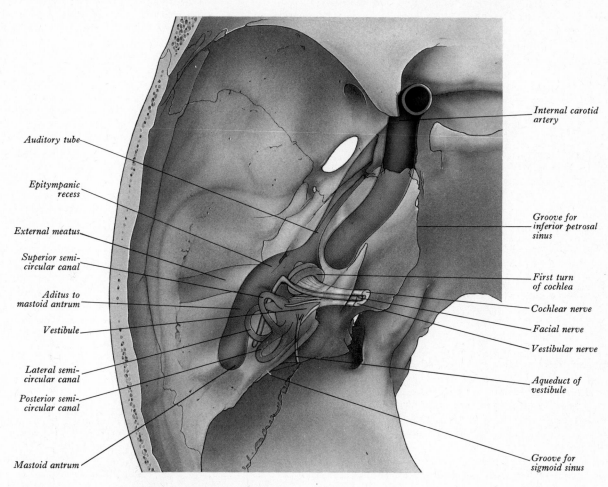

Auditory tube

Epitympanic recess

External meatus

Superior semi-circular canal

Aditus to mastoid antrum

Vestibule

Lateral semi-circular canal

Posterior semi-circular canal

Mastoid antrum

Internal carotid artery

Groove for inferior petrosal sinus

First turn of cochlea

Cochlear nerve

Facial nerve

Vestibular nerve

Aqueduct of vestibule

Groove for sigmoid sinus

**7**.285 Scheme showing the parts of the left auditory apparatus as if viewed through a semi-transparent temporal bone. Compare with **7**.283 and **7**.288.

*Applied Anatomy.* Malformations such as imperfect development of the external parts, supernumerary auricle, preauricular cysts, fistulae and sinuses, or absence of the meatus, are occasionally met with. In the child up to the age of four or five years there is a gap in the antero-inferior wall of the osseous part of the meatus, the *foramen of Huschke* (p. 296), which is filled by membrane; it may persist in the adult.

The connexions of the nerves of the meatus explain the occurrence of reflex coughing and sneezing, from implication of the vagus, when there exists any source of irritation in the meatus, and the vomiting which may follow syringing the ears of children, and the occasional heart failure similarly induced in elderly people. Probably the association of earache with toothache or with cancer of the tongue is due to involvement of the mandibular branch of the trigeminal nerve, which supplies the teeth and the tongue also. The upper half of the tympanic membrane is much more vascular than the lower half: for this reason, and also to avoid the chorda tympani nerve and ossicles,

contains a chain of movable bones, which connect its lateral to its medial wall and transmit the vibrations of the tympanic membrane across the cavity to the internal ear.

The essential functional significance of the tympanic cavity with its tympanic membrane and associated chain of ossicles, is the efficient transfer of energy from the relatively weak vibrations in the elastic, compressible medium *air* in the external acoustic meatus, to overcome the inertia in the virtually incompressible aqueous *fluids* which surround the delicate membrane-supported receptors of the internal ear. Thus the mechanical coupling between the two systems must be such that their resistances to deformation or 'flow', that is, their *impedances*, are matched as closely as possible. To this end the high-amplitude, low-force per unit area, vibrations of the air are communicated to the *tympanic membrane*, which, in surface area exceeds that of the *footplate of the stapes* (in contact with the perilymph) by 15 to 20 times. In this manner, the *force per unit area* generated by the footplate is increased by a similar amount, whilst its *amplitude* of vibration is little changed.

Protective mechanisms are also incorporated in the design of the tympanic cavity. These include the connexion via the auditory (pharyngotympanic) tube, whereby pressure is equalized on the two sides of the delicate tympanic membrane, and the protection afforded by the shape of the articulations between the ossicles, and the reflex contractions of the stapedius and tensor tympani muscles, which prevent damage due to sudden and potentially excessive excursions of the ossicles.

The tympanic cavity consists of two parts: the *tympanic cavity proper*, opposite the tympanic membrane, and the *epitympanic recess*, above the level of the membrane; the latter contains the upper half of the malleus and the greater part of the incus. Including the epitympanic recess, the vertical and anteroposterior diameters of the cavity are each about 15 mm. The transverse diameter measures about 6 mm above and 4 mm below; opposite the centre of the tympanic membrane it is only about 2 mm. The tympanic cavity is bounded *laterally* by the tympanic membrane; *medially*, by the lateral wall of the internal ear; it communicates, posteriorly, with the mastoid antrum and through it with the mastoid air cells, and anteriorly with the auditory tube (7.285).

## THE BOUNDARIES OF THE TYMPANIC CAVITY

**The roof of the tympanic cavity** (7.286) is a thin plate of compact bone, the *tegmen tympani*, which separates the cranial and tympanic cavities, and forms the greater part of the anterior surface of the petrous part of the temporal bone; it is prolonged posteriorly as the roof of the mastoid antrum, and anteriorly to cover the canal for the tensor tympani. In the young, the unossified petrosquamosal suture (p. 294) may allow direct spread of infection from the tympanic cavity to the cerebral meninges. In the adult, veins from the tympanic cavity pass through this suture to the superior petrosal sinus, or the petrosquamous sinus if present (p. 694), and may transmit infection to the intracranial sinuses.

**The floor of the tympanic cavity** is narrow, and consists of a thin, convex plate of bone which separates the cavity from the superior bulb of the internal jugular vein (7.288); in places the bone may be deficient, and then the cavity is separated from the vein by mucous membrane and fibrous tissue only. In the floor of the tympanic cavity, near the medial wall, there is a small aperture for the passage of the tympanic branch of the glossopharyngeal nerve. The floor is sometimes thick and may contain some accessory mastoid air cells.

**The lateral wall of the tympanic cavity** (7.286, 287) is formed mainly by the tympanic membrane, but partly also by the ring of bone to which this membrane is attached. There is a deficiency or notch in the upper part of the ring, close to which are three small apertures—the anterior and posterior canaliculi for the chorda tympani nerve, and the petrotympanic fissure.

The *posterior canaliculus for the chorda tympani nerve* is situated in the angle of junction between the posterior and lateral walls of the tympanic cavity immediately behind the tympanic membrane and on a level with the upper end of the handle of the malleus; it leads into a minute canal, which descends in front of the canal for the facial nerve, and ends in that canal about 6 mm above the stylomastoid foramen. Through it the chorda tympani nerve and a branch of the stylomastoid artery enter the tympanic cavity.

The *petrotympanic fissure* opens just above and in front of the ring of bone into which the tympanic membrane is inserted; in this situation it is a mere slit about 2 mm in

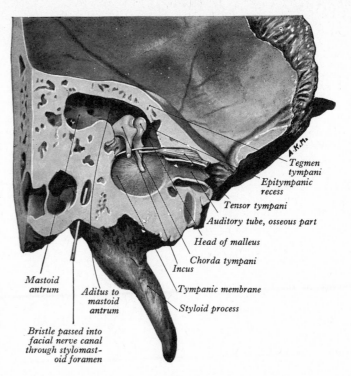

7.286 An oblique vertical section through the left temporal bone, to show the lateral wall of the middle ear and the mastoid antrum.

length. It lodges the anterior process and anterior ligament of the malleus, and transmits to the tympanic cavity the anterior tympanic branch of the maxillary artery.

The *anterior canaliculus for the chorda tympani nerve* is placed at the medial end of the petrotympanic fissure; through it the chorda tympani nerve leaves the tympanic cavity.

**The tympanic membrane** (7.286, 287) separates the tympanic cavity from the external acoustic meatus. It is thin and semi-transparent, nearly oval in form, somewhat broader above than below, and very obliquely placed, forming an angle of about 55° with the floor of the meatus. Its longest diameter is downwards and forwards, and measures from 9 to 10 mm; its shortest diameter

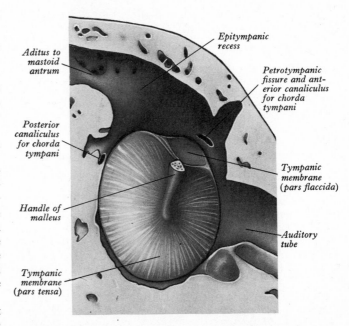

7.287 The lateral wall of the left tympanic cavity.

from 8 to 9 mm. The greater part of its circumference is thickened, and forms a *fibrocartilaginous ring* which is attached to the *tympanic sulcus* at the medial end of the meatus. This sulcus is deficient superiorly, and from the ends of the notch two bands, the *anterior* and *posterior malleolar folds*, are prolonged to the lateral process of the malleus. The small, somewhat triangular part of the membrane situated above these folds is lax and thin, and is named the *pars flaccida*; a small perforation is sometimes present. The remainder of the membrane is taut and is the *pars tensa*. The handle of the malleus is firmly attached to the inner surface of the tympanic membrane as far as its centre, which projects towards the tympanic cavity; the inner surface of the membrane is thus convex, and the point of greatest convexity is named the *umbo*. Although the membrane as a whole is convex on its inner surface, its radiating fibres (*vide infra*) are curved with their concavities directed inwards.

Structurally, the tympanic membrane is composed of three strata: an outer (cuticular), an intermediate (fibrous), and an inner (mucous). The *cuticular layer* is derived from the thin skin which lines the external acoustic meatus, and consists of stratified epithelium.

Facial nerve canal
Floor of aditus
Posterior semicircular canal
Superior semicircular canal
Lateral semicircular canal
Auditory tube
Carotid canal
Tympanic antrum
Promontory (overlying first coil of cochlea)
Stapes
Tendon of stapedius emerging from pyramid
Jugular fossa  Fenestra cochleae
Mastoid air cells

**7.288** An oblique section through the left temporal bone, to show the medial wall of the middle ear. The cochlea and the semicircular canals are in blue. Note the relationship of the first coil of the cochlea to the promontory, and the closeness of the facial nerve canal and the lateral semicircular canal to the medial wall of the aditus.

It is hairless, and the subepithelial connective tissue, which carries a number of small blood vessels, does not develop dermal papillae except for a few rudimentary ones around the periphery of the membrane. The *fibrous stratum* consists of two layers: a superficial layer of radiate fibres which diverge from the handle of the malleus, and a deep layer of circular fibres, which are plentiful around the circumference, but sparse and scattered near the centre of the membrane. Near the centre and around the margins of the membrane fine meshes of elastic fibres are said to be interspersed between the collagen fibres (but see below). The *mucous layer* is a part of the mucous membrane of the tympanic cavity; it is thickest towards the upper part of the membrane, and may be covered,

it has been claimed, by a layer of ciliated columnar epithelial cells. However, the ciliated epithelium may be present only in patches, or entirely absent, when it is replaced by a low cuboidal or simple squamous epithelium.

The foregoing traditional account of tympanic membrane structure, based on light microscopy, may well need a substantial revision, if the detailed ultrastructural and chemical studies[1275] carried out on the membrane of the guinea-pig also apply to the human membrane. In this mammal the external epithelium is approximately ten cells thick and consists of two zones, the superficial one consisting of non-nucleated squames, the deep zone resembling, in many respects, the stratum spinosum of the skin with numerous desmosomes and tight junctions between adjacent cells; the deepest cells lie on a continuous basal lamina, but lack epithelial pegs and hemidesmosomes. The internal (mucous) epithelium consists of a single layer of extremely flattened cells, with overlapping or interdigitating boundaries, which carry desmosomes and tight junctions between adjacent cells. Their cytoplasm contains only a sparse population of the usual organelles, micropinocytotic vesicles are few, and the free surfaces of these apparently metabolically inert cells bear occasional irregular microvilli and are coated with an amorphous electron-dense material. Ciliated columnar cells are not present. Most interestingly, the intermediate (fibrous) layer consists of filaments about 10 mm in diameter, with what are apparently crossbridges between adjacent filaments at 25 nm intervals. The filaments are disposed in outer radial, and inner non-radial zones, the former more profuse, and in neither situation do their ultrastructural appearance resemble collagen or elastin. In their amino acid composition, also, the filaments are quite distinctive, and it is proposed that they consist of a protein specialized for the unique function of the tympanic membrane. Similar studies in other mammals, including man, will be awaited with much interest.

Large fibroblasts lie between the outer radial fibres and the basal lamina of the external epithelium, whilst blood capillaries and their basement membranes lie immediately deep to the basal lamina of the internal epithelium. In the flaccid part of the tympanic membrane the fibrous stratum is replaced by loose connective tissue.

The *arteries* of the tympanic membrane are derived from the deep auricular branch of the maxillary artery, which ramifies beneath the cuticular stratum, and from the stylomastoid branch of the posterior auricular artery, and tympanic branch of the maxillary artery, which are distributed in the mucous surface. The *superficial veins* open into the external jugular vein; those in the *deep surface* drain partly into the transverse sinus and veins of the dura mater, and partly into the plexus of veins on the auditory tube. The *nerve supply* of the tympanic membrane is from the auriculotemporal branch of the mandibular nerve, the auricular branch of the vagus nerve, and from the tympanic branch of the glossopharyngeal nerve.

**The medial wall of the tympanic cavity** (7.288, 289) is also the lateral wall of the internal ear. Its structural features are the promontory, the fenestra vestibuli, the fenestra cochleae and the prominence caused by the underlying facial nerve canal.

The *promontory* is a rounded elevation furrowed by small grooves which contain the nerves of the tympanic plexus. It overlies the lateral projection of the basal turn of the cochlea. A minute spicule of bone frequently

---

[1275] F. R. Johnson, R. M. H. McMinn and G. N. Atfield, *J. Anat.*, **105**, 1968.

connects the promontory to the pyramidal eminence on the posterior wall. In front of the promontory the apex of the cochlea is closely related to the medial wall of the tympanum (**7.282, 288**). A depression behind the promontory, the *sinus tympani*, indicates the position of the ampulla of the posterior semicircular canal.

The *fenestra vestibuli* is a reniform opening, situated posterosuperior to the promontory, which connects the tympanic cavity to the vestibule of the internal ear; its long diameter is horizontal, and its convex border is directed superiorly. In life it is occupied by the base of the stapes, the circumference of which is fixed to the margin of the fenestra by an annular ligament.

The *fenestra cochleae* is situated below and a little behind the fenestra vestibuli, from which it is separated by the posterior part of the promontory. It lies completely under cover of the overhanging edge of the promontory in a deep hollow or niche. It is placed very obliquely, and, in the macerated bone, opens upwards and forwards from the tympanic cavity into the scala tympani of the cochlea. In life it is closed by the *secondary tympanic membrane*, which is somewhat concave towards the tympanic cavity and convex towards the cochlea, the membrane being bent so that its posterosuperior one-third forms an angle with its antero-inferior two-thirds. This membrane consists of three layers: an external, derived from the mucous lining of the tympanic cavity; an internal, from the lining membrane of the cochlea; and an intermediate, fibrous, layer.

The *prominence of the facial nerve canal* indicates the position of the upper part of the bony canal in which the facial nerve is contained; this canal, the lateral wall of which may be partly deficient, traverses the medial wall of the tympanic cavity from before backwards, immediately above the fenestra vestibuli, and then curves downwards in the posterior wall of the cavity.

**The posterior wall of the tympanic cavity** (**7.288**) is wider above than below, and its main structural features are the entrance to the mastoid antrum, the pyramid and the fossa incudis.

The *aditus to the mastoid antrum* is a large irregular aperture, which leads backwards from the epitympanic recess into the upper part of an air sinus, the *mastoid antrum*. On the medial wall of the aditus to the antrum there is a rounded eminence, situated above and behind the prominence of the facial nerve canal; it corresponds with the position of the underlying lateral semicircular canal.

The *pyramidal eminence* is situated immediately behind the fenestra vestibuli, and in front of the vertical portion of the facial nerve canal; it is hollow, and contains the stapedius; its summit projects forwards towards the fenestra vestibuli, and is pierced by a small aperture which transmits the tendon of the muscle. The cavity in the pyramidal eminence is prolonged downwards and backwards in front of the facial nerve canal, and communicates with the latter by an aperture which transmits a twig from the facial nerve to the stapedius.

The *fossa incudis* is a small depression in the lower and posterior part of the epitympanic recess; it contains the short process of the incus, which is fixed to the fossa by ligamentous fibres.

**The mastoid antrum** (**7.283, 285, 286, 287, 288, 289**) is an air sinus in the petrous part of the temporal bone, and its topographical relations are of considerable surgical importance. In the upper part of its *anterior wall* is an opening, the aditus to the mastoid antrum, which leads forwards into the epitympanic recess; medially, the aditus is related to the lateral semicircular canal. The *medial wall* of the antrum itself is related to the posterior semicircular canal (**7.285**). *Posteriorly* the antrum is closely related

to the sigmoid sinus; some of the mastoid air cells may intervene between them. The *roof* of the antrum, formed by the tegmen tympani, is related to the middle cranial fossa and the temporal lobe of the brain. The floor has a number of apertures through which the antrum communicates with the mastoid air cells. *Antero-inferiorly*, the antrum is related to the descending part of the canal for the facial nerve. The *lateral wall* of the antrum, the usual surgical approach to the cavity, is formed by the postmeatal process of the squamous part of the temporal bone. This wall is only 2 mm thick at birth, but increases in thickness at the rate of approximately 1 mm a year, attaining a final thickness of 12–15 mm. The lateral wall of the antrum in the adult corresponds to the *suprameatal triangle* on the outer surface of the skull (pp. 265, 292); it lies beneath and can be felt through the cymba conchae (p. 1135). The superior side of the triangle, formed by the supramastoid crest, is on a level with the floor of the middle cranial fossa; the antero-inferior side, formed by the posterosuperior margin of the orifice of the external acoustic meatus, lies approximately along the course of the descending part of the canal for the facial nerve; and the posterior side, formed by a vertical tangent to the

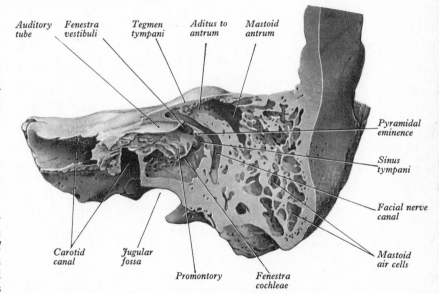

**7.289** An oblique section through the left temporal bone, showing the medial wall of the middle ear. Compare with **7.288**.

posterior margin of the meatal orifice, lies just in front of the course of the sigmoid sinus. In the adult, the mastoid antrum has a capacity of about 1 ml, each of its diameters being about 10 mm. At birth, unlike the other cranial air sinuses, it is well developed and almost the same size as in the adult; it lies at a higher level in relation to the external acoustic meatus than in the adult. In the very young child, owing to the thinness of the lateral wall of the antrum and the absence or feeble development of the mastoid process, the stylomastoid foramen and the emerging facial nerve are very superficially situated.

**The mastoid air cells** (**7.283, 288, 289**) vary considerably in number, form and size in different individuals. In general, they are a series of intercommunicating cavities, lined by mucous membrane, with a flattened squamous non-ciliated epithelium, continuous with that of the mastoid antrum and tympanic cavity. In some cases they extend throughout the mastoid process, even to its tip, and some of the cells may be separated from the sigmoid sinus and the posterior cranial fossa by extremely thin bone, which occasionally shows deficiencies. Some of the cells may lie superficial to, and even behind the sigmoid sinus, and others may lie in the posterior wall of the descending part of the canal for the facial nerve. Those contained in the squamous part of the temporal bone may sometimes be separated from the deeper cells in the petrous part by a plate of bone lying in the situation of the squamomastoid suture of early life. In other cases, the cells only extend very slightly into the mastoid process, and the process consists largely either of dense bone or of cancellous bone containing bone marrow. Many varieties of mastoid process occur, with varying mixtures of the above structures, but three types of mastoid are commonly described, namely, *pneumatic*, containing many air cells, *sclerotic*, with few or no air cells, and *mixed*, containing air cells and bone marrow. The cells may extend beyond the confines of the mastoid process. They may extend for some distance into the squamous part of the temporal bone above the supramastoid crest, and also into the posterior root of the zygoma. Others may extend forwards into the roof of the osseous part of the external acoustic meatus, lying immediately below the middle cranial fossa. Some may extend into the floor of the tympanic cavity, lying in very close relation to the superior jugular bulb. Rarely, a few cells may excavate the jugular process of the occipital bone. An important group of cells may extend medially into the petrous part of the temporal bone, even reaching as far as its tip, and they are related to the auditory tube, the carotid canal, the labyrinth and the abducent nerve. Some investigators maintain that these petrous cells are not directly continuous with the mastoid cells proper, but are independent outgrowths from the tympanic cavity. The extensions of the mastoid air cells described above are of considerable importance to the clinician. Infection of the cells may spread to the structures mentioned above as related to them. Whereas the mastoid antrum is well developed at birth, the mastoid air cells, at this time, are only just beginning to develop as tiny diverticula from the antrum. As the mastoid process begins to develop in the second year, the cells gradually extend into it, and by the fourth year they are well formed, though their greatest growth occurs at about the age of puberty. In about 20 per cent of skulls the mastoid process is not excavated by air cells.

**The anterior wall of the tympanic cavity** is constricted owing to the approximation of the medial and lateral walls of the cavity. Its inferior and larger part consists of a thin lamina of bone which forms the posterior wall of the carotid canal, and is perforated by the superior and inferior caroticotympanic nerves, and the tympanic branch or branches of the internal carotid artery. At the superior part of the anterior wall there are two parallel canals, placed one above the other; superiorly placed is the *canal for the tensor tympani*, inferiorly, the *osseous part of the auditory tube*. These canals incline anteriorly, inferiorly and medially to open in the angle between the squamous and petrous parts of the temporal bone; they are separated by a thin, bony septum. The canal for the tensor tympani and the septum run posterolaterally on the medial wall of the tympanic cavity, and end immediately above the fenestra vestibuli, where the posterior end of the septum is curved laterally to form a pulley, the *processus trochleariformis* (*cochleariformis*), over which the tendon of the tensor tympani bends in a lateral direction to reach its attachment to the upper part of the handle of the malleus.

## THE AUDITORY TUBE

The *auditory* or *pharyngotympanic* tube (7.282, 285, 286) is the channel through which the tympanic cavity communicates with the nasal part of the pharynx. Through it

air passes between pharynx and tympanic cavity thus equalizing the air pressure on the medial and lateral surfaces of the tympanic membrane. Its length is about 36 mm, and its direction is downwards, forwards and medially, forming an angle of some 45° with the sagittal plane and one of about 30° with the horizontal plane. It is formed partly of bone, partly of cartilage and fibrous tissue.

The *bony part of the tube* is about 12 mm long. It begins in the anterior wall of the tympanic cavity, and, gradually narrowing, ends at the angle of junction of the squamous and petrous portions of the temporal bone, its extremity presenting a jagged margin which serves for the attachment of the cartilaginous part; the carotid canal lies on its medial side. It is oblong in transverse section with its greater dimension lying horizontally.

The *cartilaginous part of the tube*, about 24 mm long, is formed of a triangular plate of cartilage, the greater part of which is situated in the posteromedial wall of the tube. The apex of the fibrocartilage is attached by fibrous tissue to the circumference of the medial end of the bony part of the tube, while its base lies directly under the mucous membrane of the lateral wall of the nasal part of the pharynx, where it forms the *tubal elevation*, behind the pharyngeal orifice of the tube. The superior part of the cartilage is bent laterally and downwards, and the cartilage therefore consists of a broad *medial lamina*, and a narrow *lateral lamina*. On transverse section the cartilage has the appearance of a hook; the groove or furrow produced by the bend in the cartilage is open below and laterally, and this part of the wall of the canal is completed by fibrous membrane. The cartilage is fixed to the base of the skull in the groove between the petrous part of the temporal bone and the greater wing of the sphenoid bone; this groove ends near the root of the medial pterygoid plate. The cartilaginous and bony parts of the tube are not in the same plane, the former inclining downwards a little more than the latter. The diameter of the tube is greatest at the pharyngeal orifice, least at the junction of the bony and cartilaginous parts, and again increased towards the tympanic cavity; the narrowest part of the tube is termed the *isthmus*.

The mucous membrane of the tube is continuous medially with that of the pharynx, and laterally with that of the tympanic cavity; it is covered with ciliated columnar epithelium and is thin in the bony part, while in the cartilaginous part it contains many mucous glands, and near its pharyngeal orifice a considerable aggregation of lymphoid tissue, the *tubal tonsil*.

*Relations of the auditory tube. Anterolaterally* the tensor veli palatini separates the tube from the otic ganglion, the mandibular nerve and its branches, the chorda tympani nerve and the middle meningeal artery. This muscle receives some fibres from the lateral lamina of the cartilage and from the membranous part of the tube; these fibres constitute the *dilatator tubae*. The salpingopharyngeus (p. 1249) is attached to the inferior part of the cartilage of the tube near its pharyngeal opening. *Posteromedially* the tube is related to the petrous part of the temporal bone and to the levator veli palatini, which arises partly from its medial lamina. The position and relations of the pharyngeal orifice are described with the nasal part of the pharynx (p. 1243).

The tube is opened during deglutition but the mechanism is uncertain. Some claim that the dilatator tubae, possibly aided by the salpingopharyngeus, is responsible, though others deny the existence of the dilatator tubae. It is also claimed that the levator veli palatini, by elevating the cartilaginous part of the tube, allows the tube to open passively by releasing tension on the cartilage.

In the newborn child the auditory tube is about half as

long as that of the adult. Its direction is more horizontal, and its bony part is relatively shorter, but much wider than in the adult. Its pharyngeal orifice is a narrow slit, which is on a level with the palate and is devoid of a tubal elevation.

*Vessels and nerves.* The *arteries* of the auditory tube are derived from the ascending pharyngeal branch of the external carotid artery and from two branches of the maxillary artery, namely, the middle meningeal artery and the artery of the pterygoid canal. The *veins* open into the pterygoid venous plexus. The *nerves* of the tube spring from the tympanic plexus (p. 1145) and from the pharyngeal branch of the pterygopalatine ganglion. The precise contribution from the nerves which form the plexus i.e. the glossopharyngeal, the cervical sympathetic and possibly the facial, remains uncertain in man.

## THE AUDITORY OSSICLES

The tympanic cavity contains a chain of three movable ossicles: the *malleus, incus* and *stapes.* The malleus is attached to the tympanic membrane and the base of the stapes to the circumference of the fenestra vestibuli, while the incus is placed between, and articulates with, the malleus and stapes.

**The malleus** (7.290), so named from its fancied resemblance to a mallet, is from 8 to 9 mm long, and is the largest of the auditory ossicles. It consists of a head, neck and three processes—the manubrium or handle, and the anterior and lateral processes.

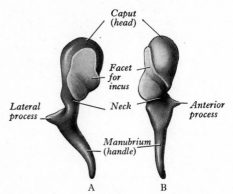

7.290   The left malleus.   A Posterior aspect.   B Medial aspect.

The *head,* which is the large upper end of the bone, is situated within the epitympanic recess; it is ovoid in shape, and articulates posteriorly with the incus, being clothed with mucous membrane over the rest of its surface. The cartilage-covered facet for articulation with the incus is constricted near the middle, and consists of an upper larger and a lower smaller part, situated nearly at right angles to each other. Opposite the constriction the lower margin of the facet projects in the form of a process which is named the *cogtooth* or *spur* of the malleus.

The *neck* is the narrow part just beneath the head; inferior to the neck there is an enlargement to which the various processes are attached.

The *manubrium mallei* is connected by its lateral margin with the tympanic membrane. It is directed downwards, medially and backwards; it decreases in size towards its free end, which is curved slightly forwards and flattened transversely. Near the upper end of its medial surface there is a slight projection, into which the tendon of the tensor tympani is inserted.

The *anterior process* is a delicate bony spicule, directed forwards from the enlargement below the neck; it is connected to the petrotympanic fissure by ligamentous

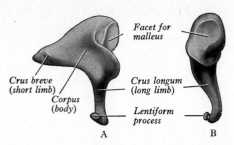

7.291   The left incus.   A Medial aspect.   B Anterior aspect.

fibres. In the fetus this is the longest process of the malleus, and it is continuous in front with the cartilage of Meckel (p. 120).

The *lateral process* is a conical projection which springs from the root of the handle of the malleus; it is directed laterally, and is attached to the upper part of the tympanic membrane and, by means of the anterior and posterior malleolar folds, to the extremities of the notch at the upper part of the tympanic sulcus.

*Ossification.* The cartilaginous precursor of the malleus is derived from near the dorsal end of the embryonic Meckel's cartilage. With the exception of its anterior process, it is ossified from a single endochondral centre, which appears near the future neck of the bone in the fourth month of fetal life. The anterior process is ossified separately, in dense connective tissue, and joins the main part of the bone about the sixth month of fetal life.

**The incus** (7.291) received its name from its supposed resemblance to an anvil, but its shape is more like that of a premolar tooth, with two widely diverging roots. It consists of a body and two processes.

The *body* is somewhat cubical, but compressed laterally. On its anterior surface there is a cartilage-covered saddle-shaped facet, for articulation with the head of the malleus.

The *long process,* rather more than half the length of the handle of the malleus, descends nearly vertically, behind and parallel to that process; its lower end bends medially, and terminates in a rounded projection, the *lentiform process,* the medial surface of which is covered with cartilage, and articulates with the head of the stapes.

The *short process,* somewhat conical in shape, projects posteriorly, and is attached by ligamentous fibres to the fossa incudis, in the postero-inferior part of the epitympanic recess.

*Ossification.* The incus has a cartilaginous precursor which is continuous with the dorsal extremity of the embryonic Meckel's cartilage. Its ossification often spreads from a single endochondral centre, which appears in the upper part of its long process in the fourth month of fetal life; the lentiform process, however, may have a separate centre of ossification.

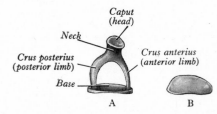

7.292   The left stapes.   A Superior aspect.   B Basal aspect.

**The stapes** (7.292), so called from its resemblance to a stirrup, consists of a head, neck, two limbs and a base.

The *head* is directed laterally, and on it there is a small cartilage-covered depression for articulation with the lentiform process of the incus.

1143

The *neck* is the constricted part adjoining the head; the tendon of the stapedius is inserted into its posterior surface.

The *limbs* diverge from the neck and are connected at their ends by a flattened oval plate, termed the *base*, which forms the footplate of the stirrup, and is fixed to the margin of the fenestra vestibuli by a ring of ligamentous fibres (the annular ligament). The anterior limb is shorter and less curved than the posterior.

*Ossification.* The stapes is preformed in the perforated dorsal moiety of the hyoid arch cartilage of the embryo. Its ossification starts from a single endochondral centre, which appears in the base of the bone in the fourth month of fetal life, and then gradually spreads through the stapedial limbs to coalesce in its body.

At birth the auditory ossicles have reached an advanced state of maturity.

### The Articulations of the Auditory Ossicles

These are typical synovial joints. The incudomalleolar joint is a saddle-shaped articulation. The incudostapedial joint is a 'ball and socket' articulation. Their articular surfaces are covered with articular cartilage, and each is enveloped by an articular capsule containing a considerable amount of elastic tissue, and lined by synovial membrane.

### The Ligaments of the Auditory Ossicles

The ossicles are connected to the walls of the tympanic cavity by ligaments: three for the malleus, and one each for the incus and stapes. Some of these 'ligaments' are mere folds of mucous membrane which carry blood vessels and nerves to and from the ossicles and their articulations. Others contain a central, strong band of collagen fibres.

The *anterior ligament of the malleus* is attached by one end to the neck of the malleus, just above the anterior process, and by the other to the anterior wall of the tympanic cavity, close to the petrotympanic fissure, some of its collagen fibres being prolonged through the fissure to reach the spine of the sphenoid bone; some fibres are continued into the sphenomandibular ligament. Both the latter ligament and the anterior ligament of the malleus are derived from the fibrous perichondrial sheath of the cartilage of Meckel (p. 120). The ligament may contain muscle fibres (the *laxator tympani* or *musculus externus mallei*).

The *lateral ligament of the malleus* is a triangular band passing from the posterior part of the border of the tympanic incisure to the head of the malleus.

The *superior ligament of the malleus* connects the head of the malleus to the roof of the epitympanic recess.

The *posterior ligament of the incus* connects the end of the short process of the incus to the fossa incudis.

The *superior ligament of the incus* is little more than a fold of mucous membrane, passing from the body of the incus to the roof of the epitympanic recess.

The vestibular surface and the circumference of the base of the stapes are covered with hyaline cartilage; that encircling the base is attached to the margin of the fenestra vestibuli by a ring of elastic fibres, termed the *annular ligament of the base of the stapes*. Its posterior part is much narrower than its anterior part, and acts as a kind of hinge on which the base of the stapes moves when the stapedius contracts.

### THE MUSCLES OF THE TYMPANIC CAVITY

The muscles of the tympanic cavity are the tensor tympani and stapedius.

**The tensor tympani** (7.282, 286), a long slender muscle, is contained in the bony canal superior to the bony part of the auditory tube, from which it is separated by a thin bony septum. It arises from the cartilaginous part of the auditory tube and the adjoining part of the greater wing of the sphenoid, as well as from the bony canal in which it is contained. Passing backwards through the canal, it ends in a slim tendon which bends laterally round the pulley-like processus trochleariformis, and is attached to the handle of the malleus, near its root.

*Nerve supply.* The tensor tympani is supplied by a branch of the nerve to the medial pterygoid, which in its turn is a branch of the mandibular nerve, and traverses the otic ganglion without interruption (p. 1007). Through this it receives both a motor and a proprioceptive innervation.[1276]

**The stapedius** arises from the wall of a conical cavity in the pyramidal eminence and from the continuation of this cavity which passes down in front of the descending part of the facial canal (p. 1141); its minute tendon emerges from the orifice at the apex of the pyramid, and, passing forwards, is inserted into the posterior surface of the neck of the stapes (7.288). This small muscle is of an asymmetric bipennate form, and consists of numerous small motor units, each containing only six to nine muscle fibres. A few neuromuscular spindles are present near the myotendinous junction.

*Nerve supply.* The stapedius is supplied by a branch of the facial nerve. (For details of the stapedius muscle and its innervation see footnote reference [1277].)

*Actions.* Under normal conditions, the tensor tympani and the stapedius contract simultaneously and reflexly in response to sounds of fairly high intensity, exerting 'a protective damping effect upon sound vibrations reaching the internal ear'.[1278] The tensor on contraction pulls inwards the tympanic membrane and renders it more tense; its action also results in the base of the stapes being pushed more tightly into the fenestra vestibuli. The stapedius opposes the latter action of the tensor. Paralysis of the stapedius muscle results in hyperacusis.

### MOVEMENTS OF THE AUDITORY OSSICLES

The manubrium faithfully follows all movements of the tympanic membrane, while the malleus and incus rotate together around an axis which runs through the short process and posterior ligament of the incus and the anterior ligament of the malleus. When the tympanic membrane and the manubrium are displaced medially, the long process of the incus also moves in the same direction and pushes the base of the stapes towards the labyrinth. This motion is communicated to the perilymph (p. 1148), the movement of which causes an outward bulging of the secondary tympanic membrane which occupies the fenestra cochleae. The conditions are reversed when the tympanic membrane moves in an outward direction, but if this movement of the membrane is exaggerated the incus does not follow the full outward excursion of the malleus but merely glides on this bone at the incudomalleolar joint, thus avoiding the danger of pulling the base of the stapes out of the fenestra vestibuli. When the manubrium is carried in a medial direction, the cogtooth on the lower margin of the head of the malleus locks the incudomalleolar joint, and this necessitates a medial movement of the long process of the incus; the joint is unlocked when the handle of the malleus is carried outwards. The three bones collectively act as a bent lever, so that the base of the stapes does not move in and out of the fenestra vestibuli like a piston, but rocks on a fulcrum which is situated on the anteroinferior border of

[1276] L. Candiollo, *Z. Zellforsch. mikrosk. Anat.*, **67**, 1965.
[1277] C. E. Blevins, *Archs otolar.*, **86**, 1967.
[1278] C. S. Hallpike, *Proc. R. Soc. Med.*, **28**, 1935.

the fenestra, and at this site the annular ligament is thickened. More complex movements of the stapes have also been described.[1279] The rocking movement around a vertical axis, which has been likened to a door opening and closing, occurs only at moderate sound intensities. With loud, low-pitched sounds, the axis becomes horizontal, the upper and lower margins of the stapedial base oscillating in opposite directions around this central axis, thus immediately and automatically preventing excessive displacement of the perilymph.

## THE TYMPANIC MUCOSA

The mucous membrane of the tympanic cavity is continuous with that of the pharynx, through the auditory tube. It invests the auditory ossicles and the muscles and nerves contained in the tympanic cavity, forms the inner layer of the tympanic membrane and the outer layer of the secondary tympanic membrane, and lines the mastoid antrum and mastoid air cells. It forms several vascular folds which extend from the walls of the tympanic cavity to the ossicles; of these, one descends from the roof of the cavity to the head of the malleus and upper margin of the body of the incus, and a second invests the stapedius; other folds invest the chorda tympani nerve and the tensor tympani. These folds separate off saccular recesses, and give the interior of the tympanic cavity a somewhat honeycombed appearance. One of these pouches, termed the *superior recess of the tympanic membrane*, lies between the neck of the malleus and the pars flaccida. Two other recesses, termed the *anterior* and *posterior recesses of the tympanic membrane*, may be mentioned: they are formed by the mucous membrane which envelops the chorda tympani nerve, and are situated, one in front of, and the other behind, the handle of the malleus. In the tympanic cavity the mucous membrane is pale, thin and slightly vascular. It is covered with ciliated columnar epithelium except over the posterior part of the medial wall, the posterior wall, often parts of the tympanic membrane, and the auditory ossicles where the cells are flatter and non-ciliated. Near the orifice of the auditory tube numerous goblet cells are present, but apart from this there are no mucous glands. The mastoid antrum and the mastoid air cells are lined by a flattened non-ciliated epithelium. Undoubtedly, there are considerable variations in the regions of the tympanic cavity and associated structures, which are lined by squamous, cuboidal, columnar, or ciliated columnar epithelium. As yet there has been no systematic exhaustive ultrastructural study of this problem. (For an account of the ultrastructure of restricted regions consult footnote reference [1280].)

It is to be noted that the tympanic cavity and mastoid antrum, the auditory ossicles and the structures comprising the internal ear are more or less fully developed by birth and undergo little subsequent alteration. In the fetus the tympanic cavity contains a jelly-like tissue, which has practically disappeared by birth, at which time the cavity is filled with a fluid that is absorbed after birth when air enters the cavity through the auditory tube.

## THE VASCULATURE OF THE TYMPANIC CAVITY

The *arteries* supplying the walls and contents of the tympanic cavity are six in number. Two of them are larger than the others—the *anterior tympanic* branch of the *maxillary artery*, which supplies the tympanic membrane, and the *stylomastoid* branch of the *posterior auricular artery*, which supplies the posterior part of the tympanic cavity and mastoid air cells. The smaller arteries are—

the *petrosal* branch of the *middle meningeal artery*, which enters through the hiatus for the greater petrosal nerve; the *superior tympanic* branch of the *middle meningeal artery*, which traverses the canal for the tensor tympani; a branch from the *ascending pharyngeal artery*, and another from the *artery of the pterygoid canal*, which accompany the auditory tube, and the tympanic branch, or branches from the *internal carotid artery*, given off in the carotid canal and perforating the thin anterior wall of the tympanic cavity. In early fetal life the *stapedial artery* passes through the ring of the stapes (p. 160). The *veins* terminate in the pterygoid venous plexus and in the superior petrosal sinus. From the mucous membrane of the mastoid antrum a small group of veins runs medially through the arch formed by the superior semicircular canal. They emerge on the posterior surface of the petrous part of the temporal bone through the subarcuate fossa, and open into the superior petrosal sinus. These small veins are the remains of the large *subarcuate veins* of the child, and constitute a pathway of infection from the mastoid antrum to the meninges of the brain. The *lymph vessels* are described on page 731.

## THE NERVES OF THE TYMPANIC CAVITY

The *nerves* constitute the *tympanic plexus*, which ramifies upon the surface of the promontory. The plexus is formed by (1) the tympanic branch of the glossopharyngeal nerve, and (2) the caroticotympanic nerves. (For details consult footnote reference [1281].) The *tympanic branch of the glossopharyngeal* enters the tympanic cavity by the *canaliculus for the tympanic nerve*, and divides into branches which ramify on the promontory and enter into the formation of the tympanic plexus. The *superior and inferior caroticotympanic nerves*, from the carotid plexus of the sympathetic, pass through the wall of the carotid canal, and join the plexus. The tympanic plexus supplies: (a) branches to the mucous lining of the tympanic cavity, auditory tube and mastoid air cells; (b) a branch which goes through an opening in front of the fenestra vestibuli and joins the greater petrosal nerve; (c) the *lesser petrosal nerve*, which may be looked upon as the continuation of the tympanic branch of the glossopharyngeal nerve through the tympanic plexus. The lesser petrosal nerve traverses a small canal below the canal for the tensor tympani, runs past, and receives a connecting branch from the genicular ganglion of the facial nerve; it emerges from the anterior surface of the temporal bone through a small opening on the lateral side of the hiatus for the greater petrosal nerve. It then passes through the foramen ovale, or through the small canaliculus innominatus (p. 289), and joins the otic ganglion. Postganglionic fibres pass from the otic ganglion, via the auriculotemporal nerve, to provide the secretomotor supply for the parotid gland.

The *chorda tympani* is a nerve derived from the facial nerve, about 6 mm. above the stylomastoid foramen. It runs anterosuperiorly in a canal, and enters the tympanic cavity through the *posterior canaliculus*. It then curves anteriorly in the substance of the tympanic membrane lying between its mucous and fibrous layers (p. 1140). After crossing the medial aspect of the upper part of the handle of the malleus it reaches the anterior wall, and enters the *anterior canaliculus*. (For its further course see p. 1014.) The other nerves which are closely related, topographically, to the tympanic cavity include the facial

[1279] G. V. Békésy, in: *Experiments in Hearing*, ed. E. G. Wever, McGraw-Hill, New York. 1960.
[1280] J. Kawabata and M. M. Paparella, *Annls. Otol. Laryngol.*, **78**, 1969.
[1281] M. Arslan, *Proc. R. Soc. Med.*, **53**, 1960.

nerve with its geniculate ganglion and stapedial and greater petrosal branches; the auricular branch of the vagus; the afferent and efferent terminals of the vestibulocochlear nerve; and the internal carotid sympathetic plexus. These are all described in greater detail elsewhere in the present section.

The *meningeal branch* (p. 1007), of the mandibular nerve, supplies branches to the mastoid air cells.

*Applied Anatomy*. Fractures of the middle fossa of the base of the skull almost invariably involve the tympanic roof, and are accompanied by a rupture of the tympanic membrane or fracture through the roof of the bony part of the external acoustic meatus. Such injuries are associated with prolonged bleeding from the ear, and, if the dura mater has also been torn, with discharge of cerebrospinal fluid.

The tympanic cavity is frequently the seat of disease, both suppurative and non-suppurative, and in practically every case the inflammation spreads upwards from the nasal cavity and nasal part of the pharynx along the auditory tube. Acute inflammation spreading up to the tympanic cavity is usually associated with much swelling of the mucous membrane of the tube, thus occluding it, and the products of inflammation, confined in the tympanic cavity, may spread directly to the mastoid antrum. In such circumstances the only means of escape for the products is by rupture of the tympanic membrane, which may occur spontaneously or be induced surgically and is followed by a free discharge of pus. Should the swelling of the walls of the auditory tube then subside, the normal drainage of the cavity will be established and the perforation in the drum will heal, but if not—as is often the case because the opening of the tube may be occluded by enlarged lymphatic aggregates in the nasal part of the pharynx or other cause—the pus may continue to accumulate in the middle ear and overflow through the perforation as a chronic otorrhoea. Several intracranial complications may result from purulent material being retained; thus an abscess may form between the bone and dura mater, (*a*) above the roof of the tympanic cavity, and immediately beneath the dura covering the temporal lobe of the brain, or (*b*) between the deep aspect of the mastoid process and the sigmoid sinus, possibly extending widely and surrounding the sinus. In this latter case thrombosis of the sinus may occur, and the infected clot tends to disintegrate and be carried into the general circulation, particles becoming lodged in the capillaries of the lungs and causing abscesses. In addition, bone disease of the tympanic cavity or mastoid antrum may be associated with severe and fatal septic meningitis, or with the formation of abscess in the brain, the most common sites being the temporal lobe of the cerebrum and the hemisphere of the cerebellum.

In some cases of chronic bone disease in the tympanic cavity, the facial nerve becomes exposed as it lies in its canal and an inflammatory process is set up in the nerve, leading to facial paralysis of the infranuclear or peripheral type (p. 1015).

## THE INTERNAL EAR

The internal ear consists of two parts—the *bony labyrinth*, a series of cavities within the petrous part of the temporal bone, and the *membranous labyrinth*, a series of communicating membranous sacs and ducts, contained within the bony cavities.

### The Bony Labyrinth

The bony labyrinth (7.285, 293) consists of three parts—the *vestibule*, the *semicircular canals* and the *cochlea*. These are cavities hollowed out of the substance of the bone, and lined by periosteum; they contain a clear fluid, known as the *perilymph*, in which the membranous labyrinth is placed. The bony labyrinth consists of harder, denser bone than the surrounding parts of the petrous portion of the temporal bone, so that it is possible, particularly in the very young skull, to separate the labyrinth from the petrous temporal by artificial dissection.

#### THE VESTIBULE

The vestibule is the central part of the bony labyrinth, and is situated medial to the tympanic cavity, posterior to the cochlea and anterior to the semicircular canals. It is somewhat ovoid in shape, but flattened transversely; it measures about 5 mm from before backwards, the same from above downwards, and about 3 mm across. In its *lateral wall* there is the opening of the fenestra vestibuli, closed in life by the base of the stapes and its annular ligament. On the anterior part of the *medial wall* there is a small *spherical recess*, containing the saccule and perforated by several minute holes, the *macula cribrosa media*. The recess corresponds to the inferior vestibular area in the bottom of the internal acoustic meatus (7.302), and the foramina transmit filaments of the vestibulocochlear nerve to the saccule. Behind this recess there is an oblique ridge, the *vestibular crest*, the anterior end of which is the *pyramid of the vestibule*; this ridge divides below to enclose a small depression, the *cochlear recess*, which is perforated by a number of holes for the passage of fibre bundles of the vestibulocochlear nerve to the vestibular end of the duct of the cochlea. Posterosuperior to the vestibular crest, and situated in the roof and medial wall of the vestibule there is an *elliptical recess* which contains the utricle. The pyramid and adjoining part of the elliptical recess are perforated by a number of holes, the *macula cribrosa superior*; the holes in the pyramid transmit the nerves to the utricle, and those in the elliptical recess the nerves to the ampullae of the superior and lateral semicircular ducts. The pyramid and the adjoining part of the elliptical recess correspond to the superior vestibular area at the bottom of the internal acoustic meatus (7.302). The orifice of the *aqueduct of the vestibule* lies below the elliptical recess. This aqueduct extends to the posterior surface of the petrous part of the temporal bone; it transmits one or more small veins, and contains a tubular prolongation of the membranous labyrinth which is termed the *endolymphatic duct*. In the posterior part of the vestibule there are the *five orifices of the semicircular canals*, in the anterior wall, an elliptical opening leading into the *scala vestibuli* of the cochlea.

#### THE SEMICIRCULAR CANALS

The semicircular canals are three in number, superior, posterior and lateral, and are situated posterosuperior to the vestibule. They are compressed from side to side, and each occupies about two-thirds of a circle. They are unequal in length, but are all about 0·8 mm in diameter; each presents a dilatation at one end, called the *ampulla*, the diameter of which is nearly twice that of the canal.

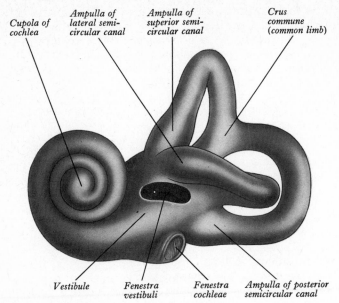

Cupola of cochlea — Ampulla of lateral semicircular canal — Ampulla of superior semicircular canal — Crus commune (common limb)

Vestibule — Fenestra vestibuli — Fenestra cochleae — Ampulla of posterior semicircular canal

7.293 A    The left bony labyrinth. Lateral aspect.

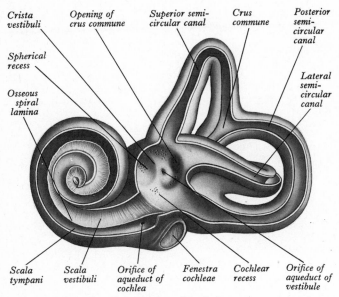

Crista vestibuli — Opening of crus commune — Superior semicircular canal — Crus commune — Posterior semicircular canal

Spherical recess

Osseous spiral lamina

Lateral semicircular canal

Scala tympani — Scala vestibuli — Orifice of aqueduct of cochlea — Fenestra cochleae — Cochlear recess — Orifice of aqueduct of vestibule

7.293 B    The interior of the left bony labyrinth.

They open into the vestibule by five orifices, one of which is common to two of the canals.

The *superior semicircular canal*, 15 to 20 mm in length, is vertical in direction, and is placed transversely to the long axis of the petrous part of the temporal bone, on the anterior surface of which its arch underlies the arcuate eminence (p. 294). Some maintain, however, that the arcuate eminence does not accurately coincide with the superior semicircular canal but is adapted to the occipitotemporal sulcus on the inferior surface of the temporal lobe of the cerebral hemisphere. The anterolateral end of the superior semicircular canal is ampullated, and opens into the upper and lateral part of the vestibule; the opposite end unites with the upper end of the posterior canal to form the *crus commune*, which is about 4 mm long, and opens into the medial part of the vestibule.

The *posterior semicircular canal*, also vertical, is directed backwards, nearly parallel with the posterior surface of the petrous bone; it is from 18 mm to 22 mm long; its ampullated end opens into the lower part of the vestibule, where there are several small holes, the *macula cribrosa inferior*, for the transmission of the nerves to this ampulla,

their position corresponding to the *foramen singulare* in the bottom of the internal acoustic meatus (7.302). Its upper end opens into the crus commune.

The *lateral* or *horizontal canal* is from 12 mm to 15 mm long, and its arch is directed horizontally backwards and laterally. Its anterior or ampullated end opens into the upper and lateral angle of the vestibule, just above the fenestra vestibuli and immediately below the ampullated end of the superior canal; its posterior end opens below the orifice of the crus commune.

The lateral semicircular canal of one ear is in the same plane as that of the other ear; while the superior canal of one ear is in a plane nearly parallel with that of the posterior canal of the other.

## THE COCHLEA

The cochlea (7.285, 293, 294, 298) resembles the shell of the common snail; it forms the anterior part of the labyrinth, is conical in form, and placed anterior to the vestibule; it measures about 5 mm from base to apex, and its breadth across the base is about 9 mm. Its apex, or *cupola*, is directed laterally towards the upper and front part of the medial wall of the tympanic cavity (7.285); its base is directed towards the bottom of the internal acoustic meatus, and is perforated by numerous apertures for the passage of the cochlear nerve. The cochlea consists of a cone-shaped central axis, the *modiolus*; of a canal, wound spirally around the central axis for roughly two turns and three-quarters; and of a delicate *osseous spiral lamina*, which projects from the modiolus into the canal, and partially divides it. In the recent state the division of the canal is completed by the *basilar membrane*, which stretches from the free border of the osseous spiral lamina to the outer wall of the bony cochlea; the two passages into which the cochlear canal is thus divided communicate with each other at the apex of the modiolus by a small opening, the *helicotrema*.

**The modiolus** is the conical, central pillar of the cochlea. Its base is broad, and appears at the lateral end of the internal acoustic meatus, where it corresponds with the *tractus spiralis foraminosus* (7.302), which is perforated by numerous orifices for the transmission of the branches of the cochlear nerve; the nerves for the first turn and a half of the cochlea pass through the foramina of the tractus spiralis; those for the apical turn, through the *foramen centrale*, in the centre of this tract. The canals of the tractus spiralis foraminosus pass through the modiolus and successively bend outwards to reach the attached margin of the osseous spiral lamina. Here they become enlarged, and by their apposition form the *spiral canal of the modiolus*, which follows the course of the attached margin of the osseous spiral lamina and lodges the *spiral ganglion*. The foramen centrale is continued into a canal which runs through the middle of the modiolus to its apex.

**The bony canal of the cochlea** takes about two turns and three-quarters round the modiolus; the first turn bulges towards the tympanic cavity and there underlies the promontory (p. 1140). It is about 30 mm long, and diminishes gradually in diameter from the base to the summit, where it ends in the *cupola*, which forms the apex of the cochlea. The beginning of this canal is about 3 mm in diameter, and in it there are three openings. One—the *fenestra cochleae*—communicates with the tympanic cavity and in life is closed by the *secondary tympanic membrane*; another is the *fenestra vestibuli* (p. 1141) occupied by the base of the stapes. The third is the aperture of the *cochlear canaliculus*, leading to a minute funnel-shaped canal which opens on the inferior surface of the petrous part of the temporal bone (p. 294). It transmits a small vein to join the inferior petrosal sinus, and establishes a communication between the subarachnoid space and the scala tympani (*vide infra*).

**The osseous spiral lamina** is a bony shelf or ledge which winds round and projects from the modiolus into the interior of the canal, like the thread of a screw. It reaches about halfway across the canal, and incompletely divides it into two passages or scalae: an upper, named the *scala vestibuli*, and a lower, the *scala tympani*. The width of the osseous spiral lamina gradually decreases from the basal to the apical coil of the cochlea, and near the summit of the cochlea the lamina ends in a hook-shaped process, the *hamulus of the spiral lamina*; this assists in forming the boundary of the *helicotrema*, through which the two scalae communicate with each other. From the spiral canal of the modiolus numerous canaliculi radiate through the osseous spiral lamina as far as its free edge and transmit branches of the cochlear nerve. In the lower part of the first turn of the cochlea a *secondary spiral lamina* projects inwards from the outer wall of the bony tube; it does not, however, reach the osseous spiral lamina, so that if the laminae be viewed from the vestibule a narrow *vestibular fissure* is seen between them.

buli and scala tympani, and throughout much of the vestibule, the perilymphatic cells which line the periosteum and cover the external surface of the membranous labyrinth are extremely flattened, with rather featureless cytoplasm. Despite occasional cytoplasmic projections into the neighbouring perilymph, in such situations the cellular arrangement approaches that of a true squamous epithelium. Over parts of the perilymphatic surface of the basilar membrane, the cells assume a cuboidal form. Closely related to the periosteal or membranous labyrinth aspect of the perilymphatic cells are bundles of collagen fibres which may, in part, be synthesized by these cells. However, in some species, fibres with a helical substructure, which differ from collagen in their ultrastructure, have been described in these situations. Their status in man remains to be determined.

**The perilymph** which occupies the perilymphatic spaces resembles cerebrospinal fluid fairly closely in its composition, although minor differences have been described.[1282] Many regard it simply as an ultrafiltrate of plasma, with perhaps some addition from the cerebrospinal fluid. Its precise source, rate of production, circu-

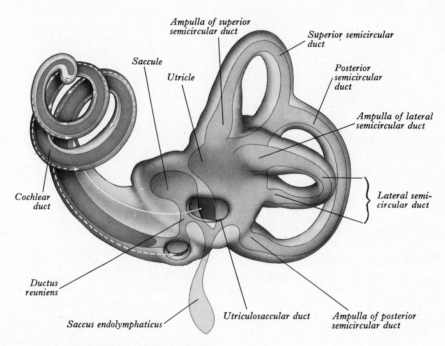

**7.294** Scheme of the membranous labyrinth (blue) projected on to the osseous labyrinth. The arrows indicate the direction of sound waves in the cochlea.

**The bony labyrinth** was classically described as being lined by a thin fibroserous membrane closely adherent to the periosteum of the neighbouring bone. The flattened epithelium of the membrane bounds the extensive *perilymphatic space*, the latter being filled with the fluid *perilymph* which bathes the external surface of the membranous labyrinth. However, ultrastructural studies have emphasized that the perilymphatic fluid-filled spaces are bounded by fibrocyte-like *perilymphatic cells*, with accompanying strands of extracellular fibres, the morphology of the cells varying in different parts of the labyrinth. Where the perilymphatic space is narrow, the cells are essentially *reticular* or *stellate* in form, their flattened sheet-like cytoplasmic extensions crossing and subdividing the perilymphatic space into a series of intercommunicating intercellular clefts of variable shapes and dimensions. Such tissue, and its accompanying spaces, occupies the cochlear canaliculus. Elsewhere, in regions where the perilymphatic space is much wider, as in the scala vesti-

lation and absorption, cannot yet be regarded as settled. The status of the connexions which exist between the perilymphatic spaces and the general subarachnoid space through the *cochlear canaliculus* has been the subject of some debate. Originally, the canaliculus was often described as containing a simple patent, epithelium-lined duct, which connected the two. Later, this suggestion was rejected by a number of workers[1283-1285] who proposed that connective tissue barriers blocked the canaliculus and separated the two fluid compartments. It seems likely, however, that extracellular crevices persist between the perilymphatic cells which occupy the canal; certainly, large-moleculed electron-dense tracers such as thorotrast, when introduced into the craniovertebral subarachnoid

[1282] F. C. Ormerod, *J. Lar. Otol.*, **74**, 1960.
[1283] J. G. Waltner, *Archs otolar.*, **47**, 1948.
[1284] S. H. Mygind, *Acta otolar.*, *Suppl.*, **68**, 1948.
[1285] M. W. Young, *Anat. Rec.*, **112** and **115**, 1952 and 1953.

space have a ready access to the perilymphatic spaces.[1286] Other investigators[1287] point out that in cats, even particulates such as india ink or avian erythrocytes, will pass into the perilymphatic spaces via the cochlear canaliculus within twenty-four hours after their introduction into the subarachnoid space of the posterial cranial fossa. The latter authors regard perilymph as probably originating from three sources: (1) a transudate from the blood vessels surrounding the spaces; (2) from the fluid spaces surrounding the sheaths of the vestibulocochlear nerve fibres; and (3) from a slow continuous flow of cerebrospinal fluid along the cochlear canaliculus. The site of removal of perilymph is uncertain.

The part of the petrous bone which immediately surrounds the labyrinth is developed from the cartilaginous ear capsule; it is denser than the rest of the petrous bone, and exhibits interglobular spaces, which contain cartilage cells (7.295). The modiolus of the cochlea, on the other hand, is formed of trabecular membrane bone.[1288]

The perilymphatic space of the vestibule communicates behind with that of the semicircular canals, and opens anteriorly into the scale vestibuli of the cochlea, which in turn opens into the scala tympani through the helicotrema, at the apex of the cochlea. The scala tympani is separated from the tympanic cavity by the secondary tympanic membrane, but is continuous with the subarachnoid space through the cochlear canaliculus (*vide supra*).

## The Membranous Labyrinth

The membranous labyrinth (7.294), while contained within, is much smaller than the bony labyrinth; it is filled with fluid unique in composition named *endolymph*, and in its walls the branches of the vestibulocochlear nerve are distributed. It includes: (*a*) the *utricle* and *saccule*, two small sacs, occupying the vestibule; (*b*) three *semicircular ducts*, enclosed within the semicircular canals; (*c*) the *duct of the cochlea*, contained within the bony cochlea. The various parts of the membranous labyrinth form a closed system of channels which, however, communicate freely with one another; the semicircular ducts open into the utricle and this into the saccule through the ductus utriculosaccularis which also joins the ductus endolymphaticus, and the saccule opens into the duct of the cochlea through the ductus reuniens.

The membranous labyrinth is fixed at certain points to the wall of the bony labyrinth, but is separated from the greater part of the bony labyrinth by a perilymphatic space (*vide supra*). For details of the fine structure of the membranous labyrinth consult footnote references [1290-1293].

### THE UTRICLE

The utricle, the larger of the two vestibular sacs, is irregularly oblong in shape, and occupies the posterosuperior region of the vestibule, lying in contact with the elliptical recess and also the area inferior to it. The part of the utricle in the elliptical recess forms a pouch or cul-de-sac; the lateral half of the floor and the adjoining lower part of the lateral wall of this pouch is thickened over an area measuring about 3 mm by 2 mm to form the *macula of the utricle* (p. 1151), which receives the utricular fibres of the vestibular nerve. The ampullae of the superior and lateral semicircular ducts open into the lateral part of the utricle, while the ampulla of the posterior duct, the crus commune and the posterior end of the lateral duct open into the medial part of the utricle. The posterior end of the lateral duct widens into a flattened cone which joins the medial end of the utricle at a right angle. From the anteromedial

part of the utricle a fine canal, named the *ductus utriculosaccularis*, is given off and opens into the ductus endolymphaticus.

### THE SACCULE

The saccule lies in the spherical recess near the opening of the scala vestibuli of the cochlea. When seen from the anterior aspect it presents a nearly globular form, but it is prolonged postero-inferiorly in the form of a cone, part of the upper surface of which is in contact with the under surface of the utricle, and the utricle and saccule have here a common wall. In its anterior wall there is an oval thickening, termed the *macula of the saccule* (pp. 1150, 1151), which lies in a plane at right angles to the macula of the utricle, and to which the saccular fibres of the vestibulocochlear nerve are distributed. Its cavity communicates indirectly through a Y-shaped tube with that of the utricle. From its posterior part the *ductus endolymphaticus* is given off and it is joined by the ductus utriculosaccularis; the ductus endolymphaticus passes medially and then inferiorly along the aqueduct of the vestibule to end in a blind pouch, the *saccus endolymphaticus*, under the dura mater on the posterior surface of the petrous portion of the temporal bone. From the lower part of the saccule a short tube, the *ductus reuniens*, passes inferiorly and gradually widens into the vestibular or basal end of the duct of the cochlea (7.294).

### THE SEMICIRCULAR DUCTS

The semicircular ducts (7.294, 295) are about one-fourth of the diameter of the semicircular canals, but are similar to them in shape and general form. Each has an ampulla at one end, which, of course, lies within the ampulla of the corresponding bony canal. The semicircular ducts open by five orifices into the utricle, one opening being common to the medial end of the superior, and the upper end of the posterior duct.

In each of the ampullae the wall is thickened, and projects into the cavity as a transverse elevation shaped somewhat like the figure 8, and named the *septum transversum*; the most prominent part of this septum being the *ampullary crest*, which projects from the wall of each ampulla that is most distant from the centre of the circle of which the semicircular duct forms an arc, a situation in which 'any movement of the endolymph would be caught by the crista to the greatest advantage'.[1289]

The utricle, saccule and semicircular ducts are held in position by fibrocellular bands which stretch across the perilymphatic space to the bony walls.

### STRUCTURE OF THE UTRICLE, SACCULE AND SEMICIRCULAR DUCTS

The walls of the utricle, saccule and semicircular ducts are commonly described as consisting of three layers. The *outer* layer is composed largely of fibrous tissue containing some blood vessels. Its superficial fibres are, in many places, clothed by flattened perilymphatic cells, and at some points this outer surface blends with the endosteum of the bony labyrinth. The *middle* layer, a more delicate vascular connective tissue, presents on its internal surface, especially in the semicircular ducts, a number of papilliform projections. The *inner* layer consists in general of a

[1286] A. J. Duvall and C. A. Quick, *Ann. Otol. Rhinol. Lar.*, **78**, 1969.
[1287] H. Silverstein, D. G. Davies and W. L. Griffin Jnr, *Ann. Otol. rhinol. Lar.*, **78**, 1969.
[1288] J. S. Fraser and J. K. M. Dickie, *J. Anat.* 49, 1914.
[1289] J. K. M. Dickie, *J. Laryngol.*, **35**, 1920.

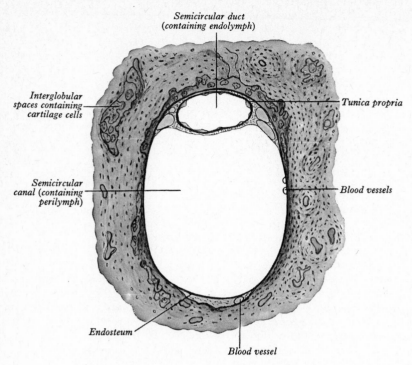

*Semicircular duct (containing endolymph)*

*Interglobular spaces containing cartilage cells*

*Tunica propria*

*Semicircular canal (containing perilymph)*

*Blood vessels*

*Endosteum*

*Blood vessel*

7.295 A transverse section through the left posterior semicircular canal and duct of an adult man. Magnification about × 50. (After Dr. J. K. Milne Dickie.)

single layer of epithelial cells, which vary from squamous to cubical or polygonal in shape, resting on a basement membrane; they exhibit a specialized arrangement in the ampullary crests of the semicircular ducts and in the maculae of the utricle and saccule (7.294, 296). In these special sites, also, the middle coat is thickened. Flanking each crest, between this and the side wall of the ampulla is an area of tall epithelium which in cross-section appears crescentic and is termed the *planum semilunatum.*

Although the non-specialized parts of the membranous labyrinth so far described have epithelia varying from squamous to tall columnar in different regions, ultrastructural studies[1290] have shown that they consist of either *light* or *dark* epithelial cells which are structurally quite dissimilar. In many regions the epithelium differs little from non-secretory simple epithelia elsewhere. The *light cells* comprising these regions contain elliptical or crenated heterochromatic nuclei, their luminal surfaces carry a few microvilli, and relatively few mitochondria, occasional ribosomes and some micropinocytotic vesicles occur in the cytoplasm. Adjacent cells show junctional complexes near their luminal borders, with also some interdigitation of neighbouring cell surfaces. Infolding of the basal plasmalemma is minimal. In contrast, some patches or strips of epithelium in the utricle and in the general and ampullated walls of the semicircular ducts consist of *dark cells.* These resemble light cells in a few respects only, their luminal surfaces carrying occasional microvilli and pinocytotic invaginations, whilst junctional complexes and interdigitations occur between adjacent cells. Their irregular nuclei are either centrally placed or situated rather near the luminal surface. The dense supranuclear cytoplasm contains numerous small coated vesicles, a profusion of larger smooth-walled vesicles, and many mitochondria, both free and membrane-attached polysomes, lipid droplets, lysosomes, lipofuscin granules, microfilaments and microtubules, and a prominent Golgi apparatus. The infranuclear part of the cell consists of numerous long cytoplasmic processes projecting towards the underlying basal lamina. Each process shows an

elongate, fusiform dilatation of its contour, completely occupied by a long narrow mitochondrion. The plasmalemma of the processes is clothed externally by electron-opaque extensions from the basal lamina. Clearly, such cells are highly active, and on general morphological grounds, and their structural similarity to cells in other ion-transporting epithelia such as those in parts of the renal tubules (p. 1322), the ciliary body, the parotid duct, and the salt-secreting glands of various sub-mammalian forms, it has been suggested that the dark cells may be involved in controlling the ionic composition of the endolymph (see also below).

In the *ampullary crests* the epithelium consists of *hair cells* and *supporting cells.* The hair cells are the sensory cells and are of two types.[1291, 1292] *Type I* is piriform with a rounded base and a short neck. Except for its free end it is surrounded by a large goblet-shaped nerve terminal or *chalice*; the apposed plasma membranes are separated by an interval of about 20–30 nm in width, but at a number of points the membranes approach each other more closely and the interval is reduced to about 5 nm. The nucleus of the hair cell is basally placed, and is surrounded by numerous mitochondria, and there is also a concentration of these organelles near the free surface of the cell. Scattered in the cytoplasm are occasional cisternae of granular endoplasmic reticulum, free polysomes, microfilaments and microtubules, numerous smooth vesicles about 20 nm in diameter, and a supranuclear Golgi apparatus is present.

The *type II* hair cell is cylindrical with its nucleus placed at varying levels, but usually more centrally placed than in the type I cell. Its cytoplasm contains similar organelles, but its population of smooth-walled vesicles is more abundant, and its supranuclear Golgi apparatus is more prominent. The basal part of the type II hair cell is not surrounded by a nerve terminal chalice, but instead is in contact with a number of bud-like synaptic *boutons.* The latter are of two varieties; both contain mitochondria and numerous small membranous vesicles, but in the *non-granulated terminals* the vesicles are clear, whereas in the *granulated terminals* many of the vesicles contain electron-dense cores. It is now generally accepted that the non-granulated terminals are those of *afferent* nerve fibres conducting sensory information towards the central nervous system. The granulated terminals are regarded as derived from efferent fibres which innervate the type II hair cells, activity in which probably modifies the effective threshold of the hair cell to sensory stimuli. Thus, the granulated and non-granulated terminals are both considered to be sites of neurochemical transmission, but of course, polarized in opposite directions; however, the details of this transmission remain uncertain. The chalice of the type I hair cell is also regarded as the terminal of an afferent vestibular fibre, but whether it operates mainly by neurochemical transmission, or whether low-resistance paths of the 'electrical synapse' type (p. 775) are extensively involved, is still to be determined. A number of granulated boutons are often present applied at points to the external aspect of the chalice, and probably these are efferent terminals which modify the transmission characteristics of the chalice.

In general, the type I hair cells may be regarded as the more discriminative variety. Their chalices are derived from the larger-diameter, faster-conducting vestibular nerve fibres, and each fibre innervates a small localized group of type I cells. In contrast, the type II cells receive boutons from a number of relatively small-diameter

[1290] R. S. Kimura, *Ann. Otol. Rhinol. Lar.,* **78**, 1969.
[1291] J. Wersäll, *Acta otolar., Suppl.,* **126**, 1956.
[1292] H. Engström and J. Wersäll, *Expl Cell Res.,* **14**, 1958.

vestibular nerve fibres, and each of the latter innervates a large number of type II cells which are distributed over a substantial area of membrane.

The apical, free surface of both types of hair cell are similar. They carry 40–100 'hairs' or stereocilia which are modified microvilli, of varying length and arranged in a regular hexagonal array when viewed from the surface. The array is, however, polarized with respect to a single long *kinocilium* which is attached to one border of the cell. The kinocilium possesses a typical basal body in the apical cytoplasm of the hair cell, and its shaft carries a ring of nine double microtubules, but the central pair of microtubules, which additionally characterize most other cilia, are sometimes less well developed and have even been claimed to be absent on occasion. Despite its name, any motile activity of this modified cilium remains uncertain. The stereocilia are non-motile microvilli, constricted at their point of attachment to the hair cell, and each contains a complement of longitudinal microfilaments which continue into a well-defined terminal web in the apical cytoplasm of the cell. On the border of the cell opposite to the kinocilium, the stereocilia are short, being about 1 $\mu$m in length, but those progressively nearer the cilium increase in length, reaching about 100 $\mu$m in the vicinity of the cilium.

In each of the specialized vestibular receptor sites, the hair cells are arranged in a precise pattern which is of great functional significance (*vide infra*). In the ampullae of the lateral semicircular ducts, the sides of the hair cells which bear a kinocilium are all directed towards the neighbouring utricular cavity, whilst in the ampullae of the superior and posterior ducts they are directed away from that cavity. In the maculae of the utricle and saccule, there is, in each, a sinuous 'parting line' which crosses the central region of the macula. The polarization of the hair cells is reversed on the opposite sides of this line. In the utricle the hair cells are arranged in curved contours with their kinocilia nearer the parting line, whilst in the saccule they are directed away from this line. For details of the complex relationship of these arrays of hair cells, to the three planes of space, consult footnote reference [1293]. The *supporting cells* are elongated and of variable diameter along their length. They rest on a basal lamina, and the nucleus is usually basal in position. The free surfaces are provided with microvilli, and the cytoplasm contains large osmiophilic granules which may be secretory in nature, in addition to a well-developed Golgi apparatus, numerous vertically running microtubules and microfilaments which enter a prominent subapical terminal web; mitochondria are plentiful. Whether the supporting cells are mainly involved in nutritive support of the hair cells, or in modifying the composition of the endolymph remains uncertain. Junctional complexes are established around the subapical parts of the hair cells and their neighbouring supporting cells. The processes of the hair cells and supporting cells project into a thick, dome shaped gelatinous protein-polysaccharide containing mass called the cupula. The precise chemical composition of the cupula is, however, undetermined. It possesses a free apical border which almost reaches the opposite ampullary wall. The whole cupula can swing from side to side in response to currents in the endolymph. After displacement in one direction, when the endolymph current ceases, an elastic recoil causes the return of the cupula towards the intermediate vertical position, but some overshoot and oscillation occurs, before it comes to rest.

The epithelial cells of the *planum semilunatum*[1294] lie adjacent to the crista on the one hand and gradually change to cuboidal epithelium of the side walls of the ampulla on the other. Their free surfaces are provided with a few microvilli. Basally they contain an abundance of parallel

smooth-walled double membranes, arranged perpendicular to the basement membrane. They are infoldings of the basal plasma membrane; they end in vesicular enlargements in the cytoplasm. Between the membrane pairs are vesicles and mitochondria arranged in a linear manner. The nucleus is placed towards the apical part of the cell where there are abundant mitochondria, endoplasmic reticulum, a well-developed Golgi apparatus, polyribosomes and vesicles, some of which contain

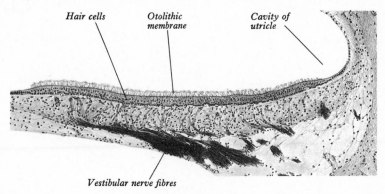

*Hair cells*   *Otolithic membrane*   *Cavity of utricle*

*Vestibular nerve fibres*

**7.296 A**   Section of the macula of the utricle of the cat. Stain—Weigert-Pal and iron haematoxylin. Magnification about ×112. (From a section kindly lent by Professor E. W. Walls.)

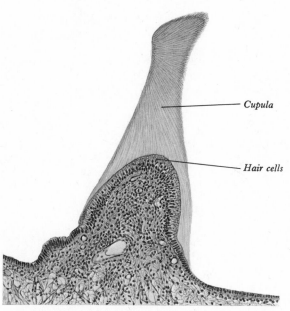

*Cupula*

*Hair cells*

**7.296 B**   Section of an ampullary crest of a six month old human fetus. Stained with haematoxylin and eosin. Magnification about ×75. (From a section kindly lent by Professor E. W. Walls, Middlesex Hospital Medical School, London.)

granules. It will be recalled that this description of the planum cells resembles that of the *dark cells* (*vide supra*) described by other investigators elsewhere in the labyrinth. The planum semilunatum is possibly concerned with the secretion of the endolymph. The *supporting* and *hair cells* of the *maculae* of the *utricle* and *saccule* are generally similar to those of the ampullary crests, but the gelatinous mass into which the cilia project is flatter and is termed an *otolithic membrane* because it contains numerous minute crystalline bodies called *otoliths* or

[1293] J. Babel, A. Bischoff and H. Spoendlin, *Ultrastructure of the Peripheral Nervous System and Sense Organs*, Churchill, London. 1970.

[1294] S. Iurato, *Submicroscopic Structure of the Inner Ear*, Pergamon Press, London, New York. 1967.

*otoconia*, which consist of calcite,[1295] and associated protein, and give the maculae, when fresh, an opaque white appearance.

The ampullary crests and the maculae of the utricle and saccule are the special end organs concerned with equilibratory vestibular reflexes influencing the position of the eyes in relation to movements of the head through the connexions of the vestibular nerves and their nuclei, via the medial longitudinal fasciculus (p. 885), with the nuclei of the third, fourth and sixth cranial nerves and influencing the general body musculature through the vestibulospinal tracts (p. 817). (The central connexions of the vestibular division of the vestibulocochlear nerve and its intimate relationship with the vestibulocerebellum are considered on pp. 852, 861, 863, 876.) Muscle activity is also influenced by the *position* of the head, and in this

The manner in which deformation of the stereocilia, consequent upon movement of the cupulae or otolithic membrane, results in alteration of the ionic conductances of the hair cell membrane is not understood. However, it has been proposed, on the basis of electrophysiological recordings, that the majority of the vestibular nerve fibres have a steady, continuous basal discharge of afferent nerve impulses when the hair cells are receiving no mechanical stimulation. Bending of the stereocilia towards the kinocilium raises the frequency of nerve impulses, whilst bending in the opposite direction lowers the frequency. Thus, the position of the head, or its state of linear or angular acceleration, is reflected by the state of balance or relative imbalance in the impulse discharge patterns from mutually cooperative pairs of receptor sites in the right and left membranous labyrinths. For

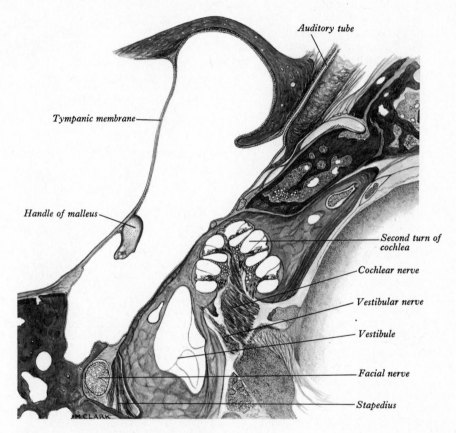

7.297   A horizontal section through the left temporal bone. (Drawn from a section prepared at the Ferens Institute and kindly lent by the late Professor J. Kirk.)

case the maculae of the utricle and saccule are the end organs concerned in that the otoliths, under the influence of gravity, exert traction on the cilia of the hair cells in varying positions of the head. The maculae are therefore often referred to as organs of static balance (statotonic reflexes), whereas the ampullary crests are called organs of kinetic balance in that they are stimulated by movement of, or pressure changes in, the endolymph caused by *angular acceleration* of the head (statokinetic reflexes) producing deviation of the cupulae. The maculae, however, may also be involved in signalling *linear acceleration* of the head. The terms static and kinetic as used above, therefore, are an oversimplification. The macula of the saccule, although it has the same histological structure as the macula of the utricle, is believed by some not to be concerned in vestibular reflexes but to be associated with the cochlea and concerned with the reception of slow vibrational (auditory) stimuli.

example, a horizontal swing of the head to the right results in an increased discharge of impulses from the ampulla of the right lateral semicircular duct, and a decreased discharge from the left. This occurs because the inertia of the endolymph causes a relative movement of this fluid to the left in both these canals. The positioning of the kinocilia and stereocilia in the ampullae is such that it results in their compression in the right ampulla, and their decompression in the left. (For further discussion of post-rotational effects, the effects of more complex movements in other planes, and methods of testing vestibular functional efficiency, see footnote reference [1296].)

[1295] D. Carlström, H. Engström and S. Hjorth, *Laryngoscope, St. Louis,* **63**, 1953.

[1296] J. Fischer, *The Labyrinth: Physiology and Functional Tests*, Grune and Stratton, N.Y. 1956.

## THE ENDOLYMPHATIC DUCT AND SAC

Throughout the endolymphatic duct, its surface cells closely resemble those lining the other non-specialized parts of the membranous labyrinth. As mentioned earlier, the duct continues into a blind-ended saccus endolymphaticus which expands under the dura mater on the posterior surface of the petrous temporal bone. Here the saccus is surrounded by a well-vascularized connective tissue, and its epithelium changes to tall columnar cells of two main types. The one variety has fairly dense cytoplasm, but is otherwise unspecialized. The other type is less dense, its luminal surface bears a profusion of long microvilli, and its cytoplasm carries numerous mitochondria, pinocytotic invaginations and vesicles, and larger smooth-walled vacuoles.

**The endolymph** which fills the different parts of the membranous labyrinth contrasts sharply in its composition with the perilymph which surrounds it externally. Whilst the latter is roughly comparable with extracellular tissue fluid or cerebrospinal fluid, the endolymph resembles intracellular fluid in its ionic composition, being rich in potassium ions, but poor in sodium ions. It is widely accepted that endolymph is a form of secretion, but its precise source is still an open question. The various structures considered to be involved in its production include the *dark cells* of the utricle and semicircular ducts, the columnar cells of the *planum semilunatum*, and the specialized epithelial cells and related blood vessels of the *stria vascularis* of the cochlear duct (*vide infra*). Whatever the relative contributions from these different sources, it is thought that the endolymph circulates and then enters the ductus endolymphaticus to be removed by the specialized epithelial cells of the saccus into the surrounding vascular plexus. Pinocytotic removal of fluid in other parts of the labyrinth is, however, not excluded.

A unique positive electrical potential exists in the endolymphatic spaces. This varies from $+77$ millivolts in the cochlear duct near the stria vascularis, to about $+4$ millivolts in the utricle, whilst it is absent or even negative in the ampullae of the semicircular ducts. Thus, a very large difference of potential of some 150 millivolts exists across the cell membrane of the cochlear hair cells, between the cochlear endolymph and the cell interior. This may account in part for the extreme sensitivity to mechanical deformation shown by these *auditory* hair cells (*vide infra*).

## THE COCHLEAR DUCT

The duct of the cochlea (7.297, 298) consists of a spirally arranged tube within the bony canal of the cochlea and lying along its outer wall.

As already stated (p. 1148), the osseous spiral lamina extends only part of the distance between the modiolus and the outer wall of the cochlea, while the *basilar membrane* stretches from the free edge of the lamina to the outer wall of the cochlea, and completes the roof of the scala tympani. The endosteum of the outer wall of the cochlea is thickened to form the *spiral ligament of the cochlea*; it projects inwards and to it is attached the outer edge of the basilar membrane. A second and more delicate *vestibular membrane*, extends from the thickened endosteum covering the osseous spiral lamina to the outer wall of the cochlea, where it is attached at some distance above the outer edge of the basilar membrane. A canal is thus shut off between the scala tympani below and the scala vestibuli above; this is the *duct of the cochlea* (7.298). It is triangular on transverse section, its roof being formed by the vestibular membrane, its outer wall by the endosteum lining the bony canal, and its floor by the basilar membrane and the outer part of the osseous spiral lamina.

The upper extremity of the duct of the cochlea is closed, and is named the *lagaena*; it is attached to the cupola (p. 1147). The lower end turns medially, and narrows into the *ductus reuniens*, through which it communicates with the saccule (7.294). The spiral organ is situated on the basilar membrane. The vestibular membrane is thin and is covered on its two surfaces by a layer of flattened epithelium. The endosteum forming the outer wall of the duct of the cochlea is greatly thickened and forms the spiral ligament. It projects inwards, inferiorly, as a triangular prominence, termed the *crista basilaris*, to which the outer edge of the basilar membrane is fixed; immediately above this there is a concavity (the *sulcus spiralis externus*), above which the periosteum is thickened, highly vascular and forms a surface projection, the *spiral prominence*, which above this again continues into a specialized periosteal zone, the *stria vascularis*.

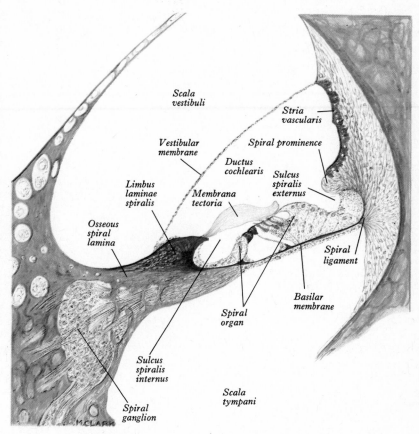

7.298 A section through the second turn of the cochlea indicated in the previous figure. (Mallory's stain.)

Ultrastructural studies have added many details concerning these different regions, including many features of the spiral organ. These can only be touched on briefly here, and the interested reader should consult footnote reference [1297] and its extensive bibliography.

## THE VESTIBULAR MEMBRANE

The vestibular membrane (of Reissner) consists of two layers of flattened epithelial cells with an intervening basal lamina. The aspect facing the scala vestibuli is clothed with perilymphatic cells which are fairly thick in their central perinuclear zone, but elsewhere the cytoplasm is extremely attenuated; adjacent cells establish zonulae occludentes between them. The endolymphatic surface is

[1297] J. Babel, A. Bischoff and H. Spoendlin, *Ultrastructure of the pheral Nervous System and Sense Organs*, Churchill, London. 1970.

covered with typical squamous epithelial cells, again joined by zonulae occludentes. Their cytoplasm contains a number of mitochondria and numerous vesicles; the basal surface is sometimes smooth but often complexly invaginated into the cell; the free surface carries numerous, short, irregular microvilli. These cells may be involved in fluid transport.

## THE STRIA VASCULARIS

The stria vascularis, as noted above, lies on the outer wall of the cochlear duct immediately above the spiral eminence. It is unique in possessing a specialized stratified epithelium which carries a rich plexus of *intraepithelial capillaries*. The epithelium consists of three cell types: (1) superficially placed *marginal, dark* or *chromophil cells*; (2) *intermediate, light,* or *chromophobe cells*; and (3) *basal cells*.

The endolymphatic surface is formed exclusively by the dark cells. The intermediate and basal cells are cytologically similar, differing merely in position. Their pale cytoplasm contains scattered mitochondria, numerous pinocytotic vesicles and a number of melanin granules. These cells send cytoplasmic processes towards the surface, where they are insinuated between and around the deeper parts of the marginal cells.

immediately dependent upon an adequate oxygenation level of the epithelial cells, provided by the blood circulation through its intra-epithelial capillaries.

## THE OSSEOUS SPIRAL LAMINA

The osseous spiral lamina consists of two plates of bone, and between these are the canals for the transmission of the filaments of the cochlear nerve. On the upper plate of that part of the lamina which is contained within the duct of the cochlea the periosteum is thickened to form the *limbus laminae spiralis* (7.298, 299); this ends externally in a concavity, the *sulcus spiralis internus*, which presents, on section, the form of the letter C; the upper part formed by the overhanging edge of the limbus is the *vestibular lip*; the lower part, prolonged and tapering, is the *tympanic lip*, and is perforated by numerous foramina for the passage of the branches of the cochlear nerve. The upper surface of the vestibular lip is intersected at right angles by a number of furrows, separated by numerous elevations; these present the appearance of teeth on the free surface and margin of the lip, the *auditory teeth* (7.299). The limbus is covered by a layer of what appears from surface view to be squamous epithelium, but only the cells covering the teeth are flattened, those in the furrows (7.299) being columnar, and occupying the intervals

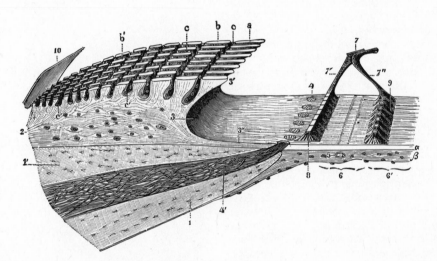

7.299 The limbus laminae spiralis and the basilar membrane. Schematic, after Testut. 1, 1'. Lower and upper lamellae of the lamina spiralis ossea. 2. Limbus laminae spiralis, with a, the auditory teeth of the first row; b, b', the teeth of the other rows; c, c', the grooves between the auditory teeth and the cells which are lodged in them. 3. Sulcus spiralis internus, with 3', its labium vestibulare, and 3", its labium tympanicum.

4. Foramina nervosa, giving passage to the nerves from the spiral ganglion. 5. Vas spirale. 6. Zona arcuata, and 6', zona pectinata of the basilar membrane, with α, its hyaline layer, β, its connective tissue layer. 7. Summit of the tunnel of Corti, with 7', its inner rod, and 7", its outer rod. 8. Bases of the inner rods, from which the cells are removed. 9. Bases of the outer rod. 10. Part of the vestibular membrane.

The marginal dark cells are highly specialized, with a dense granular cytoplasm containing many mitochondria and pinocytotic vesicles. The deep part of the cell consists of many long cytoplasmic processes separated by deep invaginations of the plasmalemma; each process contains a series of mitochondria. The intra-epithelial capillaries are closely enveloped both by descending processes from the dark cells and ascending processes from the intermediate and basal cells.

The stria vascularis is considered to be an ion transporting mechanism which maintains the unique ionic composition of the endolymph. As indicated above, however, other regions of the membranous labyrinth may also be involved in this activity. It has been established by exploration of the stria with microelectrodes that it is the source of the large positive endocochlear electrical potential. The maintenance of this potential is directly and

between the elevations. This epithelium is continuous on the one hand with that lining the sulcus spiralis internus, and on the other with that covering the under surface of the vestibular membrane. It is considered by some observers that the interdental cells secrete the material forming the tectorial membrane (*vide infra*).

## THE BASILAR MEMBRANE

The basilar membrane (7.298, 299) stretches from the tympanic lip of the osseous spiral lamina to the crista basilaris. It consists of two zones, a thin *zona arcuata*, stretching from its medial attachment, the limbus spiralis, to the bases of the outer rods and supporting the organ of Corti, and an outer thicker part, the *zona pectinata*, commencing beneath the bases of the outer rods and attached laterally to the crista basilaris. The zona arcuata is seen by electron microscopy to be composed of compact bundles of small collagen-like filaments 8–10 nm in diameter, mainly disposed radially. In the zona pectinata the membrane is three-layered with an upper layer composed of a homogeneous network of similar filaments, a lower layer of compact bundles of these filaments and an intermediate structureless layer containing a few nuclei. At its attachment to the crista basilaris, the upper and lower layers fuse and the membrane consists of one layer. The width of the basilar membrane gradually increases from 0·21 mm in the basal turn to 0·36 mm in the apical turn of the cochlea, and this increase is accompanied by a corresponding narrowing of the osseous spiral lamina, and a decrease in the thickness of the crista basilaris. The under surface of the membrane is covered by a layer of vascular connective tissue and flattened perilymphatic cells; one of the vessels in the connective tissue is larger than the rest, and is named the *vas spirale*; it lies below Corti's tunnel.

## THE SPIRAL ORGAN OF CORTI

The spiral organ[1297–1299] (7.298, 300) is composed of a series of epithelial structures placed upon the zona arcuata of the basilar membrane. The more central of these structures are two rows of rod-like bodies, the *inner and outer rods of Corti* or *pillar cells*. The bases or *foot plates* of the rods are expanded, and rest on the basilar membrane, those of the inner row at some distance from those of the outer; the two rows incline towards each other and, coming into contact above, enclose between them and the basilar membrane the *tunnel of Corti* (7.301), which is triangular in cross-section. On the medial side of the inner rods there is a single row of *inner hair cells*, and on the lateral side of the outer rods, three or four rows of *outer hair cells*, together with certain supporting cells, the *phalangeal cells of Deiters*, and the *cells of Hensen*. The free ends of the outer hair cells occupy a series of apertures in a net-like membrane, termed the *reticular lamina*, and the entire organ is covered by the *tectorial membrane*. In addition to the tunnel of Corti, sometimes termed the *inner tunnel*, described above, other spaces exist in relation to the outer hair cells which connect through intercellular crevices with each other and with the inner tunnel. These include the *outer tunnel* situated between the outermost hair cells and the inner cells of Hensen, beneath the reticular lamina, and the *space of Nuel* between the outer rods of Corti and the outer hair cells. The latter is continuous with the extracellular spaces which surround the upper two-thirds of the outer hair cells. This complex system of intercommunicating spaces is filled with a fluid termed *cortilymph* which is not continuous with either perilymph or endolymph, and is probably distinct in its chemical constitution.[1300]

**The rods or pillars of Corti** each consists of a base or foot plate, an elongated part or body, and an upper end or head; each foot plate and head is closely applied to its neighbour but the bodies are separate from each other. The nucleus lies in the triangular foot plate. The body of each rod is finely striated, but in the head there is an oval nonstriated portion which stains deeply with carmine. Electron microscopy shows many microtubules 13–15 nm in diameter, often arranged in parallel bundles, running lengthwise in the body of the rods and then diverging above to terminate in a superficial layer of dense granular cytoplasm, the *cuticle*, in the head. Below, the microtubules arise over a wide area of the limiting membrane of the foot plate from the cytoplasmic densities of an array of hemidesmosomes. Within the body of the rod, transverse sections show that the microtubules are often arranged in a regular square lattice. Detailed

analysis of the upper termination of the microtubules shows that many of them curve into the reticular lamina (*vide infra*) to end in junctional complexes (p. 6; **1.4**) established with either similar expansions from the supporting cells of Deiters or with the subapical lateral surfaces of the hair cells. The nucleated cytoplasmic zones which partly envelop the rods and extend on to the floor of Corti's tunnel, occupy the angles between the rods and the basilar membrane; these may be looked upon as the less differentiated parts of the cells from which the rods have been formed.

The *inner rods* number nearly 6,000, and their bases rest on the basilar membrane close to the tympanic lip of the sulcus spiralis internus. The body of each is sinuously curved and forms an angle of about 60° with the basilar membrane. The head resembles the proximal end of the ulna, and presents a deep concavity which accommodates a convexity on the head of the outer rod. The head plate, or portion overhanging the concavity, overlaps the head plate of the outer rod.

The *outer rods*, nearly 4,000 in number, are longer and more obliquely set than the inner, forming with the basilar membrane an angle of about 40°. Their heads are convex internally; they fit into the concavities on the heads of the inner rods, and are continued outwards as thin flattened plates, the *phalangeal processes*, which unite

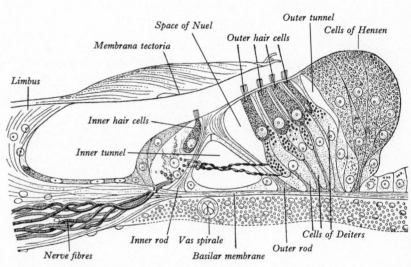

7.300 A transverse section through the spiral organ. Note that the separation shown between the stereocilia of the hair cells and the membrana tectoria is an artefact due to the preparative technique employed.

with the phalangeal processes of Deiters' cells to form the *reticular membrane* (*vide infra*).

The distances between the bases of the inner and outer rods increase from the base to the apex of the cochlea, while the angles between the rods and the basilar membrane diminish.

**The hair cells** are short columnar or piriform cells depending upon their site in the spiral organ; their free ends are on a level with the heads of the rods of Corti, and each is surmounted by about 50–100 hair-like stereocilia. The deep ends of the cells reach about halfway along the rods of Corti, and each contains a large open-faced euchromatic nucleus. The plasma membrane at the basal pole of the cell forms synaptic contacts with cochlear

[1298] C. A. Smith and E. W. Dempsey, *Am. J. Anat.*, **100**, 1957.
[1299] H. Engström and J. Wersäll, *Expl Cell Res.*, **14**, 1958.
[1300] H. Engström, in: *Neural Mechanisms of the Auditory and Vestibular Systems*, Thomas, Springfield. 1960.

nerve fibres. The cytology and supporting structures vary with the position of the hair cells, which are arranged as inner and outer groups set at an angle to each other. The *inner* hair cells, about 3,500 in number, are arranged in a single row on the inner side of the inner rods of Corti, and since their diameters are greater than those of the rods, each is related to more than one rod. The free ends of the inner hair cells are encircled by a cuticular membrane which is fixed to the heads of the inner rods (*vide infra*). Adjoining the inner hair cells there are one or two rows of columnar supporting cells, which, in turn, are continuous with the cubical cells lining the sulcus spiralis internus. The columnar supporting cells which lie adjacent to the inner rods of Corti and surround the inner hair cells are the *inner phalangeal cells*. These are succeeded medially by slender columnar *border cells* of decreasing height which gradually merge medially into the cuboidal epithelium of the sulcus mentioned above. The *outer* hair cells number about 12,000 and are nearly twice as long as the inner. In the basal coil of the cochlea they are arranged in three regular rows; in the apical coil, in four or five less regular rows.

Electron microscopy has added much about the detailed construction of the cochlear hair cells and their supporting structures (see for example footnote reference [1297]). Briefly, the **inner hair cells** resemble in some respects the type I vestibular hair cells described previously (p. 1150). Each possesses a relatively short piriform body, the expanded basal region containing a large, 'open-faced' euchromatic nucleus; this is surmounted by a constricted 'neck' which on its free apical surface carries 50–60 hairs or stereocilia, but no kinocilium. The cell cytoplasm contains free polysomes, many smooth-walled vesicles of varying diameter and subapically, a well-developed terminal web beneath which numerous mitochondria are clustered. The stereocilia resemble in structure those of vestibular hair cells; they vary in length and diameter, possess a constricted base, and their cores contain a leash of longitudinal microfilaments in a granular cytoplasm. Basally, the filaments become continuous with the terminal web. The stereocilia are clothed by an extension of the apical plasma membrane of the hair cell, and their tips enter, and are apparently tightly bound to, the tectorial membrane (*vide infra*). Although a kinocilium is absent, there is present in the surface cytoplasm near one edge of the cell a well-developed basal plate and centriole. When viewed from the surface, the stereocilia are arranged in two rows in the form of a U or flat W, the base of which is directed towards the site of the centriole. The plasma membrane at the basal pole of the cell is in synaptic contact with two types of synaptic boutons derived from cochlear nerve fibres. The terminals of *afferent* fibres contain relatively few mitochondria and microtubules, and a number of clear vesicles of varying diameter. Both the presynaptic (hair cell) and postsynaptic (bouton) membranes are thickened, the latter more markedly, and the presynaptic cytoplasm contains aggregates of both clear and dense-cored synaptic vesicles. *Accessory synaptic structures* which take the form of electron-dense rods, rings or lamellae around which synaptic vesicles are clustered, are commonly present. The bouton terminals of *efferent* fibres, in contrast, contain a number of mitochondria, microtubules and a profusion of synaptic vesicles, the majority of which are small, spherical and clear, but some are larger with dense cores. Although often described as making synaptic contact with the base of the inner hair cells, it has now been shown that the efferent terminals never make such contacts in the cat, and only infrequently in the guinea-pig and man. Much more numerous are contacts between the efferent terminal and the lateral

aspect of an *afferent fibre bouton*. Presumably activity in the efferent fibre modulates the transmission characteristics of the afferent fibre terminal. The inner hair cells are, apart from their areas of synaptic contact just described, wholly surrounded by the cytoplasm of the inner phalangeal supporting cells. The superficial rim of the latter, where it encircles the lateral margin of the apical surface of the hair cell, is joined to it by a circular zone which, in section, is seen to consist of a junctional complex (p. 6; 1.5). Similar specialized junctions exist between the outer aspect of the rim of the phalangeal cell and expansions from the inner rod of Corti. These surface specializations make up the 'cuticular membrane' of light microscopy mentioned above.

**The outer hair cells** are more highly specialized than the inner, although they have a number of features in common. They are considerably longer cells, columnar in form, with a large euchromatic basally-placed nucleus. Numerous mitochondria are found around the nucleus, along the lateral walls of the cell close to the plasmalemma, and beneath the well-defined, subapical terminal web. In the latter position there are also a number of cisternae of granular endoplasmic reticulum and scattered lysosomes. As with the inner cells there is no kinocilium, and the stereocilia have a similar structure. However, they often number about 100, and are on average longer than those of the inner cells, the longest being found near the cell margin. They usually occur in three or four rows, again arranged in surface view in the form of a flattened W, the base of which is directed towards an eccentrically placed centriole. Both the inner and outer hair cells are so arranged on the basilar membrane that their centrioles are on the side of the cell which is most distant from the central modiolus. This observation is of considerable functional significance and suggests that transverse shearing forces between the hair cells and tectorial membrane would be the most effective in stimulating the sensory receptors.

The basal pole of each outer hair cell is received into a cup-like depression on the upper end of an outer phalangeal cell of Deiters (*vide infra*), except at the synaptic contacts with cochlear nerve fibres. In this case, however, both the afferent and efferent terminals, which are structurally similar to those of the inner cells, are functionally related directly to the plasma membrane of the hair cell itself.[1301]

**The outer phalangeal cells of Deiters** (7.300), are placed between the rows of the outer hair cells; their expanded bases are planted on the basilar membrane, while the opposite end of each presents, as mentioned above, an asymmetrical cup-like region, partially enveloping the base of a hair cell, and a finger-like *phalangeal process*, which extends up between the hair cells to the reticular membrane (*vide infra*). The cytoplasm of Deiters' cells contain bundles of microtubules, which arise from basally placed hemidesmosomes, and which continue upwards into the phalangeal process. Immediately to the outer side of Deiters' cells there are five or six rows of columnar cells, the *supporting cells of Hensen* (7.300). Their free surfaces are also beset with microvilli. Near the lagaena these cells contain fat globules which decrease in number and size as the duct of the cochlea is traced towards the basal coil. It has been suggested[1302] that these globules provide a graduated loading mechanism, which tunes the region of the lagaena to low tones.

**The reticular lamina** (7.301), when viewed with a light microscope, appears as a delicate framework per-

[1301] H. Engström, H. W. Ades and J. E. Hawkins Jnr, in: *Contributions to Sensory Physiology*, ed. W. D. Neff, Academic Press, New York. 1965.
[1302] C. S. Hallpike, *J. Physiol., Lond.*, **73**, 1931.

forated by circular holes which are occupied by the free ends of the outer hair cells. It extends from the heads of the outer rods of Corti to the external row of the outer hair cells, and is formed by several rows of minute fiddle-shaped cuticular structures, called *phalanges*, between which are circular apertures containing the free ends of the hair cells. The innermost row of phalanges consists of the phalangeal processes of the outer rods of Corti; the outer rows are formed by the modified free ends of Deiters' cells. Electron microscopy has now shown that the reticular lamina consists of these horizontal expansions from the outer rods and phalangeal cells which carry bundles of microtubules in the attenuated veil of cytoplasm which they contain. The expansions encircle the upper-most rim of the hair cells, where junctional complexes are formed, and in which the microtubules end. Beneath this delicate supporting system, the upper two-thirds of the lateral surfaces of the outer hair cells are not in contact with supporting cells, but are bathed by the fluid termed cortilymph (*vide supra*).

**The membrana tectoria** (7.300) overlies the sulcus spiralis internus and the spiral organ of Corti. It consists, in fixed preparations, of delicate fibres embedded in a jelly-like matrix. In electron microscopic preparations filaments of 4 nm diameter are seen; they consist of protein which resembles keratin, associated with mucopolysaccharides. The membrana tectoria is wider and thicker in the apical than in the basal part of the cochlea. Its inner part is thin and is attached to the vestibular lip of the limbus laminae spiralis, the attachment reaching as far as the vestibular membrane. The outer part is thick and padlike, the thickness being greatest over, or slightly to the inner side of, the upper ends of the rods of Corti. The *interdental cells* of the vestibular lip to which the tectorial membrane is attached have a well-developed Golgi apparatus, numerous mitochondria, and free polysomes; it is thought that they secrete the membrane. The tips of the hair cell stereocilia are embedded in, and firmly attached to, the tectorial membrane, but this attachment is often broken during histological preparation (7.300).

**The vestibulocochlear nerve** divides near the lateral end of the internal acoustic meatus into an anterior or *cochlear*, and a posterior or *vestibular* portion. (The central connexions and proximal parts of these nerves are described on pp. 1016, 1017.)

The *vestibular nerve* supplies the utricle, the saccule and the ampullae of the semicircular ducts. The *vestibular ganglion*, from the bipolar nerve cells of which the fibres of the nerve take origin, is situated in the trunk of the nerve within the internal acoustic meatus. On the distal side of the ganglion the nerve splits into a superior, an inferior and a posterior branch. (The nerve sometimes splits on the proximal side of the ganglion, which is then also divided into three parts, one in each branch of the nerve. When this occurs, the ganglion of the posterior division is placed in the foramen singulare.) The filaments of the *superior branch* are transmitted through the foramina in the superior vestibular area, and end in the macula of the utricle and in the ampullary crests of the superior and lateral semicircular ducts; those of the *inferior branch* traverse the foramina in the inferior vestibular area, and end in the macula of the saccule. The *posterior branch* runs through the foramen singulare at the posteroinferior part of the bottom of the meatus (7.302) and divides into filaments for the supply of the ampullary crest of the posterior semicircular duct.

The *cochlear nerve*, the nerve of hearing, divides into numerous filaments at the base of the modiolus; those for the basal and middle coils pass through the foramina in the tractus spiralis foraminosus, those for the apical coil through the central canal, and the nerves bend outwards

and pass between the lamellae of the osseous spiral lamina. The *spiral ganglion* (7.298), consisting of bipolar nerve cells from which the fibres of the nerve take origin, occupies the spiral canal of the modiolus. Reaching the outer edge of the osseous spiral lamina, the nerve fibres lose their myelin sheaths and pass through the foramina in the tympanic lip; some end by arborizing around the deep ends of the inner hair cells, while others pass between the rods of Corti and across the tunnel of Corti, and end in relation to the outer hair cells. The latter pass between the cells of Deiters and are often enfolded by them. The hair cells in the basal and middle coils are more richly supplied with nerves than those in the apical coil. The cochlear nerve gives off a vestibular branch to supply the vestibular end of the duct of the cochlea; the filaments of this branch traverse the foramina in the cochlear recess (p. 1146).

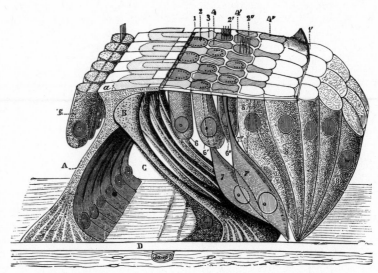

7.301 The reticular lamina and subjacent structures. Scheme based upon light microscope observations. See text for ultrastructural details. A. Inner rod of Corti, with *a*, its head. B. Outer rod (in yellow). C. Tunnel of Corti. D. Basilar membrane. E. Inner hair cells. 1, 1′. Internal and external borders of the reticular lamina. 2, 2′, 2″. The three rows of circular holes (in blue). 3. First row of phalanges (in yellow). 4, 4′, 4″. Second, third, and fourth rows of phalanges (in red). 6, 6′, 6″. The three rows of outer hair cells (in blue). 7, 7′, 7″. Cells of Deiters. 8. Cells of Hensen and Claudius.

The structure of the terminal boutons of the efferent and afferent nerve fibres was described above. The efferent nerve fibres belong to the olivocochlear system first described by Rasmussen.[1303] It is now established that this bundle contains both crossed and uncrossed components; the former start from the opposite retro-lateral olivary group of neurons, whilst the latter arise from the so-called S-shaped segment of the ipsilateral olivary complex.[1304] The pharmacology of the pathway is obscure, but it is apparently purely inhibitory in its actions, and alters the threshold level of the outer hair cells, and modifies the transmission through the afferent fibres from the inner hair cells.

The detailed distribution of nerve fibres to the inner and outer rows of hair cells is now known in considerable detail. Briefly, the vast majority of the cochlear nerve fibres are distributed to the inner hair cells. The latter each receive the terminals of a number of radially disposed afferent fibres, which are themselves in receipt of synaptic terminals from collateral branches of radially disposed

[1303] G. L. Rasmussen, *J. comp. Neurol.*, **84**, 1946.
[1304] I. C. Whitfield, *The Auditory Pathway*, Arnold, London. 1967.

inhibitory efferent fibres. The outer hair cells receive the minority of the cochlear nerve fibres. Their efferent fibres are radial in disposition and each fibre establishes inhibitory synapses with a large number of hair cells. The afferent fibres curve into a geometrically organized spiral system of fibres, each of which innervates numerous hair cells. (For proposals concerning the possible functional significance of these arrangements, consult footnote reference [1305].)

**The arteries of the labyrinth** are: (1) the labyrinthine artery (p. 644), which may arise from the basilar artery, but is more often derived from the anterior inferior cerebellar artery; and (2) the stylomastoid branch of the posterior auricular artery. The labyrinthine artery divides at the bottom of the internal acoustic meatus into cochlear and vestibular rami. The cochlear branch subdivides into twelve to fourteen twigs, which traverse the canals in the modiolus, and are distributed, in the form of a capillary network, in the lamina spiralis and basilar membrane. The vestibular branches are distributed to the utricle, saccule and semicircular ducts.

**The veins** of the vestibule and semicircular canals accompany the arteries, and, receiving the veins of the cochlea at the base of the modiolus, unite to form the labyrinthine vein, which ends in the posterior part of the superior petrosal sinus or in the transverse sinus. A small vein, from the basal turn of the cochlea, traverses the cochlear canaliculus and joins the internal jugular vein.

## THE MECHANISM OF THE AUDITORY RECEPTORS

Many elegant researches have been directed towards an understanding of the role of the different components of the ears, as analysers of the intensity and frequency patterns, and source location, of the sound wave trains which impinge upon them. These are beyond the scope of a general textbook of anatomy, and monographs and original papers should be consulted.

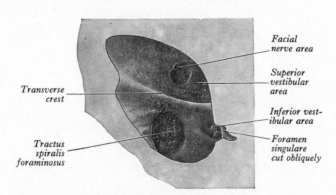

7.302 A view of the lateral end of the right internal acoustic meatus.

In outline, sound waves which reach the air column in the external acoustic meatus cause a comparable set of vibrations in the tympanic membrane, and thus in the chain of auditory ossicles. Similar vibrations occur at the foot plate of the stapes, but here the force per unit area of the oscillating surface is increased some twentyfold. These are effective in overcoming the inertia of the perilymph thus producing pressure waves within it, which are conducted almost instantaneously to all parts of the basilar membrane. The latter varies continuously in its width, mass, and stiffness from the basal to the apical end of the cochlea, but its component fibres are *not* under tension. The behaviour of such a mechanical system, when exposed to a periodic oscillating pressure wave in the neighbouring perilymph, varies with the frequency of the oscillations. At very low frequencies, for example 50 hz, the whole basilar membrane vibrates in phase, and at a similar frequency. As the frequency of the driving fluid pressure waves rises, the different parts of the basilar membrane oscillate less rapidly, and increasingly out of phase, from the basal to the apical end of the cochlea. Consequently, a series of *travelling waves* progresses along the membrane from the base towards the apex. At intermediate frequencies, the *amplitude* of these travelling waves rises slowly as they progress from the basal end, until a maximum amplitude is reached, after which point the amplitude falls rapidly on the apical side of the maximum. With increasing frequency of the driving oscillation, the *position* of the *maximum amplitude* of vibration of the basilar membrane moves progressively from the apical, towards the basal end of the cochlea. The evidence concerning such a distribution of vibration patterns in the basilar membrane stems from three main sources: (1) direct observation of the membrane in cadavers, through drill holes in the bone, using stroboscopic illumination; (2) electrophysiological recording of the *cochlear microphonic potential*, which summates the total electrical activity over short lengths of the hair cell-bearing basilar membrane; and (3) the effects of focal destructive lesions at different points along the membrane.

The vibration pattern of the basilar membrane thus varies with the intensity and frequency of the sound wave train reaching the perilymph. Because of their position and attachment, such oscillations cause a mainly transverse shearing force to be generated between the hair cells carried by the basilar membrane, and the overlying tectorial membrane in which the tips of the stereocilia are embedded. When the position of the oscillating membrane is such that the shearing force compresses the stereocilia towards the site of the centriole (p. 1156), the rate of impulse discharge in the related auditory nerve fibres increases. Since at most intermediate frequencies an appreciable length of the basilar membrane is oscillating, it follows that a specific but substantial population of the auditory nerve fibres is active, and it appears that frequency discrimination depends largely upon the topographic limits of the strip of membrane from which these fibres arise. With a just perceptible change in frequency, there is a small shift in these limits, but it must be appreciated that the majority of the nerve fibres active will be common to the two situations. Further, it is considered that at a particular frequency, an increase in the *intensity* of the stimulus is signalled by both an increased *number* of cochlear nerve fibres active, and also by their *rate of discharge* of impulses. For an extended discussion of these topics consult footnote references [1304], [1306], [1307].

---

[1305] H. Spoendlin, in: *Hearing Mechanisms in Vertebrates*, Ciba Foundation Symposium, Churchill, London. 1968.

[1306] G. v. Békésy, in: *Experiments in Hearing*, ed. E. G. Wever, McGraw-Hill, New York. 1960.

[1307] I. Tasaki, H. Davis and J.-P. Legouix, *J. acoust. Soc. Am.*, **24**, 1952. H. F. Schuknecht, in: *Neural Mechanisms of the Auditory and Vestibular Systems*, ed. G. L. Rasmussen and W. F. Windle, Thomas, Springfield. 1960.

The integument or skin is a morphologically and physiologically specialized boundary lamina which is of major importance in the life of the individual. It forms the entire external surface and is continuous with the mucosal surfaces of the respiratory, alimentary and urogenital tracts at their respective orifices, where the modified skin of the muco-cutaneous junctions occurs. It also lines the external auditory meatus, covers the lateral aspect of the tympanic membrane, and is continuous with the conjunctiva at the margins of the eyelids and with the lining of the lacrimal canaliculi at the lacrimal puncta.

at its surface good frictional properties, enhancing locomotion and manipulation by its texture and physical structure. Skin also provides a major pathway for social communication, by virtue of its vascular responses associated with signalling of emotional states, muscular responses of expression, creating a complex sign language, and by the equally subtle possibilities of tactile communication. In many primates the skin forms a signalling system related to complicated instinctive behaviour patterns which regulate aggressive, sexual, and other responses of the social group; changes in skin colour and shape in certain areas—the maxillary regions and buttocks for example—often parallel internal changes in hormonal levels, aggressive states and other factors affecting the behaviour of the individual. How far the signals mediated in man by facial expression and other alterations in skin appearance are linked to instinctive behaviour patterns rather than to conditioned behaviour is debatable in adults, although studies on children indicate the fusion of these two elements in a complex fashion.

## The Structure of the Skin

The skin is composed of two layers of distinctive structure, properties and embryological origin—the *dermis* or *corium*, a connective tissue layer of mesenchymal origin, which is covered by the *epidermis*, an epithelial layer derived from embryonic ectoderm (**7**.304). Deep to the dermis lies a layer of loose irregular connective tissue, forming the *superficial fascia, hypodermis* or *subcutaneous layer* which in turn is bound to the underlying tissues by a dense fibrous *deep fascia* corresponding to the *epimysium* of muscle blocks, or where a bony or cartilaginous surface is adjacent, to the *periosteum* or *perichondrium*.

The interface between the epidermis and the dermis shows a complex topology, being marked by peg-and-socket or ridge/groove interdigitations between the two (**7**.304). These arrangements, together with the special anchoring structures linking the epidermis and the dermis, prevent the epithelium from being stripped off the surface of the dermis by shearing forces.

Each of the two layers confers special properties on the skin as a whole. The primary barrier to mechanical damage, desiccation and microbial invasion is the epidermis, particularly the outer horny layers which are highly impermeable to water and chemically rather inert. The epidermis, moreover, has a high capacity for regeneration after damage, and is continually replacing the outer dead cells as they are abraded from the surface. The epidermis also generates the *appendages of the skin*, that is, hairs, nails, sudorific and sebaceous glands. The dermis, in contrast, gives the skin considerable mechanical strength by virtue of the high proportion of collagen fibres intermingled with fibres of elastin, and in the various cellular components, provides a reservoir of defensive and regenerative elements capable of combating infection and repairing deep wounds. The vascular supply of the skin is limited entirely to the dermis, and therefore the epidermis relies for its supply of nutrients and metabolic exchange generally on diffusion to and

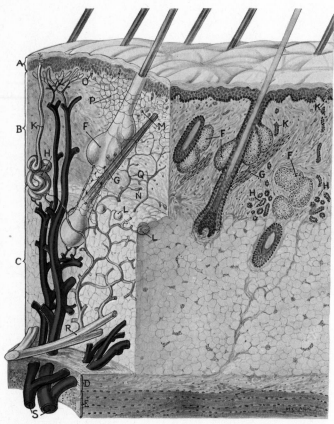

7.303 A diagrammatic scheme showing the structure of the skin. A. Epidermis. B. Dermis. C. Subcutaneous fat. D. Deep fascia. E. Muscle. F. Sebaceous glands in association with a hair follicle. G. Arrector pili muscle. H. Sweat gland. K. Duct of sweat gland. L. Bulbous corpuscle. M. Lamellated end bulb. N. Pressure corpuscle. O. Tactile corpuscle in a papilla. P. Superficial nerve plexus. Q. Deep nerve plexus. R. Cutaneous nerve. S. Cutaneous vessels.

The skin is adapted to serve many different roles, since it is the major interface between the body and its environment.[1308, 1309] It minimizes, within limits, the potentially injurious effects of mechanical, osmotic, chemical, thermal, and photic environmental stresses; it provides a barrier to invasion by micro-organisms, and it limits and regulates the exchange of heat with the environment by special neurovascular mechanisms coupled with thermally insulating properties of certain layers of the skin. The skin is a major sensory surface, containing the receptive fields of a variety of somatic sensory nerve endings; it is capable of limited absorption and excretion, and provides a surface for the conversion of precursor compounds into vitamin D by the action of ultraviolet light; it posesses

[1308] W. Montagna, *The Structure and Function of the Skin*, 2nd ed. Academic Press, New York. 1962.
[1309] W. Bloom and D. W. Fawcett, *A Textbook of Histology*, 9th ed., Saunders, Philadelphia. 1968.

from the capillaries of the most superficial regions of the dermis. The innervation of the skin, however, serves both dermis and epidermis.

Deep to the dermis lies the subcutaneous connective tissue layers of the superficial fascia. In many regions of

the body the latter is composed of loosely interwoven irregular connective tissue in the meshes of which lie numerous adipose cells, forming the *panniculus adiposus*. In addition to its mechanical properties as a shock absorber, and its energy-storing capacity, this layer is an important thermal insulator, limiting the flow of heat largely to the channels of the vascular system and thus making thermal regulation by vascular changes possible.

## THE EPIDERMIS

The external surface of the epidermis is marked by various furrows, ridges and other irregularities.[1310] Three principal varieties of surface markings exist (7.305–307), tension and flexure lines and papillary ridges. *Tension lines* form a network of linear furrows of variable size which divide the surface into a large number of polygonal or lozenge-shaped areas. In many areas, such as the back of the hand, they are faint and intersect one another at various angles. Although these lines correspond to variations in the pattern of the fibres in the dermis to some extent, they bear no special relationship to the dermal papillae. *Flexure lines* (*skin joints*) correspond to folds in the dermis associated with habitual joint movements, and to lines of attachment to the underlying deep fascia; they are conspicuous opposite the flexure of joints, particularly on the surfaces of the palms, soles and digits. *Papillary ridges* (*friction ridges*) are confined to the palmar surface of the hands and to the soles of the feet, including their digits, where they form narrow raised ridges separated by fine but distinct parallel grooves, disposed in curved arrays; the precise forms and positions of these ridges are related to the arrangement and size of the underlying dermal papillae interlocking with the base of the epidermis. In thin, hairy skin, the papillae are simple peg-like structures, scattered randomly over the dermal surface;

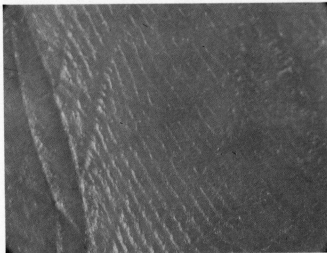

7.305 A low-power light micrograph of hairless skin, in surface view, from the palm of the hand, showing epidermal friction (papillary) ridges and larger flexure lines (left).

in thick glabrous (non-hairy) skin, the dermal papillae often show complex forms, are large, and are arranged in rows, a single row occupying the position underneath an epidermal papillary ridge. Sweat glands which open in a row along the midline of each ridge grow down during development into the gaps between papillae, dimpling the basal surface of the epithelium to form secondary epidermal pegs (*rete pegs*) or ridges which protrude into

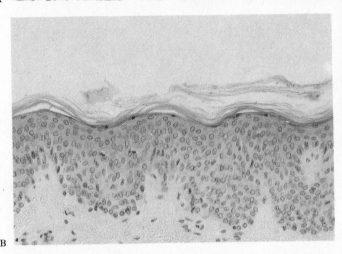

7.304A and B. A Low-power light micrograph of a vertical section through skin from the sole of the human foot: Mallory's triple stain. The finer collagen fibres of the papillary and reticular layers are stained blue, and the coarser reticular layer collagen stains red. The epidermis is differentiated into the stratum corneum and stratum lucidum above (red-brown), and the strata basale, spinosum and granulosum, which stain blue-grey. A spiral duct from a sweat gland is also seen in vertical section. The base of the epidermis is irregularly ridged. B A vertical section through the epidermis of the scalp, between hair follicles. Note the reduced karatinized layer (compare with A). Haematoxylin and eosin.

[1310] W. Montagna and W. C. Lobitz (eds.), *The Epidermis*, Academic Press, New York. 1964.

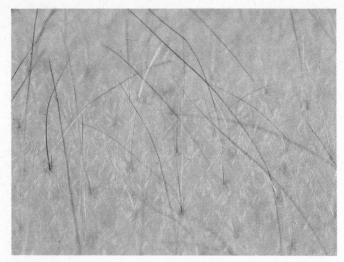

**7.306** A similar light micrograph to that shown in **7.305**, but taken from hairy skin on the extensor aspect of the forearm; note the pattern of surface grooves (tension lines) and hairs. The oblique direction of the emerging hair shafts points away from the pre-axial border of the limb.

the dermis (**7.304** A). This complex interdigitation no doubt enhances the stability of the junction between the two layers.

The pattern of papillary ridges, and particularly those of the fingers and thumbs are of considerable interest because of their morphological stability throughout life and also because they are slightly different in each individual.[1311, 1312] The use of fingerprints for purposes of identification is well known and has led to an intensive study of their variation in human populations (the subject of *dermatoglyphics*). It has become clear that only three major patterns occur in human fingerprints (**7.307**),

tion they are in the pattern of flexure lines in some cases, so that these markings may form a useful diagnostic tool in certain circumstances.[1313]

## THE MICROSCOPIC STRUCTURE OF THE EPIDERMIS

Histologically, the epidermis is composed of keratinizing stratified squamous epithelium (p. 29). In such a tissue, two distinct cellular processes are evident, the replacement of cells continually being lost from the surface, by the mitosis of deeper layers, and the transformation of polygonal living cells to dead, flattened, scale-like structures, filled with increasing amounts of the protein keratin, as they age and are moved towards the epithelial surface by the multiplication of the cells beneath them.

Considerable variation occurs over the body surface in the rate and extent of these two processes, so that in some regions, for example the eyelids, lips and other mucocutaneous junctions, the keratinizing layers and indeed the whole epithelium are extremely thin, whilst in others, particularly the palmar and plantar surfaces of the hands and feet, the keratinized layer may be 2 mm or more thick (**7.304**). In general the epidermis of the flexor surfaces of the limbs (apart from the above exceptions) are more delicate than the extensor surfaces. Because of important differences in the structure of the epidermal layers in various areas, it is customary to distinguish between the epidermis of *thin, hairy skin*, with hairs and sebaceous glands, which covers most of the body surface, and *thick, glabrous skin*, lacking hairs and sebaceous glands, which is restricted to the palms of the hands, the soles of the feet and the flexor surfaces of the digits.

The degree of keratinization is largely under genetic control, since the overall distribution of heavily and lightly keratinized areas is determined before birth.

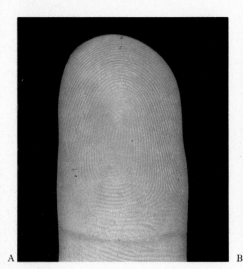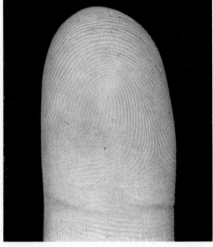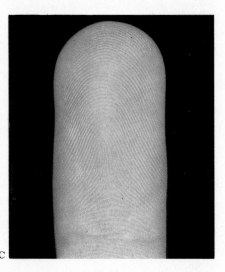

**7.307** A–C Photographs of the palmar aspect of a terminal phalanx in three different individuals, to show the major types of pattern of the finger-print ridges. The pattern in A is commonly termed a whorl; B is composed of loops; C is composed of arches. Note interphalangeal flexure lines.

consisting respectively of loops, whorls and arches, although minor pattern variations in orientation, distortion, ridge width and number, continuity, branching and anastomosing provide the enormous pool of variation which makes their precise form unique to the individual. These three major patterns, and many of the minor features, are determined genetically by multifactorial inheritance along Mendelian lines, although prenatal disturbances of metabolism may also alter their character to some extent. Certain genetic disorders may also be reflected in fingerprint and palmar markings, as, in addi-

However, intermittent mechanical pressure or abrasion stimulates the adventitious production of keratinized cells, a response of the epidermis which considerably enhances the stress-resisting properties of skin.[1314]

[1311] H. Faulds, *Nature, Lond.*, **22**, 1880.
[1312] H. Cummins and C. Midlo, *Finger-prints, Palms and Soles*, Blakiston, Philadelphia. 1943.
[1313] G. H. Valentine, *The Chromosome Disorders*, Heinemann, London. 1966.
[1314] G. E. Rogers, in: *The Biological Basis of Medicine*, vol. 6, ed. E. E. Bittar and N. Bittar, Academic Press, London. 1969.

When suitably macerated, the outer keratinized zone of the epidermis can be stripped from the underlying layers of the epithelial cells, and it has been customary to divide the layers of the epidermis, albeit in a somewhat arbitrary manner, into a deep *germinative zone* and a more superficial *horny zone* (7.304). For a more detailed treatment of the structure of these layers, the reader is referred to pp. 29, 30, and only certain special aspects of organization will be considered here.

### The Germinative Zone

This consists of living cells with little keratin precursor material visible in their cytoplasm. The deeper layers are capable of mitotic division, chiefly in a vertical direction to generate 'stacks' of epidermal cells which are continuous to the epithelial surface. This zone includes a *basal cell layer* (*stratum basale* or *stratum malpighii*) situated adjacent to a basal lamina, where mitotic activity is particularly intense. Superficial to this is a region several cells thick, the *stratum spinosum* (prickle cell layer), marked by the convoluted, interdigitating profiles of the cells, the *keratocytes* (prickle cells) which are linked by numerous desmosomes attached to internal microfilaments (tonofibrils) of the cytoplasm (7.308). This layer probably provides much of the mechanical coherence of the epithelium. Within the germinative zone three other cell types may be present, two of them with extended dendritic processes ramifying amongst the surrounding keratocytes, and one with a more rounded profile. The first two types are the epithelial *melanoblast* (*melanocyte, dendritic cell,* or *clear cell*), which synthesizes melanin (*vide infra*), and the *Langerhans cell*,[1315] the functions of which are the subject of some argument.[1318] The *melanoblasts* (7.306) are structurally distinct from the surrounding keratocytes by virtue of their lack of desmosomes, their few internal microfilaments, and the presence of specific *melanin bodies* (*melanosomes*), ellipsoidal structures up to 0·7×0·2 μm in their major and minor diameters which show, internally, a regular array of fine (5 nm) granules or fibrils, the latter with regular 5 nm striations. The *Langerhans cells*, in contrast, are devoid of melanin, but contain instead characteristic rod-like *Langerhans granules*, about 0·1 μm long by 0·01 μm wide, having a regular granular interior.[1316] Some of these granules are in continuity with the external membrane of the cell. At one time such cells were thought to be degenerating melanoblasts, but the profusion of intracellular organelles and the active DNA synthesis in their nuclei argues against this view; similar cells are known to be present in the dermis, and it is thought by some workers that they are a type of phagocytic cell, similar perhaps to the macrophages of the dermis.[1317, 1318]

There is good evidence that the melanoblasts are of neural crest origin, and that the Langerhans cells come from a different embryonic source.

The other epithelial cell type, found chiefly in hairy skin, is the *Merkel cell*,[1317] an element which lies in close association with the tactile sensory nerve endings terminating in the basal parts of the epidermis (*see* p. 799). This cell is marked by an indented nucleus, prominent Golgi complex and numerous dense-cored vesicles each about 80 nm in diameter. These cells appear to play an important role in the sensory process, but the significance of its internal contents is unclear; there is no evidence that the dense-cored vesicles contain catecholamines.

### The Keratinization Zone

In this zone occur the chief cell transformations associated with keratinization (7.304, 308). The *granular layer* (*stratum granulosum*) at its base consists of flattened cells with pyknotic nuclei, surrounded by numerous baso-philic granules of the keratin precursor *keratohyalin* (*see* pp. 29, 30). The *clear layer* (*stratum lucidum*) is situated superficially to the granular layer, and appears in sections as a homogenous, slightly striated layer composed of closely packed cells in which traces of flattened nuclei may be seen. This layer is prominent, or indeed visible, only in heavily keratinized areas such as glabrous skin, and contains the keratin precursor *eleidin*. The *cornified layer* (*stratum corneum*) consists of many thicknesses of flattened *squames*, the remnants of cells which have become completely filled with keratin and have lost all other internal structures, including nuclei. At the basal aspect of this layer the cells are closely compacted and adhere to one another strongly, but more superficially they become loosely packed and eventually flake away at the surface.

### The Pigmentation of the Skin

The final colour of the skin is determined by the presence of at least five pigments at various positions in the integument. These are: *melanin*, a brown pigment, situated chiefly in the germinative zone of the epidermis; *melanoid*, a substance similar to melanin, present diffusely throughout the epidermis; yellow to orange *carotene* in the stratum corneum and the adipose cells of the dermis and superficial fascia; and *haemoglobin* (purple) and *oxyhaemoglobin* (red), contained in the vascular supply of the skin, particularly the superficial venous plexuses (*vide infra*). The amounts of the first three of these pigments vary topographically throughout the body, chronologically with the age of the individual, and genetically between individuals. Their relative contributions determine the characteristic racial pigmentation, although considerable genetically-determined differences may occur within a single ethnic group.

*Melanin*, the brown pigment, is chemically a protein-like polymer of the amino acid *tyrosin*, and possibly of related catecholamines also.[1319-1322] Tyrosin is converted by the epidermal melanoblasts into dihydroxyphenyl-alanine (DOPA) by oxidative enzymes amongst which *tyrosinase* is important. DOPA is further converted to DOPA-quinone, commencing a series of reactions during which polymerization takes place to form the final melanoprotein (melanin). Parts of this enzyme system, and hence the identity of the dendritic melanoblasts which contain them, can be demonstrated histochemically by incubating thin pieces or sections of fresh skin with DOPA, which is converted to melanin within the cytoplasm (*the DOPA reaction*).

Complete absence of skin pigments, excepting those of the vascular system (*albinism*), is a recessive Mendelian character and may occur sporadically in any race; one or more enzymes of the DOPA pathway may be absent in this trait, which may also be associated with other disturbances of tyrosin metabolism.

Each epithelial melanoblast possesses many slender

[1315] A. S. Zelickson (ed.), *Ultrastructure of Normal and Abnormal Skin*, Kimpton, London. 1967.
[1316] A. S. Breathnach, *An Atlas of the Ultrastructure of Human Skin*, Churchill, London. 1971.
[1317] A. S. Zelickson, in: *Modern Trends in Dermatology-4*, ed. P. Borrie, Butterworth, London. 1971.
[1318] A. S. Breathnach and L. M.-A. Wyllie, in: *Advances in Biology of Skin*, ed. W. Montagna and F. Hu, vol. 7, *The Pigmentary System*, Pergamon Press, Oxford. 1967.
[1319] T. B. Fitzpatrick and W. C. Quevedo Jr., in: *Modern Trends in Dermatology-4*, ed. P. Borrie, Butterworth, London. 1971.
[1320] A. S. Breathnach, in: *Pigments in Pathology*, ed. M. Wolman, Academic Press, New York. 1969.
[1321] G. Szabó, in: *The Biological Basis of Medicine*, vol. 6, ed. E. E. Bittar and N. Bittar, Academic Press, London. 1969.
[1322] J. Duchon, T. B. Fitzpatrick and M. Seiji, in: *1967-1968 Year Book of Dermatology*, ed. A. W. Kopf and R. Andrade, Year Book Publishing Co., Chicago. 1968.

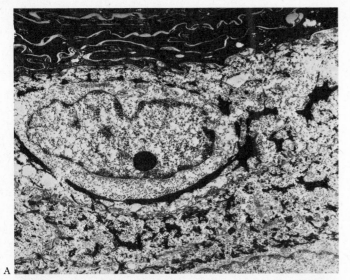

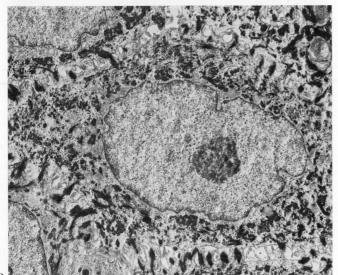

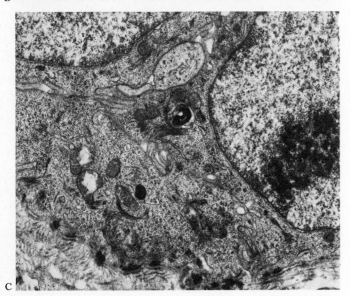

**7.308 A–C** Electron micrographs of human skin in vertical section. A This shows the transition between the stratum spinosum (below), stratum granulosum (middle), and stratum corneum (the dark laminae above). The microfilamentous bundles of the keratocytes below, become denser and more compact in the stratum granulosum, and finally the cells flatten, becoming scale-like and electron dense. B This shows keratocytes in the stratum spinosum. The cell outlines are highly convoluted and demonstrate numerous desmosomes; many cytoplasmic bundles of microfilaments are visible. C This is taken from the bases of stratum basale cells; their cytoplasm contains many ribosomes, but few microfilaments. Their bases are attached to the basal lamina of the epithelium by punctate dense hemidesmosomes; note dermal collagen (below).

branches terminating in flattened expansions applied to the surfaces of neighbouring keratocytes (7.313). The melanin granules formed in the perikaryal region of the melanoblast pass along the dendritic branches, and are either secreted at their tips, being subsequently engulfed by keratocyte cell processes and incorporated into their cytoplasm, or else phagocytosed within dendritic fragments by these cells.[1323, 1324] Similar melanoblasts sometimes occur in the dermis and may pass on their melanin to macrophages.

The degree of melanization of any particular body region may depend either upon the number of melanoblasts or on the varying activity of individual melanoblasts. Under normal conditions, melanoblasts are often more numerous at the openings of the mucous membranes, on the surface of the penis, face, and limbs than over the trunk and abdomen, varying between 800 and 2,000/mm³. In newborn infants, up to the age of five months, dermal melanoblasts in the sacral region are responsible for the bluish 'Mongolian Spot' often seen in this vicinity. Melanoblasts are also intimately associated with the bases of hair follicles and provide melanin for incorporation into the cells of hairs (7.313).

In heavily melanized races, the numbers of melanoblasts are about the same as in those with less melanin, so that the difference must lie in the rate of melanin synthesis. However, the melanin content of individual melanosomes is also higher under normal conditions of lighting. In any individual, the rate of melanin synthesis is controlled locally by the incidence of ultraviolet radiation, and systemically by the action of melanocyte stimulating hormone (MSH) from the anterior pituitary gland, amongst other normal and pathological influences. The importance of melanin in protecting the deep, mitosing layers of the epidermis against chromosomal damage by ultraviolet light is seen in the higher incidence of carcinoma of the skin found in Caucasians living in tropical and subtropical regions compared with the indigenous melanized populations. However, melanin also protects the underlying dermis against ultraviolet damage of a more direct nature, that is the inflammatory changes which typically accompany sun-burn.

The response of the melanoblasts to varying doses of ultraviolet light are interesting, since at least three distinct phases occur. With brief exposures, the melanin already present in the epidermis darkens appreciably, but later returns to its original colour; with increased exposure, melanin synthesis increases in each melanoblast, and in long exposures the melanocytes themselves increase in number. The extent to which these changes occur depends upon the genetic constitution of the individual as well as upon the dosage.

## THE DERMIS

The dermis or corium is tough, flexible and highly elastic. It is very thick in the palms of the hands and soles of the feet; thicker on the posterior than on the anterior aspect of the body, and on the lateral than on the medial sides of the limbs. It is exceedingly thin and delicate in the eyelids, scrotum, and penis.

## MICROSCOPIC STRUCTURE

The dermis consists of felted connective tissue, with a varying number of elastic fibres and numerous blood vessels, lymphatic vessels and nerves. The connective

[1323] C. N. D. Cruickshank and S. A. Harcourt, *J. invest. Derm.*, **42**, 1964.
[1324] J. Cohen and G. Szabó, *Expl Cell Res.*, **50**, 1968.

tissue is arranged in two layers: a deeper or *reticular*, and a superficial or *papillary*. Nonstriated muscular fibres occur in the superficial layers of the dermis wherever hairs are present; they are also present in the subcutaneous areolar tissue of the scrotum, penis, labia majora and nipples.

**The reticular layer** consists of strong interlacing bands, composed chiefly of white fibrous tissue, but containing some yellow elastic fibres, which vary in number in different parts. In the deeper part the fasciculi are large, and the wide intervals left by their interlacement are occupied by adipose tissue and sweat glands. Below the reticular layer is the subcutaneous areolar tissue which, except in a few situations, contains fat. The connective tissue bands in the reticular layer lie for the main part in parallel bundles, so that if a conical object is stabbed through the skin and then withdrawn it leaves a linear wound since the fibres are forced apart without much rupture. The directions taken by the parallel bundles vary in different parts of the body and constitute what are termed the *cleavage lines* of the skin. Surgical incisions made along the direction of cleavage lines heal with minimal formation of scar tissue, whereas incisions across these lines, owing to retraction of the severed fibres, lead to the formation of a broad scar. In general, the cleavage lines are arranged longitudinally in the skin of the limbs and more or less horizontally in the trunk and neck. With increasing age the yellow elastic fibres atrophy and the skin loses much of its elasticity and becomes wrinkled. If the skin becomes much stretched (as by rapidly growing tumours, fat deposition or pregnancy) the fibres in the reticular layer may undergo partial rupture, followed by scar formation; these areas may show on the surface as white streaks. These are commonly seen on the anterior abdominal wall after pregnancy and are known as *lineae gravidarum*. In many regions the skin is separated from the deep fascia or other structures by loose areolar tissue and in these sites the skin is freely movable over the deeper structures. Elsewhere, however, the skin may be firmly anchored to structures like the periosteum over 'subcutaneous' parts of bones, or to the deep fascia in regions related to movements of underlying joints. In the latter case there may be permanent creases in the skin known as *flexure lines*; they are particularly evident on the palm of the hand and flexor surfaces of the digits, where they are arranged in relation to the movements of the digits (*see* pp. 442 and 1162).

**The papillary layer** consists of numerous highly sensitive and vascular eminences, termed the *papillae*, which project perpendicularly (7.304, 310). The papillae are minute conical projections, having round or blunted apices, which may be divided into two or more parts, and are received into corresponding pits on the under surface of the epidermis. On the general surface of the body, and especially in parts endowed with slight sensibility, they are few in number and exceedingly minute; but in some situations, as upon the palmar surfaces of the hands and fingers, and upon the plantar surfaces of the feet and toes, they are large, closely aggregated together, and arranged in parallel curved lines, forming the elevated ridges seen on the surface of the epidermis. Each ridge contains two rows of papillae and between the rows the ducts of the sweat glands pass outwards to open on the summits of the ridges. Each papilla consists of very small and closely interlacing bundles of finely fibrillar tissue, with a few elastic fibres; within this tissue there is a capillary loop, and in some papillae, especially in the palms and the fingers, there are tactile corpuscles (7.31).

For a more detailed description of the cutaneous nerve terminals, and patterns of innervation, consult pp. 797–800, 1165.

## THE VASCULARIZATION OF SKIN

Within the skin, the blood supply and drainage lie along well-determined pathways (7.309) the precise form of which is related to the metabolic requirements of the various cellular components.[1325] Amongst the highly active areas of the skin are the epidermis and its cellular extensions—hair follicles, sebaceous and sudorific glands—and also the dermal papillae which contain active fibroblasts and the sensory endings of cutaneous nerves; all of these structures are closely related to rich capillary beds in the dermis. The deeper reticular layer of the dermis, in contrast, is highly fibrous and contains few active cells, and the metabolic requirements are low. Although many vessels pass through the reticular layer, they give off few capillaries and are mostly non-nutritive to this layer.

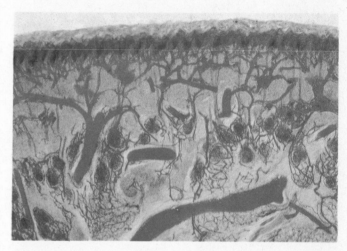

7.309 A thick vertical section through palmar skin, the arteries, arterioles and capillaries of which have been injected with red gelatin to demonstrate the pattern of dermal vascularization. At the base of the dermis a broad flat arterial plexus supplies a more superficial papillary plexus, which in turn gives off capillary loops which enter the dermal papillae. Sweat glands and their ducts are numerous in this specimen; they extend basally into the subcutaneous tissues.

Blood enters the skin through small arteries which penetrate the superficial fascia from its deep aspect and initially ramify in a sheet-like plexus, the *rete cutaneum* at the interface of the dermis and superficial fascia. From this plexus, some blood vessels run deeply to supply the subcutaneous adipose tissue and, in those regions where they are present at this depth, the bases of hair follicles and sweat glands. Other vessels arising from the rete cutaneum curve in a superficial direction, giving off capillaries around hair follicles, sebaceous glands and sudorific glands as they pass to the junction of the reticular and papillary layers of the dermis; here they form another flat plexus, the *rete subpapillare* or *superficial plexus*. Capillaries extend from this layer towards the base of the epithelium, within dermal papillae, and loop back to a flat venous plexus which lies immediately beneath the rete subpapillare; this in turn drains into a flat intermediate plexus in the middle of the reticular layer of the dermis which further connects with a deep laminar venous plexus at the dermis–superficial fascia junction. Various capillary beds situated in the dermis around glands and hair follicles drain into these three venous plexuses at appropriate levels within the skin.

In the deeper layers of the dermis, arteriovenous anastomoses are common; in glabrous skin some of these

[1325] W. Montagna, *The Structure and Function of the Skin*, 2nd ed., Academic Press, New York. 1962.

are surrounded by thick sphincter-like groups of smooth muscle and pursue a convoluted course. These vessels are termed *glomera*. Since the smooth muscle elements are under autonomic control, heat exchange at the epithelial surface can be regulated by the vasoconstriction of the afferent arterioles of the general cutaneous supply, whilst the arteriovenous anastomoses provide for a maintained deep circulation in the skin under thermal conditions which might otherwise reduce the blood supply of the integument to dangerous levels (see also p. 595).

## THE LYMPHATIC DRAINAGE OF THE SKIN

Numerous blind ending lymphatic vessels terminate in the dermis near the base of the epidermis and drain deeply first into a dermal network in the papillary layer, then into another network in the middle of the reticular layer and finally into a network at the junction of the dermis and superficial fascia. Deep to this zone, the lymph flows through wider channels provided with valves, into the main lymphatic drainage of the area. The lymphatic drainage of the skin is quite profuse, and free anastomosis appears to occur between vessels at all levels so that there is free interchange of lymph between areas of the skin which are adjacent to each other.[1326]

## THE INNERVATION OF THE SKIN

Skin is richly innervated (7.29) by myelinated and non-myelinated sensory fibres of cerebrospinal nerves, and via nonmyelinated autonomic fibres supplying blood vessels, sweat glands and smooth muscle fibres associated with the hairs (pilomotor nerves). The sensory apparatus has already been described in some cytological detail (p. 797), and will be discussed only in relation to the sensory functions of the whole skin.[1327, 1328]

The nerves associated with both efferent and afferent endings penetrate the superficial fascia and ramify through the reticular and papillary layers of the dermis. Conspicuous nerve plexuses are formed around hair follicles and in the papillary layer of the dermis beneath the epithelium where the term *dermal* or *corial plexus* is often applied. Efferent nerves ramify around blood vessels, cutaneous muscle fibres and the bases of sudorific glands. Afferent nerves usually branch to supply a limited area of the skin, or in one type of ending, the Pacinian corpuscle, they may remain unbranched; the area of innervation by a single fibre is often related to the sensitivity threshold of the fibre and inversely to the degree of spatial localization of which it is capable. Each receptive field may overlap with those of other afferent fibres, giving a complex mosaic which creates possibilities of pattern analysis (p. 800).

Since the skin forms the chief interface between the internal and external environments, the elaborate sensory apparatus which it possesses makes it the chief means of comparing physical changes in the two environments and of monitoring their interaction. Information concerning the rate of change of various effective stimuli, their duration, energy content and their spatial and temporal patterning are all being constantly provided by the array of cutaneous receptors. The interpretation and correlation of the various messages arriving in the central nervous system appear to involve the continual analysis of patterns of differential activity from a wide range of receptor types (p. 795), some of them particularly responsive to certain modalities (e.g. pressure, cold), others responding in a manner determined by their position within the skin, their intrinsic thresholds, and the mechanical characteristics of the non-nervous cells associated with their sensory terminals.

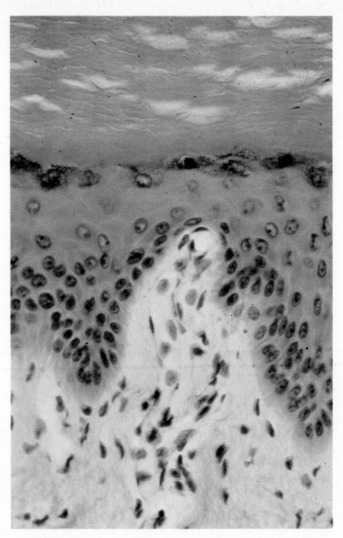

7.310 A vertical section through a dermal papilla and adjacent epidermis, showing a capillary loop. Notice the closeness of the vessel to the basal layer of the epidermis. Mallory's triple stain.

In both hairy and glabrous skin, the highly branched nonmyelinated and myelinated 'free' terminals which end within the dermis and penetrate the lower layers of the epidermis form an important sensory component. Some of these fibres are known to be responsive to heat and to cold, whilst others play a part in the signalling of pain (p. 797). In hairy skin, such fibres lie in close association with hair follicles; another type of ending, the Merkel disc is also prominent in this variety of skin, particularly around the openings of hair follicles, whereas in glabrous skin they are found at the base of the intermediate 'sweat' ridges beneath the papillary ridges of the epidermis. A single myelinated afferent fibre may give rise to several groups of such disc endings, each group corresponding to a 'touch spot' on the surface of the epithelium. Shearing forces applied to the skin surface cause such endings to respond without adapting appreciably to continued stimulation, and it seems likely that the epidermal structures—hair follicles, ridges—to which these endings are attached act as a series of levers, imparting a magnified stress to the associated expanded nerve endings. In hairless skin there are also numerous complex corpuscles, the

[1326] G. Forbes, *J. Anat.*, **72**, 1938.
[1327] D. Sinclair, *Cutaneous Sensation*, Oxford University Press, London. 1967.
[1328] D. R. Kenshalo (ed.), *The Skin Senses*, Thomas, Springfield, Illinois. 1968.

endings of Meissner, which are situated chiefly within the dermal papillae beneath the papillary ridges.[1329] Each Meissner corpuscle receives multiple innervation from the branches of as many as nine separate axons, each of which may also innervate other Meissner corpuscles, so that considerable cross innervation occurs. These endings are thought to be responsible for rapidly adapting mechanoreception, and because of their high density on the flexor surfaces of the digits for example, they may be associated with the sensing of rapidly changing, patterned tactile stimuli. Similar endings of a somewhat simpler construction are found in other areas such as the muco-cutaneous junctions, and mucous membranes (muco-cutaneous end organs, genital corpuscles, bulboid endings, lingual end-organs, etc.), where they may have similar functions. Pacinian corpuscles are present chiefly in the deeper layers of the skin, and in the superficial fascia where they are particularly prominent in the flexor surfaces of the digits. Each corpuscle is innervated only by a single axon, and may serve an entire unbranched nerve fibre. The peculiar lamellated structure of the corpuscle appears to possess important properties, making the end organ responsive to vibrations of a rather narrow range of frequencies. As with the other types of receptor endings, the position within the skin and the mechanical characteristics of adjacent non-nervous cells may create possibilities of stimulus analysis otherwise not feasible, by virtue of the action of the epidermis and dermis as filters, attenuating mechanical and thermal stimuli in different ways as they are transmitted through their successive layers. Sensory endings situated at different levels may therefore form part of a highly ordered sensory system with organization in both horizontal and vertical planes.

In addition to this minute structuring of the sensory apparatus of the skin, large-scale variation also occurs over the whole body surface. Physiologically, such variations are detectable as changes in thresholds to mechanical and thermal stimuli, in point-to-point discrimination of tactile stimuli and in the ability to identify the precise locality of a stimulus applied to the body surface. In general, both fine discrimination and location of stimuli follow similar gradients, being of a high order at the extremities of the limbs and becoming progressively cruder towards abdomen, thorax and head, although certain areas such as the lips and tongue, for example, create local reversals in this pattern. Discrimination is not entirely bilaterally symmetrical, the right side usually being more discriminative than the left, at least in dextral subjects. Other gradients, for example, of pressure thresholds, may operate in the opposite directions. Sex differences have also been shown, female subjects being generally more sensitive to pressure stimuli than men, a finding possibly related to the slightly thinner epidermis typical of female skin.

The anatomical basis of such variations is still far from being satisfactorily explained, a statement which might also be applied to the whole subject of cutaneous sensation.

[1329] T. A. Quilliam, *J. Anat.*, **109**, 1971.

## APPENDAGES OF THE SKIN

### THE NAILS

The nails (**7.311**) are flattened, elastic structures of a horny texture, placed upon the distal parts of the dorsal surfaces of the fingers and toes. The proximal part of the nail, called the *root*, is implanted into a groove in the skin; the exposed part is the *body* of the nail; the distal end forms the *free border*, and a little proximal to it the skin is attached to the under surface of the nail forming the

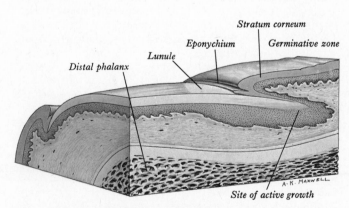

7.311   A longitudinal section through the root of a nail.

*hyponychium.* The root of the nail is overlapped by a fold of skin, the *nail fold*, the stratum corneum of which is prolonged distally as a thin cuticular fold, the *eponychium*, to cover completely or partially the white opaque crescentic part of the nail called the *lunule*. The greater part of each collateral border of the nail is overlapped by a fold of skin, termed the *nail wall*. The nail itself is analogous to the horny zone of thick skin, although the keratinized squames are hard and highly coherent;[1317, 1330] beneath it lies the germinative zone which, together with the subjacent corium, forms the *nail bed*. Under the greater part of the nail the corium is thick and raised into a series of longitudinal ridges which are very vascular, and this accounts for the pink colour seen through the translucent nail. Near the root of the nail, however, the ridges are smaller, irregularly arranged and less vascular; moreover the tissue of the nail is here more opaque, hence this part of the nail is whiter and constitutes the lunule. The lunule is usually visible in the thumb nail, but in the other digits it becomes progressively more covered by the nail fold towards the little finger, in which it is generally hidden altogether. The germinative zone of the nail bed consists functionally of two parts. The part beneath the root of the nail and the lunule (*germinal matrix*) is thicker and actively proliferative, and is concerned with the growth of the nail, the epidermal cells being gradually converted into the nail substance. On the other hand, the part beneath the rest of the nail (*sterile matrix*) is thinner and is not concerned with nail growth but provides a surface over which the growing nail glides. All growth of the nail therefore occurs at its root; the nail increases in thickness from its root to the distal edge of the lunule and the remainder is of uniform thickness. If a nail be removed without severely damaging the germinal matrix, a new nail will grow from this region. Disturbances of growth of the nails may occur in acute illnesses or local trauma, and transverse grooves may develop on the surface which move gradually distally with growth of the nails. Minute air bubbles, giving rise to white flecks, may develop in the substance of the nail. On an average nails grow about

[1330] N. Zaias and J. Alvarey, *J. invest. Derm.*, **51**, 1968.

0·5 mm a week; growth is quicker in summer than in winter, and finger nails grow about four times as fast as toe nails. In the hand, nail growth is most rapid in the longest digit (the middle finger), slowest in the little finger and intermediate in the other digits. Nails act as a rigid background for support of the digital pads of the terminal phalanges, and thus may aid tactile mechanisms. From the evolutionary point of view, nails are derived from the more elaborately structured claws which characterize many other mammals and lower tetrapods.

## THE HAIRS

The hairs are found on nearly every part of the surface of the body, but are absent from the palms of the hands, the soles of the feet, the dorsal surfaces of the distal phalanges, the umbilicus, the glans penis, the inner surface of the prepuce, the inner surfaces of the clitoris, labia majora and minora. They vary much in length, thickness and colour in different parts of the body and in different races of mankind. In some parts, as in the skin of the eyelids, they are so short as not to project beyond the follicles containing them; in others, as upon the scalp, they may be remarkably long; the eyelashes, the hairs of the pubic region, and the whiskers and beard are remarkable for their thickness. Straight hairs are stronger than curly hairs and present on transverse section a cylindrical or oval outline: curly hairs, on the other hand, are flat. (Some maintain that the form of the hair does not correspond with its shape in cross-section.)

A hair consists of a *root*, the part implanted in the skin, and a *shaft* (*scapus*), the portion projecting from the surface.

with a funnel-shaped opening, and passes inwards in an oblique or curved direction—the latter in curly hairs— to become dilated at its deep extremity, where it corresponds with the hair bulb. The ducts of one or more sebaceous glands open into the follicle near the skin surface. At the bottom of each hair follicle there is a small conical vascular eminence or papilla, similar in every respect to those found upon the surface of the skin; it is continuous with the dermal layer of the follicle, and is supplied with myelinated and nonmyelinated nerve endings. It is from the capillaries in the papilla that the hair derives its nutrition.

The hair follicle consists of two coats—an outer or dermic, and an inner or epidermic (**7**.312, 314).

The *outer coat* is formed mainly of fibrous tissue; it is continuous with the dermis, is highly vascular, and is supplied by numerous, minute nerves.

The *inner coat* is closely adherent to the root of the hair, and consists of two strata, named respectively the *outer* and *inner root sheaths*; the outer root sheath corresponds with the stratum spinosum of the epidermis, and resembles it in the rounded form and soft character of its cells; at the bottom of the hair follicle these cells become continuous with those of the root of the hair. The inner root sheath consists of: (1) a delicate cuticle next the hair, composed of a single layer of imbricated scales with atrophied nuclei; (2) one or two layers of horny flattened nucleated cells, known as *Huxley's layer*; (3) a single layer of cubical cells with clear, flattened nuclei, called *Henle's layer* (**7**.314).

The *hair bulb* is moulded over the papilla and composed of polyhedral cells. As they pass upwards into the root of the hair these cells become elongated and spindle-

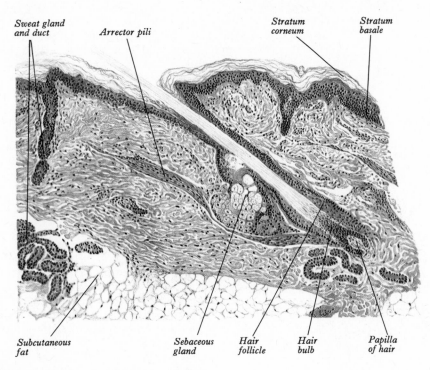

**7**.312  A section through the skin, showing the epidermis and corium (dermis), a hair in its follicle, an arrector pili muscle, and sebaceous glands opening into the hair follicle.

The *root of the hair* has a proximal enlargement, the *hair bulb*, which is set in an invagination of the epidermis and superficial portion of the corium, called the *hair follicle* (**7**.312, 313). When the hair is of considerable length the follicle extends into the subcutaneous tissue. The hair follicle commences on the surface of the skin

shaped, except those in the centre, which remain polyhedral.

The *shaft of the hair* consists, from within outwards, of the medulla, the cortex and the cuticle. The *medulla* is usually absent from the fine hairs covering the surface of the body, and commonly from these of the head. It is

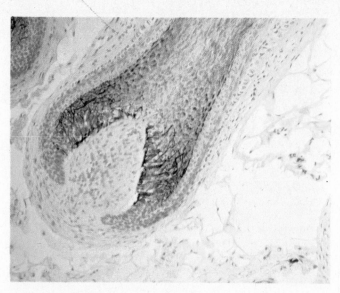

7.313 A vertical section through a hair root, showing the dermal papilla, and numerous melanocyte processes extending into the matrix of the hair. Haematoxylin and eosin.

composed of rows of polyhedral cells, with air spaces between, and sometimes within, the cells. The *cortex* constitutes the chief part of the shaft; it cells are elongated and are united to form flattened, fusiform fibres, which contain pigment granules in dark hair, and air in white hair. The *cuticle* consists of a single layer of flat scales which overlap one another from below upwards.[1317, 1331-1333]

Over most parts of the body the hairs are fine and downy and give an appearance of hairlessness. Almost the entire skin of the human at about the middle of fetal life is covered by a fine hair, called *lanugo* (primary hairs), and in fact the hairs on the back at this time are more numerous (per square centimetre) than in the gorilla or chimpanzee of corresponding fetal age. The lanugal hairs are mostly

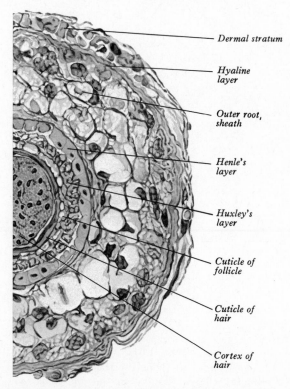

— Dermal stratum

— Hyaline layer

— Outer root, sheath

— Henle's layer

— Huxley's layer

— Cuticle of follicle

— Cuticle of hair

— Cortex of hair

7.314 Transverse section of a hair follicle from the scalp of a newborn infant. Magnification about ×600.

shed by birth and are replaced by fine hairs, termed *vellus* (secondary hairs), in the early months of post-natal life. These are retained in most regions but are replaced by the hairs (*terminal hairs*) of the scalp and eyebrows; also by the axillary and pubic hairs, and those on the face and front of the chest in the male, which appear at puberty, their development and growth being under hormonal control. In the adult the scalp hairs are more numerous (per square centimetre) than in the anthropoid apes. The lanugal and vellous hairs have no medulla. In the male the hairs in the vestibule of the nose and in the external acoustic meatus grow markedly with advancing age. In 'furry' mammals hair functions in the temperature controlling mechanism by minimizing heat loss; this function in man is served by the subcutaneous fat, and the hairs are concerned largely in the cutaneous sensation of touch (pp. 797, 834). Growth of a hair occurs at the hair bulb, where the cells capping the papilla proliferate and form the *germinal matrix* of the hair. As proliferated cells progressively move towards the surface they become keratinized to form the fibre-like cornified cells of the shaft of the hair. The duration of life of a single hair varies from about four months (eyelashes, axillary hair) to about four years (scalp hair), after which it is shed and is replaced by the sprouting of new cells from the germinal matrix. Growth of a hair varies with its texture, ranging from about 1·5 mm (fine hair) to 2·2 mm (coarse hair) a week. Greying or whitening of hair is due to the collection of minute air bubbles in the cortex (and medulla) of the shaft and to loss of pigment (melanin) formation by cells in the germinal matrix (*see* p. 1162).

Minute bundles of involuntary muscular fibres, termed the *arrectores pilorum* (7.303, 312), are connected with the hair follicles. They arise from the superficial layer of the corium, and are inserted into the outer coat of the hair follicle, below the entrance of the duct of the sebaceous gland. They are placed on the side towards which the hair slopes, and by their action diminish the obliquity of the follicle and elevate the hair. When they contract, the skin over their origin is depressed, while the skin immediately around the hair is elevated; this results in the appearance of 'goose skin' seen on exposure to cold or in emotional reactions. The sebaceous gland is situated in the angle which the arrector pili muscle forms with the superficial portion of the hair follicle, and contraction of the muscle thus tends to squeeze the sebaceous secretion out from the duct of the gland. The arrector muscles are supplied by sympathetic nerves.

## THE SEBACEOUS GLANDS

The sebaceous glands are small, sacculated, and lodged in the substance of the dermis. They are found in most parts of the skin, but are especially abundant in the scalp and face; they are also very numerous around the apertures of the ear, nose, mouth and anus, but are absent in the palms of the hands and soles of the feet. Each gland consists of a single duct, more or less capacious, which emerges from a cluster of oval or piriform alveoli, usually from two to five, but in some instances as many as twenty in number. Each alveolus is composed of a basement membrane, enclosing a number of epithelial cells. The outer or marginal cells are small and polyhedral, and are continuous with the cells lining the duct. The

[1331] A. G. Matolsty, in *The Biology of Hair Growth*, W. Montagna and R. A. Ellis (eds.), Academic Press, New York. 1958.
[1332] C. Orfanos and H. Ruska, *Arch. klin. exp. Derm.*, **231**, 1968.
[1333] M. S. C. Birbeck, in: *Progress in the Biological Sciences in Relation to Dermatology*, **2**, eds. A. J. Rock and R. H. Champion, University Press, Cambridge. 1964.

remainder of the alveolus is filled with larger cells, containing fat, but in its centre the cells are broken up, leaving a cavity filled with their debris and a mass of fatty matter, which constitutes the *sebum cutaneum*. [1317, 1334, 1335] As the sebaceous glands produce their secretion by complete fatty degeneration of their central cells they are classed as *holocrine* glands. As the central cells disintegrate, they are replaced by proliferation of marginal cells. The ducts open most frequently into hair follicles (the glands being developed as diverticula from the epithelial walls of the follicles themselves) but occasionally upon the general surface, as in the labia minora, glans penis and the free margins of the lips. On the nose and face the glands are of large size, distinctly lobulated, and often become much enlarged from the accumulation of pent-up secretion. The tarsal glands of the eyelids are elongated sebaceous glands with numerous lateral diverticula. Sebum acts as a natural lubricant of the hair and skin and protects the skin from the effects of moisture or desiccation; it also has some bacteriocidal action. The secretory activity of the sebaceous glands does not appear to be under nervous control; it is stimulated by hormonal action, particularly androgens.

## THE SWEAT GLANDS

Sudoriferous or sweat glands (7.303, 312) occur in almost every part of the skin, and have been classified into two types, *eccrine* and *apocrine*. [1317, 1336, 1337] The eccrine glands are most numerous and are found in almost every part of the skin. Each consists of a single tube, the deep part of which is coiled into an oval or spherical ball, which is situated in the deeper layers of the corium or in subcutaneous tissue and is named the *body* of the gland. The superficial part, or duct, traverses the corium and epidermis and opens on the surface of the skin by an infundibular aperture. In the superficial layers of the corium the duct is straight, but in the deeper layers it is convoluted or twisted; where the epidermis is thick, as in the palms of the hands and soles of the feet, the part of the duct which passes through it is spirally coiled. The size of the glands varies. They are especially large in those regions where the amount of perspiration is great, as in the axillae and in the groin. Their number varies. They are very plentiful on the palms of the hands and on the soles of the feet, where the orifices of the ducts are exceedingly regular, and open on the curved ridges of the epidermis; they are least numerous in the neck and back. The tube, both in the body of the gland and in the duct, consists of two layers—an outer, of fine areolar tissue, and an inner, of epithelium. The outer layer is thin and is continuous with the superficial stratum of the dermis. In the body of the gland the epithelium consists of cubical or polyhedral cells which may be classified as dark cells and clear cells; the former are rich in ribonucleic acid and

mucopolysaccharides and are the main secretory elements. The latter are mostly acidophilic and contain an abundance of glycogen. Electron microscopy reveals canaliculi between the clear cells. Between the basal aspects of these cells and the basement membrane there is an incomplete layer of longitudinally or obliquely arranged elongated, fusiform, myoepithelial cells. Electron microscopic studies show that their cytoplasm is similar to that of nonstriated muscle cells containing fine (5 nm) filaments and less frequent thicker ones (see p. 487). Desmosomes occur where their plasma membranes adjoin those of the secretory cells of the gland. The myoepithelial cells have been ascribed a contractile role in the expression of secretion from the gland. It is also suggested that they may regulate the flow of metabolites to the secretory cells. [1338] The ducts are destitute of muscular fibres and are composed of a basement membrane lined by two or three layers of polyhedral cells; the duct passes through the epidermis as a spiral channel which is simply an intercellular cleft between the epidermal cells. When the epidermis is carefully removed from the surface of the corium, the ducts may be drawn out in the form of short, thread-like processes on its deep surface. The eccrine sweat glands are *merocrine* in nature, i.e., produce their thin watery secretion without demonstrable epithelial cell disintegration.

Apocrine sweat glands occur in the axilla, eyelids, areola and nipple of the breast, in the circumanal region and in association with the external genitalia. They are larger than eccrine glands and produce a thicker secretion. In the female they show involution changes related to each menstrual cycle. They are developed in close association with hairs and their ducts sometimes open into hair follicles. The ceruminous glands of the external acoustic meatus are modified apocrine sweat glands. It should be noted that recent work, using the electron microscope, has suggested that the so-called apocrine glands do not lose superficial cytoplasm during secretion and hence all sweat glands may have a merocrine, rather than apocrine, form of secretion.

Sweat glands are concerned in the temperature control mechanism by surface evaporation of the sweat. They are supplied by sympathetic nerves, though these are cholinergic in nature (p. 1067), and no sweating occurs in a denervated area of skin. Rarely, sweat glands may be congenitally absent, in which case special means have to be adopted to prevent rise of body temperature in hot weather.

[1334] A. Charles, *J. invest. Derm.*, **35**, 1960.

[1335] R. A. Ellis, in: *Ultrastructure of Normal and Abnormal Skin*, ed. A. S. Zelickson, Kimpton, London. 1967.

[1336] R. E. Ellis in: *Handbuch der Haut und Geschlechtskrankheiten*, vol. I, eds. O. Gans and G. K. Steigleder, Springer, Berlin. 1968.

[1337] L. Biempica and L. F. Montes, *Am. J. Anat.*, **117**, 1965.

[1338] R. A. Ellis, *J. Cell Biol.*, **27**, 1965.

# Supplementary Reading List

(The main bibliographic references, totalling 1338, appear as footnotes throughout this volume. Since the text was first published, a considerable number of papers and monographs have appeared. A selection of these is here appended for the reader's convenience. They could not be included as text references).

## A

Abel, J. H. Jr., Pautler, E. L. and Hon, B. C. (1972). Cytoplasmic bridges in the photoreceptor cells of mammals and their possible relationship to disc formation. *Cytobiologie*, **6**, 115–130.

Algaba, J. and Blay, L. (1972). Estudio experimental sobre la inervacion del velo de paladar. *Revta esp. Oto-neuro-oftal. Neurocirug.*, **30**, 1–10.

Altman, J. (1972). Postnatal development of the cerebellar cortex in the rat. I. The external germinal layer and the transitional molecular layer. II. Phases in the maturation of Purkinje cells and of the molecular layer. III. Maturation of the components of the granular layer. *J. comp. Neurol.*, **145**, 353–398; 399–464; 465–514.

Altman, J. (1973). Experimental reorganisation of the cerebellar cortex. III. Regeneration of the external germinal layer and granule cell ectopia. IV. Parallel fiber reorientation following regeneration of the external germinal layer. *J. comp. Neurol.*, **149**, 153–180; 181–192.

Angaut, P. and Sotelo, C. (1973). The fine structure of the cerebellar central nuclei in the cat. II. Synaptic organisation. *Expl Brain Res.*, **16**, 431–454.

Apfelberg, D. B. and Larson, S. J. (1973). Dynamic anatomy of the ulnar nerve at the elbow. *Plast. reconstr. Surg.*, **51**, 76–81.

Armstrong, D. M., Harvey, R. J. and Schild, R. F. (1974). Topographical localization in the olivocerebellar projection: an electrophysiological study in the cat. *J. comp. Neurol.*, **154**, 287–302.

Ashton, N. and Tripathi, R. (1972). The argyrophilic mosaic of the internal limiting membrane of the retina. *Expl Eye Res.*, **14**, 49–52.

Austin, G. (Editor). (1972). *The Spinal Cord. Basic Aspects and Surgical Considerations.* 2nd ed. Thomas: Springfield, Ill.

## B

Bacsik, R. D. and Strominger, N. L. (1973). The cytoarchitecture of the human anteroventral cochlear nucleus. *J. comp. Neurol.*, **147**, 281–290.

Baldessarini, R. J. (1972). Biogenic amines and behaviour. *Ann. Rev. Med.*, **23**, 343–354.

Baldessarini, R. J. and Karobath, M. (1973). Biochemical physiology of central synapses. *Ann. Rev. Physiol.*, **35**, 273–304.

Bandaranayake, R. C. (1971). Morphology of the accessory neurosecretory nuclei and of the retrochiasmatic part of the supraoptic nucleus of the rat. *Acta anat.*, **80**, 14–22.

Bartlett Bunge, M. (1973). Fine structure of nerve fibres and growth cones of isolated sympathetic neurons in culture. *J. Cell Biol.*, **56**, 713–735.

Bellairs, R. and Gray, E. G. (Editors). (1974). *Essays on the Nervous System.* A Festschrift for Professor J. Z. Young. Clarendon Press: Oxford.

Bennett, M. R. (1972). *Autonomic Neuromuscular Transmission.* Cambridge University Press: London.

Bergstrom, B. (1973). Morphology of the vestibular nerve. II. The number of myelinated nerve fibres in man at different ages. *Acta otolar.*, **76**, 173–179.

Bijlani, V. and Keswani, N. H. (1970). The salivatory nuclei in the brainstem of the monkey (*Macaca mulatta*). *J. comp. Neurol.*, **139**, 375–384.

Bjorkland, A., Owman, C. and West, K. A. (1972). Peripheral sympathetic innervation and serotonin in the habenular region of the rat brain. *Z. Zellforsch. mikrosk. Anat.*, **127**, 570–579.

Blackwell, R. E. and Guillemin, R. (1973). Hypothalamic control of adenohypophysial secretions. *Ann. Rev. Physiol.*, **35**, 357–390.

Bondareff, W. and McLone, D. G. (1973). The external glial limiting membrane in Macaca: ultrastructure of a laminated glioepithelium. *Am. J. Anat.*, **136**, 277–296.

Borg, E. (1973). On the neuronal organisation of the acoustic middle ear reflex. A physiological and anatomical study. *Brain Res.*, **49**, 101–123.

Bowman, J. P. and Sladek, J. R. (1973). Morphology of the inferior olivary complex of the rhesus monkey (Macaca mulatta). *J. comp. Neurol.*, **152**, 299–306.

Bowman, M. H. and King, J. S. (1973). The conformation, cytology and synaptology of the opossum inferior olivary nucleus. *J. comp. Neurol.*, **148**, 491–524.

Boycott, B. B. and Kolb, H. (1973). The connections between bipolar cells and photoreceptors in the retina of the domestic cat. *J. comp. Neurol.*, **148**, 91–114.

Boycott, B. B. and Kolb, H. (1973). The horizontal cells of the rhesus monkey retina. *J. comp. Neurol.*, **148**, 115–140.

Braak, H. (1972). Uber die Kerngebiete des Menschlichen Hirnstammes. V. Das dorsale Glossopharyngeus und Vagusgebiet. *Z. Zellforsch. mikrosk. Anat.*, **135**, 415–438.

Bray, D. (1973). Branching patterns of individual sympathetic neurons in culture. *J. Cell Biol.*, **56**, 702–712.

Breipohl, W., Langwitz, H. J. and Bornfield, N. (1974). Topological relations between the dendrites of olfactory sensory cells and sustentacular cells in different vertebrates. An ultrastructural study. *J. Anat.*, **117**, 89–94.

Brightman, M. W., Hori, M., Rapoport, S. I., Reese, T. S. and Westergaard, E. (1973). Osmotic opening of tight junctions in cerebral endothelium. *J. comp. Neurol.*, **152**, 317–326.

Brodal, A. (1972). Cerebrocerebellar pathways. Anatomical data and some functional implications. *Acta neurol. scand., suppl.*, **51**, 153–195.

Brodal, A., Destombes, J., Lacerda, A. M. and Angaut, P. (1972). A cerebellar projection on to the pontine nuclei. An experimental and anatomical study in the cat. *Expl Brain Res.*, **16**, 115–139.

Brodal, A. and Szikla, G. (1972). The termination of the brachium conjunctivum descendens in the nucleus reticularis tegmenti pontis. *Brain Res.*, **39**, 337–351.

Brodal, A. and Courville, J. (1973). Cerebellar corticonuclear projection in the cat. Crus II. An experimental study with silver methods. *Brain Res.*, **50**, 1–23.

Brodal, P. (1972). Corticopontine projection from the visual cortex in the cat. I. The total projection and the projection from area 17. II. The projection from areas 18 and 19. *Brain Res.*, **39**, 297–317; 319–335.

Bunge, M. B. (1973). Fine structure of nerve fibres and growth cones of isolated sympathetic neurons in culture. *J. Cell Biol.*, **56**, 713–735.

Burton, M. and McFarland, J. J. (1973). The organisation of the seventh lumbar spinal ganglion of the cat. *J. comp. Neurol.*, **149**, 215–232.

## C

Cammermeyer, J. (1971). Median and caudal apertures in the roof of the fourth ventricle in rodents and primates. *J. comp. Neurol.*, **141**, 499–512.

Cammermeyer, J. (1972). Mast cells in the mammalian area postrema. *Z. Anat. EntwGesch.*, **139**, 71–92.

Carpenter, M. B., Harbison, J. W. and Peter, P. (1970). Accessory oculomotor nuclei in the monkey: projections and effects of discrete lesions. *J. comp. Neurol.*, **140**, 131–154.

# SUPPLEMENTARY READING LIST

Carpenter, M. B. and Peter, P. (1972). Nigrostriatal and nigrothalamic fibers in the rhesus monkey. *J. comp. Neurol.*, **144**, 93–116.

Carpenter, M. B. and Pierson, R. J. (1973). Pretectal region and the pupillary light reflex. An anatomical analysis in the monkey. *J. comp. Neurol.*, **149**, 271–300.

Cauna, N. (1973). The free penicillate nerve endings of the human hairy skin. *J. Anat.*, **115**, 277–288.

Chernyshevskaya, I. A. (1971). Morphological study of pyramidal neuron axon collaterals of mammalian cerebral cortex in ontogenesis. *J. evol. biochem. Physiol.*, **7**, 537–542.

Chiba, T. (1972). Fine structure of the baroreceptor nerve terminals in the carotid sinus of the dog. *J. Electronmicrosc. Tokyo.*, **21**, 139–148.

Chronister, R. B., Zornetzer, S. F., Bernstein, J. J. and White, L. E. (1974). Hippocampal theta rhythm: intra-hippocampal formation contributions. *Brain Res.*, **65**, 13–28.

Cloyd, M. W. and Low, F. N. (1974). Scanning electron microscopy of the subarachnoid space in the dog. I. Spinal cord levels. *J. comp. Neurol.*, **153**, 325–368.

Coates, P. W. (1973). Supra-ependymal cells in recesses of the monkey third ventricle. *Am. J. Anat.*, **136**, 533–539.

Cohen, B. (1972). Cerebellar control of the vestibular pathways to oculomotor neurons. *Prog. Brain Res.*, **37**, 411–425.

Conde, F. and Conde, H. (1973). Étude de la morphologie des cellules du noyau rouge du chat par la méthode de Golgi Cox. *Brain Res.*, **53**, 249–271.

Costa, E., Iverson, L. L. and Paoletti, R. (Editors). (1972). *Studies of Neurotransmitters at the Synaptic Level.* Advances in Biochemical Psychopharmacology, Volume 6. North Holland Publishing Company: Amsterdam.

Courville, J. and Cooper, C. W. (1970). The cerebellar nuclei of Macaca mulatta: a morphological study. *J. comp. Neurol.*, **140**, 241–284.

Courville, J., Diakiw, N. and Brodal, A. (1973). Cerebellar corticonuclear projection in the cat. The paramedian lobule: an experimental study with silver methods. *Brain Res.*, **50**, 25–45.

Cunningham, F. O. and Fitzgerald, M. J. T. (1972). Encapsulated nerve endings in hairy skin. *J. Anat.*, **112**, 93–97.

## D

Dahl, E. (1973). The innervation of the cerebral arteries. *J. Anat.*, **115**, 53–63.

Daniel, P. M. and Prichard, M. M. L. (1972). The human hypothalamus and pituitary stalk after hypophysectomy or pituitary stalk section. *Brain*, **95**, 813–824.

Davson, H., Domer, F. R. and Hollingsworth, J. R. (1973). The mechanism of drainage of the cerebrospinal fluid. *Brain*, **96**, 329–336.

Delmarcelle, Y. and Luyckx-Bacus, J. (1971). Evolution biométrique de la chambre antérieure chez l'enfant. Etude de 1960 globes. *Bull. Soc. belge. Ophtal.*, **158**, 451–465.

de Long, W. B. (1973). Anatomy of the middle cerebral artery: the temporal branches. *Stroke*, **4**, 412–418.

Denny-Brown, D., Kirk, E. J. and Yanagisawa, N. (1973). The tract of Lissauer in relation to sensory transmission in the dorsal horn of spinal cord in the Macaque monkey. *J. comp. Neurol.*, **151**, 175–199.

Denny-Brown, D. and Yonagisawa, N. (1973). The function of the descending root of the fifth nerve. *Brain*, **96**, 783–814.

de Reuck, J. (1972). The cortico-subcortical arterial angio-architecture in the human brain. *Acta neur. belg.*, **72**, 323–329.

di Carlo, V., Hubbard, J. E. and Pate, P. (1973). Fluorescence histochemistry of monoamine-containing cell bodies in the brainstem of the squirrel monkey (*Saimiri sciurus*). IV. An atlas. *J. comp. Neurol.*, **152**, 347–372.

Dublin, M. W. (1970). The inner plexiform layer of the vertebrate retina: a quantitative and comparative electron microscopic analysis. *J. comp. Neurol.*, **140**, 479–505.

Duncan, D. and Morales, R. (1973). Location of large-core synaptic vesicles in the dorsal grey matter of the cat and dog spinal cord. *Am. J. Anat.*, **136**, 123–127.

Duvernoy, H. (1972). The vascular architecture of the median eminence. In: *Brain-Endocrine Interaction. Median Eminence: Structure and Function.* pp. 79–108. Karger: Basel.

Duvernoy, H., Koritke, J. G., Monnier, G. and Jacquet, G. (1972). Sur la vascularization de l'área postrema et de la face postérieure du bulbe chez l'homme. *Z. Anat. EntwGesch.*, **138**, 41–66.

## E

Ebbeson, S. O. E. (1972). A proposal for a common nomenclature for some optic nuclei in vertebrates and the evidence for a common origin of two such nerve groups. *Brain Behav. Evol.*, **6**, 75–91.

Ebbeson, S. O. E., Jane, J. A. and Schroeder, D. M. (1972). A general overview of major interspecific variations in thalamic organization. *Brain Behav. Evol.*, **6**, 92–130.

Edwards, S. B. (1972). The ascending and descending projections of the red nucleus in the cat. *Brain Res.*, **48**, 45–63.

Ellison, J. P. and Williams, T. H. (1969). Sympathetic nerve pathways to the human heart, and their variations. *Am. J. Anat.*, **124**, 149–162.

Emery, J. L. (1972). The size and form of the cerebral aqueduct in children. *Brain*, **95**, 591–598.

Emery, J. L. and Singhal, R. (1973). Changes associated with growth in the cells of the dorsal root ganglion in children. *Dev. med. Child Neurol.*, **15**, 460–466.

Engström, H., Bergstrom, B. and Ades, H. W. (1972). Macula utriculi and macula sacculi in the squirrel monkey. *Acta otolar., suppl.*, **301**, 75–126.

Eränkö, L. (1972). Ultrastructure of the developing sympathetic nerve cell and the storage of catecholamines. *Brain Res.*, **46**, 159–175.

## F

Famiglietti, E. V. and Peters, A. (1972). The synaptic glomerulus and the intrinsic neuron in the dorsal lateral geniculate nucleus of the cat. *J. comp. Neurol.*, **144**, 285–334.

Feldman, M. L. and Peters, A. (1972). Intranuclear rods and sheets in rat cochlear nucleus. *J. Neurocytol.*, **1**, 109–127.

Feremutsch, K. and Gubser, M. (1972). Der Kernbegriff in der Neuroanatomie. *Anat. Anz.*, **131**, 324–336.

Findlay, J. M. and Daniell, G. J. (1973). A model for pattern recognition by cell networks. *J. theoret. Biol.*, **38**, 641–645.

Fisher, R. F. and Pettet, B. E. (1972). The postnatal growth of the capsule of the human crystalline lens. *J. Anat.*, **112**, 207–214.

Fisher, S. H. (1972). A somato-somatic synapse between amacrine and bipolar cells in the cat retina. *Brain Res.*, **43**, 587–590.

Foos, R. Y. and Miyamasu, W. (1973). Synaptic analysis of inner plexiform layer in human retina. *J. comp. Neurol.*, **147**, 447–454.

Fox, C. A., Andrade, A. N., Schwyn, R. C. and Rafols, J. A. (1972). The aspiny neurons and the glia in the primate striatum: a Golgi and electron microscopic study. *J. Hirnforsch.*, **13**, 341–362.

Fraher, J. P. (1972). A quantitative study of anterior root fibres during early myelination. *J. Anat.*, **112**, 99–124.

Fraher, J. P. (1973). A quantitative study of anterior root fibres during early myelination. II. Longitudinal variation in sheath thickness and axon circumference. *J. Anat.*, **115**, 421–444.

Freide, R. L. (1972). Control of myelin formation by axon caliber (with a model of the control system). *J. comp. Neurol.*, **144**, 233–252.

Freide, R. L. (1973). Dating the development of the human cerebellum. *Acta neuropath.*, **23**, 48–58.

Frigyesi, T. L., Rinvic, E. and Yahr, M. D. (1972). *Corticothalamic Projections and Sensorimotor Activities.* Raven Press: New York.

Fry, F. J. and Cowan, W. M. (1972). A study of retrograde cell degeneration in the lateral mammillary nucleus of the cat, with special reference to the role of axonal branching in the preservation of the cell. *J. comp. Neurol.*, **144**, 1–24.

Fujita, S. (1973). Genesis of glioblasts in the human spinal cord as revealed by Feulgen cytophotometry. *J. comp. Neurol.*, **151**, 25–34.

Fujita, S. (1974). DNA constancy in neurons of the human cerebellum and spinal cord as revealed by Feulgen cytophotometry and cytofluorometry. *J. comp. Neurol.*, **155**, 195–202.

Furlani, J. (1973). The anterior choroidal artery and its blood supply to the internal capsule. *Acta anat.*, **85**, 108–112.

## G

Gabella, G. (1972). Fine structure of the myenteric plexus in the guinea pig ileum. *J. Anat.*, **111**, 69–97.

Gallego, A. (1972). Conexiones centrales entre neuronas celulas moduladoras de las capas plexiformes. *Arch. Fac. med. Madrid*, **21**, 69–116.

Gamble, H. J. (1971). Electron microscope observations upon the conus medullaris and filum terminale of human fetuses. *J. Anat.*, **110**, 173–179.

Geller, M. and Barbato, D. (1972). Estudo da distribuciao nervosa terminal do nervus fibularis profundus. *Folha med.*, **64**, 911–943.

Geniec, P. and Morest, D. K. (1971). The neuronal architecture of the human posterior colliculus. *Acta otolar., suppl.*, **295**.

Gertz, S. D., Lindenberg, R. and Piavis, G. W. (1972). Structural variations in the rostral human hippocampus. *Johns Hopkins Med. J.*, **130**, 367–376.

Gillilan, L. A. (1972). Blood supply to primitive mammalian brains. *J. comp. Neurol.*, **145**, 209–222.

Gobel, S. and Purvis, M. B. (1972). Anatomical studies of the organization of the spinal V nucleus: the deep bundles and the spinal V tract. *Brain Res.*, **48**, 27–44.

Goldberg, S. J., Hull, C. D. and Buchwald, N. A. (1974). Afferent projections in the abducens nerve: an intracellular study. *Brain Res.*, **68**, 205–214.

Gosavi, V. S. and Dubey, P. N. (1972). Projection of striate cortex to the dorsal lateral geniculate body in the rat. *J. Anat.*, **113**, 75–82.

Gosling, J. A. and Dixon, J. C. (1974). Sensory nerves in the mammalian urinary tract. An evaluation using light and electron microscopy. *J. Anat.*, **117**, 133–144.

Gregg, J. M. and Dixon, A. D. (1973). Somatotopic organisation of the trigeminal ganglia in the rat. *Arch. oral Biol.*, **18**, 487–498.

Grossman, A., Lieberman, A. R. and Webster, K. E. (1973). A Golgi study of the rat dorsal lateral geniculate nucleus. *J. comp. Neurol.*, **180**, 441–468.

Gruner, J. E., Hirsch, J. C. and Sotelo, C. (1974). Ultrastructural features of the isolated suprasylvian gyrus in the cat. *J. comp. Neurol.*, **154**, 1–28.

Guillery, R. W. (1972). Binocular competition in the control of geniculate cell growth. *J. comp. Neurol.*, **144**, 117–130.

Guillery, R. W. (1973). The effect of lid suture upon the growth of cells in the dorsal lateral geniculate nucleus of kittens. *J. comp. Neurol.*, **148**, 417–422.

Guillery, R. W. and Kaas, J. H. (1971). A study of normal and congenitally abnormal retinogeniculate projection in cats. *J. comp. Neurol.*, **143**, 73–106.

Guillery, R. W. and Kaas, J. H. (1974). The effects of monocular lid suture upon the development of the lateral geniculate nucleus in squirrels (*Sciurus carolinensis*). *J. comp. Neurol.*, **154**, 433–442.

Gwyn, D. G., Wolstencroft, J. H. and Silver, A. (1972). The effect of a hemisection on the distribution of acetylcholinesterase and choline acetyltransferase in the spinal cord of the cat. *Brain Res.*, **47**, 289–301.

## H

Hall, E. (1972). The amygdala of the cat: a Golgi study. *Z. Zellforsch. mikrosk. Anat.*, **134**, 439–458.

Hamilton, B. L. (1973). Cytoarchitectural subdivisions of the peri-aqueductal grey matter in the cat. *J. comp. Neurol.*, **149**, 1–28.

Hamori, J. (1973). Developmental morphology of dendritic post-synaptic specializations. *Rec. Dev. Neurobiol., Hung.*, **4**, 9–32.

*Handbook of Sensory Physiology.* (1972). Vol III. Part 1 *Enteroceptors.* (Neil, E. ed.). Springer-Verlag: Berlin.

*Handbook of Sensory Physiology.* (1972). Vol IV. *The Chemical Senses.* Part 1 *Olfaction*; Part 2 *Taste.* (Beidler, L. M. ed.). Springer-Verlag: Berlin.

*Handbook of Sensory Physiology.* (1973). Vol VII. Part 3 *Central Processing of Visual Information.* Section A. *Integrative Functions and Comparative Data.* Section B. *Visual Centers in the Brain.* (Jung, R. ed.). Springer-Verlag: Berlin.

Harding, B. N. (1973). An ultrastructural study of the termination of afferent fibres within the ventrolateral and centre median nuclei of the monkey thalamus. *Brain Res.*, **54**, 341–346.

Harness, D., Sekeles, E. and Chaco, J. (1974). The double motor innervation of the opponens pollicis muscles: an electromyographic study. *J. Anat.*, **117**, 329–331.

Harting, J. K. (1972). Evolution of the pulvinar. *Brain Behav. Evol.*, **6**, 424–452.

Hasan, M. and Glees, P. (1973). Ultrastructural age changes in hippocampal neurons, synapses and neuroglia. *Expl Gerontol.*, **8**, 75–83.

Hashimoto, K. (1972). Fine structure of perifollicular nerve endings in human hair. *J. invest. Derm.*, **59**, 432–441.

Hashimoto, K. (1973). Fine structure of the Meissner corpuscle of human palmar skin. *J. invest. Derm.*, **60**, 20–28.

Headon, M. P. and Powell, T. P. S. (1973). Cellular changes in the lateral geniculate nucleus of infant monkeys after suture of the eyelids. *J. Anat.*, **116**, 135–145.

Heath, C. J. and Jones, E. G. (1971). An experimental study of ascending connections from the posterior group of thalamic nuclei in the cat. *J. comp. Neurol.*, **141**, 397–426.

Hendrickson, A. E., Wagoner, N. and Cowan, W. (1972). An autoradiographic and electron-microscopic study of retinohypothalamic connexions. *Z. Zellforsch. mikrosk. Anat.*, **135**, 1–26.

Henry, J. L. and Calaresu, F. R. (1972). Topography and the numerical distribution of neurons of the thoraco-lumbar intermedio-lateral nucleus in the cat. *J. comp. Neurol.*, **144**, 205–214.

Hervouet, F., George, Y., Tusques, J. and Ertus, M. (1971). Aspect de différentes structures oculaires humaines au microscope a balayage. *Bull. Soc. fr. Ophtal.*, **84**, 603–620.

Heuser, J. E., Reese, T. S. and Landis, D. M. D. (1974). Functional changes in frog neuromuscular junctions studied with freeze-fracture. *J. Neurocytol.*, **3**, 109–131.

Heym, C. (1972). Development of the human Gasserian ganglion and its relation to the meninges. *Z. mikrosk.-anat. Forsch.*, **86**, 50–80.

Hillebrand, A. (1972). Is there a homologon of the central oculomotor nucleus in the chicken and turkey? *Anat. Anz.*, **132**, 24–31.

Hinds, J. W. and Hinds, P. L. (1972). Reconstruction of dendritic growth cones in neonatal mouse olfactory bulb. *J. Neurocytol.*, **1**, 169–187.

Hirsch, W. and Schweichel, J. U. (1973). Morphological evidence concerning the problem of skin ridge formation. *J. ment. Defic. Res.*, **17**, 58–72.

Hubbard, J. E. and di Carlo V. (1973). Fluorescence histochemistry of monoamine-containing cell bodies in the brain stem of the squirrel monkey (Saimiri sciurus). I. The locus coeruleus. *J. comp. Neurol.*, **147**, 553–566.

Hubbard, J. E. and di Carlo, V. (1974). Fluorescence histochemistry of monoamine-containing cell bodies in the brain stem of the squirrel monkey (Saimiri sciurus). II. Catecholamine-containing groups. II. Serotonin-containing groups. *J. comp. Neurol.*, **153**, 369–384; 385–398.

Hubel, D. H. and Wiesel, T. N. (1972). Laminar and columnar distribution of geniculo-cortical fibers in the Macaque monkey. *J. comp. Neurol.*, **146**, 421–450.

## I

Iqbal, K. and Telleznagel, I. (1972). Isolation of neurons and glial cells from normal and pathological human brains. *Brain Res.*, **45**, 296–301.

## J

Jabbur, S. J., Baker, M. A. and Towe, A. L. (1972). Wide field neurons in thalamic nucleus ventralis posterolateralis of the cat. *Expl Neurol.*, **36**, 213–238.

Jack, R. L. (1972). Ultrastructure of the hyaloid vascular system. *Archs Ophthal., N.Y.*, **87**, 555–567.

Jacob, M. S., Morgane, P. J. and Willard, L. M. (1971). The anatomy of the brain of the bottlenose dolphin (Tursiops truncatus). Rhinic lobe. I. The paleocortex. *J. comp. Neurol.*, **141**, 205–272.

Jacobs, M. J. (1970). The development of the human motor trigeminal complex and accessory facial nucleus and their topographic relations with the facial and abducens nuclei. *J. comp. Neurol.*, **138**, 161–194.

Jacobson, M. (1970). *Developmental Neurobiology.* Holt, Rinehart and Winston: New York.

Jain, P., Shukla, P. L., Bajpai, R. N. and Tewari, S. P. (1973). A metrical study of human spinal cord. *J. Anat. Soc. Ind.*, **22**, 130–136.

Johnstone, B. M. and Sellick, P. M. (1972). The peripheral auditory apparatus. *Q. Rev. Biophys.*, **5**, 1–57.

Jones, E. G. and Burton, H. (1974). Cytoarchitecture and somatic sensory connectivity of thalamic nuclei other than the ventrobasal complex in the cat. *J. comp. Neurol.*, **154**, 395–432.

Jones, E. G. and Leavitt, R. Y. (1974). Retrograde axonal transport and the demonstration of non-specific projections to the cerebral cortex and striatum from thalamic intralaminar nuclei in the rat, cat and monkey, *J. comp. Neurol.*, **154**, 349–378.

Jordan, H. (1973). The structure of the medial geniculate nucleus (MGN): a cyto- and myelo-architectonic study in the squirrel monkey. *J. comp. Neurol.*, **148**, 469–480.

## K

Kaas, J. H., Guillery, R. W. and Allman, J. M. (1972). Some principles of organisation in the dorsal lateral geniculate nucleus. *Brain Behav. Evol.*, **6**, 253–299.

Kaas, J. H., Hall, W. C. and Diamond, I. T. (1972). Visual cortex of the grey squirrel (*Sciurus carolinensis*): architectonic subdivisions and connections from the visual thalamus. *J. comp. Neurol.*, **145**, 273–305.

Kaas, J. H., Guillery, R. W. and Allman, J. M. (1973). Discontinuities in the dorsal lateral geniculate nucleus corresponding to the optic disc: a comparative study. *J. comp. Neurol.*, **147**, 163–180.

Kanagasuntheram, R., Krishnamurti, A. and Wong, W. C. (1973). The termination of optic fibres in the lateral geniculate nucleus of some primates. An ultrastructural study. *Acta anat.*, **84**, 76–84.

Karten, H. J., Hodos, W., Nauta, W. J. H. and Revzin, A. M. (1973). Neural connections of the "visual Wulst" of the avian telencephalon. Experimental studies in the pigeon (Columba livia) and owl (Speotyto cunicularia). *J. comp. Neurol.*, **150**, 253–278.

Kawamura, K. and Brodal, A. (1973). The tectopontine projection in the cat: an experimental anatomical study with comments on pathways for teleceptive impulses to the cerebellum. *J. comp. Neurol.*, **149**, 371–390.

Kemp, J. M. and Powell, T. P. S. (1971a). The site of termination of afferent fibres in the caudate nucleus. *Phil. Trans. R. Soc. B.*, **262**, 413–427.

Kemp. J. M. and Powell, T. P. S. (1971b). The structure of the caudate nucleus of the cat: light and electron microscopy. *Phil. Trans. R. Soc. B.*, **262**, 383–401.

Kemp, J. M. and Powell, T. P. S. (1971c). The synaptic organisation of the caudate nucleus. *Phil. Trans. R. Soc. B.*, **262**, 403–412.

Kemp, J. M. and Powell, T. P. S. (1971d). The termination of fibres from the cerebral cortex and thalamus upon dendritic spines in the caudate nucleus: a study with the Golgi method. *Phil. Trans. R. Soc. B.*, **262**, 429–439.

Kemper, T. L., Wright, S. J. Jr. and Locke, S. (1972). Relationship between the septum and the cingulate gyrus in Macaca mulatta. *J. comp. Neurol.*, **146**, 465–478.

Kerr, F. W. L. (1972). Central relationships of trigeminal and cervical primary afferents in the spinal cord and medulla. *Brain Res.*, **43**, 561–572.

King, J. S., Schwyn, R. C. and Fox, C. A. (1971). The red nucleus in the monkey (*Macaca mulatta*): a Golgi and electron microscopic study. *J. comp. Neurol.*, **141**, 75–107.

Kiss, A. and Tombol, T. (1972). Golgi analysis and degeneration studies of the nucleus centralis lateralis and ventralis medialis in the cat thalamus. *Brain Res.*, **47**, 303–315.

Kornguth, S. E. and Scott, G. (1972). The role of climbing fibers in the formation of Purkinje cell dendrites. *J. comp. Neurol.*, **146**, 61–82.

Kostyuk, P. G. and Maisky, V. A. (1972). Propriospinal projections in the lumbar spinal cord of the cat. *Brain Res.*, **39**, 530–535.

Kozlovski, A. P. (1972). Effects of gravitational stresses on the state of spinal ganglion neurons. *Arkh. anat. gistol. embriol.*, **62**, 55–59.

Kranz, H., Adorjani, C. and Baumgartner, G. (1973). The effect of nociceptive cutaneous stimuli on human motoneurons. *Brain*, **96**, 571–590.

Krechowiecki, A., Goscicka, D. and Samulak, S. (1972). Der Nervus phrenicus von Macaca mulatta. *Acta anat.*, **82**, 565–573.

Krishnamurti, A., Kanagasuntheram, R. and Wong, W. C. (1972). Functional significance of the fibrous laminae of the ventrobasal complex of the thalamus of the slow loris. *J. comp. Neurol.*, **145**, 515–523.

Kristensson, K. and Olsson, Y. (1973). Uptake and retrograde axonal transport of protein tracers in hypoglossal neurons. Fate of the tracer and reaction of the nerve cell bodies. *Acta neuropath.*, **23**, 43–47.

Künzle, H. (1973). The topographic organisation of spinal afferents to the lateral reticular nucleus of the cat. *J. comp. Neurol.*, **149**, 103–116.

Kuo, J-S. and Carpenter, M. B. (1973). Organization of pallidothalamic projections in the rhesus monkey. *J. comp. Neurol.*, **151**, 201–236.

Kurylcio, L. (1972). Galezie koncowe pni blednych u czlowieka. *Folia morph.*, **31**, 255–282.


### L


Landis, D. M. D. and Reese, T. S. (1974). Differences in membrane structure between excitatory and inhibitory synapses in the cerebellar cortex. *J. comp. Neurol.*, **155**, 93–126.

Lange, W. (1972). Uber regionale Unterschiede in der Myeloarchitektonik der Kleinhirnrinde. I. Der Plexus supraganglionaris. *Z. Zellforsch. mikrosk. Anat.*, **134**, 129–142.

Larsell, O. and Jansen, J. (1972). *The Comparative Anatomy and Histology of the Cerebellum. Vol 3. The Human Cerebellum, Cerebellar Connections and Cerebellar Cortex.* Oxford University Press: London.

Lentz, T. L. (1972). Development of the neuromuscular junction. III. Degeneration of motor end plates after denervation and maintenance in vitro by nerve explants. *J. Cell Biol.*, **55**, 93–103.

LeVay, S. (1973). Synaptic patterns in the visual cortex of the cat and monkey. Electron microscopy of Golgi preparations. *J. comp. Neurol.*, **150**, 53–86.

Lieberman, A. R. (1971). The axon reaction: a review of the principal features of perikaryal responses to axon injury. *Int. Rev. Neurobiol.*, **14**, 49–124.

Lieberman, A. R. (1973). Neurons with presynaptic perikarya and presynaptic dendrites in the rat lateral geniculate nucleus. *Brain Res.*, **59**, 35–59.

Lim, D. J. (1972). Fine morphology of the tectorial membrane. Its relationship to the organ of Corti. *Archs Otolar.*, **96**, 199–215.

Ling, E. A., Paterson, J. A., Privat, A., Mori, S. and Leblond, C. P. (1973). Investigation of glial cells in semithin sections. I. Identification of glial cells in the brains of young rats. II. Variation with age in the numbers of the various glial cell types in rat cortex and corpus callosum. III. Transformation of sub-ependymal cells into glial cells as shown by radio-autography after ³H-thymidine injection into the lateral ventricle of the brains of young rats. *J. comp. Neurol.*, **149**, 43–72; 73–82; 83–102.

Lloyd, D. P. (1970). Action in primary afferent fibers in the spinal cord. *Int. J. Neurosci.*, **1**, 1–25.

Locke, S. and Kerr, C. (1973). The projection of nucleus lateralis dorsalis of monkey to basomedial temporal cortex. *J. comp. Neurol.*, **149**, 29–42.

Loewy, A. D. (1972). The effects of dorsal root lesions on Clarke neurons in cats of different ages. *J. comp. Neurol.*, **145**, 141–164.

Loewy, A. D. (1973). Transneuronal changes in the gracile nucleus. *J. comp. Neurol.*, **147**, 497–510.

Lucas, D. (1972). Uber die postnatale Entwicklung der Neuroglia im corpus callosum des Kanichens. *Z. mikrosk.-anat. Forsch.*, **85**, 341–352.

Lukáš, Z. and Buriánek, P. (1971). Unmyelinized nerve fibres in the ganglion Gasseri. *Z. mikrosk.-anat. Forsch.*, **84**, 340–346.

Lund, J. S. (1973). Organisation of neurons in the visual cortex, area 17, of the monkey (Macaca mulatta). *J. comp. Neurol.*, **147**, 455–496.


### M


McDonald, W. I. and Olrich, G. D. (1971). Quantitative anatomical measurements on single isolated fibres from the cat spinal cord. *J. Anat.*, **110**, 191–202.

McLaughlin, B. J. (1972). The fine structure of neurons and synapses in the motor nuclei of the cat spinal cord. *J. comp. Neurol.*, **144**, 429–460.

McLaughlin, B. J. (1972). Dorsal root projections to the motor nuclei in the cat spinal cord. *J. comp. Neurol.*, **144**, 461–474.

Magalhães, M. M., Coimbra, A. and Silva, P. (1973). Aspects anatomophysiologiques de la cellule de Muller. *Bull. Ass. Anat., Paris*, **57**, 1–34.

Magyar, P., Szechenyi, B. and Palkovits, M. (1972). A quantitative study of the olivocerebellar connexions. *Acta morph. Hung.*, **20**, 71–75.

Mann, R. M. A. and Yates, P. O. (1973). Polyploidy in the human nervous system. II. Studies of the glial cell populations of the Purkinje cell layer of the human cerebellum. *J. neurol Sci.*, **18**, 197–205.

Manni, E., Palmieri, G. and Marini, R. (1972). Pontine trigeminal termination of proprioceptive afferents from the eye muscles. *Expl Neurol.*, **36**, 310–318.

Manni, E., Palmieri, G. and Marini, R. (1972). Mesodiencephalic representation of eye muscle proprioception. *Expl Neurol.*, **37**, 412–421.

Manuelli, G. F., Carella, G. and Ghisolfi, A. (1972). Ultrastructure, histoenzymologie et microangiotectonique de l'iris humain. *Archs Ophthal. Rev. gén. Ophthal.*, **32**, 633–652.

Marks, A. F. (1972). Regenerative reconstruction of a tract in a rat's brain. *Expl Neurol.*, **34**, 455–464.

Marsh, R. C. (1972). Comparative cytoarchitecture of the spinal and grey matter in the pig and cat: does Rexed's scheme apply to the pig? *Acta anat.*, **83**, 435–439.

Mathers, L. H. (1972). Ultrastructure of the pulvinar of the squirrel monkey. *J. comp. Nuerol.*, **146**, 15–42.

Mathers, L. H. (1972). The synaptic organization of the cortical projection to the pulvinar of the squirrel monkey. *J. comp. Neurol.*, **146**, 43–60.

Matsushita, M. and Ikeda, M. (1973). Propriospinal fiber connexions of the cervical motor nuclei in the cat: a light and electron microscope study. *J. comp. Neurol.*, **150**, 1–32.

Matsushita, M. and Ueyama, T. (1973). Ventral motor nucleus of the cervical enlargement in some mammals; its specific afferents from the lower cord levels and its cytoarchitecture. *J. comp. Neurol.*, **150**, 33–52.

Matthews, M. A. (1973). Death of the central neuron: an electron microscopic study of thalamic retrograde degeneration following cortical ablation. *J. Neurocytol.*, **2**, 265–288.

Matthews, M. R. and Raisman, G. (1972). A light and electron microscopic study of the cellular response to axonal injury in the superior cervical ganglion of the rat. *Proc. R. Soc. B.*, **181**, 43–79.

Matthews, P. B. C. (1973). *Mammalian Muscle Receptors and Their Central Actions.* Arnold: London.

Maurizi, M., Campora, E. and Frenguelli, A. (1972). Rilievi sull'origine apparente della corda del timpano. *Valsalva*, **48**, 186–194.

Maw, A. R. (1973). Further morphological modifications of the concept of efferent cochlear innervation at an ultrastructural level. *J. Laryngol.*, **87**, 619–638.

May, M. (1973). Anatomy of the facial nerve (spatial orientation of fibers in the temporal bone). *Laryngoscope*, **83**, 1311–1329.

Mayhew, T. M. and Momoh, C. K. (1973). Contribution to the quantitative analysis of neuronal parameters: the effects of biased sampling procedures on estimates of neuronal volume, surface area and packing density. *J. comp. Neurol.*, **148**, 217–228.

Mayr, R. (1971). Structure and distribution of fibre types in the external eye muscles of the rat. *Tissue & Cell*, **3**, 433–462.

Mazza, J. P. and Dixon, A. D. (1972). A histological study of chromatolytic cell groups in the trigeminal ganglion of the rat. *Archs oral Biol.*, **17**, 377–387.

Mehta, A. C. (1972). The blood vessels of the spinal cord (a review). *Neurol. India*, **20**, 190–205.

Mensah, P. and Deadwyler, S. (1974). The caudate nucleus of the rat: cell types and the demonstration of a commissural system. *J. Anat.*, **117**, 281–294.

Miller, R. A. and Strominger, N. I. (1973). Efferent connexions of the red nucleus in the brainstem and spinal cord of the rhesus monkey. *J. comp. Neurol.*, **152**, 327–346.

Millhouse, O. E. (1973). Certain ventromedial hypothalamic afferents. *Brain Res.*, **55**, 89–105.

Mlonyeni, M. (1973). The number of Purkinje cells and inferior olivary neurones in the cat. *J. comp. Neurol.*, **147**, 1–10.

Møller, A. R. (1972). Coding of sounds in lower levels of the auditory system. *Q. Rev. Biophys.*, **5**, 59–155.

Molliver, M. E., Kostović, I. and van der Loos, H. (1973). The development of synapses in cerebral cortex of the human fetus. *Brain Res.*, **50**, 403–407.

Monagle, R. D. and Brody, H. (1974). The effects of age upon the main nucleus of the inferior olive in the human. *J. comp. Neurol.*, **155**, 61–66.

Moore, R. Y. (1973). Retinohypothalamic projection in mammals: a comparative study. *Brain Res.*, **49**, 403–409.

Morris, V. B. (1970). Symmetry in a receptor mosaic demonstrated in the chick from the frequencies, spacing and arrangement of the types of retinal receptor. *J. comp. Neurol.*, **140**, 359–398.

Mosko, S., Lynch, G. and Cotman, C. W. (1973). The distribution of septal projections to the hippocampus of the rat. *J. comp. Neurol.*, **152**, 163–174.

Moskowitz, N. and Liu, J-C. (1972). Central projections of the spiral ganglion of the squirrel monkey. *J. comp. Neurol.*, **144**, 335–344.

Murphy, J. T., MacKay, W. A. and Johnson, F. (1973). Differences between cerebellar mossy and climbing fibre responses to natural stimulation of forelimb muscle proprioceptors. *Brain Res.*, **55**, 263–289.

**N**

Nakamura, S. and Sutin, J. (1972). The pattern of termination of pallidal fibres upon cells of the subthalamic nucleus. *Expl Neurol.*, **35**, 254–264.

Nathan, H. and Goldhammer, Y. (1973). The rootlets of the trochlear nerve. Anatomical observations in human brains. *Acta anat.*, **84**, 590–596.

Nauta, H. J. W., Butler, A. B. and Jane, J. A. (1973). Some observations on axonal degeneration resulting from superficial lesions of the cerebral cortex. *J. comp. Neurol.*, **150**, 349–360.

Nauta, H. J. W., Pritz, M. B. and Lasek, R. J. (1974). Afferents to the rat caudoputamen studied with horseradish peroxidase. An evaluation of a retrograde neuroanatomical research method. *Brain Res.*, **67**, 219–238.

Nguyen, H. (1972). Observations sur l'ultrastructure de l'épithelium pigmentaire de la rétine. *Acta anat.*, **83**, 606–618.

Norgren, R. and Leonard, C. M. (1973). Ascending central gustatory pathways. *J. comp. Neurol.*, **150**, 217–238.

**O**

Ochoa, J., Fowler, T. J. and Gilliat, R. W. (1972). Anatomical changes in peripheral nerves compressed by a pneumatic tourniquet. *J. Anat.*, **113**, 433–455.

Odutola, A. B. (1972). The organisation of cholinesterase-containing systems of the monkey spinal cord. *Brain Res.*, **39**, 353–368.

Ogden, T. E. (1974). The morphology of retinal neurons of the owl monkey (Aotes). *J. comp. Neurol.*, **153**, 399–428.

Olmos, J. S. de and Ingram, W. R. (1972). The projection field of the stria terminalis in the rat brain. An experimental study. *J. comp. Neurol.*, **146**, 303–334.

Olson, M. and Bunge, R. P. (1973). Anatomical observations on the specificity of synapse formation in tissue culture. *Brain Res.*, **59**, 19–33.

Olsson, Y. and Reese, T. S. (1971). Permeability of vasa nervorum and perineurium in mouse sciatic nerve studied by fluorescence and electron microscopy. *J. Neuropath. exp. Neurol.*, **30**, 105–119.

O'Neal, J. T. and Westrum, L. E. (1973). The fine structural synaptic organisation of the cat lateral cuneate nucleus. *Brain Res.*, **51**, 97–124.

Orgel, M., Aguayo, A. and Williams, H. B. (1972). Sensory nerve regeneration: an experimental study of skin grafts in the rabbit. *J. Anat.*, **111**, 121–135.

Osen, K. K. (1972). Projection of the cochlear nuclei on the inferior colliculus in the cat. *J. comp. Neurol.*, **144**, 355–372.

Ouaknine, G. and Nathan, H. (1973). Anastomotic connexions between the eleventh nerve and the posterior root of the first cervical nerve in humans. *J. Neurosurg.*, **38**, 189–197.

Ovalle, W. K. Jr. (1972). Motor nerve terminals on rat intrafusal muscle fibres, a correlated light and electron microscopic study. *J. Anat.*, **111**, 239–252.

**P**

Palay, S. L. and Chan Palay, V. (1973). High voltage electron microscopy of the central nervous system in Golgi preparations. *J. Microsc.*, **97**, 41–47.

Palay, S. L. and Chan Palay, V. (1974). *Cerebellar Cortex–Cytology and Organisation*. Springer: Berlin.

Palkovits, M., Magyar, P. and Szentágothai, J. (1972). Quantitative histological analysis of the cerebellar cortex in the cat. IV. Mossy fibre Purkinje cell numerical transfer. *Brain Res.*, **45**, 15–29.

Pannese, E., Bianchi, R., Calligaris, B., Ventura, R. and Weibel, E. R. (1972). Quantitative relationships between nerve and satellite cells in spinal ganglia. An electron microscopical study. I. Mammals. *Brain Res.*, **46**, 215–234.

Pappas, G. D. and Purpura, D. D. (1972). *Structure and Function of Synapses*. North Holland Publishing Company: Amsterdam.

Passingham, R. E. (1973). Anatomical differences between the neocortex of man and other primates. *Brain Behav. Evol.*, **7**, 337–359.

Paul, E. and Hundeiker, M. (1972). Aminergen Nerven und Capillaren im Ductus deferens. *Arch. dermatol. Forsch.*, **243**, 188–198.

Peach, R. (1972). Fine structural features of light and dark cells in the trigeminal ganglion of the rat. *J. Neurocytol.*, **1**, 151–160.

Perrachia, C. (1973). Low resistance junctions in crayfish. I. Two arrays of globules in junctional membranes. *J. Cell Biol.*, **57**, 54–65.

Perrachia, C. (1973). Low resistance junctions in crayfish. II. Structural details and further evidence for intercellular channels by freeze-fracture and negative staining. *J. Cell Biol.*, **57**, 66–76.

Peters, A. (1974). The surface fine structure of the choroid plexus and ependymal lining of the rat lateral ventricle. *J. Neurocytol.*, **3**, 99–108.

Petras, J. M. and Cummings, J. F. (1972). Autonomic neurons in the spinal cord of the rhesus monkey: a correlation of the findings of cytoarchitectonics and sympathectomy with fiber degeneration following dorsal rhizotomy. *J. comp. Neurol.*, **146**, 189–218.

Petrovický, P. (1971). Structure and incidence of Gudden's tegmental nuclei in some mammals. *Acta anat.*, **80**, 273–286.

Pfaff, F. and Keiner, M. (1973). Atlas of estradiol-concentrating cells in the central nervous system of the female rat. *J. comp. Neurol.*, **151**, 121–157.

Pfenninger, K., Akert, K., Moor, H. and Sandri, C. (1972). The fine structure of freeze-fractured presynaptic membranes. *J. Neurocytol.*, **1**, 129–149.

Phillips, D. D., Hibbs, R. G., Ellison, J. P. and Shapiro, H. (1972). An electron microscopic study of central and peripheral nodes of Ranvier. *J. Anat.*, **111**, 229–238.

Pickel, V. M., Segal, M. and Bloom, F. E. (1974). A radioautographic study of the efferent pathways of the nucleus locus coeruleus. *J. comp. Neurol.*, **155**, 15–42.

Plante, S. (1972). The comparative anatomy of the interpeduncular nucleus in the brain of the rat, cat and monkey. *J. neurol. Sci.*, **18**, 155–163.

Potts, A. M., Hodges, D. and Shelman, C. B. (1972). Morphology of the primate optic nerve. I. Method and total fiber count. II. Total fiber size distribution and fiber density distribution. III. Fiber characteristics of the foveal outflow. *Invest. Ophthal.*, **11**, 980–988; 989–1003; 1004–1016.

Powell, E. W. (1973). Limbic projections to the thalamus. *Expl Brain Res.*, **17**, 394–401.

Price, J. L. and Powell, T. P. S. (1971). Certain observations on the olfactory pathway. *J. Anat.*, **110**, 105–126.

Privat, A., Drian, M. J. and Mandon, P. (1974). Synaptogenesis in the outgrowth of rat cerebellum in organized culture. *J. comp. Neurol.*, **153**, 291–308.

Pubols, B. H. and Pubols, L. H. (1971). Somatotopic organization of spider monkey somatic sensory cortex. *J. comp. Neurol.*, **141**, 63–75.

**R**

Raisman, G. (1972). An experimental study of the projection of the amygdala to the accessory olfactory bulb and its relationship to the concept of a dual olfactory system. *Expl Brain Res.*, **14**, 395–408.

Rakhawy, M. T. (1972). Phosphatases in nervous tissue. (The nature of the ganglionic nerve cells in the tongue). *Acta anat.*, **83**, 356–366.

Rakhawy, M. T., Shehata, S. H. and Badawy, Z. H. (1972). Experimental and histological study of the mesencephalic nucleus of the fifth cranial nerve and its relation to the muscles of mastication in the rat. *Acta anat.*, **81**, 586–601.

Rakic, P. (1971). Neuron-glia relationship during granule cell migration in developing cerebellar cortex. A Golgi and electron microscopic study in Macacus rhesus. *J. comp. Neurol.*, **141**, 283–312.

Rakic, P. (1972). Mode of cell migration to the superficial layers of fetal monkey neocortex. *J. comp. Neurol.*, **145**, 61–84.

Rakic, P. (1972). Extrinsic cytological determinants of basket and stellate cell dendritic pattern in the cerebellar molecular layer. *J. comp. Neurol.*, **146**, 335–354.

Rakic, P. (1973). Kinetics of proliferation and latency between final cell division and onset of differentiation of cerebellar stellate and basket cells. *J. comp. Neurol.*, **147**, 523–546.

Ralston, H. J. and Chow, K. L. (1973). Synaptic reorganisation in the degenerating lateral geniculate nucleus of the rabbit. *J. comp. Neurol.*, **147**, 321–350.

Ramon Moliner, E. (1973). Presynaptic perikarya in olfactory bulb of guinea pig. *Brain Res.*, **63**, 351–356.

Raviola, E. and Gilula, N. B. (1973). Gap junctions between photoreceptor cells in the vertebrate retina. *Proc. natn. Acad. Sci. U.S.A.*, **70**, 1677–1681.

Rawlins, F. A. (1973). A time-sequence autoradiographic study of the in vivo incorporation of [1, 2-³H] cholesterol into peripheral nerve myelin. *J. Cell Biol.*, **58**, 42–53.

# SUPPLEMENTARY READING LIST

Rees, E. L. (1971). Nucleolar displacement during chromatolysis. A quantitative study on the hypoglossal nucleus of the rat. *J. Anat.*, **110**, 463–475.

Réthelyi, M. (1972). Cell and neuropil architecture of the intermediolateral (sympathetic) nucleus of cat spinal cord. *Brain Res.*, **46**, 203–213.

Ringvold, A. (1972). The ultrastructure of the extracellular components of the limbal conjunctiva in the human eye. *Acta ophthal.*, **50**, 393–404.

Robertson, R. T., Lynch, G. S. and Thompson, R. F. (1973). Diencephalic distributions of ascending reticular systems. *Brain Res.*, **55**, 309–322.

Rockel, A. J. and Jones, E. G. (1973). The neuronal organization of the inferior colliculus of the adult cat. I. The central nucleus. *J. comp. Neurol.*, **147**, 11–60.

Rockel, A. J. and Jones, E. G. (1973). Observations on the fine structure of the central nucleus of the inferior colliculus of the cat. *J. comp. Neurol.*, **147**, 61–92.

Rockel, A. J. and Jones, E. G. (1973). Observations on complex vesicles, neurofilamentous hyperplasia and increased electron density during terminal degeneration in the inferior colliculus. *J. comp. Neurol.*, **147**, 93–118.

Rockel, A. J. and Jones, E. G. (1973). The neuronal organisation of the inferior colliculus of the adult cat. II. The precentral nucleus. *J. comp. Neurol.*, **149**, 301–334.

Rogers, L. A. and Owman, W. M. (1973). The development of the mesencephalic nucleus of the trigeminal nerve in the chick. *J. comp. Neurol.*, **147**, 291–320.

Rohrschneider, I., Schinko, I. and Wetzstem, R. (1972). Der Feinbau der Area Postrema der Maus. *Z. Zellforsch. mikrosk. Anat.*, **123**, 251–276.

Rosén, L. (1972). Projection of forelimb group I muscle afferents to the cat cerebral cortex. *Int. Rev. Neurobiol.*, **15**, 1–25.

Rosenhall, U. (1972). Vestibular macular mapping in man. *Ann. Otol. Rhinol. Lar.*, **81**, 339–351.

Rubel, F. W. (1971). A comparison of somatotopic organization in sensory neocortex of newborn kittens and adult cats. *J. comp. Neurol.*, **143**, 447–480.

Rustioni, A. (1973). Non-primary afferents to the nucleus gracilis from the lumbar cord of the cat. *Brain Res.*, **51**, 81–95.

Ruttkay Nedecka, E., Cierny, G., Osvaldova, M. and Zlatos, J. (1972). Localization of the motor cells of the median nerve in the cat. *Folia morphol.*, **20**, 241–242.


S

Saban, R. (1972). Le cartilage annulaire de l'oreille externe chez les Mammifères. *C.r. Ass. Anat.*, **154**, 1152–1163.

Sakata, H., Takaoka, Y., Kawarasaki, A. and Shibutani, H. (1973). Somatosensory properties of neurons in the superior parietal cortex (area 5) of the rhesus monkey. *Brain Res.*, **64**, 85–102.

Sanderson, K. J. (1971). The projection of the visual field to the lateral geniculate and medial intralaminar nuclei in the cat. *J. comp. Neurol.*, **143**, 101–118.

Sanderson, K. J. (1974). Lamination of the dorsal lateral geniculate nucleus in carnivores of the weasel (Mustelidae), racoon (Procyonidae) and fox (Canidae) families. *J. comp. Neurol.*, **153**, 239–266.

Sando, I., Black, F. O. and Hemenway, W. G. (1972). Spatial distribution of the vestibular nerve in internal auditory canal *Ann. Otol. Rhinol. Laryngol.*, **81**, 305–314.

Scalia, F. (1972). The termination of retinal axons in the pretectal region of mammals. *J. comp. Neurol.*, **145**, 223–258.

Scheibel, M. E. and Scheibel, A. B. (1973). Dendrite bundles in the ventral commissure of cat spinal cord. *Expl Neurol.*, **39**, 482–488.

Schmitt, F. O. and Worden, F. G. (Editors). (1974). *The Neurosciences Third Study Program*. M.I.T. Press: Cambridge, Mass., London.

Schoultze, T. W. and Swett, J. E. (1972). The fine structure of the Golgi tendon organ. *J. Neurocytol.*, **1**, 1–26.

Scott, D. E., Paull, W. K. and Dudley, G. K. (1972). A comparative scanning electron microscopic analysis of the human cerebral ventricular system. I. The third ventricle. *Z. Zellforsch. mikrosk. Anat.*, **132**, 203–215.

Scott, D. E., Kozlowski, G. P. and Paull, W. K. (1973). Scanning electron microscopy of the human cerebral ventricular system. II. The fourth ventricle. *Z. Zellforsch. mikrosk. Anat.*, **139**, 61–68.

Seguchi, H. (1971). Studies on the brain stem of Orang Utan. *Acta anat. nippon.*, **46**, 375–399.

Shabo, A. L. and Maxwell, D. S. (1972). The structure of the trabecular meshwork of the primate eye: a light and electron microscopic study with peroxidase. *Microvasc. Res.*, **4**, 384–398.

Shepherd, G. M. (1972). Synaptic organisation of the mammalian olfactory bulb. *Physiol. Rev.*, **52**, 864–917.

Sidman, R. L. and Rakic, P. (1973). Neuronal migration, with special reference to developing human brain: a review. *Brain Res.*, **62**, 1–35.

Sinclair, D. (1973). The nerves of the skin. In: *The Physiology and Pathophysiology of the Skin.* (Jarret, A. ed.). Vol 2. Academic Press: New York, London.

Sklenska, A. (1972). Contribution to the ultrastructure of the Golgi tendon organ. *Folia morph.*, **20**, 195–197.

Sloper, J. J. (1972). Gap junctions between dendrites in the primate cortex. *Brain Res.*, **44**, 641–646.

Sloper, J. J. (1973). An electron microscopic study of the neurons of the primate motor and somatic sensory cortices. *J. Neurocytol.*, **2**, 351–359.

Sloper, J. J. (1973). An electron microscope study of the termination of afferent connections to the primate motor cortex. *J. Neurocytol.*, **2**, 369–381.

Smart, I. H. M. (1972a). Proliferative characteristics of the ependymal layer during the early development of the spinal cord in the mouse. *J. Anat.*, **111**, 365–380.

Smart, I. H. M. (1972b). Proliferative characteristics of the ependymal layer during the early development of the mouse diencephalon as revealed by recording the number, location and plane of cleavage of mitotic figures. *J. Anat.*, **113**, 109–129.

Smart, I. H. M. (1973). Proliferative characteristics of the ependymal layer during the early development of the mouse neocortex: a pilot study based on recording the number, location and plane of cleavage of mitotic figures. *J. Anat.*, **116**, 67–91.

Smith, P. J. (1972). Cortical projection of the human pulvinar. *J. Anat.*, **111**, 510P.

Smith, R. B. (1970). The development of the intrinsic innervation of the human heart between the 10 and 70 mm. stage. *J. Anat.*, **107**, 271–279.

Snell, R. S. (1972). An electron microscopic study of melanin in the hair and hair follicles. *J. invest. Derm.*, **58**, 218–228.

Sobrino, J. A. and Gallego, A. (1972). Cytology of the granular layer of the bulbar cochlear nuclei. *J. comp. Neurol.*, **145**, 179–193.

Sobusiak, T., Zimny, R. and Matlosz, Z. (1971). Primary glossopharyngeal and vagal afferent projection into the cerebellum in the dog. *J. Hirnforsch.*, **13**, 117–134.

Sobusiak, T., Zimny, R. and Zabel, J. (1972). Comparative pattern of the primary afferent projection from the 8th, 9th and 10th cranial nerves to the accessory cuneate nucleus. *Anat. Anz.*, **131**, 248–258.

Sotelo, C. and Angaut, P. (1973). The fine structure of the cerebellar central nuclei in the cat. I. Neurons and neuroglial cells. *Expl Brain Res.*, **16**, 410–430.

Spatz, W. B. and Tigges, J. (1972). Experimental-anatomical studies on the "middle temporal visual area (MT)" in Primates. *J. comp. Neurol.*, **146**, 451–464.

Spencer, P. S. and Schaumberg, H. H. (1973). An ultrastructural study of the inner core of the Pacinian corpuscle. *J. Neurocytol.*, **2**, 217–235.

Spicer, S. S., Martin, B. J. and Simson, J. V. (1972). The junctional complex associated body of human eccrine sweat gland. *J. Cell Biol.*, **53**, 582–586.

Spicer, S. S. and Prioleau, W. H. (1972). Ultrastructure of lipid inclusions and dense bodies in the human sweat gland. *Lab. Invest.*, **27**, 1–8.

Spicer, S. S. and Prioleau, W. H. (1972). Cytochemical studies of lipid and acid phosphatase in the human eccrine sweat gland. *Lab. Invest.*, **27**, 9–16.

Spira, A. W. and Hollenberg, M. J. (1973). Human retinal development: ultrastructure of the inner retinal layers. *Dev. Biol.*, **31**, 1–21.

Spoendlin, H. (1971). Inervationsmuster als Grundlage der Schnecken funktion. *Mschr. Ohrenheilk. Lar.-Rhinol.*, **105**, 317–328.

Steinberg, R. H., Reid, M. and Lacy, P. A. (1973). The distribution of rods and cones in the retina of the cat (Felis domesticus). *J. comp. neurol.*, **148**, 229–248.

Stevens, J. C., Lofgren, E. P. and Dyck, P. J. (1973). Histometric evaluation of branches of the peroneal nerve; I. Technique for combined biopsy of muscle nerve and cutaneous nerve. *Brain Res.*, **52**, 37–59.

Stewart, G. R., Mountain, J. C. and Colcock, B. P. (1972). Non-recurrent laryngeal nerve. *Br. J. Surg.*, **59**, 379–381.

Stone, J., Leicester, J. and Sherman, S. M. (1973). The naso-temporal division of the monkey's retina. *J. comp. Neurol.*, **150**, 333–348.

Strick, P. L. (1973). Light microscopic analysis of the cortical projection of the thalamic ventrolateral nucleus in the cat. *Brain Res.*, **55**, 1–24.

Strominger, N. L. (1973). The origins, course and distribution of the dorsal and intermediate acoustic striae in the rhesus monkey. *J. comp. Neurol.*, **147**, 209–234.

Strominger, N. L. and Strominger, A. I. (1971). Ascending brain stem projections of the anteroventral cochlear nucleus in the rhesus monkey. *J. comp. Neurol.*, **143**, 217–242.

Sulman, F. G. (1970). Hypothalamic control of lactation. *Mongr. Endocrinol.*, **3**, 1–235.

Svedburgh, B. and Bill, A. (1972). Scanning electron microscopic studies of the corneal endothelium in man and monkeys. *Acta ophthal.*, **50**, 321–336.

Swash, M. and Fox, K. P. (1972). Muscle spindle innervation in man. *J. Anat.*, **112**, 61–80.

Symington, R. B., Marks, S. M. and Ryan, P. M. (1972). Secretory cells of the human hypothalamus. *S. Afr. med. J.*, **46**, 1484–1487.

**T**

Tamura, T. and Smelser, G. K. (1973). Development of the sphincter and dilator muscles of the iris. *Archs Ophthal., N.Y.*, **89**, 332–339.

Tani, E., Ikeda, K. and Nishiura, M. (1973). Freeze-etching images of central myelinated nerve fibres. *J. Neurocytol.*, **2**, 305–314.

Tanishama, T. (1972). Fine structure of Edinger Westphal nucleus of the cat. *Acta Soc. ophthal. jap.*, **26**, 950–957.

Tarlov, E. (1972). Anatomy of the two vestibulo-oculomotor projection systems. *Prog. Brain Res.*, **37**, 471–491.

Tasker, R. R., Richardson, P. and Rewcastle, B. (1972). Anatomical correlation of detailed sensory mapping of the human thalamus. *Confin. Neurol.*, **34**, 184–196.

Tasman, W. (1973). The retina and optic nerve. *Archs Ophthal., N.Y.*, **89**, 422–436.

Torack, R. M., Stranaham, P. and Hartman, B. K. (1973). The role of norepinephrine in the function of the area postrema. I. Immunofluorescent localization of dopamine-$\beta$ hydroxylase and electron microscopy. *Brain Res.*, **61**, 235–252.

Torebjörk, H. E. and Hallin, R. G. (1974). Identification of afferent C units in intact human skin nerves. *Brain Res.*, **67**, 387–403.

Toshida, M. (1971). Uber die Ultrastruktur der Nervenzellen des Ganglion ciliare beim Affen (*Macacus irus* F. Cuvier). *Kobe J. med. Sci.*, **17**, 65–73.

Tower, D. B. and Young, O. M. (1973). Interspecies correlations of cerebral cortical oxygen consumption, acetylcholinesterase activity and chloride content: studies on the brains of the fin whale (Balaenoptera physalus) and the sperm whale (Physeter catodon). *J. Neurochem.*, **20**, 253–267.

Tower, D. B. and Young, O. M. (1973). The activities of butyrylcholinesterase and carbonic anhydrase, the rate of anaerobic glycolysis and the question of a constant density of glial cells in cerebral cortices of various mammalian species from mouse to whale. *J. Neurochem.*, **20**, 269–277.

Tredici, G., Pizzini, G. and Miani, A. (1973). The ultrastructure of the red nucleus of the cat. *J. submicrosc. Cytol.*, **5**, 29–48.

Tripathi, R. C. (1973). Ultrastructure of the arachnoid mater in relation to outflow of cerebrospinal fluid. A new concept. *Lancet*, **819**, 8–11.

Tripathi, R. C. and Tripathi, B. (1974). Vacuolar transcellular channels as a drainage pathway for cerebrospinal fluid. *J. Physiol., Lond.*, **239**, 195–206.

Trontelj, M. and Trontelj, J. V. (1973). First component of human blink reflex studied on single facial motoneurones. *Brain Res.*, **53**, 214–217.

**V**

van Buren, J. M. and Borke, R. C. (1971). A re-evaluation of the 'nucleus ventralis lateralis' and its cerebellar connections. A study in man and chimpanzee. *Int. J. Neurol.*, **8**, 155–177.

van Buren, J. M. and Borke, R. C. (1972). *Variations and Connections of the Human Thalamus. Part 1. The Nuclei and Cerebral Connections of the Human Thalamus. Part 2. Variations of the Human Diencephalon.* Springer-Verlag: Berlin.

van der Loos, H. and Glaser, E. M. (1972). Autapses in neocortex cerebri: synapses between a pyramidal cell's axon and its own dendrites. *Brain Res.*, **48**, 355–360.

Veale, J. L. and Rees, S. (1973). Renshaw cell activity in man. *J. Neurol. Neurosurg. Psychiat.*, **36**, 674–683.

Vlahovitch, B. and Fuentes, J. M. (1972). Les homologies insulaires données de l'anatomie comparée chez les Mammifères. *Neuro-chirurg.*, **18**, 511–520.

von Bonin, G. (1973). About quantitative studies on the cerebral cortex. *J. Microsc.*, **99**, 75–83.

**W**

Walberg, F. (1972). Cerebellovestibular relations: anatomy. *Prog. Brain Res.*, **37**, 361–376.

Warr, W. B. (1972). Fiber degeneration following lesions in the multipolar and globular cell areas in the ventral cochlear nucleus of the cat. *Brain Res.*, **40**, 247–270.

Watson, W. E. (1972). Some quantitative observations upon the responses of neuroglial cells which follow axotomy of adjacent neurons. *J. Physiol., Lond.*, **225**, 415–435.

Waxman, S. G. and Pappas, G. D. (1971). An electron microscopic study of synaptic morphology in the oculomotor nuclei of three inframammalian species. *J. comp. Neurol.*, **143**, 41–72.

Webster, K. E. (1973). Thalamus and basal ganglia in reptiles and birds. *Symp. zool. Soc. Lond.*, **33**, 169–203.

Weiss, P. A. (1972). Neuronal dynamics and axonal flow: axonal peristalsis. *Proc. natn. Acad. Sci. U.S.A.*, **69**, 1309–1312.

Welker, W. I. (1973). Principles of organisation of the ventrobasal complex in mammals. *Brain Behav. Evol.*, **7**, 253–336.

Westheimer, G. and Blair, S. M. (1973). The parasympathetic pathways to the internal eye muscles. *Invest. Ophthal.*, **12**, 193–197.

Whitsel, B. L., Dreyer, D. A. and Roppolo, J. R. (1971). Determinants of body representation in postcentral gyrus of macaques. *J. Neurophysiol.*, **34**, 1018–1034.

Willey, T. J. (1973). The ultrastructure of the cat olfactory bulb. *J. comp. Neurol.*, **152**, 211–232.

Williams, M. A. (1969). The assessment of electron microscopic autoradiographs. In: *Advances in Optical and Electron Microscopy.* (Barer, R. and Cosslett, V. E. eds.). Vol 3. pp. 219–272. Academic Press: New York, London.

Williams, M. A. (1973). Electron microscopic autoradiography: its applications to protein biosynthesis. In: *Techniques in Protein Biosynthesis.* (Campbell, P. N. and Sargent, J. R. eds.). Vol 2. pp. 125–190. Academic Press: New York, London.

Williams, P. L. and Hall, S. M. (1971). Chronic Wallerian degeneration: an in vivo and ultrastructural study. *J. Anat.*, **109**, 487–503.

Williams, T. H., Jew, J. and Palay, S. L. (1973). Morphological plasticity in the sympathetic chain. *Expl Neurol.*, **39**, 181–293.

Williams, W. J., BeMent, S. L., Yin, T. C. T. and McCall, W. D. (1973). Nucleus gracilis responses to knee joint motion: a frequency response study. *Brain Res.*, **64**, 123–140.

Wilson, V. J. (1972). Physiological pathways through the vestibular nuclei. *Int. Rev. Neurobiol.*, **15**, 27–81.

Winick, M. and Rosso, P. (1973). Effects of malnutrition on brain development. In: *Biology of Brain Dysfunction.* (Gaull, G. E. ed.), Vol. 1. Plenum Press: London.

Wirth, F. P. (1973). Insular-diencephalic connexions in the macaque. *J. comp. Neurol.*, **150**, 361–392.

Wong-Riley, M. T. T. (1972). Terminal degeneration and glial reactions in the lateral geniculate nucleus of the squirrel monkey after eye removal. *J. comp. Neurol.*, **144**, 61–92.

Wulle, K. G. (1972). Electron microscopy of the fetal development of the corneal endothelium and Descemet's membrane of the human eye. *Invest. ophthal.*, **11**, 897–904.

**Y**

Yamauchi, A. and Lever, J. D. (1971). Correlations between formol fluorescence and acetylcholinesterase (AChE) staining in the superior cervical ganglion of normal rat, pig and sheep. *J. Anat.*, **110**, 435–443.

Young, J. Z. (1971). *An Introduction to the Study of Man.* Clarendon Press: Oxford.

Young, R. F. and King, R. B. (1973). Fiber spectrum of the trigeminal sensory root of the baboon determined by electron microscopy. *J. Neurosurg.*, **38**, 65–72.

**Z**

Zeki, S. M. (1973). Comparison of the cortical degeneration in the visual regions of the temporal lobe of the monkey following section of the anterior commissure and the splenium. *J. comp. Neurol.*, **148**, 167–176.

# INDEX

# INDEX

# INDEX

# INDEX

Printed by T. & A. Constable Ltd., Edinburgh